PLASTIC SURGERY

Editor

JOSEPH G. McCARTHY, M.D.

Lawrence D. Bell Professor of Plastic Surgery and
Director of the Institute of Reconstructive Plastic Surgery
New York University Medical Center
New York, New York

Editors, Hand Surgery Volumes

JAMES W. MAY, JR., M.D.

Director of Plastic Surgery and Hand Surgery Service
Massachusetts General Hospital
Associate Clinical Professor of Surgery
Harvard Medical School
Boston, Massachusetts

J. WILLIAM LITTLER, M.D.

Past Professor of Clinical Surgery
College of Physicians and Surgeons
Columbia University, New York
Senior Attending Surgeon
The St. Luke's–Roosevelt Hospital Center
New York, New York

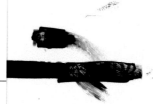

PLASTIC SURGERY

VOLUME 4
CLEFT LIP & PALATE
AND
CRANIOFACIAL ANOMALIES

W.B. SAUNDERS COMPANY
A Division of Harcourt Brace & Company
Philadelphia ▪ London ▪ Toronto
Montreal ▪ Sydney ▪ Tokyo

W.B. SAUNDERS COMPANY
A Division of
Harcourt Brace & Company

The Curtis Center
Independence Square West
Philadelphia, PA 19106

Library of Congress Cataloging-in-Publication Data

Plastic surgery.
    Contents: v. 1. General principles—v. 2–3.
The face—v. 4. Cleft lip & palate and craniofacial
anomalies—[etc.]
    1. Surgery, Plastic.   I. McCarthy, Joseph G., 1938–
[DNLM: 1. Surgery, Plastic. WO 600 P7122]

RD118.P536   1990   617'.95   87–9809

ISBN 0–7216–1514–7 (set)

25/7/94

Editor: W. B. Saunders Staff
Designer: W. B. Saunders Staff
Production Manager: Frank Polizzano
Manuscript Editor: David Harvey
Illustration Coordinator: Lisa Lambert
Indexer: Kathleen Garcia
Cover Designer: Ellen Bodner

Volume 1 0–7216–2542–8
Volume 2 0–7216–2543–6
Volume 3 0–7216–2544–4
Volume 4 0–7216–2545–2
Volume 5 0–7216–2546–0
Volume 6 0–7216–2547–9
Volume 7 0–7216–2548–7
Volume 8 0–7216–2549–5
8 Volume Set 0–7216–1514–7

Plastic Surgery

Printed in the United States of America.

Last digit is the print number: 9   8   7   6   5   4   3

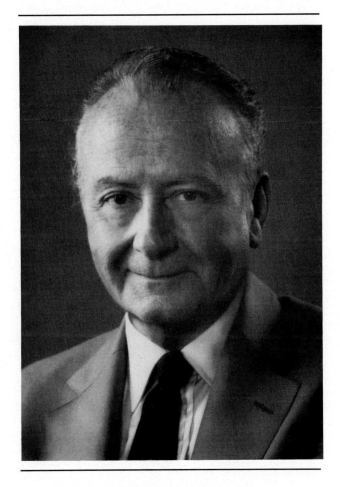

John Marquis Converse
(1909–1981)

This book is dedicated to John Marquis Converse. His enthusiasm for plastic surgery was unrivaled and his contributions to the field were legendary. Through his many writings he not only educated and inspired the plastic surgeon in the era after World War II, but also helped to define modern plastic surgery. This book is a testimony to his professional accomplishments.

Contributors

A. D. BAGNALL, L.C.S.T., M.A.A.S.H.
Speech Pathologist, South Australia Cranio-Facial Unit, Adelaide Children's Hospital, Adelaide, South Australia.

SAMUEL I. BERKOWITZ, D.D.S.
Clinical Professor of Pediatrics, University of Miami School of Medicine; Orthodontist, Dental Clinic, Miami Children's Hospital, Miami, Florida.

PETER T. BRONSKY, D.M.D., M.S.
Visiting Scientist, Department of Orthodontics and the Dental Research Center, University of North Carolina at Chapel Hill, North Carolina.

PETER J. COCCARO, D.D.S.
Formerly Associate Professor of Orthodontics, New York University School of Dentistry, and Research Professor of Clinical Surgery (Orthodontics), New York University School of Medicine, New York, New York.

ERNEST D. CRONIN, M.D.
Clinical Assistant Professor of Plastic Surgery, Baylor College of Medicine; Chief of Plastic Surgery, St. Joseph Hospital, Houston, Texas.

THOMAS D. CRONIN, M.D.
Clinical Professor of Plastic Surgery, Baylor College of Medicine; Attending Surgeon, St. Joseph Hospital, Houston, Texas.

COURT B. CUTTING, M.D.
Assistant Professor of Surgery (Plastic Surgery), New York University School of Medicine; Attending Surgeon, New York University Medical Center and Bellevue Hospital; Chief of Plastic Surgery, Manhattan Veterans Administration Hospital, New York, New York.

DAVID J. DAVID, F.R.C.S., F.R.A.C.S.
Head, South Australian Cranio-Facial Unit, Adelaide Children's Hospital; Head, Department of Plastic and Reconstructive Surgery, Royal Adelaide Hospital, Adelaide, South Australia.

DONALD H. ENLOW, PH.D.
Thomas Hill Distinguished Professor of Oral Biology, Case Western Reserve University School of Dentistry, Cleveland, Ohio.

FRED J. EPSTEIN, M.D.
Professor of Neurosurgery, New York University School of Medicine; Attending Surgeon, University Hospital, Bellevue Hospital Center, and St. Vincent's Medical Center, New York, New York.

MIROSLAV FÁRA, M.D.
Professor of Plastic Surgery, Charles University; Head, Clinic of Plastic Surgery and Burn Unit, Prague, Czechoslovakia.

MICHAEL C. FASCHING, M.D.
Minneapolis, Minnesota.

BARRY H. GRAYSON, D.D.S.
Associate Professor of Clinical Surgery (Orthodontics), New York University School of Medicine; Associate Professor of Clinical Orthodontics, New York University School of Dentistry, New York, New York.

V. MICHAEL HOGAN, M.D.
Clinical Professor of Surgery (Plastic), New York University Medical Center, New York, New York.

IAN T. JACKSON, M.B., CH.B., F.R.C.S., F.A.C.S.
Director, Institute for Craniofacial and Reconstructive Surgery, Providence Hospital, Southfield, Michigan.

MALCOLM C. JOHNSTON, D.D.S., M.Sc.D., Ph.D.
Professor of Orthodontics, School of Dentistry; Professor of Cell Biology and Anatomy, School of Medicine, University of North Carolina at Chapel Hill, North Carolina.

HENRY K. KAWAMOTO, Jr., M.D., D.D.S.
Associate Clinical Professor, UCLA Division of Plastic Surgery, Los Angeles, California.

PETER P. KAY, M.B., B.Ch., F.R.C.S.
Assistant Professor of Plastic and Reconstructive Surgery, Mayo Medical School; Consultant, Division of Plastic and Reconstructive Surgery, and Co-Director, Craniofacial Unit, Mayo Clinic, Rochester, Minnesota.

DON LaROSSA, M.D.
Associate Professor of Surgery (Plastic Surgery), University of Pennsylvania School of Medicine; Director, Cleft Palate Program, Children's Hospital of Philadelphia, Philadelphia, Pennsylvania.

R. A. LATHAM, B.D.S., Ph.D.
Clinical Instructor in Orthodontics, University of Western Ontario; Assistant Professor of Plastic Surgery, University of Miami School of Medicine; Staff Member, Victoria Hospital Corporation, London, Ontario, Canada.

GOTTFRIED LEMPERLE, M.D.
Professor of Surgery (Plastic Surgery), Johann Wolfgang Goethe University; Chief of the Department of Plastic and Reconstructive Surgery, St. Markus Krankenhaus, Frankfurt-am-Main, Germany.

JOSEPH G. McCARTHY, M.D.
Lawrence D. Bell Professor of Plastic Surgery, New York University School of Medicine; Director, Institute of Reconstructive Plastic Surgery, New York University Medical Center; Attending Surgeon, University Hospital, Bellevue Hospital, Manhattan Eye, Ear and Throat Hospital, and Veterans Administration Hospital, New York, New York.

HAROLD McCOMB, F.R.A.C.S.
Clinical Lecturer, University of Western Australia; Plastic Surgeon, Princess Margaret Hospital for Children, Perth, Western Australia.

D. RALPH MILLARD, Jr., M.D.
Light-Millard Professor and Chief of the Division of Plastic Surgery, University of Miami School of Medicine; Attending Surgeon, Jackson Memorial Hospital, Miami Children's Hospital, and Mount Sinai Hospital, Miami, Florida.

GUILLERMO MILLICOVSKY, Ph.D.
Director of Research, International Craniofacial Institute, Humana Advanced Surgical Institutes, Dallas, Texas.

IAN R. MUNRO, M.D.
Director, Humana International Craniofacial Institute, Humana Hospital, Dallas, Texas.

G. WESLEY PRICE, M.D.
Clinical Assistant Professor of Plastic Surgery, Georgetown University School of Medicine; Clinical Instructor of Plastic Surgery, George Washington University School of Medicine; Attending Surgeon, Sibley Memorial Hospital, Washington, D.C., and Fairfax Hospital, Falls Church, Virginia.

PETER RANDALL, M.D.
Professor of Plastic Surgery, University of Pennsylvania School of Medicine; Senior Surgeon, Children's Hospital of Philadelphia, Philadelphia, Pennsylvania.

PAMELA ROPER, M.D., Ph.D.
Attending Staff, St. Joseph Hospital, Women's Hospital of Texas, Park Plaza Hospital, and Hermann Outpatient Surgery Center, Houston, Texas.

R. BRUCE ROSS, D.D.S.
Assistant Professor, Faculty of Dentistry, University of Toronto; Director, Craniofacial Treatment and Research Centre, and Head, Division of Orthodontics, Department of Dentistry, The Hospital for Sick Children, Toronto, Ontario, Canada.

GREGORY L. RUFF, M.D.
Assistant Professor of Plastic Surgery, Duke University School of Medicine, Durham, North Carolina.

JOHN W. SIEBERT, M.D.
Assistant Professor of Surgery, New York University Medical Center; Chief of Plastic Surgery, Bellevue Hospital, New York; Director of Microsurgery, New York University Medical Center and Bellevue Hospital, New York, New York.

JAMES M. STUZIN, M.D.
Attending Surgeon, Mercy Hospital, Cedars Medical Center and Mount Sinai Medical Center, Miami; Clinical Instructor, Department of Plastic Surgery, University of Miami School of Medicine, Miami, Florida.

CHARLES H. M. THORNE, M.D.
Assistant Professor of Surgery (Plastic Surgery), New York University School of Medicine; Attending Surgeon, Manhattan Eye, Ear & Throat Hospital, University Hospital, Bellevue Hospital, and Manhattan Veterans Administration Hospital, New York, New York.

AUGUSTUS J. VALAURI, D.D.S.
Professor of Surgery (Maxillofacial Prosthetics), New York University School of Medicine; Clinical Professor of Removable Prosthodontics and Occlusion, New York University School of Dentistry; Chief of the Maxillofacial Prosthetics Service, Institute of Reconstructive Plastic Surgery, New York University Medical Center, New York, New York.

S. ANTHONY WOLFE, M.D.
Clinical Professor of Plastic and Reconstructive Surgery, University of Miami School of Medicine; Chief of Plastic Reconstructive Surgery, Miami Children's Hospital and Victoria Hospital, Miami, Florida.

DONALD WOOD-SMITH, M.D., F.R.C.S.E.
Professor of Surgery (Plastic Surgery), New York University School of Medicine; Chairman, Department of Plastic Surgery, New York Eye & Ear Infirmary; Attending Surgeon (Plastic Surgery), Bellevue Medical Center; Attending Surgeon, New York University Hospital, New York Veterans Administration Hospital, and Manhattan Eye, Ear & Throat Hospital, New York, New York.

Preface

Where does a book begin? Initially, I think of a warm September afternoon in a hotel in Madrid when I first organized an outline of the chapters while waiting for an international surgery meeting to begin. However, a scientific book is only an extension of earlier publications. This text is descended from *Reconstructive Plastic Surgery*, edited in 1964 by my predecessor John Marquis Converse, and reedited in 1977. I had been Assistant Editor of the latter. Many of the ideas and principles, if not the exact words, that were integral to the teaching and writing of Dr. Converse live on in the present volumes. *Reconstructive Plastic Surgery* in turn was derived from his earlier collaboration with V. H. Kazanjian, *The Surgical Treament of Facial Injuries*, published in 1949, 1959, and 1974.

Earlier textbooks by Nélaton and Ombrédanne (1904), Davis (1919), Gillies (1920), and Fomon (1939) had played a germinal role in the development of modern plastic surgery. However, even these books represented only a continuum of publications extending back over the centuries to Tagliacozzi and Sushruta. Indeed, there are also the many surgeons who never published but who by their teachings contributed greatly to the body of knowledge that is represented in the present publication. Their concepts, too, have found their way into the plastic surgery literature for the edification of another generation of students.

My own career has been greatly influenced by my teachers, and their spirit has remained an integral part of my personal and professional life. This heritage of the plastic surgeon–teacher represents the spirit of this book.

The title defines the subject—*Plastic Surgery*. Adjectives such as *reconstructive* or *esthetic* are misleading and redundant and represent artificial divisions of this surgical specialty. The parents of the infant undergoing cleft lip repair are more interested in the *esthetic* aspects of the procedure, which traditionally has been regarded as *reconstructive*. The contemporary face lift, long perceived as an *esthetic* operation, represents a surgical reconstruction of the multiple layers of the soft tissues of the face. Plastic surgery, a term first popularized by Zeis in 1838, is preferred.

With the deliberate exception of parts of Chapters 1 and 35, originally written by Dr. Converse and revised through subsequent editions of various books, few paragraphs in these volumes remain unchanged from the 1977 edition. Many of the authors, however, have used material from the previous editions. Line drawings prepared for these editions by Daisy Stillwell have been reproduced again where appropriate. With the death of Ms. Stillwell, I was fortunate to recruit yet another outstanding medical artist, Craig Luce, to draw hundreds of new illustrations to reflect the continuing developments in this specialty.

The purpose of this book is to define the specialty of plastic surgery. To accomplish this goal, contributions have been sought from the acknowledged leaders of this discipline in all of its ramifications. The clinical applications of plastic surgery, practiced over the whole of the human anatomy, range from skin grafting to the management of uncommon craniofacial clefts, to replantation of the lower extremity. Its practice varies from uncomplicated procedures to sophisticated multistage reconstructions that ally the plastic surgeon with other specialists. The chapters that follow vary in the same way from the short and direct to the lengthy and complex. More than any other, this type of surgery strives for the restoration or improvement of form as well as the restoration of function. The teaching of plastic surgery thus lends itself to illustration. The contributors to this book have been encouraged to use drawings and photographs liberally as an enhancement of the principles and techniques described in the text. Special attention has been given to the sizing and placement of more than 5000 illustrations submitted in accordance with this plan. The contributors and publisher have also made every effort to acknowledge and cite the work of other authors. In a text of this magnitude any omission, while understandable, is regrettable.

In Volume 1 will be found discussions of the essential principles basic to all plastic surgery: wound healing, circulation of the skin, microneurovascular repairs, skin expansion, and grafting of tendons, nerves, and bone, as well as their associated methods of repair. This is the largest of the volumes and testifies to the broadening scope of the field. Much of what is now fundamental to the training of a plastic surgeon was only imagined a generation ago.

After the discussion of general principles in Volume 1, the organization of the text is by anatomic regions. Volumes 2 and 3 are devoted to the face; here, as throughout the book, each chapter draws upon the expertise of acknowledged master surgeons particularly experienced in the subjects on which they have written.

Clefts of the lip and palate as well as severe craniofacial anomalies make up Volume 4. In addition to plastic surgery, these chapters incorporate contributions from the allied fields of embryology, craniofacial growth and development, orthodontics, prosthodontics, speech pathology, and neurosurgery.

Volume 5 covers tumors of the skin and head and neck and Volume 6 the trunk, lower extremity, and genitourinary system. Of particular note, the text details recent advances in reconstruction that involve newly developed flaps of ingenious design and considerable sophistication.

The application of plastic surgical principles and techniques of the upper extremity are discussed in Volumes 7 and 8 under the editorship of Drs. James W. May, Jr., and J. William Littler. The latter, one of the most esteemed and influential hand surgeons of the modern era, edited the upper extremity section in 1964 and 1977. He has been joined in this edition by Dr. May, who is qualified in both hand surgery and microsurgical reconstruction. Both, who are my personal friends, brought their usual enthusiasm, experience, and equanimity to bear on this project. Because surgery of the upper extremity is practiced so extensively, ample space has been afforded for the comprehensive description of the reconstructive procedures specifically designed for the restoration of injured parts. Much of the current progress in plastic surgery of the upper extremity has been made possible by the gradual perfection of microvascular techniques, and these newer developments have been incorporated into the text.

Continuing change, the hallmark of all medical and surgical practice, dictates the need for a reference book such as this and makes its accomplishment a challenging task for everyone involved. With the writing of these words the lengthy process of revising, updating, and improving is ended. The book is committed to the press with the promise that it is both complete and current, in the belief that readers will find it an invaluable resource, and with the hope that it makes a contribution to the body of plastic surgery knowledge and to the education of tomorrow's plastic surgeon.

JOSEPH G. MCCARTHY, M.D.

Acknowledgments

The authors or contributors, all with heavy clinical responsibilities and demands, have contributed greatly and are responsible for this text. In addition to outlining their personal views, they have conducted exhaustive literature searches and have organized their illustrative material. They represent the heart and soul of the book.

I wish also to acknowledge my fellow faculty members at the Institute of Reconstructive Plastic Surgery, since their work and concepts, as well as their encouragement, have been so important in the development of this text: Sherrell J. Aston, Donald L. Ballantyne, Robert W. Beasley, Phillip R. Casson, David T.W. Chiu, Peter J. Coccaro, Stephen R. Colen, Court B. Cutting, Barry H. Grayson, V. Michael Hogan, Glenn W. Jelks, Frances C. Macgregor, Thomas D. Rees, Blair O. Rogers, William W. Shaw, John W. Siebert, Charles H. M. Thorne, Augustus J. Valauri, Donald Wood-Smith, and Barry M. Zide. Dr. Frank Cole Spencer, George David Stewart Professor of Surgery and Chairman of the Department of Surgery at the New York University Medical Center, has always championed the goals of the Institute and has especially encouraged development in the newer areas of craniofacial surgery and microsurgery.

I should also pay tribute to Ms. Karen Singer, who did so much of the bibliographic study, and Wayne Pearson and Harry Weissfisch, who provided photographic support. I must also acknowledge my associates at the Institute, Robert E. Bochat, Linda Gerson, Donna O'Brien, Caren Crane, Marilyn Deaton, Margy Maroutsis, Marjorie Huggins, and others for acts of kindness and support during the years of preparation of this book.

Mr. Albert Meier, Senior Editor at Saunders, had a major share in the organization and editing of this book. A friend and colleague since 1974 when we began the Second Edition, I have benefited immensely from his advice and counsel. He has also shown an unusual sense of understanding throughout this project. Special thanks are also due to David Harvey, Frank Polizzano, and Richard Zorab of the W. B. Saunders Company for their support.

I am also grateful to the residents and fellows at the Institute of Reconstructive Plastic Surgery, whose boundless enthusiasm is ever encouraging and who have given generously of their time to proofread manuscripts and galleys: Christopher Attinger, Constance Barone, Richard Bartlett, P. Craig Hobar, William Hoffman, Armen Kasabian, Gregory LaTrenta, George Peck, Rosa Razaboni, Gregory Ruff, John Siebert, R. Kendrick Slate, Henry Spinelli, Michael Stevens, Charles Thorne, and Douglas Wagner.

Special thanks are also due to my colleagues and friends at the National Foundation for Facial Reconstruction, whose support and encouragement have provided a unique environment at the Institute that is conducive to writing and research.

Finally, I want to thank my family, Karlan, Cara, and Stephen, for their love and understanding during the demanding years of this project, especially those times spent at a desk when I may have appeared distracted or lost in thought. They remain my main support and life focus.

I also want to thank my friends, especially Charles and Heather Garbaccio, who had the ability to offer those special moments of lightheartedness, good cheer, and camaraderie.

JGM

Contents

Volume *4*

Cleft Lip & Palate and Craniofacial Anomalies

PLASTIC SURGERY

45

Joseph G. McCarthy, M.D.
Court B. Cutting, M.D.
V. Michael Hogan, M.D.

Introduction to Facial Clefts

HISTORY

CLASSIFICATION

EPIDEMIOLOGY AND GENETICS

Rehabilitation of the patient with cleft lip and palate includes many of the appealing features of plastic surgery: the need to understand the etiopathogenesis or pathomechanics, being a member of a multidisciplinary diagnosis and treatment team, the opportunity for continued treatment of the patient during growth and development (the "fourth dimension"), and the execution of surgical procedures that involve the skeletal and soft tissues and demand technical finesse.

HISTORY

Each of the following chapters dealing with information to assist the plastic surgeon in the rehabilitation of the patient with facial clefting contains relevant historical information. There are excellent historical reviews of the subject of cleft lip and palate by Dorrance (1933), Rogers (1971), and Millard (1976). This introduction will be concerned only with outlining the historical trends associated with investigative studies and the treatment of facial clefts.

The Age of Empiricism

Surgeons through the ages have attempted to correct the abnormal anatomic arrangement of the cleft lip and palatal tissues and achieve a "normal" appearance. In ancient times many congenital deformities, including cleft lip and palate, were considered to be evidence of an evil spirit in the afflicted child. These children were often removed from the tribe or cultural unit and left to die in the surrounding wilderness.

Boo-Chai (1966) reported a case of successful closure of a cleft lip in approximately 390 A.D. in China, although the surgeon's name is not mentioned. In Europe many surgical techniques were used for the treatment of wounds during the early Christian era. Hot cautery was a special feature of Arabian surgery, whereas the scalpel was favored by Greek and Roman surgeons. Yperman (1295–1351) was a Flemish surgeon who appears to have written the first fully documented description of cleft lip and its surgical repair. He closed the freshened borders of the cleft lip with a triangular needle armed with a twisted wax suture, a common method of suture at the time. In order to approximate the internal and external wound edges, he reinforced the closure with a long needle passed through the lip some distance from the edges of the cleft; the needle was held in place by a wrap-around figure-of-eight thread. A similar technique of lip closure was still being performed by Pancoast in 1844.

Palatal deformities caused by syphilis and gunshot wounds interested Jacques Houllier (cited by Gurlt, 1898), who appears to have been the first to propose direct suture of palatal perforations. However, the failure rate was high, and he suggested that when surgery failed the region could be occluded with wax or a sponge. Franco (1556) wrote: "... cleft lips are sometimes cleft without a cleft of the jaw or palate, sometimes the cleft is only slight, and at times the cleft is as long and as wide as the lip" (Rogers, 1967). In 1561 he wrote: "Those who have cleft palates are more difficult to cure: and they always speak through their nose. If the palate is only slightly cleft, and if it can be plugged with cotton, the patient will speak more clearly, or perhaps even as well as if there were no cleft: or better, a plate of silver or lead can be applied by some means and retained there" (Rogers, 1967). Palatal occlusion by plates of gold or silver was also described in 1564 by Paré, who designated such a plate as an "obturateur"; Paré (1575) was also the first to use the term "bec-de-lièvre" ("harelip").

Tagliacozzi (1597) described a lip closure that employed mattress sutures passed through all layers of the lip tissue. This was a departure from the prevailing technique of needle closure and figure-of-eight suture material reinforcement. Thus, in the sixteenth century, closure of cleft lip to improve appearance was widely practiced, and the need for closure of the cleft palate to improve speech was appreciated in more limited surgical circles.

Treatment of the protruding premaxilla using a head bandage to achieve external compression of the premaxillary segment, thereby reducing it to a more favorable position for lip closure, was introduced by Desault and Bichat (1798). Over the years, various combinations of intraoral and extraoral devices were developed in order to reduce the protruding premaxillary segment and also to maintain the lateral arch segments in adequate anatomic relationship with the lower jaw. At the present time, there is renewed interest in orthodontic (pin) appliances inserted into infants' mouths to recess the protruding premaxilla and expand the collapsed maxillary segments (see Chap. 57).

The origins of the present techniques for successful closure of the secondary cleft palate are found in the early work of Graefe and Roux, who in 1817 and 1819, respectively, closed the cleft of the *soft palate* with interrupted twine sutures. In Roux's patient, a dramatic change of voice was immediately noted and described.

Direct closure of the *hard palate* followed in 1826. Dieffenbach (1828) recommended that clefts of the hard palate could be closed by separating palatal mucosa from the bone. He also recommended lateral relaxing osteotomies to close clefts of the secondary palate, but did not employ these until 1828. This technique continued to be practiced well into the twentieth century.

Early closure of the soft palate to induce a narrowing of a wide cleft of the hard palate was mentioned in 1828 by Warren. This approach to wide clefts of the hard palate was repopularized by Schweckendiek in 1962 and is currently the subject of much debate because of associated speech problems. Langenbeck in 1859 and 1861 introduced the concept of subperiosteal dissection to elevate the periosteum with the palatal mucosa, thus forming bilateral mucoperiosteal flaps. This technique is still in use in some centers today. Veau drew attention to the fact that palatal lengthening was not achieved by this technique, and launched a full-scale attack on the technique in the Deutsche Zeitschrift für Chirurgie in 1936 (Converse, 1962). He converted Langenbeck's bipedicle flaps into single pedicle flaps based on the descending palatine vessels. Modifications of Veau's basic techniques were made by Wardill (1937), Kilner (1937), and Peet (1961), resulting in a pushback technique for closure of clefts of the secondary palate that is widely used today. Simultaneous lengthening of the nasal surface of the velum can be accomplished by the Cronin modification (1957) (see Chap. 53). Furlow (1986) advocated a double Z-plasty type of cleft palate closure.

Mirault introduced the modern crossflap technique of lip closure in 1844, and since that time nearly every conceivable type of flap—triangular, rectangular, and curvilinear—has been attempted. Mirault's technique remained popular and was advocated during the twentieth century by Blair and Brown (1930). Further modification of cleft lip closure was described in 1884 by Hagedorn, who devised a rectangular flap technique to prevent linear contracture. This procedure appears to have led to the operation of LeMesurier in 1949. During this period Z-plasty techniques were also used in various guises to relieve the tendency of linear scars to contract. This line of endeavor led to the Tennison (1952) low triangular flap technique and the high Z-plasty rotation flap of Millard

(1958) (see Chap. 52). Over the years there have been periodic advocates of correction of the nasal deformity at the time of primary lip repair. Currently, there has been a reawakening of interest in this (McComb, 1986).

Throughout the evolution of the techniques of treatment for cleft lip and palate, therapy for ancillary problems such as dentoalveolar arch deformities, nasal abnormalities, maxillary hypoplasia, and speech difficulties had also progressed to a point at which, in modern times, teams of specialists have been formed to manage the total problem, which has grown too complicated for one or two disciplines alone. This concept of the multidisciplinary team for treatment and evaluation is especially important in the case of the more complex craniofacial anomalies (McCarthy, 1976; Munro, 1981).

Management of the dentoalveolar arch deformity in the patient with cleft lip or palate by techniques of banding and prosthetic stabilization failed to achieve the goal of an adequate upper-lower dental arch relationship after early therapeutic approaches to this problem. Orthodontic therapy proceeded during the period of the eruption of the permanent teeth, and usually during the period of mixed dentition, and often, after years of treatment, a Class III malocclusion with significant crossbite remained.

This led dental innovators such as McNeil (1954) and Burston (1958) to advocate orthodontics in the first year of life in an attempt to establish proper arch relationships. These authors postulated that early alignment of arch segments would aid normal development of the maxilla. Arch position was maintained by appliances, initially a combination of internal and external appliances and finally a simple internal appliance. However, removal of the retaining appliance before puberty often resulted in recurrence of the original arch deformity. It was then thought that perhaps primary bone grafts might (1) stabilize the arch and (2) either grow or promote growth of the uninhibited maxilla. These speculations, however, had no scientific basis (see Chap. 55).

Primary bone grafting in the treatment of cleft alveolar arch deformities has lost many of its enthusiastic supporters. Initially, surgeons attempted bone grafting in the region of the incisive foramen in an effort to improve their statistics on successful palatal closure (Lexer, 1908; Drachter, 1914). Establishment of adequate bone continuity between the premaxilla and lateral bone segments appeared to some surgeons such as Axhausen (1952) to be the "final problem in the repair of complete clefts at the present time." The mere presence of the bone gap was enough to inspire a surgical rush to fill it. However, as will become apparent in Chapter 55, filling the gap was not the end of the matter. Bone grafts appear to be unable on their own to "hold apart" any arch that has a tendency to collapse; the bone graft absorbs under pressure. Also, primary bone grafts do not grow as was originally postulated, but instead hinder growth with a significant limitation of maxillary development and a dramatic increase in crossbite malocclusion and pseudoprognathism (Kling, 1964).

Moreover, as the story of primary bone grafting in cleft palate surgery unfolded, it tended to confirm the prescience of Pruzansky, who in 1964 condemned the unscientific and unsubstantiated use of primary bone grafting when bone graft fever was sweeping many surgical circles. Nevertheless, there are still some advocates of primary bone grafting (Rosenstein and associates, 1982) and most surgeons recommend bone grafting of dentoalveolar clefts at approximately the time of permanent canine eruption (see Chap. 55).

In retrospect, however, we must marvel at the ingenuity of surgeons of the past who made major progress using the trial and error method in an era when corollary scientific information was virtually nonexistent. Nevertheless, there have been surgeons throughout history who attempted to apply their knowledge of anatomy and physiology and use scientific discipline in the design of their surgical procedures.

The Scientific Approach

The nineteenth century witnessed a blossoming of scientific surgical studies in western Europe. The design of a surgical procedure came to be based on precise anatomic studies. The anatomic observations of Pancoast (1844) led him to design a specific operation, in which he divided the insertion of the palatal muscles "so as to prevent their straining the sutured edges of the palate asunder." Fergusson (1844–1845), noting that most palatal repairs disrupted, conducted a series of anatomic studies leading him to propose an operation that divided the levator veli palatini muscles, the posterior tonsillar pillars, and sometimes the anterior tonsillar pillars. The incisions provided relaxation to the muscles and tissues of the palate in order to prevent lateral pull.

The father of modern surgery of cleft lip and palate, Victor Veau, spent many hours studying embryologic specimens. His contributions to the study of cleft lip and palate in and outside of the operating room are significant.

With regard to surgery of the cleft lip, Veau (1931, 1938) pointed out the paucity of muscle fibers in the medial aspect of the unilateral cleft and also in the prolabial segment of the bilateral cleft lip (Converse, 1962):

The median border of the cleft lip is sterile. This anatomic fact, the inadequacy of the musculature of the median aspect, should provide us with a surgical directive: Demand nothing from the inner aspect which is sterile, utilize to the maximum the muscles of the lateral aspect which is fertile, sacrifice all of the mucosa of the inner aspect, but preserve carefully all of the mucosa of the lateral aspect.

The principal cause of the mediocre results obtained in bilateral cleft lip repair is the absence of muscle in the prolabial segment of the lip. One can hope for contour and shape approaching the normal only if the lip contains muscle. I have long emphasized this fact: The muscular sterility of the prolabial segment.

In the treatment of the bilateral cleft lip, Veau was one of the first to take advantage of the pressure resulting from the lip repair to recess the premaxilla:

We are operating on faces in full evolution. The profile of the face will be submitted to a dual transformation. In the nose, the vomer will grow on condition that it has not been altered and it will increase the projection of the nose. In the lip, the reconstituted muscular ring in front of the premaxilla will push it backward. The operation of the cleft lip in the newborn is not an ordinary definitive operation of the type one does in plastic surgery in the patient in whom growth is completed. Our role, in the newborn, is to create conditions of development as close to the normal as possible.

In considering surgical intervention on the vomer to recess the premaxilla, Veau wrote:

In order that the face of the newborn becomes a normal adult face, a series of unknown factors must come into play. All of these factors have their role in the distribution of forces which create the definitive form. They are the instrumental contributions the assembly of which makes the harmony we know. Eliminate the violins and you will no longer recognize a Beethoven symphony. That is what we have done (by sectioning the vomer) in the treatment of bilateral cleft lip: We have done away with the axial beam supporting the evolution of the face.

It was in embryology, however, that Veau made his greatest contribution. His career as an embryologist started when he was over 60 years of age.

I am only a surgeon, yet circumstances have led me to play the role of an embryologist. ... Yesterday, everyone said "cleft lip is caused by the absence of coalescence of the processes of the face." Tomorrow, they will say, "cleft lip is caused by the persistence of the subnarial epithelial membrane."

This concept is not my own; it is the concept of Professor A. Fleischmann, who is still living in Erlangen, where he spent his entire academic career as Professor of Zoology. I have been, however, the gardener who has been responsible for the growth of the small plant, once it was germinated. The embryologists ignored Fleischmann, or only referred to his hypothesis with irony. I showed that Fleischmann's hypothesis could be applied to all clinical varieties of the cleft lip malformation and, in addition, I have supported the hypothesis by embryological findings outlined in drawings of the stages of development of the subnarial region.

I would like to relate the set of circumstances that led me to explore an area that was not my own. Until 1930, I had never looked at an embryo. I knew of the development of the embryo only by what is found in books. I was searching for an operative method for the treatment of cleft lip and I was trying out various methods; I ascertained the fact that the only productive methods were those which approximated normal development: surgery of malformations is experimental biology. In 1926, I wrote a paper on "The role of the prolabial segment in the formation of the face." The theory of the coalescence of the processes led me to a method that I thought to be a good one because it had an embryological basis. I experienced a series of disasters. I was deeply distressed. What was wrong? Was it the surgical technique that was not successful or was embryology providing the wrong directives? I did not understand that I should look at the embryo as a surgeon instead of searching for new ideas in surgical techniques. I was encouraged to go to Vienna to see Professor Fischel who had the famous collection of embryos. There I heard the name of Professor Fleischmann and I began to have some precise idea of the evolution of the face.

The ideas of Fleischmann tallied with what I know of the various types of the cleft lip malfor-

mation; but I had difficulty in understanding the work of the German author; his pictures were poorly demonstrative. I wrote to him asking for explanations. Since that time, we have not ceased to be in touch with each other. We have written volumes of letters to each other.

In 1935, I wrote a paper entitled: "Hypothesis of the initial malformation of the cleft lip." I did not try to do the work of an embryologist. Staying on clinical grounds, I showed that the theory of the facial processes fitted poorly with what I observed in the cleft lip; the theory of Fleischmann, on the other hand, appeared to be the key to all the anatomical details and clinical varieties of the deformity. This was an indirect attack on the classical theory. Fleischmann had sent me diagrams drawn from cat embryos for this paper. These drawings were necessary, I felt, to provide a visual explanation of the theory of the professor from Erlangen.

I sent this paper to Professor Hochstetter, whom I did not know. I admired his work: he had been the first to describe the oronasal membrane, which is an incomprehensible finding according to the theory of the facial processes. Hochstetter did not go as far as to denounce the theory of the facial processes, but his own research, in addition to what I had observed in Fischel's laboratory, convinced me that the facial process theory was a "myth" that has vitiated the study of embryology of the face.

Hochstetter answered my letter, "I have had two specimens of cleft lip embryos put away in a drawer for many years; I have never discussed these specimens because I do not understand them. I am sending them to you." You can imagine how joyful, but at the same time, how anxious, I was when I looked at these specimens. There I found the indisputable proof of the Fleischmann theory. These specimens were embryos of 22 mm (unilateral cleft) and 23.3 mm (bilateral cleft).

I then returned to Vienna. With Hochstetter, I discussed the embryos at great length and in great detail. In Fischel's laboratory, I worked with his first assistant, Professor Politzer. We wrote a paper entitled: "The primary palate. Formation. Anomalies." This is a work of pure embryology: we studied 140 embryos from 5 to 25 mm in size at which the definitive form of the face is constituted.

While I was working on this paper (April, 1935), I went to Heidelberg to operate on cleft palate patients in the service of Professor Kirschner. I visited the embryological laboratory of Professor Keibel, who had just recently died. I arrived when they were finishing the staining of a specimen of a 22 mm embryo with a cleft. It showed renewed proof of Fleischmann's theory. Professor Hoepke, the first assistant, to whom I explained my idea, was not convinced.

Embryologically, the oronasal membrane which plays a role in the cleft lip is constituted by two fundamentally different formations: (A) The floor of the nose between the integument and the naso-palatine canal. This region is formed by the primary palate, a very precocious embryonic structure (5 mm, 2nd week) which appears when the mesoderm has invaded the epithelial wall (7 mm) and is definitively constituted when bone has commenced to differentiate into the undifferentiated mesenchyme (11 mm, 5th week). (B) The hard and soft palate. This long partition is constituted by the secondary palate, a relatively late embryonic formation, definitively constituted when the palatine processes have achieved their fusion (30 mm, 12th week). The malformation in the secondary palate is the congenital cleft of the palate. Most often (6 out of 10) the malformation of the primary palate, the true cleft lip, is associated with a malformation of the secondary palate and the two deformities form a teratologic entity which is dissociable because of its embryonic origins, but which forms, nevertheless, a clinical and surgical entity.

The gist of Fleischmann's hypothesis consists in the following: The cleft palate is the arrest of the disappearance of the epithelial membrane which remains intact, not penetrated by the adjacent mesoderm. Figure [45–1] is the diagram which Politzer and I arrived at in 1936. It summarizes the formation of the subnarial region. The legends explain the 5 stages. We used 108 drawings of normal embryos to represent these stages. We made an effort to eliminate the role of our imagination. We avoided making any comments on our illustrations for fear that these comments might be prejudiced. We did not allow ourselves to define the process of evolution ... In our paper the word "process" does not appear.

The work of Veau has been quoted at length in order to demonstrate his awareness of other scientific disciplines and his dedication to scientific objectivity. He employed information from outside his own narrow field. His style and approach can be an inspiration to those who continue to manifest an interest in cleft lip and palate.

Fára's study of the anatomy of cleft lip and palate (1968); Kriens' (1969) research on the anatomy of the cleft palate and velopharyngeal region; the investigation by Lubker of the physiology of the velopharyngeal mechanism (1968); the work of Warren and Devereux on the aerodynamics of the velopharyngeal region (1966); the acoustical analysis of speech and velopharyngeal incompetence by Isshiki, Honjow, and Morimoto (1968); the embryologic studies of Avery (1962); the anatomic studies of Stenström and Öberg (1960) on cleft lip-nose deformity; the analysis of the anatomy of the columella by Latham (1970); and Johnston's studies of the etiopathogenesis of clefting (see Chap. 48) provide the kind

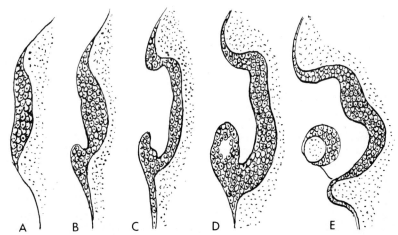

Figure 45–1. Formation of the primary palate. *A,* The plaque is the initial stage. It is formed by the localized thickening of the ectodermal covering (5 mm embryo). *B,* The fossa is produced by the raising of the edges of the plaque and the formation of a spur on the caudal aspect. *C,* The epithelial wall is the result of the increase in height of the spur by the drawing together of the edges of the fossa. *D,* The disappearance of the wall coincides with the spread of the mesoderm. It is not possible to say whether the primary role is played by the ectoderm, which becomes hollow, or by the mesoderm, which perforates it. *E,* The primary palate is formed by the extension of the mesoderm, whose progressive growth leads to the formation of the subnarial region (16 mm embryo). (Redrawn after Veau, V., and Politzer, J.: Le palais primaire. Formation. Anomalies. Ann. Anat. Pathol., *13:*275, 1936.)

of information that must be sought if the surgeon is to continue the strong heritage of the past in seeking the final goal: to make the abnormal as normal as possible.

Contemporary Theories

Throughout the historical development of the treatment of cleft lip and cleft palate, different aspects of the problem have alternately received priority. At the time of publication of this book, there appears to be an emphasis on the role of nasal correction at the time of primary lip repair, a revival of a procedure attributed to Blair (Holdsworth, 1951). This surgical concept had been earlier criticized as interfering with subsequent nasal development, but present advocates (McComb, 1986) have emphasized that, properly executed, primary nasal surgery restores nasal form without having a deleterious effect on normal development (see Chap. 53).

A second area of contemporary interest concerns the use of orthodontic appliances in infants for repositioning of the dentoalveolar segments in order to achieve a gingival repair as well as an optimal, tension-free lip repair (see Chaps. 53 and 57).

Another area of interest for the surgeon today is the problem of crossbite and malocclusion resulting from cleft palate repair. Combined orthodontic-orthognathic surgical programs are discussed in Chapter 29.

Treatment of the anterior palatal deformity has been modified after the publication by Walker and associates (1966) of data indicating the deleterious effect of extensive lateral undermining to facilitate the lip repair. The authors suggested that the technique of lip adhesion, followed in several months by lip closure without lateral periosteal or soft tissue undermining, significantly reduces the incidence of crossbite and malocclusion.

In addition, early complete closure of the primary and secondary palates can also produce significant dental deformities. Ross and Johnston (1972) suggested that surgery should not be performed on the hard palate in areas adjacent to or abutting on teeth during the years of growth and development. An alternative approach is the Schweckendiek (1962) technique of simple closure of the soft palate, followed by obturation of the hard palate cleft and delay of repair of the latter until age addresses this problem. However, longitudinal studies (Cosman and Falk, 1980) demonstrated significantly impaired speech when this therapeutic program is followed.

CLASSIFICATION

Various classification systems have been proposed, but only a few have found wide clinical acceptance.

In the classification of Davis and Ritchie (1922), congenital clefts were divided into

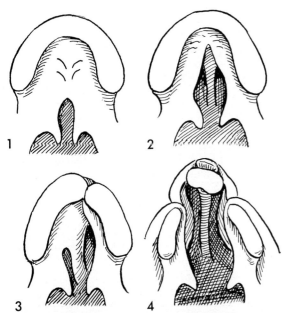

Figure 45–2. The Veau classification of the clefts of the lip and palate. Group 1: cleft of the soft palate only. Group 2: cleft of the soft and hard palate as far forward as the incisive foramen. Group 3: complete unilateral alveolar cleft, usually involving the lip. Group 4: complete bilateral alveolar cleft, usually associated with bilateral clefts of the lip. (After Veau, 1931.)

three groups according to the position of the cleft in relation to the alveolar process:

Group I: Prealveolar clefts, unilateral, median, or bilateral.

Group II: Postalveolar clefts involving the soft palate only, the soft and hard palates, or a submucous cleft.

Group III: Alveolar clefts, unilateral, bilateral, or median.

Veau (1931) suggested a classification divided into four groups (Fig. 45–2):

Group 1: Cleft of the soft palate only.

Group 2: Cleft of the hard and soft palate extending no further than the incisive foramen, thus involving the secondary palate alone.

Group 3: Complete unilateral cleft, extending from the uvula to the incisive foramen in the midline, then deviating to one side and usually extending through the alveolus at the position of the future lateral incisor tooth.

Group 4: Complete bilateral cleft, resembling Group 3 with two clefts extending forward from the incisive foramen through the alveolus. When both clefts involve the alveolus, the small anterior element of the palate, commonly referred to as the premaxilla, remains suspended from the nasal septum.

Kernahan and Stark (1958) recognized the need for a classification based on embryology rather than morphology. The roof of the mouth—from the incisive foramen or its vestige, the incisive papilla, to the uvula—is termed the secondary palate. It is formed after the primary palate (premaxilla, anterior septum, and lip). The incisive foramen is the dividing line between the primary and secondary palates (Fig. 45–3).

A cleft of the secondary palate is further classified as incomplete or complete, depending on its extent. An incomplete cleft is the common cleft of the velum, while a complete cleft includes both the velum and the hard palate as far as the incisive foramen. To this classification must be added the cleft of the mesoderm of the palate, or submucous cleft, which may be camouflaged unless the uvula is cleft. It may not be easy to detect dehiscence of the velum musculature, but the presence of velopharyngeal incompetence and palpation of a notching of the posterior nasal spine aid in the diagnosis.

Kernahan (1971) subsequently proposed a

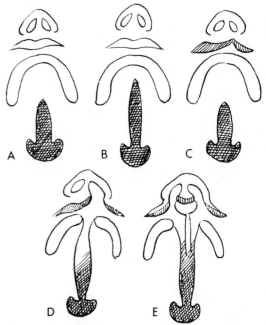

Figure 45–3. Classification of cleft palate. The division between primary palate (prolabium, premaxilla, and anterior septum) and secondary palate is the incisive foramen. *A,* Incomplete cleft of the secondary palate. *B,* Complete cleft of the secondary palate (extending as far as the incisive foramen). *C,* Incomplete cleft of the primary and secondary palates. *D,* Unilateral complete cleft of the primary and secondary palates. *E,* Bilateral complete cleft of the primary and secondary palates. (After Kernahan and Stark, 1958.)

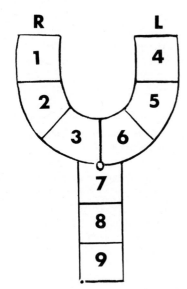

Figure 45-4. The striped Y classification. The involved area is filled in by pen and provides graphic demonstration of the site and extent of cleft involvement. (From Kernahan, D. A.: The striped Y–A symbolic classification for cleft lip and palate. Plast. Reconstr. Surg., 47:469, 1971.)

striped Y classification (Fig. 45–4). As in the previous classification, the incisive foramen is the reference point. With stippling of the involved portion of the Y, the system provides rapid graphic presentation of the original pathologic condition and lends itself to computergraphic presentation.

Harkins and associates (1962) presented a classification of facial clefts based on the same embryologic principles used by Kernahan and Stark (1958). A modified version follows:

1. Cleft of Primary Palate
   A. Cleft Lip
      (1) Unilateral: right, left
         (a) Extent: one-third, two-thirds, complete
      (2) Bilateral: right, left
         (a) Extent: one-third, two-thirds, complete
      (3) Median
         (a) Extent: one-third, two-thirds, complete
      (4) Prolabium: small, medium, large
      (5) Congenital scar: right, left, median
         (a) Extent: one-third, two-thirds, complete
   B. Cleft of Alveolar Process
      (1) Unilateral: right, left
         (a) Extent: one-third, two-thirds, complete
      (2) Bilateral: right, left
         (a) Extent: one-third, two-thirds, complete
      (3) Median
         (a) Extent: one-third, two-thirds, complete
      (4) Submucous: right, left, median
      (5) Absent incisor tooth

2. Cleft of Palate
   A. Soft Palate
      (1) Posteroanterior: one-third, two-thirds, complete
      (2) Width: maximum (mm)
      (3) Palatal shortness: none, slight, moderate, marked
      (4) Submucous cleft
         (a) Extent: one-third, two-thirds, complete
   B. Hard Palate
      (1) Posteroanterior
         (a) Extent: one-third, two-thirds, complete
      (2) Width: maximum (mm)
      (3) Vomer attachment: right, left, absent
      (4) Submucous cleft
         (a) Extent: one-third, two-thirds, complete

3. Mandibular Process Clefts
   A. Lip
         (a) Extent: one-third, two-thirds, complete
   B. Mandible
         (a) Extent: one-third, two-thirds, complete
   C. Lip Pits: Congenital lip sinuses

4. Naso-ocular: Extending from the narial region toward the medial canthal region.

5. Oro-ocular: Extending from the angle of the mouth toward the palpebral fissure.

6. Oro-aural: Extending from the angle of the mouth.

Spina (1974) modified and simplified the above classification as follows:

Group I: Preincisive foramen clefts (clefts lying anterior to the incisive foramen). Clefts of the lip with or without an alveolar cleft.
   A. Unilateral
      (1) right { total when they reach the alveolar arcade or partial
   B. Bilateral
      (1) total
      (2) partial { on one or both sides
   C. Median
      (1) total
      (2) partial

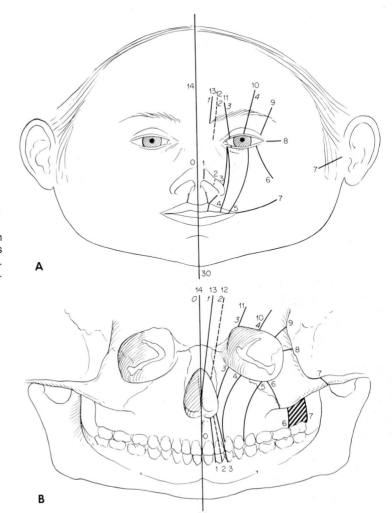

Figure 45–5. Tessier classification of facial clefts. *A,* Location of the clefts on the face. *B,* Skeletal pathways. (Courtesy of Drs. P. Tessier and H. Kawamoto.)

Group II. Transincisive foramen clefts (clefts of the lip, alveolus, and palate).
A. Unilateral $\begin{cases} \text{right} \\ \text{left} \end{cases}$
B. Bilateral
Group III: Postincisive foramen clefts.
A. Total
B. Partial
Group IV: Rare facial clefts.

Tessier (1976) introduced a classification system for the more complex orbitofacial clefts, which have attracted the attention of the surgeon since the introduction of craniofacial surgical techniques. Discussed in detail in Chapter 59, the system (Fig. 45–5) classifies the clefts in a circumferential manner around the orbit with cranial extensions. All components of an individual cleft add up to 14.

EPIDEMIOLOGY AND GENETICS

Clefts of the lip, with or without clefts of the palate (CL/P), must be distinguished from isolated clefts of the hard and soft palates (CP) because of different embryologic, etiologic, and epidemiologic factors (Fogh-Andersen, 1942; Fraser and Calnan, 1961).

Clefts of the secondary palate can be induced in the mouse by teratogens after the primary palate has completely formed. Moreover, clefting of the secondary palate in association with clefts of the primary palate probably represents a secondary (tongue positioning) rather than a primary defect (Trasler and Fraser, 1963).

Family studies have also shown that siblings of patients with CL/P have an increased incidence of CL/P, but the same is not true of isolated CP; conversely, siblings of patients with CP have an increased frequency of CP but not of CL/P (Fogh-Andersen, 1942; Woolf, Woolf, and Broadbent, 1963a, b). There is a male excess in CL/P and a female excess in CP.

In general, the collection of epidemiologic data is associated with many problems. The surveys are traditionally conducted from three sources: birth certificates, hospital records, and treatment (habilitation) or surgical records. The most accurate data are collected from the records of well-organized hospitals. Birth certificates are often hastily completed and lacking in detail. Treatment or surgical records tend to be biased toward a certain segment of the cleft lip and palate population. Other factors to be considered in evaluating the data include the percentage of ascertainment, the racial and socioeconomic composition of the population segment under study, the quality of the records, and the absence of details such as the degree of clefting and the presence of associated anomalies.

The reader is referred to the publications of Fraser (1970), Ross and Johnston (1972), and Bixler (1981) for a more complete discussion of the epidemiology of cleft lip and palate.

Incidence

In the classic studies of Fogh-Andersen (1942), the overall frequency of cleft lip and palate in Denmark was reported as 1.47 per 1000 live births; the incidence of CL/P was 1.16 and that of CP 0.34 per 1000 live births. A similar overall incidence was reported by Woolf, Woolf, and Broadbent (1963a) for a geographic section of the United States and by Wilson (1972) for a region in Great Britain. Racial differences are discussed later in this chapter.

In more recently reported series, cleft lip with palate involvement is reported to be 1.5 to 3.0 times as frequent as isolated cleft lip.

One review gave the following birth incidence of posterior cleft palate (CP): one of every 1500 to 3000 whites, one of every 2000 to 5000 blacks, one of every 1600 to 4200 Asians, and one of 1700 native Americans. For CL/P the estimates are as follows: one of every 775 to 1000 whites, one of every 1370 to 5000 blacks, one of every 470 to 850 Asians,

and one of every 230 to 1000 native Americans (Aylsworth, 1985).

In a follow-up study of the Danish statistical data, Fogh-Andersen (1961) noted an increase in the number of patients operated on from 1.31 per 1000 live births (period from 1938 to 1942) to 1.64 per 1000 live births (period from 1953 to 1957). In a German study (Tünte, 1969) confined to CL/P, an increased incidence of approximately 50 per cent over a 50 year interval was observed, and it was thought that the rise could not be attributed to underreporting alone. Fára (1975) in a Czech study also noted an increased incidence of cleft lip and palate.

Many factors could account for the observed increased frequency of cleft lip and palate: a fall in the postnatal mortality rate, and/or a decrease in operative mortality associated with improvements in anesthesia. In addition, contemporary rehabilitative and surgical efforts yield results so favorable that many more affected individuals marry and transmit the genetic potential for clefting.

Fogh-Andersen (1942) noted a distribution according to type of cleft of 25 per cent cleft lip alone, 50 per cent CL/P, and 25 per cent isolated CP. Ingalls, Taube, and Klinberg (1964) reported a respective frequency of 16, 30, and 54 per cent; Fraser and Calnan (1961) reported 21, 46, and 33 per cent, respectively. Unilateral left-sided clefting, unilateral right-sided clefting, and bilateral clefting occur in a 6:3:1 relationship (Wilson, 1972).

As noted by Fogh-Andersen (1942) and confirmed by other studies (Fraser and Calnan, 1961; Ingalls, Taube, and Klinberg, 1964; Fraser, 1970; Wilson, 1972), there is a left-sided preponderance of cleft lip; in addition, there is a male excess in CL/P and a female excess in isolated CP. Cleft palate is more often associated with bilateral (86 per cent) than with unilateral (68 per cent) clefts of the lip (Fraser, 1970), and this finding is consistent with the concept that cleft palate is seen in the more severe type of lip deformities (Fogh-Andersen, 1942).

Racial Influences

Although the Caucasian race has been the most extensively studied, statistics are also available for the incidence of cleft lip and cleft palate in the black and Oriental races.

The mean incidence of CL/P in Caucasians is approximately one per 1000 population (Fraser, 1970). A higher frequency of CL/P among Japanese infants was reported as approximately 2.1 per 1000; the incidence rate for CP was 0.00055 (Neel, 1958). The data of Fujino, Tanaka, and Sanui (1963) also support the findings of an increased frequency among Orientals.

Blacks in the United States have been extensively studied, and it was noted that blacks are at considerably lower risk of CL/P than are Caucasians (Aylsworth, 1985). In a large collaborative survey of births in several university hospitals, the frequency of CL/P per 1000 births was 1.34 for whites and 0.41 for blacks (Chung and Myrianthopoulos, 1968). A review of birth records in two Washington hospitals serving mainly black patients (Altemus and Ferguson, 1965) and in a similar hospital in New Orleans (Longenecker, Ryan, and Vincent 1965) showed a decreased frequency of CL/P in blacks. Ivy (1962) reported similar data from Philadelphia.

Unlike the data for CL/P, there is less evidence to show racial variation in the incidence of isolated CP between blacks and whites (Altemus and Ferguson, 1965; Chung and Myrianthopoulos, 1968; Aylsworth, 1985).

Thus, there is supporting evidence that racial heterogeneity exists in the frequency of CL/P in a descending order of frequency among Orientals, Caucasians, and blacks. There appears to be no such heterogeneity in the incidence of isolated CP among the three races: it is approximately 0.5 per 1000 births.

Sex Ratio

In whites there is an excess of males with CL/P, the proportion ranging from 60 to 80 per cent (Drillien, Ingram, and Walkinson, 1966). Fogh-Andersen (1942) noted that male preponderance is more marked in the more severe or complete CL/P defects and in bilateral rather than unilateral clefts. Male excess in CL/P is less pronounced among the Japanese (Fujino, Tanaka, and Sanui, 1963).

Female excess has been reported in isolated CP (Fogh-Andersen, 1942; Fraser and Calnan, 1961). In addition, those clefts extending more anteriorly toward the incisive foramen are far more frequent in females.

Parental Age

Birth order appears to play no role in the development of either CL/P or CP.

There is some evidence that the risk of producing an affected child is decreased in younger parents and increased in older parents (Woolf, 1963). Fraser and Calnan (1961) considered that the most important factor was elevated parental and not maternal age.

A significant positive relationship between parental age and isolated CP could not be demonstrated in a study of Caucasians (Woolf, Woolf, and Broadbent, 1963b).

Genetic Factors

As discussed earlier, there is a significant increase of CL/P among relatives of CL/P propositi, but isolated CP occurs in a frequency expected in the general population. Conversely, there is an increased frequency of CP among relatives of patients with CP without an increased incidence of CL/P (Fogh-Andersen, 1942; Woolf, Woolf, and Broadbent, 1963a).

Fogh-Andersen (1942) described the inheritance of CL/P as of "variable expressivity," and Roberts (1964) suggested that it had a "multifactorial etiology" dependent on multiple genes and environmental factors. In affected females with CL/P there is a higher frequency of affected offspring than in affected males with CL/P (Woolf, Woolf, and Broadbent, 1964).

On the basis of the data of Fogh-Andersen (1942); Curtis, Fraser, and Warburton (1961); and Woolf, Woolf, and Broadbent (1963b), the following table of risk figures was established (Ross and Johnston, 1972):

Affected Relatives	Predicted Recurrence (%)	
	CL/P	CP
One sibling	4.4	2.5
One parent	3.2	6.8
One sibling, one parent	15.8	14.9

The risk to siblings born of unaffected parents rises from 4.4 per cent to approximately 9 per cent after two affected children have been born (Curtis, Fraser, and Warburton, 1961).

Bixler (1981) cautioned against pooling together all cleft population data in counseling families. For example, an affected parent should not be told he or she carries a 5 per cent risk of having affected offspring if there are other affected near-relatives. In that situation, the risk is considerably higher (at least 16 per cent or higher).

Syndromic Clefting

A few patients with clefts do not fall into the "multifactorial inheritance" category,* and these individuals usually make up approximately 3 per cent of a clinic cleft population (Fraser, 1970). Most of this group of patients have identifiable syndromes or a "pattern of multiple anomalies thought to be pathogenetically related" (Aylsworth, 1985).

The syndromal etiologic factors can be classified (Pashayan, 1983) into one of the following categories: (1) major mutant genes usually with a known mendelian inheritance pattern such as the Treacher Collins, Stickler, or van der Woude syndrome; (2) chromosomal aberrations such as the more common trisomies D, E, and G; and (3) teratologic syndromes secondary to drug and alcohol ingestion.

---

*Many genes, each with a relatively small effect, interact with the environment to determine whether the developing embryo reaches a threshold of abnormalities. The cases show a strong familial tendency without mendelian inheritance patterns (Pashayan, 1983).

REFERENCES

Altemus, L. A., and Ferguson, A. D.: Comparative incidence of birth defects in Negro and white children. Pediatrics. 36:56, 1965.

Avery, J. K.: The Nasal Capsule in Cleft Palate. Jena, Gustav Fisher Verlag, 1962, p. 722.

Axhausen, G.: Technik und Ergebnisse der Spaltplastiken. München, Hanser, 1952.

Aylsworth, A. S.: Genetic considerations in clefts of the lip and palate. Clin. Plant. Surg., 12:533, 1985.

Bixler, D.: Genetics and clefting. Cleft Palate J., 18:10, 1981.

Blair, V. P., and Brown, J. B.: Mirault's operation for single harelip. Surg. Gynecol. Obstet., 51:81, 1930.

Boo-Chai, K.: An ancient Chinese text on a cleft lip. Plast. Reconstr. Surg., 38:189, 1966.

Burston, W. R.: The early orthodontic treatment of cleft palate conditions. Dent. Pract., 9:41, 1958.

Chung, C. S., and Myrianthopoulos, N. C.: Racial and prenatal factors in major congenital malformations. Am. J. Hum. Genet., 20:44, 1968.

Converse, J. M.: Victor Veau (1871–1949): the contributions of a pioneer. Plast. Reconstr. Surg., 30:225, 1962.

Cosman, B., and Falk, A. S.: Delayed hard palate repair and speech deficiencies: a cautionary report. Cleft Palate J., 17:27, 1980.

Cronin, T. D.: Method of preventing raw area on the nasal surface of the soft palate in push-back surgery. Plast. Reconstr. Surg., 20:474, 1957.

Curtis, E., Fraser, F. C., and Warburton, D.: Congenital cleft lip and palate: risk figures for counseling. Am. J. Dis. Child., 102:853, 1961.

Davis, J. S., and Ritchie, H. P.: Classification of congenital clefts of the lip and palate. J.A.M.A., 79:1323, 1922.

Desault, P. J., and Bichat, X.: Sur l'opération du bec-de-lièvre. In Oeuvres Chirurgicales ou Exposé de la Doctrine et de la Plastique. Vol. 2. Paris, Megengnon, 1798.

Dieffenbach, J. F.: Beitraege zur Gaumennath. Litt. Ann. Ges. Heilk., 10:322, 1828.

Dorrance, G. M.: The Operative Story of Cleft Palate. Philadelphia, W. B. Saunders Company, 1933.

Drachter, R.: Die Gaumenspalte und deren operative Behandlung. Dtsch. Z. Chir., 131:1, 1914.

Drillien, C. M., Ingram, T. T. S., and Walkinson, E. M.: The Causes and Natural History of Cleft Lip and Palate. Edinburgh, E. & S. Livingstone, 1966.

Fára, M.: Anatomy and arteriography of cleft lips in stillborn children. Plast. Reconstr. Surg., 42:29, 1968.

Fára, M.: The anatomy of cleft lip. Clin. Plast. Surg., 2:205, 1975.

Fára, M., and Brousilova, M.: Experiences with early closure of velum and later closure of hard palate. Plast. Reconstr. Surg., 44:134, 1969.

Fergusson, W.: Observations on cleft palate and on staphylorrhaphy. Med. Time Gaz., 2:256, 1844–1845.

Fogh-Andersen, P.: Inheritance of Harelip and Cleft Palate. Copenhagen, Nyt Nordisk Forlag, Arnold Busck, 1942.

Fogh-Andersen, P.: Incidence of cleft lip and palate: constant or increasing? Acta Chir. Scand., 122:106, 1961.

Franco, P.: Bec-de-lièvre. In Nicaise, E. (Ed.): Chirurgie Composée en 1561. Paris, Alcan, 1985, p. 313.

Fraser, F. C.: The genetics of cleft lip and palate. Am. J. Hum. Genet., 22:336, 1970.

Fraser, G. R., and Calnan, J. S.: Cleft lip and palate: seasonal incidence, birth weight, birth rank, sex, site, associated malformations and parental age. Arch. Dis. Child., 36:420, 1961.

Fujino, H., Tanaka, K., and Sanui, Y.: Genetic study of cleft lips and cleft palates based on 2828 Japanese cases. Kyushu J. Med. Sci., 14:317, 1963.

Furlow, L. T., Jr.: Cleft palate repair by double opposing Z-plasty. Plast. Reconstr. Surg., 78:724, 1986.

Georgiade, N. G., and Latham, R.: Ideals in the treatment of the protruding bilateral cleft with rapid intraoral premaxillary retraction and a one stage bilateral lip repair. Second International Congress of Cleft Palate. August 26–31, Copenhagen, 1973.

Graefe, C. F., von: Kurze Nachrichten und Auszuge. J. D. Pract. Arznek. u. Wundarzk., 44(Part 1):116, 1817.

Hagedorn, W.: Ueber eine Modifikation der Hasenscharten Operation. Zentralbl. Chir., 11:756, 1884.

Harkins, C. S., Berlin, A., Harding, R. L., Longacre, J. J., and Snodgrasse, R. M.: A classification of cleft lip and cleft palate. Plast. Reconstr. Surg., 29:31, 1962.

Holdsworth, W. G.: Cleft Lip and Palate. London, William Heinemann Medical Books, 1951.

Houllier, J.: Cited by Gurlt, E. J.: Geschichte der Chirurgie und ihrer Ausübung. Berlin. Hirschwald, 1898.

Ingalls, T. H., Taube, I. E., and Klinberg, M. A.: Cleft lip and cleft palate: epidemiologic considerations. Plast. Reconstr. Surg., 34:1, 1964.

Isshiki, N., Honjow, I., and Morimoto, M.: Effects of velopharyngeal incompetence upon speech. Cleft Palate J., 5:297, 1968.

Ivy, R. H.: The influence of race on the incidence of certain congenital anomalies, notably cleft lip–cleft palate. Plast. Reconstr. Surg., 30:581, 1962.

Kernahan, D. A.: The striped Y—a symbolic classification for cleft lip and palate. Plast. Reconstr. Surg., 47:469, 1971.

Kernahan, D. A., and Stark, R. B.: A new classification for cleft lip and cleft palate. Plast. Reconstr. Surg., 22:435, 1958.

Kilner, T. P.: Cleft lip and palate repair technique. St. Thomas Hosp. Rep., 2:127, 1937.

Kling, A.: Evaluation of results with reference to the bite. In Hotz, R. (Ed.): Early Treatment of Cleft Lip and Palate. Bern, Switzerland, Hans Huber, 1964.

Kriens, O. B.: An anatomical approach to veloplasty. Plast. Reconstr. Surg., 43:29, 1969.

Langenbeck, B. R. C., von: Beitraege zur Osteoplastik. Dtsch. Klinik, 11:471, 1859.

Langenbeck, B. R. C., von: Die Uranoplastik mittels Ablösung des mucös-periostalen Gaumenuberzuges. Arch. Klin. Chir., 2:205, 1861.

Latham, R. A.: Maxillary development and growth: the septo-premaxillary ligament. J. Anat., 107:471, 1970.

LeMesurier, A. B.: A method of cutting and suturing the lip in the treatment of complete unilateral clefts. Plast. Reconstr. Surg., 4:1, 1949.

Lexer, E.: Die Verwendung der freien Knochenplastik Lenktransplantation. Langenbecks Arch. Klin. Chir., 86:939, 1908.

Lindsay, W. K.: In Georgiade, N. G. (Ed.): Symposium of Management of Cleft Lip and Cleft Palate and Associated Deformities. St. Louis, MO., C. V. Mosby Company, 1974, p. 163.

Longenecker, C. G., Ryan, R. F., and Vincent, R. W.: Cleft lip and cleft palate. Incidence at a large charity hospital. Plast. Reconstr. Surg., 35:548, 1965.

Lubker, J. F.: An electromyographic-cinefluorographic investigation of velar function during normal speech production. Cleft Palate J., 5:1, 1968.

McCarthy, J. G.: The concept of a craniofacial anomalies center. Clin. Plast. Surg., 3:611, 1976.

McComb, H.: Primary repair of the bilateral cleft lip nose: a 10-year review. Plast. Reconstr. Surg., 77:701, 1986.

McNeil, C. K.: Oral Facial Deformity. London, Pitman & Sons, 1954.

Millard, D. R., Jr.: A radical rotation in single harelip. Am. J. Surg., 95:318, 1958.

Millard, D. R., Jr.: Cleft Craft: The Evolution of Its Surgery. Boston, Little, Brown & Company, 1976.

Mirault, G.: Deux lettres sur l'opération du bec-de-lièvre considéré dans ses divers états de simplicité. J. Chir. (Paris), 2:275, 1844.

Munro, I. R.: Current surgery of craniofacial anomalies. Otolaryngol. Clin. North Am., 14:157, 1981.

Neel, J. V.: A study of major congenital defects in Japanese infants. Am. J. Hum. Genet., 10:398, 1958.

Pancoast, J. A.: A Treatise on Operative Surgery. Philadelphia, Carey & Hart, 1844, p. 234.

Paré, A.: Les Oeuvres de M. Ambroise Paré. Paris, G. Buon, 1575.

Pashayan, H. M.: What else to look for in a child born with a cleft of the lip and/or palate. Cleft Palate J., 20:54, 1983.

Peet, E.: The Oxford technique of cleft palate repair. Plast. Reconstr. Surg., 28:282, 1961.

Pruzansky, S.: Pre-surgical orthopedics and bone grafting for infants with cleft lip and palate: a dissent. Cleft Palate J., 1:164, 1964.

Roberts, J. A. F.: Multifactorial inheritance and human disease. In Steinberg, A. G., and Bearn, A. G. (Eds.): Advances in Medical Genetics. New York, Grune & Stratton, 1964.

Rogers, B. O.: Palate surgery prior to von Graefe's pioneering staphylorrhaphy (1816): an historical review of the early causes of surgical indifference in repairing the cleft palate. Plast. Reconstr. Surg., 39:1, 1967.

Rogers, B. O.: History of cleft lip and palate treatment. In Grabb, S. W., Rosenstein, S. W., and Bzoch, K. R. (Eds.): Cleft Lip and Plate. Boston, Little, Brown & Company, 1971.

Rosenstein, S. W., Monroe, C. W., Kernahan, D. A., Jacobson, B. N., Griffith, B. H., and Bauer, B. S.: The case of early bone grafting in cleft lip and cleft palate. Plast. Reconstr. Surg., 70:297, 1982.

Ross, R. B., and Johnston, M. C.: Cleft Lip and Palate. Baltimore, Williams & Wilkins Company, 1972.

Roux, P. J.: Observation sur une division congénitale du voile du palais et de la luette, guérie au moyen d'une opération analogue à celle du bec-de-lièvre, pratiquée par M. Roux. J. Universal Sci. Med., 15:356, 1819.

Schweckendiek, W.: Die Ergebnisse der Kieferbildung und die Sprache nach der primaen Veloplastik. Arch. Ohren-Heilk, 180:541, 1962.

Spina, V.: A proposed modification for the classification of cleft lip and cleft palate. Cleft Palate J., 10:251, 1974.

Stenström, S. J., and Öberg, T. R. H.: The nasal deformity in unilateral cleft lip. Plast. Reconstr. Surg., 28:295, 1960.

Tagliacozzi, G.: De Curtorum Chirurgia per Insitionem. Venetiis, G. Bindonus, 1597.

Tennison, C. W.: The repair of unilateral cleft lip by the stencil method. Plast. Reconstr. Surg., 9:115, 1952.

Tessier, P.: Anatomical classification of facial, craniofacial and latero-facial clefts. J. Maxillofac. Surg., 4:69, 1976.

Tolarova, M., Havlova, Z., and Ruzickova, J.: The distribution of characters considered to be microforms of cleft lip and/or palate in a population of normal 18–21 year old subjects. Acta Chir. Plast., 9:1, 1967.

Trasler, D. G., and Fraser, F. C.: Role of the tongue in producing cleft palate in mice with spontaneous cleft lip. Dev. Biol., 6:45, 1963.

Tünte, W.: Is there a secular increase in the incidence of cleft lip and palate? Cleft Palate J., 6:430, 1969.

Veau, V.: Division Palatine. Paris, Masson et Cie, 1931.

Veau, V.: Bec-de-Lièvre. Paris, Masson et Cie, 1938.

Veau, V., and Politzer, J.: Embryologie du bec-de-lièvre. Ann. Anat. Pathol., *13:*278, 1936.

Walker, J. C., Collito, M. B., Mancusi-Ungaro, A., and Meijer, R.: Physiologic considerations in cleft lip closure: the C-W technique. Plast. Reconstr. Surg., *37:*552, 1966.

Wardill, W. E. M.: Technique of operation for cleft palate. Br. J. Surg., *25:*117, 1937.

Warren, D. W., and Devereux, J. L.: An analog study of cleft palate speech. Cleft Palate J., *3:*103, 1966.

Warren, J. C.: On an operation for the cure of natural fissure of the soft palate. Am. J. Med. Sci., *3:*1, 1828.

Wilson, M. E. A. C.: A ten-year survey of cleft lip and cleft palate in the South West region. Br. J. Plast. Surg., *25:*224, 1972.

Woolf, C. M.: Paternal age effect for cleft lip and palate. Am. J. Hum. Genet., *15:*389, 1963.

Woolf, C. M., Woolf, R. M., and Broadbent, T. R.: A genetic study of cleft lip and palate in Utah. Am. J. Hum. Genet., *15:*209, 1963a.

Woolf, C. M., Woolf, R. M., and Broadbent, T. R.: Genetic and nongenetic variables related to cleft lip and palate. Plast. Reconstr. Surg., *32:*65, 1963b.

Woolf, C. M., Woolf, R. M., and Broadbent, T. R.: Cleft lip and heredity. Plast. Reconstr. Surg., *34:*11, 1964.

46

Malcolm C. Johnston

Embryology of the Head and Neck

In recent years the understanding of both normal and abnormal craniofacial development has increased dramatically. The probable pathogenesis of some of the more common, surgically important malformations has been clarified by the detailed correlation of experimentally induced malformations with those caused in humans by identical terato- gens or by genetic defects. Technical advances in methods used to study the normal regula- tion of development have provided informa- tion about the normal mechanisms, even at the molecular level, and this in turn is mak- ing it possible to determine the primary ac- tions of abnormal genetic and environmental factors.

New information on normal developmental mechanisms and on malformations in hu- mans and experimental animals necessitates reassessment of the pathogenesis of some human malformations.

The chapter begins with a brief overview of normal development and proceeds to a more detailed consideration of the progressive stages of normal development, with discus- sions of abnormal alterations at each stage. This format should permit the reader to un- derstand better how later development is changed following a primary alteration at an earlier stage. The embryogenesis of cleft lip and palate will be covered only briefly, since this subject is discussed in considerable detail in Chapter 48.

NORMAL DEVELOPMENT: AN OVERVIEW

The surface changes observed in the devel- opment of the human embryo are illustrated in Figure 46–1. Underlying developmental changes, such as cell migrations and rates of cell proliferation, have been determined from studies conducted on subhuman vertebrates, but the fact that their surface morphologic changes are similar (at least for the higher vertebrates) through the sensitive stages of development permits extrapolation with a

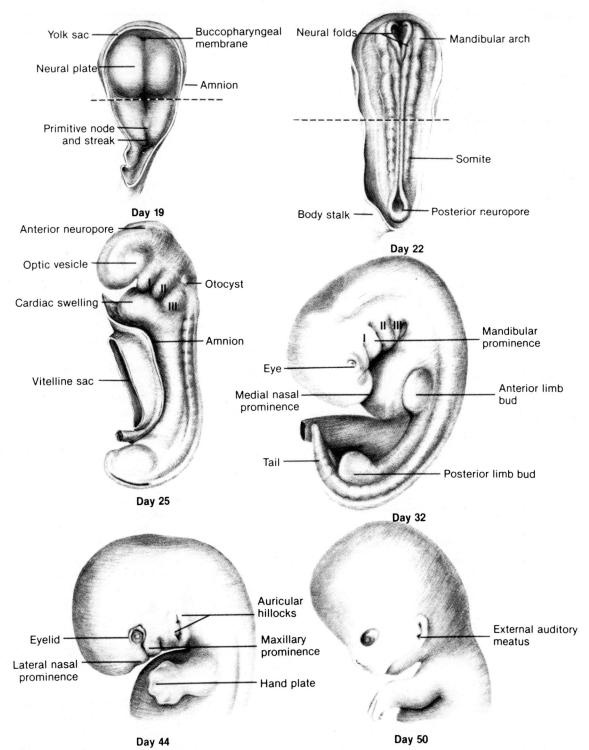

Figure 46–1. Development of the human embryo from the germ layer stage (day 19) to near the end of the embryonic period (day 50). The visceral arches are labeled by Roman numerals. Up to day 32, surface features of the human embryo are similar to those of other higher vertebrates, indicating similar developmental mechanisms. Most major craniofacial malformations have occurred by this time (day 32). (From Johnston, M. C., and Sulik, K. K.: Development of the face and oral cavity. *In* Bhaskar, S. N. (Ed.): Orban's Oral Histology and Embryology. 9th Ed. St. Louis, C. V. Mosby Company, 1980.)

considerable degree of confidence. Although many of these changes are complex, the division of craniofacial development into a step by step sequence simplifies its understanding.

The earliest sequence of changes is illustrated in Figure 46–2. Fertilization is followed by a series of cell divisions and the formation of a fluid-filled cavity. Only some of the cells (the inner cell mass) in the resulting vesicle go on to form the embryo; the remaining cells serve support functions (e.g., the formation of the placenta). The cells of the inner cell mass separate into two layers; migration of cells from the upper layer (epiblast) initiates formation of the middle germ layer. This particular migration is termed "gastrulation." It is usually accepted that the lower layer (hypoblast) forms the endoderm, but at least a portion of it may be formed from cells migrating from the epiblast. All the mesoderm (middle germ layer) is formed by the migrating cells, while unmigrated epiblast cells remain on the surface to become the ectoderm.

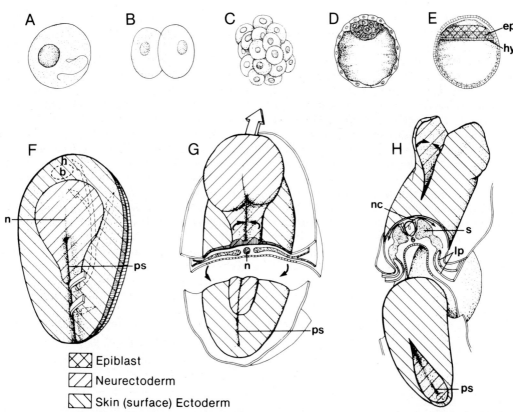

Epiblast
Neurectoderm
Skin (surface) Ectoderm

Figure 46–2. Development of the human embryo from fertilization *(A)* through neural tube formation *(H)*. After several divisions, fluid accumulation within the interior leads to formation of the blastocyst *(D)*. Only a portion of the blastocyst (the inner cell mass = *dark stipple*) forms the embryo, while the remainder forms support tissues such as the placenta. The inner cell mass separates into two cell layers (the epiblast or ep and hypoblast or hy in *E*). During gastrulation *(F)*, cells from the epiblast migrate through the midline primitive streak (ps) into the space between the epiblast and hypoblast *(arrow)*. They form the mesoderm and at least some of the endoderm. The notochord (n) appears to be formed by cells being deposited from the caudally regressing primitive streak. The remaining mesoderm is formed by migrating primitive streak cells that penetrate between the ectoderm (formerly hypoblast) *(arrow* in *F)* and endoderm at all points except the buccopharyngeal plate (b), which later separates the developing oral and pharyngeal cavities. The portion of the epiblast that remains on the surface is termed "ectoderm," completing formation of the three germ layers. The anterior portion of the neural plate (neuroectoderm and outlined in *F)* rapidly overgrows *(open arrow* in *G)* the future facial region and heart. Folding movements (solid arrows in *G* and *H)* lead to neural tube and gut formation. In the last stage illustrated *(H)*, three mesodermal areas—notochord (nc), somites (s), and lateral plate (lp)—are recognizable, and neural crest cells (nc) are beginning their migrations from the neural folds ("crests"). (Modified from Johnston, M. C. and Sulik, K. K.: Embryology of the head and neck. *In* Serafin, D., and Georgiade, N. (Eds.): Pediatric Plastic Surgery. St. Louis, C. V. Mosby Company, 1984.)

Such cell migrations bring different cell populations together, permitting interactions between them. In the first of many such interactions, *primary embryonic induction,* a portion of the mesodermal cells induce the overlying ectodermal cells to form the neural plate. Induction is an exclusively embryonic interaction in which, once the message is transferred, the inducing cell population is no longer required. On explantation of the induced neural plate to culture, it is capable of going through further differentiation and other developmental changes on its own. The ability to respond is termed "competence." There is some evidence that definable chemical substances are involved in inductive interactions, but the underlying mechanisms are poorly understood.

The induced neural plate thickens and rolls up to form the neural tube (Fig. 46–2F to H). At the same time, the lateral body walls fold under the embryo to form the gut and associated structures (Fig. 46–2G, H), and the forebrain overgrows (*open arrow* in G) the buccopharyngeal membrane and heart (b and h in F) that were initially in front of it.

Usually at about the time when the neural folds make contact, or slightly before, neural crest cells migrate from them (Fig. 46–2H). These cells often follow long and complicated migrations, interacting with local tissues to form a spectacular array of derivatives, including those of the peripheral nervous system, the pigment cells of the skin, and almost all of the skeletal and connective tissues of the face and anterior neck and considerable portions of the cranium. These tissues are formed by mesoderm elsewhere; trunk crest cells cannot form such tissues in higher vertebrates. The peculiar role of cranial crest cells in the head and neck provides the key to understanding a number of craniofacial malformations.

When crest cells leave the neural folds, they became dissociated and migrate as individuals, forming a loosely arranged mesenchyme. The term "mesenchyme" is used to describe loosely organized embryonic tissue as contrasted with more compactly arranged epithelia, such as those found in the neural plate. These terms describe the histologic appearance of the two principal embryonic tissues and should not be confused with terms used to describe the germ layers from which they are derived (Fig. 46–3). The loosely arranged mesoderm itself is a mesenchymal tissue while it is migrating from the epiblast. Later it organizes itself into compactly arranged epithelial structures such as somites, which again break down to form loosely arranged migrating mesenchyme cells such as myoblasts (embryonic muscle cells).

Cranial neural crest cells reach the facial region by migrating under the surface ectoderm (Fig. 46–4). At the completion of their migration, the crest cells surround the mesodermal cores in the visceral arches and form all the mesenchyme of the rest of the face.

The initial mesodermal cores of the visceral arches are involved in the formation of vascular elements. Endothelial buds from this tissue invade and vascularize the surrounding crest cell mesenchyme. After vascularization of the mesenchyme, the remaining cells in the core degenerate and are replaced

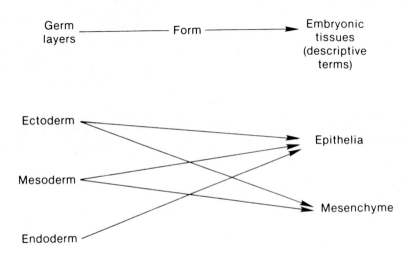

Figure 46–3. The terms "epithelia" and "mesenchyme" are descriptive and used by embryologists to describe compactly and loosely organized embryonic tissues, respectively. Neither germ layer origins nor derivatives are considered. (From Johnston, M. C., and Sulik, K. K.: Embryology of the head and neck. *In* Serafin, D., and Georgiade, N. (Eds.): Pediatric Plastic Surgery. St. Louis, C. V. Mosby Company, 1984.)

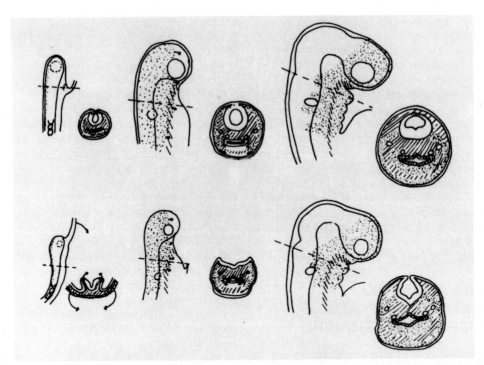

Figure 46–4. Migrations and destinations of cranial neural crest cells *(stipple)* in chick and rat embryos as determined by ³H-thymidine labeling of the cells. Although the neural tube closes later in the rat, the migrations and distributions of crest cells are similar. Comparison of the scanning electron micrographic morphology of neural crest cells in chick, rodent, and human embryos indicates similar developmental patterns. (From Johnston, M. C., Vig, K. and Ambrose, L.: Neurocristopathy as a unifying concept: clinical correlations. Adv. Neurol., 29:97, 1981.)

by other mesodermal cells migrating from locations close to the neural tube. The new core cells are myoblasts that will eventually form the contractile cells in most of the voluntary (skeletal) muscles in the face and anterior neck. In order to reach their final destinations, they must sometimes undergo long secondary migrations.

Another peculiar feature of the head that appears to be critical for an understanding of at least one craniofacial malformation (the Treacher Collins syndrome) is the fact that major contributions to the peripheral nervous system are made by ectodermal thickenings (placodes) that are not part of the neural plate.

At the completion of crest cell migration, facial (and anterior neck) development enters a phase dominated by the establishment of "growth centers" in which high rates of cell proliferation are maintained. Three of these growth centers, the medial and lateral nasal prominences and the maxillary prominence, give rise to the primary palate, which, upon contact, forms the initial separation of the

oral and nasal cavities. Morphogenetic movements of the medial and lateral nasal prominences appear also to play a major role. Failure of contact and fusion between these prominences leads to both common and rare forms of cleft lip. At a later stage, the palatal shelves form from the medial (inner) aspect of the maxillary prominences. Their failure to unite in the midline results in clefts of the hard and soft palate. Normal development of the primary and secondary palates, and cleft lip and palate formation, is covered in detail in Chapter 48. Also considered in some detail in Chapter 48 is the mechanism by which growth in these and other centers may be regulated through epithelial mesenchymal interactions, possibly involving a mesenchymal cell process meshwork.

The distal portions of the first and second visceral arches reorganize and appear to develop further as more or less free-ended growth centers, eventually uniting in the midline through a process of merging in which the underlying mesenchyme becomes confluent, as opposed to the fusions involved in primary and secondary palate formation in which breakdown of contracting epithelia is required. Other growth centers are involved in formation of the external ear.

It is only at the time of secondary palate formation that skeletal tissues begin to form. These include cartilages, bones, and teeth, each of which has its own developmental problems.

The onset of skeletal formation is sometimes considered to signal the end of the embryonic period and the onset of the fetal period. However, some types of embryonic phenomena, such as cell migrations and interactions, are still taking place in the central nervous system.

GASTRULATION AND ORGANIZATIONAL PLANS OF ECTODERM AND MESODERM

Much of the "blueprint" of the head is determined during or immediately after gastrulation. The structural relationships of the upper face are dependent on the organizational plans of the mesoderm and anterior neural plate.

The mesoderm first induces the overlying ectoderm to differentiate into neural tissues. Although neural plates removed to culture will continue to form neural ectoderm, the degree of organization is increasingly improved as the period between induction and explanation is lengthened. Although this function of the mesoderm is not inductive, its apparent ability to organize the ectoderm is responsible for the name *organizer* given to a portion of the gastrulating mesoderm.

The induced neural plates have considerable ability to "self-organize," even when completely artificial inducers (such as toxic substances) are used in culture, and the prospective ectoderm has never "seen" any mesoderm. The specificity for derivatives such as eyes and olfactory placodes is in the competent ectoderm, but the quantity and positioning of derivatives is erratic (Holtfreter and Hamburger, 1955). Areas of prospective neural plate structures, such as the eye, are said to constitute fields, which become progressively more committed to form that particular structure. The mechanisms underlying field formation are poorly understood. However, recent findings on the role of retinoic acid in regulating pattern formation

in limb development indicate the type of regulation that may be involved (Thaller and Eichele, 1988).

The underlying organizer mesoderm is required for a high level of organization in the neural plate. This mesoderm has two major components: the notochord and the paraxial mesoderm. A third major mesodermal component, the lateral plate, seems to provide little more than angiogenic (blood and blood vascular) tissue in the head.

A cranial extension from the notochord reaches forward to the future oral plate. Although this structure, sometimes called "prechordal plate," never forms notochord, it appears to have organizing abilities similar to those of the notochord. Both notochord and prechordal plate are initially firmly attached to or inserted into the endoderm, but that attachment is lost (at about 5 or 6 somites in amphibia—Adelmann, 1934) when paraxial mesoderm becomes confluent across the midline.

Much of the mesodermal organization is inherent to that tissue and not dependent on the neural plate. This was clearly shown many years ago by experiments in which the formation of "exogastrulas" was caused by excessively high salt concentrations in solutions used for the culture of developing amphibian embryos (Holtfreter, 1934). Instead of gastrulating mesodermal cells moving into the interior of the embryo, they ballooned outward to form a mass connected to the ectoderm by only a stalk. The mass of mesodermal and endodermal cells is able to form notochord. Incomplete (partial) gastrulation results in cyclopic eyes (Holtfreter and Hamburger, 1955).

Other experiments by Holtfreter (1934) and Adelmann (1937) are helpful to an understanding of head organization and the problems of cyclopia and the holoprosencephalies (see below). Explants of developing neural tubes adjacent to notochords thin out in that region (as in the thin floor plates of the neural tube and brain), while somitic material stimulates a thickening of the adjacent neural plate. Adelmann found that removal or inhibition of formation of the prechordal plate resulted in failure of the thinning in the midline neural plate and a relatively large cyclopic eye. Removal of adjacent paraxial mesoderm was less effective. Adelmann did not rule out primary defects in the anterior neural plate as a cause of cyclopia, but thought they were probably very rare.

The relationship of the neural plate to other ectodermal placodes ("thickenings") is somewhat controversial. There is some evidence (Couly and Le Douarin, 1985, 1987) that the olfactory placodes are derived from the neural folds, supporting the above observation that explanted neural plates are capable of forming olfactory placodes. The otic placodes also develop in close relation to the neural plate and tube. Ganglionic placodes are formed at some distance from the neural plate and tube. They contribute neurons to the cranial sensory ganglia.

Organization of the mesoderm, in turn, is at least partly dependent on the neural plate and tube and, possibly, the notochord. Variable combinations of these tissues in culture have shown that the formation of cartilage is dependent on neural tube and notochord, while the formation of muscle is dependent on the presence of neural tube (Fig. 46–5).

The organization of occipital somites in the hindbrain region forms a pattern similar to that found in the cervical and trunk regions. The dermatomes contribute to the dermis of the skin immediately overlying the somite; the myotome forms the contractile cells of voluntary (skeletal) muscle; while the sclerotome forms skeletal and connective tissues, including most of the cranial base and vault.

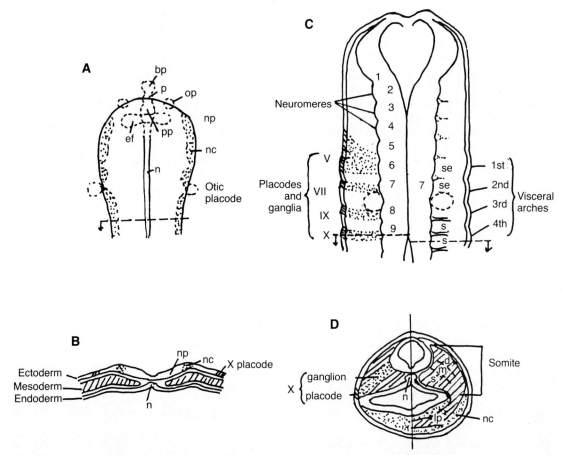

Figure 46–5. Organizational plan of the ectoderm and mesoderm. At the postgastrulation stage, many ectodermal structures are already "determined" although they cannot yet be recognized morphologically. Much segmentation and further pattern formation is recognizable at the post-tubulation stage. The neural tube is segmented into neuromeres (C). Ganglionic placodal cells will add neuroblasts to the developing cranial sensory ganglia (Roman numerals in C and left side of post-tubulation section, D). Contact occurs between the endoderm and ectoderm at the location of all ganglionic placodes except the trigeminal. These contacts occur between the visceral arches. Segmentation in the mesoderm gives rise to well-defined somites (s) in the postotic region and poorly defined somitomeres (se) in the preotic region. Somites are further divided into dermatomes (d), myotomes (m), and sclerotomes (s). Somitomeres do not have dermatomes. The lateral plate (right side of post-tubulation section, D) becomes segmented to form cores in each of the visceral arches. These cores become surrounded by neural crest cells. Other structures are as follows: bp, buccal plate; p, anterior pituitary anlage; ef, eye field; pp, prechordal plate; n, notochord; nc, neural crest; op, olfactory placode.

The lateral plate forms many skeletal and connective tissues in the trunk (including the dermis of the skin), but in the head and anterior neck the lateral plate forms only the cores of the visceral arches. Their function appears to be almost exclusively the formation of endothelial cells that contribute the linings of blood vessels. Initially, the lateral mesoderm in the visceral arch region is a continuous sheet, but later it becomes segmented by pinching in of the endoderm and ectoderm between the prospective arches. Apart from the dermis of the skin immediately overlying the occipital somites, this tissue is formed exclusively by neural crest and sclerotomes in the head and anterior neck. Somite-like somitomeres anterior to the otic placode do not have dermatomes. In the trunk region, there is an intermediate segment of mesoderm between the somites and lateral plate that forms the kidney.

Variable degrees of deficiency of the medial portion of the anterior neural plate lead to a series of malformations termed the "holoprosencephalies." The name is derived from the partial or complete failure of the anterior neural tube to form cerebral hemispheres with ventricles, so that there is only one (holo) forebrain (prosencephaly) cavity in severe cases.

One of the mildest forms of holoprosencephaly is the fetal alcohol syndrome (or, more correctly, fetal alcohol embryopathy). Webster, Walsh, and Lipson (1980) showed that acute administration of ethanol at the time of gastrulation leads to midfacial defects. Others (Sulik, Johnston, and Webb, 1981; Sulik and Johnston, 1982, 1983) showed that such malformations are characteristic of the fetal alcohol syndrome (FAS), and detailed the pathogenesis of the syndrome. The well-defined loss of midline tissues in the face is striking (Fig. 46–6). Midline deficiency of the anterior neural plate leads to more closely approximated olfactory placodes (Fig. 46–7), and this in turn leads to small medial nasal prominences. Comparable midline defects are seen in the developing brain (Sulik, Lauder, and Dehart, 1984). Contact of the placode has been shown to lead to failure of medial nasal prominence formation and to arhinencephaly in human embryos (Johnston and Sulik, 1980) and in ethanol-induced malformations.

Almost all the holoprosencephalies can be induced by ethanol in experimental animals (Sulik, Cook, and Webster, 1988). In humans, they may also result from trisomy 13 (Gorlin, Pindborg, and Cohen, 1976) or, with the exception of cyclopia, from single gene defects (Ardinger and Bartley, 1988). Only very rudimentary cyclopic eyes are found in specimens from the ethanol experiments (Sulik, Cook, and Webster, 1988). Over the spectrum of holoprosencephaly, eye size decreases progressively as the malformations become more severe (see Fig. 46–9). Cyclopia perfecta (more "typical" cyclopia with a large median eye) cannot therefore be part of the spectrum.

More typical cyclopic eyes were found in malformed salamander embryos after removal (by extirpation) of the prechordal plate (see Fig. 46–2F) underlying the medial portion of the anterior neural plate (Adelmann, 1934). The overlying medial neural plate did not develop further, with the result that the two developing eye fields failed to separate. Although Adelmann noted that removal of paraxial mesoderm adjacent to the prechordal

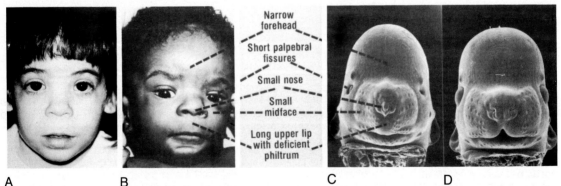

A   B   C   D

Figure 46–6. *A, B,* Children with the fetal alcohol syndrome (FAS). *C,* FAS mouse embryo. *D,* Control mouse embryo. The affected structures are indicated. The above changes are remarkably consistent. (From Sulik, K. K., Johnston, M. C., and Webb, M. A.: Fetal alcohol syndrome: embryogenesis in a mouse model. Science, *214*:936, 1981. Copyright 1981 by the American Association for the Advancement of Science.)

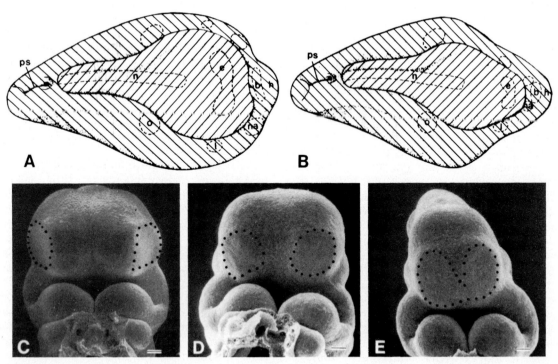

Figure 46–7. *A*, Schematic drawing of a human embryo. *B*, Altered development in an embryo removed from an ethanol-treated mother. *C* to *E*, Scanning electron micrographs of mouse embryos. Note the relations of the nasal placodes (na) to the neural plate and developing facial prominences during normal development. Structures illustrated include the nasal (na), lens (l), and otic (o) placodes; heart (h); buccopharyngeal membrane (b); eye field (e); notochord (n); prechordal mesoderm (pm); and primitive streak (ps). The opening into the cavity of the invaginating lens epithelium is indicated by the arrow on the scanning electron micrograph on the far right. The developing oral (buccal) cavity (b) is also shown. The nasal placodes are positioned much more closely to the midline in both the sketch and scanning electron micrograph. (Modified from Johnston, M. C., and Sulik, K. K.: Embryology of the head and neck. *In* Serafin, D., and Georgiade, N. G. (Eds.): Pediatric Plastic Surgery. St. Louis, C. V. Mosby Company, 1984.)

plate was less effective in producing cyclopia, he did not comment on the size of the cyclopic eye. Since induction would have long since taken place, it would presumably be some supportive function of the mesoderm that is lost, at least in the case of partial mesoderm removal. Removal of the midline portion of the anterior neural plate resulted in two small eyes. Ethanol administration leads to cell death in the medial portion of the anterior neural plate and in other areas. Prospec-

tive prechordal mesoderm normally penetrates between the endoderm and overlying medial anterior neural plate at a late stage in mice (at least in C57B1/6J mice) and its involvement in the pathogenesis of the holoprosencephalies (with the apparent exception of cyclopia) remains unclear. The mesoderm was severely reduced in embryos from ethanol-treated mothers (Sulik, Johnston, and Webb, 1981).

A defect in the programming of the mesoderm is apparently responsible for the oto-cephaly (literally "ear head") spectrum (Fig. 46–8). The least severe cases (mandibular loss or agnathia, Fig. 46–8A) are associated with breakdown of the mesodermal cores in the first visceral arch in a mouse mutant (Juriloff, Sulik, and Roderick, 1980). Neural crest cells appeared to be normal in this study, but apparently failure of vascularization from the mesodermal core leads to complete arch breakdown. The mesodermal core cells normally break down after vascularization of the neural crest cell mesenchyme (Johnston and Listgarten, 1972). The next most severe cases include malformations similar to those of the fetal alcohol syndrome through cyclopia (with rudimentary eyes only). One of the most severe is the typical "ear head" form shown in Figure 46–8B, which is associated with more widespread (angiogenic?) mesodermal cell death, including that in mesoderm underlying the developing fore- and midbrains, which fail to develop further. In retrospect, a primary role for mesoderm makes much more sense than the neural crest hypothesis put forward by Wright and Wagner (1934) and Johnston (1965). There are even more severe specimens in Wright and Wagner's guinea pigs in which there is virtually no head at all (acephaly).

EMBRYO FOLDING (TUBULATION)

Folding movements lead to the formation of two embryonic tubes: the neural tube and the endodermally lined gastrointestinal tube (Fig. 46–2G, H). The mechanism of neural tube closure has been studied intensively and seems to involve, primarily, the coordinated contraction of a filamentous actin-myosin meshwork (terminal web), which is just beneath the luminal lining cell surfaces (Sadler and associates, 1982). Terminal webs are involved in many epithelial foldings, including morphogenetic movements of the olfactory placode (see Chap. 48). Cell proliferation and matrix formation in the mesenchymal tissue underlying the neural plate and folds seem also to be involved.

Failure of complete neural tube closure leads to a variety of neural tube defects (NTDs) including anencephaly (Fig. 46–9) in the head and spina bifida in the cervical and trunk regions. Severe closure defects in the brain lead to eversion of the brain with degeneration of all but the brain stem portion. Thus, the term "anencephaly" is a misnomer since the brain is not entirely absent.

Anencephaly can also be experimentally caused by postclosure rupture of the dorsal brain, an event usually associated with prior degeneration. Weakening with failure to rupture in such cases might account for meningomyeloceles in which there is a protrusion of the brain into the surrounding tissue. As the name implies, meningomyeloceles are fluid-filled cavities with walls consisting of both brain tissue and meninges. Meningocele walls that contain only meninges presumably are the outcome of closure of the meninges only, with failure of complete closure or secondary opening of the underlying brain.

Failure of neural tube closure associated with cell death can be induced in guinea pigs

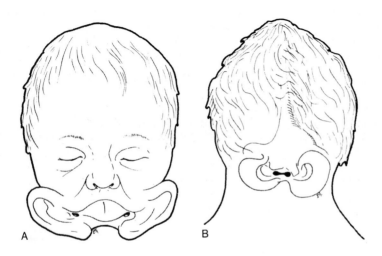

Figure 46–8. Otocephaly. A, In the milder form, the derivatives of the distal portions of the first arch (mandible, etc.) are absent. B, In the more severe form, little more than the external ears are apparent—hence the name oto-cephaly (ear head). (From Duhamel, B.: Morphogenese pathologique. Paris, Masson, 1966.)

A   B

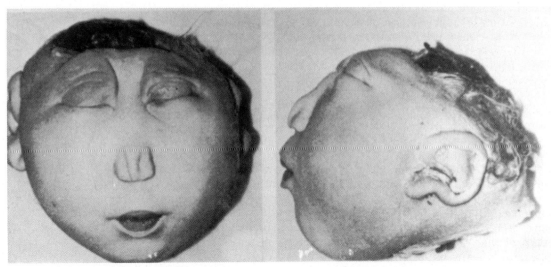

Figure 46–9. Anencephaly. Although the name implies "no-brain," most subjects have intact functional brain stems in spite of the fact that both cerebral and cerebellar hemispheres are absent. The facial characteristics of this individual are typical of fairly severe holoprosencephaly (microphthalmos). (From Lemire, R. J., Cohen, M. M., Jr., Beckwith, J. B., Kokich, V. G., and Siebert, J. R.: The facial features of holoprosencephaly in anencephalic human specimens. Teratology, 23:297, 1981.)

by modest elevations of body temperature of only a few degrees centigrade (Edwards, Warner, and Mulley, 1976). Such elevations in temperature are often associated with infections such as those caused by influenza virus. When such infections occur around day 26, the time of cranial neural tube closure, it is suggestive. Pleet, Graham, and Smith (1981) provided evidence that in addition to effects on the brain (principally mental retardation), hyperthermia affects neural crest and placodal cells in humans.

Taken together, the evidence that vitamin supplementation dramatically reduces the incidence of NTDs is now convincing (Smithells and associates, 1981; Lawrence, 1984; Mulinare and associates, 1988). Large doses of vitamins are usually employed, but even regular ("one-a-day") vitamins appear to be helpful. There is some evidence that folate supplementation alone provides at least some protection. This vitamin is involved in nucleotide synthesis, and the demands of the embryo and fetus are so great that maternal plasma levels fall during the latter part of pregnancy. It would presumably be the cell proliferation aspects of neural tube closure that are being promoted. Vitamin supplementation may also be effective in reducing the incidence of cleft lip and palate (see Chap. 48).

NEURAL CREST

Enormous advances in the understanding of both normal and abnormal neural crest development have taken place in recent years. Most of these advances have been related to the cranial neural crest, which plays such a dominant role in the embryonic development of the face and anterior neck.

Cranial neural crest arises from virtually all but the most anterior margins (folds) of that portion of the neural plate that will give rise to the brain. In preparation for migration, the crest cells separate from the neural plate and from each other as they lose cell adhesion molecules and develop surface receptors for fibronectin, which they will use for make-and-break attachments to fibronectin, a prominent component of the extracellular matrix through which they migrate (Duband and Thiery, 1982, 1987; Edelman and Thiery, 1985). Fibronectin is a glycoprotein that forms an open meshwork along which the crest cells apparently pull themselves. Occupying the space within the fibronectin meshwork is a highly hydrated polysaccharide called hyaluronic acid, which provides a sort of watery gel through which the cells move (Pratt, Larson, and Johnston, 1975).

Migrating crest cells usually adopt a bipolar configuration and are usually oriented in the direction of migration (see Fig. 46–4) as they "glide" through the matrix (Bard and Hay, 1975). Apart from the attachment mechanism, little is known about the mechanisms involved in cell movement. One model hypothesizes that there is an actin-myosin meshwork that results in movement of the cell membrane over the subsurface cytoplasm (Fig. 46–10). Also, little is known about what determines the direction of movement. The presence of retinoic acid–binding protein in migrating crest cells presumably has something to do with regulating their movements. It has been known for many years that excess levels of retinoids interfere with the movements of many embryonic cells. Crest cells appear to lose the binding protein as soon as they have reached their destinations. The mechanisms of crest cell migration have recently been reviewed by a number of authors (Erickson, 1986; Tucker and associates, 1988; Bronner-Fraser, Stern, and Fraser, in press).

During their migration into the facial region, the crest cells primarily follow a path beneath the surface ectoderm. They surround the mesodermal cores in the visceral arches and constitute all of the mesenchyme between the surface ectoderm and underlying brain and eye in the rest of the face. Figure 46–4 also illustrates the cords of crest cells that maintain contact with the neural tube to form the initial primordia of each of the cranial sensory ganglia, except that of the eighth nerve, which is a special case.

While they are migrating, and when they reach their final destination, crest cells come into contact with other cells and tissues. As with other cell migration systems, production of hyaluronidase after migrations are completed apparently allows the crest cells to condense and come into closer contact with inducing tissues and with each other (Toole and Trelstad, 1971; Toole, 1973) in order to foster these interactions. For example, there is experimental evidence that such close contact of crest cells with visceral arch endoderm permits the endoderm to induce the formation of cartilages such as Meckel's cartilage. Cranial neural crest cell interactions and derivatives are summarized in Figure 46–11. Of overwhelming significance for both normal and abnormal craniofacial development are the large contributions to the skeletal and connective tissues (Fig. 46–12).

The type of cell (e.g., chondrocyte) is largely determined by interactions between crest cells and other cell populations, but later development is largely dependent on the initial anteroposterior (cephalocaudal) positioning of the crest cells in the neural folds (Noden, 1988). The specificity for organizing

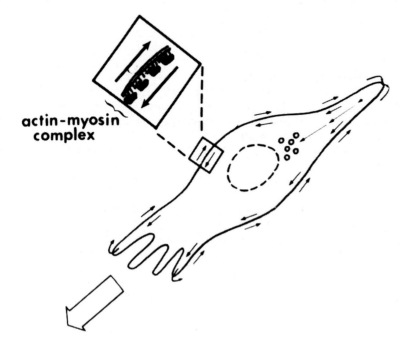

actin-myosin complex

Figure 46–10. The mechanisms by which cells move are still poorly understood. It is known that crest cells glide through their matrix making (and breaking) attachments to fibrinectin. There is forward movement of the cytoplasm relative to the surface membrane (arrows in box). There is also evidence (J. Holtfreter, personal communication) that membrane components are internalized at the trailing tip of the cell and wind up in the Golgi apparatus (behind the nucleus in the illustration). They are then presumably transported to the leading edge of the cell to be reincorporated into the plasma membrane. (From Johnston, M. C., and Sulik, K. K.: The neural crest. In Shields, E. D., Burzynsky, N. J., and Melnick, M. (Eds.): Craniofacial Dysmorphology: Genetics, Etiology, Diagnosis and Treatment. Littleton, MA, John Wright/PSG, 1983.)

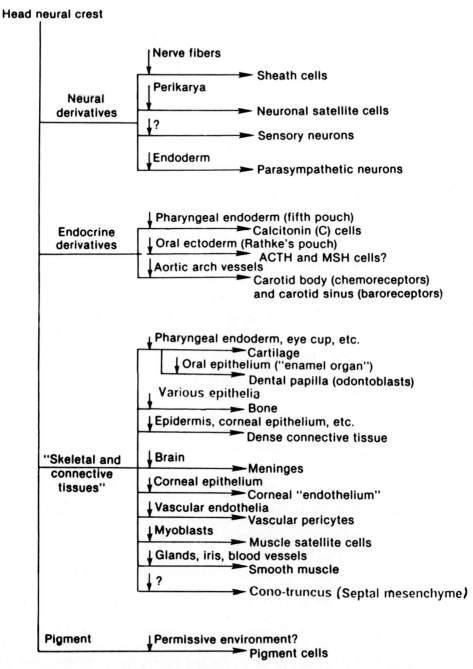

Figure 46–11. The number of derivatives of head (cranial) neural crest cells has been considerably expanded through the use of recently developed cell-marking techniques. Known or presumed inductive interactions with various structures are indicated by arrows. (From Johnston, M. C., and Sulik, K. K.: Embryology of the head and neck. *In* Serafin, D., and Georgiade, N. G. (Eds.): Pediatric Plastic Surgery. St. Louis, C. V. Mosby Company, 1984.)

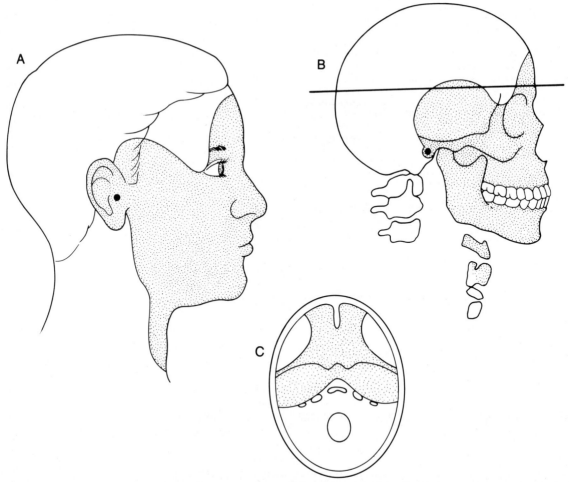

Figure 46–12. The apparent distribution *(stipple)* of connective *(A)* and skeletal *(B, C)* tissues of crest origin in the head and neck. C, The distribution in the floor and walls of the cranial cavity (top of skull removed as indicated in *B*). Of the skeletal tissues in the face, only the enamel of the teeth is not of crest origin. The distribution of crest-derived connective tissues (dermis and subcutaneous tissues, voluntary muscle, glands, eyes, meninges, blood vessels, and so forth) roughly corresponds to that of the skeletal tissues. The distribution is roughly coincident with crest cell distribution at the end of migration (see Fig. 46–4). (Modified from Johnston, M. C., Bhakdinaronk, A., and Reid, Y. C.: An expanded role for the neural crest in oral and pharyngeal development. *In* Bosma, J. F. (Ed.): Oral Sensation and Perception—Development in the Fetus and Infant. Washington, D.C., U.S. Govt. Printing Office, 1974, pp. 37–52.

the first arch jaw apparatus is resident in the first arch crest before it migrates. Also, crest cells from a very small portion, and only that portion, of the postotic neural folds give rise to most of the mesenchyme in the developing septa that divide the conotruncus of the embryonic heart into the proximal portions of the aortic arch and pulmonary artery (Kirby, Gale, and Stewart, 1983).

Extirpation of these cells prior to migration leads to the so-called conotruncal outflow tract defects, which include some types of interventricular septal defects and abnormalities of the great vessels. These types of cardiovascular malformation are often seen as components of syndromes that may have, as

their common denominator, abnormalities of neural crest cell development.

Another major insight has been provided by human malformations caused by inadvertent use of the acne drug Accutane (isotretinoin, 13-cis-retinoic acid, 13-cis-RA) during pregnancy. Accutane is the first effective drug for the treatment of severe cystic acne and has gained wide popularity since it was introduced in 1982. Since the drug is a retinoid, a group of compounds including vitamin A (retinol) and related compounds, and because retinoids have long been known to be teratogenic (Cohlan, 1953), it was marketed as a category X drug (not to be taken during pregnancy). However, large numbers of exposures have occurred (probably 500 to 1000 in the U.S.) and, when pregnancies are permitted to come to term, about one-quarter of the infants have severe craniofacial and cardiovascular malformations as well as deficiencies or absence of the thymus. Most of the severely affected children do not survive beyond the first year of life. This is perhaps the most serious example of a drug-induced malformation since the thalidomide disaster of the early 1960's. Many of the malformations resulting from thalidomide were similar to those induced by the 13-cis-RA–induced malformations.

13-cis-RA differs from all-transretinoic acid (all-trans-RA), which is now known to play a major role in normal embryonic development, only in the orientation of the carboxyl group on the side chain. While it is, itself, capable of producing characteristic malformations in whole embryo culture (Webster, 1985; Goulding and Pratt, 1986), much of its activity in vivo may result from derived all-trans-RA (Kochhar and Penner, 1987) to which it spontaneously isomerizes.

One of the main reasons for the severe teratogenicity of 13-cis-RA in humans is that its 4-oxo metabolite accumulates to approximately three to five times the level of the parent compound (Brazzell and associates, 1983). The 4-oxo metabolite is equally teratogenic with the parent compound in whole embryo culture (Webster, 1985; Goulding and Pratt, 1986). The drug has almost no effect on the embryo when used at the same levels as found in the serum of patients being treated with 13-cis-RA, but if equal amounts of the 4-oxo metabolite are added, the combination is severely teratogenic. This is still only half the combined levels of the two compounds in the sera of patients undergoing 13-cis-RA treatment.

There has long been evidence that retinoids (particularly retinol and all-trans-RA) cause craniofacial malformations somewhat similar to those of the retinoic acid syndrome (RAS) described above (Morriss, 1972; Poswillo, 1975; Fantel and associates, 1977). Doses used in the last-named study, which was conducted on monkeys, were relatively low: about ten times the human 13-cis-RA dose. Most of the structures affected were of neural crest origin, providing indirect evidence for crest cell involvement. Direct evidence was also provided by studies on the intact embryo (Hassell, Greenberg, and Johnston, 1977) and

on neural crest cells in vitro (Thorogood and associates, 1982).

Malformations in the human RAS have been studied fairly extensively (Lammer and associates, 1985). With the possible exception of the brain, cells of the affected tissues are derived partly or almost entirely from neural crest cells. There are moderate effects on the mandible and moderate to severe effects on the middle and external ear. The thymus, whose connective tissue components are largely derived from crest cells, is also deficient or absent. Brain malformations are largely limited to the hindbrain region, particularly the cerebellum and rhombic lip. The entire rhombic lip is essentially derived from neural folds. Although a number of rhombic lip (presumably neural crest) cells migrate ventrally into the brain stem, where they give rise to the inferior olivary nucleus and other structures, the possible involvement in RAS malformations is unknown. The most affected portion of the cerebellum is the midline vermis, which is a neural fold derivative. Other cells from the rhombic lip contribute at least some cells to the external granular layer, which presumably migrate into deeper locations within the cerebellum, as do other cells from this layer. In any case, the RAS hindbrain malformations appear to be far too extensive for crest involvement alone, and there are other reasons supporting effects on noncrest cells.

The reason for the particular vulnerability of cranial neural crest cells to retinoic acid is apparently at least partly related to a normal role for all-trans-RA in crest cell development. Even before migration, crest cells take up large amounts of radiolabeled all-trans-RA and react positively to an immunohistochemical stain for all-trans-RA binding protein, as do cells in the neural plate at this stage of development (Dencker, 1979; Dencker and associates, 1987; Dencker and associates, in press). These characteristics, which are maintained during the entire migration of cranial neural crest cells, are lost temporarily, only to reappear later in selected populations of crest cells such as those in the primary palate. The role of all-trans-RA in these cells is unknown, but it may be involved in the establishment of fields or pattern formations, as is apparently the case for developing limb buds.

The pathogenesis of 13-cis-RA–induced malformations has been studied fairly exten-

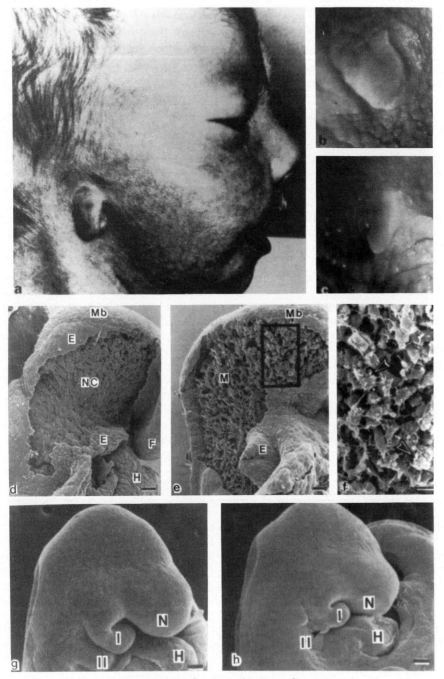

Figure 46–13 *See legend on opposite page*

sively in mouse models in which the resulting malformations are virtually identical to those in humans (Goulding and Pratt, 1986; Pratt, Goulding, and Abbott, 1987; Sulik, Cook, and Webster, 1988). The most affected crest cell population appears to be that of the hyoid arch crest, which appears to undergo complete cell death before ever leaving the neural folds (Sulik, Cook, and Webster, 1988). For some reason there is a considerable amount of cell death in this portion of the hindbrain neural plate in controls, presumably making crest cells in this region more vulnerable to 13-cis-RA. It appears that many cell populations undergoing programmed (normal) cell death are particularly vulnerable. There are a number of possible reasons why cell populations undergoing programmed cell death display such vulnerability, including possible normal developmental regulation by 13-cis-RA and the fact that retinoids may destabilize the membranes of lysosomes, a prominent feature of such cell populations. Release of cytolytic enzymes would then lead to cell death.

There also appear to be major effects on migrating crest cells. Surface blebbing is a major feature and is especially prominent at higher doses (Fig. 46–13). All-trans-RA and retinol are normal constituents of cell membranes, where they are involved in the transfer of sugar molecules across the membrane (e.g., from the inside of the surface membrane to the outer surface, where they are incorporated into cell surface glycoproteins). Excessive amounts of retinoid in this membrane could lead to its destabilization and ballooning out of the cell membrane. Such effects, or even much less severe effects, could disturb the intricate mechanism of cell migration. Presumably, the all-trans-RA binding protein and consequent concentration of 13-cis-RA would make the crest cells even more vulnerable.

The effects of 13-cis-RA treatment on facial and visceral arch development are illustrated in 27 somite mouse embryos (developmental age is roughly equivalent to day 30 human embryos) (Fig. 46–13). While the frontonasal and maxillary prominences and the mandible arch are moderately affected, only a distal rudiment of the hyoid arch is observed. It seems probable that the hyoid crest is eliminated entirely and the distal rudiment mesenchyme has migrated from the first arch at a point where the two mesenchyme populations are normally confluent. The break in the arch would prevent somitomeric myoblasts (see below) from entering the arch and would presumably abort further development of the seventh nerve musculature. Absence of facial muscle activity in the human RAS syndrome therefore may not actually be facial nerve paresis, as it has been termed (Lammer and associates, 1985). Since most of the pinna of the ear and two of the three middle ear ossicles are derived from the second arch, it is not surprising that there are major effects on the external and middle ears. For reasons yet to be determined, the altered development is often largely limited to one (usually the right) side. Almost identical developmental alterations can be produced in whole embryo culture with either 13-cis-RA or its 4-oxo metabolite (Webster, 1985).

Maternal ethanol administration at the time of crest cell migration also produces malformations similar to the RAS, including

Figure 46–13. Craniofacial alterations in the retinoic acid syndrome (RAS). Craniofacial malformations (upper panel) include severe abnormalities of the brain (particularly in the cerebellar region), external and middle ear abnormalities, mandibular underdevelopment, and cleft palate. Thymus deficiency or absence, and cardiovascular defects of the outflow tract type, are frequently found. Apart from the brain defects, virtually all the abnormalities involve structures with major components of neural crest origin. Most of these children die within the first year. Almost identical malformations can be induced in a mouse model by administering the compound just before or during the early stages of crest cell migration (approximately day 22 in humans). The scanning electron micrographic morphology of crest cells migrating to the facial region is shown in the 8 somite control embryo in the middle panel. The crest cells (NC) form a fairly compact layer, with the cells frequently bipolar and oriented in the direction of migration. In embryos from a mother treated with a high dose of Accutane, the crest cell population is thinned and many cells show severe blebbing (arrowheads). A relatively normal crest cell (arrow) is also shown. Crest cells (arrowheads) normally destined for the second (hyoid) visceral arch are seen at the edge of the neural plate. These cells apparently undergo cell death before leaving the neural plate. The latter finding probably accounts for the almost complete failure of second arch development (compare the control and treated embryos). Lower panel, 27 somite mouse embryos show the effects of drug treatment on facial and visceral arch development. The abnormalities are often unilateral, more frequently on the right side. Other abbreviations: Mb = midbrain; E = surface ectoderm; M = mesoderm; N = nasal (olfactory) placode; H = heart; I and II = first and second visceral arches. (From Webster, W. S., Johnston, M. C., Lammer, E. J., and Sulik, K. K.: Isotretinoin embryopathy and the cranial neural crest: an in vivo and in vitro study. J. Craniofac. Genet. Dev. Biol., 6:211, 1986.)

ear and facial defects and cardiovascular defects of the outflow tract type (Daft, Johnston, and Sulik, 1986; Sulik and associates, 1986). These malformations are also similar to DiGeorge's syndrome in which, in at least one case, severe maternal alcoholism was documented (Ammann and associates, 1982; Sulik and associates, 1986). Here the ethanol is rapidly lethal for migrating crest cells, and again membrane labilization has been proposed as the mechanism underlying crest cell injury (Sulik and associates, 1986).

Thalidomide has effects on facial, brain, cardiovascular and limb development in both humans and experimental animals that are virtually identical to those induced by 13-cis-RA when administered at the same developmental times, suggesting direct effects on crest cells. Human maternal hyperthermia also appears to produce similar malformations at the same developmental ages (Pleet, Graham, and Smith, 1981), although this has not been documented experimentally.

A number of syndromes that consistently, or frequently, have combinations of facial, auditory, and cardiovascular system defects include craniofacial microsomia, the velocardiofacial syndrome, and the CHARGE association.

DEVELOPMENT OF THE VISCERAL ARCHES AND TONGUE

The development of the lower face and anterior neck is dominated by the visceral arches. Each arch has its own complement of blood vessel, voluntary muscle, nerve, and skeletal elements (Table 46–1).

The term "branchial" is often used to describe the arches, instead of "visceral" or "pharyngeal." This term is technically incorrect. It is correctly used to describe those arches that have gill branches in fish and in amphibian larvae. The mandibular and hyoid arches never have gill branches.

The arches initially contain only angiogenic mesoderm. Crest cells migrating into the arches surround the mesoderm. The aortic arch vessel endothelium is derived from the mesoderm, while other cells of the vessel wall (e.g., pericytes) are derived from the neural crest. Other mesodermal capillary endothelial buds grow into and vascularize the surrounding crest cell mesenchyme.

The structural relations and changing morphology of the visceral arches and tongue are illustrated in Figure 46–14. The initial mesoderm becomes partially segmented by the ingrowth of pharyngeal cleft ectoderm and the outgrowth of pharyngeal pouch endoderm (Fig. 46–14B). The two epithelia contact each other between the proximal portions of the arches, and in amphibians and fish the contact breaks down to form the gill slits. Occasionally, abnormal breakdown of the contacting epithelia occurs in the human embryo.

One of the first signs of tongue formation is the appearance of the lingual swellings (Fig. 46–14E), which presumably result from the ingress of hypoglossal cord myoblasts that will form the contractile components of the muscle of the tongue. Connective tissue com-

Table 46–1. Visceral Arch–Derived Craniofacial Structures

Visceral Arch	Cranial Nerve	Muscles	Skeletal Structures
First	V (mandibular branch)	Muscles of mastication (temporal, masseter, medial and lateral pterygoid), mylohyoid and anterior belly of digastric; tensor muscle of tympanic membrane and palatine curtain	Meckel's cartilage, malleus and incus, mandible, sphenomandibular ligament
Second	VII	Muscles of facial expression (cheek, occipitofrontal, auricular, platysma, orbicular), stapedius, stylohyoid, posterior belly of digastric	Reichert's cartilage, stapes, styloid process, lesser cornu of hyoid, upper part of body of hyoid bone, stylohyoid ligament
Third	IX	Stylopharyngeal and upper pharyngeal	Greater cornu of hyoid, lower part of body of hyoid bone
Fourth, fifth, and sixth	X (superior laryngeal and recurrent laryngeal branch)	Pharyngeal and laryngeal	Thyroid, arytenoid, corniculate, and cuneiform cartilages

From Johnston, M. C., and Sulik, K. K.: Embryology of the head and neck. *In* Serafin, D., and Georgiade, N. G. (Eds): Pediatric Plastic Surgery. St. Louis, C. V. Mosby Company, 1984.

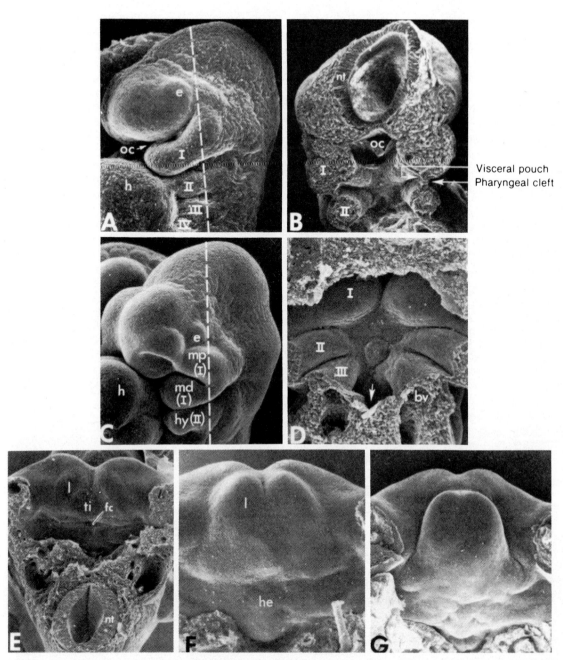

Visceral pouch
Pharyngeal cleft

Figure 46–14. Scanning electron micrographs of the developing visceral arches and tongue in mouse embryos. The planes of section for the specimens in *B* and *D* are shown in *A* and *C*. *B* and *D* (equivalent to day 30 and day 35 human embryos, respectively) are dorsal views of the visceral arches and floor of the pharynx. The visceral arches in *A* to *D* are indicated by Roman numerals. In *A* the first arch (I) is already separating from the heart (h) but the second aortic arch vessel is still carrying blood from the heart (see bv in *D*). Other abbreviations: e = eye; oc = oral cavity; mp = maxillary prominence; md = mandibular arch; hy = hyoid arch. The entrance to the lower pharynx is indicated by the arrow in *D*. The development of the tongue is illustrated in *E* to *G*. The developmental ages of these embryos are roughly equivalent to those of day 40 and day 50 human embryos. The lingual swellings (l) in *E* presumably represent arrival of the hypoglossal cord myoblasts. The tuberculum impar (ti) also contributes to the tongue, and the foramen cecum (fc) represents both the invaginating thyroid epithelium and the junction between the anterior one-third and posterior two-thirds of the tongue. The posterior one-third is formed by contributions from the third and fourth arches. More advanced stages are shown in *F* and *G*. Other abbreviations: nt = neural tube; he = hypobranchial eminence. (From Johnston, M. C., and Sulik, K. K.: Embryology of the head and neck. *In* Serafin, D., and Georgiade, N. G. (Eds.): Pediatric Plastic Surgery. St. Louis, C. V. Mosby Company, 1984.)

ponents in the anterior two-thirds of the tongue are provided by first arch neural crest cells, and the endothelia of blood vessels by the mesodermal cores of the first arch. Sensory innervation is provided by the lingual branch of the first arch (mandibular) nerve. Noncontractile elements of the posterior third of the tongue behind the foramen cecum (fc in Fig. 46–14*E*) are provided by the second and third visceral arches.

VASCULAR DEVELOPMENT

Development of the facial arteries and great vessels involves three major phases (Fig. 46–15). The origin of the aortic arch vessels has already been noted. During the initial phase (the 3½ week specimen in Fig. 46–15), the visceral arches serve as little more than conduits carrying blood from the heart to the rest of the embryo. By six weeks the first two arches have lost their connec-

tions with the heart, and the first aortic arch vessel has been essentially replaced. The portion of the second aortic arch artery adjacent to the internal carotid artery (dorsal aorta) persists as the stem of the stapedial artery, which for a temporary period in the human embryo supplies virtually all the facial region. The proximal portion of the third aortic arch vessel that is adjacent to the internal carotid (six week specimen) grows forward and upward and by nine weeks has fused with the stapedial artery. Only a small portion of the stem of the stapedial artery persists (nine week specimen in Fig. 46–15), and the external carotid and its branches form the definitive vascular system for most of the face.

As already discussed, there is evidence suggesting that the fusion between the external carotid and stapedial arteries may constitute a developmental weakpoint predisposed to hemorrhages which may be responsible for at least some aspects of unilateral craniofacial

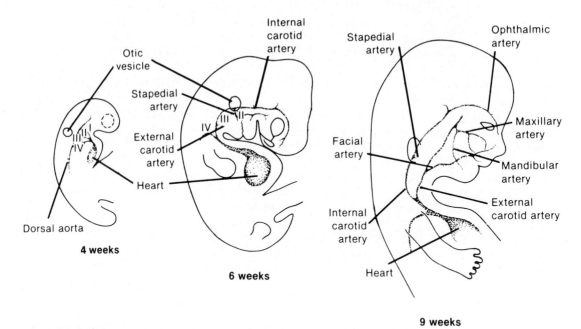

Figure 46–15. Development of the arteries of the face. The main function of the visceral arches in the 3½ week embryo is to carry blood from the heart to the rest of the embryo through the aortic arch vessels, one of which is contained in each arch (numbered by Roman numerals). By six weeks, the first and second arches have lost their connections with the heart. The proximal portion of the second aortic arch vessel persists as the stem of the stapedial artery, which temporarily (in humans) supplies the facial region. The proximal portion of the third aortic arch vessel persists as the stem of the external carotid. Finally, the fourth aortic arch vessel on the right side forms the arch of the aorta. By nine weeks, the definitive vascular system is present. The external carotid has fused with the stapedial and takes over the blood supply of the face. Only part of the proximal portion of the stapedial artery survives and this forms only a small local vessel. (From Ross, R. G., and Johnston, M. C.: Cleft Lip and Palate. Baltimore, Williams & Wilkins Company, 1972.)

microsomia and related malformations. The fact that this evidence was clouded by previous developmental changes has been emphasized.

The conotruncus is the conical-shaped outflow segment of the embryonic heart. Longitudinal septa form on opposite sides of the conotruncus, grow toward each other, and fuse. The septum is lined up and fuses with the developing interventricular septum. The conotruncal septum then splits so that the conotruncus becomes divided into two vessels: the stems of the arch of the aorta and the pulmonary artery (nine week specimen).

Extremely important findings related to abnormalities of the interventricular septum and great vessels (the so-called outflow tract defects) and a host of associated craniofacial malformations have been reported by Kirby, Gale, and Stewart (1983). They found that most of the mesenchyme in the conotruncal septum originates from a small group of neural crest cells originally found in hindbrain neural folds behind the otic placode. Extirpation of this small segment of neural fold in the chick leads to a typical array of outflow tract defects, the mildest expressions of which are interventricular septal defects. Since neural crest cells do not contribute to the interventricular septum, the latter defects are presumably secondary to adjacent abnormalities of the conotruncal septum with which the developing interventricular septum normally lines up and fuses.

The associated craniofacial malformations (e.g., RAS, DiGeorge's syndrome, the velocardiofacial syndrome, unilateral craniofacial microsomia and related first and second arch defects, CHARGE association) have already been discussed in the neural crest section above. Although many aspects of these syndromes are obviously not of neural crest origin, those aspects involving neural crest derivatives associated with outflow tract defects are highly suspect.

ORIGINS OF VOLUNTARY MUSCLES

With the apparent exception of those contributing to the extrinsic ocular muscles, all voluntary (skeletal) myoblasts throughout the body appear to arise from the myotomes of somites (Fig. 46–16), or from comparable structures (dermatomes) in the preotic region.

Their migrations have been followed, primarily, by various cell-marking procedures in submammalian vertebrates. Antibodies to a Z-disc protein, desmin, have also been used for the immunohistochemical identification of myoblasts in chick embryos (Solursh, 1984) and it appears that the stain also works on mouse embryos, so that it should be possible to track myoblast migrations in mammals.

A ^{3}H-thymidine cell marker was used by Hazelton (1970) to follow hypoglossal cord myoblasts as they migrated from the occipital somites to the tongue region in chick embryos. The results of further studies using transplants of quail paraxial mesoderm (somites and somitomeres) were reported for the extrinsic ocular muscles by Johnston and associates (1979). These results have been considerably extended by Noden (1982, 1983a, b, 1986), especially for older stages. Noden (1988) also transplanted trunk somites into the head region and found that their myoblasts contributed in a normal fashion to facial muscles, indicating that local mesenchyme dictates the final morphology.

Apart from the musculature associated with the vertebrae and posterior neck muscles, the (voluntary) myoblasts undergo long and sometimes spectacular migrations. In general, the migrations occur in two distinct phases. During the first phase (primary migration), they move in a tightly packed array, especially in the hypoglossal cord. The mechanisms involved are unknown.

As noted previously, the visceral arch myoblasts move into the core of the visceral arches, replacing the angiogenic mesoderm, the last cells of which undergo massive degeneration (Johnston and Listgarten, 1972). After midline merging of mandibular and hyoid arches, the myoblast cores of the visceral arches (sometimes called muscle plates) from the two sides meet each other in the midline. The migrations of cords of cells that form the extrinsic ocular muscles can be easily followed by ordinary H & E–stained histologic sections in the chick. Migration paths can be long and tortuous. This is especially true for the sixth nerve cord, which forms the lateral rectus, and this may at least partly account for the high incidence of internal strabismus.

During their primary migrations, the cords of myoblasts "bring" their nerve supply with them. These fibers eventually penetrate through the center of the visceral arch myoblast cores, ultimately reaching the ventral

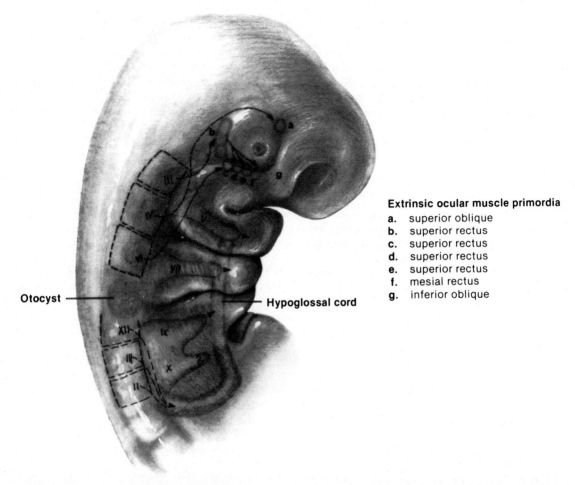

Extrinsic ocular muscle primordia

a.　superior oblique
b.　superior rectus
c.　superior rectus
d.　superior rectus
e.　superior rectus
f.　mesial rectus
g.　inferior oblique

Otocyst

Hypoglossal cord

Figure 46–16. The visceral arches play a major role in the development of the voluntary (skeletal) muscles of the head and neck. The original mesoderm forming the cores of the visceral arches is replaced by presumptive myoblasts that migrate into the arches (*arrowheads*) from proximally located mesoderm, the mytotomes of postotic somites, or, in the preotic region, from structures that are apparently homologous with the myotomes of postotic somites. The myotomes of the first three postotic somites give rise to the hypoglossal cord, which supplies the myoblasts of the tongue and other muscles supplied by the 12th cranial nerve. The myoblasts of the extrinsic ocular muscle are derived from poorly defined myotomes supplied by the third, fourth, and sixth cranial nerves. (Adapted from Johnston, M. C., and Sulik, K. K.: Development of face and oral cavity. *In* Bhaskar, S. N. (Ed.): Orban's Oral Histology and Embryology. 9th Ed. St. Louis, MO, C. V. Mosby Company, 1980.)

midline, where they appear to unite with fibers from the opposite nerve bundle.

Some myoblasts fuse together to form myotubes in which typical actin-myosin arrays appear almost immediately after the primary migration, but other myoblasts seem to remain as single cells, or small groups of cells, and then undergo secondary migrations to the definitive locations of the muscles, "bringing" along with them branches of the appropriate nerve. These secondary migrations have been documented by only a few descriptive studies such as that of Gasser (1967). They may cover incredibly long distances, given the large size of the embryo at the time that the migrations begin (e.g., those of the hyoid arch myoblasts that form the occipitalis, a muscle at the back of the head that moves the scalp, and those from the first arch that form the temporalis muscle).

When the myoblasts reach their final location, they fuse together to form myotubes. Since the myotube nuclei can no longer divide, further growth regulation must be by other mechanisms, which must sometimes be very extensive, since muscle cells (fibers) frequently extend through the entire length of a muscle. These other mechanisms include additions of nuclei derived from associated satellite cells, by addition at the ends of the myotubes that occurs at least into early postnatal life, and by hypertrophy (as with exercise) that does not involve increased numbers of nuclei.

Muscle spindles that monitor muscle length and whose innervation is from proprioceptive neurons are modified muscle fibers and so presumably have the same origins. Other components of the muscle are derived from other sources. Endothelial cells are derived from angiogenic mesoderm (Johnston and associates, 1979) and other connective tissue elements (e.g., fibroblasts) from crest mesenchyme or mesodermal mesenchyme (Le Lièvre and Le Douarin, 1975; Johnston and associates, 1979; Noden, 1982, 1983a, b), depending on the location of the particular muscle. The origins of muscle fiber satellite cells are unknown. They may be derived from crest cells, which might explain the occasional presence of quail crest nuclei in myotubes seen in the Le Lièvre and Le Douarin (1975) study. Johnston and associates (1979) were unable to find crest nuclei in myotubes (see also Noden, 1983b).

Abnormalities in muscle development can apparently result from alterations at almost any developmental stage. As noted earlier in discussions related to the retinoic acid syndrome (RAS), failures of hyoid crest and hyoid arch formation appear to prevent the primary migration of paraxial mesoderm myoblasts into the arch, thereby aborting further development of the second arch muscles of facial expression and leading to the so-called facial paresis seen in human RAS. Extra hypoglossal myoblast divisions prior to fusion have been postulated as being responsible for the excessively large tongue size in human cleft palate (see Chap. 48).

DEVELOPMENT OF PERIPHERAL NERVOUS SYSTEM

There are a number of unique features in the development of the peripheral nervous system of the head, particularly with respect to the sensory and autonomic components. The organs of special sense are not discussed here (the ocular and acoustic-vestibular systems are dealt with later in this chapter, and the olfactory system in Chap. 48). Much of the peripheral nervous system in the neck develops according to the trunk pattern.

The first elements of the peripheral nervous system to form in the head are the primordia of the cranial (general) sensory ganglia, which consist of cords of neural crest cells that remain attached to the neural tube. Most of the neurons of these ganglia (V, VII, IX, and X) have general sensory functions. In contrast to the neck and trunk, where most prospective proprioceptive neurons migrate from the neural folds with the rest of the crest cells, most of the prospective proprioceptive neurons in the head remain in the neural tube. Those of the dominating trigeminal system remain in the mesencephalic nucleus, which later migrates to the ventral brain stem on mammals but remains in a dorsal position in birds (Fig. 46–17). Although it is known that proprioceptive fibers from the mesencephalic nucleus eventually travel with motor nerve branches, it is not clear whether they leave the brain stem with motor division of the fifth nerve (which is immediately medial to the ganglion) or whether they first travel through the ganglion. There are no muscle spindles in the muscles of facial

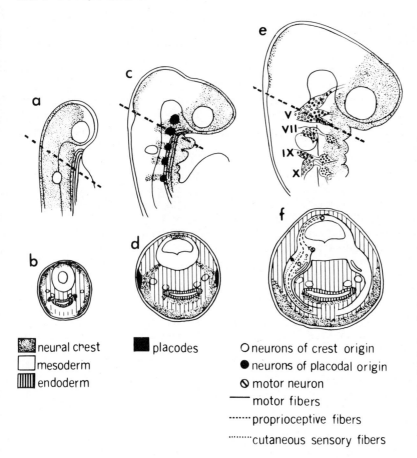

neural crest
mesoderm
endoderm

placodes

○ neurons of crest origin
● neurons of placodal origin
Ø motor neuron
— motor fibers
······· proprioceptive fibers
·········· cutaneous sensory fibers

Figure 46–17. The migratory (*a*) and postmigratory pattern (*c* and *e*) distributions of neural crest cells (*stippled*) and the origins of the cranial sensory ganglia. The initial ganglionic primordia are formed by cords of neural crest cells that remain attached to the neural tube. The section plane in *c* and *e* passes through the primordium of the trigeminal ganglion. Ectodermal "thickenings," termed placodes, form adjacent to the distal ends of the ganglionic primordia—two for the trigeminal (V) and one each for the facial (VII), glossopharyngeal (IX), and vagal (X) ganglia. They contribute presumptive neuroblasts that migrate into the previously purely crest primordia. (Adapted from Johnston, M. C., and Hazelton, R. B.: Embryonic origins of facial structures related to oral sensory and motor function. *In* Bosma, J. F. (Ed.): Oral Sensory Perception: The Mouth of the Infant. Springfield, IL, Charles C Thomas, 1972, pp. 76–97.)

expression. There is some evidence that twelfth nerve proprioceptive neuron cell bodies are also located in the brain stem.

Another feature peculiar to the head region, and not found in the neck and trunk of any vertebrates, is the placodal origins of many of the neurons in the cranial sensory ganglia. As noted previously, placodes are thickenings of any surface or lining epithelium. The ganglionic placodes of higher vertebrates are (with the exception of the trigeminal placodes) closely related to contacting endodermal pouches that are extensions of the pharyngeal endoderm. They appear to induce or concentrate prospective placodal neurons. No obvious contact of pharyngeal endoderm with surface ectoderm occurs for trigeminal placode induction, and the trigeminal placodes are thinner and spread over a greater area. Cells of the trigeminal placodes move into the distal end of the ophthalmic and maximandibular portions of the trigeminal ganglia individually or in small clusters, while those of other ganglion placodes migrate into the distal ends of their ganglia more as solid cords. The histologic appearance

and early migrations of cells from ganglion placodes are similar in all vertebrates studied, including mice (Nichols, 1986) and humans (Gasser, 1967), except that the two trigeminal placodes appear to be confluent in mammals.

Available information indicates that placodal cells are partly differentiated into neurons. At least some of them have overt characteristics of neuroblasts at the time they begin their migrations. In contrast, crest cells in the ganglia are much less mature and do not begin to differentiate into neurons for perhaps two days in chicks (about eight to ten days in humans). There is a comparable population of differentiating neurons in spinal ganglia in the neck and trunk, and although they may originate from surface ectoderm adjacent to the neural plate, they certainly migrate with the crest cells. All supporting cells (Schwann's sheath cells for the nerve fibers and satellite cells for the neuronal cell bodies) are provided by the neural crest.

Apart from their probably being the first functional neurons in the head, no specific functions have ever been identified for placodal neurons. The close relation of the seventh, ninth, and tenth nerve placodes to pharyngeal endoderm suggests that they might subserve taste functions. The neurons of the fifth nerve do not have taste functions, although its branches carry fibers from the seventh nerve; e.g., seventh nerve fibers reaching the lingual nerve via the chorda tympani to eventually innervate taste buds in the anterior two-thirds of the tongue, while taste buds of the posterior third are supplied by the ninth nerve. Placodal neurons of the tenth nerve provide general sensory innervation for most of the gastrointestinal tract.

Little information is available with respect to the manner in which the nerve fibers of ganglionic neurons find their way either back into the neural tube or out into the peripheral tissues. Perhaps 50 per cent of the fibers traveling through the myoblast cores of the first visceral arches, as identified in silver-stained preparations, can be traced back to neuronal cell bodies in the trigeminal ganglion. While a few proprioceptive neurons may be present in this ganglion (as noted before, most of them are in the brain), it seems likely that many of them are general sensory in function and that this is merely an organizational phenomenon, with the sensory fibers reaching their final destination after break-up of the myoblast core. Although some observations have been made on silver-stained fibers beginning to form the ophthalmic and maxillary nerves (Hamburger, 1961), their outgrowth seems to be very diffuse, and factors determining the pathways are altogether unknown.

Considerable information has now accumulated on ganglionic cell survival and the possible role of pathfinder neurons. As with the neurons of sympathetic ganglia, it appears that sensory neurons depend for their survival on the retrograde transport of nerve growth factor (NGF), which appears to be synthesized by the target tissue. Once the target (NGF-producing) sites are occupied, there is no possibility for new fibers growing into the area to occupy such sites, and these neurons undergo cell death. It has been estimated that approximately 70 per cent of the neurons in spinal sensory ganglia undergo cell death.

Although normal cell death in the mouse trigeminal ganglion peaks on day ten, it has already been initiated on day nine. Accutane (13-cis-RA) administration on day nine greatly accelerates the cell death. Dead cells in the ganglion were found to have the same distributions as marked ganglionic placodal cells (Johnston and Hazelton, 1972; D'Amico-Martel and Noden, 1983). Also, dead cells that are assumed to be of placodal origin accumulate in a mass under the placode. This mass extends somewhat toward the first arch, and many of the surrounding (presumably crest) cells are seen engulfing the pyknotic debris (Fig. 46–18).

The distribution of the dead cells noted above and presumed secondary effects on neural crest cells can account for almost all features of the resulting malformation, which is uncannily similar to the malformations of the Treacher Collins syndrome (Sulik, Cook, and Webster, 1988). These malformations include a high incidence of wide posterior palatal clefts (often the soft palate only) that are typical of those found in about 35 per cent of patients with this malformation. Treacher Collins patients have never been studied for sensory deprivations, although such information would be very important.

Autonomic innervation of the head also has a number of peculiar features. Differentiation of neural crest cells requires interaction with somitic mesoderm. Trunk crest cells enter the anterior halves of the somites (Bronner-Fraser, Stern, and Fraser, in press). Apparently occipital somites do not perform this function, as the first ganglion in the sympathetic chain is the superior cervical ganglion. As with other sympathetic ganglia, the superior cervical is intimately related to major arteries, in this case the common carotid. Postganglionic fibers from the superior cervical neurons travel throughout the head by following the vascular tree. In addition to innervating blood vessels, they supply the autonomic innervation for salivary and lacrimal glands, ciliary and iris muscle of the eye, and so forth.

Almost all parasympathetic neurons arise from cranial neural crest. The exceptions are the small number that are derived from the most caudal trunk neural crest. These neurons innervate the lowest portion of the gastrointestinal tract and other structures in that region. In the cranial region, prospective parasympathetic neurons reach the face and anterior neck by migrating with the crest cells traveling under the surface ectoderm. They apparently interact with pharyngeal endoderm and other epithelia, taking up final positions that are usually close to or within

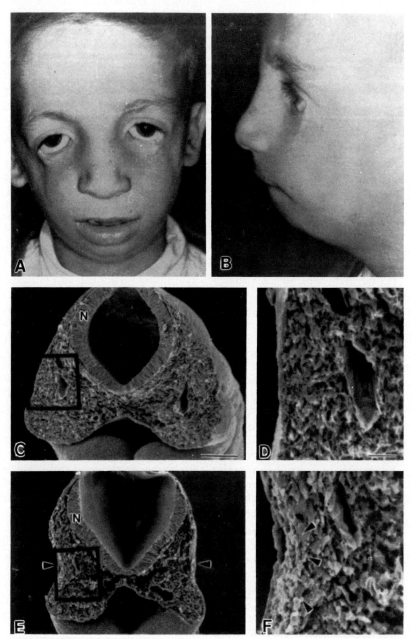

Figure 46–18. Treacher Collins syndrome. *A, B,* In the Treacher Collins malformation, there are bilateral abnormalities of the external and middle ear, mandibular underdevelopment, and deficiency or absence of the zygomatic bone. Approximately one-third of patients have cleft palate as well as generalized underdevelopment in the oropharyngeal region. Studies on mouse models indicate that the primary defect is excessive death of trigeminal placodal cells, with secondary involvement of regional crest cell mesenchyme. (From Ross, R. B., and Johnston, M. C.: Cleft Lip and Palate. Baltimore, Williams & Wilkins Company, 1972.) *C, D,* Control mouse embryo SEM (scanning electron micrograph) specimen sectioned from the corner of the mouth through the hindbrain. Although not distinguishable here, the section passes through the trigeminal placode and ganglion. *E,* Specimen similar to *C* but removed from a murine mother treated with 13-cis-retinoic acid (animal model for Treacher Collins syndrome). A scalloped out depression (*arrowheads* in *E*) is characteristic of severely affected cases. The depression is lined with the trigeminal placode epithelium, which is underlain with debris (*arrowheads* in *F*). *F,* The histologic section in *E* is through a specimen similar to *E* but not as severely affected. Pyknotic cell debris is present in the placode and distributed through the relatively huge trigeminal ganglion (TG) in a pattern similar to that of placodal cells with a ^{3}H-thymidine or quail chromatin markers.

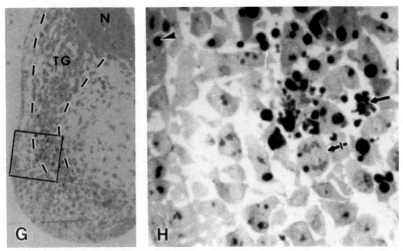

Figure 46–18 *Continued G, H,* Higher magnification of area indicated by box in *E*. Much of the pyknotic debris *(arrows)* is seen to have been phagocytosed by presumed crest cells in the area. (From Sulik, K. K., Johnston, M. C., Smiley, S. J., Speight, H. S., and Jarvis, B. E.: Mandibulofacial dysostosis (Treacher Collins syndrome): a new proposal for its pathogenesis. Am. J. Med. Genet., *27:*359, 1987.)

the organs that they innervate. Thus, postganglionic neuronal fibers (e.g., those of the otic, submaxillary, and sublingual ganglia) usually have only a short distance to travel. Parasympathetic ganglia that are not particularly close to the organs they innervate are the pterygopalatine and ciliary ganglia. The greatest migrators are the vagal prospective parasympathetic neuroblasts that migrate from the fourth visceral arch almost to the caudal end of the gastrointestinal tract.

Specialized sensory receptors develop from local tissues; for example, taste buds develop directly from epithelia. Their maintenance, however, depends on continued innervations.

PITUITARY AND PHARYNGEAL GLANDS

The epithelial components of the pituitary gland originate from two primordia. The first is derived from an invagination of the oral ectoderm (Rathke's pouch) that is intimately related to the undersurface of the overlying forebrain (Fig. 46–19). An extension from this forebrain tissue, termed the infundibulum, develops into the posterior pituitary (pars nervosa), while the remaining epithelial components are derived from Rathke's pouch and form the anterior pituitary (anterior lobe and pars intermedia in Fig. 46–19). The an-

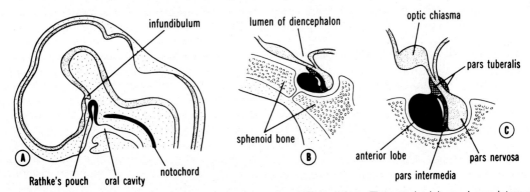

Figure 46–19. Development of the pituitary gland as seen in sagittal sections. The anterior lobe and pars intermedia develop from Rathke's pouch while the pars nervosa is an extension from the forebrain. (From Sadler, T. W.: Langman's Medical Embryology. 5th ed. Baltimore, Williams & Wilkins Company, 1985.)

terior pituitary gland lies just within neural crest cell mesenchyme, and the connective tissues are derived from this mesenchyme. Pearse (1969) postulated that on the bases of biochemical characteristics, ACTH and MSH cells in the anterior pituitary should be of neural crest origin, but there is still no experimental evidence to support this suggestion. The functional relations (sometimes via blood vessels) between cells in the anterior pituitary and the pars nervosa (and between the pars nervosa and overlying hypothalamus) are now beginning to be much better understood.

The ectoderm that gives rise to Rathke's pouch is initially closely associated with the anterior neural folds (Couly and Le Douarin, 1985, 1987, 1988). This may be the reason why deficiencies of the median portion of the anterior neural plate in the holoprosencephalies frequently lead to pituitary deficiencies. The only manifestations of the milder forms of holoprosencephaly may consist of pituitary hypoplasia and a single central incisor, or pituitary hypoplasia alone.

With the exception of the calcitonin (C) cells (which are derived from neural crest), the epithelial components of the pharyngeal glands are derived from endoderm (Fig. 46–20). Although the final distribution of the glands in avian species (in which most of the experimental work has been conducted) and mammalian species is somewhat different, the initial locations in the embryo are virtually identical.

The origins of different cell populations have been clearly demonstrated by cell-marking procedures in avians. When the epithelial buds of the pharyngeal glands invaginate from the pharyngeal endoderm between the visceral arches, they become invested with crest cell mesenchyme. The connective tissue components of the glands are derived from this crest mesenchyme, as are the C cells that invade the epithelium invaginating from the fourth pouch. In submammalian species, the gland containing C cells remains as a separate unit termed the "ultimobranchial body," while in mammals it fuses with the thyroid, where the C cells eventually reside in the peripheral portions of the follicles.

Deficiencies in or absence of the crest cell mesenchyme into which pharyngeal glands invaginate are presumably responsible for their hypoplasia or absence in the retinoic acid and DiGeorge syndromes. The thymus and parathyroids are particularly susceptible. No information on C cells is available. The thyroid gland apparently is not affected to any great extent.

CAROTID AND AORTIC BODIES AND SINUSES

Crest cells also make major contributions to the carotid and aortic bodies and sinuses (Fig. 46–20), where they appear to function as chemo- and baroreceptors, respectively. Crest cells contributing to the aortic sinus are presumably the same crest cells (shown by Kirby, Gale, and Stewart, 1983) that form the mesenchyme of the conotruncal septum. As noted earlier, this longitudinal septum eventually splits, the two halves of the truncus forming the proximal portions of the aortic arch and pulmonary aorta. Although one would therefore expect abnormalities of the chemo- and baroreceptors in the retinoic acid and DiGeorge syndromes, none appears to have been documented.

DEVELOPMENT OF THE EYE AND ASSOCIATED STRUCTURES

The general features of eye development are presented in Figure 46–21. An outpouching of the forebrain forms the optic vesicle, which induces formation of the lens placode when contact is made with the surface ectoderm. The lens then invaginates with the invaginating optic vesicle, eventually pinching off to form the lens. The inner layer of the now bilaminar optic vesicle forms the neural retina, while the outer layer forms the pigmented retina, whose primary function is light absorption. The sensing capacity of the eye lies entirely within the inner (neural) retina, whose cells form the receptor rods and cones and the neurons that send fibers back through the optic stalk. These fibers find their way to the visual cortex at the posterior poles of the cerebral hemispheres, many of them crossing over at the optic chiasm to travel through the opposite hemisphere. They carry nerve impulses generated at synapses with the rods and cones. Most of the iris, including the iridial muscles, is formed by cells from the edge of the optic vesicle. Melanoblasts,

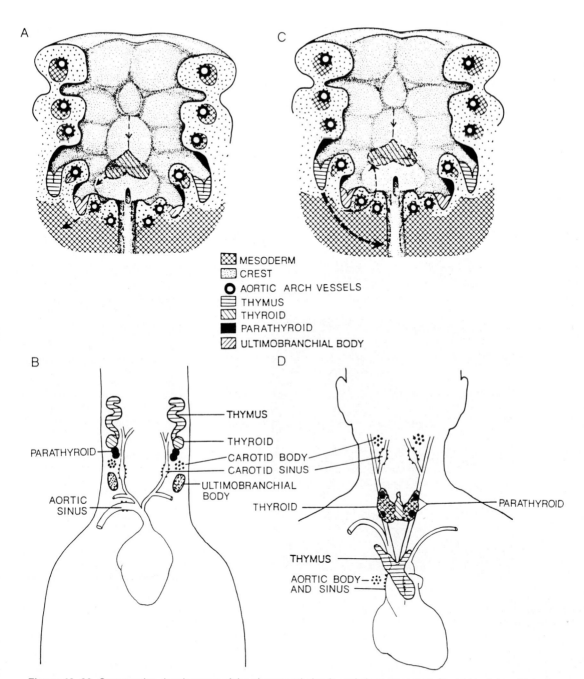

Figure 46–20. Comparative development of the pharyngeal glands and chemoreceptors (carotid body) and baroreceptors in avian *(A, B)* and human embryos *(C, D)*. In *A* and *C* the primordia in the two classes are virtually identical.
Migrations of the primordia in later development *(B* and *D)* display a tendency for the primordia to develop laterally in
avians and medially in humans. Note the fusion of the ultimobranchial body with the thyroid in the human, which is
responsible for bringing the neural crest calcitonin cells into the thyroid. The exact neural crest–mesodermal interface in
the lower (caudal) pharyngeal region is poorly documented. (Modified from Johnston, M. C., Bhakdinaronk, A., and Reid,
Y. C.: An expanded role for the neural crest in oral and pharyngeal development. *In* Bosma, J. F. (Ed.): Fourth Symposium
on Oral Sensation and Perception. Washington, D.C., U.S. Government Printing Office, 1974.)

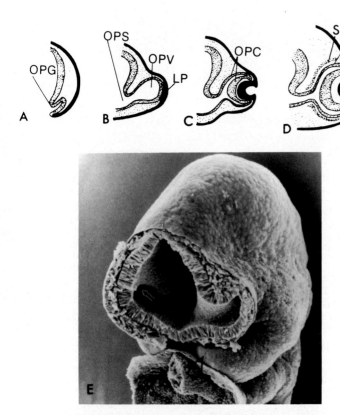

Figure 46–21. Development of the eye as seen in frontal sections. The optic groove (OPG) in *A* is the initial outpouching of the forebrain, which leads to optic vesicle formation (OPV) in *B,* which remains connected to the forebrain by the optic stalk (OPS). On contact of the optic vesicle with the overlying epithelium, the vesicle induces the epithelium to differentiate into the thickened lens placode (LP in *B*). The lens placode invaginates with the invaginating optic cup (OPC in *C*). Finally, the lens vesicle (LV in *D*) pinches off from the overlying ectoderm and separates from the optic cup. The inner layer of the optic vesicle (I in *D*) forms the neural retina, while the outer layer forms the pigmented retina. Almost all the sclera and all of the corneal stroma (CS) are of neural crest origin. The sectioned scanning EM specimen in *E* is slightly less advanced than the frontal section in *B*. The section is asymmetric, cutting in front of the eye vesicle on the embryo's right side. A solid arrow indicates the opening into the cavity of the otic stock. The open arrow indicates the tip of the developing mandibular process. (*A* to *D* modified from Waterman, R. E., and Meller, S. M.: Prenatal development of the oral cavity and paraoral structures in man. *In* Shaw, J. H., Sweeney, E. A., Cappuccino, C. C., and Meller, S. M. (Eds.): Textbook of Oral Biology. Philadelphia, W. B. Saunders Company, 1978. *E* from Johnston, M. C., and Sulik, K. K.: Embryology of the head and neck. *In* Serafin, D., and Georgiade, N. G. (Eds.): Pediatric Plastic Surgery. St. Louis, C. V. Mosby Company, 1984.)

which are derived from the neural crest, change the color of the iris from blue to green to brown, depending on their density. The blood vessels that cross over the retinal surface reach the interior of the eye through the choroid fissure before it closes.

Contributions of neural crest and paraxial mesoderm to the developing eye have been studied fairly extensively (Johnston and associates, 1979). Crest cells make very extensive contributions to the eye, forming virtually all of the sclera, all of the corneal stroma and endothelium (the inner lining of the cornea), and the ciliary muscles that change the shape of the lens. Most of the other periocular connective tissue, including that of the extrinsic ocular muscles, is derived from crest cells. Paraxial mesoderm forms the myoblasts of the extrinsic ocular muscles and the endothelia of the blood vessels, but *not* the corneal endothelium (which should probably be termed "mesothelium").

A wide variety of earlier developmental alterations lead to microphthalmia (frequently accompanied by retinal colobomas) and anophthalmia. Perhaps the most common of the previous alterations is underdevelopment of the anterior neural plate, including that seen in the holoprosencephalies. Peters' anomaly appears to result from failure of the lens to separate completely from the corneal endothelium. Ocular abnormalities are sometimes associated with unilateral craniofacial microsomia and related syndromes. These abnormalities include microphthalmos and anophthalmos in severe cases, and the epibullar dermoids of the Goldenhar variant.

GROWTH CENTERS IN THE FACE AND VISCERAL ARCHES

At the completion of neural crest migration, a new phase of development begins in which regional growth centers predominate (see Fig. 48–6). Epithelial-mesenchymal interactions appear to be the primary regulators.

Explants of epithelia and mesenchyme from the facial prominences (Hall, in press; Minkoff, in press) and from limb buds and the flank region (Solursh, 1984) have shown that continued proliferation and organization of the mesenchyme depends on the presence of associated epithelium. How this regulation is achieved is still unclear. Evidence for the production or concentration of the primitive neurotransmitter serotonin in the facial epithelium and the presence of serotonin binding protein in the underlying basement membrane region has been provided by Lauder, Tannir, and Sadler (1988). It is known that serotonin stimulates cell proliferation in vitro; other growth factors may also be involved (Solursh, 1984).

Directed outgrowth of facial prominences (including the visceral arches) appears to be similar to that of limb buds, which have been much more extensively studied. In the limb bud, directed outgrowth and sequential (progressive) organization are regulated by the apical ectodermal ridge (AER). It is not just the thickened apical ectoderm that provides the organizational capability, but rather the combination of this epithelium and the underlying mesenchyme. As growth of the limb bud continues, this regulatory unit first organizes, in the case of the forelimb, the proximal scapula; then the femur, radius, and ulna; and finally the bones of the hand, including the digits. Disruption of this regulatory unit can occur at any time with failure to form distal segments (e.g., digits as in ectrodactyly) or the more proximal portion as in phocomelia. In the case of phocomelia, the more proximal units may undergo secondary degeneration.

The maxillary prominences and visceral arches appear to develop in a similar manner. After the completion of crest cell migration and its vascularization, the remaining mesodermal core cells degenerate and are replaced by paraxial mesoderm myoblasts. At about the same time, the first and second aortic arch vessels shut down and the arches largely separate from the heart. At the tip of the arches, growth centers are organized (presumably somewhat similar to the AER) and the arches grow ventrally over the surface of the heart (see Fig. 48–6). They eventually contact each other in the ventral midline and merge. The mesodermal cores also contact each other across the ventral midline.

Midline clefts of the mandible may or may not involve the lip and soft tissue of the chin. Often, the most medial structures such as the incisor teeth are absent, suggesting that final stages of mandibular arch formation were never completed.

The maxillary prominence (MxP) grows in a similar manner but has no mesodermal core. It is first organized from mesenchyme and epithelia in the proximal portion of the first arch and behind the eye. The prominence grows under the eye and continues forward until it contacts the developing medial nasal (MNP) and lateral nasal (LNP) prominences. Most growth is at the tip, which remains fused with the underlying epithelium except when it "jumps" a groove between it and the LNP, leaving the primordium of the lacrimal duct underneath. The MxP is capable of developing as a free-ended structure, as was sometimes observed after crest cell extirpation (Johnston, 1965) or after retinol administration to chick embryos in culture.

Development of the MNP and LNP is covered in Chapter 48 and will be considered only briefly here. The prominences are organized around the olfactory placode. Radial symmetry of the placode is lost early as its lateral edge curls forward, initiating LNP formation. Rapid growth along the medial edge leads to distinct MNP formation. The lower edge of the MNP fuses with the MxP at an early stage (approximately day 30 in the human embryo). The LNP appears to sweep over the MxP with which it is now confluent, contacting the MNP at about day 35, thereby completing formation of the bilaminar epithelial seam. Breakdown of a portion of this contacting epithelium permits the mesenchymes of the two sides to become confluent. Behind the area of confluence, the epithelium hollows out to form the nasal passage connecting the nasal and oral cavities. All three prominences continue to grow forward, and continued merging enlarges the area of mesenchymal confluence. Primary palate formation is completed by about day 37 in the human embryo.

Normal primary palate and cleft formation is considered in much greater detail in Chapter 48. One syndrome that includes clefting is worth noting here: the EEC (ectodermal dysplasia-ectrodactyly-clefting) syndrome (Bixler and associates, 1972). The combination of cleft lip with absent digits (ectrodactyly) in this syndrome indicates an abnormal developmental step common to both primary palate and limb development, and the inclusion of deficient sweat glands and abnormal tooth formation indicates a fairly broad defect in epithelial-mesenchymal interactions.

The palatal shelves also appear to develop in a limb bud–like fashion with the medial edge of the shelf functioning in a manner similar to the AER. There are syndromes in which there appear to be multiple failures of this aspect of development, because mandibular clefts (with missing incisors), clefts of the palate, and ectrodactyly are combined in the same patients.

The significance of multiple secondary and tertiary growth centers (and so forth) in facial development is not entirely clear. However, failure of their coalescence may explain a number of developmental abnormalities. Normally, these centers coalesce through the phenomenon of merging.

After the merging of the mandibular and hyoid prominences in the ventral midline, a number of centers appear on their lateral surfaces, most of which are auricular hillocks that form the external ear. Initially, the part of the mandibular arch between the hillocks is rudimentary, but this region undergoes incredible growth to form the mandible and associated structures. Any deficiencies in this growth result in the ears remaining relatively close to the ventral midline. Although such ears are often described as being "low set," they are usually in their normal position relative to the rest of the face and the cranium.

Two of the centers contributing to rapid growth of the arch are adjacent to the midline and sometimes termed "md'" to distinguish them from the rest of the arch. Growth is predominantly outward from the surface of the arch, and the groove between these centers and the rest of the mandibular arch normally becomes quite deep before finally being smoothed out through merging. Failure of the merging phenomenon is probably responsible for the bilateral clefts seen in the whistling face syndrome, and incomplete merging may be responsible for the formation of the lip pits in Van der Woude's syndrome. Variable combinations with clefts of the lip or palate in this dominantly inherited syndrome indicate that there is a more generalized problem of fusion or merging.

A secondary growth center similar to md[1] is seen at the growing tip of the MxP. The globular process of His at the end of the MNP probably represents another growth center, although it appears to be complicated by a morphogenetic movement.

Conditions in which there are apparent multiple merging (as opposed to merging-fusion) problems in the facial area are the orofacial-digital (OFD) syndromes. There are usually medial clefts of the upper lip. The nose may be bifid and there is almost invariably hypertelorism. The latter can be severe and, rarely, is associated with partial agenesis of the corpus callosum. The soft palate (the portion of the secondary palate that undergoes midline coalescence exclusively by merging), is almost invariably cleft. Midline clefts of the tongue in the OFD syndromes are presumably also merging problems, but occasional lateral clefts of the tongue may not be. Distinctive features are clefts of the maxillary and mandibular alveolar processes from which frenula extend to the adjacent lip (Fig. 46–22). Sometimes two cuspids are found on either side of the maxillary cleft. In most instances the teeth in the cleft region are missing, especially in the mandibular arch. These clefts are in approximately the location of the Mx-Mx^1 and Md-Md^1 junctions (Fig. 46–22) and this may be somehow related to their pathogenesis, perhaps involving some tissue destruction. The digital defects sometimes include partial duplications, which could involve additional areas of cell death, but more characteristically distortions of digits are found, and these are hard to relate to the facial defects.

Finally, some comments should be made about disruptions, which may sometimes be associated with amniotic bands, a highly controversial subject. Fragments or large pieces of amniotic bands are sometimes found attached to bizarre facial clefts and other areas of tissue disruption. It is usually thought that the bands cause the defects following premature amnion disruption, but it is also possible that some adhesions relate to lesions already present. Amniotic bands seem to be the possible causative factor for some bizarre clefts involving little or no tissue destruction.

DEVELOPMENT OF THE EAR

The ear consists of three major components, all of which develop more or less independently. This is particularly true for the inner ear. These differences account for much of the great variability in ear abnormalities.

The Inner Ear

Otic placode formation is the initial stage of ear development. It initially forms as a thickened epithelium whose dorsal half is in close contact with the neural tube at the junction of the prospective anterior and posterior hindbrain (see Fig. 46–5A). It has been shown experimentally (Jacobson, 1966) that its induction is dependent on both neural tube and mesoderm. Crest cells migrate around its anterior and posterior margins as they make their way into the second and third visceral arches, respectively.

Eventually, the placode lifts off the neural tube, becomes underlaid with mesodermal mesenchyme, and begins to invaginate. It later pinches off from the surface ectoderm to become the otocyst (see Fig. 46–16). The otocyst undergoes a complex series of evaginations, fusions, and breakdown to eventually form the epithelial linings of the semicircular canals, and the common vestibule of the vestibular (balance) component and the long spiral cochlea of the acoustic (auditory) component.

The surrounding mesodermal layer (the otic capsule) is very important for these morphologic changes and subsequent development of sensory (hair) cells (Noden and van de Water, 1986). Eventually, the otocyst induces capsular cells to form cartilage, which later undergoes endochondrial ossification to form the bulk of the petrous portion of the temporal bone. Although crest cells form some of the outer capsular chondrocytes, it has been shown that the otic epithelium is incapable of eliciting chondrocyte differentiation directly from neural crest mesenchyme (Noden and van de Water, 1986).

Although development of the sensory cells is dependent on the surrounding mesoderm, it is not dependent on innervation (van de Water, 1988). The ends of the stereocilia (hairs) of these cells become buried in a gelatinous matrix that becomes mineralized in the vestibule, adding the weight that is critical for sensing changes in head position. Other sensors in the vestibular canals sense movement by monitoring fluid movements. In the acoustic component, the hair cells monitor sound-induced vibrations in the cochlear endolymphatic fluid.

Unlike the eye, where all the neurons remain in the sensory epithelium, or the olfactory epithelium, where some of them do, all the neurons of the ear sensory epithelia leave to form the neurons of the acousticovestibular (eighth) nerve ganglion (D'Amico-Martel and Noden, 1983; Noden and van de Water, 1986). All the supporting cells and a few neurons

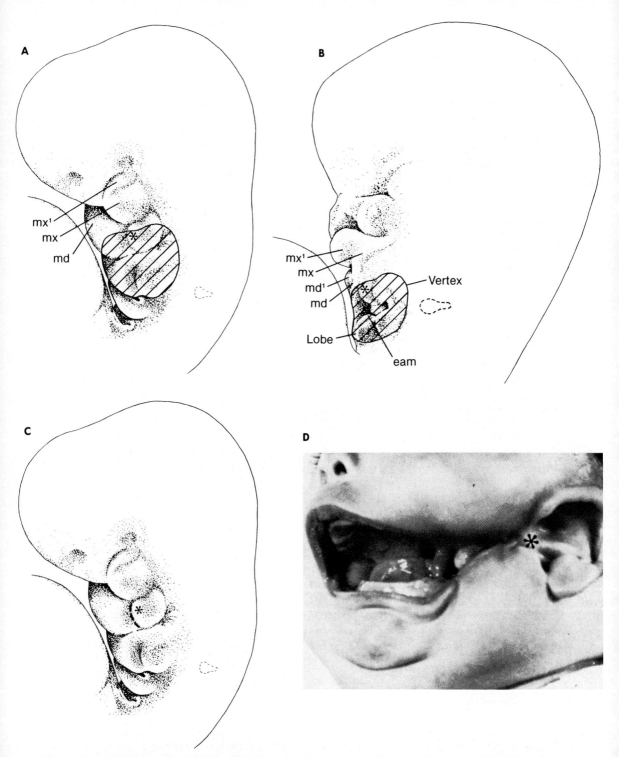

Figure 46–22. Lateral aspect of facial growth centers with particular emphasis on the development of the external ear (oblique hatching indicates pinna and external auditory meatus) in day 30 *(A)* and day 40 *(B)* human embryos. The otocyst *(broken outline)* is relatively closer to the external ear in the older embryo, but the hillocks of the external ear are still close to the ventral midline. They will be further separated by developing mandibular and anterior neck structures. The pinna also undergoes considerable reorientation in later development. Failure of merging of the growth centers in *C* apparently is responsible for the lateral facial cleft in *D*. Abbreviations: mx¹ and mx are growth centers of the maxillary prominence; md and md¹ are growth centers of the mandibular arch; eam is external auditory meatus. (*A, B,* and *C* from Johnston, M .C., and Sulik, K. K.: Embryology of the head and neck. *In* Serafin, D., and Georgiade, N. G., (Eds.): Pediatric Plastic Surgery. St. Louis, C. V. Mosby Company, 1984. *D* from Gorlin, R. J., Pindborg, J. J., and Cohen, M. M.: Syndromes of the Head and Neck. New York, McGraw-Hill Book Company, 1976.)

were found by these investigators to be derived from the neural crest, presumably from the seventh nerve ganglion with which the acousticovestibular ganglion is fused in early development. The sensory epithelium also receives motor fibers that modulate the activity of the sensory cells.

Although the 13-cis-RA–treated embryos have not been directly examined for evidence of neuronal cell death related to acousticovestibular ganglion formation, it appears almost certain that this will be the case. Inner ear abnormalities, including deafness, are common when thalidomide is administered at the time when these cells are migrating in monkeys (Newman and Hendrickx, 1981) and humans (Livingstone, 1965). Similar abnormalities are seen in the Treacher Collins syndrome.

In addition to forming the neural support cells, presumed crest cells (which contain melanin granules) are found related to the inner ear vasculature (stria vascularis) and in close apposition to epithelial cells adjacent to the sensory epithelium that appear to have a secreting (endolymph-forming?) function. In the dancer mouse, absence of these pigment cells in the stria is associated with structurally and functionally abnormal vestibular sensory epithelia (Doel, 1970). This mutant mouse has other pigmentation defects and

cleft lip, rather similar to Waardenburg's syndrome, in which the inner ear defect is deafness and the incidence of cleft lip is about 6 per cent. The nature of the presumed crest cell defect is unknown, although a proliferation defect is a strong possibility.

The Middle Ear

The major function of the middle ear is to conduct noise vibrations from the tympanic membrane through a chain of ossicles to the membrane in the oval window of the inner ear (Fig. 46–23). The inner face of this membrane is in contact with cochlear endolymph, which then carries the vibrations to the cochlear sensory epithelium.

The evolution and development of the middle ear ossicles and temporomandibular joint are of considerable interest (Crompton and Parker, 1978). In most submammalian species, only the equivalent of the second arch stapes is present as the columella. In higher reptiles the formation of a new, more anterior jaw (temporomandibular) joint "frees up" the two posterior bones of the lower jaw, which become the malleus and incus, inserted between the tympanic membrane and the columella, now termed the stapes. To form the new joint a new (condylar) cartilage forms

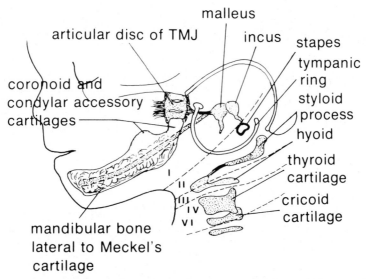

Figure 46–23. Cartilaginous skeletal components of the visceral arches (Roman numerals) and their relationships with the developing mandible and temporomandibular joint (TMJ). (From Waterman, R. E., and Meller, S. M.: Prenatal development of the oral cavity and paraoral structures in man. *In* Shaw, J. H., Sweeney, E. A., Cappuccino, C. C., and Meller, S. M. (Eds.): Textbook of Oral Biology. Philadelphia, W. B. Saunders Company, 1978.)

MOUSE

HUMAN

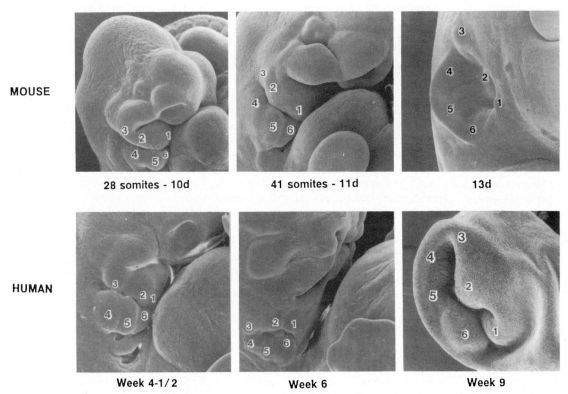

28 somites - 10d   41 somites - 11d   13d

Week 4-1/2   Week 6   Week 9

Figure 46–24. Comparison of external ear development in the mouse *(upper panel)*, on which most experimental studies have been conducted, and the human *(lower panel)*. The various growth centers (auricular hillocks, which are six in number) are virtually the same in the two species. (From Jarvis, B. L., Sulik, K. K., and Johnston, M. C.: Congenital malformations of the external, middle and inner ear produced by isotretinoin exposure in fetal mice. Otol. Head Neck Surg., submitted.)

from the mesenchyme between the most anterior jawbone (now termed the mandible) with which it fuses as it does in the human embryo. This peculiar origin of the condylar cartilage may help explain the regeneration of the condyle sometimes seen after injury and resorption of the original condyle in young children.

The cartilaginous models of the inner ear ossicles first form in mesenchyme and are secondarily enveloped by the middle ear epithelium, which is an extension of the endodermal lining of the first pharyngeal pouch. The remainder of the first pharyngeal pouch endoderm persists as the epithelial lining of the eustachian tube.

The External Ear

The development of the pinna of the external ear of mouse and human embryos is illustrated in Figure 46–24. The initial primordium consists of six auricular hillocks (growth centers) located on the sides of the mandibular and hyoid arches near the ventral midline. The hillocks continue to increase in size and eventually merge with one another to form characteristic components of the pinna. The author finds no evidence for the contention that much of the anterior pinna is derived through late forward rotation of the hyoid arch hillocks.

Since avian species do not have pinnas, the neural crest origin of the external ear mesenchyme has never been directly demonstrated. However, all the mesenchyme in the visceral arches of the region where the hillocks initially form is known to be of crest origin. The mesenchyme of the external ear canals and the tympanic rings of birds are also of crest origin.

DEVELOPMENT OF SKELETAL TISSUES

Some of the earliest skeletal structures are of a temporary nature. The embryonic origins of the visceral arch skeletal components are illustrated in Figure 46–25. The anterior portion of Meckel's cartilage becomes incorporated into the developing mandible, and it now appears that at least some of the chondrocytes redifferentiate into osteoblasts and osteocytes. Only the perichondrium of the posterior portion persists in the form of the sphenomandibular segment (Fig. 46–25). Similarly, the perichondrium of Reichert's

Figure 46–25. In this schematic drawing, the visceral arch cartilages are designated by oblique hatching while the cranial base cartilages are heavily stippled and outlined by broken (dashed) lines. The remaining skeletal elements are the intramembranous bones of the face and cranial vault. (From Hamilton, W. J., and Mossman, H.: Human Embryology. 4th Ed. Cambridge, England, W. Heffer & Sons, 1972.)

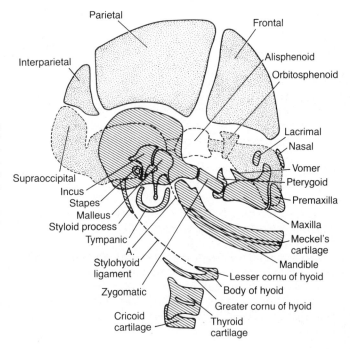

cartilage gives rise to the stylohyoid ligament, styloid process, and stapes.

Much of the cranial base is initially formed as a cartilaginous model, as is also the nasal capsule, which includes the nasal septum. Most of this cartilage undergoes endochondral ossification, and only small amounts remain in the sphenoethmoidal and sphenooccipital synchondroses and the nasal septum. The synchondroses persist through the growth period, providing much of the growth force in the cranial base.

Growth of cartilage may be deficient in genetically determined conditions such as achondroplasia. Such defects result in characteristic craniofacial malformations. They are superficially similar to those of Crouzon's disease.

The formation of both cartilage and bone from crest cells requires previous interaction with epithelia (Thorogood, 1988; Hall, in press). In vivo these interactions must occur very early, because at later stages differentiation of these tissues in subepithelial mesenchyme is found.

The onset of bone formation is sometimes considered as marking the end of the embryonic period. Although some embryonic development still continues in the brain, the fetus is generally much more resistant to the effects of common teratogens.

Intramembranous (i.e., nonendochondral) bones are common in the head. Usually there is one ossification center for each bone, and bone formation stops before contact and fusion of the centers, with sutures remaining between the bones. Bone growth occurs by apposition at the sutures and is apparently secondary to expansive growth forces exerted by soft tissues. If premature closure of sutures (synostosis) occurs, growth is inhibited. Premature closure may be genetically determined, such as in Crouzon's disease (craniofacial dysostosis), or may result from premature contact and fusion of (cranial vault) bones because of excessive intrauterine pressure secondary to oligohydramnios (Graham, deSaxe, and Smith, 1979). Excessive intrauterine pressure may also result in deformations (Greer-Walker, 1958).

In Crouzon's disease, both cranial and facial sutures are affected. Involvement of cranial vault sutures may be somewhat variable in both time of onset (prenatal life through the fifth year) and location (Gorlin, Pindborg, and Cohen, 1976). Exophthalmos readily distinguishes Crouzon's disease from achondroplasia. It is primarily related to deficient growth of the periorbital bones but may be partially due to downward pressure from the developing brain, leading to remodeling of the orbital roof. Increased intracranial pressure in unoperated cases may be associated with mental retardation. Although the basic nature of the developmental defect is unknown, it is inherited as an autosomal dominant trait (see also Chap. 61).

Although most of the craniofacial manifestations seen in Apert's syndrome are similar to those in Crouzon's disease, it appears that the two conditions are etiologically different. The developmental disturbances in Apert's syndrome are always present at birth, more widespread, and, in addition to premature suture closure, include syndactyly and clefts of the soft palate in about 30 per cent of cases (Gorlin, Pindborg, and Cohen, 1976). There are other palatal abnormalities. Although few patients reproduce successfully, it appears that most cases result from abnormal autosomal dominant genes.

Tooth development has been studied in much detail (Lumsden, 1988; Kollar and Mina, in press). Interactions between crest cell mesenchyme and oral ectoderm are involved. It now appears that the original specifications for tooth form (e.g., incisor versus molar form) are in the oral ectoderm but the responding mesenchyme must be of neural crest origin. However, once the dental papilla begins to form, it can dictate tooth form even in foreign ectoderm.

The initial primordia of the teeth (the dental laminae and associated mesenchyme) form at about the time of fusion of the medial nasal, lateral nasal, and maxillary prominences (Fig. 46–26). Failure of fusion of these prominences leads to cleft lip, and alters further development of teeth in the fusion area with a peculiarly wide spectrum of supernumerary and missing teeth and unusual structures of those teeth that are present (Ross and Johnston, 1972). Tooth abnormalities may be associated with a wide variety of craniofacial malformations (Gorlin, Pindborg, and Cohen, 1976) or there may be abnormalities of structure, form, size, or numbers not associated with other malformations. Since enamel and dentin do not undergo remodeling, as do other mineralized tissues, they may

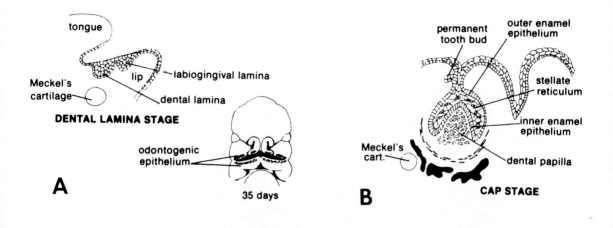

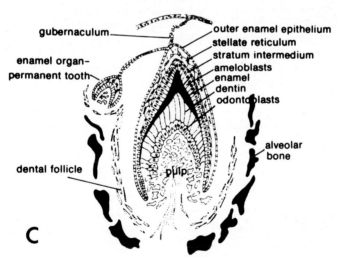

Figure 46–26. The first evidence of tooth formation is the formation of the dental lamina *(A)* in the oral ectoderm, which is associated with condensation of the surrounding crest cell mesenchyme. Only these tissues are capable of forming teeth (see text). Initially independent portions of the dental lamina are formed on the medial nasal prominence and the two halves of the mandibular arch. Localized epithelial proliferation leads to formation of the tooth bud, which develops into characteristically shaped enamel organs that will form the enamel and organize root development *(B and C)*. The enamel organ is associated with the mesenchymal dental papilla *(B),* which forms the pulp and dentin *(C).* The surrounding mesenchymal dental follicle *(C)* is responsible for formation of the periodontal ligament and the root cementum in which the fibers of the periodontal ligament become embedded. (Adapted from Waterman, R. E., and Meller, S. M.: Prenatal development of the oral cavity and paraoral structures in man. *In* Shaw, J. H., Sweeney, E. A., Cappuccino, C. C., and Meller, S. M. (Eds.): Textbook of Oral Biology. Philadelphia, W. B. Saunders Company, 1978.)

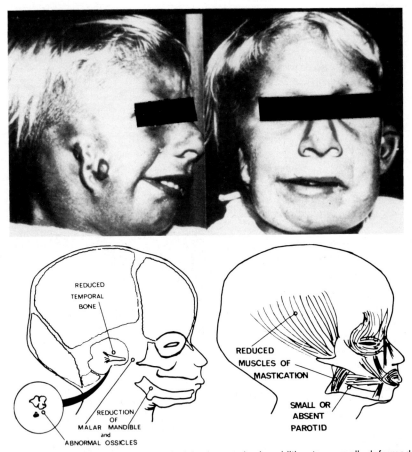

Figure 46–27. Major features of unilateral craniofacial microsomia. In addition to a small, deformed pinna (external ear), there is generalized hypoplasia of the adjacent soft tissue and skeleton: temporomandibular joint, middle ear ossicles, muscles of mastication, and parotid gland. (Modified from Poswillo, D.: Oral Surg., *35*:302, 1973.)

provide evidence of the timing of more generalized developmental disturbances, such as those occurring at birth.

REEXAMINATION OF PATHOGENESIS OF CRANIOFACIAL MICROSOMIA AND RELATED MALFORMATIONS

A number of observations since Poswillo (1973) suggested that craniofacial microsomia resulted from focal hemorrhage indicate that this mechanism is unlikely to be the primary defect.

Craniofacial microsomia (Fig. 46–27) is a complex malformation usually associated with abnormalities in other systems. The minimal anomaly is usually considered to be a deficient dysplastic ear, although the ear may be normal while other features (e.g., epibulbar dermoids) may be present (see Chap. 62). Features usually present include abnormalities of the middle ear and underdevelopment of the mandibular ramus and condyle. The condition is usually unilateral, but if bilateral it is usually asymmetric.

It is unclear how much heterogeneity of etiology and pathogenesis is present. Some investigators separate the cases according to associated malformations. Goldenhar considered craniofacial microsomia associated with epibulbar dermoids-lipodermoids to constitute another syndrome; most (75 to 85 per cent) of Goldenhar's syndrome cases have associated vertebral (usually cervical) and occasional rib abnormalities. Gorlin, Pindberg, and Cohen, 1976, included these as part of the syndrome, which they name the oculoauricular-vertebral syndrome. When patients are carefully examined, approximately 50 per cent have associated cardiovascular defects, and virtually all of these may be of the conotruncal (outflow tract) type. The incidence of cardiovascular defects seems to be about the same in Goldenhar's syndrome and other variants of craniofacial microsomia. Associated cleft lip with or without associated cleft palate and, less frequently, (isolated) cleft palate are found with variable frequency (7 to 25 per cent) in all types of craniofacial microsomia. Renal anomalies are found in approximately 5 to 6 per cent, and this com-

bination is sometimes called branchio-otorenal syndrome. Limb anomalies (almost invariably minor) are found in as many as 50 per cent of cases.

Whether the large number of associated malformations indicates heterogeneity is problematic. Many investigators feel that most represent variable expressions of the same basic defect.

Recent studies suggesting a reassessment of the pathogenesis of craniofacial microsomia include the findings that postotic crest cells form much of the mesenchymal septum of the conotruncal portion of the heart and that extirpation of these cells leads to a wide range of cardiovascular defects. These defects are not limited to conotruncal derivatives (i.e., portions of the great vessels) but include other cardiovascular defects, particularly interventricular septal defects. Some of these may be secondary to abnormal flow resistance caused by narrowing of the great vessels, which leads to distention of the embryonic heart and abnormalities of septation.

Two other advances relate to retinoic acid. One is the increasing awareness that all-trans-RA plays major and multiple roles in regulating normal development. Crest cells have large amounts of RA binding protein both before and during their migration. Accutane (13-cis-RA) kills many crest cells before they migrate and interferes with crest cells during their migration. The resultant malformations have many similarities to craniofacial microsomia. When Accutane is administered later, it kills ganglionic placodal cells and results in malformations similar to the Treacher Collins syndrome.

Another major advance has been the gradual realization that thalidomide produces a wide range of malformations that are virtually identical to those produced by RA. This is especially useful because of the large amount of work that has been done on resulting malformations in both humans and experimental animals. The use of thalidomide in most countries as a drug for nausea in pregnancy meant that most exposures were too late for the critical developmental stages. However, in Germany it was used as a nonprescription antidepressant. It has been estimated that its early use there resulted in 1000 to 3000 infants with ear malformations similar to craniofacial microsomia and the Treacher Collins syndrome.

Many of the exposures to thalidomide were

for well-documented brief periods, and the resulting malformations have been described in considerable detail. There were two periods of sensitivity for ear malformations: the first before and during preotic crest cell migration when severe ear malformations ("anotia") resulted, and the second before and during migrations of ganglionic placodal cells when less severe ear "deformations" occurred. Sensitivity to cardiovascular malformations (usually of the conotruncal outflow tract type) occurred after exposures mostly during the second period and later.

Recognizing the sensitivity of the ear malformations to craniofacial microsomia, Poswillo (1973) treated monkeys during the second period and concluded that he was producing malformations comparable with craniofacial microsomia. Newman and Hendrickx (1981) repeated the experiments and concluded that the malformations more closely resembled those of the Treacher Collins syndrome, chiefly on the basis of major inner ear involvement, which is more typical of the latter (Livingstone, 1965). Examination of the embryos described in the Poswillo (1973) paper showed developmental changes closely resembling the mouse 13-cis-retinoic acid model for the Treacher Collins syndrome, where this compound was administered at the same developmental age (Jarvis, Sulik, and Johnston, in press).

In a second model for craniofacial microsomia (Poswillo, 1973), azetidine was administered to pregnant mice at a slightly later stage of development, the time of primary palate (lip) development. Frank hemorrhages occurred, but not until four days after administration of the drug. The most severe hemorrhages occurred in the region of the ear and could certainly be responsible for the associated regional malformations, which were similar to those of craniofacial microsomia.

An alternative model, at least for some variants of craniofacial microsomia, is the retinoic acid syndrome (RAS) model described earlier. Not only do the malformations (e.g., those of the external and middle ear and the cardiovascular system) closely resemble those of craniofacial microsomia but they also are similar to the vertebral anomalies. The malformations involving the craniofacial region involve almost exclusively structures of neural crest origin. These include the squa-mous portion of the temporal bone, which is often severely affected, while other portions of the temporal bone that receive only minor contributions from crest cells show only minor defects.

Undoubtedly, there will be true heterogeneity with respect to craniofacial microsomia (as is apparently the case for nonsyndromic cleft lip with or without associated cleft palate—see Chap. 48) in terms of both etiology and pathogenesis. Also, the different animal models may be applicable to at least some aspects of related malformations such as the CHARGE association and the velocardiofacial syndrome (Shprintzen and associates, 1978).

REFERENCES

Adelmann, H. B.: The embryological basis of cyclopia. Am. J. Ophthalmol., *17:*890, 1934.

Adelmann, H. B.: The problem of cyclopia. Q. Rev. Biophys., *11:*61, 284, 1937.

Ammann, A. J., Wara, D. W., Cowan, A. J., Barrett, D. J., and Stechm, E. R.: The DiGeorge syndrome and the fetal alcohol syndrome. Am. J. Dis. Child., *136:*906, 1982.

Ardinger, H. H., and Bartley, J. A.: Microcephaly in familial holoprosencephaly. J. Craniofac. Genet. Dev. Biol., *8:*53, 1988.

Ardinger, H. H., Clark, E. B., and Hanson, J. W.: Cardiovascular anomalies in craniofacial disorders: pathogenetic and epidemiologic implications. Proc. Greenwood Genet. Center, *4:*80, 1985.

Arvystas, M., and Shprintzen, R. J.: Craniofacial morphology in the velocardiofacial syndrome. J. Craniofac. Genet. Dev. Biol., *4:*39, 1984.

Bard, J. B., and Hay, E. D.: The behavior of fibroblasts from the developing avian cornea: their morphology and movement in situ and in vitro. J. Cell Biol., *67:*400, 1975.

Bixler, D., Spivack, J., Bennett, J., et al.: The ectrodactyly-ectodermal dysplasia-clefting (EEC) syndrome. Report of 2 cases and review of the literature. Clin. Genet., *3:*43, 1972.

Brazzell, R. K., Vane, F. M., Ehmann, C. W., and Colburn, W. A.: Pharmacokinetics of isotretinoin during repetitive dosing to patients. Eur. J. Pharmacol., *24:*695, 1983.

Bronner-Fraser, M., Stern, C. D., and Fraser, S.: Analysis of neural crest cell lineage and migration. J. Craniofac. Genet. Dev. Biol. (Suppl.) (in press).

Cohlan, S. Q.: Excessive intake of vitamin A as a cause of congenital anomalies in the rat. Science, *117:*535, 1953.

Cook, C. S., and Sulik, K. K.: Keratolenticular dysgenesis (Peters' anomaly) as a result of acute embryonic insult during gastrulation. Pediatric Ophthalmol. Strabis (in press).

Couly, G. F., and Le Douarin, N. M.: Mapping of the early neural primordium in quail-chick chimeras. I.

Developmental relationships between placodes, facial ectoderm, and prosencephalon. Dev. Biol., 110:422, 1985.

Couly, G. F., and Le Douarin, N. M.: Mapping of the early neural primordium in quail-chick chimeras. II. The prosencephalic neural plate and neural folds: implications for the genesis of cephalic human congenital abnormalities. Dev. Biol., 120:198, 1987.

Couly, G., and Le Douarin, N. M.: The fate map of the cephalic neural primordium at the presomitic to the 3-somite stage in the avian embryo. Development (Suppl.), 103:101, 1988.

Crompton, A. W., and Parker, P.: Evolution of the mammalian masticatory apparatus. Am. Sci., 66:192, 1978.

Daft, P. A., Johnston, M. C., and Sulik, K. K.: Abnormal heart and great vessel development following acute ethanol exposure in mice. Teratology, 33:93, 1986.

D'Amico-Martel, A., and Noden, D. M.: Contributions of placodal and neural crest cells to avian cranial peripheral ganglia. Am. J. Anat., 166:445, 1983.

Dencker, L.: Embryonic-fetal localization of drugs and nutrients. In Persaud, T. V. (Ed.): Advances in the Study of Birth Defects. Vol. 1. Lancaster, MTP Press, 1979, pp. 1–8.

Dencker, L., Annerwall, E., Busch, C., and Eriksson, U.: Retinoid-binding proteins in craniofacial development. J. Craniofac. Genet. Dev. Biol. (Suppl.) (in press).

Dencker, L., D'Argy, R., Danielsson, B. R., Ghantous, H., and Sperber, G. O.: Saturable accumulation of retinoic acid in neural and neural crest derived cells in early embryonic development. Dev. Pharmacol. Ther., 10:212, 1987.

Doel, M. S.: The relationship between abnormalities of pigmentation and the inner ear. Proc. R. Soc. (Lond.), 175:201, 1970.

Dryburgh, L. C.: Epigenetics of early tooth development in the mouse (abstract). J. Dent. Res., 46:1264, 1967.

Duband, J. L., and Thiery, J. P.: Distribution of fibronectin in the early phase of avian cephalic neural crest cell migration. Dev. Biol., 93:308, 1982.

Duband, J. L., and Thiery, J. P.: Distribution of laminin and collagens during avian neural crest development. Development, 101:461, 1987.

Edelman, G. M., and Thiery, J. P.: The Cell in Contact: Adhesion and Junctions as Morphogenetic Determinants. New York, John Wiley & Sons, 1985.

Edwards, M. J., Warner, R. A., and Mulley, R. C.: Exencephaly in fetal hamsters following exposure of hyperthermia. Teratology, 14:3203, 1976.

Erickson, C. A.: Morphogenesis of the neural crest. In Browder, L. W. (Ed.): Developmental Biology. A Comprehensive Synthesis. Vol. 2, New York, Plenum Press, 1986, pp. 481–543.

Fantel, A. G., Shepard, T. H., Newell-Morris, L. N., and Moffett, B. C.: Teratogenic effects of retinoic acid in pigtail monkeys (Macaca nemestrina). Teratology, 15:65, 1977.

Gasser, R. F.: The development of the facial muscles in man. Am. J. Anat., 120:367, 1967.

Gorlin, R. J., Pindborg, J. J., and Cohen, M. M.: Syndromes of the Head and Neck. New York, McGraw-Hill Book Company, 1976.

Goulding, E. H., and Pratt, R. M.: Isotretinoin teratogenicity in mouse whole embryo culture. J. Craniofac. Genet. Dev. Biol., 6:99, 1986.

Graham, J. M., deSaxe, M., and Smith, D. W.: Sagittal craniostenosis: fetal head constraint as one possible cause. J. Pediatr., 95:747, 1979.

Greer-Walker, D.: Malformations of the Face. Edinburgh, E. & S. Livingstone, 1958.

Hall, B. K.: Cellular interactions during cartilage and bone development. J. Craniofac. Genet. Dev. Biol. (Suppl.) (in press).

Hamburger, V.: Experimental analysis of the dual origin of the trigeminal ganglion in the chick embryo. J. Exp. Zool., 148:91, 1961.

Hassell, J. R., Greenberg, J. H., and Johnston, M. C.: Inhibition of cranial neural crest cell development by vitamin A in the cultured chick embryo. J. Embryol. Exp. Morphol., 39:267, 1977.

Hazelton, R. D.: A radioautographic analysis of the migration and fate of cells derived from the occipital somites of the chick embryo with specific reference to the hypoglossal musculature. J. Embryol. Exp. Morphol., 24:455, 1970.

Holtfreter, J.: Formative Reize in der Embryoanalentwicklung der Amphibien, dargestellt an Explantationsversuchen. Arch. f. exp. Zellf., 15:281, 1934.

Holtfreter, J., and Hamburger, V.: Amphibians. In Willier, D. H., Weiss, P. A., and Hamburger, B. (Eds.): Analysis of Development. Philadelphia, W. B. Saunders Company, 1955, pp. 230–296.

Jacobson, A. G.: Indictive processes in embryonic development. Science, 152:25, 1966.

Jarvis, B. L., Sulik, K. K., and Johnston, M. C.: Congenital malformations of the external, middle and inner ear produced by isotretinoin exposure in fetal mice. Otolaryngel. Head Neck Surg. (in press).

Johnston, M. C.: The neural crest in vertebrate cephalogenesis. Ph.D. Thesis, University of Rochester, 1965.

Johnston, M. C., Bhakdinaronk, A., and Reid, Y. C.: An expanded role for the neural crest in oral and pharyngeal development. In Bosma, J. F. (Ed.): Oral Sensation and Perception—Development in the Fetus and Infant. Washington, D.C., U.S. Govt. Printing Office, 1974, pp. 37–52.

Johnston, M. C., and Hazelton, R. B.: Embryonic origins of facial structures related to oral sensory and motor function. In Bosma, J. F. (Ed.): Oral Sensory Perception: The Mouth of the Infant. Springfield, IL, Charles C Thomas, 1972.

Johnston, M. C., and Listgarten, M. A.: The migration interaction and early differentiation of oro-facial tissues. In Slavkin, H. S., and Bavetta, L. A. (Eds.): Developmental Aspects of Oral Biology. New York, Academic Press, 1972, pp. 55–80.

Johnston, M. C., Noden, D. M., Hazelton, R. D., Coulombre, J. L., and Coulombre, A. J.: Origins of avian ocular and periocular tissues. Exp. Eye Res., 29:27, 1979.

Johnston, M. C., and Sulik, K. K.: Development of the face and oral cavity. In Bhaskar, S. V. (Ed.): Orban's Oral Histology and Embryology. 9th Ed. St. Louis, C. V. Mosby Company, 1980, pp. 1–23.

Johnston, M. C., and Sulik, K. K.: The neural crest. In Shields, E. D., Burzynsky, N. J., and Melnick, M. (Eds.): Craniofacial Dysmorphology: Genetics, Etiology, Diagnosis and Treatment. Littleton, John Wright, PSG, 1983.

Juriloff, D. M., Sulik, K. K., and Roderick, T. H.: Morphogenesis of spontaneously occurring otocephaly in a newly developed mouse mutant (abstract). Teratology, 21:47, 1980.

Kirby, M. L.: Role of extracardia factors in heart development. Experientia, 44:944, 1988.

Kirby, M. L., Gale, T. F., and Stewart, D. E.: Neural

crest cells contribute to normal aorticopulmonary septation. Science, *220:*1059, 1983.

Kochhar, D. M.: Transplacental passage of label after administration of (^{3}H) retinoic acid (vitamin A acid) to pregnant mice. Teratology, *14:*53, 1976.

Kochhar, D. M., and Penner, J. D.: Developmental effects of isotretinoin and 4-oxo-isotretinoin: the role of metabolism in teratogenicity. Teratology, *36:*67, 1987.

Kollar, E. J., and Mina, M.: The role of the early epithelium in the patterning of the teeth and Meckel's cartilage. *In* Townsley, J., and Johnston, M. C. (Eds.): Research Advances in Prenatal Craniofacial Development. New York, Alan R. Liss (in press).

Lammer, E. J., Chen, D. T., Hoar, R. M., Agnish, N. D., Benke, P. J., et al.: Retinoic acid embryopathy. N. Engl. J. Med., *313:*837, 1985.

Lauder, J. M., Tannir, H., and Sadler, T. H.: Serotonin and morphogenesis. I. Sites of serotonin uptake and binding protein immunoreactivity in the midgestation mouse embryo. Development, *102:*709, 1988.

Lawrence, K. M.: Causes of neural tube malformation and their prevention by dietary improvement and perconceptional supplementation with folic acid and multivitamins. *In* Briggs, M. (Ed.): Recent Vitamin Research. Boca Raton, CRC, 1984.

Le Lièvre, C., and Le Douarin, N. M.: Mesenchymal derivatives of the neural crest: analysis of chimeric quail and check embryos. J. Embryol. Exp. Morphol., *34:*125, 1975.

Livingstone, G.: Congenital ear abnormalities due to thalidomide. Proc. R. Soc. Med., *58:*493, 1965.

Lumsden, A. G.: Spatial organization of the epithelium and the role of neural crest cells in the initiation of the mammalian tooth germ. Development (Suppl.), *103:*155, 1988.

Minkoff, R.: Cell proliferation during formation of the embryonic facial primordia. J. Craniofac. Genet. Dev. Biol. (Suppl.) (in press).

Morriss, G.: Morphogenesis of the malformation induced in rat embryos by maternal hypervitaminosis A. J. Anat. (Lond.), *113:*241, 1972.

Morriss, G.: Abnormal cell migration as a possible factor in the genesis of vitamin A–induced craniofacial anomalies. *In* Neubert, D. (Ed.): New Approaches to the Evaluation of Abnormal Mammalian Embryonic Development. Stuttgart, Georg Thieme, 1976.

Mulinare, J., Cordero, H. F., Erickson, J., and Berry, R.: Periconceptional use of multivitamins and the occurrence of neural tube defects. J.A.M.A., *260:*3141, 1988.

Newman, L. M., and Hendrickx, A. G.: Fetal ear malformations induced by maternal ingestion of thalidomide in the bonnet monkey (Macaca radiata). Teratology, *23:*351, 1981.

Nichols, D. H.: Mesenchyme formation from the trigeminal placodes of the mouse embryo. Am. J. Anat., *176:*19, 1986.

Nicolet, G.: Analyse autoradiographique de la localisation des différentes ébauches présomptives dans la ligne primitive de l'embryon de Poulet. J. Embryol. Exp. Morphol., *23:*79, 1970.

Noden, D. M.: Patterns and organizations of craniofacial skeletogenic and myogenic mesenchymes. *In* Dixon, A., and Sarnat, B. (Eds.): Factors and Mechanisms Influencing Bone Growth. New York, Alan R. Liss, 1982.

Noden, D. M.: The role of the neural crest in patterning of avian cranial skeletal, connective, and muscle tissue. Dev. Biol., *96:*144, 1983a.

Noden, D. M.: The embryonic origins of avian craniofa-

cial muscles and associated connective tissues. Am. J. Anat., *186:*257, 1983b.

Noden, D. M.: Patterning of avian craniofacial muscles. Dev. Biol., *116:*3477, 1986.

Noden, D. M.: Interactions and fates of avian craniofacial mesenchyme. Development (Suppl.), *103:*121, 1988.

Noden, D. M., and van de Water, T. R.: The developing ear: tissue origins and interactions. *In* Ruben, R. J., and van de Water, T. R. (Eds.): The Biology of Change in Otolaryngology. Amsterdam, Elsevier/North Holland, 1986, pp. 15–46.

Pearse, A. G.: The cytochemistry and ultrastructure of polypeptide hormone producing cells of the APUD series, and the embryologic, physiologic and pathologic implications of the concept. J. Histochem. Cytochem., *17:*303, 1969.

Pleet, H., Graham, J. M., Jr., and Smith, D. W.: Central nervous system and facial defects associated with maternal hyperthermia at four to 14 weeks' gestation. Pediatrics, *67:*785, 1981.

Poswillo, D.: The pathogenesis of the first and second branchial arch syndrome. Oral Surg., *35:*302, 1973.

Poswillo, D.: The pathogenesis of the Treacher-Collins syndrome (mandibulofacial dysostosis). Br. J. Oral Surg., *13:*1, 1975.

Pratt, R. M., Goulding, E. H., and Abbott, B. D.: Retinoic acid inhibits migration of cranial neural crest cells in the cultured mouse embryo. J. Craniofac. Genet. Dev. Biol., *7:*205, 1987.

Pratt, R. M., Larson, M. H., and Johnston, M. C.: Migration of cranial neural crest cells in a cell-free, hyaluronate-rich space. Dev. Biol., *44:*298, 1975.

Ross, R. B., and Johnston, M. C.: Cleft Lip and Palate. Baltimore, Williams & Wilkins Company, 1972.

Sadler, T. W., Greenberg, D., Doughlin, P., and Lessard, J. L.: Actin distribution patterns in the mouse neural tube during neurulation. Science, *215:*172, 1982.

Shprintzen, R. J., Goldberg, R. B., Lewin, H. L., Sidoti, E. J., Berkman, M. D., et al.: A new syndrome involving cleft palate, cardiac anomalies, typical facies, and learning disabilities: velocardio-facial syndrome. Cleft Palate J., *15:*56, 1978.

Siebert, J. R., Graham, J. M., and MacDonald, C.: Pathological features of the "CHARGE" association: support for involvement of the neural crest. Teratology, *31:*331, 1985.

Smithells, R. W., Sheppard, S., Schorah, C. J., Seller, M. J., Nevin, N. C., et al.: Apparent prevention of neural tube defects by periconceptional vitamin supplementation. Arch. Dis. Child., *56:*911, 1981.

Solursh, M.: Ectoderm as a determinant of early tissue pattern in the limb bud. Cell Differ., *15:*17, 1984.

Solursh, M., Jensen, K. L., and Reiter, R. S.: Patterning of myogeneic cells in the early chick limb bud. *In* Slavkin, H. C. (Ed.): New Discoveries and Technologies in Developmental Biology. New York, Alan R. Liss, 1985.

Streeter, G. L.: Developmental horizons in human embryos, description of age groups XV, XVI, XVII, and XVIII. Contrib. Embryol., *32:*133, 1948.

Sulik, K. K., Cook, C. S., and Webster, W. S.: Teratogens and craniofacial malformations: relationships to cell death. Development (Suppl.), *103:*213, 1988.

Sulik, K. K., and Johnston, M. C.: Cleft palate investigations in T1Wh mice. Anat. Rec., *190:*555, 1978.

Sulik, K. K., and Johnston, M. C.: Embryonic origin of holoprosencephaly: interrelationship of the developing brain and face. Scan. Elect. Microsc., *1:*309, 1982.

Sulik, K. K., and Johnston, M. C.: Sequence of developmental changes following ethanol exposure in mice: craniofacial features of the fetal alcohol syndrome (FAS). Am. J. Anat., 166:257, 1983.

Sulik, K. K., Johnston, M. C., Daft, P. A., and Russell, W. E.: Fetal alcohol syndrome and DiGeorge anomaly: critical ethanol exposure periods for craniofacial malformations as illustrated in an animal model. Am. J. Med. Genet., 2:191, 1986.

Sulik, K. K., Johnston, M. C., and Webb, M. A.: Fetal alcohol syndrome: embryogenesis in a mouse model. Science, 214:936, 1981.

Sulik, K. K., Lauder, J. M., and Dehart, D. B.: Brain malformations in prenatal mice following acute maternal ethanol administration. Int. J. Dev. Neurosci., 2:203, 1984.

Tam, P. P., and Meier, S.: The establishment of a somitomeric pattern in the mesoderm of the gastrulating mouse embryo. J. Anat., 164:209, 1982.

Thaller, C., and Eichele, G.: Characterization of retinoid metabolism in the developing chick limb bud. Development, 103:473, 1988.

Thorogood, P. V.: The developmental specification of the vertebrate skull. Development (Suppl.), 103:141, 1988.

Thorogood, P. V., Smith, L., Nicol, A., McGinty, R., and Garrod, D.: Effects of vitamin A on the behavior of migratory neural crest cells in vitro. J. Cell Sci., 57:1, 1982.

Toole, B. P.: Hyaluronate and hyaluronidase in morphogenesis and differentiation. Am. Zool., 13:1961, 1973.

Toole, B. P., and Trelstad, R. L.: Hyaluronate production and removal during corneal development in the chick. Dev. Biol., 26:28, 1971.

Tucker, G. C., Duband, J. L., Dufour, S., and Thiery, J. P.: Cell-adhesion and substrate-adhesion molecules: their instructive roles in neural crest cell migration. Development (Suppl.), 103:82, 1988.

van de Water, T.: Tissue interactions and cell differentiation; neurons–sensory cell interaction during optic development. Development (Suppl.), 103:185, 1988.

Webster, W. S.: Isotretinoin embryopathy: the effects of isotretinoin and 4-oxo-isotretinoin on postimplantation rat embryos in vitro. Teratology, 31:59A, 1985

Webster, W. S., Johnston, M. D., Lammer, E. J., and Sulik, K. K.: Isotretinoin embryopathy and the cranial neural crest: an in vivo and in vitro study. Submitted to J. Craniofacial Genet. Dev. Biol., 6:211, 1986.

Webster, W. S., Walsh, D. A., and Lipson, A. H.: Teratogenesis after acute alcohol exposure in inbred and outbred mice. Neurobehav. Toxicol. Teratol., 2:227, 1980.

Willhite, C., Hill, R. M., and Irving, D. W.: Isotretinoin-induced craniofacial malformations in humans and hamsters. J. Craniofacial Genet. Dev. Biol. (Suppl.), 2:193, 1986.

Wright, S., and Wagner, K.: Types of subnormal development of the head from inbred strains of guinea pigs and their bearing on the classification and interpretation of vertebrate monsters. Am. J. Anat., 54:383, 1934.

47

Donald H. Enlow

Postnatal Craniofacial Growth and Development

CHARACTERISTICS OF CRANIOFACIAL DEVELOPMENT

The face of a young child is not simply a miniature of the adult face; moreover, it does not have the same proportions among the various regions and parts. Progressive facial enlargement is a *differential* growth process. Some parts or regions increase in size earlier or later than others, at different rates and directions, and to different extents (Fig. 47–1). Growth involves a maturation sequence leading eventually to the establishment of adult dimensions, angles, and relationships. The conventional title *growth and development* is proper and descriptive.

The child has a distinctly bulbous forehead because brain and neurocranial growth are precocious relative to facial development. The face appears small in proportion, especially in vertical size. The eyes appear quite wide set because vertical facial growth normally lags, whereas the side to side facial dimension is established earlier to maintain maxillofacial sutural and mandibular condylar articulations with the basicranium. The ears appear to be low for the same reason; i.e., the downward enlargement of the face lags considerably relative to the basicranium, and as the vertical facial dimension gradually increases, the relative position of the ears rises.

The mandible is normally retrusive in early childhood, as is the lower lip. Unless a Class II malocclusion develops, the lower jaw later catches up with maxillary growth and development. In a young child the face appears quite flat and wide because the superstructures of the face have not yet become fully protrusive. The upper orbital rim is still on or behind a vertical plane in line with the lower orbital rim. The nose is vertically short, and the palate is at a level just inferior to the orbital floor. The characteristic pug nose of the infant has a low nasal bridge, and the breadth of the nose at the nasal alae scarcely exceeds the width of the interorbital compartment.

Throughout childhood the face assumes considerably different regional proportions. The entire midfacial area of the infant is occupied by a massive pallisade of unerupted tooth buds in varying stages of formation. As the primary and then the secondary dentition come into full occlusion, a corresponding expansion of the whole middle and lower face takes place. The progressively increasing size of the lungs, and the body in general, is accompanied by a proportionate enlargement of the facial and pharyngeal airway. The size of the nasopharynx is increased by the enlargement of the middle endocranial fossa (this part of the basicranium forms the roof of the pharynx and essentially establishes its

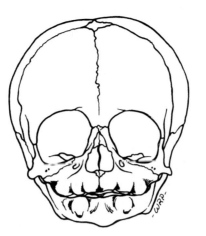 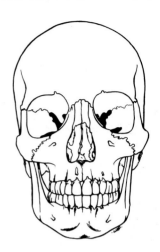

Figure 47–1. By enlarging the neonatal skull to match that of the adult, we can visualize the marked differences in the regional proportions between the two. (From Enlow, D. H.: Handbook of Facial Growth. 2nd Ed. Philadelphia, W. B. Saunders Company, 1982, p. 13.)

horizontal dimension). The nose becomes much more protrusive, thus enlarging the airway entrance, and the width of the nose at the level of the alae increases noticeably. The vertical dimension of the paired nasal chambers lengthens markedly. Downward nasal enlargement, eruption of the primary and secondary dentition, growth of the musculature, and proportionate enlargement of the supporting bone of the maxillary arch and mandible produce a considerable composite expansion of the vertical dimension of the entire face.

In a newborn the tips of the tiny nasal bones have not yet reached the forward point of the hard palate. With continued postnatal enlargement of the nasal region the bony nasal tip eventually protrudes somewhat beyond the palate (nasal spine) in the Caucasian face. The sizable extent of nasal protrusion and the expansion of the nasal chambers bring about a massive anterior enlargement of the entire upper facial region. This raises the nasal bridge and carries the outer table of the frontal bone forward with it. A separation of the inner from the outer tables of the frontal bone occurs. The inner table remains fixed to the dura of the frontal lobe, which ceases growth at about 5 or 6 years of age, whereas nasal protrusion results in the remodeling of the outer table of the forehead in an anterior direction as long as airway growth continues. A progressively enlarging frontal sinus and a more sloping forehead are thereby produced (the extent varies among different population groups and between the sexes).

A chin is virtually nonexistent in the infant. As a result of divergent remodeling changes in the alveolar and basal bone regions, the mental protuberance gradually takes form and enlarges through the childhood years.

The cheekbone region actually grows backward in the face (although the whole face, including the malar protuberances, becomes displaced anteriorly, as explained later). The forward growth of the forehead and nasal region, together with the backward growth movement of the cheek area, results in a distinct and characteristic rotation of alignment interrelationships (Fig. 47–2). In an adult the upper orbital rim has come to lie well forward of the inferior rim and malar protuberance, in contrast to the position of these parts in the young child. This change is especially remarkable in the male face because of the larger nose.

The horizontal length of the cranium is about 90 per cent complete by 5 years, and the width has been largely established by about the second year. The fontanels of the calvaria have all been reduced to sutures by about 18 months (some earlier), and all the various suture lines slowly begin to assume the sharply serrated and interlocking form characteristic of the adult skull. By the second year the metopic suture has usually closed, but most of the other sutural junctions throughout the face and neurocranium remain intact well into the adult or old age period, and some may never close. The fusion of the right and left halves of the mandible at the symphysis is usually complete by about the first year. The mastoid process, largely unformed at birth, becomes distinct by the first year, and the bony acoustic ring, which faces downward at birth, rotates into a ver-

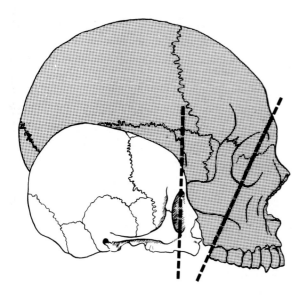

Figure 47–2. Rotation of the vertical orbital plane during growth and development. See text for description.

tical position. The styloid process may not become fully formed and fused with the basicranium until about puberty. The spheno-occipital synchondrosis has closed by about the 20th year, although its growth activity has largely ceased by the 14th or 15th year (earlier in the female). As the bony regions housing the various cranial and facial sinuses enlarge, the sinuses correspondingly increase in size. A sinus occupies some area not otherwise functionally used or genetically programed, and provides for size increase in that skeletal region without adding weight or sacrificing strength (the hollow cylinder concept of biomechanics). The other various functions often ascribed to sinuses are entirely secondary.

Until the time of puberty, boy and girl faces are comparable. Facial growth in the female, however, essentially ceases shortly after puberty, but considerable growth continues in the male face into the 20's. For example, forward nasal and eyebrow ridge expansion continues beyond the female level to the point that forehead overhang in the male constitutes one of the major dimorphic features of the face. Because of the greater extent of male nasal protrusion, particularly in the upper part, the nose of the male has a greater tendency for a convex or aquiline configuration than the female nose. When straight rather than convex, the nasal profile of the male tends to be more vertical in alignment because of greater forward growth in the upper part. Nasal size is usually greater in the male to accommodate a larger lung capacity.

GROWTH CONCEPTS

Skeletal growth and development involve two separate but closely interrelated morphogenic processes: (1) displacement and (2) remodeling growth. *Displacement* (also termed *translation*) constitutes whole bone movements away from one another at their articular junctions (movable joints, sutures, occlusal plane, and synchondroses). As all the various growing soft tissues undergo progressive expansion, each bone becomes carried away from the other bone(s) with which it articulates. This, in effect, creates a space into which the bones, virtually simultaneously, enlarge intramembranously and/or endochondrally (Fig. 47–3). Current theory holds that the displacement movement is primary, and that actual bone growth is secondarily responsive to this movement and presumably triggered by it owing to changes in biomechanical equilibrium (and/or numerous other physiologic balance factors) in the area of joint contact.

Cartilage is a tissue that has a special capacity to function and grow in regions involving direct surface pressure. The phenomenon occurs because it (1) can exist without a surface connective tissue membrane, (2) has a nonvascular matrix, (3) has a noncalcified matrix, and (4) can grow interstitially. All four of the features are functionally interrelated. Cartilage provides for a bone's growth by the endochondral bone replacement process whenever high level pressure bears directly on a bone's surface. Conversely, periosteum is a vascular membrane that cannot

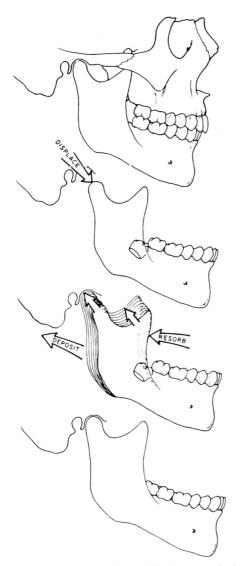

Figure 47–3. As the whole mandible becomes displaced anteriorly and inferiorly away from the basicranium, an equivalent amount of remodeling (resorption and deposition) occurs that retains the ramus and condyle in their proper anatomic positions. This same process also widens and lengthens the ramus, as well as increases the horizontal size of the corpus. (From Enlow, D. H.: Handbook of Facial Growth. 2nd Ed. Philadelphia, W. B. Saunders Company, 1982.)

withstand any undue amount of pressure but rather is adapted to surface tension, as exerted by muscles, tendons, and ligaments. In all nonpressure sites of a bone, therefore, osteogenesis takes place by the intramembranous (periosteal and endosteal) mode of growth. Pressures and tensions, in this regard, refer specifically to biomechanical forces affecting either the covering membrane

or the cartilage. It is important to understand that other types of forces are involved as well. Body weight and muscle actions, for example, cause bendings of bones or parts of bones by creating bioelectric reactions (the piezoelectric effect and perhaps others). The resultant positive and negative potentials are believed to trigger osteoclastic and osteoblastic responses, respectively. It is necessary, therefore, to specify to which particular tissue target any given pressure and tension relate, i.e., to the membranes and cartilage or to the calcified part of the bone.

The enlargement of a bone by the osteogenic activity of the periosteum and endosteum is termed *remodeling growth* because the same depository and resorptive processes that produce overall enlargement also carry out remodeling at the same time. Indeed, remodeling *is* the growth enlargement process; for a bone to grow, it must necessarily remodel at the same time. The term *remodeling* is often used with other, different meanings, e.g., biochemical remodeling, pathologic remodeling, and haversian remodeling. *Growth remodeling* is a separate and distinct process from the others, and an exceedingly basic one.

As pointed out earlier, skeletal growth is a differential process in which different areas or parts of a given bone enlarge at different rates, amounts, and directions. It is important to understand that any given bone does *not* grow in the uniform manner illustrated in Figure 47–4. A bone does *not* enlarge merely by a process of external surface (periosteal) deposition of bone coupled with inner (endosteal) resorption. Rather, a bone grows by a continuous remodeling process. This requires that about half the periosteal surface undergo resorption, a circumstance that is always surprising to new students of facial growth. In Figure 47–5 the pattern of distribution of surface resorptive and depository growth fields on the face is shown. How can a bone enlarge if half of its outside surface is actually resorptive? Why does a bone undergo remodeling as it enlarges? These key questions are answered in the following section.

First, it is helpful to keep in mind that a bone grows by adding new bone tissue on the particular surface facing the direction of growth in any region of a given bone. The opposite side of that same bony cortex is usually resorptive. A given part of a bone does not necessarily grow in an outward direction. About half the surfaces of any given

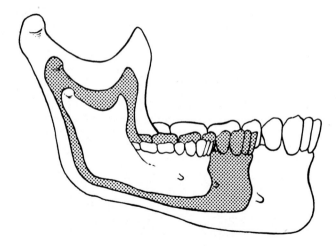

Figure 47–4. Enlargement of each individual bone in the face and cranium does not take place in the oversimplified manner shown here. Rather, the growth process involves extensive regional remodeling. (From Cohen, B., and Kramer, I. R. N.: Scientific Foundations of Dentistry. London, England, William Heinemann Medical Books, Ltd., 1975, p. 30.)

bone actually grow in an inward direction, and thus such areas are characterized by a periosteal cortical surface that is resorptive and an endosteal cortical surface that is depository. About half (or more) of the compact bone tissue in the skeleton is of endosteal origin. Beginning students always presume, incorrectly, that the bone tissue of the cortex is necessarily produced by the periosteum.

Second, a principal function of the remodeling process is not to actually change the shape of a bone, as the term itself might imply, but rather to sustain its shape throughout the enlargement process. As the bone grows in all its various regional direc-

tions, the same osteoblastic and osteoclastic activities producing growth also simultaneously carry out remodeling. This provides for the *relocation* of the bone's regional parts. To explain the rationale for the relocation process and the remodeling changes needed to perform it, the manner of vertical growth of the nasomaxillary complex is briefly summarized. In Figure 47–6, note that the vertical level of the hard palate in the young child is very close to the inferior orbital rim. In the adult the palate has grown downward to a level considerably below the orbit. Part of this inferior palatal movement is produced by remodeling growth. That is, the bony cortex

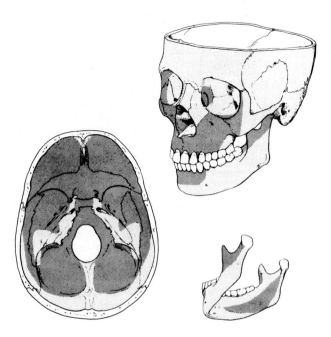

Figure 47–5. Fields of surface bone *deposition* are represented by the light areas, and fields of surface *resorption* by the dark areas. (From Enlow, D. H., and Moyers, R. E.: J. Am. Dent. Assoc., 82:764, 1971. Copyright by the American Dental Association. Reprinted by permission.)

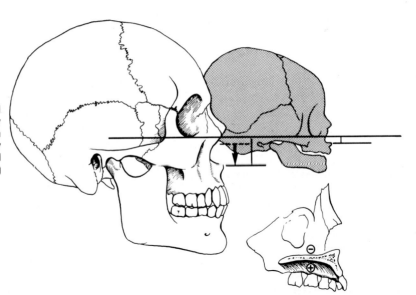

Figure 47–6. As the palate and maxillary arch grow inferiorly by deposition (+) and resorption (−), the regions once held by these parts in the younger child are *remodeled* Into the enlarging nasal chambers of the adult.

on the nasal side of the palate has a resorptive periosteal surface together with a depository endosteal surface, and the bony cortex on the oral side has a depository periosteal surface with a resorptive endosteal surface (Fig. 47–7). The cortical bone tissue of the hard palate is thus about half endosteal and half periosteal in origin. About half the outer surfaces are resorptive and half depository. By this remodeling process the whole hard palate undergoes relocation in a progressively inferior direction; the morphogenetic reason is to provide for nasal chamber expansion. The area occupied by the maxillary arch in a

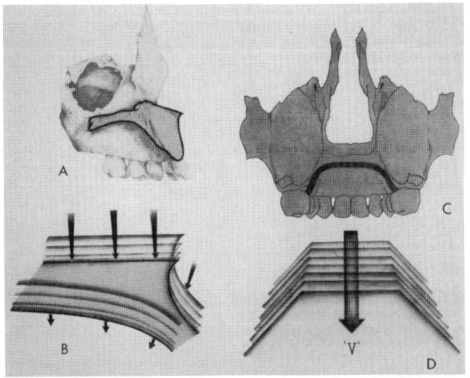

Figure 47–7. Inferior growth of the palate and maxillary arch. (From Enlow, D. H., and Bang, S.: Am. J. Orthod., *51*:446, 1965.)

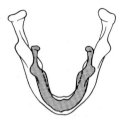

Figure 47–8. As the mandibular ramus becomes relocated posteriorly by growth (resorption and deposition), former parts of the ramus are converted by remodeling into new additions for the body of the mandible. (From Enlow, D. H.: Handbook of Facial Growth. 2nd Ed. Philadelphia, W. B. Saunders Company, 1982.)

young child later becomes occupied by the enlarged nasal region in an adult. What was formerly bony maxillary arch and palate become *remodeled* into additions for the nasal area as the palate and arch undergo downward *relocation.*

The growth of the mandible provides another example of the concepts of remodeling and relocation (Fig. 47–8). The mandible enlarges predominantly posteriorly and superiorly, and the entire ramus becomes *relocated* in these directions by combinations of deposition and resorption on its anterior, posterior, superior, buccal, and lingual surfaces. This process takes place continuously throughout the growth period, and successive areas once occupied by the posterior-moving ramus become sequentially occupied by the lengthening body of the mandible. What was once ramus becomes converted into additions for the posterior part of the mandibular corpus by *remodeling.* Thus, the ramus growth movement provides the space for mandibular arch lengthening, and both the relocation movement and the structural changes required to alter a former part of the ramus into a new part for the corpus are carried out by the remodeling process.

GROWTH OF BASICRANIAL, NASOMAXILLARY, AND MANDIBULAR COMPLEXES

The various major component parts of the cranial base, ethmomaxillary region, and the lower jaw are not independently assembled; rather, they have a close structural interrelationship. They follow a number of equivalent growth changes and share several key growth perimeters. The basicranium, in ad-

dition to housing the underside of the brain, functions as the platform from which the facial complex is suspended. The relationship between the cranial base and the ethmomaxillary complex is closely bound because of the direct union by shared sutures between them. The mandible, while conforming to growth fields established by the basicranium, is much less constrained by the boundaries of these fields because it is a separate bone not sharing direct articulation by common sutures.

There are distinct structural and morphogenic counterparts among the anterior cranial floor, nasomaxillary region, and mandible (Fig. 47–9). Note that the ethmomaxillary complex relates specifically to the anterior cranial fossa. (This term refers to the actual fossae housing the frontal lobes of the cerebrum, not the anterior cranial base. The latter is a cephalometric term designating the span from sella to nasion and is not a discrete anatomic unit.) The fossa circumscribes the posterior, anterior, and lateral boundaries of

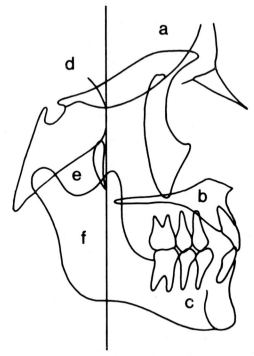

Figure 47–9. "Counterpart" relationships among the parts of the face and cranium. The anterior cranial fossa (*a*), the palate and maxillary arch (*b*), and the mandibular corpus (*c*) are structural counterparts to one another, as are the middle cranial fossa (*d*), the postmaxillary (pharyngeal) compartment (*e*), and the mandibular ramus (*f*). (From Cohen, B., and Kramer, I. R. N.: Scientific Foundations of Dentistry. London, England, William Heinemann Medical Books, Ltd., 1975, p. 45.)

the field within which the midface grows and develops. The *body* of the mandible relates specifically to the corpus of the maxilla and in turn to the anterior cranial fossa. The paired *rami* of the mandible relate specifically to the postmaxillary space (the pharynx), the horizontal dimension of which is established by the middle cranial fossae housing the temporal lobes of the cerebrum. A principal function of the ramus (in addition to providing insertion for masticatory muscles) is to bridge the span across the pharyngeal space to place the lower arch in proper juxtaposition with the upper arch. In this sense the ramus is a counterpart to the middle cranial fossa. The horizontal growth of the two should approximate each other in a balanced craniofacial composite, just as growth among the anterior cranial fossa, palate, bony maxillary arch, and bony mandibular arch should be approximately equal. These basic developmental relationships help to define the important concept of morphologic and morphogenic balance (Enlow, 1982).

Horizontal Craniofacial Growth

With the continued growth of the paired anterior cranial fossae (until ceasing at about age 5 or 6 years), the template for the contiguous ethmomaxillary complex becomes enlarged and thereby provides the space for subsequent enlargement of the midface. The latter does not fully catch up with horizontal anterior cranial fossa expansion until long after cranial growth essentially ceases.

Until the child is approximately 2 or 3 years of age, the horizontal growth of the hard palate and the bony maxillary arch proceeds both anteriorly and posteriorly (mesially and distally) within the compartment established by the anterior cranial fossae. After age 3 years, continued palatal and maxillary arch horizontal enlongation occurs almost entirely in a posterior direction. The series of changes is believed to conform to the following sequence. First, the expansion of the frontal lobes of the cerebrum is simultaneously accompanied by a corresponding enlargement of the anterior cranial fossae. This development establishes the anteroposterior and lateral dimensions of the field within which the ethmomaxillary complex can grow to achieve a balanced anatomic and functional relationship. Second, the entire eth-

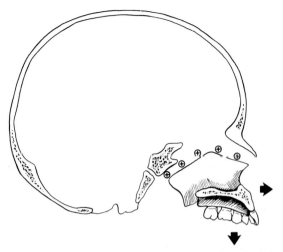

Figure 47–10. As the whole nasomaxillary complex becomes displaced away from the basicranium (*arrows*), bone is laid down at the various sutural articulations (+), thus enlarging the maxilla in proportion to the amount of displacement and sustaining bone-to-bone contacts.

momaxillary complex becomes *displaced anteriorly* within the growth field (Fig. 47–10). Growth then proceeds (essentially simultaneously) posteriorly to keep the posterior aspect of the maxilla in line with its prescribed anatomic boundary, which is the middle-anterior endocranial fossae junction. The extent of backward growth approximately equals the amount of forward displacement.

The source of the biomechanical force that is responsible for the displacement movement has long been a controversial issue among investigators. The old pterygoid buttress and sutural push theories have long been discarded because it is now realized that sutural and periosteal membranes cannot withstand the high level pressures that would be required to push (thrust) the entire nasomaxilla forward. Another explanation holds that the growth expansion of the pressure tolerant cartilaginous nasal septum (Scott, 1953) causes traction on the septopremaxillary ligaments (Latham, 1970), which in turn pull the maxillae anteriorly and inferiorly. Although this theory was popular for many years, some researchers now believe this process may be operative only at earlier age levels (Latham, 1970), and other investigators have abandoned the idea entirely. The problem is that it is difficult to design controlled laboratory studies in which built-in experimental variables can be effectively eliminated to the point that clear interpretations of results can be made.

Another theoretical explanation for the maxillary displacement movement holds that the composite expansion of all the facial soft tissues (the functional matrix) acts to carry the entire midface downward and forward (Moss, 1969). The introduction of this concept had great significance because it emphasized the point that the genetic determinants of skeletal growth do not reside within the actual bony part itself. In other words, the "pacemakers" of the displacement process, and the bony remodeling process as well, occur in *other,* surrounding soft tissue parts (epigenetic control). A basic point to understand with regard to the functional matrix concept is that it describes essentially *what* happens during displacement and remodeling growth activities, but is not intended to explain *how* it happens or what the regulating process actually is at the tissue and cellular levels. Much has yet to be learned with regard to the local growth control mechanism (Enlow, 1973).

After age 2 or 3 years, as previously pointed out, the palate and bony maxillary arch lengthen horizontally only in a posterior direction (except for some alveolar lengthening in relation to permanent incisor eruption). The whole overlying nasal region, however, continues to enlarge anteriorly as well as posteriorly. Because of this development, progressive nasal protrusion occurs relative to the maxillary arch. Thus, the facial part of the airway is expanded in conjunction with lung and whole body growth. The extent is greater in boys, and the male nose thereby tends to be more protrusive and convex in shape.

When the horizontal growth of the paired maxillae is complete, a structural balance with their earlier-growing counterparts, the anterior endocranial fossae, has been attained. Just as the maxilla lags in growth relative to the cranium, another counterpart more distant to the anterior cranial fossae, the mandibular corpus, normally lags relative to the maxilla. Although growth timing differs, mandibular arch development mirrors that of the maxillary arch. After age 2 or 3 years the growth of the mandible also proceeds largely posteriorly (and superiorly). Just as the maxilla lengthens horizontally by backward growth at the maxillary tuberosity, the mandibular arch lengthens posteriorly at its counterpart structure, the lingual tuberosity (Figs. 47–10 and 47–11). The latter

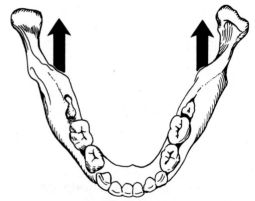

Figure 47–11. The mandibular corpus lengthens posteriorly by remodeling conversions from the posterior growing ramus and new bone additions at the lingual tuberosity. (Adapted from Enlow, D. H.: Handbook of Facial Growth. 2nd Ed. Philadelphia, W. B. Saunders Company, 1982.)

represents the effective boundary between the corpus and ramus, although the anterior edge of the ramus overlaps this functional junction to provide insertion for the temporal muscle. One basic structural difference between the maxilla and mandible is the presence of the ramus joined onto the mandibular arch. Although backward growth of the maxilla takes place by direct bone deposition on its posterior-facing tuberosity, posterior lengthening of the bony mandibular arch must necessarily proceed by continuous remodeling conversions from the ramus. To do this, the whole ramus moves backward by combinations of deposition on its various posterior-facing surfaces and resorption from anterior-facing surfaces (including all buccal and lingual surfaces, not merely the posterior and anterior edges). As the entire ramus grows and relocates posteriorly, areas once occupied by the ramus in succession become *remodeled* into new additions, thereby lengthening the body of the mandible (Fig. 47–12).

In the meantime the temporal lobes of the cerebrum have continued to expand (for several years after frontal lobe growth ceases). This cerebral expansion increases the anteroposterior breadth of the underlying pharyngeal space. Because one principal function of the ramus is to bridge this enlarging space, the breadth of the ramus increases commensurate with middle endocranial fossa enlargement by having the extent of posterior deposition exceed slightly the amount of anterior resorption. Thus, the width of the ramus increases by several millimeters during the

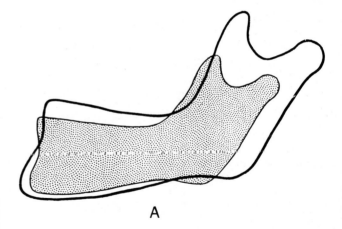

A

Figure 47–12. Upper overlay (*A*) illustrates the *remodeling* growth of the mandible by regional combinations of surface deposition and resorption of bone. Lower overlay (*B*) illustrates the downward and forward *displacement* of the mandible. (From Cohen, B., and Kramer, I. R. N.: Scientific Foundations of Dentistry. London, England, William Heinemann Medical Books, Ltd., 1975, p. 31.)

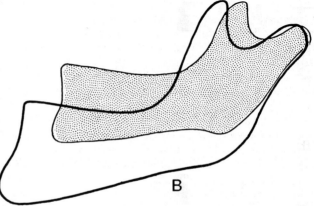

B

five to 15 year age period as it simultaneously *relocates* posteriorly to allow for mandibular arch lengthening (Enlow, 1982).

Condylar Growth Process

The backward (and upward) enlargement and the posterior relocation of the mandibular ramus is customarily referred to simply as condylar growth. It is to be understood, however, that the entire ramus participates in this remodeling process. It is not merely the condyle that is growing backward and/or upward but rather a movement that involves the ramus as a whole. The condylar component of ramus growth has historically received special emphasis because it was once believed that the cartilage of the condyle represented the pacemaker of mandibular growth and thereby provided a region of un-

usual importance. Current theory, although still highly controversial, assigns considerable significance to the condylar growth mechanism for quite different reasons.

The condylar cartilage is not a master center responsible for regulating overall mandibular growth and development. Its genes do not appear to control the entirety of its own growth, much less all other parts of the entire lower jaw. The condyle is *not* now believed (by most but not all investigators) to represent the source of the mechanical thrust producing the anteroinferior displacement of the mandible. Rather, this bone as a whole is believed to behave in a manner essentially analogous to the maxilla. Thus, as the mandible becomes displaced in continued forward and downward directions, it grows in response in opposite upward and backward directions (Fig. 47–12). The extent of growth is determined by the amount of displacement. Displacement creates the space into which the mandible enlarges; displacement is believed to be primary and enlargement secondary. As with the maxillae, many investigators support the theory that mandibular displacement is carried out by the expanding functional matrix.

If the condylar growth apparatus does not function in a primary pace-setting capacity, what is its special significance? The answer appears to lie in at least two unique functions served by the condylar cartilage. First, the presence of cartilage is an adaptation to levels of pressure that would exceed the capacity of a periosteum to provide for posterosuperior growth at the condylar articulation; the cartilage covering, in effect, substitutes for a periosteum. In fact, what is now the condylar part of the mandible, phylogenetically, was originally a membranous type of bone, and its periosteal covering was supplanted by ectopic cartilage when the original mandibular articular bone (endochondral in type) became converted into an ear ossicle. The new condylar cartilage is secondary in origin as well as in growth behavior. The presence of this cartilage and the endochondral mechanism of growth it provides represent a *regional* adaptation to a localized functional and developmental circumstance, i.e., a pressure type of bone to bone articulation. Elsewhere throughout the mandible, growth is largely carried out by the membranous (periosteal-endosteal) mode of ossification because surface pressure is not involved.

The second key role provided by the condylar cartilage relates to the special construction and growth potential of the cartilage itself. The prechondroblasts appear to be genetically programmed to undergo continued cell divisions but no more than this (Koski, 1971). The timing, rate, and directions of the cell divisions are now believed to be controlled largely by a composite of extrinsic factors (levels of articular pressure, muscle action, occlusal forces and sensory feedbacks, tissue induction, and many other possible input factors). Chondrogenic proliferation takes place in a manner that basically differs from most of the various other growth cartilages in the skeleton (epiphyseal plates, synchondroses). The daughter cells do not divide in a linear, unidirectional manner. The continued growth of the condyle is not committed to a one direction course. It can significantly alter the route of its growth to provide the best compromise fitting for its multifaceted

junctions with the cranial base, the maxillary dentition, and the masticatory muscles. During the extended period of childhood growth the condyle is required to alter its growth directions to adapt to continued expansions and complex rotations occurring in the basicranium and the maxillae. The ramus to corpus angle, for example, becomes more acute to accommodate ongoing, long-term vertical nasal enlargement. Vertical ramus lengthening continues throughout the facial growth period, long after horizontal ramus enlargement has ceased. Because the condylar cartilage can proliferate and provide for endochondral bone growth in almost any direction needed to accommodate these situations, it thereby provides the exceedingly important function of secondary (i.e., responsive) growth adaptation. This is in direct contrast to the old presumption that its principal role was to provide primary, pacemaking growth regulation. Not only is the new conceptual meaning no less important than the old, it is actually far more noteworthy in biologic significance.

Synchondroses

The synchondroses of the basicranium, particularly the spheno-occipital synchondrosis, have similarly been presumed to represent primary control sites serving to regulate the development of the cranial base. It was believed that the chondrocytes exert direct genetic control over the rate, amount, and directions of progressive basicranial growth. This theory may or may not be the case, and the subject is currently controversial in the same sense that direct genetic versus indirect epigenetic control is argued for other cartilages and bones in the skeleton. One important point, however, is that the role of the synchondroses has been overemphasized and largely misplaced in the general literature. A synchondrosis has been customarily designated as *the* site of growth for the cranial floor. Actually, the contribution of its endochondral bone is quite small in terms of the total bone mass in the basicranium, and the regions involved are limited (Fig. 47–13). The bony tissues produced in conjunction with synchondrosis proliferation and bony replacement are restricted to the cancellous medullary core of parts only in the midventral axis of the cranial base. Similarly, endochondral

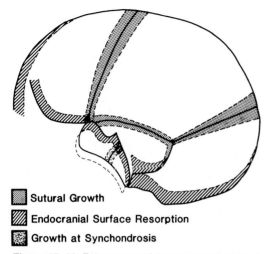

Sutural Growth

Endocranial Surface Resorption

Growth at Synchondrosis

Figure 47–13. Enlargement of the neurocranium involves endochondral growth at the synchondroses, sutural bone growth, and remodeling at endocranial and ectocranial surfaces.

bone formation by the mandibular condyle is restricted to the medulla of the condylar neck. Other parts, constituting the major expanse of the basicranium, are produced intramembranously by periosteal-endosteal activity. The dura functions as a periosteum on the endocranial side of both the basicranium and the calvaria. As with other growth cartilages (i.e., cartilages involved with bone growth), a synchondrosis provides for the elongation of a bone in areas where pressure levels exceed that in which a vascular periosteum can function; chondroblasts rather than osteoblasts develop from mesenchyme because presumably compression on the tissue results in hypoxia. As shown by Hall (1970), such a tissue environment triggers cartilage rather than bone development. All other areas subject to surface membrane tension rather than pressure (or subject at least to low level pressure) grow by membrane activity. The latter constitutes the principal expanse of the cranial floor as well as the calvaria.

Like most other growth cartilages, but unlike the mandibular condyle, the chondrocyte cell divisions within a synchondrosis occur in linear columns, and growth is constrained to an essentially unidirectional course on each side of the cartilage plate.

The greater part of the basicranium is produced by direct remodeling growth, as just noted, and this involves growth fields active in both resorption and deposition (see Fig.

47–5). Sutural growth is also directly involved. Unlike the calvaria (described later), the bone surfaces in many parts of the basicranium on the *endocranial* side are resorptive in nature because expansion of the topographically complex cranial floor containing endocranial fossae would not be possible by sutural growth activity alone. Extensive remodeling provided by combinations of endocranial resorption and bone deposition allows for the enlargement of the cranial floor in conjunction with progressive increases in brain size. Basicranial remodeling also provides for the progressive placement of the passageways for the cranial nerves and the major blood vessels. This would not be possible by a sutural growth mechanism alone.

In the calvaria, however, the growth process is different. One still encounters in the literature the mistaken presumption that the expansion of the lateral walls and roof of the skull is brought about by resorption on the inside of the cranium together with deposition on the outside. In reality, the endocranial and ectocranial surfaces of the calvaria are both depository in nature, in contrast to the greater part of the more complex basicranium. This phenomenon serves to thicken the flat bones of the cranial vault and, with resorption on the endosteal (medullary) surface, increase the thickness of the diploë. The enlargement of the perimeter of each of the separate flat bones is produced by sutural bone growth. In other words, the enlargement of the brain separates the bones at their various sutural junctions, and this apparently acts as a stimulus for the simultaneous deposition of new bone in the spaces created (Fig. 47–14). Remodeling growth in the bones of the calvaria is not extensive, and is usually limited to relatively minor curvature adjustments on the ectocranial and endocranial surfaces adjacent to the sutures.

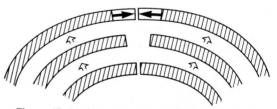

Figure 47–14. As the bones of the calvaria are displaced outward in conjunction with the enlarging brain, new bone is deposited by the sutural membranes.

Vertical Facial Growth

As with all other bones in the skeleton, there are two basic parts to the vertical growth process of the midfacial bones (just as there are for horizontal midfacial growth): (1) displacement movement and (2) remodeling growth.

Sutural bone growth in the maxillary complex relates specifically to the displacement movement. Many experimental studies have demonstrated that the process of bone deposition at sutural interfaces does not produce displacement by pushing the enlarging bones away from one another. Rather, the displacement movement is the primary act, and sutural bone formation follows (virtually simultaneously) by enlarging the perimeter of the bone by the amount of separation at the sutural interfaces (Fig. 47–15).

The same displacement movements that carry the midface and mandible anteriorly function to move them inferiorly as well. The individual bones within the ethmomaxillary complex also become separated by the displacement process, and sutural bone growth provides for their enlargement by amounts that equal the extent of the individual displacements.

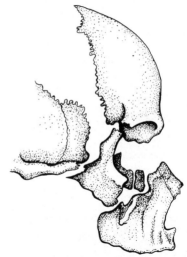

Figure 47–15. The separate bones of the nasomaxillary complex are displaced away from one another and from the basicranium. Sutural bone growth simultaneously enlarges each bone by an amount that equals the displacement.

Remodeling takes place throughout all parts of each bone making up the midfacial complex, and this process occurs at the same time as the bones undergo displacement movements and sutural growth (Fig. 47–16). As mentioned, the maxilla grows downward

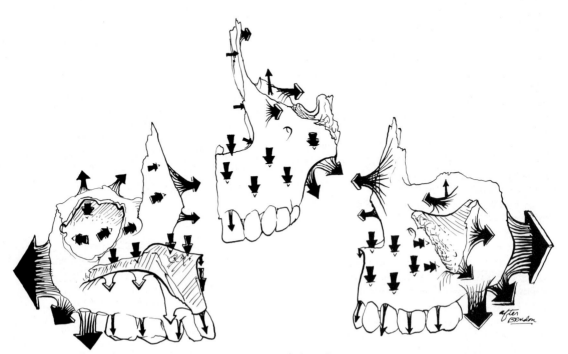

Figure 47–16. Multidirectional manner of *remodeling* growth throughout all parts of the maxilla. Arrows penetrating the bone surface represent fields of resorption; arrows leading away from the surface indicate fields of surface deposition. (From Enlow, D. H.: The Human Face. New York, Harper & Row, 1968.)

by displacement with consequential sutural bone growth. Remodeling growth also produces an inferior direction of enlargement, and the total extent of downward growth movement of the maxillary arch is the sum of the separate but simultaneous displacement and remodeling movements.

Remodeling growth in the nasomaxillary complex, just as in all other skeletal units, involves the relocation of its component parts into successively new positions by progressive deposition of new bone on those surfaces facing toward the growth directions, and resorption from bone surfaces facing away from these regional directions. For the nasal region the lining bone surface of each nasal chamber is thus largely resorptive in nature, thereby expanding the size of the airway. As the internal side of the lateral nasal walls and superior side of the hard palate undergo removal, the oral side of the palate and external surfaces of the nasal protuberance (including the nasal bones and the lateral nasal component of the maxilla) receive continuing bone deposits. The maxillary sinuses expand in all directions, except medially, by a similar combination of internal bone removal and external addition.

Structurally the paired maxillae are complex bones. In addition to providing most of the floor for the nasal chambers, the maxillae contribute to the orbital floors. The nasal and orbital components, however, remodel in contrasting directions: the nasal part remodels downward, whereas the orbital part remodels upward (Fig. 47–17). Because they are of the same bone, both areas become *displaced* inferiorly in conjunction with sutural bone growth. For the hard palate, inferior remodeling adds to the total, composite amount of downward palatal movement. For the orbits, however, the extent of inferior maxillary displacement movement exceeds the extent of orbital increase needed. The orbital floor thus remodels superiorly as the whole maxilla becomes displaced inferiorly to maintain its constant position contiguous with the eyeball.

In Figure 47–5 one can observe that the muzzle of the maxilla has an external surface that is resorptive. This is a situation unique to the human face. In all other species, including anthropoids, the labial and buccal surfaces of the maxilla anterior to the orbits are depository in nature. The human face, however, is characterized by bimaxillary reduction to the extent that, after approxi-

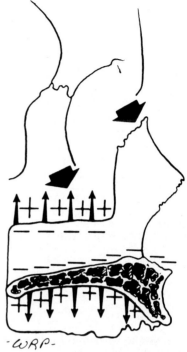

Figure 47–17. Palatal and orbital growth. (From Enlow, D. H.: Handbook of Facial Growth. 2nd Ed. Philadelphia, W. B. Saunders Company, 1982.)

mately age 2 or 3 years, the maxillae enlarge in the posteroanterior dimension in only a posterior direction. In contrast, the maxillae in other species lengthen horizontally in anterior (mesial) as well as posterior (distal) directions. The characteristic surface resorptive nature of the anterior region of the human upper jaw is a feature adapted to its *vertical* growth. The anterior parts of the bony maxillary arch and palate grow essentially straight downward. The combination of resorptive and depository fields producing this directional growth is schematized in Figure 47–18. The buccal and labial surfaces of alveolar bone anterior to the cheekbones are oriented so that they face upward, and the straight downward growth of this whole area of concavity is thereby brought about by outer surface resorption combined with deposition on the opposite, inferior-facing cortical surfaces.

As seen in Figure 47–19, the anterior surface of the malar protuberance is also resorptive. The entire cheekbone and lateral orbital rim grow posteriorly, and the posterior-facing surfaces of bone within the temporal fossa behind the malar protuberance and lateral rim of the orbit are correspondingly deposi-

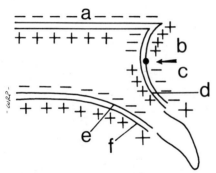

Figure 47–18. Surface *a* is the nasal side of the palate and is resorptive (−). Part *b* is the nasal spine and has a depository inferior surface (+). The arrow indicates a reversal and coincides with cephalometric A point. The alveolar bone is deposited by the periodontal membrane at *d* and has a resorptive labial surface at *c*. On the oral side surface, *e* is resorptive and *f* is depository. The composite of these remodeling combinations produces a downward growth movement of the palate and maxillary arch. (From Enlow, D. H.: Handbook of Facial Growth. 2nd Ed. Philadelphia, W. B. Saunders Company, 1982.)

tory. Because the bony maxillary arch lengthens posteriorly, the malar region must also grow in a like direction to sustain its anatomic position relative to the remainder of the enlarging maxilla. Of course, the entire maxillary complex, including the zygomatic region, undergoes forward displacement at the same time, as previously described.

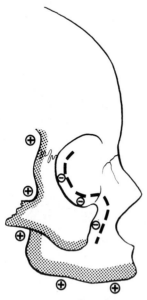

Figure 47–19. As the maxilla enlarges posteriorly, the malar protuberance and lateral orbital rim also remodel in a correspondingly posterior direction.

The backward remodeling of the cheekbone region together with the forward remodeling growth of the nasal area produces considerable expansion of the topographic contours and the depth of the midface. As the upper, nasal part of the face, supraorbital rims, and forehead grow forward and each malar protuberance and lateral orbital rim grow backward, a facial rotation occurs (see Fig. 47–2). The nose becomes much more protrusive relative to the cheekbones, and the supraorbital rims come to lie well anterior to the lower rims (particularly in the male face).

The inferior displacement of the mandibular arch is accompanied by a vertically upward growth of the ramus, and the remodeling that is required involves the ramus as a whole. Condylar growth, as previously mentioned, is just one part of this process. As seen in Figure 47–20, the various upward- (and backward-) facing surfaces of the ramus receive continued bone deposits. Thus, for example, the coronoid process has a lingual surface that is depository and a buccal surface that is resorptive (Fig. 47–21). The margin of the mandibular (sigmoid) notch is depository, as is the superior surface of the condylar neck.

The vertical lengthening of the ramus provides for the progressively downward placement of the mandibular corpus to accommodate (1) the vertical enlargement of the nasal chambers, (2) the successive eruption of the deciduous and permanent dentition, and (3) the expansion of the musculature. Although most of the descent of the mandibular corpus is produced by this displacement movement, the vertical enlargement of the middle endocranial fossae also functions to separate the mandible from the maxilla; the amount of ramus lengthening must adjust to this. For the descent of the maxillary arch, in contrast, only about half the total extent of vertical growth is produced by the displacement type of movement (associated with bone growth at sutures). As described earlier, there is also a considerable amount of direct downward remodeling as the palate and maxillary arch grow inferiorly by composite resorptive and depository activity.

As the maxilla moves inferiorly by both remodeling growth and displacement, the mandibular dentition and supporting alveolar bone grow upward at the same time. In the human face the lower anterior teeth characteristically move into an overbite-overjet relationship. This is produced by a lingual

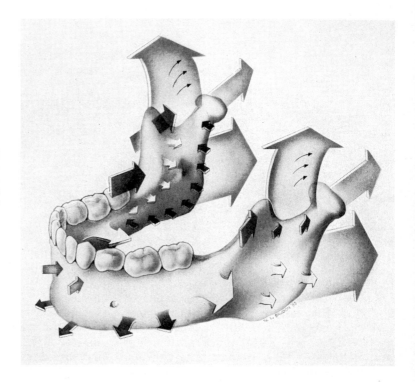

Figure 47–20. Multidirectional manner of mandibular enlargement. (From Enlow, D. H., and Harris, D. B.: A study of the postnatal growth of the human mandible. Am. J. Orthod., *50*:25, 1964.)

tipping and uprighting of the mandibular incisors. They drift *posteriorly* as well as superiorly (Fig. 47–22). Whereas the outer surface of the chin itself is depository in nature, the periosteal surface of the overlying alveolar bone on the labial side is resorptive; the alveolar lingual side is depository. This combination brings about a gradual, progressive increase in chin size and protrusion.

The phrase *working with growth* is often used with regard to many orthodontic and surgical procedures. As can be appreciated from the foregoing descriptions, there are different *kinds* of growth, and to be able to

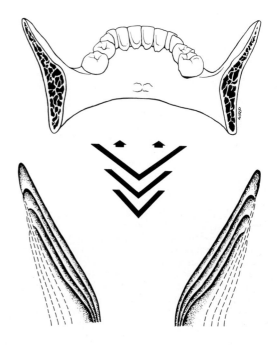

Figure 47–21. Upward and backward growth of the coronoid processes is produced by the combination of bone deposition on the lingual surfaces and resorption from the buccal surfaces. (From Enlow, D. H.: Handbook of Facial Growth. 2nd Ed. Philadelphia, W. B. Saunders Company, 1982.)

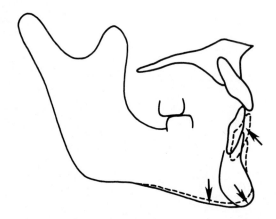

Figure 47–22. Mandibular incisors drift into an overbite and overjet relationship by the combination of alveolar bone deposition on the lingually facing surfaces and resorption from the labially facing surfaces. Note that, although only incisor drift is shown, the other mandibular teeth have similarly drifted in a generally superior direction. (From Enlow, D. H.: Handbook of Facial Growth. 2nd Ed. Philadelphia, W. B. Saunders Company, 1982.)

understand the rationale for using each requires a sound understanding of the biologic basis for all.

One must be aware of the various principal directions and amounts of (1) displacement and (2) remodeling growth in every major part of the entire face and cranium. For example, one would quite naturally but mistakenly presume that the premaxillary and cheekbone areas grow forward. This notion is inaccurate on two counts. First, the important distinction between growth movements produced by displacement and by remodeling is not taken into account. (An example of why this is significant is outlined below.) Second, the actual tissue that *produces* the bone is incorrectly presumed. For the maxillary (and mandibular) alveolar bone housing the anterior teeth, it is the periodontal membrane that lays down the bone on the labial side of each tooth. The outer periosteum is engaged in bone resorption, not deposition. It is therefore emphasized that the concept of forward and downward growth must be approached with great caution (Fig. 47–23) because this oversimplified old notion has caused great confusion and misunderstanding.

In Figure 47–24 the downward remodeling growth of the palate and maxillary dentition is illustrated. Each tooth is moved individually and separately from level *1* to level *2*, and it is the *periodontal membrane* of each tooth and alveolar socket that paces and pro-

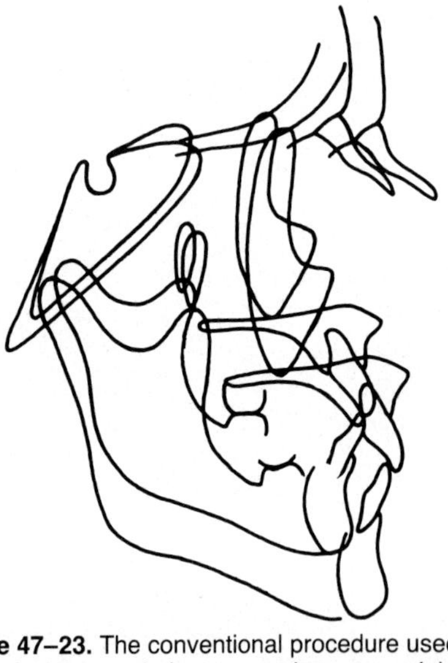

Figure 47–23. The conventional procedure used to demonstrate facial growth is to superimpose serial headfilm tracings on the cranial base (e.g., sella). The resultant forward and downward expansion of the face as a whole can then be seen. This method, however, does not show either the actual remodeling growth (deposition and resorption) or the displacement of each of the various component bony parts. It shows, rather, the composite effect of both and the resultant *location* of each part relative to the sella.

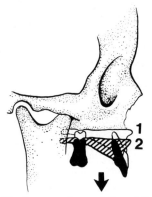

Figure 47–24. Downward remodeling of the palate and maxillary arch.

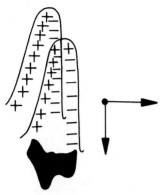

Figure 47–25. Combination of alveolar resorption and deposition that produces mesial drift also provides the important *vertical* drifting movements of each tooth. (From Enlow, D. H.: Handbook of Facial Growth. 2nd Ed. Philadelphia, W. B. Saunders Company, 1982.)

duces this movement. Each bony socket also grows downward, and the alveolar remodeling required is carried out by the periodontal membrane. The teeth are drifting downward. The same deposition and resorption of bone that produce mesial drift also provide for the process of vertical drift. Every first year dental student has heard of mesial drift, but somehow the very important process of vertical drifting had escaped attention until recently. Because the tooth and its socket move downward together, the vertical movement is properly termed *drift* rather than *eruption* or *extrusion*. The tooth's vertical drifting move-

ment is one that takes place *in addition* to its eruption. Furthermore, the tooth is not becoming extruded out of its socket; the tooth and socket move downward as a composite unit (Fig. 47–25).

As the maxillary teeth drift downward, the mandibular teeth drift superiorly at the same time (see Fig. 47–22). However, the extent of vertical drift movement by the lower teeth is less than that of the uppers. There is more available growth in the maxilla (considering here only remodeling growth). The maxillary arch is thus often attacked for Class II orthodontic treatment rather than the mandibular arch, even though it is usually the mandible that is retrusively positioned.

In Figure 47–26 the inferior movement of the palate and maxillary dentition produced by the in toto downward displacement of the nasomaxillary complex is illustrated. The *entire* maxillary dental arch and palate are carried inferiorly from level *2* to level *3* as the whole maxilla moves downward in association with bone deposition at all the various ethmomaxillary sutures. This is a passive movement of the arch, and all the teeth are moved with it. The maxilla may rotate during the displacement process; the anterior part of the arch may become displaced inferiorly to a greater or lesser extent than the posterior part, thus producing a rotation of the palate and occlusal plane. Remodeling growth may compensate for such rotations or in some cases add to their extent. Note that although the remodeling movement from level *1* to *2* and the displacement movement from *2* to *3* are shown separately in Figure 47–26, the growth changes take place simultaneously.

When the orthodontist moves an *individual* tooth, it is the growth movement associated specifically with remodeling growth that is considered. The periodontal membrane for each tooth and its alveolar bone is the direct target. In contrast, movements of the whole nasomaxillary complex and maxillary arch (surgical movements) use the displacement process rather than remodeling growth, and the sutural membranes are the primary targets. For the mandible a comparable situation exists. Movements of individual teeth are directed at individual periodontal membranes, whereas mandibular surgical repositioning uses the displacement growth process. Ramus and condylar growth are the primary targets for the latter.

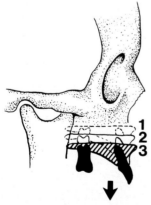

Figure 47–26. Movements of the palate, maxillary arch, and dentition from level *1* to *2* are accomplished by *remodeling* (Fig. 47–24). The movement from *2* to *3* is produced by the inferior *displacement* of the entire maxilla.

REFERENCES

Enlow, D. H.: The Human Face. New York, Harper & Row, 1968.

Enlow, D. H.: Growth and the problem of the local control mechanism. Am. J. Anat., *178*:2, 1973.

Enlow, D. H.: Postnatal growth of the face and cranium. *In* Cohen, G., and Kramer, I. R. N. (Eds.): Scientific Foundations of Dentistry. London, Heinemann, 1975.

Enlow, D. H.: Handbook of Facial Growth. 2nd Ed. Philadelphia, W. B. Saunders Company, 1982.

Enlow, D. H., and Bang, S.: Growth and remodeling of the human maxilla. Am. J. Orthod., *51*:446, 1965.

Enlow, D. H., and Harris, D. B.: A study of the postnatal growth of the human mandible. Am. J. Orthod., *50*:25, 1964.

Enlow, D. H., and Moyers, R. E.: Growth and architecture of the face. J. Am. Dent. Assoc., *82*:763, 1971.

Hall, B. K.: Differentiation of cartilage and bone from common germinal cells. J. Exp. Zool., *173*:383, 1970.

Koski, K.: Some characteristics of cranio-facial growth cartilages. *In* Moyers, R. E., and Krogman, W. M. (Eds.): Cranio-facial Growth in Man. Oxford, England, Pergamon Press, 1971.

Latham, R. A.: Maxillary development and growth: the septopremaxillary ligament. J. Anat. (Lond.), *107*:471, 1970.

Moss, M. L.: The primary role of functional matrices in facial growth. Am. J. Orthod., *55*:566, 1969.

Sarnat, B. G.: Clinical and experimental considerations in facial bone biology: growth, remodeling, and repair. J. Am. Dent. Assoc., *82*:876, 1971.

Sarnat, B. G.: Surgical experimentation and gross postnatal growth of the face and jaws. J. Dent. Res., *50*:1462, 1971.

Scott, J. H.: The cartilage of the nasal septum. Br. Dent. J., *95*:37, 1953.

48

Malcolm C. Johnston
Peter T. Bronsky
Guillermo Millicovsky

Embryogenesis of Cleft Lip and Palate

Although clefts of the lip, palate, or both are by far the most common major facial malformations (Fig. 48–1), the mechanisms underlying their embryogenesis are only now beginning to be understood. This is due to the complexity of primary and secondary palate development and the fact that appropriate methods for study have only recently been developed. Combinations of new and older techniques are permitting the resolution of long-standing controversies and facilitating the development of new concepts concerning the underlying mechanisms. Such combinations are also making possible detailed extrapolations from the embryos of experimental animals (in which most studies related to underlying mechanisms are conducted) to the human embryo.

Because of its obvious relevance to cleft lip and palate, much of the details of normal development of the primary and secondary palate are addressed in this chapter rather than in Chapter 46.

EARLY CRANIOFACIAL DEVELOPMENT

The primary palate forms the initial separation between the developing oral and nasal cavities. It eventually gives rise to much of the upper lip, the associated dentoalveolar ridge, and that portion of the hard palate in front of the incisive foramen (Fig. 48–1A). It appears that almost all cases of human cleft lip, with or without associated cleft palate [CL(P)], are caused by failure of the medial nasal prominence or process (MNP) to make contact with the lateral nasal process (LNP) and maxillary process (MxP) (see Fig. 48–8C).

The secondary palate (see Fig. 48–25) completes the separation between the oral and nasal cavities by forming most of the hard palate and all of the soft palate. Almost all palatal clefts appear to result from the failure of the palatal shelves to make contact with each other.

Owing to their relevance, or possible relevance, to certain types of CL(P) and cleft palate (CP), two aspects of earlier facial development, anterior neural plate (and olfactory placode) development and the origins of craniofacial tissues, will be described. More detailed descriptions of these events are presented in Chapter 46.

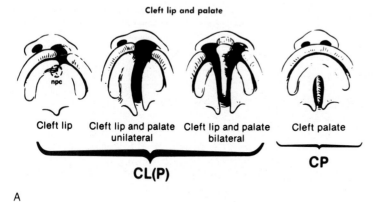

Cleft lip and palate

| Cleft lip | Cleft lip and palate unilateral | Cleft lip and palate bilateral | Cleft palate |

CL(P)   CP

A

MAJOR FACIAL MALFORMATIONS – FREQUENCY

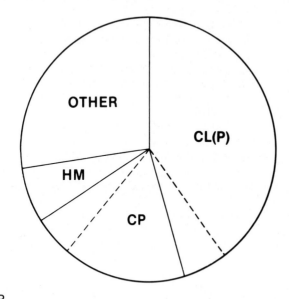

B

Figure 48–1. *A,* The etiology and embryogenesis of clefts of the lip with or without cleft palate [CL(P)] are distinctly different from those of isolated cleft palate (CP). Only "complete" clefts are shown. Isolated clefts of the lip extend as far posteriorly as the incisive foramen (nasopalatine canal, npc), while isolated clefts of the palate extend anteriorly as far as this landmark. *B,* Clefts of the lip and/or palate (CL/P) make up almost two-thirds of all major facial malformations. The broken lines separate the less common syndromic clefts from the more common nonsyndromic clefts. The third most common malformation is craniofacial microsomia (HM). (From Johnston, M. C.: Animal models for craniofacial disorders: a critique. Prog. Clin. Biol. Res., *46:*33, 1980.)

Anterior Neural Plate Development and Positioning of Olfactory (Nasal) Placodes

Malformations in the holoprosencephaly series include underdeveloped forebrain derivatives, including a tendency to form only one ventricle, as implied by the name. Facial defects range from mild midfacial underdevelopment, fairly typical CL(P), and more severe defects (see Chaps. 46 and 60). The deficiencies appear to be almost exclusively limited to derivatives of the midline region of the anterior neural plate (Fig. 48–2).

Much of the "blueprint" for midfacial development is laid down very early (by gesta-

tional day 17 in the human embryo) at the time of anterior neural plate formation. A key element is the position of the olfactory placodes (Fig. 48–2). Placodes are epithelial thickenings that play a dominant role in midfacial development. Their positioning is determined by the anterior neural plate. There is evidence (Couly and Le Douarin, 1985, 1987) that the olfactory placodes are derived directly from the anterior margin of the neural plate (Fig. 48–2), separating from this margin in later development. Midline deficiencies in the anterior neural plate would consequently lead to the prospective placodes being too close to the midline. As discussed later, placode positioning may be involved in CL(P) predisposition.

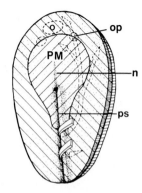

���Neuroectoderm
���Skin (surface) Ectoderm

Figure 48–2. The middle germ layer (mesoderm) is formed by cells migrating from the upper layer of a two layer embryo through the primitive streak (ps) into the intermediate space (*broken arrows*). After completion of the migration and the deposition of cells from the anterior end of the primitive streak to form the notochord (n), a midline mesodermal structure, the upper and lower layers (now called ectoderm and endoderm, respectively) are separated by mesoderm at all points except the oropharyngeal plate (o). Mesodermal cells are responsible for inducing a portion of the overlying ectoderm to form the neural plate (neuroectoderm), which later forms most of the brain and spinal cord. In turn the anterior neural plate is at least partially responsible for the induction of the olfactory placodes (op) if not contributing directly to them (see text). In the midline between the oropharyngeal plate and the notochordal mesoderm is the prechordal mesoderm (PM), which, unlike the midline notochordal mesoderm, is formed by cells migrating through the primitive streak (*broken arrows*). Deficiency of the portion of the anterior neural plate over the prechordal mesoderm leads to a particular type of craniofacial malformation (holoprosencephaly) that often includes clefts of the lip and palate. (From Johnston, M. C., and Sulik, K. K.: Embryology of the head and neck. *In* Serafin, D., and Georgiade, N. G. (Eds.): Pediatric Plastic Surgery. St. Louis, C. V. Mosby Company, 1984, pp. 184–215.)

Origins of Craniofacial Tissues

Neural Crest Origins of Facial Mesenchyme. Neural crest cells originate from the lateral edges of the neural plate and migrate into subepithelial locations, either laterally under the surface epithelium or down beside the neural tube (Fig. 48–3). In the head region of the human embryo, the migrations are initiated at approximately gestational day 22. As the crest cells leave the compact epithelial arrangement of the ectoderm, they adopt a loosely arranged mesenchymal appearance.[*] Crest cells migrating beside the neural tube form primarily components of the peripheral nervous system; those migrating under the surface ectoderm in the trunk region form exclusively pigment cells, while in the head and anterior neck region they also form skeletal and connective tissues (Fig. 48–4) (see Chap. 46) (Noden, 1983; Le Douarin, 1983).

As discussed later in the chapter, it is possible to produce fairly typical CL(P)s by extirpating or killing crest cells before or at the beginning of their migration, thereby reducing the facial mesenchyme and the size of the facial prominences. Consequently, the latter do not contact to form the lips and associated structures. However, this may have little or no relevance to nonsyndromic human CL(P). On the other hand, a much

---

[*]It should again be emphasized (see Chap. 46) that "epithelia" and "mesenchyme" are terms used to describe the histologic appearance of embryonic tissues and are not to be confused with the terms "ectoderm" and "mesoderm," which are names of embryonic germ layers.

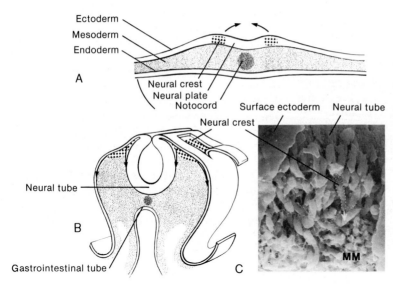

Figure 48–3. Cross sections through embryos before (*A*) and after (*B*) the onset of crest cell (diamond pattern) migration. The ectoderm in *C* has been peeled back (as indicated in *B*), permitting direct visualization with scanning electron microscopy of the underlying mouse embryo neural crest cells. Like crest cells in other species, the cells in *C* are frequently bipolar and oriented (*arrow*) in the direction of migration. Mesodermal mesenchyme (MM) cells over which the crest cells will migrate are also visible. (From Johnston, M. C., and Sulik, K. K.: Development of face and oral cavity. *In* Bhaskar, S. N. (Ed.): Orban's Oral Histology and Embryology. 10th Ed. St. Louis, MO, C. V. Mosby Company, 1985.)

Figure 48–4. The migratory (*a*) and postmigratory pattern (*c* and *e*) distributions of neural crest cells (*stippled*) and the origins of the cranial sensory ganglia. The initial ganglionic primordia are formed by cords of neural crest cells that remain attached to the neural tube. The section plane in *c* and *e* passes through the primordium of the trigeminal ganglion. Ectodermal "thickenings," termed placodes, form adjacent to the distal ends of the ganglionic primordia—two for the trigeminal (V) and one each for the facial (VII), glossopharyngeal (IX), and vagal (X) ganglia. They contribute presumptive neuroblasts that migrate into the previously purely crest primordia. (Adapted from Johnston, M. C., and Hazelton, R. B.: Embryonic origins of facial structures related to oral sensory and motor function. *In* Bosma, J. F. (Ed.): Oral Sensory Perception: The Mouth of the Infant. Springfield, IL, Charles C Thomas, 1972, pp. 76–97.)

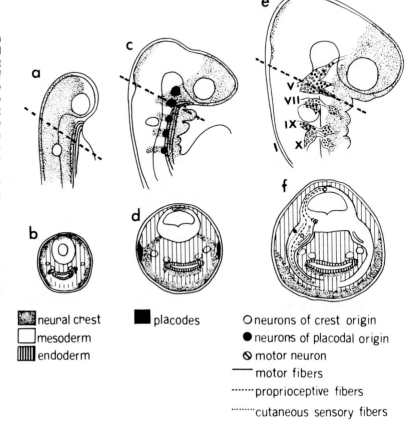

stronger case can be made for CL(P)s associated with Waardenburg's syndrome, which apparently involves only crest cell derivatives.

Placodal Contributions to Sensory Ganglia. Another unique feature of craniofacial development is the origin of a large number of sensory ganglionic neurons from surface ectodermal placodes (Fig. 48–4). In the trunk region, all the neurons of the peripheral nervous system originate from neural crest cells.

As described in Chapter 46 and later in this chapter, a complicated sequence of developmental events initiated by experimentally induced cell death in the above placodal cell population at a very early age (equivalent to roughly day 27 in the human embryo) leads to, at a much later stage (roughly days 55 to 60 in the human), CP associated with a malformation complex essentially identical to the Treacher Collins syndrome.

Origins and Migration of Myoblasts of Voluntary Muscles

The myoblasts that form the contractile elements of skeletal voluntary muscle originate from somites or somite-like structures adjacent to the neural tube. Somites are blocks of mesoderm that form beside the neural tube (see Chap. 46), the middle layer of which forms the myoblasts of voluntary muscles. The myoblasts have a two-stage migration. The first brings the cells into the facial region as single groups related to the individual cranial nerves (Fig. 48–5). During the second stage, the myoblasts migrate as smaller subgroups of cells, which may travel long distances to the final locations of individual muscles. The connective tissue of the muscle is derived from local mesenchyme, almost invariably of neural crest origin.

It now appears that many, if not most, cases of CP are caused by excessive size of the tongue. The manner in which these and other muscle masses are determined is largely unknown.

NORMAL DEVELOPMENT OF THE PRIMARY PALATE

At the completion of migration, crest cells surround the mesodermal cores in the visceral arches (Fig. 48–6A) and constitute the entire facial mesenchymal cell population above the developing oral cavity. Endothelial capillary buds from the mesodermal cores and other mesoderm invade and vascularize the crest mesenchyme, which in turn forms all of the vessel wall except the endothelial lining.

At this time (human gestational day 35) facial development enters a new phase with the regional growth of the facial prominences and visceral arches (Fig. 48–6). High rates of proliferation in these structures (Minkoff and Kuntz, 1977, 1978) may be maintained by an epithelial-mesenchymal interaction. A mesenchymal cell process meshwork (CPM) is found in close contact with the underside of the epithelial areas (Sulik and associates 1979, 1980), and the mesenchymal cells are connected by gap junctions (Minkoff, 1986). Both of these features may mediate the epithelial-mesenchymal interaction. This possibility has been supported by the findings of serotonin uptake by the epithelium and by the demonstration of serotonin binding protein in the underlying basement membrane that contains the CPM (Lauder, Tannir, and Sadler, 1988). It is known that the epithelium is necessary for the normal development of facial prominence mesenchyme in vitro (Minkoff, in press) and it is tempting to speculate that epithelia are involved in growth regulation mediated by serotonin via the CPM.

The maxillary prominence is formed by the proximal half of the first visceral (mandibular) arch, which bends so that its more proximal part ends up facing forward under the eye (Fig. 48–6A, B, see Fig. 48–8A). It then grows forward at its tip (Patterson and Minkoff, 1985), which eventually contacts the MNP (medial nasal process) and LNP (lateral nasal process). These prominences then coalesce through the phenomenon of fusion and merging (Fig. 48–7), to be described in detail later.

Development of the MNP and LNP is complicated by a series of morphogenetic movements (Smuts, 1981; Bronsky and associates, 1989). Initially, the olfactory placode sits over the corner of the forebrain, so that its medial edge is more forward (ventral) than its lateral edge (Fig. 48–8). A curling forward of its lateral margin initiates formation of the LNP and causes it to "grow"* forward rapidly and

---

*The term "growth" is defined simply as an increase in size. In the case of the facial prominences, contributing factors are cell proliferation, matrix accumulation and hydration, and morphogenetic movements.

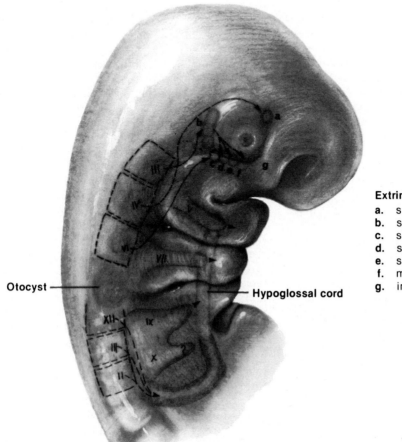

Extrinsic ocular muscle primordia

a. superior oblique
b. superior rectus
c. superior rectus
d. superior rectus
e. superior rectus
f. mesial rectus
g. inferior oblique

Otocyst

Hypoglossal cord

Figure 48–5. The visceral arches play a major role in the development of the voluntary (skeletal) muscles of the head and neck. The original mesoderm forming the cores of the visceral arches is replaced by presumptive myoblasts that migrate into the arches (*arrowheads*) from proximally located mesoderm, the mytotomes of postotic somites, or, in the preotic region, from structures that are apparently homologous with the myotomes of postotic somites. The myotomes of the first three postotic somites give rise to the hypoglossal cord, which supplies the myoblasts of the tongue and other muscles supplied by the 12th cranial nerve. The myoblasts of the extrinsic ocular muscle are derived from poorly defined myotomes supplied by the third, fourth, and sixth cranial nerves. (Adapted from Johnston, M. C., and Sulik, K. K.: Development of face and oral cavity. *In* Bhaskar, S. N. (Ed.): Orban's Oral Histology and Embryology. 9th Ed. St. Louis, MO, C. V. Mosby Company, 1980.)

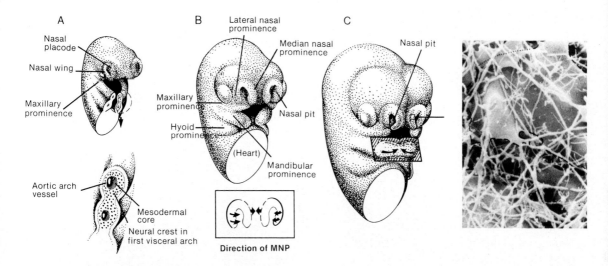

Figure 48–6. Embryonic development from the completion of major crest cell migrations to fusion of the facial prominences. The heart and contiguous portions of the visceral arches have been removed in *A*. The relations of the aortic arch blood vessels and the crest and mesodermal core are indicated in the enlarged sketch of *A*. Arrows in *B* (*inset*) illustrate the growth directions of the facial prominences primarily related to morphogenetic movements (considered in greater detail in Fig. 48–9). *C*, The scanning electron micrograph illustrates the subepithelial mesenchymal cell process meshwork (after removal of the overlying epithelium) that may be involved in epithelial-mesenchymal interactions, possibly including the maintenance of high rates of mesenchyme cell proliferation. (Modified from Johnston, M. C., and Sulik, K. K.: Development of face and oral cavity. *In* Bhaskar, S. N. (Ed.): Orban's Oral Histology and Embryology. 10th Ed. St. Louis, MO, C. V. Mosby Company, 1985.)

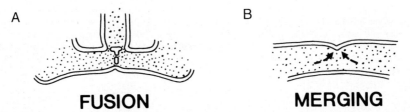

Figure 48–7. *A,* Fusion of the palatal shelves to each other and to the nasal septum (see Fig. 48–26). *B,* Merging as in the developing mandibular arch. *Fusion* involves contact of essentially "free-ended" structures, adhesion, epithelial breakdown, and mesenchymal consolidation as between the palatal shelves and nasal septum. Epithelial breakdown between the septum and palatal shelves has been initiated in *A*. *Merging* is the coalescence of growth centers whose already confluent mesenchyme appears to "push out" (*arrows*) and to smooth intervening epithelial grooves (*B*). (From Johnston, M. C., and Sulik, K. K.: Embryology of the head and neck: *In* Serafin, D., and Georgiade, N. G. (Eds.): Pediatric Plastic Surgery. St. Louis, MO, C. V. Mosby Company, 1984, pp 184–215.)

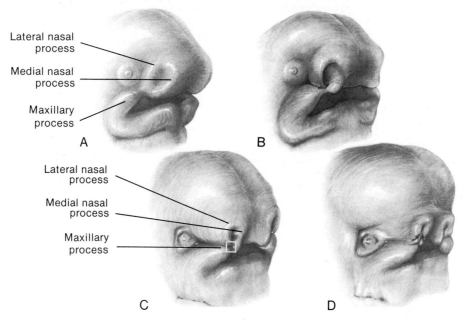

Lateral nasal
process

Medial nasal
process

Maxillary
process

A

B

Lateral nasal
process

Medial nasal
process

Maxillary
process

C

D

Figure 48–8. Progressive stages of primary palate development. Morphogenetic movements of the olfactory placode appear to play a major role. The lateral portion of the placode curls forward (*A, B*). An epithelial seam is formed between the prominences that breaks down deep to the area indicated by the square (*C*). Mesenchymal penetration through this area of breakdown consolidates the three prominences, while ''hollowing out'' of the epithelial seam behind this region leads to an open communication between the nasal pit and the roof of the primitive oral cavity (see also Figs. 48–11*B*, 48–25*C,D*). The fusion area is further broadened by merging (*arrows* in *D*). (From Johnston, M. C., and Sulik, K. K.: Development of face and oral cavity. *In* Bhaskar, S. N. (Ed.): Orban's Oral Histology and Embryology. 10th Ed. St. Louis, MO, C. V. Mosby Company, 1980.)

"catch up" with the MNP, which forms at the medial edge of the placode (Figs. 48–8, 48–9, see Fig. 48–20—normoxia diagrams). The curling forward of the lateral portion of the placode involves a major translocation of both epithelia and mesenchyme (Patterson, Johnston, and Minkoff, 1984; Patterson and Minkoff, 1985). The above placodal movement and other movements involved in primary palate formation (Fig. 48–9) appear to be mediated by a contractile terminal web system (Fig. 48–10), similar to that involved in neural tube closure.

Upon contact, the epithelia fuse to form the "epithelial seam," which undergoes partial degeneration (Gaare and Langman, 1977) and mesenchymal consolidation (Fig. 48–11, see Fig. 48–13). Behind this region of fusion, spaces appear between the epithelial cells, which eventually coalesce to form the initial nasal cavity connecting the nasal pit with the primitive oral cavity (stomodeum).

Most research related to normal and abnormal primary palate development has been conducted on the mouse. The mechanisms involved are fundamentally the same, but

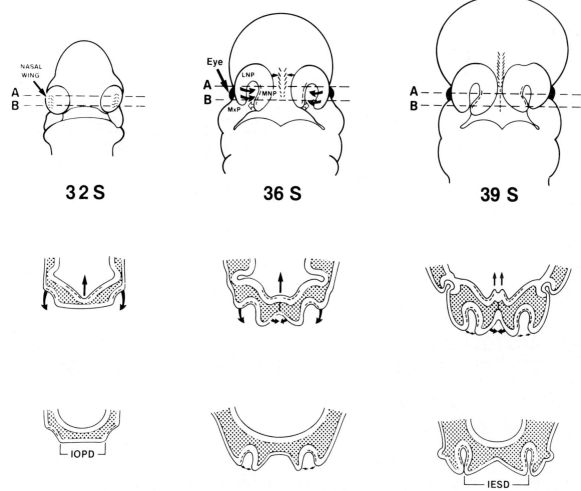

Figure 48–9. Primary palate development in 32, 36, and 39 somite mouse embryos. The horizontal section planes pass through the upper (A) and lower (B) portions of the developing primary palate. Morphogenetic movements are initiated by a curling forward of the lateral portion of the olfactory placode to form the nasal wing or early lateral nasal prominence (LNP) in the 32S embryo. Primary palate closure (nearing completion in the 39S embryo) is dependent on the medial nasal prominence (MNP) making contact with the lateral nasal prominence (LNP) and maxillary prominence (MxP). The arrows represent the directions of growth and/or morphogenetic movements. The forebrain invagination appears to draw the MNPs toward the midline. The force-generating component for these morphogenetic movements is apparently the terminal web ("active" portions indicated by broken lines—see also Fig. 48–10). (From Bronsky, P. T., and Johnston, M. C.: Craniofacial morphogenetic movements: normal development and alterations leading to cleft lip. In preparation.)

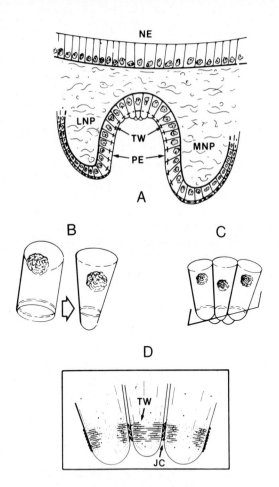

Figure 48–10. The major components involved in the morphogenetic movement of the nasal placodal epithelium. *A,* Section similar to the horizontal sections in Figure 48–9 (36S embryo). It depicts normal structure and relations of the placodal epithelium (PE), which lines the inner surfaces of the lateral nasal (LNP) and medial nasal (MNP) prominences and is separated from the neuroepithelium (NE) by mesenchyme (scroll). The location of the terminal web (TW), a structure believed to be primarily responsible for the morphogenetic "force," is indicated by the broken line. *B,* Changes in the shape of a cell resulting from contraction of the terminal web. *C,* The conical shape of placodal cells in the deepest region of the olfactory pit is evident. The position of the terminal web is indicated by broken lines. *D,* Components of the terminal web (TW) and the junctional complex (JC) to which the filaments of the web are anchored are seen in this section (plane indicated in *C*). The junctional complexes anchor the apical portions of the placodal cells together. The terminal web therefore forms a network whose contraction reduces the diameter of the apical portions of the placodal cells. The force generated by web contraction apparently causes the placodal epithelium to "curve" forward, resulting in the nasal pit or groove. Massive regional cell death, as observed in the studies to be described (see Fig. 48–19*D* to *F*), would grossly interfere with the integrity of the web and normal placodal morphogenesis (From Bronsky, P. T., Johnston, M. C., Moore, N. B., Dehart, D. B., and Sulik, K. K.: Lateral nasal placodal morphogenesis in mice: normal development and alterations leading to hypoxia-induced cleft lip. Submitted.)

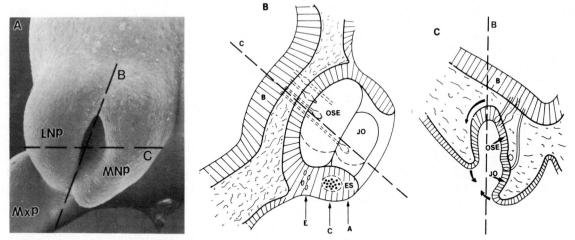

Figure 48–11. Components of the olfactory placode. *A,* Scanning electron micrograph of right side lateral nasal (LNP), medial nasal (MNP), and maxillary (MxP) facial prominences of a normal 39 somite embryo, indicating section planes for diagrams in *B* and *C. B,* Diagram indicating the cut surfaces and medial wall of the nasal pit. Many neurons of the olfactory sensory epithelium (OSE) and Jacobson's organ (JO, vomeronasal organ) have already differentiated and sent processes into the brain (B). Some neuronal cell bodies have moved into the olfactory nerve. The epithelial seam (ES), formed by contact of the MNP with the LNP and MxP, is breaking down in one area (*stippled*) where mesenchyme will consolidate the primary palate, and is cavitating in another area (*open circles*) where union of the cavities will open direct communication between the nasal and oral cavities. *C,* "Horizontal" section showing that the curling forward (*arrows*) of the lateral portion of the placode (with associated LNP) is nearing completion. Largely because of this morphogenetic movement the olfactory sensory epithelium will be finally located at the top of the nasal cavity. The medial nasal prominence appears to bend laterally (*arrow*) in the horizontal plane as well as in the lateral plane, as illustrated in the 36S embryo in Figure 48–9. (From Bronsky, P. T., and Johnston, M. C.: Morphogenetic movements involved in normal primary palate development and cleft lip formation. In preparation.)

there are minor differences between the mouse and human primary palate (Fig. 48–12) that need to be addressed. Initially, the olfactory placodes and the beginning LNPs and MNPs of both species are quite separate from the MxPs. The forward curling of the lateral margins of the olfactory placodes forming the initial LNPs, the nasal wings of Streeter (1948), is similar (compare *A* and *D*

in Fig. 48–12). As the morphogenetic movements continue, the LNPs become progressively more developed and sweep forward over the underlying maxillary prominence (Fig. 48–12*B, E*). The MxP has already made contact with the MNP in both mouse and human embryos (between the arrows in Fig. 48–12*B* and 48–12*E*, respectively). The position of the future opening from the primitive

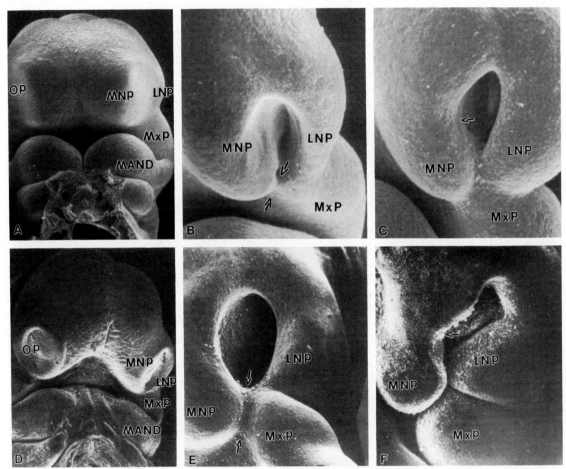

Figure 48–12. Scanning electron micrographs comparing the three major stages of primary palate development in mouse (*A* to *C*) and human (*D* to *F*) embryos. In the initial stage (*A,D*), the edges of the olfactory placodes (OP) elevate somewhat asymmetrically with the lateral portions of the placodes showing a pronounced curling forward to initiate formation of the lateral nasal prominences (LNP, nasal wing). The medial nasal prominences (MNP) have formed at the medial edges of the placodes while the maxillary prominences (MxP) are growing forward from the proximal portions of the mandibular arches (MAND). At this stage the MxPs appear to be essentially independent of the developing placodes. By the second stage (*B,E*), the MNPs and LNPs have increased greatly in size, partly through cell proliferation and, especially in the case of the LNPs, partly through morphogenetic movements. The MxPs have contacted the MNPs, and epithelial seams (between arrows) have formed. The LNPs are attached to the underlying MxPs by confluent mesenchyme and have not yet reached the MNP. In the third stage (*C,F*), the LNPs have reached the MNPs, with which they form the upper parts of the epithelial seams (see Fig. 48–13*B,D*). By this stage, epithelial breakdown has advanced considerably in the lower parts of the seams (portions formed by MNP:MxP contact in Fig. 48–13*B*), and breakdown has been initiated in the upper MNP:LNP portion. (*A* to *C* from Sulik, K. K., and Schoenwolf, G. C.: Highlights of craniofacial morphogenesis in mammalian embryos as revealed by scanning electron microscopy. Scanning Electron Microscopy, 1985. *D* to *F* from Jirasek, J. E.: Atlas of Human Prenatal Morphogenesis. Hingham, MA, Kluwer Martinus, 1983.)

oral cavities into the nasal cavities is behind the lower arrows. With continued development, mostly growth in a forward direction, the LNP comes into contact with the MNP. The maxillary prominences in the mouse become somewhat "overwhelmed" (Fig. 48–12C) because the LNPs and MNPs are extremely well developed; this presumably is related to the highly developed sense of smell in the mouse. Similar disproportions are related to the large eyes in the chick embryo and the large brains in the human embryo. In all three species, the MNPs fuse with the conjoined lateral nasal and maxillary prominences (Fig. 48–13). On the lateral side, the fusion epithelium (which breaks down to permit mesenchymal penetration) is found at the junction of the LNP and MxP (Fig. 48–13D) (Johnston, Sulik, and Minkoff, 1981). Further development of the primary palate is primarily by merging with the LNP, and the MNP also continues to make major contributions in both mouse and human embryos.

EMBRYOGENESIS OF CLEFT LIP WITH OR WITHOUT ASSOCIATED CLEFT PALATE [CL(P)]

There are many types of clefts of the primary palate. The common (lateral) cleft lip, with or without associated cleft palate [CL(P)] (see Fig. 48–1), may be divided into syndromic and nonsyndromic subgroups, depending on whether there are associated malformations. As will be seen below, nonsyndromic clefts may also be divided into subgroups.

CL(P) Variability and its Relation to Normal Primary and Secondary Palate Development. The authors believe that the initial contact and fusion between the MxP and MNP (see Fig. 48–12B, E) may be normal in many embryos that will develop CL(P), and that the critical problem is failure of the LNP to make contact with the MNP (Fig. 48–14A, B). The initial MxP-MNP fusion remains intact during the early stages of cleft formation (Fig. 48–14A, B), but in approximately 90 per cent of cases later ruptures. The Simonart's band illustrated in Figure 48–14C may represent persistence of the initial MxP-MNP fusion. Another possible developmental alteration leading to Simonart's band formation has been proposed by Sulik and associates (1979).

Another variant (Fig. 48–14D, E) may account for a number of incomplete cleft lips

(Fig. 48–14F). In the embryo shown in Figure 48–14D, E, the initial MxP-MNP fusion and the LNP-MNP fusion (and possibly the previous initial MxP-MNP fusion) have taken place but the MxP becomes somewhat disconnected with the MNP during its later forward growth, resulting in an incomplete cleft.

Little is known of the reason why palatal clefts are associated with some clefts and not with others. After the formation of a complete cleft of the primary palate in A/J mice, the tongue remains wedged in the cleft and presumably is responsible for the more rapid increase in maxillary width that is observed (Smiley, Vanek, and Dixon, 1971). The increased width could in itself account for the cleft because of the failure of the palatal shelves to contact each other when they elevate (see Fig. 48–26), but they do not, in fact, elevate at all, presumably because of the tongue remaining wedged in the cleft. Tongue protrusion with downward deflection by an intact primary palate may be helpful for its removal from a position between the shelves. The association between "tongue-tie" (ankyloglossia—persistent attachment of the tongue tip to the floor of the mouth) and cleft palate in an extended Icelandic family (Moore and associates, 1987) suggests that such movement may be necessary. The fact that the shelves frequently elevate in humans in the presence of complete primary palate clefts is indicated by the relatively high incidence of cleft lip without cleft palate (CL).

In addition to the above specific instances, the many degrees of severity of CL(P), from lip scarring or notching to complete bilateral CL(P), indicate that the process of contact and fusion may cease at any point.

Many Different Development Alterations Lead to CL(P). Normal contact and fusion of the embryonic facial prominences may be considered to be a developmental weak point, with a wide variety of developmental alterations leading to its failure and CL(P). Most of the developmental alterations lead to CL(P) through failure of prominence contact.

Studies of facial morphology in monozygotic (MZ) twins discordant for CL(P) (Johnston and associates, in preparation) suggest that approximately two-thirds of the CL(P) cases are caused by underdevelopment of the MNPs, which leads to contact failure. The twin studies indicated that many of the remaining one-third of CL(P) cases result from underdevelopment of the maxillary prominences.

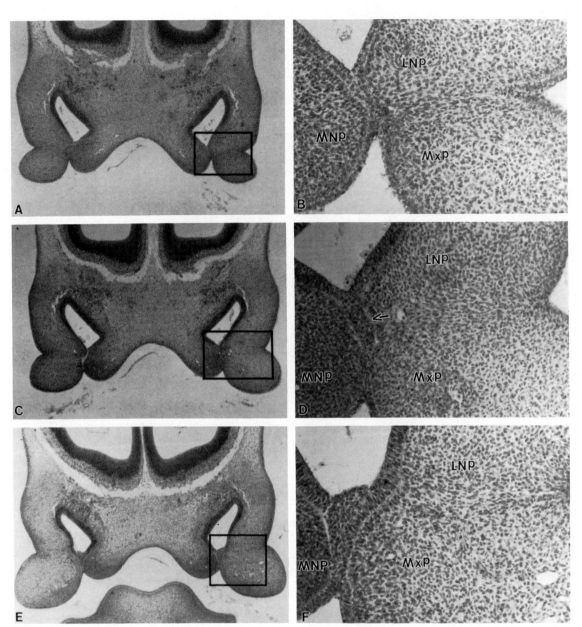

Figure 48–13. Coronal sections through the primary palate of a human embryo at a stage of development comparable with that of the embryos in Figures 48–11 and 48–12F. Boxes in A, C, and E indicate the enlarged areas of B, D, and F. The section plane in A and B is through the anterior portions of the prominences (arrow labeled A in Fig. 48–11B and in the same plane as Fig. 48–12F). Contact of the LNP with the MNP is more dominant than that of the MxP with the MNP at this level. Sections (C,D) at the intermediate level (arrow labeled C in Fig. 48–11B) show complete breakdown of the portion of the epithelial seam derived from the MNP:MxP contact with mesenchymal penetration. The portion of the seam derived from the MNP:LNP contact shows degenerative changes and will shortly be replaced by mesenchyme. The deepest (most posterior) section (arrow labeled E in Fig. 48–11B) (E,F) is through the portion of the seam that will persist, eventually "hollowing out" to form a portion of the nasal cavity epithelium. Most or all of the epithelial seam at this level is derived from the initial MNP:MxP contact (see Fig. 48–12E). As contact and fusion progress, the LNP makes a progressively larger contribution to the epithelial seam (see Figs. 48–12F, 48–13C,D) until it plays a dominant role (Fig. 48–13E,F). (From Diewert, V. M.: Normal primary palate development and cleft lip in human embryos. In preparation.)

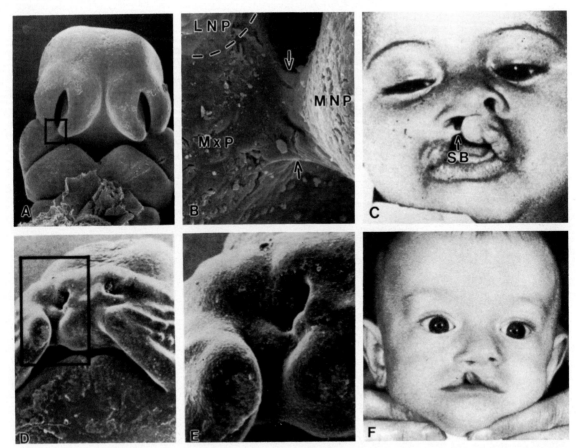

Figure 48–14. Postulated causes of Simonart's band and other incomplete CL(P)s. *A,B,* Persistence of MNP:MxP contact or bridge (between arrows in *B*) following reduced LNP development caused by maternal hypoxia (which leads to CL(P) formation in almost all embryos). Mesenchymal penetration through the bridge should have already occurred at this stage of development, and the epithelium behind the penetration region will later cavitate to form a passage connecting the back of the nasal pit to the primitive oral cavity. This bridge is in the correct position to give rise to Simonart's band, which is far posteriorly and superiorly (SB in *C*). Growth of the primary palate beyond the stage illustrated in *A* and *B* would be forward and downward from the area of the bridge illustrated in *B*. *D,E,* Spontaneous incomplete CL(P) in a CL/Fr mouse embryo. In this case, fusion between the MNP and LNP has taken place while MNP:MxP fusion has failed to occur, at least in the anterior regions. This might result if the MNP were vertically too short to make contact with the MxP as it did in Figure 48–12*E,F,* or if the MxP grew in an excessively lateral direction, failing to continue contacting the MNP and LNP. Such developmental alterations could explain certain types of incomplete CL(P) such as that shown in *F*. (*A* and *B* from Bronsky, P. T.: Effects of hypoxia on facial prominence development in CL/Fr mice. M.S. Thesis, University of North Carolina, 1985. *C* from Millard, D. R.: Cleft Craft: The Evolution of its Surgery. I. The Unilateral Deformity. Boston, Little, Brown & Company, 1976. Copyright 1976, Little, Brown & Company. *D* and *E* modified from Millicovsky, G., Ambrose, L. J. H., and Johnston, M. C.: Developmental alterations associated with spontaneous cleft lip and palate in CL/Fr mice. Am. J. Anat., *164*:29, 1982. *F* from Ross, R. B., and Johnston, M. C.: Cleft Lip and Palate. Baltimore, Williams & Wilkins Company, 1978, pp. 17–20. Copyright 1978, Williams & Wilkins Company.)

Little is known about the other types of developmental alterations that may lead to human CL(P) cases. Töndury (1961) described a human embryo just after the time of cleft formation that had an underdeveloped LNP, which would be comparable with many experimentally induced CL(P)s, in which it appears that environmental factors interfere with the major morphogenetic movement critical to LNP formation. Diewert and Shiota (1988) observed hemorrhages in the primary palate fusion region in human Japanese embryos, a finding suggesting a rupture during or after fusion. Hematomas in the fusion line of A-strain and related mice have occasionally been observed (Steiniger, 1939; Millicovsky, Ambrose, and Johnston, 1982). Steiniger (1939) proposed that post-closure opening after hemorrhage was the primary mechanism in this A-strain subline.

Many experimental manipulations lead to contact failure and CL(P). Extirpation of any one of the three prominences causes CL(P) in mouse embryos growing in culture (Ohbayashi and Eto, 1986). Insertion of a sable hair probe loaded with tunicamycin (which digests glycoproteins) into the LNP of mouse embryos reduced its size, leading to CL(P) (Eto and associates, 1981). Underdevelopment and contact failure of the prominences result from extirpation or killing of crest cells before their migration in the chick embryo (Johnston, 1964; van Lienborgh, Lieuw Kie Song, and Been, 1983), and administration of agents (cadmium, x-irradiation) that are lethal for crest cells in the mouse (Kushner and associates, unpublished; Eto, King, and Johnston, 1976) leads to CL(P) in the mouse and homologous clefts in the chick. There are numerous brain, eye, and other malformations associated with these clefts and it is doubtful whether this is an important mechanism for human CL(P).

Nonsyndromic CL(P)

The following discussion concerning different types of developmental alteration predisposing to cleft lip is organized into genetic factors, environmental factors, and interactions between them. As noted earlier, almost all these factors cause developmental alterations that lead to contact failure between the facial prominences.

Genetic Factors. Some progress has been made concerning the developmental abnormalities caused by genetic factors. The most extensively studied experimental animal has been the A-strain mouse (Kalter, 1975), with publications dating back to the 1930's (Reed and Snell, 1931; Steiniger, 1939) and more recent studies (Davidson, Fraser, and Schlager, 1969; Biddle and Fraser, 1986). The incidence of spontaneous cleft lip varies from near zero to 25 per cent, depending on the subline and other factors. One observation was that some genetic effects are peculiar to the mother; i.e., the environment she provides for the embryo predisposes the embryo to CL(P) (Davidson and Fraser, 1969). It also appears that a single major recessive gene is primarily responsible for the genetic predisposition (Biddle and Fraser, 1986). Little evidence for such maternal effects has been found in humans (Niswander, 1970). Otherwise, A-strain mice appear to be satisfactory animal models for many cases of human CL(P).

With respect to the A/J subline, Trasler (1968) proposed that differences in the observed growth direction of the MNPs in A/J mice, as compared with the genetically resistant C57Bl/6J mouse (Fig. 48–15), could make the A/J embryo more susceptible to cleft lip. This difference would make it necessary for the LNP to migrate further medially in order to make contact, thus predisposing the embryo to contact failure. In the A/J embryos in which contact and fusion occur, the medial wall of the LNP would be closer to the midline. Since this mechanism dictates the position of the lateral wall of the nasal cavity, it would be consistent with the narrow nasal cavities (piriform fossae) in the unaffected human twins of MZ pairs when the affected twin has CL(P) (Johnston and associates, in preparation). The unaffected twins were used in the study because they would be expected to have just avoided having a cleft (see below) and their subsequent growth would not be altered by a cleft. They were compared with controls that had no close relatives with clefts. Not all the unaffected cotwins have narrow nasal cavities, a finding indicating that other developmental alterations lead to CL(P) in other twins.

The narrow nasal cavities of the twins are also consistent with underdeveloped MNPs related to olfactory placodes being positioned too close to the midline. The abnormal placode positioning appears to be a key feature of malformations in the holoprosencephaly series (see Chap. 46) (Johnston and Sulik, 1984). Subsequent deficiencies of the MNPs lead to a number of malformations, including those of the fetal alcohol syndrome and, possibly, cleft lip. Such "holoprosencephaly" malformations are associated with ethanol exposure in mice at very early stages of development (Sulik, Johnston, and Webb, 1981; Sulik and Johnston, 1983; Webster and Ritchie, in press) and with trisomy 13 (Gorlin, Pindborg, and Cohen, 1976). Most of the facial malformations in trisomy 13 are clefts of the lip and palate. The fact that the premaxillary segments of these individuals are small (Gorlin, Pindborg, and Cohen, 1976) suggests that they are part of the series. CL(P) was not observed in the fetal alcohol syndrome study, but this may be related to the use of the CL(P)-resistant C57Bl/6J strain for the study.

Factors of possible relevance to this problem are racial differences in facial morphology and CL(P) susceptibility. In Oriental peo-

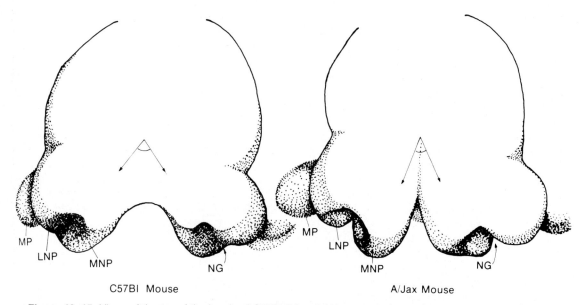

C57Bl Mouse   A/Jax Mouse

Figure 48–15. Views of the top of the heads of C57BL/6J and A/J mouse embryos demonstrate that the MNPs of A/ Jax (A/J) embryos grow more parallel and close to the midline than the MNPs of C57Bl/6J embryos, possibly making the A/J strain more susceptible to CL(P) since the LNPs would have to come further medially in order to make contact. On the other hand, the widely spaced MNPs of the C57Bl/6J strain may be responsible for its predisposition to induced median clefts. (From Meller, S. M., and Waterman, R. E.: Congenital craniofacial anomalies. *In* Shaw, J. H., Sweeney, E. A., Cappuccino, C. C., and Meller, S. M. (Eds.): Textbook of Oral Biology. Philadelphia, W. B. Saunders Company, 1978, as adapted from Trasler, 1968.)

ple there is noted underdevelopment of MNP derivatives, a high incidence of class III malocclusion (deficient maxillary components), and an incidence of cleft lip that is double that of Caucasians. Infants born with arhinencephaly (missing premaxillary segments) and a moderately severe degree of holoprosencephaly resemble Orientals in overall facial appearances. At the opposite end of the spectrum are blacks, who have broad and well-developed MNP derivatives and an incidence of CL(P) that is one-half that of Caucasians and one-quarter that of Orientals.

As noted above, the twin studies have shown that many of the unaffected twins of MZ pairs discordant for CL(P) have nasal cavity widths within the normal range. It is probable that they have a wide variety of other types of problems. Another type of developmental alteration predisposing to CL(P) was observed in CL/Fr mice (Millicovsky, Ambrose, and Johnston, 1982). In normal primary palate development there is a great deal of epithelial activity between the MNP and LNP as they approach one another (Fig. 48–16*A*) (Millicovsky and Johnston, 1981a). This may help to bring the prominences together and/or promote adhesion once contact is achieved. The CL/Fr strain was developed by Fraser (1967) by crossing A/J mice with

another strain carrying a mutant gene that gave rise to a condition termed "migratory spot lesion of the retina." In offspring produced by the cross there was a higher incidence of CL(P) than in the A/J mice, and after backcrossing and selection for CL(P) the incidence reached a high level (36 per cent in the authors' laboratory versus 0 to 7 per cent in the A/Js). Presumably the mutant gene is responsible for the fact that the epithelial activity is absent, or virtually absent, in CL/ Fr embryos (Fig. 48–16*B*). Although the A/J embryo has apparent problems with facial prominence growth direction, the above activity is normal. Thus, it appears that the CL/ Fr mouse has at least two major genes predisposing to CL(P). Since they both work against prominence contact, their combined effects presumably account for the high incidence of CL(P) in this mouse strain. Clefts similar to the incomplete clefts illustrated in Figure 48–14 are also seen in A/J embryos and do not seem to be related to the problems of epithelial activity. Presumably many other abnormal genes affect primary palate development. It must be hoped that only a few will account for the genetic predisposition in most nonsyndromic CL(P) cases.

Environmental Factors. The number of known environmental factors affecting CL(P)

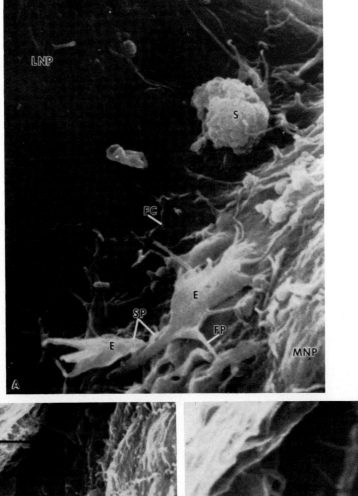

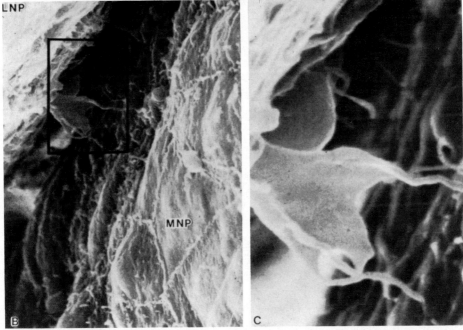

Figure 48–16. Epithelial activity may assist in bringing the facial prominences together. *A,* Epithelial activity is first seen in the epithelia between the approaching LNPs and MNPs in the area approximating that under the square in Figure 48–8C. Various cell processes extend from one prominence to the other, including the edges of flattened cells (FC), secondary projections (SP) with enlargements (E), and filopodia (FP). Spheroidal particles (S) and other apparent cell debris are believed to be derived from sloughed surface peridermal cells. (From Millicovsky, G., and Johnston, M. C.: Active role of embryonic facial epithelium: new evidence of cellular events in morphogenesis. J. Embryol. Exp. Morphol., *65*:153, 1981. By permission of Company of Biologists Ltd.) *B,* The above activity is almost entirely absent in CL/Fr strain mouse embryos and this may account for their much higher spontaneous cleft lip incidence compared with the A/J strain. Intact peridermal cells with junctional microvilli are observed (MNP label is over such a cell in *B*). Occasionally, individual cell processes are seen apparently attempting to bridge the gap (*B, C*). (From Millicovsky, G., Ambrose, J. L., and Johnston, M. C.: Developmental alterations associated with spontaneous cleft lip and palate in CL/Fr mice. Am. J. Anat., *164*:129, 1982.)

formation is increasing at a modest rate. As discussed later, even if much less important than genetic factors, they are the factors that can be manipulated and that therefore offer hope of prevention. The environmental factors considered below are selected primarily because there is evidence of their relevance to CL(P) in humans, and because animal experiments have provided information on how they alter development.

Environmental factors that inhibit the electron transport chain (and consequent ATP production) are potent inducers of CL(P) in mammals and comparable clefts in the chick embryo (Fig. 48–17). Electrons mostly enter the chain via the NAD⁺–NADH dehydrogenase enzyme complex, and as they travel down the chain to progressively lower energy states, ATP is generated. Oxygen is the final acceptor of the electrons. Of the environmental factors affecting the NADH dehydrogenase complex, 6-aminonicotin-amide (6-AN) has been the most extensively studied (Pinsky and Fraser, 1959; Landauer and Sopher, 1970; Trasler, Reardon, and Rajchgot, 1978; Trasler and Ohannessian, 1983). Where studied, the effects on development appear to be consistent with those resulting from hypoxia (see below). An interesting observation was provided by the experiments of Landauer and Sopher (1970) in which they bypassed the 6-AN–induced block at the NADH dehydrogenase complex through the use of a high energy intermediate such as ascorbate (vitamin C) that donates the electron farther down the chain beyond the block. The incidence of 6-AN–induced clefts was dramatically decreased. There is some evidence that phenytoin (Dilantin), a potent inducer of CL(P) (see below), may exert some of its teratogenic activity at the NADH dehydrogenase level (Fig. 17) (Mackler and associates, 1975).

Factors operating at the other end of the

Site of Action of Teratogens in Electron Transport

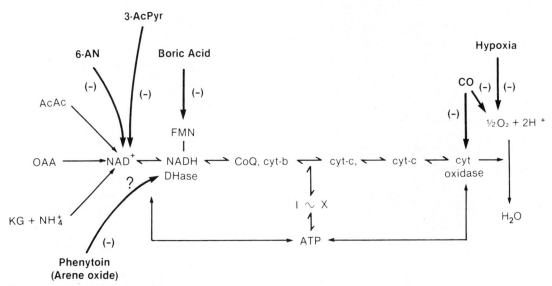

Figure 48–17. Teratogens that block ATP production by interference with electron transport. Nicotinic acid analogues (6-AN) and 3-acetyl-pyridine (3-AcPyr) block electron transport (−) by interfering with NAD+ function. Boric acid, and possibly phenytoin via its arene oxide intermediates, block electron transport (−) by binding to NADH dehydrogenase. Carbon monoxide (CO) blocks electron transport (−) by inhibiting cytochrome oxidase, and also decreases the oxygen supply to tissues by preventing the binding of oxygen to hemoglobin and the release of oxygen from oxyhemoglobin. Hypoxia blocks electron transport (−) because of the decreased amount of oxygen available to act as the final electron acceptor in this chain of reactions. AcAc = acetoacetate; ATP = adenosine triphosphate; CoQ = cooenzyme Q (ubiquinone); cyt = cytochrome; I and X denote hypothetical energy-transfer carriers; KG = ketoglutarate; NAD+ = nicotinamide adenine dinucleotide oxidized; OAA = oxaloacetate; 6-AN = 6-aminonicotinamide; 3-ACPyr, 3 acetyl-pyridine; CO = carbon monoxide; FMN = flavin mononucleotide. (From Bronsky, P. T.: Effects of hypoxia on facial prominence development in CL/Fr mice. M.S. Thesis, University of North Carolina, 1985.)

chain impeding the flow of electrons include hypoxia and carbon monoxide (CO). Although its action is complex, it appears that most of the teratogenic effect of CO is also through embryonic tissue hypoxia. The relevant human factor is cigarette smoking, which appears to double the incidence of CL(P) (Erickson, Kallen, and Westerholm, 1979; Khoury and associates, 1987). The administration of CO at roughly the same level as that in cigarette smoke (180 ppm) to pregnant A/J mice also roughly doubles the incidence of CL(P) (Bailey and Johnston, 1988). Maternal respiratory hypoxia (10 per cent O_2 vs roughly 22 per cent in air) dramatically increases the incidence of CL(P) in both CL/Fr (Millicovsky and Johnston, 1981b; Bronsky, Johnston, and Sulik, 1986) and A/J mice (Bailey and Johnston, 1988). Although there have been anecdotal reports of increased CL(P) in children born to mothers living at high altitude (the 12,000 foot level, approximately equivalent to 10 per cent O_2, or higher), no controlled studies have been conducted.

By the time that the primary palate begins to develop in the mouse, the chorioallantoic placenta is functioning and the embryo's requirements for oxygen (in whole embryo culture) have risen dramatically.

Although the mechanism of neural tube closure is similar to that of olfactory placodal morphogenesis, almost all the ATP is generated by anaerobic glycolysis at this earlier time, as opposed to only about 45 per cent at the time of primary palate development (Hunter and Sadler, in press). Moreover, the embryo's requirements for oxygen in whole embryo culture are low. Such differences in oxygen requirements in humans may explain why there is neither an apparent relation betweeen cigarette smoking and neural tube closure defects (anencephaly and spina bifida) nor even anecdotal reports linking neural tube defects to altitude.

The pathogenesis of hypoxia-induced CL(P) has been extensively studied (Bronsky, Johnston, and Sulik, 1986; Bronsky and associates, submitted, 1989; Bronsky and Johnston, in preparation; Bronsky and associates, unpublished). The most vulnerable aspect of craniofacial development related to hypoxia appears to be the morphogenetic movements described earlier (Fig. 48–18). As illustrated, the principal movements affected are the curling forward of the lateral portion of the olfactory placode, the bringing together of the MNPs in the midline (apparently mediated

primarily by forebrain invagination), and the lateral flexure of the distal portion of the MNP (see Fig. 48–9, open arrow in 36S embryo, and Fig. 48–12C, F). A large amount of cell death is associated with the inhibition of lateral olfactory placodal morphogenesis (Figs. 48–19, 48–20) owing to apparent uncoupling of the terminal web contraction. Edema and minor hemorrhage may also play a role (Grabowski, 1970); however, the authors were unable to find much supporting evidence.

Another CL(P)-inducing environmental factor in which the pathogenesis has been studied is the anticonvulsant drug phenytoin (Dilantin). The incidence of CL(P) in the children of epileptic mothers receiving phenytoin appears to be approximately ten times that in controls. After treatment of pregnant A/J mice with phenytoin, the overall growth of the embryo, including the facial prominences, is reduced (Fig. 48–21) (Sulik and associates, 1979), as reflected by a reduction in the rate of mesenchymal cell proliferation in facial prominences to approximately 50 per cent that of controls (Hicks, Johnston, and Banes, 1983). The LNP is much more severely affected (Fig. 48–21D), a finding possibly reflecting interference with oxidative metabolism (see Fig. 48–17), reduced placodal morphogenetic movements, and/or a phenytoin-induced reduction of the epithelial activity between the facial prominences (see Fig. 48–16A). The latter is a developmental alteration similar to that occurring spontaneously in CL/Fr mice (Millicovsky, unpublished). As noted in the section on normal primary palate development, it is known from tissue culture studies of facial prominences that a covering epithelium is necessary for the maintenance of the underlying mesenchyme.

It was also noted that growth of the mesenchyme may normally be regulated by epithelial serotonin via the mesenchymal cell process meshwork, which presumably contains the serotonin binding protein found in that area (Lauder, Tannir, and Sadler, 1988). The anticonvulsant drugs are thought to function therapeutically through interference with neurotransmitters, and it is possible that at least part of their teratogenic activity may result from interference with neurotransmitter regulation of development.

Although not well documented, there appears to be a high incidence of CL(P) associated with prenatal ethanol (alcohol) exposure (Jones and associates, 1974). In most cases,

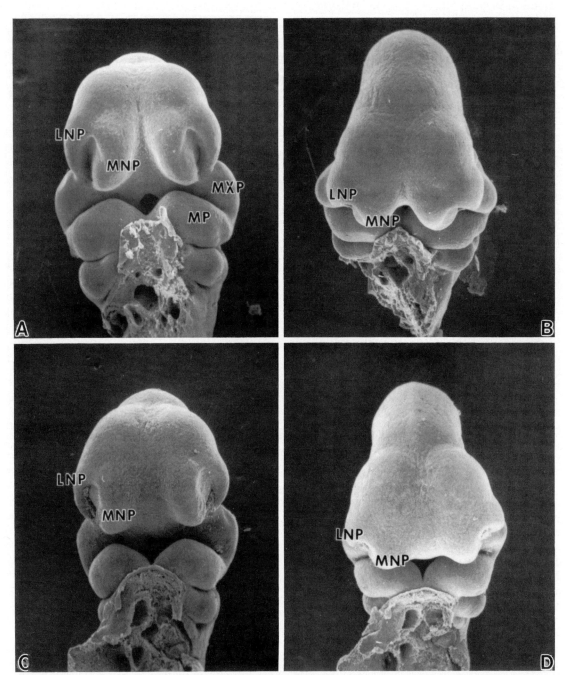

Figure 48–18. Scanning electron micrographs of 36 somite normoxic (*A,B*) and hypoxic (*C,D*) embryos. Overall retardation of morphogenetic movements is seen in the hypoxic embryo compared with the normoxic embryo. Note the wide separation between the MNPs and the smaller sized LNPs (related to retarded placodal morphogenesis) in the hypoxic embryo compared to the normoxic embryo. (From Bronsky, P. T.: Effects of hypoxia on facial prominence development in CL/Fr mice. M.S. Thesis, University of North Carolina, 1985.)

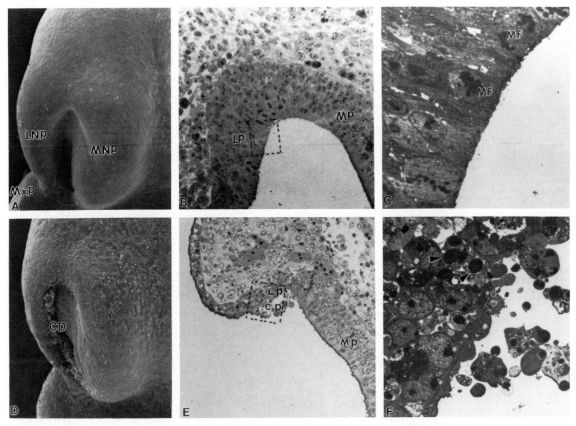

Figure 48–19. Combined scanning electron micrograph (EM), light microscopy, and transmission EM of the right side of the same primary palates of 36 somite control (*top panel*) and hypoxic (*bottom panel*) mouse embryos. Section planes are illustrated in *A* and *D*. The transmission EMs are from the region indicated by the boxes in *B* and *E*. The debris in the deepest portion of the olfactory pit in *D* is shown to be cellular in nature in *E* and *F*. Pyknotic bodies (*arrowheads* in *F*) are seen throughout the lateral placode, completely disrupting the terminal web system. The medial placode (MP in *E*), which has not begun its morphogenetic movements at this time, is intact. (From Bronsky, P. T., Johnston, M. C., Moore, N. B., Dehart, D. B., and Sulik, K. K.: Lateral nasal placodal morphogenesis in mice: normal development and alterations leading to hypoxia-induced cleft lip. Submitted.)

it is associated with fairly typical fetal alcohol syndrome (FAS), features suggesting that it may result from the same basic defect (i.e., closely set olfactory placodes and small MNPs), as suggested for trisomy 13. This idea was supported by the small premaxillary segments of bilaterally clefted trisomy 13 cases, and it would be interesting to examine these segments in bilateral CL(P) FAS cases. It should be pointed out that CL(P) was not observed in the CL(P)-resistant C57BL/6J FAS model (Sulik, Johnston, and Webb, 1981; Sulik and Johnston, 1983). The CL(P)-sensitive A/J has not been tested at the FAS-sensitive stage. There is a moderate increase in CL(P) when pregnant A/Js are treated at the time of primary palate formation (Sanzone, unpublished).

A great deal of interest is currently being generated about the possible use of vitamins

in CL(P) prevention. Although studies in vitamin supplements related to CL(P) prevention actually predated those related to neural tube defects (NTDs) (Briggs, 1976), the work on NTDs has progressed much more rapidly and there is now overwhelming evidence that the recurrence rates for NTDs (Lawrence, 1984) can be drastically reduced by such supplements.

In theory, one would expect such supplements to be more effective for NTD prevention than for CL(P) prevention, since there is evidence of a much greater role for environmental factors in NTDs. For example, the incidence of NTDs is much higher in wet climates than in dry climates, even when the genetic background is the same. There has also been a fairly steady drop in NTDs over time, an observation that correlates with overall improvement in nutrition. There is

Normoxia   **Hypoxia**

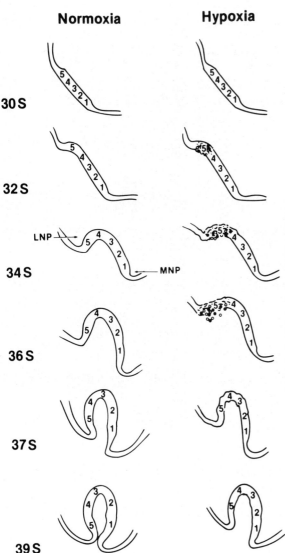

30 S

32 S

LNP

34 S   MNP

36 S

37 S

39 S

Figure 48–20. Comparison of nasal placodal morphogenesis of normoxic and hypoxic embryos between 30 and 39 somites in developmental age (section plane *B* in Fig. 48–9). Different mediolateral points in the placodes are designated by number in order to show the shift in position related to the curling forward of the lateral portion of the placode. Between 36 and 37 somites in the hypoxic embryos, cell debris (compare with Fig. 48–19*E,F*) is sloughed and the placode begins to reorganize. In almost all hypoxic embryos the reorganization occurs too late for the attainment of contact and fusion. (From Bronsky, P. T., Johnston, M. C., Moore, N. B., Dehart, D. B., and Sulik, K. K.: Lateral nasal placodal morphogenesis in mice: normal development and alterations leading to hypoxia-induced cleft lip. Submitted.)

now some evidence that the incidence of CL(P) in Oriental individuals living in the United States is beginning to decrease (Tyan, 1982), presumably because of dietary improvements.

Little is known about the optimal levels of vitamins in pregnancy. There is evidence that deficiencies of key vitamins such as folic acid, which is involved in nucleotide (DNA and RNA) synthesis and thus critical for cell proliferation, can cause CL(P) experimentally (Asling, 1961). Folate supplements alone may also reduce the incidence of NTDs in humans (Lawrence, 1984). There is a general feeling that it is difficult to exceed an upper limit of tolerance for water-soluble vitamins (e.g., folic acid and vitamin C) in that excess amounts are easily eliminated through the

kidneys. However, a number of side effects have been noted (Pauling, 1976). Blood levels for folate may reach five times those of controls in pregnant women being supplemented with this vitamin for NTD prevention (Lawrence, 1984). On the other hand, vitamin A, a fat-soluble vitamin that is difficult to clear, may be teratogenic at high levels (Cohlan, 1953).

The first major study in the use of vitamins for the prevention of cleft lip was reported by Briggs in 1976. This was a multicenter study in which some pregnancies following the birth of a child with CL(P) or CP were supplemented with high levels of folate and vitamin B_6 and moderately high levels of other vitamins (Stresstabs). Vitamin A was not included. The incidence of CL(P) in the sup-

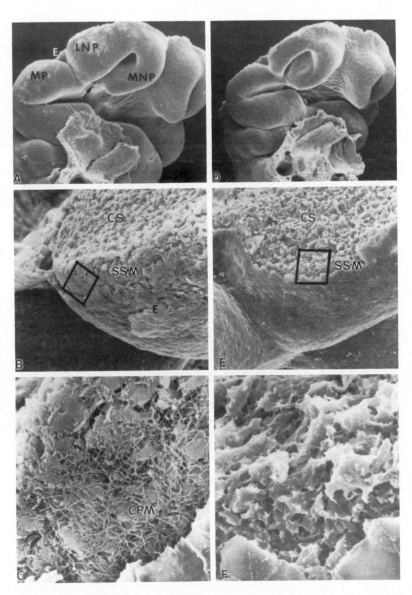

Figure 48–21. Scanning electron micrographs (EMs) of embryos removed from control and phenytoin-treated A/J mice. The embryos have been sectioned through the eye, which serves for orientation. Although all the facial prominences of the embryo (D) from the treated mother have been reduced in size compared with the control embryo (A), the LNP is much more severely affected. The specimens are tilted in the remaining photomicrographs to reveal the cut surfaces (CS) and the areas of the subsurface mesenchyme (SSM) where the covering epithelium has pulled away (B,E). Examination at higher magnification (C,F) of the area indicated in B and E reveals that the mesenchymal cell process meshwork (CPM) that normally underlies the epithelium in the control (C) is essentially absent in the embryo from the treated mother. (Adapted from Sulik, K. K., Johnston, M. C., Ambrose, L. J. H., and Dorgan, D.: Phenytoin (Dilantin)-induced cleft lip: a scanning and transmission electron microscopic study. Anat. Rec., 195:243–256, 1979.)

plemented group was one-third that of the nonsupplemented group (borderline statistical significance). A second study of similar design was reported by Tolarova (1982, 1987), in which the incidence of clefting was reduced to two-fifths that of the controls. An unpublished study in Britain apparently had similar success (Ferguson, 1988). Finally, a study currently being conducted at the Centers for Disease Control (CDC) indicates that ordinary vitamin supplements can reduce the clefting incidence by more than 20 per cent (Erickson, 1989). The long-range picture for such methods is further discussed below.

There are many drugs and other environmental factors that appear to predispose to CL(P). It is expected that their identification will eventually lead to substantial progress in cleft prevention.

Gene-Environment Interactions. A number of gene-environment interactions have already been discussed. Use of the CL/Fr mouse in hypoxia studies provides an example in which there appear to be two major genes affecting primary palate development. In Figure 48–22 the embryo depicted in A has a normally fusing primary palate, while bilateral spontaneous clefts have formed in B. An environmental factor (hypoxia) was added for the embryo in C and this presumably contributed to the development of its clefts. Although histologic exam-

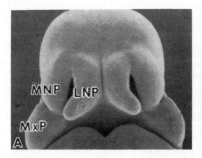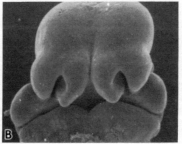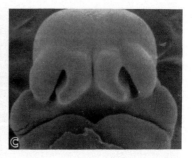

Figure 48–22. Normal development of the primary palate of a CL/Fr mouse is depicted in *A*. The spontaneous cleft in the CL/Fr embryo in *B* is similar to the cleft associated with hypoxia in the CL/Fr embryo in *C*. Both show similar size reductions and changes in growth direction. (From Bronsky, P. T.: Effects of hypoxia on facial prominence development in CL/Fr mice. M.S. Thesis, University of North Carolina, 1985.)

ination of the embryo in *C* would probably demonstrate decreased thickness of the lateral olfactory placode, the remarkable feature is its similarity to the embryo in *B*. Some of the differences between the cleft and the noncleft embryos (e.g., the short "globular" prominences) may be secondary to the clefting.

There is considerable evidence that most cases of human CL(P) have multifactorial causes as in the above example. Perhaps the most important evidence is that relatives of CL(P) patients who have similar percentages of genes in common (e.g., both siblings and offspring would have 50 per cent of their genes in common with the cleft case) should show the same recurrence rates (incidence). For CL(P) this appears to be the case, the recurrence rate being about 4 to 5 per cent for both siblings and offspring. If a single major recessive gene were involved, the recurrence rates in the offspring would be expected to be roughly twice the recurrence

rates in siblings. If a single dominant gene were involved, half the offspring and siblings would have the gene, and one would expect to see greater decreases in nasal cavity width in studies (Kurisu and associates, 1974) in which this dimension was measured in children and siblings of CL(P) patients. Infinite numbers of genes could be involved, but it seems more likely that there are probably only a few (perhaps 2 to 4) with major impact in each individual case, such as in the CL/Fr example above (Carter, 1977).

The multifactorial threshold model depicted in Figure 48–23 is useful. It shows a theoretical distribution of the genetic and environmental factors for a particular abnormality [e.g., CL(P)] in the general population. The sum of these factors determines the liability of each individual for the abnormalities in that population. If the liability for that individual crosses a threshold (failure of the prominences to contact), the abnormality [CL(P)] would be expressed. For "rare" ab-

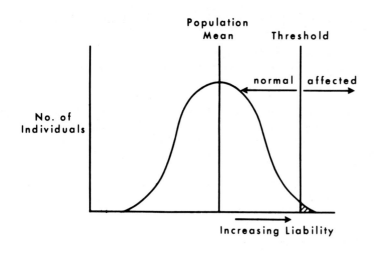

Figure 48–23. The multifactorial threshold concept developed by Falconer and Carter. It illustrates a population of individuals following the normal population curve with liability for a particular disease, such as cleft lip, increasing to the right. With individuals having increasing liability due to combinations of genetic and environmental factors predisposing to cleft lip, a threshold (complete or partial failure of contact and fusion of the facial prominences for cleft lip) is eventually exceeded beyond which normal development is no longer possible, and clefting results. Embryos with CL(P) cannot be far over the threshold, and minor improvements in the pregnancy should bring substantial numbers back to the normal side of the threshold. (From Ross, R. B., and Johnston, M. C.: Cleft Lip and Palate. Baltimore, Williams & Wilkins Company, 1982. Copyright 1982, Williams & Wilkins Company.)

normalities, the area under the curve (which indicates the number of individuals) beyond the threshold is small. It is virtually impossible to be far beyond (to the right of) the threshold. Thus, the facial prominences of individuals with CL(P) would have barely missed making contact, and slight improvements in the conditions affecting the pregnancy (e.g., elimination of cigarette smoking or the use of vitamin supplements) could substantially improve the chances of contact and prevent an appreciable number of clefts from occurring. The fact that so many clefts are incomplete (when contact is insufficient for complete fusion) indicates that a large number of embryos are sitting squarely on the threshold.

The multifactorial threshold model also helps in the interpretation of the high discordance rate (53 per cent) for CL(P) in MZ twins (Falconer, 1965). As noted earlier, a twin study (Johnston and associates, in preparation) suggests that in many such pairs of twins, abnormal genes would have placed the contact portions of the MNPs so far medially that the LNP and maxillary prominences would have difficulty in making contact. Because of the genetic factors (and shared environmental factors), the embryos would be virtually sitting on the threshold (Fig. 48–23), and minor differences in the environments of the two embryos would place some of them on the normal side of the threshold (contact and no cleft) and others on the abnormal side (contact failure and a cleft).

There is considerable evidence of an association between CL(P) and excess embryonic death. The high incidence at early stages of pregnancy, as seen in electively aborted embryos (Nishimura and associates, 1966), may largely be attributed to syndromic clefts (Ross and Johnston, 1972), including chromosomally abnormal embryos. However, there are peculiarities in the sex ratios of the remaining siblings (Niswander and associates, 1972; Dronamraju and Bixler, 1983) that suggest that the effects of the abnormal genetic and environmental factors predisposing to CL(P) may sometimes be lethal.

A peculiar association between CL(P) and atrial septal defects is worth noting. This includes an observation by Fraser and Rosen (1974) that spontaneous CL(P) in A/J newborns is always associated with retarded development of the interatrial septum. Fasel (1981) has also shown that the phenytoin treatment that induces CL(P) in A/J mice

also causes atrial septal defects. In both cases, there seems to be the possibility of a causal relationship, with a circulatory disturbance predisposing to CL(P). Arguing against the possibility that the atrial septal defect may also be lethal in some cases is the low resorption rate associated with high phenytoin treatment doses (Johnston, Sulik, and Dudley, 1978). Finally, it should be noted that there may be a modest elevation in atrial septal defects in patients with CL(P).

Syndromic CL(P)

At birth, in approximately 14 per cent of CL(P) patients, CL(P) is part of a syndrome (Ross and Johnston, 1972). As discussed below, this is a much lower percentage than for CP.

Chromosomal Anomalies. Most of the syndromic CL(P) cases at birth are trisomic, and almost all of these die within the first year or two of life. Trisomy 13 has been discussed in relation to the holoprosencephaly. CL(P) incidence is also elevated in trisomy 21 (Down syndrome), which, like trisomy 13, involves underdevelopment of the MNP derivatives, with affected individuals resembling Orientals in facial appearance as indicated by its former name (mongolism).

Waardenburg's Syndrome. In perhaps 1 per cent of CL(P) patients at birth, the cleft is associated with Waardenburg's syndrome in which the incidence of CL(P) is approximately 7 per cent. The primary problem in this syndrome is abnormal development of neural crest cells, judging from the defects of crest derivatives in animal models (e.g., Dancer mutant in the mouse). Defects include abnormalities (patchy absence) of pigmentation in the hair, iris, and skin. There are abnormalities of the inner ear (deafness in humans and abnormal vestibular function in animal models). Studies of ear development in animal models demonstrate an associated absence of pigment cells (Deol, 1970) whose function is unknown. Studies on the Dancer mutant show underdevelopment of the initial (crest) facial nerve ganglion (Deol, 1970; Trasler, 1968) and decreased proliferation of crest cells (Trasler and Leong, 1982). One possible explanation for the patchy loss of pigment cells is the absence of progenitor cell populations.

Van Der Woude's Syndrome. Van der Woude's (1954) syndrome, an autosomal recessive condition, constitutes virtually the only example in which CL(P)s are mixed with CPs. Lip pits are caused by abnormal salivary glands, which are often found and may be the only abnormality. Less than 1 per cent of all cases of CL(P) are in this category. One suggestion concerning the pathogenesis of the developmental abnormality is failure of regression of the fusion epithelia.

Other Syndromes. CL(P) is also a component of many other syndromes (Gorlin, Pindborg, and Cohen, 1976). Although individually unimportant (see Chap. 46), they provide insights into the variety of developmental abnormalities that lead to CL(P).

Rare Clefts of the Primary Palate

A section in Chapter 46 deals with the embryogenesis of rare facial clefts. However, because normal morphogenetic movements are dealt with in this chapter and because of their possible relevance to some types of median facial "clefts," these types of clefts will also be considered here. Oblique facial clefts will also be briefly discussed. The clinical aspects of rare craniofacial clefts are discussed in Chapter 59.

Medial Facial Clefts/Orbital Hypertelorism. The face begins its development as two essentially independent halves (see Figs. 48–6, 48–8, and 48–9). Neural crest cells migrating into the face never cross the midline, apparently blocked by acellular connective tissue membranes (Johnston and associates, 1979). In later development the upper portions of the MNPs appear to be drawn together, at least partly, by forebrain invagination (see Fig. 48–9) (Smuts, 1981; Bronsky and associates, submitted). Medial growth of the MNPs obviously contributes to the midline coalescence. The visceral arches also grow from the two sides to coalesce (merge) in the midline (see Fig. 48–6).

Failure of the two halves of the upper and middle face to reach their normal relations to the midline results in a wide variety of facial malformations. In orbital hypertelorism, unusually wide but normal tissues may be found between the orbits (Greig, 1924; Converse and associates, 1974). In other cases, abnormal tissue may be found between such widely separated orbits (Converse and associates, 1974), suggesting the possibility that the tissues prevented midline approximation. A more common situation is that

found in "frontonasal dysplasia" (Fig. 48–24A) (Sedano, Jirasek, and Gorlin, 1970) where the only tissues between widely separated facial halves are skin and underlying meninges. These latter malformations might be more appropriately termed "medial facial clefts." Another variation is midline facial clefts involving only the lip or extending into the nose and higher facial structures (Fig. 48–24B) (Iregbulem, 1978, 1982). Some clefts in the latter studies were associated with only minor increases in facial width.

Midline clefts can be experimentally produced by a wide variety of procedures. Burk and Sadler (1983) used 6-diazo-5-oxo-L-norleucine (DON), a drug that interferes with nucleotide (DNA and RNA) and glycoprotein synthesis in mice. Excessive cell death in the MNPs was found. Darab and associates (1987) used the antifolate drug methotrexate, and the developmental alterations were associated with midline hemorrhage. Another drug, 6-aminonicotinamide (6-AN), also produces midline clefts when used on day 9 in C57BL/6J mice, and lateral (typical) clefts when used a day later at the beginning of primary palate formation (Trasler, Reardon, and Rajchgot, 1978). Reductions in mitotic indices were reported (Trasler and Leong, 1982). All the above clefts seem to involve little increase in facial width at later (fetal) stages of development. Bronsky, Johnston, and Sulik (1986) observed greatly increased width between MNPs in mouse embryos with maternal hypoxia treatments designed to produce CL(P) in CL/Fr mice (see Fig. 48–18), but have neither followed them into late stages of development nor looked for increases in interorbital width. Possibly, treatment one day earlier of C57BL/6J mice, which already have increased separation of their MNPs (see Fig. 48–15) (Trasler, Reardon, and Rajchgot, 1978), might be effective in producing increased interorbital width in association with medial facial clefts.

Oblique Facial Clefts. These are rare facial clefts resulting from lack of fusion between the LNPs and MxPs. Fusion of these prominences is similar to fusion of the MNP with the LNP and MxP. The earliest epithelia to make contact become buried in the cleft of an epithelial seam, a finding not unlike the situation between the MNP and the LNP and MxP. This too persists, eventually hollowing out to form the epithelial lining of the lacrimal duct. The more superficial epithelium breaks down, followed by mesenchymal pen-

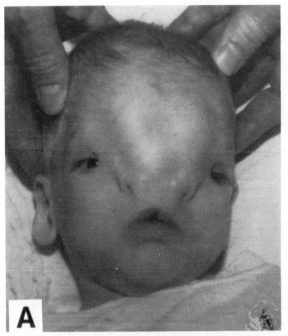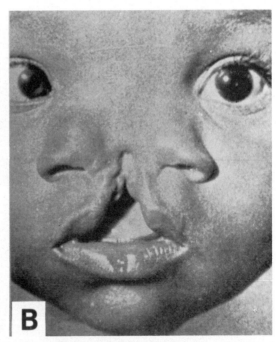

Figure 48–24. Median facial clefts and orbital hypertelorism. These defects (split face, orbital hypertelorism, frontonasal dysplasia) result from failure of the two facial halves to unite in the midline. On occasion, the cleft involves the skin (*A*) and sometimes it involves only structures deep to the skin (*B*). In the patient in *A* the major site of clefting is high, while that in the patient in *B* is low at the vermilion border of the lip. Most experimentally induced median clefts are similar to that shown in *A*. (*A* from Iregbulem, L. M.: Midline clefts of the upper lip. Br. J. Plast. Surg., *31*:63, 1978; *B* from Sedano, H., Cohen, M. M., Jirasek, J., and Gorlin, R. J.: Frontonasal dysplasia. Pediatrics *76*:906, 1970.)

etration. Apart from the fact that oblique facial clefts are sometimes associated with amniotic bands, virtually nothing is known about their embryogenesis.

NORMAL DEVELOPMENT OF SECONDARY PALATE

Experimental (animal) research on both normal development of the secondary palate and on cleft palate (CP) formation has been much more extensive than animal research on primary palate development and cleft lip [CL(P)] formation. Consequently, more is known about the embryogenesis of the secondary palate and developmental alterations leading to CP. In contrast, less research has been conducted on the genetics and development of human CP.

The initial stages of secondary palate formation are illustrated in Figure 48–25. Primary palate development has been completed and the secondary palatal shelves are beginning to form on the medial aspects of the maxillary processes. Before these stages, an

inductive epithelial-mesenchymal interaction has already specified many of the later characteristics of the developing secondary palate (Tyler and Koch, 1974).

As the shelves grow medially, they encounter the tongue and are deflected downward (Fig. 48–26*A*, *C*, *E*). The growth of the shelves is apparently regulated by an epithelial-mesenchymal interaction at the shelf edges, perhaps not unlike that taking place at the end of the limb bud where the apical ectodermal ridge epithelium interacts with the underlying mesenchyme (the so-called "progress zone").

When the shelves have reached a size sufficient for contact after elevation, they begin the process of reorientation. In the hard palate region they appear to hinge upward, while in the posterior region they apparently undergo a remodeling process (Fig. 48–26). The shelves undergo the reorientation phenomenon if the tongue is experimentally removed (Walker and Quarles, 1973). The nature of the "intrinsic shelf force" is unknown. Evidence has been put forward for concerted contraction of mesenchyme cells (Zimmerman and Wee, 1984) and for selective hydration of

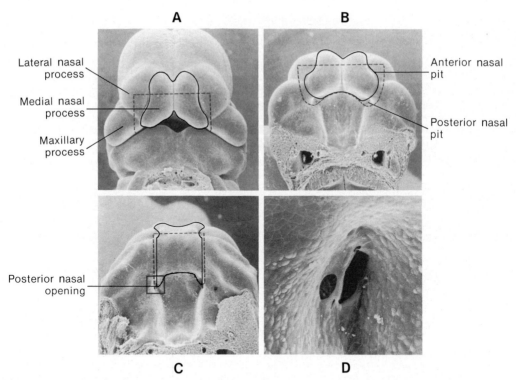

Figure 48–25. Upper midfacial development of mouse embryos at the end of primary palate formation and the beginning of secondary palate formation. *A* to *C,* The intermaxillary segment is outlined by solid lines and the primary palate by broken lines. *B, C,* The palatal shelves are beginning to grow from the medial aspect of the maxillary prominences. *C, D,* The "hollowing out" or stretching and disruption of the epithelial connection between the base of the nasal pit and the roof of the primitive oral cavity has reached an advanced stage in the older specimen. (From Johnston, M. C., and Sulik, K. K.: Embryology of the head and neck. *In* Serafin, D, and Georgiade, N. G. (Eds.): Pediatric Plastic Surgery. St. Louis, MO, C. V. Mosby Company, 1984, pp. 184–215.)

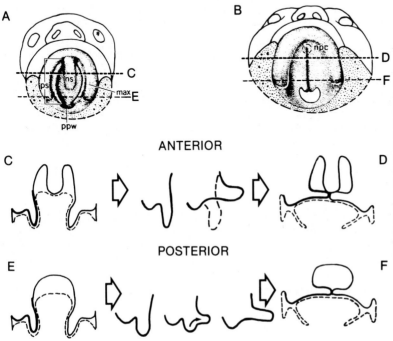

Figure 48–26. *A* to *F,* Secondary palatal shelf elevation in human embryos. It appears that shelf elevation is somewhat different in the anterior (hard palate) and posterior (soft palate) regions, as is the case also in rodent embryos. Shelf elevation in the posterior region appears to involve a remodeling process. ns = nasal septum; ps = palatal shelf; max = maxillary alveolus; ppw = posterior pharyngeal wall; npc = region of the nasopalatine canal. (Modified from Johnston, M. C., et al: The embryology of cleft lip and cleft palate. Clin. Plast. Surg., 2:195, 1975.)

extracellular matrix components (Brinkley and Morris-Wiman, 1984).

The factors involving removal of the tongue from between the shelves have also been extensively studied. The tongue is attached to the anterior end of the mandible and rapid mandibular growth may assist in bringing the tongue down and forward from between the shelves (Diewert, 1980). In addition mouth-opening movements (Walker, 1969; Humphrey, 1969) and possibly even tongue movements appear to be involved.

The shelf edge epithelium undergoes a sequence of developmental alterations that begin even before contact is made. Unlike the other covering epithelia that differentiate into mucus-secreting (nasal surface) and keratinizing (oral surface) epithelia, the shelf edge epithelia cease proliferation and undergo partial breakdown and other changes. The covering peridermal cells are sloughed (Fig. 48–27) (Waterman and Meller, 1974). The underlying cells become active in the contact and adhesion through extended cell processes and the production of adhesive glycoproteins. Desmosomes form rapidly between the contacting epithelial cells (Waterman and Meller, 1974) to complete the adhesion.

The events of further development of the epithelial seam are less clear. There appears to be at least some additional cell death but it is possible that the pyknotic elements may simply be trapped debris. In any case, the seam fragments, with at least some individual epithelial cells, apparently undergo transformation to connective tissue cells, principally fibroblasts (Fitchette and Hay, 1988). Mesenchyme consolidates the union and palatal bone formation is initiated at approximately the same time.

The above sequence of changes in the epithelium goes on whether or not contact is made. This is shown by A/J mouse palatal shelves that remain vertical after primary palatal clefting (Smiley, Vanek, and Dixon, 1971) and by shelves grown in culture (Pourtois, 1972; Ferguson and Honig, 1984). The responsibility for the programming apparently resides in the mesenchyme, as shown by reciprocal recombinations of epithelia and mesenchyme from the palatal shelves of mouse and chick embryos grown in culture (Koch and Smiley, 1981; Ferguson and Honig, 1984).

Information regarding the biochemical controls regulating the epithelial events is also accumulating. For example, the cessation of proliferation in the epithelium is regulated through cyclic AMP (Pratt and Martin, 1975), which is produced by the mesenchyme (Greene and associates, in press).

Not only does the soft palate region of the secondary palate horizontalize by a different mechanism (remodeling) than the more anterior portion, but it also consolidates in the midline by merging rather than fusion (Burdi and Faist, 1967; Russell, 1987). Sexual differences in the timing of shelf elevation will be considered later in relation to CP formation.

EMBRYOGENESIS OF CLEFT PALATE (CP)

As with CL(P), there are major subtypes of CP, a relatively high number of human CPs being of the syndromic variety (i.e., as components of a syndrome). Animal models are available for many of the syndromic clefts, but the suitability of animal models for nonsyndromic clefts is more open to question. Studies of twins and single birth CPs are beginning to show some insight regarding heterogeneity in nonsyndromic clefts.

As seen below, syndromic CPs occasionally show distinctive cleft morphology (e.g., the posterior wide clefts of the Treacher Collins syndrome and the wide "horseshoe" clefts of the Pierre Robin sequence). The increased incidence of submucous CPs (deficient bone and muscle in the midline) and bifid uvulas in families with CP (Meskin, Gorlin, and Isaacson, 1965; Niswander, 1968) indicates that at least some of these abnormalities are microforms of CP.

CPs can be produced experimentally in a variety of ways: (1) through interference with shelf elevation (as in corticosteroid-induced CP) (Diewert and Pratt, 1981); or (2) through amniotic sac puncture (Poswillo, 1966) and interference with palatal shelf growth, either directly (as in retinol-induced CP) (Shah, 1984) or by earlier interference with maxillary prominence development as in retinoic acid–induced CP (Sulik and associates, 1987, 1988). In dioxin-induced CP (Dencker and Pratt, 1981) and other types of induced CP (Goldman and associates, in press), the shelves make contact and pull apart. As seen below, with the possible exception of the last mechanism, these may be the more common mechanisms for human CP formation, but the variety is probably much greater.

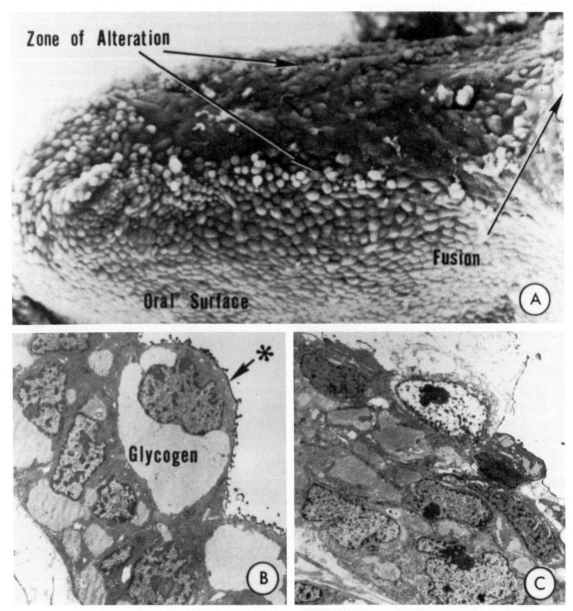

Figure 48–27. Scanning and transmission electron micrographs of the human palatal shelf before the time of contact and fusion. The area marked Zone of Alteration will eventually make contact with and adhere to a similar epithelium on the opposite palatal shelf. The transmission electron micrographs in *B* and *C* are made by embedding and sectioning the specimen shown in *A*. The heavy metal coating (necessary for scanning electron microscopy) over the specimen is indicated by the asterisk over the glycogen-containing cell in *B*. In *C* a number of epithelial cells are undergoing degenerative changes. (Adapted from Waterman, R. E., and Meller, S. M.: Scanning microscope study of secondary palate formation in the human. Anat. Rec., *180*:11, 1974.)

Nonsyndromic CP

Although the overall incidence of CP is similar in different racial groups (approximately 0.5 in 1000 live births), there is considerable variation with respect to etiologic heterogeneity in different populations. For example, in Finland there appears to be a large group of CP patients largely limited to one part of the country that is distinctly different from other nonsyndromic CPs (Saxen and Lahti, 1973). This group is so large that it doubles the incidence of CP in Finland to about 1 in 1000 live births. Another possible example is the high incidence of CP in the Hallowar Indians of North Carolina (Witkop, 1989).

Genetic Factors. Studies on monozygotic (MZ) twins discordant for CP are, as in the case of CL(P), helpful (Johnston, Hunter, and Niswander, in preparation). In this case the lower facial dimensions of the unaffected members (who presumably just missed getting a CP but would be expected to grow in a manner similar to that of the controls) indicate an average increase in tongue size of 30 to 40 per cent over that of controls who have no close relatives with CP. Although the numbers are small (N = 8), these dimensions are virtually the same in the twin with the cleft, a finding indicating that the dimensions are not affected by the presence of the cleft or subsequent treatment. Similar alterations were observed in a study of single birth CP cases compared with controls (Shibasaki and Ross, 1969). Thus, it should be possible to expand the study using readily available cephalometric radiographs of single birth cases.

A large tongue would be expected to interfere with shelf elevation by protruding further into the nasal cavities (see Fig. 26C, E). A larger tongue would also push apart the midfacial halves, a finding consistent with increased facial widths in the twins. This would move the bases of the palatal shelves further apart, thereby decreasing the chances of their making contact after elevation (see Fig. 48–26).

It is expected from the twin, Finnish, and other studies that there will be a considerable amount of etiologic heterogeneity among CP cases. In three of the eight twin pairs, the lower facial dimensions were within the normal range, indicating a different mechanism, or mechanisms, for these cases. Genetically determined broader faces have been suggested for the unusually large subgroup in Finland (Saxén and Lahti, 1973).

Unlike CL(P), where more than one major gene appears involved in the etiology of most cases, an argument can be made for a single major gene in most CP patients. This possibility is discussed further below under Gene-Environment Interactions.

Little work has been conducted on the developmental alterations related to genetic factors in experimental animals such as the SW/Fr mouse, which has a spontaneous CP rate of about 5 per cent. Alterations such as tongue size may have been overlooked.

Some observations regarding timing of palatal shelf elevation in male and female embryos (Burdi and Silvey, 1969) may be highly relevant to the preponderance of females (4:1 over males) with CP. These investigators found that palatal shelf elevation occurs several days later in female embryos. The late elevation could put the female embryos at greater risk for ever attaining shelf elevation, or otherwise could make the embryo more susceptible to other errors in position, size, or fusion that might jeopardize normal contact and fusion.

Environmental Factors. The secondary palate and brain are among the last structures undergoing "embryonic" stages of development (such as differentiation). Because of this, they are among the few structures sensitive to late environmental factors affecting developmental phenomena. Since abnormalities of these structures do not affect prenatal viability, it is possible, for example, to utilize a wide variety of environmental factors to produce experimentally almost 100 per cent CP without increasing resorptions. Fraser and Fainstat (1951) pioneered in this area, producing nearly 100 per cent CP with cortisone in mice. The ability to conduct such "clean-out" experiments greatly stimulated work in this area, and far more than 200 different chemical agents and other factors are now known to produce CP. Many studies have also been conducted concerning the mechanisms by which these agents produce CP.

Since the Fraser and Fainstat (1951) publication, a great deal of attention has been focused on steroids and CP. It appears that endogenous corticosteroids function as morphogens in normal development in a manner somewhat similar to retinoic acid (Eichele and Thaller, 1987). The gene responsible for the synthesis of the intracellular receptors for corticosteroids (cortisol in the human, corticosterone in the mouse) and retinoic acid appears to be derived from the same ancestral gene, as are those for other apparent morphogens such as thyroxin. The level of corticosteroid receptors is also elevated in human (Yoneda and Pratt, 1981) and mouse (Salomon and Pratt, 1976) palatal mesenchyme cells, and there are considerable interstrain differences that correlate well with their sensitivity for corticosteroid-induced CP (Salomon and Pratt, 1976; Kim and associates, 1984). The possible relation between the H-2 locus and sensitivity to steroid-induced CP has attracted much attention since it was first suggested by Bonner and Slavkin (1975), but it remains a complex problem (Vekemans, and Biddle, 1984; Goldman, Herald, and Piddington, in press; Gasser and associates, in press).

Steroids cause major reductions in cell proliferation (Shah, 1984) and inhibit palate shelf elevation (Diewert and Pratt, 1981). Even when the shelves elevate they often make little or no contact (Diewert and Pratt, 1981), presumably because of the reduced cell proliferation and subsequent decreased size.

There is little evidence to indicate that steroids play a major role in the cause of human CP (Fraser, 1967), although there have been anecdotal reports of associations between maternal cortisone therapy and births of children with CP (Harris and Ross, 1955). The possibility that stress could sufficiently raise cortisone levels to increase the incidence of CP receives little support from human studies (Fraser and Warburton, 1964), although interesting results have been derived from animal studies using various types of stress (Peters and Strassburg, 1968; Brown, Johnston, and Niswander, 1972).

Among vitamin deficiencies known to induce CP experimentally are deficiencies of vitamin A (retinol) (Hale, 1935), riboflavin (Walker and Crain, 1960), and folic acid (Evans, Nelson, and Asling, 1951). Excess levels of retinol also increase CP incidence (see below), and Sulik (1978) determined an optimal level for minimizing the incidence of cortisone-induced CP in A/J strain mice. Unfortunately, human diets are generally far less optimal, and more recent evidence (Erickson, 1987) indicates that it may also be possible to reduce the incidence of CP by means of vitamin supplements.

In a study by Khoury and associates (1987), maternal cigarette smoking was associated with a 2.5 times increase in the incidence of CP, which is similar to that noted for CL(P) earlier in this chapter. A more recent study by Khoury and associates (1988) indicates an even greater effect on CP, and a comparison of cigarette smoking by mothers of CL(P) and CP children indicates that it may be as much as twice as high for mothers of CP children (Ham, unpublished). CPs have also been induced experimentally with fetal anoxia (Ingalls, Curley, and Prindle, 1952; Ingalls, Taube, and Klingberg, 1964) and hypoxia (Bailey and Johnston, unpublished). Morphogenetic movements are also involved in secondary palate morphogenesis, a finding suggesting a possible explanation of the parallel effects concerning agents that interfere with oxidative metabolism. By this stage of development, almost all ATP is generated by oxidative metabolism (Hunter and Sadler, in press), which apparently may explain the greater sensitivity of CP formation to maternal smoking.

A host of other environmental agents appear to increase the incidence of CP. Some of them have human relevance and some also increase the incidence of CL(P). These include phenytoin (Hanson and Smith, 1975) and ethanol (Jones and associates, 1974). Both phenytoin (Massey, 1966; Finnell, 1981) and ethanol produce CP in experimental animals, but little is known about the pathogenesis. There is some evidence (Goldman, 1984) that at least part of the effect of phenytoin on secondary palate development is through interference with the steroid receptor.

Dioxin, a contaminant of Agent Orange and a widely distributed toxin, is a potent producer of CP in mice (Dencker and Pratt, 1981). Although there is no evidence that it causes CP in humans, the mouse embryo pathogenesis is of considerable interest in that it demonstrates a unique mechanism for CP formation. It is thought to alter DNA function (Dencker and Pratt, 1981) and it must be administered before the 12th day of gestation, which is the time of the initiation of palate shelf formation. It is not known whether the preceding inductive interaction is the primary target.

Gene-Environment Interactions. The multifactorial threshold model of Figure 48–23 is just as applicable to the problem of CP as it is to CL(P). As with CL(P), most cases of CP appear to be threshold phenomena requiring contact and fusion of embryonic primordia. For both CP and CL(P) the discordance rate of MZ twins is approximately 50 per cent, indicating that both twins are close to the threshold and that minor differences in the environment determine on which side of the threshold they will fall. Although the evidence for reduced incidence through vitamin supplementation is weaker, it is still suggestive. Similar considerations to those for CL(P) apply to cessation of cigarette smoking during pregnancy.

Syndromic CP

As discussed in greater detail below, the percentages of all CPs that are syndromic are much higher than those for CL(P)s. The variety of syndromes is also much greater.

Chromosomal Anomalies. CP is associated with a wide variety of chromosomal aberrations, including trisomies D, E, and G (Down syndrome). Detailed studies (Schutt, 1966) searching for minor chromosomal anomalies in CP patients with associated malformations have been conducted, and the incidence has been found to be high.

Treacher Collins Syndrome. This syndrome (see also Chap. 63) is caused by a single dominant gene (Gorlin, Pindborg, and Cohen, 1976). It consists of severe underdevelopment or absence of the zygomatic bone, a micrognathic mandible, external and middle ear defects, and CP in approximately 36 per cent of the cases. The clefts are wide and often involve only the soft palate region.

A mouse model in which the teratogenic agent is a retinoid (13-*cis*-retinoic acid, Accutane) produces essentially an identical syndrome when administered just before the migration of placodal cells into the trigeminal ganglion (see Fig. 48–4) (Sulik and associates, 1987). The following describes the apparent pathogenesis. The massive amount of placodal cell debris interferes with regional development, primarily of crest cells that become secondarily involved. The resultant underdevelopment of the proximal portions of the maxillary prominence and mandibular arch leads to malformation of the derived structures, mostly deficiencies such as those of the palatal shelves (posterior portions), which lead to CP.

Pierre Robin Sequence. This syndrome (see Chap. 63) consists of severe mandibular micrognathia, glossoptosis (in which the tongue blocks the airway), and variable other malformations including CP (in approximately 25 per cent), cardiac defects, and eye defects (Gorlin, Pindborg, and Cohen, 1976). The pathogenesis is usually considered to be decreased amniotic fluid that allows the fetal membranes to press the head down onto the chest wall and inhibit mandibular growth and movement. The resulting tongue interference with shelf elevation causes CP. Suitable animal models have been developed (Poswillo, 1966).

Van der Woude's Syndrome. This syndrome has already been discussed in relation to CL(P). It consists of variable combinations of CL(P), CP, and lip pits (abnormal salivary glands) and is autosomally inherited (Gorlin, Pindborg, and Cohen, 1976). Nothing is known about the pathogenesis, but an epithelial abnormality, possibly affecting breakdown and fusion, is a possibility.

Klippel-Feil Syndrome. In this syndrome the neck is short, with anomalous and missing cervical vertebrae (see Chap. 63). The associated CPs are thought to result from interference with mandibular movements (Ross and Johnston, 1972).

Although CP is also associated with many other syndromes, the following syndromes alone account for perhaps 17% of all CP cases:

Subgroup	% of total CP
Chromosomal anomalies	5
Klippel-Feil syndrome	2
Van der Woude syndrome	1
Treacher Collins syndrome	1
Pierre Robin sequence	8
Total	17

The reasons for the high incidence of associated malformations are not entirely clear, but several possibilities have been suggested. Since this is such a late-developing structure, most other craniofacial malformations have already occurred, and growth distortions, therefore, could secondarily interfere with secondary palate development. In addition, clefts of the secondary palate are not life threatening during prenatal development.

REFERENCES

Adelmann, H. B.: The embryological basis of cyclopia. Am. J. Ophthalmol., *17*:890, 1934.

Asling, C. W.: Congenital defects of the face and palate following maternal deficiency of pteroylglutamic acid. *In* Pruzansky, S. (Ed.): Congenital Anomalies of the

Face and Associated Structures. Springfield, IL, Charles C Thomas, 1961.

Bailey, L. J., and Johnston, M. C.: Carbon monoxide effects on cleft lip development in mice. J. Dent. Res., 67 (Special Issue):194, 1988.

Bailey, L. J., Minkoff, R., and Koch, W. E.: Relative growth rates of maxillary mesenchyme in the chick embryo. J. Craniofac. Genet. Dev. Biol. (in press).

Been, W., and Lieuw Kie Song, S. H.: Harelip and cleft palate conditions in chick embryos following local destruction of the cephalic neural crest: a preliminary note. Acta Morphol. Neerl. Scand., 16:245, 1978.

Biddle, F. G., and Fraser, F. C.: Major gene determination of liability to spontaneous cleft lip in the mouse. J. Craniofac. Genet. Dev. Biol. (Suppl.), 2:67, 1986.

Bonner, J. J., and Slavkin, H. C.: Cleft palate susceptibility linked to histocompatibility-2 (H-2) in the mouse. Immunogenetics, 2:213, 1975.

Briggs, R. M.: Vitamin supplementation as a possible factor in the incidence of cleft lip/palate deformities in humans. Clin. Plast. Surg., 3:647, 1976.

Brinkley, L. L., and Morris-Wiman, J.: The role of extracellular matrices in palatal shelf closure. Curr. Top. Dev. Biol., 19:17, 1984.

Bronsky, P. T., and Johnston, M. C.: Craniofacial morphogenetic movements: normal development and alterations leading to cleft lip (in preparation).

Bronsky, P. T., Johnston, M. C., Moore, N. B., Dehart, D. B., and Sulik, K. K.: Lateral nasal placodal morphogenesis in mice: normal development and alterations leading to hypoxia-induced cleft lip (submitted).

Bronsky, P. T., Johnston, M. C., and Sulik, K. K.: Morphogenesis of hypoxia-induced cleft lip in CL/Fr mice. J. Craniofac. Genet. Dev. Biol. (Suppl.), 2:113, 1986.

Brown, K. S., Johnston, M. C., and Niswander, J. D.: The effects of transportation by air on the production of isolated cleft palate in mice. Teratology, 5:119, 1972.

Burdi, A. R., and Faist, K.: Morphogenesis of the palate in normal human embryos with special emphasis on the mechanisms involved. Am. J. Anat., 120:149, 1967.

Burdi, A. R., and Silvey, R. G.: Sexual difference inclosure of the human palatal shelves. Cleft Palate J., 6:1, 1969.

Burk, D., and Sadler, T. W.: Morphogenesis of median facial clefts in mice treated with diazo-oxo-norleucine (DON). Teratology, 27:385, 1983.

Carter, C. O.: Principles of polygenic inheritance. Birth Defects, 13:69, 1977.

Chung, C. S., Mi, M. P., and Beechert, A. M.: Genetic epidemiology of cleft lip with or without cleft palate in the population of Hawaii. Genet. Epidemiol., 4:415, 1987.

Cohlan, S. O.: Excessive intake of vitamin A as a cause of congenital anomalies in the rat. Science, 117:535, 1953.

Coleman, R. D.: Development of the rat palate. Anat. Rec., 151:107, 1965.

Converse, J. M., Wood-Smith, D., McCarthy, J. G., and Coccaro, P. J.: Craniofacial surgery. Clin. Plast. Surg., 1:499, 1974.

Couly, G. F., and Le Douarin, N. M.: Mapping of the early neural primordium in quail-chick chimeras. I. Developmental relationships between placodes, facial ectoderm, and prosencephalon. Dev. Biol., 110:422, 1985.

Couly, G. F., and Le Douarin, N. M.: Mapping of the early neural primordium in quail-chick chimeras. II.

The prosencephalic neural plate and neural folds: implications for the genesis of cephalic human congenital abnormalities. Dev. Biol., 120:198, 1987.

D'Amico-Martel, A., and Noden, D. M.: Contributions of placodal and neural crest cells to avian sensory ganglia. Am. J. Anat. (in press).

Darab, D. J., Minkoff, R., Sciote, J., and Sulik, K. K.: Pathogenesis of median facial clefts in mice treated with methotrexate. Teratology, 36:77, 1987.

Davidson, J. G., Fraser, F. C., and Schlager, G.: A maternal effect on the frequency of spontaneous cleft lip in the A/J mouse. Teratology, 2:371, 1969.

Dencker, L., Annerwall, E., Busch, C., and Eriksson, U.: Retinoid-binding proteins in craniofacial development. In Townsley, J. D., and Johnston, M. C. (Eds.): Research Advances in Prenatal Craniofacial Development. J. Craniofac. Genet. Dev. Biol. (Suppl.) (in press).

Dencker, L., and Pratt, R.M.: Association of the presence of the Ah receptor in embryonic tissues from mice sensitive to TCDD-induced cleft palate. Teratogen. Carcinogen. Mutagen; 1:399, 1981.

Deol, M. S.: The relationship between abnormalities of pigmentation and the inner ear. Proc. R. Soc. Lond., 175:201, 1970.

Deol, M. S., and Lane, P. W.: A new gene affecting the morphogenesis of the vestibular part of the inner ear in the mouse. J. Embryol. Exp. Morphol., 16:543, 1966.

Diewert, V. M.: Differential changes in cartilage cell proliferation and cell density in the rat craniofacial complex during secondary palate development. Anat. Rec., 198:219, 1980.

Diewert, V. M., and Pratt, R. M.: Cortisone-induced cleft palate in A/J mice: failure of palatal shelf contact. Teratology, 24:149, 1981.

Diewert, V. M., and Shiota, K.: Morphology of human cleft lip embryos. Teratology, 37:452, 1988.

Dronamraju, K. R.: Cleft Lip and Palate: Aspects of Reproductive Biology. Springfield, IL, Charles C Thomas, 1986.

Dronamraju, K. R., and Bixler, D.: Fetal mortality and cleft lip with or without cleft palate. Clin. Genet., 23:38, 1983.

Eichele, G. and Thaller, C.: Characterization of concentration gradients of a morphogenetically active retinoid in the chick limb bud. J. Cell Biol., 105:1917, 1987.

Erickson, A., Kallen, B., and Westerholm, P.: Cigarette smoking as an etiologic factor in cleft lip and palate. Am. J. Obstet. Gynecol., 135:348, 1979.

Erickson, J. D.: Personal communication, 1989.

Eto, K., Figueroa, A., Tamura, G., and Pratt, R. M.: Induction of cleft lip in cultured rat embryos by localized administration of tunicamycin. J. Embryol. Exp. Morphol., 64:1, 1981.

Eto, K., King, C. T. G., and Johnston, M. C.: Developmental effects of teratogens influencing the incidence of cleft lip. J. Dent. Res., 55 (Special Issue):B203, 1976.

Evans, H. M., Nelson, M. M., and Asling, C. W.: Multiple congenital abnormalities resulting from acute folic acid deficiency during gestation (abstr.). Science, 114:479, 1951.

Falconer, D. S.: The inheritance of liability to certain diseases, estimated from incidence among relatives. Ann. Hum. Genet., 29:51, 1965.

Fasel, A. R.: Cardiac malformations in A/J mice and induced by phenytoin. Pediatr. Res., 15:643, 1981.

Ferguson, M. W. J.: Personal Communication, 1988.

Ferguson, M. W. J., and Honig, L. S.: Epithelial-mesenchymal interactions during vertebrate palatogenesis. Curr. Top. Dev. Biol., 19:137, 1984.

Finnell, R. H.: Phenytoin-induced teratogenesis: a mouse model. Science, 211:483, 1981.

Fitchette, J. E., and Hay, E. D.: Medial edge epithelium (MME) transfer to mesenchyme after embryonic palatal shelves fuse. J. Dent. Res., 62 (Special Issue):165, 1988.

Fraser, F. C.: Cleft lip and palate. Science, 158:1603, 1967.

Fraser, F. C., and Fainstat, T. D.: The production of congenital defects in the offspring of pregnant mice treated with cortisone: a program report. Pediatrics, 8:527, 1951.

Fraser, F. C., and Rosen, J.: Association of cleft lip and strial septal defects in mice: a preliminary report. Teratology, 11:321, 1974.

Fraser, F. C., and Warburton, D.: No association of emotional stress or vitamin supplement during pregnancy to cleft lip or palate in man. Plast. Reconstr. Surg., 33:395, 1964.

Gaare, J. D., and Langman, J.: Fusion of nasal swellings in the mouse embryo: surface coat and initial contact. Am. J. Anat., 150:461, 1977.

Gasser, D. L., Goldner-Sauve, A., Katsumata, M., and Goldman, A. S.: Restriction fragment length polymorphisms, glucocorticoid receptors, and phenytoin-induced cleft palate in congenic strains of mice with steroid susceptibility differences. In Townsley, J. D., and Johnston, M. C. (Eds.): Research Advances in Prenatal Craniofacial Development, J. Craniofac. Genet. Dev. Biol. (Suppl.) (in press).

Goldman, A. S., Herald, R., and Piddington, R.: Inhibition of embryonic palatal shelf horizontalization and medial edge epithelial breakdown by cortisol in the mouse. Role of H_2. J. Craniofac. Genet. Dev. Biol. (in press).

Gorlin, R. J., Pindborg, J. J., and Cohen, M. M.: Syndromes of the Head and Neck. New York, McGraw-Hill Book Company, 1976.

Grabowski, C. T.: Embryonic oxygen deficiency—a physiological approach to analysis of teratological mechanisms. Adv. Teratol., 4:125, 1970.

Greene, R. M., and Garbarino, M. P.: Role of cyclic AIP, prostaglandins, and catecholamines during normal palate development. Curr. Top. Dev. Biol., 19:65, 1984.

Greene, R. M., Linask, K. K., Pisano, M. M., and Lloyd, M. R.: Transmembrane and intracellular signal transduction during palatal ontogeny. In Townsley, J. D., and Johnston, M. C. (Eds.): Research Advances in Prenatal Craniofacial Development. J. Craniofac. Genet. Dev. Biol. Suppl. (in press).

Greene, R. M., and Pratt, R.: Developmental aspects of secondary palate formation. J. Embryol. Exp. Morphol., 36:225, 1976.

Greig, D. M.: Hypertelorism: a hitherto undifferentiated congenital craniofacial deformity. Edinburgh Med. J., 31:560, 1924.

Hale, F.: The relation of vitamin A to anophthalmus in pigs. J. Ophthalm. Otolaryngol., 18:1087, 1935.

Hanson, J. W., and Smith, D. W.: The fetal hydantoin syndrome. J. Pediatr., 87:285, 1975.

Harris, J. W. S., and Ross, I. P.: Cortisone therapy in early pregnancy; relation to cleft palate. Lancet, 1:1045, 1955.

Hicks, H. E., Johnston, M. C., and Banes, A. J.: Maternal phenytoin administration affects DNA and protein synthesis in embryonic primary palates. Teratology, 28:389, 1983.

Humphrey, T.: The relation between human fetal mouth opening reflexes and closure of the palate. Am. J. Anat., 125:317, 1969.

Hunter, E. S., and Sadler, T. W.: Embryonic metabolism of fetal fuels in whole embryo culture. Toxicology In Vitro (in press).

Igawa, H. H., Yasuda, M., Nakamura, H., and Ohura, T.: Changes in the subepithelial mesenchymal cell process meshwork in developing facial prominences in mouse embryos. J. Craniofac. Genet. Dev. Biol., 6:27, 1986.

Ingalls, T. H., Curley, F. J., and Prindle, R. A.: Experimental production of congenital anomalies. N. Engl. J. Med., 247:758, 1952.

Ingalls, T. H., Taube, I. E., and Klingberg, M. A.: Cleft lip and cleft palate: epidemiologic considerations. Plast. Reconstr. Surg., 34:1, 1964.

Iregbulem, L. M.: Midline clefts of the upper lip. Br. J. Plast. Surg., 31:63, 1978.

Iregbulem, L. M.: The incidence of cleft lip and palate in Nigeria. Cleft Palate J., 19:201, 1982.

Jackson, I. T.: Orbital hypertelorism. In Serafin, D., and Georgiade, N. G. (Eds.): Pediatric Plastic Surgery. St. Louis, MO, C. V. Mosby Company, pp. 467–498, 1984.

Jirasek, J. E.: Atlas of Human Prenatal Morphogenesis. Hingham, MA, Kluwer Martinus, 1983.

Johnston, M. C.: Facial malformations in chick embryos resulting from removal of neural crest. Preprinted Abstrs., Ann. Meeting, Int. Assoc. Dental Res., Los Angeles, CA. J. Dent. Res., 43 (Special Issue):822, 1964.

Johnston, M. C., and Hazelton, R. B.: Embryonic origins of facial structures related to oral sensory and motor function. In Bosma, J. F. (ed.): Oral Sensory Perception: The Mouth of The Infant. Springfield, IL, Charles C Thomas, 1972.

Johnston, M. C., Hunter, W. S., and Niswander, J. D.: Facial morphology in twins discordant for clefts of the lip and palate; a pilot study. (In preparation.)

Johnston, M. C., and Millicovsky, G.: Normal and abnormal development of the lip and palate. Clin. Plast. Surg., 12:521, 1985.

Johnston, M. C., Noden, D. M., Hazelton, R. D., Coulombre, J. L., and Coulombre, A. J.: Origins of avian ocular and periocular tissues. Exp. Eye Res., 29:27, 1979.

Johnston, M. C., and Sulik, K. K.: Embryology of the head and neck. In Serafin D., and Georgiade, N. G. (Eds.): Pediatric Plastic Surgery. St. Louis, MO, C. V. Mosby Company, 1984, pp. 184–215.

Johnston, M. C., Sulik, K. K., and Dudley, K. H.: Phenytoin (diphenylhydantoin, Dilantin)-induced cleft lip and palate in mice. Teratology, 17:20A, 1978.

Johnston, M. C., Sulik, K. K., and Minkoff, R.: Embryogenesis of the craniofacial complex. In Barrer, P. (Ed.): Proceedings of the International Conference in Orthodontics. Philadelphia, University of PA Press, 1981, pp. 275–288.

Jones, K. L., Smith, D. W., Hall, B. D., et al.: A pattern of craniofacial and limb defects secondary to aberrant tissue bands. J. Pediatr., 84:90, 1974.

Kalter, H.: Prenatal epidemiology of spontaneous cleft lip and palate, open eyelid, and embryonic death in A/J mice. Teratology, 12:245, 1975.

Khoury, M. J., Gomez-Farias, M., Mulinare, J., and Boring, J.: Does maternal cigarette smoking during pregnancy cause cleft lip and palate in offspring? Preprinted abstract. Society of Epidemiology Research Annual Meeting, Vancouver, 1988.

Khoury, M. J., Weinstein, A., Panny, S., Holtzman, N. A., Lindsay, P. K., et al.: Maternal cigarette smoking and oral clefts: a population-based study. Am. J. Public Health, 77:623, 1987.

Kim, C. S., Lauder, J. M., Joh, T. H., and Pratt, R. M.: Immunocytochemical localization of glucocorticoid receptors in midgestation murine embryos and human embryonic cultured cells. J. Histochem. Cytochem., 32:1234, 1984.

Koch, W. E., and Smiley, G. R.: In-vivo and in-vitro studies of the development of the avian secondary palate. Arch. Oral Biol., 26:181, 1981.

Kosaka, K., and Eto, K.: Appearance of a unique cell type in the fusion sites of facial processes. J. Craniofac. Genet. Dev. Biol. (Suppl.), 2:45, 1986.

Kurisu, K., Niswander, J. D., Johnston, M. C., and Mazaheri, M.: Facial morphology as an indicator of genetic predisposition to cleft lip with or without palate. Am. J. Hum. Genet., 26:702, 1974.

Landauer, W. J., and Sopher, D.: Succinate, glycerophosphate and ascorbate as sources of cellular energy and as antiteratogens. J. Embryol. Exp. Morphol., 24:187, 1970.

Lauder, J. M., Tannir, H., and Sadler, T. H.: Serotonin and morphogenesis. I. Sites of serotonin uptake and binding protein immunoreactivity in the mid-gestation mouse embryo. Development, 102:709, 1988.

Lawrence, K. M.: Causes of neural tube malformation and their prevention by dietary improvement and preconceptional supplementation with folic acid and multivitamins. In Briggs, M. (Ed.): Recent Vitamin Research. Boca Raton, FL, CRC, 1984.

Le Douarin, N.: The Neural Crest. Cambridge, Cambridge University Press, 1983.

Longo, L. D.: Environmental pollution and pregnancy: risks and uncertainties for the fetus and infant. Am. J. Obstet. Gynecol., 137:162, 1980.

Mackler, B., Grace, R., Trippit, D. F., Lemire, R. J., Shepard, T. H., and Kelley, V. C.: Studies of the developmental anomalies in rats. III. Effects of inhibition of mitochondrial energy systems on embryonic development. Teratology, 12:291, 1975.

Massey, K. M.: Teratogenic effect of diphenylhydantoin sodium. J. Oral Ther. Pharmacol., 2:380, 1966.

McKee, G. J., and Ferguson, M. W.: The effects of mesencephalic neural crest cell extirpation on the development of chicken embryos. J. Anat., 139:491, 1984.

Meskin, L. H., Gorlin, R. J., and Isaacson, R. J.: Abnormal morphology of the soft palate. II. The genetics of cleft uvula. Cleft Palate J., 2:40, 1965.

Millicovsky, G., Ambrose, L. J. H., and Johnston, M. C.: Developmental alterations associated with spontaneous cleft lip and palate in CL/Fr mice. Am. J. Anat., 164:29, 1982.

Millicovsky, G., and Johnston, M. C.: Active role of embryonic facial epithelium: new evidence of cellular events in morphogenesis. J. Embryol Exp. Morphol., 63:53, 1981a.

Millicovsky, G., and Johnston, M. C.: Hyperoxia and hypoxia in pregnancy: simple experimental manipulation alters the incidence of cleft lip and palate in CL/Fr mice. Proc. Natl. Acad. Sci. USA, 78:5722, 1981b.

Millicovsky, G., and Johnston, M. C.: Maternal hyperoxia greatly reduces the incidence of cleft lip and palate in A/J mice. Science, 212:671, 1981c.

Minkoff, R.: Cell proliferation during formation of the embryonic facial primordia. In Townsley, J. D., and Johnston, M. C. (Eds.): Research Advances in Prenatal Craniofacial Development. J. Craniofac. Genet. Dev. Biol. (Suppl.) (in press).

Minkoff, R.: Cell communication among mesenchymal cells of the embryonic facial primordia. J. Dent. Res., 65:(Special Issue):762, 1986.

Minkoff, R., and Kuntz, A. J.: Cell proliferation during morphogenetic change: analyses of frontonasal morphogenesis in the chick embryo explaining DNA labeling indices. J. Embryol. Exp. Morphol., 40:101, 1977.

Minkoff, R., and Kuntz, A. J.: Cell proliferation and cell density of mesenchyme in the maxillary process and adjacent regions during facial development in the chick embryo. J. Embryol. Exp. Morphol., 46:65, 1978.

Moore, G. E., Ivens, A., Chambers, J., Farrall, M., Williamson, R., et al.: Linkage of an X-chromosome cleft palate gene. Nature, 326:91, 1987.

Moore, G. E., Williamson, R., Jensson, O., Chambers, J., Takakubo, F., et al.: Localization of a mutant gene for cleft palate and ankyloglossia in an X-linked Icelandic family. In Townsley, J. D., and Johnston, M. C. (Eds.): Research Advances in Prenatal Craniofacial Development. J. Craniofac. Genet. Dev. Biol. (Suppl.) (in press).

Nishimura, H., Takano, K., Tanimura, T., Yasuda, M., and Uchida, T.: High incidence of several malformations in the early human embryos as compared with infants. Biol. Neonate, 10:93, 1966.

Niswander, J. D.: Laminographic x-ray study in families with cleft lip and cleft palate. Arch. Oral Biol., 13:109, 1968.

Niswander, J. D.: Personal communication, 1970.

Niswander, J. D., MacLean, C. J., Chung, C. S., and Dronamraju, K.: Sex ratio and cleft lip with or without cleft palate. Lancet, 2:858, 1972.

Noden, D. M.: The role of the neural crest in patterning of avian cranial skeletal, connective, and muscle tissues. Dev. Biol., 96:144, 1983.

Ohbayashi, N., and Eto, K.: Relative contributions of the facial processes to facial development: a microsurgical assay. J. Craniofac. Genet. Dev. Biol. (Suppl.), 2:41, 1986.

Patterson, S. B., Johnston, M. C., and Minkoff, R.: An implant labeling technique employing sable hair probes as carriers for ^{3}H-thymidine: applications to the study of facial morphogenesis. Anat. Rec., 210:525, 1984.

Patterson, S. B., and Minkoff, R.: Morphometric and autoradiographic analysis of frontonasal development in the chick. Anat. Rec., 212:90, 1985.

Pauling, L.: The Common Cold and The Flu. San Francisco, W. H. Freeman, 1976.

Peters, S., and Strassburg, M.: Erzeugung von Gaumspalten durch Lärm und Hunger. Dtsch. Zahnaertzl. Z., 23:843, 1968.

Pinsky, L., and Fraser, F. C.: Production of skeletal malformations in the offspring of pregnant mice treated with 6-aminonicotinamide. Biol. Neonat., 1:106, 1959.

Poswillo, D.: Observations of fetal posture and causal mechanisms of congenital deformity of the palate, mandible, and limbs. J. Dent. Res., 45:584, 1966.

Pourtois, M.: Morphogenesis of the primary and secondary palate. In Slavkin, H. C., and Bavetta, L. A. (Eds.): Developmental Aspects of Oral Biology. London, Academic Press, 1972, pp. 81–108.

Pratt, R. M., Dencker, L., and Diewert, V. M.: TCDD-induced cleft palate in the mouse: evidence for alterations in palatal shelf fusion. Teratogenesis Carcinogen, Mutagen, 4:427, 1984.

Pratt, R. M., and Martin, G. R.: Epithelial cell death and cyclic AMP increase during palatal development. Proc. Natl. Acad. Sci. U.S.A., 72:874, 1975.

Reed, S. C., and Snell, G. D.: Harelip, a new mutation in the house mouse. Anat. Rec., 51:43, 1931.

Ross, R. B., and Johnston, M. C.: Cleft Lip and Palate. Baltimore, Williams and Wilkins Company, 1972.

Russell, M. M.: Comparative morphogenesis of the secondary palate in murine and human embryos. Ph.D. Thesis. University of North Carolina, Chapel Hill, 1987.

Salomon, D. S., and Pratt, R. M.: Glucocorticoid receptors in murine embryonic facial mesenchyme cells. Nature, 264:174, 1976.

Salomon, D. S., Gift, V. M., and Pratt, R. M.: Corticosterone levels during midgestation in the maternal plasma and fetus of cleft palate sensitive and -resistant mice. Endocrinology, 104:154, 1979.

Saxen, I.: Cleft lip and palate in Finland: parental histories, course of pregnancy and selected environmental factors. Teratology, 3:263, 1973.

Saxen, I.: Associations between oral clefts and drugs taken during pregnancy. Int. J. Epidemiol., 4:37, 1975.

Saxen, I., and Lahti, A.: Cleft lip and palate in Finland: incidence, secular, seasonal, and geographical variations. Teratology, 9:217, 1973.

Schutt, W. H.: Chromosomal and single gene defects in children with clefts of lip and palate. In Drillien, C. M., Ingram, T. T. S., and Wilkinson, E. M. (Eds.): The Causes and Natural History of Cleft Lip and Palate. Edinburgh, London, E. & S. Livingston, 1966, pp. 217–228.

Sedans, H., Jirasek, J., and Gorlin, R. J.: Frontonasal dysplasia. Pediatrics, 76:966, 1970.

Shah, R. M.: Morphological, cellular, and biochemical aspects of differentiation of normal and teratogentreated palate in hamster and chick embryos. Curr. Top. Dev. Biol., 19:108, 1984.

Shah, C. V., Pruzansky, S., and Harris, W. S.: Cardiac malformations with facial clefts. Am. J. Dis Child., 119:238, 1970.

Shibasaki, Y., and Ross, R. B.: Facial growth in children with isolated cleft palate. Clin. Chem. 6:290, 1969.

Smiley, G. R., Vanek, R. J., and Dixon, A. D.: Width of the craniofacial complex during formation of the secondary palate. Cleft Palate J., 8:371, 1971.

Smuts, M. K.: Rapid nasal pit formation in mouse stimulated by ATP-containing medium. J. Exp. Zool., 216:409, 1981.

Steiniger, F.: Neue Beobachtungen an der erblichen Hausenscharte der Maus. Z. Mensch. Vererb., 23:427, 1939.

Streeter, G. L.: Developmental horizons in human embryos. Contrib. Embryol. Carnegie Inst., 32:133, 1948.

Sulik, K. K.: Personal communication, 1978.

Sulik, K. K., and Johnston, M. C.: Sequence of developmental alterations following ethanol exposure in mice: craniofacial features of the fetal alcohol syndrome (FAS). Am. J. Anat., 166:275, 1983.

Sulik, K. K., Johnston, M. C., Ambrose, L. J., and Dorgan, D.: Phenytoin (Dilantin)-induced cleft lip and palate in A/J mice: a scanning and transmission electron microscopic study. Anat. Rec., 195:243, 1979.

Sulik, K. K., Johnston, M. C., Ambrose, L. J., and Dorgan, D. R.: Mechanism of phenytoin (PHT)-induced malformations in a mouse model. In Hassell, T. M.,

Johnston, M. C., and Dudley, K. H. (Eds.): Phenytoininduced Teratology and Gingival Pathology. New York, Raven Press, 1980, pp. 67–74.

Sulik, K. K., Johnston, M. C., Smiley, J., Speight, H. S., and Jarvis, E.: Mandibulofacial dysostosis (Treacher Collins syndrome): a new proposal for its pathogenesis. Am. J. Med. Genet., 27:359, 1987.

Sulik, K. K., Johnston, M. C., and Webb, M. A.: Fetal alcohol syndrome: embryogenesis in a mouse model. Science, 214:936, 1981.

Sulik, K. K., Smiley, S. J., Turvey, T. A., Speight, H. S., and Johnston, M. C.: Pathogenesis involving the secondary palate in mandibulofacial dysostosis and related syndromes. Cleft Palate J., 1988 (in press).

Thaller, C., and Eichele, G.: Characterization of retinoid metabolism in the developing chick limb bud. Development, 103:473, 1988.

Tolarova, M.: Periconceptional supplementation with vitamins and folic acid to prevent recurrence of cleft lip. Lancet, 2:217, 1982.

Tolarova, M.: Orofacial clefts in Czechoslovakia. Scand. J. Plast. Reconstr. Surg., 21:19, 1987.

Töndury, G.: On the mechanism of cleft formation. In Pruzansky, S. (Ed.): Congenital Anomalies of the Face and Associated Structures. Springfield, IL, Charles C Thomas, 1961.

Trasler, D. G.: Pathogenesis of cleft lip and its relations to embryonic face shape in A/J and C57BL mice. Teratology, 1:33, 1968.

Trasler, D. G., and Leong, S.: Mitotic index in mouse embryo with 6-aminonicotinamide-induced inherited cleft lip. Teratology, 25:259, 1982.

Trasler, D. G., and Ohannessian, L.: Ultrastructure of initial nasal process cell fusion in spontaneous and 6-aminonicotinamide-induced mouse embryo cleft lip. Teratology, 28:91, 1983.

Trasler, D. G., Reardon, C. A., and Rajchgot, H.: A selection experiment for distinct types of 6-aminonicotinamide-induced cleft lip in mice. Teratology, 18:49, 1978.

Tyan, M. L.: Differences in the reported frequencies of cleft lip plus cleft lip and palate in Asians born in Hawaii and the continental United States. Proc. Soc. Exp. Biol. Med., 171:41, 1982.

Tyler, M. S., and Koch, W. E.: Epithelial-mesenchymal interactions in the secondary palate of the mouse. J. Dent. Res., 53:64, 1974.

Van der Woude, A.: Fistula labii inferioris congenita and its association with cleft lip and palate. Am. J. Hum. Genet., 6:244, 1954.

Van Lienborgh, J., Lieuw Kie Song, S. H., and Been, W.: Cleft lip and palate due to deficiency of mesencephalic neural crest cells. Cleft Palate J., 20:251, 1983.

Vekemans, M. J. J., and Biddle, F. G.: Genetics of palate development. Curr. Top. Dev. Biol., 19:165, 1984.

Walker, B. E.: Correlation of embryonic movement with palate closure in mice. Teratology, 2:191, 1969.

Walker, B. E., and Crain, B.: Effects of hypervitaminosis A on palate development in two strains of mice. Am. J. Anat., 107:49, 1960.

Walker, B. E., and Fraser, F. C.: Closure of the secondary palate in three strains of mice. J. Embryol. Exp. Morph., 4:176, 1956.

Walker, B. E., and Patterson, A.: Induction of cleft palate in mice by tranquilizers and barbiturates. Teratology, 10:159, 1974.

Walker, B. E., and Quarles, J.: Palate closure in embryonic mice after excising the tongue. Teratology, 7:4, 1973.

Waterman, R. E., and Meller, S. M.: Alterations in the epithelial surface of human palatal shelves prior to and during fusion: a scanning microscopic study. Anat. Rec., *180*:11, 1974.

Webster, W. S., and Ritchie, H. E.: The teratological effects of isotretinoin on craniofacial development: an analysis of animal models. *In* Townsley, J. D., and Johnston, M. C. (Eds.): Research Advances in Prenatal Craniofacial Development. J. Craniofac. Genet. Dev. Biol. (Suppl.) (in press).

Wedden, S. E.: The effects of retinoids on chick face development. *In* Townsley, J. D., and Johnston, M. C. (Eds.): Research Advances in Prenatal Craniofacial Development. J. Craniofac. Genet. Dev. Biol. (Suppl.) (in press).

Witkop, C.: Personal communication, 1989.

Yoneda, T., and Pratt, R. M.: Glucocorticoid receptors in palatal mesenchymal cells from the human embryo: relevance to human cleft palate formation. J. Craniofac. Genet. Dev. Biol., *1*:411, 1981.

Zimmerman, E. F., and Wee, E. L.: Role of neurotransmitters in palate development. Dev. Biol., *19*:37, 1984.

49

R. Bruce Ross

Facial Growth in Cleft Lip and Palate

The surgeon or orthodontist who deals with a clinical population of children with clefts of the lip and palate is well aware that facial growth is often unsatisfactory, and that these children present with esthetic and functional problems that are difficult to overcome. The clinical findings are confirmed by virtually every comparative cephalometric study published. For example, the average 16 year old male with a complete unilateral cleft lip and palate has a profile and skeletal pattern that deviates from the noncleft individual, as illustrated in Figure 49–1 (Ross, 1987a). Equally abnormal facial morphology is found in bilateral cleft lip and palate and in isolated cleft palate.

There are several factors to account for the poor facial morphology, and it may be instructive to consider them separately. This approach may lead to a better understanding of facial growth problems and the potential success of therapeutic methods to overcome them.

The major factors in facial growth are:

1. *Intrinsic* factors, including the initial development and growth potential of the face.

2. *Functional* activity, which may cause distortions of normal as well as abnormal parts.

3. *Iatrogenic* factors, usually the effects of treatment on facial growth.

INTRINSIC DEFICIENCIES

The malformation that consists of an orofacial cleft not only interferes with the development and morphology of the affected areas, but also causes alterations in contiguous structures that are developmentally normal. The anatomic arrangement of muscles, nerves, arteries, veins, skin, and mucous membranes is distorted. These are described in Chapter 51.

It would be helpful in treatment planning if one could distinguish between structures that are intrinsically abnormal and those that only appear to be abnormal because they have become distorted by secondary environmental disturbances. The former are resistant to correction; the latter may be self-correcting if the proper environment can be provided.

It is currently accepted that cleft lip and cleft palate have a multifactorial etiology.

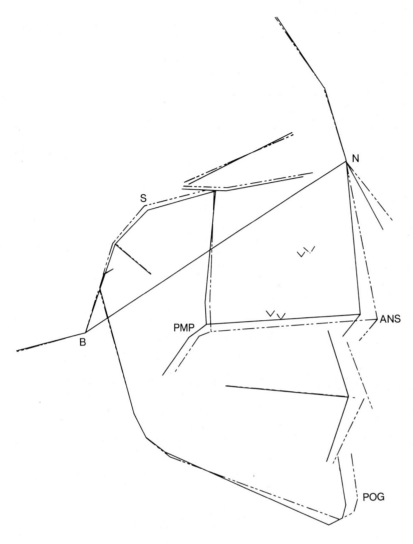

Figure 49–1. Comparison of the mean cephalometric tracings of males with complete unilateral cleft lip and palate (*solid line*) and noncleft males (*interrupted line*) at 16 years of age. N = nasion; ANS = anterior nasal spine; POG = pogonion; S = sella; B = basion; PMP = posterior maxillary point. The diagrams are superimposed on the nasion-basion plane, and the size is adjusted so that nasion to basion lengths are equal. See text for discussion.

One of the predisposing factors is a deficiency of midface mesenchyme at the critical embryonic stages (see Chap. 48). This does not appear to be a simple genetic trait, since parents of children with orofacial clefts do not have a small maxilla (Coccaro, D'Amico, and Chavoor, 1970; Karout and Ross, 1974).

Before examining the maxillary complex in detail, it might be well to establish a frame of reference by considering the other components of the facial skeleton. With the occasional exception of the mandible and the orbits, there is no evidence that any other bone is primarily affected to any significant degree by the presence of a cleft of the lip or palate.

In most cases the mandible, although slightly smaller, is normal in size and shape at birth. There are as many variations as in the noncleft population, presumably because the mandible usually is not directly involved in the production of a cleft and the normal genetic variation is expressed. The one notable exception to this statement is the group of children with Pierre Robin sequence, in which the mandible is small or retruded (see Chap. 63). There appear to be several variants of the Pierre Robin sequence, as regards etiology. The mandible and its subsequent growth are discussed later in this chapter.

The orbital complex is affected, exhibiting a slight tendency toward increased interorbital distance (Psaume, 1957; Graber, 1964; Moss, 1965; Ross and Coupe, 1965; Farkas and Lindsay, 1972), although this is hardly sufficient to warrant the term orbital hypertelorism. This finding may be a secondary characteristic induced by environmental forces. The zygomatic bones (Harvold, 1954; Subtelny, 1955; Coupe and Subtelny, 1960), the pterygoid plates of the sphenoid (Van Limborgh, 1964; Atkinson, 1966), and the cranial base (Ross, 1965; Bishara and Iverson, 1974) are essentially normal.

For all practical purposes one may conclude that the embryo with a cleft of the lip or palate has an *intrinsically normal facial framework to which is attached a mildly deficient maxillary complex.*

PRENATAL ENVIRONMENTAL INFLUENCES

By the time of birth the face of the infant with cleft lip or palate has developed enormously from the embryonic condition. It has been subjected to many environmental forces in utero that influence the shape of the parts and their relation to each other. The reaction of the facial skeleton to external forces depends largely on the type of cleft that is present.

Complete Unilateral Cleft Lip and Palate. The infant with a complete unilateral cleft lip and palate (Fig. 49–2) has a maxilla with deficiencies of the alveolar and palatal bones and the maxillary basal bone (Coupe, 1962). Alveolar bone deficiencies are partly related to the absence or abnormality of tooth development adjacent to the cleft, since growth of the alveolar bone is dependent on the presence of teeth (edentulous individuals have virtually no alveolar bone). The size of the palatal shelves at birth is difficult to ascertain, since many conflicting reports are available. One can assume that a deficiency in shelf width is not clinically significant in most cases, and the shelves grow at a normal rate thereafter. The tongue may intrude between the shelves and inhibit medial growth, causing a "clubbing" at the medial margin

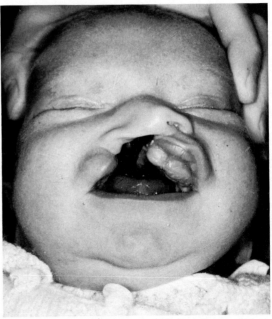

Figure 49–2. Newborn with complete unilateral cleft lip and palate on the right side. The deformity is typical of the condition, with severe displacement of the left (noncleft) segment of the maxilla away from the midline of the face. The nose accompanies the maxillary base, causing the stretching and straightening of the right alar cartilages.

(Subtelny, 1955) and a changing shelf angulation.

The most striking characteristic of the infant with complete unilateral cleft lip and palate is the severe deviation of the noncleft side of the maxilla away from the cleft (Figs. 49–2, 49–3), carrying with it the nasal structures, including the nasal septum. This distortion is the response of inadequately supported bone structures to pressure. In complete unilateral cleft lip and palate, the abnormal insertion of the cheek muscles on the maxilla at the base of the nose causes a rotating force on the larger segment during

Figure 49–3. The forces that cause maxillary displacement in a complete unilateral cleft lip and palate. The major factors are the lateral pull of the lip and cheek muscles abnormally inserted into the anterior maxilla, and the normal tongue pressure expanding the maxillary segments laterally and anteriorly.

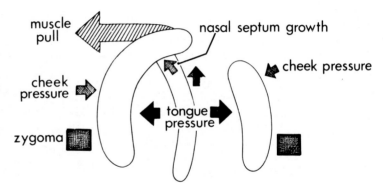

muscle contraction (Fig. 49–3). This action is reinforced by tongue protrusion (Ross and Johnston, 1972). There may also be a relatively unrestrained nasal septum growth (Latham and Burston, 1964). The smaller segment on the cleft side is exposed to less expanding force, and has a mild contracting force exerted by the base of the nasal ala on this side.

Since the nose is deviated toward the normal side, except for the alar base on the cleft side, the nostril on the cleft side is stretched and straightened. This configuration is established very early in the embryo (Atherton, 1967; Latham, 1969), and the alar cartilages develop and grow in a deformed matrix. The deformity is so well established by birth that the surgeon has great difficulty recontouring the nose to a satisfactory symmetry.

Measurements of dental models of the newborn (Peyton, 1931; Harding and Mazaheri, 1972) indicate that arch width is greater in cleft conditions. This finding confirms work on other facial widths (Subtelny, 1955; Ross and Coupe, 1965) showing that the entire face is slightly wider in children with extensive clefts. This finding likely represents a secondary response to the expanding forces detailed above.

Complete Bilateral Cleft Lip and Palate. Although infants with complete bilateral cleft lip and palate have a significantly different maxillary complex from that of infants with unilateral clefts, the differences would probably be minimal except for the activity of attached muscles. The major morphologic characteristics are the result of an altered response of the skeletal element to muscular deformation tendencies. The premaxilla, relatively unsupported on the nasal septum, is not able to resist the force of the active tongue, and tilts forward (Fig. 49–4). The base (anterior nasal spine) is somewhat supported by the septum and by the nose, so that excessive protrusion of the base is limited. If the tongue habitually protrudes through one side, the premaxilla is protruded and forced to the opposite side, giving the asymmetry pictured in Figure 49–5. Some authors (Latham, 1969, 1973; Pruzansky, 1971) believe that an intrinsic excessive nasal septum growth is responsible for protrusion of the premaxilla (see also Chap. 50).

The smaller posterior segments of the maxilla respond to their environment in the same way as in the unilateral condition; i.e., there is an increase in maxillary width.

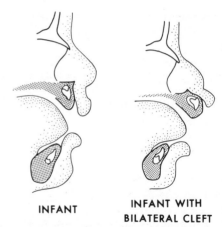

INFANT   INFANT WITH BILATERAL CLEFT

Figure 49–4. Displacement of the premaxillary area in a complete bilateral cleft lip and palate. The major movement is a forward tilt induced by tongue pressure on the poorly supported bone. The anterior nasal spine is only slightly advanced. (From Ross, R. B., and Johnston, M. C.: Cleft Lip and Palate. Copyright 1972, The Williams & Wilkins Company, Baltimore.)

The anterior bone of the maxilla in humans is not a premaxilla as in other species. Although one refers to the "premaxilla" for convenience in bilateral cleft lip and palate,

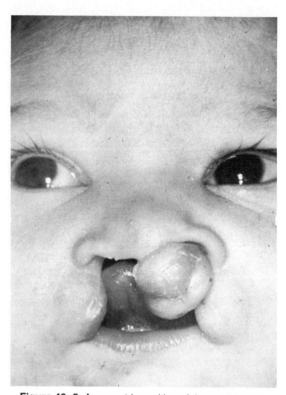

Figure 49–5. Asymmetric position of the premaxilla in an infant with complete bilateral cleft lip and palate. This finding is probably solely due to a tongue thrust into the right cleft rather than to an intrinsic deformity.

this area is abnormal in complete bilateral cleft lip and palate, because the clefts have prevented mesenchyme from the maxillary processes from migrating into the midline during embryonic development. The result is a premaxilla grossly deficient in basal bone. The bulk of the bone present is alveolar bone, which develops in response to the development of teeth. This is apparent when teeth are removed in later life and the premaxilla is soon reduced to a tiny mass of bone under the anterior nasal spine. The great variation in size of the premaxilla at birth in bilateral cleft lip and palate is frequently a reflection of the number and size of teeth present.

Other Types of Clefts. Facial morphology in other types of clefts varies, but the same principles of deficiency and distortion apply. Isolated cleft palate presents no gross disturbance in form, although there is greater width than normal in the area of the posterior tuberosity. Clefts of the lip and anterior maxilla may show distortions in the alveolus and nasal structures similar to those of unilateral cleft lip and palate; however, these are localized and the overall morphology of the face is close to normal. The explanation is simple: if there is continuity of bone in any area, the resistance to distortion is sufficient to prevent major problems. This principle applies to incomplete unilateral or bilateral cleft lip and palate, where part of the palate or part of the anterior maxilla is intact and less distortion is possible. Even a bridge of tissue across the cleft (Simonart's band) prevents many of the expected morphologic changes from occurring, particularly those of the nose. The maxilla in these cases, however, may be rotated, since the tongue and cheek muscles are exerting abnormal forces.

GENERAL GROWTH

The stature of children with cleft lip or palate, or both, is smaller than that of children without clefts (Johnson, 1960; Drillien, Ingram, and Wilkinson, 1966) and they may have retarded skeletal age (Menius, Largent, and Vincent, 1966; Przezdziak, 1969). Shibasaki and Ross (1969) found evidence that the pubertal growth spurt of facial structures is delayed in patients with isolated cleft palate. Ross (1965) found that, although the proportions in the cranial base of children with cleft lip and palate were identical, the entire cranial base was smaller, indicating that the children were smaller.

Initial growth retardation could be explained by the preoperative feeding difficulties and trauma associated with surgical procedures. One would expect these adverse environmental influences to have only a temporary effect, yet the study of Dahl (1970) indicated that young adults with all types of cleft were shorter than a similar control group by several inches. This suggests that an intrinsic deficiency is present, and "catch-up" growth does not occur. Thus, at any age, smaller facial structures can be expected.

NORMAL FACIAL GROWTH

Before proceeding to a discussion of postnatal facial growth in children with cleft lip or palate, it is helpful to have some understanding of normal facial growth (see also Chap. 47). This is a complex subject, incompletely understood at present, but there is sufficient available evidence to permit some relevant conclusions to aid in the analysis of abnormal facial growth. This chapter limits discussion to three important skeletal elements: mandibular basal bone, maxillary basal bone, and the dentoalveolar component of each.

Mandibular Basal Bone

Many of the bones of the body are not single morphologic units. The mandible, for example, has many components that develop relative to specific functions, all somewhat independently of each other. The major components of the mandible are a central core, termed the basal bone, which is dependent on strong genetic control; a coronoid process, which is dependent for its size and shape on temporal muscle function and the position of the mandibular basal bone; a gonial area, which is dependent on the masseter and medial pterygoid muscles; and a dentoalveolar process, which is dependent on the development of teeth.

The central core or basal bone of the mandible appears to be genetically determined in size and shape. Growth occurs only at the posterior portion of the bone, primarily at the condyle. Orthodontists have attempted to alter the size of the mandible by applying forces in a variety of ways, but with limited success.

Consequently, a disproportionately large or small mandible must be altered surgically.

The position of the mandible, however, is the result of all the muscular, soft tissue, and external forces that act on it, since the bone is not firmly attached to other bones, but only indirectly attached through the temporomandibular joints. Thus, a change in the surrounding soft tissues or an external appliance such as the Milwaukee brace (Weinstein, 1967) easily induces rotation to a new position. Rotations over a long period, such as with continuous mouth breathing, are accompanied by alterations in the bony muscle attachments and dentoalveolar component, so that the shape of the mandible can be dramatically changed without affecting the shape or size of the central core. Alterations in mandibular position and shape occur in cleft lip and palate (discussed later in this chapter).

Maxillary Basal Bone

The delineations between the various functional components are less obvious in the maxilla. There are orbital, nasal, palatal, zygomatic, and dentoalveolar processes, all of which are relatively independent in the normal child. The basal bone (that which remains when the other processes are removed) is probably the result of a genetic blueprint, but with some critical differences from the mandible.

Despite the apparently firm attachment of the maxilla to the skull, strong environmental forces can alter the position of the maxilla, and interference with the sutures or nasal septum can alter maxillary size. The maxilla is thus more easily influenced in its growth than the mandible (Wieslander, 1963; Jakobsson, 1967; Droschl, 1973).

Essentially all maxillary growth in a forward direction occurs by apposition of bone to the posterior surfaces (Enlow and Bang, 1965; Bjork, 1966). Figure 49–6 diagrammatically shows the areas in which bone is laid down to increase maxillary length. During growth, there is actually resorption of bone in the anterior basal area to permit remodeling of the surface (see Chap. 47).

Koski (1968) and others concluded that the areas of growth in the face are not primary growth centers that would force the maxilla forward. The role of the nasal septum is not completely understood, although its importance in directing maxillary growth is currently held to be of minor significance (Moss and associates, 1968; Stenstrom and Thilander, 1970). The sutures are adjustment areas that provide bone to maintain skeletal continuity.

Ross and Johnston (1972) concluded that there is no major skeletal force driving the maxilla forward, that it seems rather to move

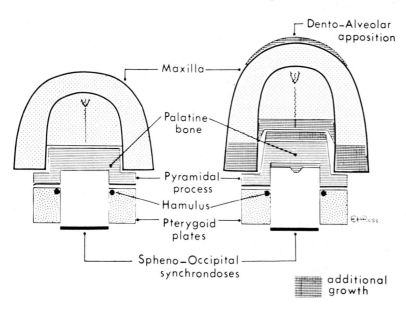

Figure 49–6. Growth in length of the maxillary basal bone is achieved by apposition to the posterior tuberosity area, with little or no contribution from the anterior maxilla, the pyramidal process of the palatine bone, or the pterygoid plates of the sphenoid. (From Ross, R. B., and Johnston, M. C.: Cleft Lip and Palate. Copyright 1972, The Williams & Wilkins Company, Baltimore.)

forward as part of the overall genetic pattern of growth, and that, as the maxilla moves forward, bone is laid down in convenient places (i.e., in the sutures and on the maxillary tuberosity).

Increase in width of the basal maxilla occurs in infancy in conjunction with activity in the midpalatine suture. The contribution of this suture is considerably reduced after the second year of life, and the width in the anterior region of the maxilla remains virtually constant from this time. The apparent increase in maxillary width is due to greater posterior width accompanying apposition on the tuberosity.

Dentoalveolar Processes

The dentoalveolar processes are truly remarkable adaptive mechanisms. Alveolar bone develops in response to the presence of teeth and disappears if the teeth are absent or lost in later life. Teeth do not erupt at predetermined distances along a predetermined path into occlusion. If they did, a precise meshing of maxillary and mandibular teeth would be extremely rare. Nature has provided a mechanism to compensate for minor disharmonies between the maxilla and mandible.

A tooth erupts until it meets resistance. In the normal course, this resistance is the tooth in the opposing arch, although the tongue, thumb, or lip may interfere with full eruption. Once contact is made, an equilibrium is established.

A force exerted against a tooth is transmitted to the alveolar bone through the fibers of the periodontal ligament (as compression on one side of the tooth socket and tension on the other). The bone resorbs in response to pressure and builds in response to tension on the fibers. Thus, the tooth moves away from pressure. An erupting tooth is guided into position by the gentle pressure of the soft tissues, principally the tongue, lip, and cheek muscles. The orthodontist uses this normal biologic mechanism to correct malocclusion by applying artificial forces to move teeth.

It is essential for the attainment of a satisfactory occlusion that the dentoalveolar mechanism be free to respond to the guiding forces in the mouth. This principle is important in the later discussion on the occlusion in the operated and nonoperated cleft lip and palate.

GROWTH POTENTIAL IN CLEFT LIP AND PALATE

The true growth potential of the cleft maxilla can be determined only when growth can be observed in the absence of other extrinsic influences. Since surgical repair of the cleft is a major influence affecting growth, such data are difficult to accumulate.

There have been numerous reports in the literature of older children and adults with cleft lip and palate who have not received the benefits of surgical repair. Their facial form is the result of the interaction of an intrinsic defect, subsequent normal and abnormal environmental influences, and the expression of the growth potential of the facial skeleton. Careful study of these individuals should provide answers to many questions regarding the disturbed facial morphology frequently encountered in a cleft palate clinic.

In individuals with unrepaired cleft lip and palate there is evidence that the face is wider in all areas, probably as a result of environmental forces that cause a decrease in the *restraining* factors (loss of lip continuity, loss of skeletal continuity) while maintaining the *expansive* factors (tongue pressure, facial growth processes). There is also the possibility that an increased width is inherent and may even be an etiologic factor in the formation of a cleft. In any case, the areas of the facial skeleton responsible for increasing width appear to function normally in the growing child with cleft lip and palate. Areas of bone apposition and suture growth can be neither deficient nor inhibited if the end result is as satisfactory as is found in all studies on unoperated clefts of the lip and palate.

The facial growth parameter of most concern in cleft lip and palate is undoubtedly midface depth. Studies by Graber (1951, 1954), Ortiz-Monasterio and associates (1959, 1966), Mestre, DeJesus, and Subtelny (1960), Hagerty and Hill (1963), and Boo-Chai (1971) indicate that the basal maxilla achieves normal relationships with the remainder of the face in the unoperated adult with cleft lip and palate. Again, it must be concluded that the areas of bone growth are not inhibited by the presence of a cleft.

Data on facial height are not adequate to permit firm conclusions. The available evidence indicates, however, that vertical height is normal, and there is no evidence of a deficiency of midface height. Most of the increase in the normal maxilla is related to dentoalveolar growth and the downward migration of the hard palate by means of an apposition-resorption mechanism (Enlow and Bang, 1965). Obviously the palate migrates in the cleft lip and palate condition, in spite of the gross disturbance of structure.

Finally, and most significantly, the dentoalveolar structures accommodate to the basal jaw relations almost exactly as they do in the normal child. The maxillary teeth are positioned in an essentially normal relation to the mandibular teeth, with local disturbances in the area of the alveolar cleft. This observation indicates that, even when a gross morphologic disturbance involves the maxilla and its alveolar ridge, teeth erupt until they contact opposing teeth, and they can be guided into a satisfactory functional relationship through the influence of the adjacent soft

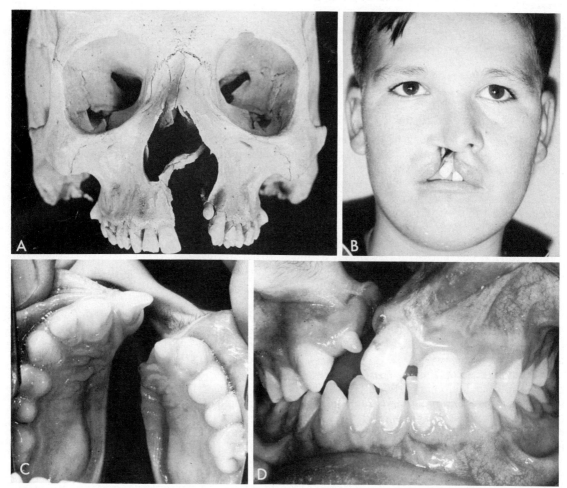

Figure 49–7. *A,* Adult skull with complete unilateral cleft of the anterior maxilla and palate. Presumably the lip was also completely cleft. Facial growth has been essentially normal, except for the deviation of the nasal bones, the nasal septum, and the noncleft segment of the maxilla; a deficiency of bone in the nasal floor on the cleft side; and a mild vertical deficiency in the position of the teeth on the cleft side. The morphologic features are remarkably similar to those of the newborn condition, indicating that the initial deformity is maintained. Note that the left central incisor has been lost, but indications are that it had been sharply angled toward the cleft. The facial and dental features of this individual must have been strikingly similar to those of the 14 year old boy in *B.* The dental arch form was excellent in this boy (*C*), with regular tooth alignment. The width of the cleft appears to be as much due to expansion of the segments as to deficiency of adjacent tissue. *D,* The occlusion of the teeth is, in general, excellent. The smaller segment shows normal relations except for a slight vertical opening in the cuspid region. The larger segment is displaced away from the cleft, resulting in an excessive overlap of the upper teeth with the lower teeth. Note that the incisors tilt toward the cleft to establish more normal relations with the lower incisors. (*A* from Atkinson, R. W.: Jaws out of balance. Am. J. Orthod., *52:*371, 1966. *B* to *D* from Ross, R. B., and Johnston, M. C.: Cleft Lip and Palate. Copyright 1972, The Williams & Wilkins Company, Baltimore.)

tissues (i.e., tongue, cheek, and lip muscles). The discrepancy of bone in the cleft area is sufficient to prevent complete dentoalveolar adaptation.

The conclusions to be drawn from the foregoing are clear: the midface is not extensively damaged by the embryonic disturbance concomitant with cleft formation. After the cleft has developed, additional growth proceeds in a reasonably normal manner, with some environmentally induced distortions remaining. The maxilla, which must advance freely during growth to permit apposition at the posterior aspect and sutural adjustment growth, advances with little inhibition. The teeth and alveolar bone, which must be free to adapt to the jaw relations and the soft tissue environment, adapt without inhibition except in the area of the cleft (Fig. 49–7).

Several studies (Dahl, 1970; Bishara and Iverson, 1974) that include unoperated cases appear to contradict some of these findings. The prosthetic management of these patients and the variable completeness of the clefting, plus a slightly different interpretation of the data, could affect the conclusions. It appears to the author that the weight of evidence favors the conclusion that the child with an unoperated cleft lip and palate is capable of developing a functionally normal facial skeleton except for the presence of the local bony defect.

FACIAL GROWTH FOLLOWING SURGICAL REPAIR

In spite of the compensating mechanisms available, as noted above, most children with a repaired cleft lip and palate show facial growth deficits that can present severe functional and esthetic problems. There is enormous variation related to the racial and familial genetic background, the type of cleft, and the type of surgical and orthodontic management received. However, the conclusion that surgery has been mainly responsible for the facial and dental problems is inescapable. Occasional incidents such as the one illustrated in Figure 49–8 reinforce this conclusion. Data from cephalometric studies invariably confirm this observation.

Mandibular Growth

The size of the basal bone of the mandible is determined by genetic factors. It appears that only a severe environmental influence can alter the genetic blueprint, but evidence of the subtle interplay of genetic and environmental forces is inadequate at present. Studies on cleft lip and palate have usually noted that the mandible is essentially normal in length (Ross and Johnston, 1967; Dahl, 1970; Narula and Ross, 1970; Nakamura, Savara, and Thomas, 1972; Smahel, 1984), although a more recent report (Ross, 1987a) indicates that the mandible is reduced in length.

Cephalometric studies consistently show, however, that there is a change in the position of the mandible (Fig. 49–9). The chin is usually retruded and is lower; i.e., there is greater facial height in spite of normal or decreased maxillary height. The change in vertical height is mild in younger children but is especially noticeable in older children. The condyle is positioned slightly upward and forward.

The explanation for these differences seems obvious: the mandible is more open than in the normal individual. As the mandible opens, the chin point moves downward and backward. The mandibular plane becomes steeper. The gonial area should also move back and down, but generally the position of gonion is normal or higher. The reason is that altering the position of the mandible does not permanently alter muscle length; instead, the bony attachment remodels to permit the muscles to maintain their correct length for optimal function. Thus, the gonial angle (the angle formed by the mandibular body and ramus) is found to be more obtuse (open) in groups of individuals with cleft lip and palate, and it increases with age (Narula and Ross, 1970), in contrast to the normal decrease with age (Munroe, 1966).

The observation that gonion is even higher in cleft lip and palate individuals than in noncleft individuals may relate to the fact that most cephalometric assessments are made with the teeth in occlusion rather than with the mandible in rest position. In the latter state there is a greater freeway space in individuals with cleft lip and palate, which would decrease the differences in the gonion position. There may also be intrinsic shortening of the muscles, an altered insertion on the pterygoid plates, or an interference with their growth as a result of palatal surgery (Ross and Johnston, 1972).

In the Pierre Robin sequence the mandible is extremely small and remains small throughout life. There is a strong likelihood

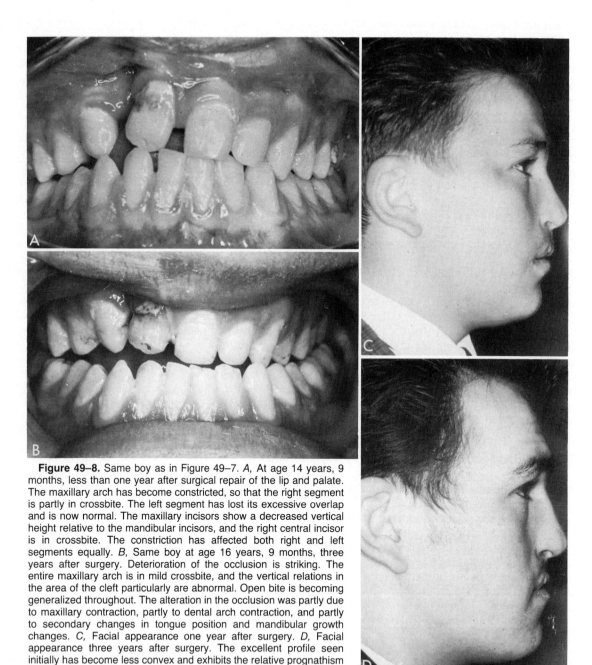

Figure 49–8. Same boy as in Figure 49–7. *A,* At age 14 years, 9 months, less than one year after surgical repair of the lip and palate. The maxillary arch has become constricted, so that the right segment is partly in crossbite. The left segment has lost its excessive overlap and is now normal. The maxillary incisors show a decreased vertical height relative to the mandibular incisors, and the right central incisor is in crossbite. The constriction has affected both right and left segments equally. *B,* Same boy at age 16 years, 9 months, three years after surgery. Deterioration of the occlusion is striking. The entire maxillary arch is in mild crossbite, and the vertical relations in the area of the cleft particularly are abnormal. Open bite is becoming generalized throughout. The alteration in the occlusion was partly due to maxillary contraction, partly to dental arch contraction, and partly to secondary changes in tongue position and mandibular growth changes. *C,* Facial appearance one year after surgery. *D,* Facial appearance three years after surgery. The excellent profile seen initially has become less convex and exhibits the relative prognathism so frequently observed in individuals with cleft lip and palate.

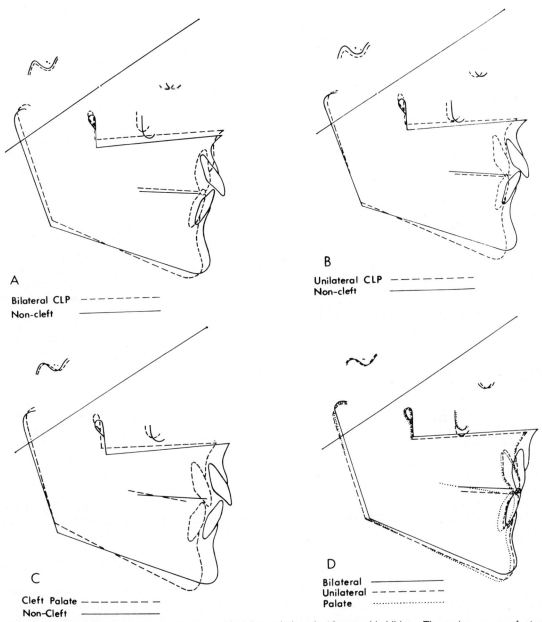

Figure 49–9. *A* to *D,* Cephalometric tracings of facial morphology in 12 year old children. The major common features of the three main cleft types are: (1) maxillary vertical underdevelopment in the posterior region, (2) maxillary underdevelopment in length (not apparent in the bilateral condition because of the protrusion of the premaxilla), (3) normal mandibular length, (4) more open mandible in cleft cases with a down-and-back rotation of the chin, and (5) acceptable jaw and tooth relations resulting from chin retrusion. (From Ross, M. B., and Johnston, M. C.: Cleft Lip and Palate. Copyright 1972, The Williams & Wilkins Company, Baltimore.)

that the cleft palate associated with the Pierre Robin sequence is secondary to the mandible and tongue relationship and is caused by a mechanical blockage of palatal shelf elevation and fusion. A similar mechanical explanation has also been advanced for the high incidence of cleft palate in the Klippel-Feil syndrome (Ross and Lindsay, 1965).

Maxillary Growth

Cleft Lip. Children with only a cleft of the lip and anterior maxilla have a minimal disturbance in facial form. There are dental irregularities in the region of the cleft, of course, and the anterior nasal spine shows some positional differences (Harvold, 1954; Coupe, 1962; Graber, 1964; Ross and Coupe, 1965; Dahl, 1970). In bilateral cleft of the lip and alveolus, particularly when the premaxilla is isolated from the remainder of the maxilla, many features of the bilateral cleft lip and palate are present, but to a lesser degree.

Cleft Palate. Facial form in individuals with isolated clefts of the hard and soft palate is characterized by a deficiency in maxillary length and a retruded position of the anterior region of the maxilla relative to the cranial base (Graber, 1954; Jolleys, 1954; Ross and Coupe, 1965; Osborne, 1966; Shibasaki and Ross, 1969; Dahl, 1970; Bishara and Iverson, 1974). These characteristics become accentuated as growth continues to maturity (Osborne, 1966; Shibasaki and Ross, 1969). The posterior vertical development of the maxilla is deficient. Figure 49–9C illustrates the morphologic differences from the normal.

Complete Unilateral Cleft Lip and Palate. Most studies noted that the anterior maxilla is retruded relative to the cranial base and becomes more retruded during growth. This is partly due to a decreased length of the maxilla and partly to a retropositioning of the maxilla. Anterior vertical development is normal or slightly less than normal, but posterior development is deficient. Studies in the literature include Graber (1954), Jolleys (1954), Foster (1962), Ross and Coupe (1965), Osborne (1966), Ross and Johnston (1967), Dahl (1970), Smahel and Brejcha (1983), and Ross (1987a). Figures 49–1 and 49–9B illustrate the morphologic differences from the normal.

Bilateral Cleft Lip and Palate. Most of the maxillary complex in bilateral cleft lip and palate is retruded, as it is in the other cleft types. The presence of a separate premaxillary area, however, results in a different growth pattern. As mentioned previously, the mild protrusion of the basal portion of the premaxilla and the severe protrusion of the dentoalveolar portion present at birth are reduced, rapidly at first after lip reconstruction, then more slowly as facial growth proceeds. Studies demonstrated that the protrusion of the premaxilla relative to the cranial base at ages 6, 8, 12, and 16 years is greater than the normal value by 8°, 4.4°, 2°, and 1.5° respectively (Ross and Johnston, 1972; Narula and Ross, 1970). In the adult the premaxillary position is normal (Birch, Ross, and Lindsay, 1967). Other studies (Friede and Pruzansky, 1972) give slightly different values, but the pattern is similar, modified by the type of surgery as well as by individual variations. In many cases the growth inhibition is excessive, and at the completion of facial growth the premaxilla is retruded relative to the remainder of the face. In almost no instance does the early protrusion persist into adulthood. Figure 49–9 illustrates the morphologic differences from the normal.

Some clinicians feel that initial surgical repositioning of the basal premaxilla to a more retruded position is desirable in many cases. Surgical intervention at an early age is unnecessary, since natural growth accomplishes the same result in time (Fig. 49–10). The experience of most clinicians is that these procedures may interfere with growth so that an apparently successful result in a young child may become a severe deformity in later years (Friede and Pruzansky, 1985). Modern management of difficult cases by presurgical orthopedics offers a less dangerous alternative, since the initial reduction of premaxillary protrusion can be accomplished quickly and easily, with no long-term effect on sensitive growth areas.

Narula and Ross (1970) have shown that the posterior segments of the maxilla, although retruded, are of normal size.

Jaw and Tooth Relations

The retrusion of the maxillary basal bone in cleft palate and unilateral cleft lip and palate is somewhat balanced by the rotation of the mandible and consequent retrusion of the chin (see Fig. 49–9). Anteroposterior jaw relations are usually found to be satisfactory

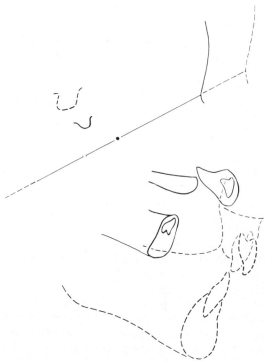

Figure 49–10. Cephalometric tracings of a child with a complete bilateral cleft lip and palate. The grossly protrusive premaxilla at age 2 months is molded back by the repaired lip. The relationship at age 7 years is greatly improved, and further reduction in premaxillary protrusion occurs as the face matures. (From Ross, R. B., and Johnston, M. C.: Cleft Lip and Palate. Copyright 1972, The Williams & Wilkins Company, Baltimore.)

in young children, but become progressively worse in older children (Ross, 1987g) and in patients who have had more traumatic surgical procedures.

The occlusal relationship is satisfactory in the primary dentition, although there is a high incidence of incisor crossbite, but there is a deterioration in the permanent dentition, with incisor crossbite and a flattening back of the incisors in both arches. In bilateral conditions the maxillary incisors are frequently inclined palatally; thus, incisor crossbite may occur even when the premaxilla is protrusive.

Maxillary width varies, but in general there is a narrowing of the dental arch following surgery, and posterior crossbites are frequent.

The increased vertical face height due to the more open mandible is compensated for by overeruption of the teeth, particularly the maxillary posterior teeth and the mandibular anterior teeth (see Fig. 49–9).

CAUSES OF ABNORMAL FACIAL GROWTH

Discussion of the actual causes of abnormal facial growth remains speculative. The au-

thor presented in detail (Ross and Johnston, 1972) one hypothesis that appears to fit the available data, and it stands as a plausible explanation of the abnormal growth and development of the face. The remainder of this chapter attempts a detailed cause and effect discussion.

Failure of adequate growth of the maxilla in length must be considered partly a basal bone problem, partly a dentoalveolar problem. The basal bone probably has an intrinsic defect caused by a general deficiency of mesenchyme in the embryonic maxillary region. The maxillary deficiency observed in any population of operated older children or adults, however, is more than could be expected and more than that observed in individuals with unoperated cleft lip and palate. The evidence is almost overwhelming that surgical repair of the lip and palate has induced a maxillary basal underdevelopment as well as the dentoalveolar distortion and the alteration in mandibular posture.

The various surgical procedures are considered separately below.

Effect of Lip Reconstruction

The effects of surgical reconstruction of the lip are generally beneficial. Continuity of the orbicularis oris and the buccinator muscles is established, providing a more normal functional matrix to influence maxillary growth.

Many of the unoperated patients reported in the literature had undergone cleft lip repair. The reports indicated that lip surgery had little adverse influence on facial growth and minimal influence on dental occlusion (Davies, 1951; Innis, 1962; Herfert, 1958; Ortiz-Monasterio and associates, 1966; Bernstein, 1968; Pitanguy and Franco, 1968; Boo-Chai, 1971). A repaired lip exerts a force on the anterior teeth that apparently is not usually sufficient to disrupt the tongue-lip guidance of the incisor teeth, although incisor crossbite can occur.

The influence of lip repair on the growth of the maxillary complex must be considered in terms of its effect on the two somewhat independent components of the maxilla: the basal bone and the alveolar bone. Reconstruction of the nasal floor and upper portion of the lip initiates pressure on the maxillary basal bone and nasal septum. Reconstruction of the lower portion of the lip establishes pressure on the dentoalveolar structures (Fig. 49–11).

Lip repair is undertaken over a maxilla that has widely separated segments. Thus, the tension produced by repair serves to bring the segments together, and maxillary width becomes normal (Harding and Mazaheri, 1972). By the time the segments contact, lip tension has stabilized and is usually close to normal. A modern, well-designed lip repair does not involve any growing area of the maxilla, nor does it interfere with the dentoalveolar adjustment mechanism. Thus, midfacial growth and adjustment proceed with no more than a mild, generalized inhibition. Ross (1987b) came to this conclusion in a study on partly repaired cases. There was no evidence that the age at which lip surgery was performed had any appreciable effect on the results.

There are occasions when lip repair can cause interference with maxillary development. An increased pressure on the basal maxilla, because of either tissue deficiency or poor surgical technique, may inhibit forward drift of the maxilla, producing a slow, progressive retrusion of the midface. A tight lower portion of the upper lip molds the dentoalveolar structures posteriorly to an excessive degree. If there is a severe bony deficiency in the cleft area, the segments may be brought together by lip pressure, resulting in a small maxilla.

Lip Reconstruction in Unilateral Cleft Lip and Palate. In complete unilateral cleft lip and palate, the major (noncleft) segment following surgery is subjected to lip muscle pull toward the midline of the face, reversing the previous pull away from the midline. The result is a rapid improvement in its position. The outward rotation of the premaxillary area is molded back, and a slight medial movement of the small segment occurs. These three factors result in reasonably normal maxillary arch shape, and apposition of the alveolar margins occurs in a large percentage of cases. The maxillary dental arch is usually well related to the mandibular dental arch as the teeth erupt.

In spite of the rotation of the noncleft segment, the midline of the maxilla (anterior nasal spine) invariably remains deviated from the midline of the face (Harvold, 1954). The nasal septum, which was bowed toward the noncleft side, is brought back after surgery and assumes the shape so characteristic of unilateral cleft lip and palate (Fig. 49–12).

The repair of the floor of the nose narrows the base of the cleft nostril to match the noncleft nostril, and the columella returns to the midline of the face. Distortion of the nasal cartilages, however, persists to some extent.

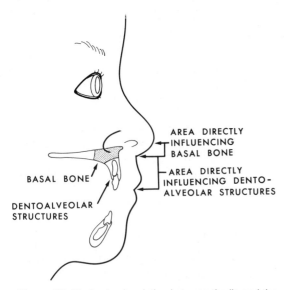

Figure 49–11. Anatomic relation between the lip and the maxilla. The lower part of the lip presses on the teeth and alveolar bone and can cause retrusion of these structures if the pressure is excessive. The basal bone of the maxilla is not directly affected by this pressure. The nasal floor and upper portion of the lip can directly influence basal bone growth.

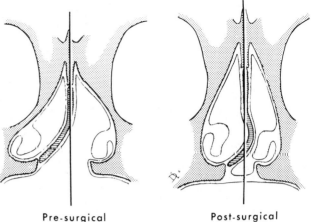

Figure 49–12. Displacement of the larger segment of the maxilla in a complete unilateral cleft lip and palate causes displacement of the attached nasal septum, especially in the anterior region. Following surgical repair of the lip and palate, the maxillary segment is positioned close to the midline of the face, and the nasal septum assumes a characteristic configuration. (From Ross, R. B., and Johnston, M. C.: Cleft Lip and Palate. Copyright 1972, The Williams & Wilkins Company, Baltimore.)

Pre-surgical   Post-surgical

Subsequent improvement in alar form does not usually occur, and asymmetries persist throughout life unless reconstructive surgery is undertaken.

Lip Reconstruction in Bilateral Cleft Lip and Palate. The morphologic features of a bilateral cleft lip and palate are quite different from those of the unilateral; there are entirely different considerations in evaluating the sequelae of lip reconstruction. The basal component of the premaxilla is reduced in this condition, since the contributions from the maxillary processes are absent. Like all basal bone, it is resistant to environmental influences. Thus, the position of the anterior nasal spine is only slightly forward at birth, and it is only slowly inhibited or displaced posteriorly by upper lip pressure. In most cases the basal bone of the premaxilla responds by becoming progressively less protrusive than at birth.

The dentoalveolar component attached to the basal bone is extremely sensitive to environmental forces. Lip repair, which restores a soft tissue–muscle balance to this area, contains the protrusive alveolus and molds it back without directly affecting the basal bone. When there is severe protrusion (anterior rotation) of the premaxilla, together with a deficiency of prolabium and lateral lip tissue, it becomes difficult to achieve an ideal lip repair. In such cases, presurgical orthopedics are valuable in rotating the premaxilla posteriorly (see Chap. 57).

If the lower portion of the lip exerts excessive pressure, there is a dentoalveolar retrusion that may have almost no effect on the position of the anterior nasal spine (Fig. 49–13). Lip repair that joins lateral lip tissue under the prolabium may result in a tight

lip. The use of the prolabium for the entire midsection of the lip usually stimulates its growth, and an adequate lip size usually

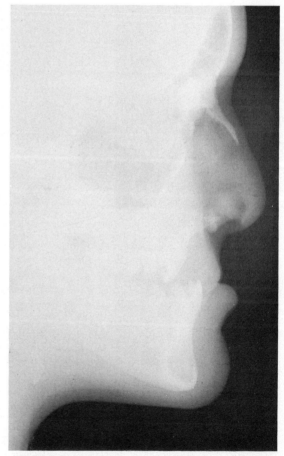

Figure 49–13. Boy with complete bilateral cleft lip and palate. The upper lip was thick and tight, exerting excessive pressure on the teeth and alveolar process. Note that the basal maxilla (anterior nasal spine) was not affected. There was also mouth breathing, which eliminated the support of the tongue and mandibular teeth.

results. If the lip is so short that it is incapable of molding back the alveolar process, severe protrusion of the alveolus remains, and the teeth erupt without anterior support. In this situation the lower lip falls behind the maxillary teeth, encouraging further protrusion of the teeth. Since teeth erupt until they encounter resistance from the lower teeth or the lip, and since this resistance is almost completely lacking, a great deal of excessive eruption of the teeth may occur in these cases (Fig. 49–14).

Dentoalveolar distortions due to either inadequate or excessive lip pressures are extremely difficult to correct at a later age. It is incumbent upon the surgeon to provide the young child with a lip that will reverse the prenatal distorting influences. At the same time, the reconstructed lip should encourage

a growth pattern that results in the establishment of normal skeletal relationships at maturity and guides the upper teeth into a satisfactory relationship with the lower teeth.

Effect of Repair of Cleft Alveolus

Many surgeons repair the alveolus with soft tissue flaps of various kinds while repairing the lip. This maneuver closes off the anterior oral cavity from the nasal, and subsequent hard and soft palate repair completes the reconstruction.

The early proponents of presurgical orthopedics followed by bone grafting to the alveolus reasoned that, by fusing the segments in a much more normal configuration than at birth, collapse of the maxilla would

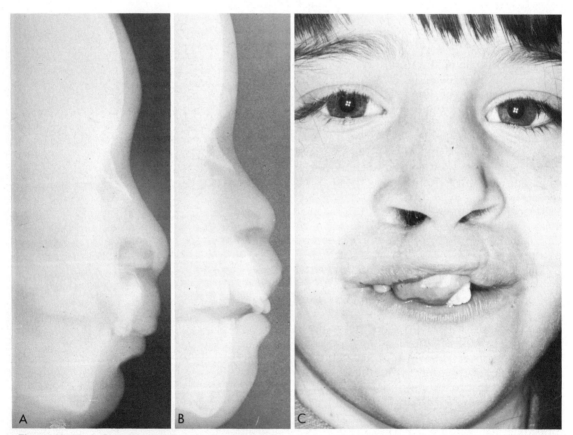

Figure 49–14. *A,* Complete bilateral cleft lip and palate in a young child in whom the lip had been repaired by bringing the lateral segments together under the prolabium. The result is a long lip that molds the erupted incisors and alveolus posteriorly. An adequate dental relationship is established in spite of the severe premaxillary protrusion. *B,* Complete bilateral cleft lip and palate in a young child in whom the prolabium was used for the entire lip length. A short lip has resulted, with no pressure on the erupted incisors and no molding of the teeth and alveolus. The lower lip falls behind the maxillary teeth and causes incisor protrusion. Note that the unerupted permanent incisors are in identical positions in both cases. As the permanent incisors erupt in *B,* however, they will produce an unsatisfactory facial appearance, as in the older girl in *C.* (From Ross, R. B., and Johnston, M. C.: Cleft Lip and Palate. Copyright, 1972, The Williams & Wilkins Company, Baltimore.)

be prevented and improved growth and dental occlusion would follow. Different kinds of bone in various configurations have been used to fill partially or completely the alveolus, the basal bone to the pyriform fossa, and even part of the hard palate. Skoog (Hellquist and Ponten, 1979) developed a periosteoplasty procedure that induced bone to bridge the alveolar gap. Koberg (1973) and Witsenburg (1985) published excellent reviews of the use of bone grafts to fill the alveolar cleft.

The results were variable. Friede and Johanson (1982) reported well-documented studies showing that patients who had received their type of alveolar bone graft in infancy developed a severe maxillary retrognathia and vertical deficiency that worsened with age. These authors discontinued the procedure and later noted that 50 per cent of the patients required orthognathic surgery to achieve satisfactory occlusion and facial appearance. Robertson and Jolleys (1983) had a similar experience, noting in addition that the grafts deteriorated to a small strut of bone, with no evidence of tooth migration into it.

Rosenstein and associates (1982) and Nordin and associates (1983) continued to use primary bone grafts and were not dissatisfied with the maxillary growth that resulted. The Nordin study indicated that the "T-traction" orthopedic device improved the results considerably.

Ross (1970) pointed out that the alveolus and area of the maxilla in which the bone graft is placed is not a site of maxillary growth (Enlow, 1968). Consequently, anteroposterior maxillary development should not be affected if grafts are confined to the alveolar area. Grafting could prevent medial collapse of the bony segments, but would have no effect on the dentoalveolar medial collapse caused by residual scar tissue from the palate surgery. The additional scar tissue from the bone graft, however, could interfere with vertical development of the adjacent alveolar process and alter the eruptive direction of the teeth. Friede and Johanson (1982) were of the opinion that the poor development they observed was caused by interference with the maxillary-vomerine suture. Dahl, Hanusardottir, and Bergland (1981) found that some techniques of vomeroplasty did cause an increased incidence of crossbites in the primary dentition.

Ross (1987c), in a large, multicenter study, determined that alveolar repair resulted in a reduced vertical height of the anterior maxilla (Fig. 49–15). If a bone graft were used, the effect was exaggerated and anteroposterior inhibition was also noted (Fig. 49–16). Later bone grafting after the age of 9 years also affects vertical growth of the maxilla but does not inhibit anteroposterior growth. Ross (1987c) suggested that alveolar repair in unilateral clefts be postponed until the age of 9 years or later if there is any intimation of a vertical disproportion.

Effect of Palate Reconstruction on Maxillary Complex

In the reconstruction of a cleft palate, the surgeon must obtain tissue to bridge the cleft. Many techniques are employed, but they usually involve raising mucoperiosteal flaps from the palate and relocating them medially and posteriorly, leaving a denuded area of bone adjacent to the alveolar process (see Chap. 54). The filling in of the denuded area produces scar tissue, which exerts an initial contracting force on adjacent tissues (Kremenak, 1984). Following the early stages of contraction, however, there is only a mild reduction in arch width (Dixon, 1966; Kremenak, Huffman, and Olin, 1970; Harding and Mazaheri, 1972). If maxillary growth could proceed normally from this point on (as it does in unoperated clefts), the dentoalveolar structures could easily cope with the mild discrepancy, and a normal occlusion would result.

Growth in length of the maxilla requires that the entire maxilla move forward freely so that bone can be deposited on the tuberosity. If during palatal repair there is undermining of tissues and hamulus fracture in the area of the pterygo-palato-maxillary junction, scar tissue may form across this sensitive growth area and inhibit the forward movement of the maxilla. It is not necessary that the inhibition of growth be severe, because even a fraction of a millimeter of inhibition each year would create a severe problem by the time of facial maturity. The cited evidence indicates that maxillary underdevelopment is indeed progressive, and Figure 49–17 illustrates the type of problem encountered clinically.

Vertical growth of the posterior maxilla may be inadequate owing to an intrinsic deficiency or surgical interference with growth.

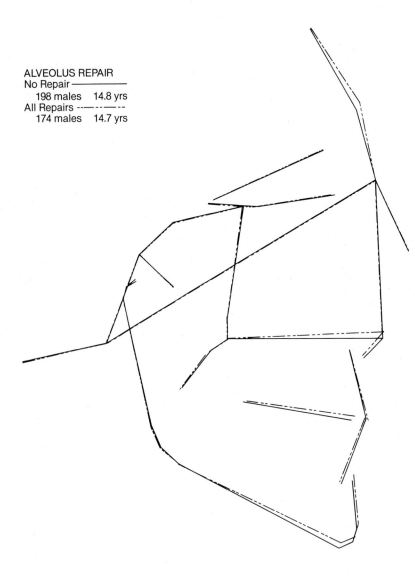

ALVEOLUS REPAIR
No Repair ————————
   198 males   14.8 yrs
All Repairs ——–··——··
   174 males   14.7 yrs

Figure 49–15. The effect of early repair of the alveolar cleft is illustrated by a comparison of the mean facial diagrams of males with complete unilateral cleft lip and palate. The repaired group (*interrupted lines*) have a decreased anterior maxillary height compared with the nonrepaired group (*solid line*).

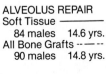

ALVEOLUS REPAIR
Soft Tissue ————
   84 males   14.6 yrs.
All Bone Grafts -- —--
   90 males   14.8 yrs.

Figure 49–16. The major difference in midface growth between samples with soft tissue alveolus repair (*solid line*) and with a bone graft (*interrupted line*) is a decreased anteroposterior growth in the bone grafted cases.

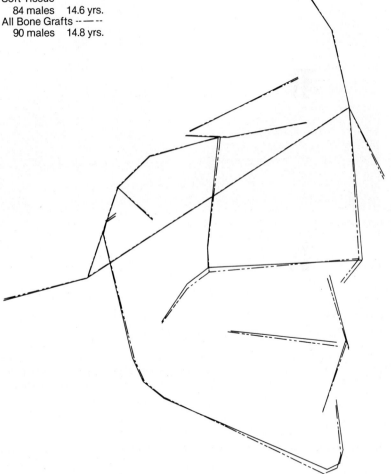

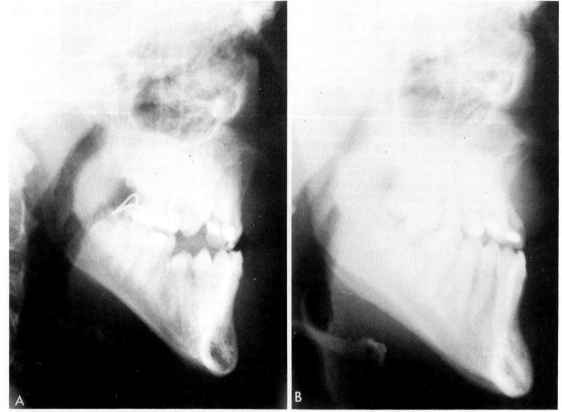

Figure 49–17. Cephalometric radiographs of a boy with surgical repair of a complete unilateral cleft lip and palate, illustrating the progressive nature of the midface underdevelopment. *A,* At age 12 years the skeletal relations are adequate to achieve a balanced face and dental occlusion. *B,* In spite of extensive orthodontic treatment, which advanced the maxillary incisors and retracted the mandibular incisors, by 16 years of age the skeletal relations have become unbalanced. There is now a severe midface retrusion with poor dental relationships.

The width of the basal maxilla probably is not appreciably reduced in most patients with cleft lip and palate (Coupe and Subtelny, 1960; Dahl, 1970; Nakamura, Savara, and Thomas, 1972). The apparent narrowing is mainly in dental arch width and may also be related to the decreased length of the maxilla, which places a narrower portion of the dental arch in contact with a wider portion of the mandibular dental arch. There are, of course, many patients with a true deficiency in maxillary width.

The dentoalveolar component of the maxilla is more certainly affected by surgery and is probably an even more important factor in abnormal facial development, at least from the orthodontist's viewpoint. Surgical procedures on the palate result in scar tissue adjacent to the alveolus (Fig. 49–18). The initial scar tissue contraction during healing causes a movement of the maxillary segments until, in most cases, contact between the segments is achieved. There probably is con-striction of the dental arch also, since the suspensory mechanism of the teeth, the periodontal ligament, sends fibers into the surrounding mucosa that are caught up in the scar tissue. More important, the scarred palatal mucosa resists further growth to some extent, and tension on the periodontal fibers during subsequent tooth eruption causes a

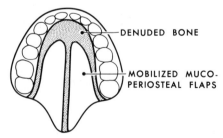

Figure 49–18. After palate repair that involves extensive flap mobilization, there is a continuum of scar tissue created in the palate adjacent to the alveolar process. The entire dentition is induced to develop in a more palatal direction by the inhibiting influence of the scarred mucosa.

posterior and medial deflection of the teeth (Figs. 49–19, 49–20) by the continuum of scar tissue from the pterygoid plates to the incisor region. Thus, the satisfactory relationship of the primary teeth progressively worsens by the time of full permanent dentition.

Multiple procedures to effect palate closure cause severe maxillary inhibition (Slaughter and Brodie, 1949; Graber, 1951; Chapman and Birch, 1965). One often sees repaired palates with irregular contours and a lowered vault. This appears to be the result of movement of the flaps after surgery because of poor fixation, hemorrhage, and hematoma formation, or contraction during healing, which tends to pull the flaps away from the vault. It is likely that callus-like bone forms under the flaps. The lowered, irregular vault impinges on the space available for the tongue and interferes with tongue posture and function.

Many secondary factors act to alter facial growth. Normal tongue posture in the palatal

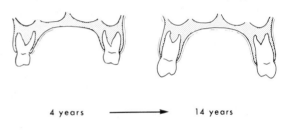

NON-CLEFT

4 years ——————▶ 14 years

CLEFT

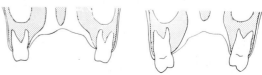

Figure 49–20. The teeth in the buccal segments of the maxilla normally erupt in a downward, forward, and lateral direction. As is the case with the incisor teeth, scar tissue adjacent to the alveolar process deflects these teeth medially and posteriorly during eruption by causing tension on the periodontal fibers that extend into the palatal mucosa. (From Ross, R. B., and Johnston, M. C.: Cleft Lip and Palate. Copyright 1972, The Williams & Wilkins Company, Baltimore.)

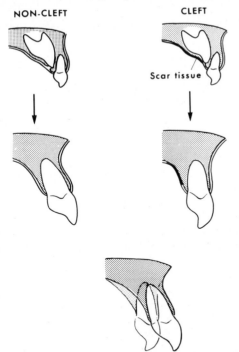

NON-CLEFT   CLEFT

Scar tissue

Figure 49–19. The maxillary incisor teeth normally erupt in a downward and forward direction. In a child in whom scar tissue has been created in the palate close to the alveolar process, the incisor teeth are deflected palatally by tension on the periodontal fibers that extend into the palatal mucosa. Free movement of the teeth to adjust to the mandibular incisors is prevented, and crossbite may develop in cases in which the skeletal relations are adequate. (From Ross, R. B., and Johnston, M. C.: Cleft Lip and Palate. Copyright 1972, The Williams & Wilkins Company, Baltimore.)

vault is particularly important for resistance to abnormal growth tendencies. The frequent occurrence of mouth breathing in children with cleft lip and palate is related to the deviated nasal septum and the high incidence of upper respiratory infections that interfere with breathing and cause enlarged tonsils and adenoids.

Mouth breathing causes a lowered tongue posture, out of the palatal vault. This is compounded by the decreased size of the palatal vault (constricted dental arch and postsurgical vault shape), which inhibits proper tongue placement. Enlarged tonsils mechanically induce a forward tongue position. The altered tongue posture, with or without mouth breathing, causes two problems. First, it removes some of the essential tongue support of the maxillary arch, encouraging further constriction (Linder-Aronson, 1970; Paul and Nanda, 1973). Second, it forces the mandible to open and accounts for the altered position of the mandible discussed previously (Linder-Aronson, 1970; Dunn, Green, and Cunat, 1973; Paul and Nanda, 1973). If the mandible is held excessively open at rest, the mandibular incisors do not support the maxillary teeth adequately, and they are less able to resist the constricting tendency. Figure 49–21 summarizes the role of many of these factors.

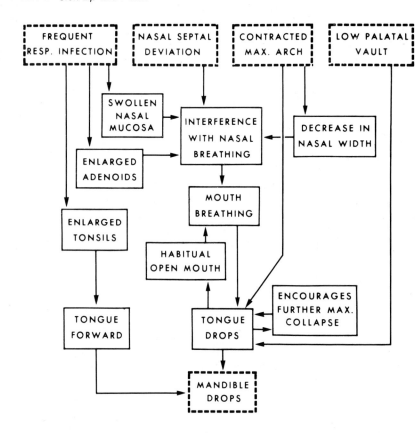

Figure 49–21. Many of the factors that cause the mandible in children with cleft lip and palate to assume a more open position than in the normal child. (From Ross, R. B., and Johnston, M. C.: Cleft Lip and Palate. Copyright 1972, The Williams & Wilkins Company, Baltimore.)

As mentioned earlier, vertical development of the dentoalveolar process is not inhibited in the early years. Even cases with an excess freeway space are characterized by normal molar eruption; the excess freeway is caused by an excessive amount of mandibular opening (Fig. 49–22). A vertical problem frequently occurs in the incisor region during the final stages of mandibular growth. Growth normally ceases in the maxilla before it does in the mandible, but compensatory dentoalveolar development maintains the occlusion. In cleft lip and palate, the maxillary incisors often are unable to make this compensation, and an open bite results (Fig. 49–23).

To encourage less traumatic surgery, many authors suggested that the soft palate be repaired early to facilitate speech, but that surgical correction of the hard palate be deferred for a later repair (Gillies and Fry, 1921; Coursin, 1950; Graber, 1951; McNeil, 1950; Rosenthal, 1951, 1964; Slaughter and Pruzansky, 1954; Trusler, Bauer, and Tondra, 1955; Webster and associates, 1958; Lewin and Ship, 1962; Lewin, 1964; Penkava, 1967).

Ross (1987a) noted that the portion of his sample with the soft palate repaired, but without hard palatal repair, showed excellent maxillary growth in length and anteroposterior position, even when compared with the totally unoperated sample. There was, however, a deficiency in posterior vertical height. His conclusion was that repair of the soft palate did not inhibit facial growth in any clinically significant way.

It was often noted that if only the soft palate is repaired at the initial phase of palatal surgery, the palatal shelves grow and the cleft narrows almost to obliteration. The second phase of repair thus becomes a simple midline closure at a later date. The advantage of this technique is the avoidance of surgery in the periphery of the palate. Since there is no scar tissue near the teeth, there is no interference with the dentoalveolar adjustment, and deformation of the dental arch should not occur. Schweckendiek delayed hard palatal repair into the adolescent years (Schweckendiek, 1978). Robertson and Jolleys (1974) reported the results of a delayed hard palatal repair, and Hotz and associates (1978) made it an acceptable practice to delay hard palatal repair until the time of early mixed dentition. It is interesting that the similar delayed hard palatal repair adopted

HIGH AND LOW FREEWAY CASES

Figure 49–22. Diagrams from a cephalometric study of children with cleft lip and palate, comparing cases with a large freeway space between the teeth in rest position to cases with a small freeway space between the teeth in rest position. Note that the relationship in the occlusal contact position (teeth together) is not too different. The cause of the excessive freeway space, therefore, is not undereruption of the teeth but rather the excessive opening of the mandible. It appears that the mandible is more open in cases in which the maxilla is most underdeveloped. (From Cohen E.: Skeletal variations in cleft palate individuals with excessive interocclusal clearance. *In* Ross, R. B., and Johnston, M. C.: Cleft Lip and Palate. Copyright 1972, The Williams & Wilkins Company, Baltimore.)

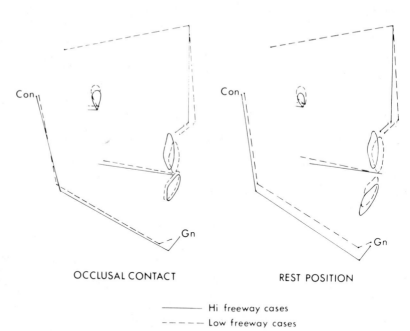

OCCLUSAL CONTACT   REST POSITION

———— Hi freeway cases

– – – – Low freeway cases

by Jolleys and Robertson (1972) and by Hotz and associates (1978) apparently achieved very different results. The technique had long been abandoned by the former as being unsatisfactory, while being enthusiastically promoted by the latter group.

Evidence for the value of these procedures has been scanty, although Olin (Bardach, Morris, and Olin, 1984) provided data that facial growth using the Schweckendiek procedure was excellent. Blijdorp and Egyedi (1984) found no difference between repair of the hard palate at 3 years or 6 years of age. Late repair in theory should be less damaging than early repair, on the assumption that the more growth that has occurred, the less there remains to interfere with. There has, however, been no adequate evidence to support the theory that growth is improved by delaying surgery for several years (Witzel, Salyer, and Ross, 1984). Meanwhile, many speech scientists have been less than enthusiastic, particularly in North America, about the results of delaying surgery past the age of early speech development (Dorf and Curtin, 1982; Witzel, Salyer, and Ross, 1984).

Repair of the hard palate probably accounts for the major growth interference in clefts. As noted in Figure 49–24, the group with palatal repair shows decreased posterior maxillary vertical height, restricted maxillary

forward positioning (shallow pharynx), and little or no restriction in maxillary basal bone length, but restriction in forward development of the teeth and alveolar process. The jaw and incisor relations were also much less satisfactory with palatal repair.

Ross (1987e) reported that the timing of hard palatal repair did not matter within the first decade. Early repair (before 12 months of age) gave at least as satisfactory results as delayed hard palatal repair. Similarly, the particular technique used to accomplish palatal repair does not affect the growth of the facial skeleton (Ross, 1987f). The conclusions on palatal repair were that it does inhibit maxillary growth, and that the principal variant is the surgeon performing the operation, not the timing or type of technique.

Effect of Orthopedics and Orthodontics

Despite the popularity of presurgical infant orthopedic procedures, they appear to have no effect on facial growth (Ross, 1987b). This is also true for early orthodontic treatment during periods of primary or mixed dentition (Ross and Johnston, 1967). The potential exists for altering jaw growth, but the orthopedic procedures currently in use have not

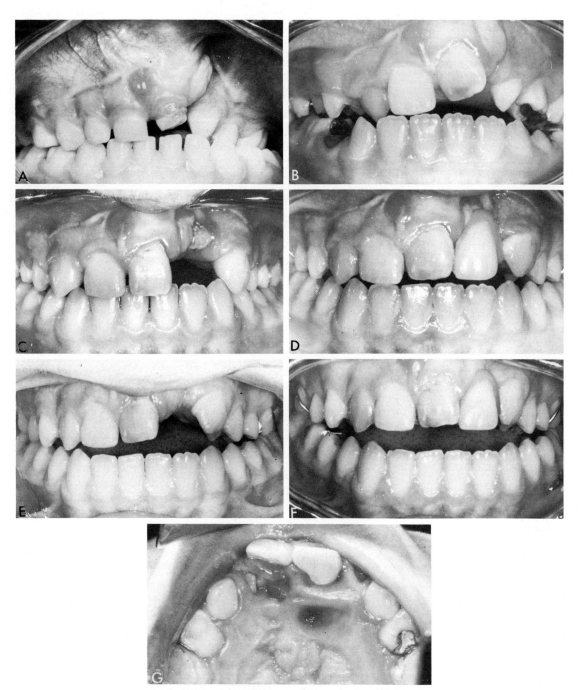

Figure 49–23. Development of the dental occlusion in a boy with repaired complete unilateral cleft lip and palate. The malocclusion in the primary dentition at age 5 (*A*) was limited to segmental contraction on the left side. At age 11 (*B*) there was some indication of mild open bite development. At age 13 (*C*), following orthodontic treatment, the occlusion was excellent, and a temporary prosthesis was inserted. Opening of the bite occurred within four months (*D*) and progressively worsened to 15 years (*E*) and 17 years (*F*). A major factor was the abundance of scar tissue in the palate adjacent to the anterior teeth (*G*), which interfered with vertical eruption of the teeth. The effect of the interference became most obvious during adolescence with the increase in the vertical dimension of the face. At this time the maxilla grows less than the mandible, and the maxillary and mandibular teeth must erupt to maintain the occlusal relations. (From Ross, R. B., and Johnston, M. C.: Cleft Lip and Palate. Copyright 1972, The Williams & Wilkins Company, Baltimore.)

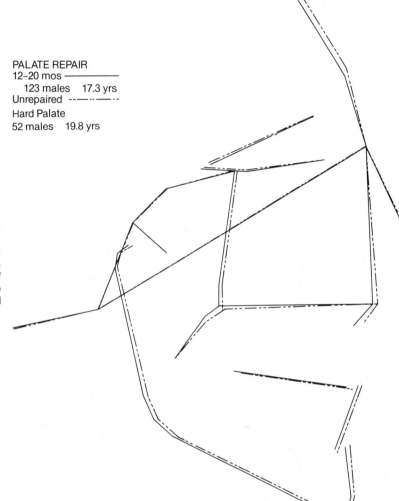

PALATE REPAIR
12–20 mos ————
   123 males 17.3 yrs
Unrepaired --—--—··
Hard Palate
52 males 19.8 yrs

Figure 49–24. A comparison of two samples of males with unilateral cleft lip and palate, one having hard palate repair at the traditional 12 to 20 months of age (*solid line*) and the other with no hard palate repair (*interrupted line*). The deficiency of midface growth is apparent in the operated group.

been shown to produce permanent increased basal bone growth.

DISCUSSION

The surgeon who undertakes the habilitation of an infant with cleft lip and palate has four major goals: to reconstruct a functional speech mechanism, to reconstruct the features of the lip and nose for maximal esthetics, to separate the nasal and oral cavities, and to encourage adequate growth of the facial skeleton.

An explanation has been presented for the abnormal growth and development of the facial skeleton and dentition. To recapitulate the major points covered:

1. The intrinsic defect in an individual with cleft lip and palate is mild, except in the immediate area of the cleft.

2. The potential for growth of the maxillary complex is adequate to produce harmonious skeletal relationships.

3. The teeth and alveolar bone have the capacity to overcome minor deficiencies in the maxillary complex and produce a satisfactory occlusion.

4. Surgery produces scar tissue that interferes with maxillary growth. It is not necessary that this be a severe restriction; any reduction in maxillary growth can be significant for children with cleft lip and palate.

5. Surgery produces scar tissue in the palate that prevents the free adjustment of the teeth and causes distortion of the dental arch by deflecting the eruption of the teeth.

6. Secondary changes in tongue position

cause displacement and deformation of the mandible.

7. Early repair of the alveolus, with or without bone grafting, is detrimental to facial growth.

8. The most important variable in cleft palate surgery is the surgeon; the traditional techniques do not exert appreciably different influences on facial growth.

9. The timing of hard palatal repair within the first decade is not critical. There is no advantage in delaying repair to 4 to 7 years of age.

REFERENCES

Abyholm, F. E., Bergland, O., and Semb, G.: Secondary bone grafting of alveolar clefts. Scand. J. Plast. Reconstr. Surg., 15:127, 1981.

Atherton, J. D.: Morphology of facial bones in skulls with unoperated unilateral cleft palate. Cleft Palate J., 4:18, 1967.

Atkinson, S. R.: Jaws out of balance. II. Am. J. Orthod., 52:371, 1966.

Bardach, J., Morris, H. L., and Olin, W. H.: Late results of primary veloplasty: the Marburg Project. Plast. Reconstr. Surg., 73:207, 1984.

Bariana, G., Ross, R. B., and Lindsay, W. K.: A comparison of maxillary growth in two types of palate repair. Unpublished manuscript, 1972.

Bernstein, L.: The effect of timing of cleft palate operations and subsequent growth of the maxilla. Laryngoscope, 78:1510, 1968.

Bill, A. H., Moore, A. W., and Coe, H. E.: The time of choice for repair of cleft palate in relation to the type of surgical repair and its effect on bony growth of the face. Plast. Reconstr. Surg., 18:469, 1956.

Birch, J., Ross, R. B., and Lindsay, W. K.: The end result of growth and treatment in bilateral complete cleft lip and palate. Panminerva Med., 9:391, 1967.

Bishara, S. E., and Iverson, W. W.: Cephalometric comparisons on the cranial base and face in individuals with isolated clefts of the palate. Cleft Palate J., 11:162, 1974.

Bjork, A.: Sutural growth of the upper face studied by the implant method. Acta Odontol. Scand., 24:109, 1966.

Blijdorp, P., and Egyedi, P.: The influence of age at operation for cleft on the development of the jaws. J. Maxillofac. Surg., 12:193, 1984.

Boo-Chai, K.: The unoperated adult bilateral cleft of the lip and palate. Br. J. Plast. Surg., 24:250, 1971.

Boyne, P. J., and Sands, N. R.: Secondary bone grafting of residual alveolar and palatal clefts. J. Oral Surg., 30:87, 1972.

Chapman, J. H., and Birch, D. A.: An orthodontic and otolaryngological review of thirty-four cleft-lip and cleft-palate patients. Br. J. Surg., 52:646, 1965.

Coccaro, P. J., D'Amico, R., and Chavoor, A.: Craniofacial morphology of parents with and without cleft lip and palate children. Cleft Palate J., 9:28, 1970.

Coupe, T. B.: A study of the morphology and growth of the nasal septum in children with clefts of the lip and palate. M.Sc. thesis, University of Toronto, 1962.

Coupe, T. B., and Subtelny, J. D.: Cleft palate—deficiency or displacement of tissue. Plast. Reconstr. Surg., 26:600, 1960.

Coursin, D. B.: Treatment of the patient with cleft palate. Am. J. Dis. Child., 80:442, 1950.

Dahl, E.: Craniofacial morphology in congenital clefts of the lip and palate. Acta Odontol. Scand., 28(Suppl. 57):11, 1970.

Dahl, E., Hanusardottir, B., and Bergland, O.: A comparison of occlusions in two groups of children whose clefts were repaired by three different surgical procedures. Cleft Palate J., 18:122, 1981.

Davies, A. D.: Unoperated bilateral complete cleft lip and palate in the adult. Plast. Reconstr. Surg., 7:482, 1951.

Dixon, D. A.: Abnormalities of the teeth and supporting structures in children with clefts of lip and palate. In Drillien, C. M., Ingram, T. T. S., and Wilkinson, E. M. (Eds.): The Causes and Natural History of Cleft Lip and Palate. Edinburgh, E. & S. Livingstone, 1966, pp. 178–205.

Dorf, D. S., and Curtin, J. W.: Early cleft palate repair and speech outcome. Plast. Reconstr. Surg., 70:74, 1982.

Dorrance, G. M., and Bransfield, J. W.: Studies in the anatomy and repair of cleft palate. Surg. Gynecol. Obstet., 84:187, 1947.

Drillien, C. M., Ingram, T. T. S., and Wilkinson, E. M. (Eds.): The Causes and Natural History of Cleft Lip and Palate. Edinburgh, E. & S. Livingstone, 1966.

Droschl, H.: The effect of heavy orthopedic forces on the maxilla in the growing Saimiri sciureus (squirrel monkey). Am. J. Orthod., 63:449, 1973.

Dunn, G. F., Green, L. J., and Cunat, J. J.: Relationships between variation of mandibular morphology and variation of nasopharyngeal airway size in monozygotic twins. Angle Orthod., 43:129, 1973.

Enlow, D. H.: The Human Face. New York, Harper & Row, 1968.

Enlow, D. H., and Bang, S.: Growth and remodeling of the human maxilla. Am. J. Orthod., 51:446, 1965.

Farkas, L. G., and Lindsay, W. K.: Morphology of the orbital region in adults following the cleft lip-palate repair in childhood. Am. J. Phys. Anthropol., 37:65, 1972.

Foster, T. D.: Maxillary deformities in repaired clefts of the lip and palate. Br. J. Plast. Surg., 15:182, 1962.

Friede, H., and Johanson, B.: Adolescent facial morphology of early bone-grafted cleft lip and palate patients. Scand. J. Plast. Reconstr. Surg., 16:41, 1982.

Friede, H., and Pruzansky, S.: Longitudinal study of growth in bilateral cleft lip and palate, from infancy to adolescence. Plast. Reconstr. Surg., 49:392, 1972.

Friede, H., and Pruzansky, S.: Long-term effects of premaxillary setback on facial skeletal profile in complete bilateral cleft lip and palate. Cleft Palate J., 22:97, 1985.

Gillies, H. D., and Fry, K. W.: A new principle in the surgical treatment of congenital cleft palate. Br. Dent. J., 42:293, 1921.

Graber, T. M.: A study of the congenital cleft palate deformity. Ph.D. thesis, Northwestern University, Chicago, 1951.

Graber, T. M.: The congenital cleft palate deformity. J. Am. Dent. Assoc., 48:375, 1954.

Graber, T. M.: A study of craniofacial growth and development in the cleft palate child from birth to six years of age. In Hotz, R. (Ed.): Early Treatment of Cleft Lip and Palate. Bern, Hans Huber, 1964, pp. 30–43.

Hagerty, R. F., and Hill, M. J.: Facial growth and dentition in the unoperated cleft palate. J. Dent. Res., *42*:412, 1963.

Harding, R. L., and Mazaheri, M.: Growth and spatial changes in the arch form in bilateral cleft lip and palate. Plast. Reconstr. Surg., *50*:591, 1972.

Harvold, E.: Cleft lip and palate. Morphologic studies of the facial skeleton. Am. J. Orthod., *40*:493, 1954.

Hellquist, R., and Ponten, B.: The influence of infant periosteoplasty on facial growth and dental occlusion from five to eight years of age in cases of complete unilateral cleft lip and palate. Scand. J. Plast. Reconstr. Surg., *13*:305, 1979.

Herfert, O.: Fundamental investigations into problems related to cleft palate surgery. Br. J. Plast. Surg., *11*:97, 1958.

Herfert, O.: Two-stage operation for cleft palate. Br. J. Plast. Surg., *16*:37, 1972.

Hotz, M. M., Gnoinski, W. M., Nussbaumer, H., and Kistler, E.: Early maxillary orthopedics in CLP cases: guidelines for surgery. Cleft Palate J., *15*:405, 1978.

Huddart, A. G., MacCauley, F. J., and Davis, M. E.: Maxillary arch dimensions in normal and unilateral cleft palate subjects. Cleft Palate J., *6*:471, 1969.

Innis, C. O.: Some preliminary observations on unrepaired harelips and cleft palates in adult members of the Dusan tribes of North Borneo. Br. J. Plast. Surg., *15*:173, 1962.

Jakobsson, S. O.: Cephalometric evaluation of treatment effect on Class II, Division I malocclusions. Am. J. Orthod., *53*:446, 1967.

Johnson, R.: Physical development of cleft lip and palate children. *In* Cox, M. A. (Ed.): Five Year Report (1955–1959) of the Cleft Lip and Palate Research and Treatment Centre. Toronto, Hospital For Sick Children, 1960, pp. 104–108.

Jolleys, A.: A review of the results of operations on cleft palates with reference to maxillary growth and speech function. Br. J. Plast. Surg., *7*:229, 1954.

Jolleys, A., and Robertson, N. R.: A study of the effects of early bone-grafting in complete clefts of the lip and palate—a five year study. Br. J. Plast. Surg., *25*:229, 1972.

Karout, G. G., and Ross, R. B.: Facial characteristics of parents of children with bilateral cleft lip and palate. M.Sc. thesis, University of Toronto, 1974.

Koberg, W. R.: Present view on bone grafting in cleft palate. J. Maxillofac. Surg., *1*:185, 1973.

Koski, K.: Cranial growth center: facts or fallacies. Am. J. Orthod., *54*:566, 1968.

Kremenak, C. R.: Physiological aspects of wound healing: contraction and growth. Otolaryngol. Clin. North Am., *17*:437, 1984.

Kremenak, C. R., Huffman, W. C., and Olin, W. H.: Maxillary growth inhibition by mucoperiosteal denudation of palatal shelf bone in non-cleft beagles. Cleft Palate J., *7*:817, 825, 1970.

Latham, R. A.: The pathogenesis of the skeletal deformity associated with unilateral cleft lip and palate. Cleft Palate J., *6*:404, 1969.

Latham, R. A.: Development and structure of the premaxillary deformity in bilateral cleft lip and palate. Br. J. Plast. Surg., *26*:1, 1973.

Latham, R. A., and Burston, W. R.: The effect of unilateral cleft of the lip and palate on maxillary growth pattern. Br. J. Plast. Surg., *17*:10, 1964.

Lewin, M. L.: Management of cleft lip and palate in the United States and Canada. Plast. Reconstr. Surg., *33*:383, 1964.

Lewin, M. L., and Ship, A. G.: Management of patients with cleft lip and palate. N. Y. J. Med., *62*:2523, 1962.

Linder-Aronson, S.: Adenoids. Acta Otolaryngol. (Stockh.), [Suppl.] *265*:1, 1970.

McNeil, K.: Orthodontic procedures in the treatment of congenital cleft. Dent. Rec., *70*:126, 1950.

Menius, J. A., Largent, M. D., and Vincent, C. J.: Skeletal development of cleft palate children as determined by hand-wrist roentgenographs; a preliminary study. Cleft Palate J., *3*:67, 1966.

Mestre, J., DeJesus, J., and Subtelny, J. D.: Unoperated oral clefts at maturation. Angle Orthod., *30*:78, 1960.

Moss, M. L.: Hypertelorism and cleft palate deformity. Acta Anat. (Basel), *61*:547, 1965.

Moss, M. L., Bromberg, B. E., Song, I. C., and Eisenman, G.: The passive role of nasal septal cartilage in midfacial growth. Plast. Reconstr. Surg., *41*:536, 1968.

Munroe, N.: Radiographic cephalometric study of mandibular morphology at gonion and its relation to tongue posture in cleft palate and normal individuals (abstract). J. Can. Dent. Assoc., *32*:478, 1966.

Nakamura, S., Savara, B., and Thomas, D.: Facial growth of children with cleft lip and/or palate. Cleft Palate J., *9*:119, 1972.

Narula, J., and Ross, R. B.: Facial growth in children with complete bilateral cleft lip and palate. Cleft Palate J., *7*:239, 1970.

Nordin, K. E., Larson, O., Nylen, B., and Eklund, G.: Early bone grafting in complete cleft lip and palate cases following maxillofacial orthopedics. I. The method and the skeletal development from seven to thirteen years of age. Scand. J. Plast. Reconstr. Surg., *17*:33, 1983.

Ortiz-Monasterio, F., Rebeil, A. F., Valderrama, M., and Cruz, R.: Cephalometric measurements on adult patients with nonoperated cleft palates. Plast. Reconstr. Surg., *24*:53, 1959.

Ortiz-Monasterio, F., Serrano, A., Barrera, G., and Rodriquez-Hoffman, H.: A study of untreated adult cleft palate patients. Plast. Reconstr. Surg., *38*:36, 1966.

Osborne, H. A.: A serial cephalometric analysis of facial growth in adolescent cleft palate subjects. Angle Orthod., *36*:211, 1966.

Paul, J. L., and Nanda, R. S.: Effect of mouth breathing on dental occlusion. Angle Orthod., *43*:201, 1973.

Penkava, J.: Treatment of patients with cleft in CSSR. Cleft Palate J., *4*:115, 1967.

Peyton, W. T.: Dimensions and growth of the palate in the normal infant and in the infant with gross maldevelopment of the upper lip and palate. Arch. Surg., *22*:704, 1931.

Pitanguy, I., and Franco, T.: Facial clefts in nonoperated adults (abstract). Plast. Reconstr. Surg., *41*:187, 1968.

Pruzansky, S.: The role of the orthodontist in a cleft palate team. Plast. Reconstr. Surg., *14*:10, 1954.

Pruzansky, S.: The growth of the premaxillary-vomerine complex in complete bilateral cleft lip and palate. Tandlaegebladet, *75*:1157, 1971.

Przezdziak, B.: Somatic development of children with cleft palate. Pediatr. Pol., *44*:1279, 1969.

Psaume, J.: A propos des anomalies faciales associées à des divisions palatines. Ann. Chir. Plast., *2*:3, 1957.

Robertson, N. R. E., and Jolleys, A.: The timing of hard palate repair. Scand. J. Plast. Reconstr. Surg., *8*:49, 1974.

Robertson, N. R. E., and Jolleys, A.: An 11-year follow-up of the effects of early bone grafting in infants born with complete clefts of the lip and palate. Br. J. Plast. Surg., *36*:438, 1983.

Rosenstein, S. W., Munroe, C. W., Kernahan, D. A., Jacobson, B. N., Griffith, B. H., and Bauer, B. S.: The case for early bone grafting in cleft lip and cleft palate. Plast. Reconstr. Surg., 70:297, 1982.

Rosenthal, W.: Postoperative maxillary deformities after hare lip and cleft palate operations. Chirurg., 22:483, 1951.

Rosenthal, W.: The development of cleft surgery. *In* Hotz, R. (Ed.): Early Treatment of Cleft Lip and Palate. Bern, Hans Huber, 1964, pp. 52–58.

Ross, R. B.: Cranial base in children with lip and palate clefts. Cleft Palate J., 2:157, 1965.

Ross, R. B.: The clinical implications of facial growth in cleft lip and palate. Cleft Palate J., 7:37, 1970.

Ross, R. B.: Treatment variables affecting facial growth in complete unilateral cleft lip palate: Part 1. Cleft Palate J., 24:5, 1987a.

Ross, R. B.: Treatment variables affecting facial growth in complete unilateral cleft lip palate: Part 2, Presurgical orthopedics. Cleft Palate J., 24:24, 1987b.

Ross, R. B.: Treatment variables affecting facial growth in complete unilateral cleft lip palate: Part 3, Alveolar repair and bone grafting. Cleft Palate J., 24:33, 1987c.

Ross, R. B.: Treatment variables affecting facial growth in complete unilateral cleft lip palate: Part 4, Cleft lip repair. Cleft Palate J., 24:45, 1987d.

Ross, R. B.: Treatment variables affecting facial growth in complete unilateral cleft lip palate: Part 5, Timing of cleft palate repair. Cleft Palate J., 24:54, 1987e.

Ross, R. B.: Treatment variables affecting facial growth in complete unilateral cleft lip palate: Part 6, Techniques of cleft palate repair. Cleft Palate J., 24:64, 1987f.

Ross, R. B.: Treatment variables affecting facial growth in complete unilateral cleft lip palate: Part 7, An overview. Cleft Palate J., 24:71, 1987g.

Ross, R. B., and Coupe, T. B.: Craniofacial morphology in six pairs of monozygotic twins discordant for cleft lip and palate. J. Can. Dent. Assoc., 31:149, 1965.

Ross, R. B., and Johnston, M. C.: The effect of early orthodontic treatment on facial growth in cleft lip and palate. Cleft Palate J., 4:157, 1967.

Ross, R. B., and Johnston, M. C.: Cleft Lip and Palate. Baltimore, Williams & Wilkins Company, 1972.

Ross, R. B., and Lindsay, W. K.: The cervical vertebrae as a factor in the etiology of cleft palate. Cleft Palate J., 2:273, 1965.

Schweckendiek, W.: Primary veloplasty: long-term results without maxillary deformity. A twenty-five year report. Cleft Palate J., 15:268, 1978.

Shibasaki, Y., and Ross, R. B.: Facial growth in children with isolated cleft palate. Cleft Palate J., 6:290, 1969.

Skoog, T.: The management of the bilateral cleft of the primary palate (lip and alveolus). Plast. Reconstr. Surg., 35:34, 1965.

Slaughter, W. B., and Brodie, A. G.: Facial clefts and their surgical management. Plast. Reconstr. Surg., 4:311, 1949.

Slaughter, W. B., and Pruzansky, S.: The rationale for velar closure as a primary procedure in the repair of cleft palate defects. Plast. Reconstr. Surg., 13:341, 1954.

Smahel, Z.: Craniofacial morphology in adults with bilateral complete cleft lip and palate. Cleft Palate J., 21:159, 1984.

Smahel, Z., and Brejcha, M.: Differences in craniofacial morphology between complete and incomplete unilateral cleft lip and palate in adults. Cleft Palate J., 20:113, 1983.

Stenstrom, S. J., and Thilander, B. L.: The effects of nasal septal cartilage resections on young guinea pigs. Plast. Reconstr. Surg., 45:160, 1970.

Subtelny, J. D.: Width of the nasopharynx and related anatomic structure in normal and unoperated cleft palate children. Am. J. Orthod., 41:889, 1955.

Trusler, H. M., Bauer, T. B., and Tondra, J. M.: The cleft lip–cleft palate problem. Plast. Reconstr. Surg., 16:174, 1955.

Van Limborgh, J.: Some aspects of the development of the cleft-affected face. *In* Hotz, R. (Ed.): Early Treatment of Cleft Lip and Palate. Bern, Hans Huber, 1964, pp. 25–29.

Vargervik, K.: Growth characteristics of the premaxilla and orthodontic treatment principles in bilateral cleft lip and palate. Cleft Palate J., 20:289, 1983.

Webster, R. C., Quigley, L. F., Coffey, R. J., and Querze, R. H.: Pharyngeal flap staphylorrhaphy and speech aid as means of avoiding maxillofacial growth abnormalities in patients with cleft palate: a preliminary report. Am. J. Surg., 96:820, 1958.

Weinstein, S.: Minimal forces in tooth movement. Am. J. Orthod., 53:881, 1967.

Wieslander, L.: The effect of orthodontic treatment on the concurrent development of the craniofacial complex. Am. J. Orthod., 49:15, 1963.

Witsenburg, B.: The reconstruction of anterior residual bone defects in patients with cleft lip, alveolus and palate: a review. J. Maxillofac. Surg., 13:197, 1985.

Witzel, M. A., Salyer, K., and Ross, R. B.: Delayed hard palate closure: the philosophy revisited. Cleft Palate J., 21:263, 1984.

50

R. A. Latham

Anatomy of the Facial Skeleton in Cleft Lip and Palate

The anatomic studies of Veau laid the foundation for our present understanding of cleft lip and palate (Veau, 1926, 1931, 1935). His embryologic research into the pathogenesis of cleft lip and palate in the human is a classic study (Veau and Politzer, 1936). Veau recognized that unilateral and bilateral cleft conditions showed a characteristic skeletal deformity that was consistently uniform in each cleft type, and he regarded the skeletal deformity as a product of abnormal growth subsequent to the initial embryonic failure of palate formation. It was his opinion that the protrusion of the anterior premaxillary segment seen in the unilateral and bilateral conditions was caused by uninhibited growth of the bony part of the septal stem, consisting of the vomer and premaxillary bones. The premaxillovomeral suture was regarded as

having growth potential similar to that of long bone epiphyseal plates. Consideration of numerous details of the anatomic analysis presented in this chapter may render untenable the hypothesis of growth thrust from the bony septal stem. A synthesis of the available material, in keeping with present concepts of growth and development, is proposed to which scrutiny is invited, both to test the facts and to prompt appraisal of treatment principles.

In man, except for a brief period in the embryo, the premaxilla does not exist as a separate entity. The term has been retained with reference to cleft lip and palate conditions because of its descriptive convenience and homology with experimental animals. In man, the term premaxilla is used to define that part of the upper jaw anterior to the incisive suture and the canine teeth. A cleft of the primary palate is usually thought to divide the premaxillary bone from that of the maxilla.

BILATERAL CLEFT LIP AND PALATE

Premaxilla

The complete bilateral cleft at birth shows a distinct premaxillary malformation characterized by a protrusion of the entire premaxillary bone with respect to the cartilaginous nasal septum and a protrusion of the tooth-bearing alveolar process. The protrusive premaxillary bone obliterates the columellar area of the nose so that the lip attaches directly to the nasal tip (Fig. 50–1). The total protrusion seen clinically is the summation of three factors: the abnormal forward posi-

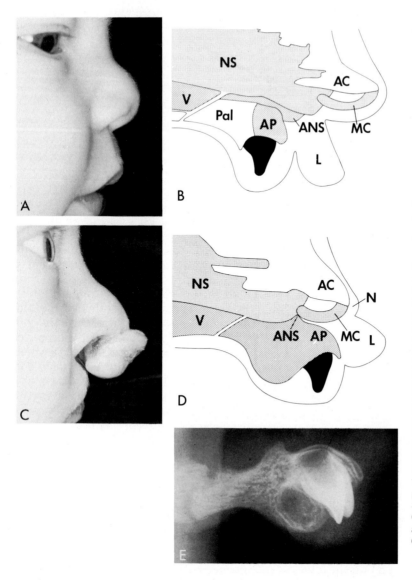

Figure 50–1. *A*, Nasolabial profile of a normal 1 month old male infant. *B*, Relationship of skeletal and soft tissues of a normal neonatal infant, drawn from a reconstruction. Medial crura (MC) of alar cartilages (AC) support the columella and nose (N). The lip lies inferior to the exposed anteroinferior angle of the nasal septum (NS); the anterior nasal spine (ANS) and alveolar process (AP) are posterior to the septal angle. Cut surface of palatal bone (Pal); vomer (V). *C*, Profile of a 2 month old male infant with complete bilateral cleft lip and palate. (Courtesy of Dr. M. L. Kasdan and Dr. H. W. Sorensen.) *D*, The protrusion of the premaxillary basal and alveolar bone in a newborn infant with bilateral cleft lip and palate. Drawn from reconstruction. The alveolar process (AP) is superimposed upon the medial crura (MC) with the lip (L) displaced anteriorly. The anterior nasal spine (ANS) is in the fork of the medial crura and adapted to the anterior border of the nasal septum (NS). *E*, Lateral radiograph of the infant in *C*, showing the premaxillary deformity. (Courtesy of Dr. M. L. Kasdan and Dr. H. W. Sorensen. From Latham, R. A., and Workman, C.: Anatomy of the philtrum and columella: the soft tissue deformity in bilateral cleft lip and palate. *In* Georgiade, N. G. (Ed.): Symposium on Management of Cleft Lip and Palate and Associated Deformities. St. Louis, MO, C. V. Mosby Company, 1974.)

tion of the premaxillary alveolar bone; an abnormally advanced position of the premaxillary basal bone; and possible underdevelopment of the maxillary segments as a whole, including some degree of anteriorly localized hypoplasia at the site of the canine tooth.

Alveolar bone supports or contains the incisor teeth, while the basal bone has a skeletal function. The basal bone articulates with the cartilaginous septum superiorly and the vomer posteriorly. It is normally continuous with the body of the maxilla laterally. In normal structure the alveolar process is directly inferior to the basal bone, but in the bilateral cleft condition the alveolar bone is anterior to the basal bone in horizontal arrangement (Fig. 50–1*C* to *E*). The basal bone

and the anterior nasal spine normally lie posterior to the anteroinferior point of the nasal septum, whereas the basal bone of the bilateral cleft premaxillae is anteriorly advanced and adapted around this septal point, and the anterior nasal spine ascends the anterior septal border (Fig. 50–1*D*, *E*). The contributions of the alveolar and basal protrusions to the overall premaxillary protrusion appear to be approximately equal.

In profile view the primary central incisor teeth lie anterior to the cartilaginous nasal septum. Part of the profile of the nasal septum may be seen in a lateral radiograph of the premaxillary segment, where it corresponds to the posterior slope of the anterior nasal spine. The incisors are not rotated forward and upward, as might be thought, but have a relatively normal vertical orientation (Fig. 50–1*E*). They are supported by a thin protruding alveolar process, which commences at the level of the anterior nasal spine, passes forward over the developing incisor roots, inferior to the medial crura of the alar cartilages, and turns inferiorly for a short distance in relation to the labial surface of the teeth.

Lip and Columella

The normal form of the upper lip, in particular the philtrum, philtrocolumellar angle, and Cupid's bow, is determined mainly by the underlying musculature (Latham and Deaton, 1976). Labial muscle fibers insert densely, into the skin lateral to the philtrum, which, not receiving such support, presents as the median philtral dimple (see also Chapter 51). The inferior border of the orbicularis oris muscle inserts closely along the vermilion border and, together with the other labial muscles, appears to give rise to the tubercle, which is inferior to the philtrum. The labial musculature inserts thickly into the skin at the base of the columella and on the nostril floors, attaching this skin to the underlying bone. This anatomic arrangement is clearly a main factor in the development of the philtrocolumellar angle.

The medial part of the bilaterally cleft upper lip is conspicuously everted. This gives the erroneous impression that the premaxillary segment is rotated anterosuperiorly on the nasal septum. The eversion of the lip and, to some extent, the hypoplasia of the columellar skin appear to be caused by the premaxillary protrusion. However, it is also possible that the tethered lip induces forward growth of the alveolar process into a protrusive position. Other important factors contributing to the malformation must also be considered. The medial lip moiety contains no muscular tissue (Veau, 1926; Latham, 1973). It is therefore grossly deficient in bulk and lacks features of form normally produced by muscle (see Chapter 51). Extrinsic factors such as the tongue, mandible, and lower lip play a variable role.

The columella may be clinically absent, but it is not anatomically absent. By definition the columella is the fleshy external termination of the septum of the nose, supported by the medial crura of the alar cartilages and covered by skin. A preliminary study of the reconstructed nasopremaxillary region of a full term infant with bilateral cleft lip and palate showed that the medial crura of the alar cartilages occupied a normal position in relation to the nose and the cartilaginous nasal septum and were of relatively normal proportions (Latham and Workman, 1974). They were almost totally obscured by the protruding alveolar process, and the columellar skin was correspondingly hypoplastic (Fig 50–1*C, D*). Unfortunately, rapid retraction of the premaxillary bones does not serve to uncover the medial crura, because columellar skin is not available to cover them, and the result is a depression of the nasal tip.

Nasal Septum, Premaxillae, and Vomer

In the bilateral cleft condition the inferior border of the cartilaginous nasal septum is reinforced by bone, which provides a stemlike support for the premaxillary segment. This stem consists mainly of the vomer, its anterior part being formed by the premaxillae. The premaxillovomeral joint is located at a point approximately one-third of the septal length posterior to the premaxillary alveolar process. The premaxillary segment consists of paired premaxillary bones jointed in the midline by the interpremaxillary suture, which represents the anterior third of the normal midpalatal suture. Posteriorly the premaxillary stem consists of paired processes joined by the suture and termed the infravomerine processes of the premaxillae. These overlap the single vomer, whose tapering anterior edge adapts closely to the nasal septum (Fig. 50–1*D, E*). The premaxillovomeral joint is, therefore, of a tongue-and-groove type, the vomer being the tongue and the oblique groove being formed by the infravomerine processes of the premaxillae.

The vomer adapts to the inferior border of the cartilaginous nasal septum and articulates posteriorly with the sphenoid bone. In cross section the vomer of prenatal specimens is "U"shaped, but after birth resorption occurs on its lateral surfaces to give a thin "V" shaped cross section with a notable edge inferiorly (Fig. 50–2).

A slight swelling frequently occurs on the inferior border of the septum just posterior to the alveolar process at a position corresponding with the location of the premaxillovomer suture. The most likely reason for this is the

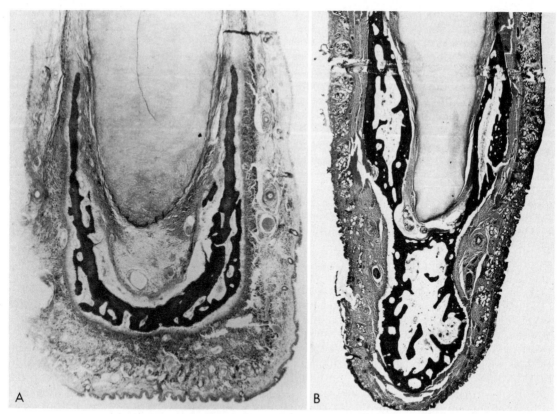

Figure 50–2. *A,* Vomer in cross section from a 20 week fetus with CCLP (bilateral cleft lip and palate) showing a rounded "U" shape. *B,* Vomer from a 6 month old postnatal CCLP infant. Lateral resorption commences after birth to reduce the vomer width, producing an inferior edge.

presence of the paraseptal cartilages, bilateral finlike structures that articulate with the inferior border of the septal cartilage and diverge inferiorly in lateral relation to the vomer. The premaxillovomer stem, in the vicinity of the suture, is flanked for a short distance by the paraseptal cartilage plates. It is improbable that the premaxillovomer suture itself produces the swelling.

Maxillary Segments

The gum pads of the maxillary segments of the infant with bilateral cleft are covered with gingival mucosa. They are demarcated from the palatal mucosa on their medial aspect by a groove corresponding with the position of the palatal alveolar process, to which the oral epithelium has fibrous connections. The developing teeth are situated lateral to this groove; the area medial to it corresponds to the horizontal process of the maxilla and palatine bones, which are covered by the thick palatal mucosa (Fig. 50–3A).

The shape and size of the maxillary palatal processes occasionally show evidence of intrauterine molding by the tongue. Figure 50–3B shows a transverse section through the palatine bone of the same specimen shown in Figure 50–3A. The horizontal process of the palatine bone is deflected superiorly, suggesting that the embryonic palatal processes actually reached a horizontal orientation and that inferior pressure from the tongue then molded the processes superiorly. Despite the presence of the cleft and severed relations with the nasal septum and vomer, the growth pattern of the palatal bone appears to be unaffected in that bone resorption occurs on the nasal aspect and bone formation on the oral aspect. It is the usual finding that the palatal mucosa has been molded or deflected superiorly, and the level of the horizontal process of the maxilla (palatal bone) tends to lie superior to the inferior border of the nasal septum.

The arch form of the maxillary segments generally appears normal soon after birth. However, the position of the maxillary seg-

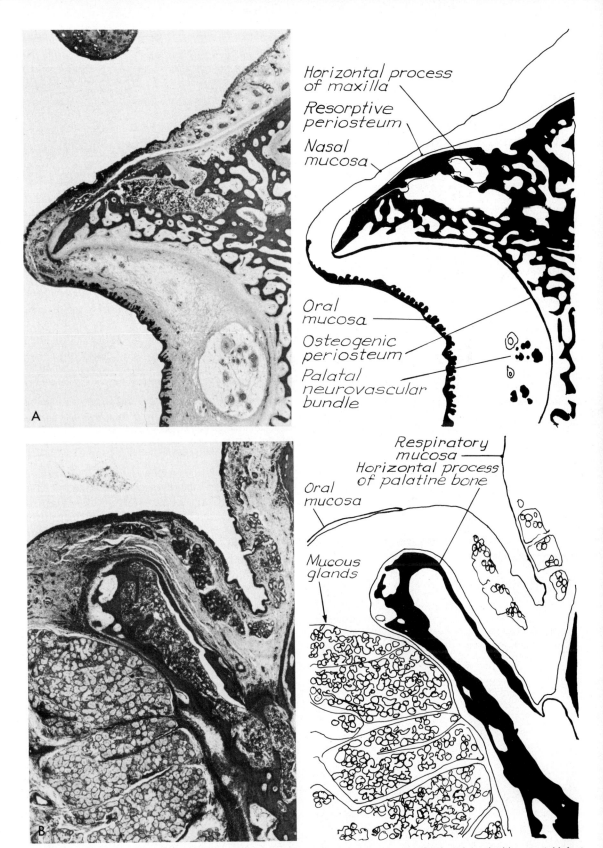

Figure 50–3. *A,* Cleft horizontal process of the maxilla and soft tissues in cross section in a 6 week old postnatal infant with bilateral cleft lip and palate. *B,* Coronal section through the palatine bone of the same specimen to show the superior deflection of the palatal process, probably secondary to tongue pressure.

ments is subject to intrauterine molding, particularly by the tongue, so that at birth they may be asymmetric. The tongue may have been wedged superiorly into one nasal cavity or the other, deflecting the septum a little and displacing a maxillary segment considerably in a lateral direction, so as to enlarge that nasal cavity (Fig. 50–4). After birth both maxillary segments tend to collapse medially.

Development of the Deformity

Human embryos with bilateral clefts of the primary palate have been illustrated by Kraus, Kitamura, and Latham (1966); two embryos aged 41 and 43 days showed no sign of premaxillary protrusion. However, in a 47 day specimen, protrusion of the premaxilla was beginning to appear, and it was conspicuous in a 9-week specimen. Veau and Politzer (1936) illustrated the palatal view of Hochstetter's 41 day specimen (23 mm C.R.), which showed protrusion of the premaxillary segment. Stark (1954) illustrated a well-preserved embryo of approximately 8½ weeks' ovulation age (46 mm C.R.) with bilateral clefts that showed advanced skeletal deformity. A 13 week specimen demonstrated extreme premaxillomaxillary malrelation (Fig. 50–5).

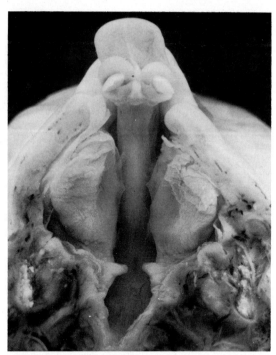

Figure 50–5. The palate of a 13 week fetus with bilateral cleft. Note that extreme relative protrusion of the premaxillary segment is already established. (Specimen courtesy of Dr. J. Li and Dr. M. L. Lewin.)

From these observations it appears that the premaxillary protrusion of the bilateral condition arises after original cleft formation in the embryo. The primary palate is normally formed by 35 days, and clefts would be apparent by that time. In a matter of days palatal malrelationships would begin to show, subsequently developing rapidly to reach, at ten weeks, proportions comparable with those seen after birth.

The deformity seen in the 13 week fetus (Fig. 50–5) represents the failure and abnormal activity of embryonic growth mechanisms. The maxillary segments lose some of their normal forward displacement because of their isolation from the nasal septum. The premaxillary bones are held at the anteroinferior point of the nasal septum by the septopremaxillary ligament (Latham, 1971, 1973), so that protrusion of the basal premaxillary bone is fully established in the 13 week fetus.

In older fetuses the gradual forward growth of the labial alveolar process as teeth develop has been observed. In a sagittal section through the premaxillary segment of a 17 week fetus (Fig. 50–6), the labial alveolar process shows a little convexity anteriorly, a

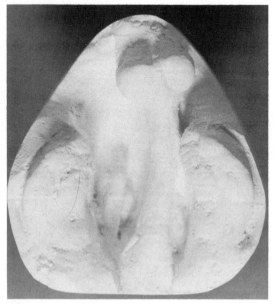

Figure 50–4. Model of the upper jaw in a newborn with bilateral cleft lip and palate. Note the asymmetric displacement of the maxillary segments due to the intrauterine molding effect of the tongue. (Courtesy of Dr. E. S. Beason.)

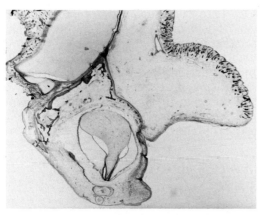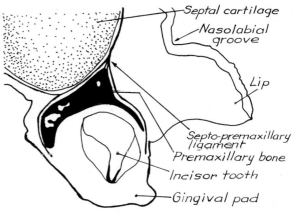

Figure 50–6. Sagittal section of the premaxillary segment of a 17 week fetus with bilateral cleft lip and palate. The basal premaxillary bone is adapted to the anteroinferior point of the nasal septal cartilage and held by the septopremaxillary ligament. Tooth and alveolar bone show a commencing tendency to grow forward, with consequent eversion of the lip. (From Latham, R. A.: Development and structure of the premaxillary deformity in bilateral cleft lip and palate. Br. J. Plast. Surg., 26:1, 1973.)

finding indicative of its early forward growth pattern. The position of the premaxillary segment at the anteroinferior point of the cartilaginous nasal septum is also clearly demonstrated. The septopremaxillary ligament, arising from the anterior septal border, inserts onto the anterior nasal spine and into the interpremaxillary suture. The anterior nasal spine develops in a superior direction under the influence of its ligamentous attachment. Eversion of the lip is already established and may be attributed, in part, to the protruded position of its mucosal attachment to the labial alveolar bone. This section also demonstrates the absence of muscle in the lip (Fig. 50–6).

The protrusion of the basal premaxillary bone is evidently established by the age of approximately 10 weeks in utero. The dentoalveolar protrusion is a slowly progressing feature over a period of about seven months in utero and continues for some months after birth until the crowns of the primary incisor teeth reach a mature size.

Causes of Premaxillary Protrusion

It was Veau's opinion that the premaxillary segment was driven forward by excessive growth of the bony premaxillary stem (Veau, 1934). However, his concept of a forward growth force generated within the developing vomeropremaxillary stem is no longer in keeping with concepts of facial growth and

bone maturation (see also Chapter 47). Bone cannot grow interstitially, so the presumed growth force would have to be a function of the premaxillovomeral suture. Since this suture still has not formed by the tenth week of fetal life, when protrusion of the premaxillary basal bone is almost complete, it is clear that another explanation must be sought.

The evidence indicates that the septopremaxillary ligament plays a key role. In the normal situation, premaxillary bone is kept in place by its early fusion with the maxilla to form one bone, and the developing dental arch is controlled by continuity of the mucogingival arch. The alveolar process develops inferiorly from the basal bone in relation to the developing teeth, which in turn are affixed to the gingiva by their fibrous follicles. The lip also influences dentoalveolar form.

The complete cleft condition never develops continuity of bony, gingival, or labial structure between the premaxillary and maxillary regions, so that the developing premaxillary segment is under no lateral restraint from any of these structures. Consequently, its attachment to the nasal septum by the septopremaxillary ligament becomes a dominant factor. Commencing as early as the sixth week of embryonic life, the ligament tends to shorten, drawing the premaxillary segment into the protrusive position with respect to the nasal septum and position in which it remains.

In the unaffected individual, there is differential growth between the nasal septum and the upper jaw; the cartilaginous septum slides forward relative to the bone, overshooting to the extent shown in Figure 50–1A, B. The bilateral cleft premaxillae are carried forward by the growing nasal septum at an identical rate, since the ligament prevents their relative posterior movement. Septal growth stimulates equal elongation at the premaxillovomeral suture, so that the premaxillovomeral stem becomes much longer than normal. The additional protrusive growth of the alveolar process increases the deformity considerably, and by growing forward it may give the erroneous impression that the entire segment is being pushed by growth of the premaxillary stem.

Given the absence of normal relationships due to clefts, the causative factors contributing to the deformity may be summarized thus: protrusion of the premaxillary basal bone is determined by the septopremaxillary ligament; elongation or excessive growth of the premaxillovomeral stem derives its motivation from the nasal septum; and the alveolar process becomes protrusive by growing in the direction of least resistance.

UNILATERAL CLEFT LIP AND PALATE

Unilateral cleft lip and palate consistently shows an associated skeletal deformity, of which the prominent features are lateral dis-

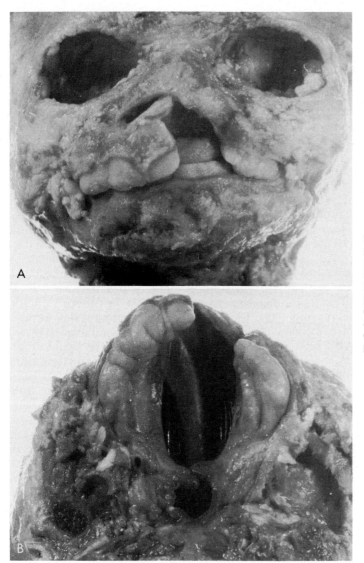

Figure 50–7. *A,* Face of a newborn infant with unilateral cleft lip and palate; soft tissues removed to show the skeletal deformity. *B,* Palatal view after removal of the lower jaw of the same specimen. Note the lateral displacement of the noncleft maxillopremaxillary segment and lateral dislocation of the nasal septum. (From Latham, R. A., and Burston, W. R.: The effect of unilateral cleft of the lip and palate on maxillary growth pattern. Br. J. Plast. Surg., *17*:10, 1964.)

placement of the noncleft maxillopremaxillary part of the upper jaw, malformation of the nose, and lateral distortion of the nasal septum (Fig. 50–7).

Premaxillary Segment and Nasal Septum

The premaxillary segment, in frontal view, tilts upward into the cleft. The interpremax-

illary suture is also rotated markedly, as seen in coronal sections (Fig. 50–8), a finding that indicates that the upturning of the premaxillary segment is due to bodily rotation of the entire segment and not solely to a local alveolar deficiency. The cartilaginous nasal septum is very much bent laterally and upward with the noncleft segment, to which it is attached in the region of the anterior nasal spine. The incisor teeth within the uptilted premaxillary segment later erupt with their

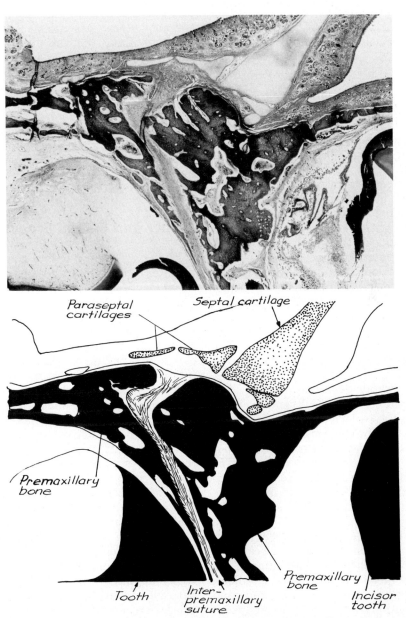

Figure 50–8. Coronal section through the premaxillary segment of the specimen in Figure 50–7, showing the structural detail of the septopremaxillary deformity. Note the obliquity of the interpremaxillary suture, indicating that the entire segment is rotated upward into the cleft.

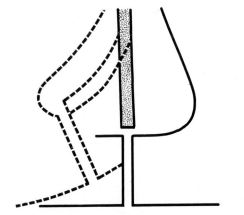

Figure 50–9. When the normally straight nasal septum is deviated to one side, a vertical shortness results.

crowns tilted and their occlusal plane sloping upward into the cleft. In an older patient this malocclusion indicates persistence of the original skeletal deformity present at birth.

The deviated nasal septum and displaced premaxillary region have significant implications with regard to the height of the middle third of the face. Normally the full height of the upper face is realized when the nasal septum is straight and located in the median plane. If one regards the nasal septum of the infant with unilateral cleft as being of normal size and proportions, the fact that it is bent means that it must also be shorter vertically (Fig. 50–9). Thus the premaxillary segment to which it is connected suffers a decreased vertical dimension as long as the cartilaginous nasal septum remains deviated. The same observation may be made for the anteroposterior dimension when the nasal septum is considerably deviated (see Fig. 50–7B). If straightened the nasal septum would extend further anteriorly, and a corresponding advance of the premaxillary segment would be necessary owing to the ligamentous connection between these two structures. The depressed middle third of the face occasionally seen in the 10 to 12 year old may represent a residuum of the original skeletal deformity.

The nostril on the noncleft side is constricted and may be functionally occluded. The constriction results from deviation of the cartilaginous nasal septum into the floor, with the effect of raising the skin, and from the approximation of the alar base and columella. The ala nasi of the cleft side is usually stretched and flattened.

Lip and Columella

If it were presumed that the labial muscle on the noncleft side is normal in bulk and attachments, there would be reason to expect that part of Cupid's bow and the philtral ridge on that side might be identifiable. However, the lip over the premaxillary segment is subjected to a unilateral muscle pull, which tends to retract it from the gingival pad over the incisor tooth of the cleft side, thus contributing to lip distortion. The latter finding can be attributed to the fact that the muscle band of the orbicularis oris inserts at the border of the cleft along the vermilion border, which turns superiorly at the cleft (see Chapter 51).

A columella may be identified in relation to the noncleft nostril, but on the cleft side it is merged with the stretched ala nasi. The columellar skin is more developed than in the bilateral cleft condition, but the deviated nasal septum and asymmetric alar cartilages jeopardize the prospects of normal development of a symmetric columella and adequate support for the nose.

Vomer and Palatal Process

In the secondary palate the cleft may be unilateral or bilateral with respect to the nasal septum. When the cleft condition is bilateral, the vomer has a structure like that described above for the complete bilateral cleft lip and palate. It is symmetrically attached to the inferior border of the septal cartilage, tending to thin laterally in later infancy to develop a sharp inferior edge. In either case, since the deformity of the primary palate is similar, the middle third of the nasal septum distends into the nasal cavity corresponding to the side of the cleft lip.

In the event of unilateral union between the nasal septum and a secondary palatal process, the nasal floor thus formed is stretched laterally owing to the two factors dilating the nasal cavity. The noncleft maxilla is displaced away from the cleft, the cartilaginous septum is distended into the nasal cavity on the cleft side, and the horizontal palatal process is stretched so that the vomer is pulled into the nasal floor (Fig. 50–10). The suture between the vomer and the palatal process of the maxilla is thus located in the center of the floor of the nasal cavity. The mucosa covering the oral aspect of the

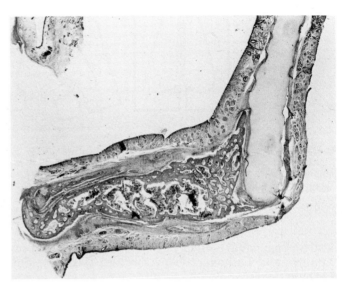

Figure 50–10. Histologic section through the nasal septum and vomer from the specimen illustrated in Figure 50–7. The vomer is deformed horizontally.

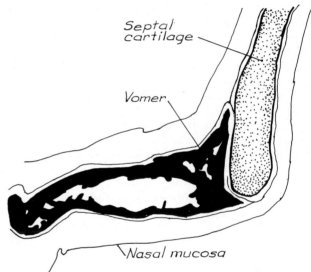

vomer where it contributes to the palate in this way is lined by ciliated columnar epithelium. The vomer makes a remarkable right-angle junction with the cartilaginous nasal septum, which remains upright.

The intact side of the secondary palate, where the vomer is joined to the palatal process, always corresponds with the side of the intact primary palate. In the 6 to 7 week embryo, in the developmental stage at which palate formation normally takes place, the unilateral cleft of the primary palate favors secondary palate fusion on the noncleft side because the septum is bent and displaced toward that side. It antagonizes fusion on the cleft side when conditions for fusion are unfavorable because of the increased distance between the palatal process and both the nasal septum and fellow palatal process.

At birth, both nasal cavities are functionally obstructed—the noncleft side anteriorly at the nostril, and the cleft side posteriorly at the conchal level.

Development of the Deformity

Interest in the cause of the skeletal deformity has been prominently featured in some of the principles on which surgical treatment has been based. Related information such as the time of onset and the rate of development of the skeletal deformity has had important clinical applications in the past. The following account is based on the anatomic study of six human specimens personally collected and reported and five additional fetal specimens that have been illustrated in the liter-

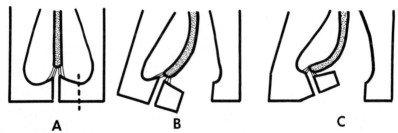

Figure 50–11. Development of the unilateral cleft lip and palate deformity. *A,* The nasal septum and bone at the time of their first differentiation before the deformity arises at 37 to 39 days. *B,* Drawn from a coronal section of the Hochstetter embryo, 41 day, 23 mm C. R., to show the early stage of the septal bending of the premaxillary displacement. (From Veau, V., and Politzer, G.: Embryologie du bec-de-lièvre. Le palais primaire. Ann. Anat. Pathol., *13:*275, 1936.) *C,* Nature of the deformity at birth. Rotation of the premaxillary segment is the reverse of that seen initially; the cleft premaxilla tilts upward.

ature (Veau and Politzer, 1936; Kraus, Kitamura, and Latham, 1966; Atherton, 1967; Latham, 1969).

Two distinct phases were identified in the development of the deformity, as seen in coronal sections through the premaxillary region. Illustrations of the youngest known human embryos with complete unilateral cleft of the primary palate (6 weeks) were published by Veau and Politzer (1936). These specimens showed a deformity different from that seen at birth in some important details. Deviation of the nasal septum toward the noncleft side is of mild degree and similar in nature to that found later; however, the interpremaxillary suture is tilted toward the cleft, and there is inferior displacement of the cleft-side premaxilla (Fig. 50–11*A, B*). At approximately 12 weeks in fetal life, the direction of rotation of the premaxillary region is reversed. The interpremaxillary suture becomes tilted toward the noncleft side, and the premaxillary segment is rotated upward into the cleft (Fig. 50–11*C*). In the horizontal plane, lateral displacement of the premaxillary segment toward the noncleft side is well established by the age of 8½ weeks (Atherton, 1967). Such displacement is accompanied by bending of the anterior part of the nasal septum to the noncleft side. Once the nasal septum becomes bent anteriorly, its middle third begins to distend into the nasal cavity on the cleft side. This is seen in specimens of 12 weeks and may occur earlier. In this manner the septal bending results in a narrowing of the nasal cavity on the cleft side and a widening of the noncleft nasal cavity. The distention of the nasal septum also disrupts its articulation with the vomer and, anteriorly, with the interpremaxillary suture (see Fig. 50–8). Normally the nasal

septum is situated directly superior to the midpalatal suture. However, since the suture is displaced toward the noncleft side and the septum is distended in the opposite direction, except in the vicinity of the anterior nasal spine where the septum and bone have a strong attachment, a dislocation of the septal keel away from the interpremaxillary suture occurs.

Onset and Rate of Development

Evidence from the youngest known human embryos with unilateral cleft supports the view that, at the crucial time of initial cleft formation, the primordial face is symmetric (at 33 to 35 days) and that the deformity arises in the period immediately following, when the skeletal structures of the face begin to appear. Either the deformity is present at the beginning in miniature and simply enlarges, or it is not part of the original affliction but rather is superimposed upon the facial structure during subsequent development. In embryos of 41 days, a mild degree of deformity was noted, a finding consistent with the view that the skeletal deformity was present at a very early stage of formation. It may be said, therefore, that the deformity arises in the latter part of the sixth week, soon after initial cleft formation.

The skeletal deformity is well established by 12 weeks of fetal life, although the fetus does not exhibit the upturned premaxillary segment at this stage. The latter feature is seen in all specimens older than 12 weeks. The skeletal deformity develops rapidly in the embryonic and early fetal periods, and subsequently increases slowly in severity as the fetus approaches full term.

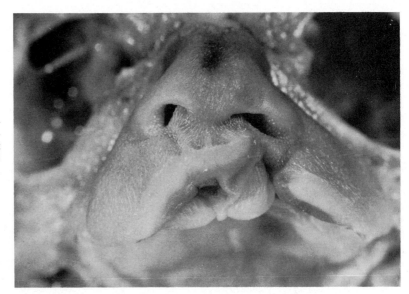

Figure 50–12. Unilateral incomplete cleft of the primary palate in an 18 week fetus. The cleft is bridged by a Simonart's band of soft tissue containing arterioles, nerves, and muscle fibers.

Simonart's Band

It is frequently found that a cleft of the primary palate is bridged by a bar of lip tissue, referred to as Simonart's bar or band (Fig. 50–12). Depending on its size, such a connection of soft tissue across a cleft may prevent the development of much of the skeletal deformity present in complete clefts. Substantial bridging bars usually pass from lip tissue to lip tissue. Narrow bridging bars may pass from the lip laterally to the alveolar mucosa medially, and this is associated with some protrusion of the premaxillary segment with malalignment of the alveolar arch.

Histologic examination of Simonart's band shows that it may be composed of muscle fibers and a substantial number of arterioles and nerves (see also Chapter 51). These vessels may be of such size as to warrant a surgical effort to preserve them (Fig. 50–13).

Simonart's band has been the focus of attention in the discussions of the pathogenesis of the cleft primary palate. Maurer (1936) regarded Simonart's band as the result of a healing process after breakdown had occurred. Veau and Politzer (1936), in a well-documented study, explained that the connecting bridge was the result of only partial penetration of the epithelial wall or nasal fin, which at first separates the maxillary and frontonasal processes and which is then normally penetrated by mesoderm to establish the primary palate. This subject was reviewed briefly by Töndury (1961), who suggested that Simonart's band may result from only partial formation of the epithelial wall in the first instance.

CLEFT PALATE

A cleft of the secondary palate involves both the hard palate and the soft palate from the uvular processes posteriorly to the junction with the primary palate anteriorly; the junction corresponds with the position of the incisive foramen on an intact skull. Normal fusion of the palatal processes first occurs in the anterior third at about 47 days and progresses posteriorly to complete uvular fusion by about 54 days. The variation in severity of palatal clefts reflects the anteroposterior progress of development, and the cleft invariably affects the uvular area, which is the last to fuse. Deficiency of the bony palate varies from a midline notch in the posterior border at the normal site of the posterior nasal spine to a "V"-shaped defect extending throughout the hard palate to the anterior limit of the secondary palate. At birth the uvular processes are usually shortened and distorted in an anterior direction, presumably as a result of the contraction of the musculus uvulae, which originate in part from the posterior border of the horizontal process of the palatine bone.

The tongue exercises great influence over

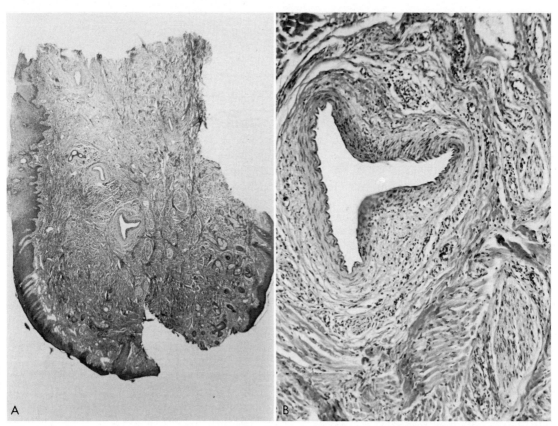

Figure 50–13. *A,* Histologic section through a Simonart's band of a 2 month old infant. *B,* Photomicrograph at higher magnification showing artery, nerves, and muscle fibers. Such structures pass over the cleft, varying in size and in proportion to the size of the bridging band of tissue. (Specimen courtesy of Dr. N. G. Georgiade.)

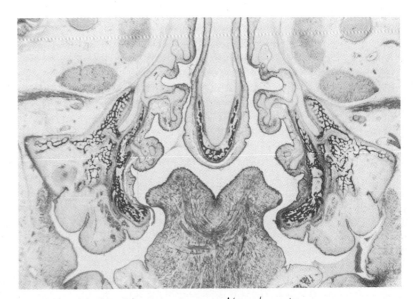

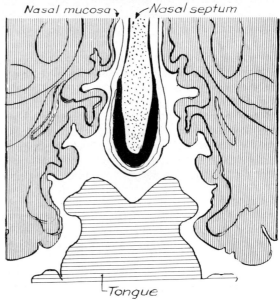

Nasal mucosa   Nasal septum

Tongue

Figure 50–14. Coronal section through the head of a 17 week fetus with mandibular retrognathia and cleft palate to show the "tongue in the nose" condition. In this disorder, clinically described as the Pierre Robin sequence, impaction of the tongue into the nose causes respiratory obstruction. (From Latham, R. A., Smiley, G. R., and Gregg, J. M.: The problem of tissue deficiency in cleft palate: an experiment in mobilising the palatine bones of cleft dogs. Br. J. Plast. Surg., *26*:252, 1973.)

the size and shape of the cleft palatal shelves and does so most obviously in some patients with the Pierre Robin sequence (Latham, 1966). The syndrome comprises mandibular hypoplasia, paroxysmal respiratory obstruction due to glossoptosis, and cleft palate (see Chapter 63). The cleft palate is not necessary for recognition of the Pierre Robin sequence. Occasionally there is a cleft of the entire secondary palate with impaction of the tongue into the nasal cavities (Fig. 50–14). In this case the palatal shelves tend to slope inferiorly; this finding is strongly suggestive of the mode of failure of palatal formation. Underdevelopment of the lower jaw may have forced the tongue to remain between the secondary palatal processes at the time when the latter normally elevate to a horizontal position and subsequently fuse in the midline (Davis and Dunn, 1933). It is thought that intrauterine pressure, possibly due to oligohydramnios, could cause such developmental embarrassment of both the tongue and the lower jaw. The mandibular hypoplasia is frequently severe, and in such cases it is more likely to have an intrinsic cause, residing primarily in the mandibular arch cartilage (Meckel's cartilage). In the pathogenesis of the hypoplasia of the mandibular arch cartilage, the origin may lie in the cells of the neural crest. Whatever its cause, an underdeveloped mandibular arch cartilage must result in an underdeveloped mandible. The resulting mandible, while initially small, need have no impairment of growth rate at the mandibular condyles, which develop later at about 12 weeks' ovulation age.

Deficiency of mucosal tissue and bone is the main characteristic of the cleft hard palate. In the soft palate, deficiency of mucosal tissue is combined with shortening of the velar musculature, which has abnormal insertion sites (Latham, Long, and Latham, 1980) (see Chapter 51). Deficiency of palatal tissue entails two factors. There may have been a deficiency of palatal mesenchyme at the time of normal palatal formation. On the other hand, a significant deficiency evidently results from the fact that the palatal processes failed to fuse. If it is postulated that normal growth of the palate is dependent to some extent on the continuity of palatal tissue across the midline, then a cleft palate will always incur some degree of subsequent underdevelopment of the palatal processes.

Absence of Midpalatal Suture

In normal development the midpalatal suture between the horizontal processes of the maxillae is established at about 12 weeks of embryonic life; the interpremaxillary part of the midpalatal suture forms in the primary palate at about 6½ weeks (Latham, 1971). In regard to the role of the midpalatal suture in the growth in width of the upper jaw, it must first be recalled that present teaching does not support the concept that these sutures generate the kind of growth force that would result in growth in palatal width. Bone formation in the midpalatal suture must be seen as a response to the tendency of the maxillae to move apart secondary to forces originating elsewhere and not in the midpalatal suture. The five week time lag between the development of bony support in the primary and secondary palates is another indication that growth of the hard palate in the midpalatal suture represents a secondary fill-in process rather than a mechanism of basic importance to overall jaw growth.

Therefore, a cleft of the secondary palate does not disrupt a basic growth mechanism of the upper jaw. The main skeletal function of the secondary hard palate appears to be one of mechanical support for the partition between the oral and nasal cavities with regard to masticatory function. A second function involves bracing the molar segments against medial and lateral forces. The latter aspect becomes understandable when the continuity of the primary palate is breached by a cleft and a tendency toward maxillary collapse is observed. In such an event, an intact secondary palate counters the collapse tendency.

REFERENCES

Atherton, J. D.: A descriptive anatomy of the face in human fetuses with unilateral cleft lip and palate. Cleft Palate J., 4:104, 1967.

Davis, A. D., and Dunn, R.: Micrognathia. A suggested treatment for correction in early infancy. Am. J. Dis. Child., 45:799, 1933.

Kraus, B. S., Kitamura, H., and Latham, R. A.: Atlas of Developmental Anatomy of the Face. New York, Harper & Row, 1966, p. 248.

Latham, R. A.: The pathogenesis of cleft palate associated with the Pierre Robin syndrome: an analysis of a seventeen week human foetus. Br. J. Plast. Surg., 19:205, 1966.

Latham, R. A.: The pathogenesis of the skeletal deformity associated with unilateral cleft lip and palate. Cleft Palate J., 6:404, 1969.

Latham, R. A.: The development, structure and growth pattern of the human mid-palatal suture. J. Anat. (Lond.), 108:31, 1971.

Latham, R. A.: Development and structure of the premaxillary deformity in bilateral cleft lip and palate. Br. J. Plast. Surg., 26:51, 1973.

Latham, R. A., and Burston, W. R.: The effect of unilateral cleft of the lip and palate on maxillary growth pattern. Br. J. Plast. Surg., 17:10, 1964.

Latham, R. A., and Deaton, T. G.: The structural basis of the philtrum and the contour of the vermilion border: a study of the musculature of the upper lip. J. Anat. (Lond.), 121:151, 1976.

Latham, R. A., Long, R. E., and Latham, E. A.: Cleft palate velopharyngeal musculature in a five-month-old infant: a three-dimensional histological reconstruction. Cleft Palate J., 17:1, 1980.

Latham, R. A., and Workman, C.: Anatomy of the philtrum and columella: the soft tissue deformity in bilateral cleft lip and palate. In Georgiade, N. G. (Ed.): Symposium on Management of Cleft Lip and Palate and Associated Deformities. St. Louis, MO, C. V. Mosby Company, 1974, pp. 10–12.

Latham, R. A., Smiley, G. R., and Gregg, J. M.: The problem of tissue deficiency in cleft palate. An experiment mobilising the palatine bones of cleft dogs. Br. J. Plast. Surg., 26:252, 1973.

Maurer, H.: Die Entstehung der Lippen-Kieferspalte bei einem Keimling von 22mm. SSL. Z. Anat. Entwicklungsgesch., 105:359, 1936.

Stark, R. B.: The pathogenesis of harelip and cleft palate, Plast. Reconstr. Surg., 13:20, 1954.

Töndury, G.: On the mechanism of cleft formation. In Pruzansky, S. (Ed.): Congenital Anomalies of the Face and Associated Structure. Springfield, IL, Charles C Thomas, 1961, pp. 85–101.

Veau, V.: Le rôle du tubercule médian dans la constitution de la face. Ann. Anat. Pathol. Anat. Normale, 3:305, 1926.

Veau, V.: Division Palatine, Anatomie, Chirurgie Phonétique. Paris, Masson & Cie, 1931.

Veau, V.: Le sequelette du bec-de-lièvre. Ann. Anat. Normale Medico-Chirurgicale, 11:873, 1934.

Veau, V.: Bec-de-lièvre: hypothèses sur la malformation initiale. Ann. Anat. Pathol. Anat. Normale, 12:389, 1935.

Veau, V., and Politzer, G.: Embryologie du bec-de-lièvre. Le palais primaire. Ann. Anat. Pathol. Anat. Normale, 13:275, 1936.

51
Miroslav Fára

The Musculature of Cleft Lip and Palate

The anatomic differences in the structural arrangement of the muscles in the cleft lip and palate are characterized by the fact that the muscles, during their embryonic growth in a lateromedial direction, fail to meet in the midline, and thus seek other attachments. The substitute attachments prevent the muscles from becoming fully functional, and their development is incomplete. Atypical insertions and varying degrees of hypoplasia constitute the main pathologic features of the cleft lip and palate musculature.

On the basis of this knowledge, detachment of the muscle stumps from their substitute insertions becomes a prime requisite for any successful operation on the cleft lip and cleft palate. Such a maneuver joins the muscle fibers in an end to end fashion and ensures satisfactory development and function of the musculature in subsequent years.

MUSCLES OF THE LIP

The principal muscle of the lip is the orbicularis oris muscle (Fig. 51–1). It passes partially around the entire oral fissure and is in intimate contact anteriorly with the skin and posteriorly with the mucous membrane. The orbicularis oris muscle consists anatomically and functionally of two parts, the superficial and the deep layers.

In the upper lip, these fibers decussate in the midline to insert into the opposite philtral column. The orbicularis is joined by the muscles of facial expression, which intermingle with it and participate in its function by their dilating or stabilizing effect, or both. The superficial portion of the orbicularis oris muscle also brings the lips together, and its fibers contract independently to provide fine shades of expression.

The deep layers of the muscles encircle the orifice of the mouth and function solely as mouth constrictors.

Latham and Deaton (1976) performed a Plexiglas study of the structural basis of the philtrum and vermilion border. This presentation of the musculature of the upper lip demonstrated that the basic three muscles of the upper lip (Fig. 51–1*B*) were the *orbicularis oris,* the *levator labii superioris,* and the *nasalis (depressor septi).* This study demonstrated that the orbicularis oris muscle (superior portion) is actually decussated in the midline and continues from one side to the other to insert into the skin lateral to the philtral groove. The philtral groove itself has a muscle free zone beneath it; there are no muscles that, per se, insert into the philtral

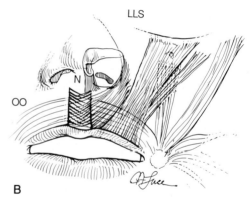

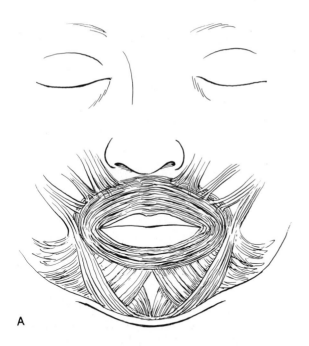

A

Figure 51–1. *A,* The muscles of the mouth. *B,* Details of the muscles of the upper lip. OO = orbicularis oris; N = nasalis; LLS = levator labii superioris. (Redrawn from Latham, R. A., and Deaton, T. G.: The structural basis of the philtrum and the contour of the vermilion border: a study of the musculature of the upper lip. J. Anat., *121*:151, 1976.)

dimple. The muscles from each side decussate in the midline to insert and form part of the bulk of the philtral columns. In fact, the philtral columns are actually fortresses of muscle that occur as a result of an increase in muscle bulk. The lower portion of this increase in muscle bulk consists of the orbicularis oris and the levator labii superioris. The upper portion is the orbicularis and the nasalis muscle.

The nasalis muscle arises from the alveolar bone over the central and lateral incisors, and courses anterior and medially to mingle with the overlying fibers of the orbicularis oris. They also decussate in the midline to a degree and insert into the skin of the columella. These muscles actually insert into the footplates of the medial crura (Zide, 1985). Vogt (1983) has noted that some fibers may actually continue between the medial crura to insert into the tip of the nose. It is this muscle, when contracted, that depresses the tip of the nose via its pull on the medial footplates as well as through some of the more extensive fibers inserting directly on the tip.

The lower portion of the philtral columns is formed not only by the decussating fibers of the orbicularis oris but also by some of the fibers of the levator labii superioris, which course superiorly above the surface of the orbicularis oris. These muscle fibers insert into the lower philtral columns and also into the vermilion border as far medially as the peak of the Cupid's bow.

The tubercle of the lip is caused by eversion of a specific portion of the orbicularis oris muscle called the pars marginalis, which is found along its lower border (Latham and Deaton, 1976). The pars marginalis is that portion of the orbicularis oris found closest to the vermilion.

There are no strictly vertical fibers observed running the entire length of the philtral columns. The medial fibers of the oblique muscles, specifically the levator labii superioris, enter the lower third of the philtral ridges to contribute to the above. As stated before, the inferior portion of the orbicularis oris (pars marginalis) inserts so close to the vermilion border that by its protrusion anteriorly it everts the median tubercle inferior to the philtrum, and thus produces the tubercle. In summary, the key muscles of the normal philtral ridge are the orbicularis oris, the levator labii, and the nasalis, whose fibers form the bulk of the columns. The orbicularis oris fibers decussate in the midline to insert into the opposite philtral column, and help to form the bulk of the philtral column. Inferiorly the levator labii superioris muscle contributes to the bulk of the lower philtral columns and inserts partially into the Cupid's bow. The upper portion of the philtral col-

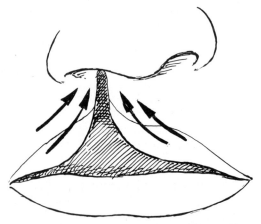

Figure 51–2. The changes in the direction of the orbicularis oris muscle in a complete unilateral cleft lip.

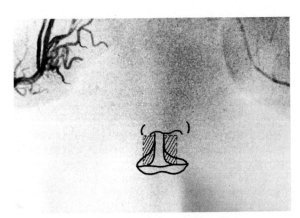

Figure 51–4. Typical arteriogram in a complete right-side cleft. The main branch of the superior labial artery passes along the edge of the cleft on both sides but is much more developed in the lateral segment. Inset shows the orientation of the radiograph.

umns is formed by the bulk of the nasalis muscle, specifically the depressor septi portion. Latham and Deaton (1976) did not observe fibers of the orbicularis oris extending completely from one modiolus to the other; the fibers, however, decussated in the midline. The opinion of Nairn (1975) that the muscle of the orbicularis oris simply encircles the mouth appears to be inconsistent with this study.

Unilateral Cleft Lip

In a *complete unilateral cleft,* the fibers of the orbicularis muscle, proceeding horizontally from the commissure toward the midline, turn upward along the margins of the cleft. They terminate laterally beneath the

base of the ala of the nose and medially beneath the base of the columella, where most of them attach to the periosteum of the maxilla, a few disappearing in the subcutis (Figs. 51–2 to 51–5).

In the *more advanced forms of incomplete cleft,* in which only narrow bridges are formed, the muscle has similar characteristics.

In the *lesser forms of incomplete cleft,* in which the cleft does not exceed two-thirds of the lip height, the muscle fibers reach over the tip of the cleft and pass from the lateral to the medial lip segments (Figs. 51–6, 51–7). The muscle within the cleft, however, is interspersed by the trabeculae of the collagenous connective tissue (Figs. 51–8, 51–9).

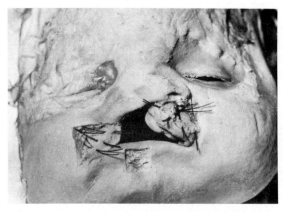

Figure 51–3. Dissection of a complete right-side cleft lip. The main muscle bundles are more clearly shown by the length of black nylon. The muscles pass along the edge of the cleft.

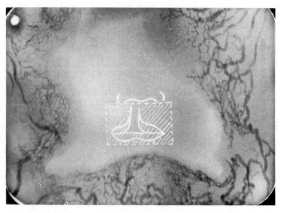

Figure 51–5. Arteriogram in another complete unilateral cleft lip, demonstrating an unusually dense anastomotic network between the superior labial artery and the angular artery in both lip segments.

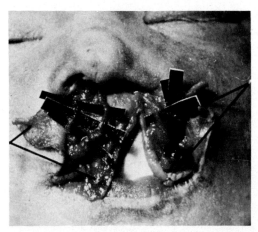

Figure 51–6. Dissection of the orbicularis oris muscle in an incomplete left-side cleft with a narrow bridge. Some dissected muscle bundles have been placed on strips of black paper for better demonstration. On the lateral side, the transition of muscle fibers into the bridge can be seen. On the philtral (medial) side, however, the stronger muscle bundles only reach the central line of the lip.

A protrusion of excess muscle may be seen and palpated on the lateral aspect of the cleft in complete as well as incomplete clefts. This is caused by the contraction or heaping up of the muscle, which was prevented from developing to its normal length. The musculature on the medial side, on the other hand, is underdeveloped and does not extend as far forward to the edge of the cleft as it does on the lateral side. This observation was originally made by Veau (1938), who wrote: "la berge interne est sterile" (the medial border is sterile). In autopsies and during cleft lip operations, one can observe a striking thin-ning of the muscle layer in the entire half of the philtrum adjacent to the cleft.

In the lesser form of incomplete cleft, characterized by a small coloboma in the lower part of the lip, a groove on the skin passes upward to the threshold of the nostril. This external finding is always manifest on the muscle ring, which is depressed beneath the cutaneous groove (Fig. 51–10).

Lehman and Artz (1976) noted that minimal clefts of the lip have a deformity that is more extensive than previously reported. The skin overlying this area is devoid not only of hair but also of sweat glands. Beneath any lip groove that might be present, there is a break in the continuity of the lip musculature that can be confirmed histologically.

Similar findings have been seen in the arterial network (see Figs. 51–4, 51–5). The superior labial artery on the lateral side of the cleft follows the course of the orbicularis muscle bundles and the edge of the cleft upward to the nasal ala, where it anastomoses with the lateral nasal or angular artery. In incomplete clefts, the artery in the form of a thin, terminal branch passes through the bridge (see Fig. 51–7). On the medial side of the cleft, the artery behaves in a similar way, but its diameter is visibly smaller and its branches are fewer than on the lateral side. The lesser degree of arterial development corresponds to the lesser degree of musculature development on the medial aspect of the cleft. Its terminal branches extend into the columella, where they anastomose mainly with the posterior septal arteries.

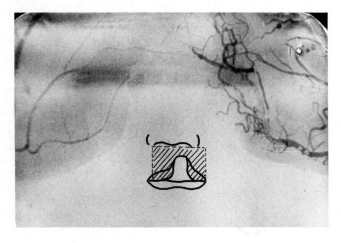

Figure 51–7. Arteriogram of an incomplete left-side cleft (see Fig. 51–6). Injected with barium-formalin. Note the distinct difference in the caliber of the arteries in the lateral and medial segments. From the lateral side, a strong arterial branch penetrates into the bridge.

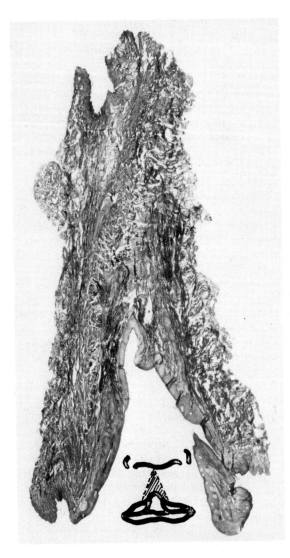

Figure 51–8. Specimen excised during operation for correction of an incomplete right-side cleft (frontal view). The muscle bundles follow the margin of the cleft. Inset shows the orientation of the specimen.

Figure 51–9. Specimen excised during operation for correction of an incomplete right-side cleft. The horizontal section was taken from just above the cleft. The muscle bundles change direction at this point; they deviate above the cleft and extend above it from one side to the other.

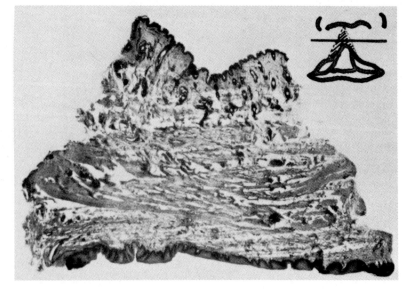

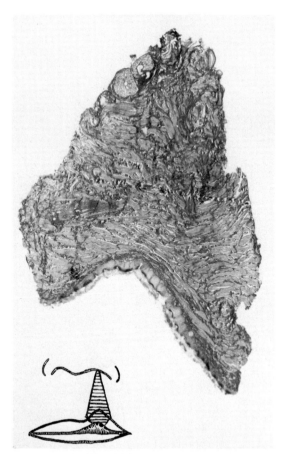

Figure 51–10. Specimen resected during operation for correction of a lesser form of incomplete left-side cleft. Note the depression on the muscle groove.

Bilateral Cleft Lip

In the *complete bilateral cleft lip,* the muscle stumps and arterial network of the lateral segments of the lip are similar to those of the unilateral cleft (Figs. 51–11 to 51–16). The medial lip segment or prolabium, on the other hand, is composed only of collagenous connective tissue; this is penetrated, however, by a rich vascular network originating in the septal and columellar arteries.

In order to ascertain possible postoperative changes in the prolabium after its fusion with the lateral segments, a threefold histologic examination of 30 children was undertaken (Figs. 51–17 to 51–19). During the suture of the first side of the lip, performed in infants aged 5 to 7 months by means of rotating the muscle stump downward into the margin of the prolabium, only collagenous, fibrillar connective tissue was found in the excised parts of the prolabial tissue (Fig. 51–20). During the suture of the contralateral side, performed after an interval of six weeks to six months, proliferation of muscle fibers from the lateral into the medial lip segment appeared to be active (Figs. 51–21, 51–22).

The greatest number of more or less differentiated muscle fibers proliferating from the lateral muscle stump into the prolabium was found in the vicinity of the previous repair. Toward the center of the prolabium, the number of fibers decreased, until finally only isolated fibers were discerned. The number of

Text continued on page 2608

Only rarely (in two of the 28 dissected specimens) did the muscle fibers show a tendency to run horizontally, entering the edge of the cleft and disappearing in the connective tissue. The blood supply in these specimens was also atypical, as can be noted in the arteriogram of a complete right-sided cleft (see Fig. 51–5).

The underdevelopment of the muscles and the reduced blood supply in the medial portion of the lip, extending to the midline of the philtrum, suggest that the ability of the muscular stump of the orbicularis muscle to grow across the midline of the lip (which ontogenetically represents its anatomic midline border) is limited. It is as though the orbicularis musculature of one-half of the lip is incapable of supplying musculature to the contralateral side.

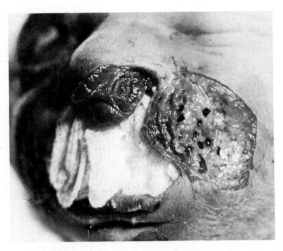

Figure 51–11. Dissection of muscle bundles (placed over black paper strips) in a complete bilateral cleft.

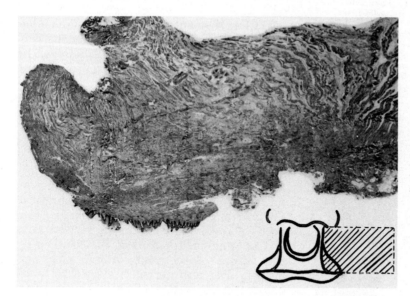

Figure 51–12. Frontal section of the lateral segment in a complete bilateral cleft (Van Gieson). The muscle fiber bundles pass upward along the edge of the cleft. At the corner of the mouth, they merge with the muscles of facial expression.

Figure 51–13. Frontal section from a prolabium; cartilages of the nasal septum are seen in the upper part. Note the absence of muscle fibers (Van Gieson).

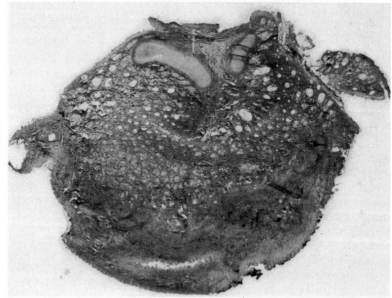

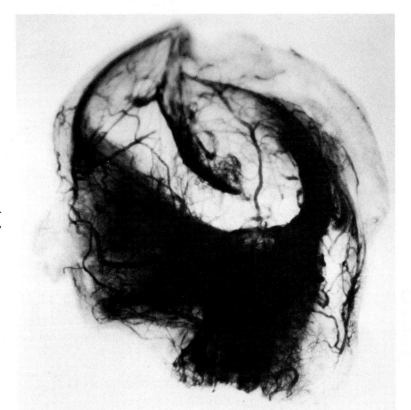

Figure 51–14. Lateral arteriogram of a complete bilateral cleft, after barium-formalin injection.

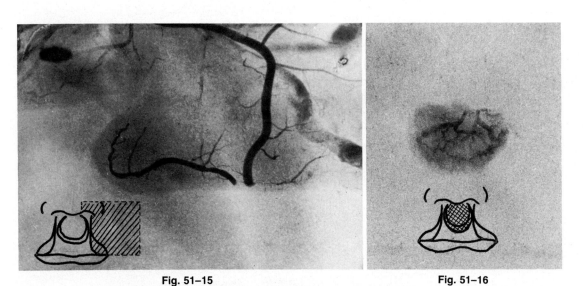

Fig. 51–15   Fig. 51–16

Figure 51–15. Arteriogram of the lateral segment of a stillborn with complete bilateral cleft. The lip was severed just above the beginning of the superior labial artery. In the left upper edge of the picture, a branch for the nasal ala can be seen.

Figure 51–16. Arteriogram of an isolated prolabium of a stillborn with a complete bilateral cleft. Note that well-developed vessels originate from the nasal septum.

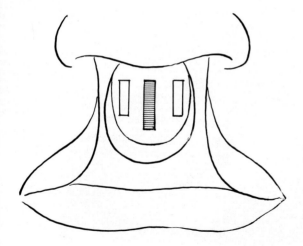

Figure 51–17. Histologic sections prior to repair of the first side.

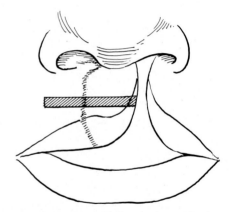

Figure 51–18. Section removed after repair of one side.

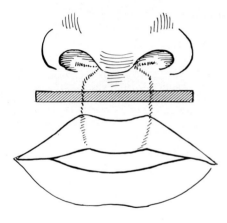

Figure 51–19. Section removed following repair of both sides.

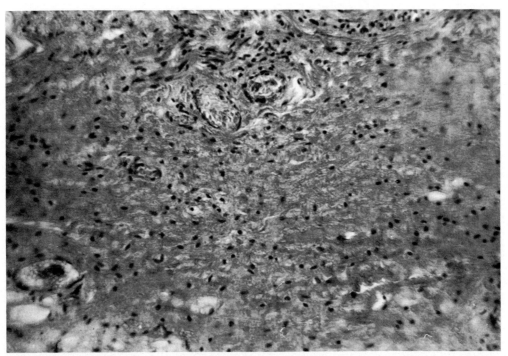

Figure 51–20. Histologic section from a prolabium at the time of repair of the first side: collagenous connective tissue without any muscular fibers, either mature or in any stage of development.

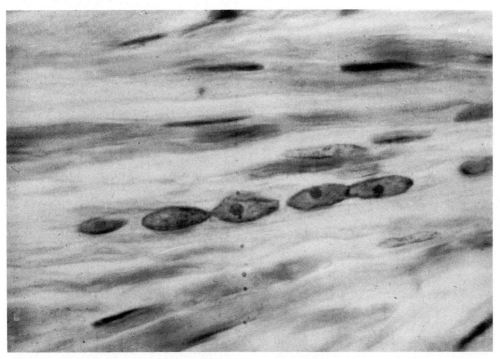

Figure 51–21. Histologic section from a prolabium three months after the above repair. Note the sarcoblast with vesicular nuclei in a row. Masson, × 640.

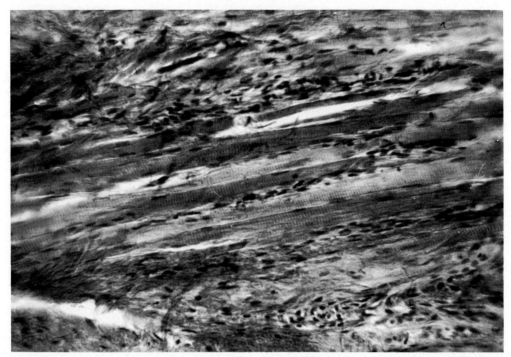

Figure 51–22. Histologic section from a prolabium three months after surgery. Striated muscle fibers embedded in collagenous connective tissue. Masson, × 250.

muscular fibers and the degree of penetration into the prolabium differed in each case. In order to obtain an overall orientation of the muscle, the distance between the cleft line and the furthest extent of ingrowth of the muscle fibers was measured by a millimeter scale placed on the slide after previously fixing the starting line; it was noted that the fibers had penetrated an average distance of 2 to 5 mm, a distance representing one-fourth to one-third of the width of the average prolabium at each side. Twenty patients of the original series of 30 required secondary reconstruction, i.e., deepening of the labial buccal sulcus, one to ten years after primary lip closure. Biopsies of the contents of the repaired lip at the same time revealed that many muscle fibers had been gradually replaced by connective tissue (Fig. 51–23). The fibers of the collagenous connective tissue were mostly parallel to the longitudinal axis of the lip and at some points suggested a tendon-like arrangement, particularly in the central part of the prolabium. Many muscle fibers, however, were preserved, and these, together with the collagen fibers, were collected into horizontal rows, providing a favorable elastic link between the contractile ends of the orbicularis muscle.

In this way the restoration of the oral constrictor is satisfactorily achieved in the wide bilateral cleft, even when the approximation and suture of muscle stumps from each side without excessive tension are impossible.

In the incomplete bilateral cleft, the muscle bundles of the lateral segments cross the bridge above the cleft into the medial lip segment and completely fill it (Figs. 51–24 to 51–27).

There is a striking difference between the soft tissue bridges in unilateral and bilateral incomplete clefts. In the incomplete unilateral cleft, the muscles do not, as a rule, cross the cleft unless the bridge occupies at least one-third of the height of the lip (Fig. 51–28). In contradistinction, in an incomplete bilateral cleft the bridges are usually well filled with muscle fibers, even when the bridges are narrow. The muscle fibers penetrate from the lateral to the medial portion of the lip, where they expand in a fanlike fashion. Such bridges in incomplete bilateral clefts tend to be cylindric in shape; in unilateral clefts they are generally flat.

A possible explanation for the different behavior of the musculature in the incomplete bilateral cleft is the fact that the central

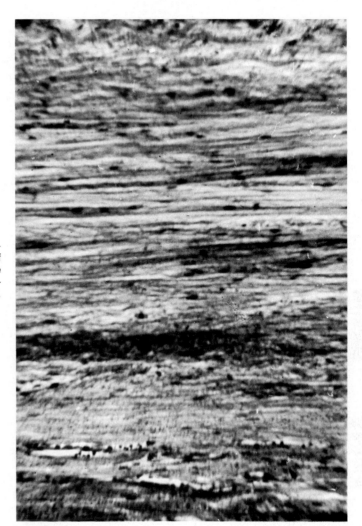

Figure 51–23. Histologic section of the middle portion of the lip ten years after repair of a bilateral cleft lip. Note that much of the muscle has been replaced by a parallel arrangement of collagen fibers. Masson, × 80.

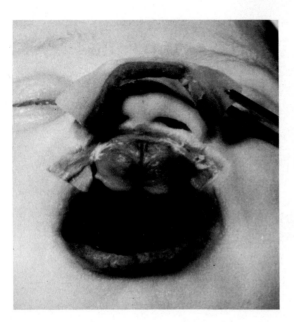

Figure 51–24. In a stillborn with incomplete bilateral cleft, the main part of the upper lip was excised and examined histologically. It was noted that the muscle fibers passed through the wide bridges into the central segment. Note the excised specimen held by a surgical clamp.

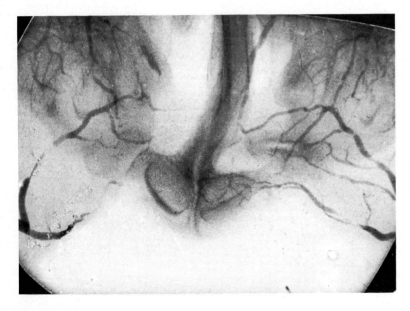

Figure 51–25. Arteriogram of the upper lip and premaxilla in an incomplete bilateral cleft, taken from a semiaxial angle. Branches of the superior labial artery pass through the soft tissue bridges into the central part of the lip. Intraoral view.

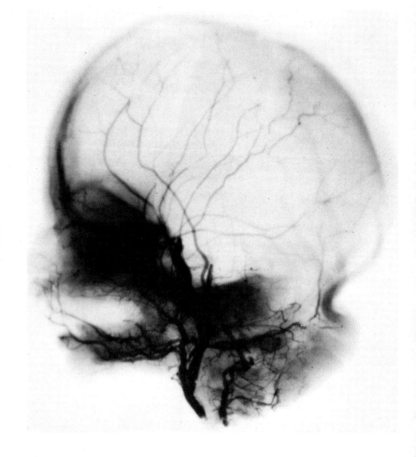

Figure 51–26. Lateral arteriogram of an incomplete bilateral cleft after barium-formalin injection. Note that the branches of the labial vessels pass into the prolabial segment.

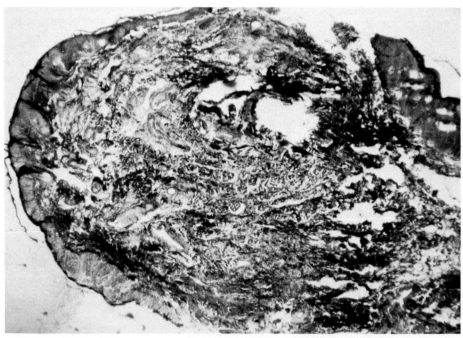

Figure 51–27. Cross section of the thin, soft tissue bridge from an operated incomplete bilateral cleft. Numerous muscle fiber bundles penetrate the collagenous tissue from the lateral segment to the central part (Van Gieson).

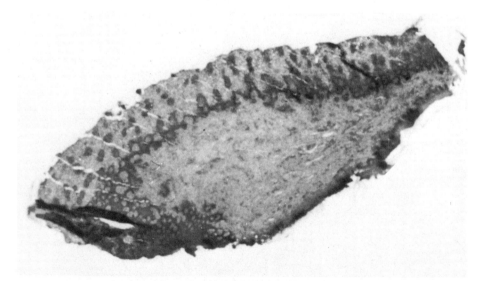

Figure 51–28. Cross section of a bridge from an operated incomplete unilateral cleft. Only collagenous tissue is seen; muscle fibers are absent (Van Gieson).

or prolabial segment of the lip, partially isolated by the cleft and originally without any muscle fibers, is capable of receiving the necessary tissue for each half of the segment from the ontogenetically corresponding lateral segment, which is rich in musculature.

MUSCLES OF THE PALATE

To become acquainted with the anatomy of the cleft palate and to determine common deviations from the normal, autopsies were performed by the author on the palatopharyngeal region in 26 mature stillborn children with all types of palatal clefts. Four stillborn children without clefts served as controls. Twenty-two autopsies were performed on fresh bodies, four after fixation in 10 per cent formalin.

Tensor Veli Palatini

The tensor is a flat muscle (Figs. 51–29, 51–30) arising from the *scaphoid fossa* at the base of the medial pterygoid plate, from the spina angularis of the sphenoid, and from the anterolateral aspect of the cartilage of the eustachian tube. It runs anteroinferiorly and narrows toward the hamulus, where some of its bundles become attached. However, most of the bundles pass into a tendon that turns at a right angle around the hamulus and widens like a fan toward the center of the palate. It terminates either on the oral side of the aponeurosis, which occupies the whole anterior third of the velum, or directly into it.

The morphology and origin of the tensor veli palatini are normal in cleft patients (Latham, Long, and Latham, 1980). As noted by Maue-Dickson (1979), there is evidence that

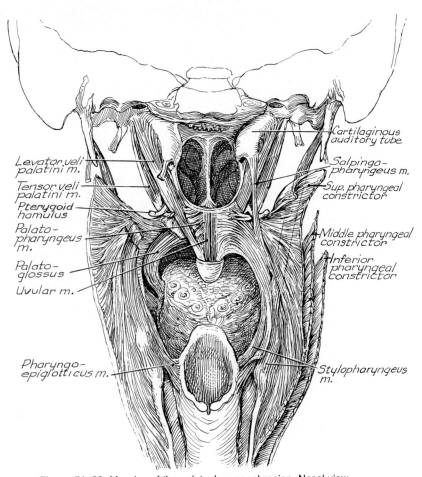

Figure 51–29. Muscles of the palatopharyngeal region. Nasal view.

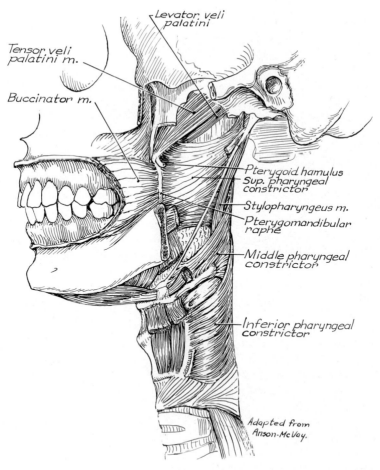

Figure 51–30. Muscles of the palatopharyngeal region. Lateral view.

the tensor veli palatini and tensor tympani muscles share a common innervation. In fact, the latter has fibers that originate from the former. It has been hypothesized that these muscles act together in auditory tube clearance by direct action on the auditory tube: tensor veli palatini contraction and simultaneously tensor tympani contraction on the malleolus. Kamerer (1978) performed an electromyographic study of these muscles, and found that the tensor tympani muscle consistently responded during swallowing and that the two tensor muscles had similar latency response times. These data suggest that the equalization of pressure between the middle ear and nasopharynx may be accomplished via a reflex contraction of the tensor veli palatini and tensor tympani muscles. In short, the tensor veli palatini has no palatal role. It serves primarily to dilate the eustachian tube (Honjo and associates, 1979a).

Electromyographic studies show the muscle to be active during swallowing, blowing, sucking, and the inspiration of air (Hairston and Sauerland, 1981).

Autopsies in Newborns with Cleft Palate. The tensor was somewhat thinner than in a normal newborn child. By pulling on it, it was observed that a few bundles attached to the hamulus, and the tendon itself (appearing atypical) was clearly identified. The front part of its bundles extended along the rudimentary palatine aponeurosis toward the posterior nasal spine or ran laterally to the posterior edge of the palatine bone. Some of the tensor fibers radiated into the aponeurosis. The main part of the tendon, however, arched backward to the cleft edge of the soft palate, where it terminated in two different manners: (1) the tendon occasionally became partly dispersed, and a triangular portion passed into the anterior bundles of the levator

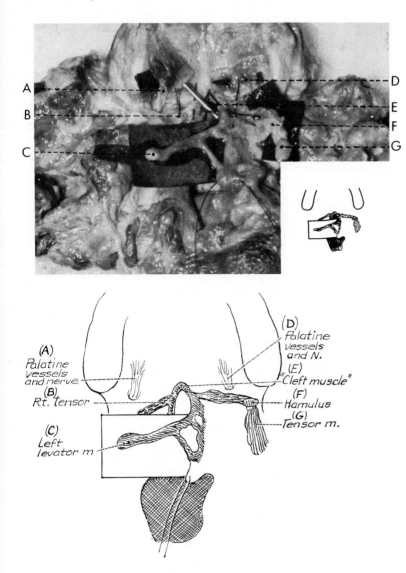

Figure 51–31. Cleft of the soft palate, fresh specimen. On the left side of the specimen (*reader's right*) are the following: *D,* the major (descending) palatine vessels and nerve; *F,* the hamulus; *G,* the tensor muscle freed from its bed and placed on a black strip; *C,* the left levator freed from its bed and turned over the cleft (lying on a black rectangle), all of its three insertions clearly visible. At the top of the cleft, the "cleft muscle" is labeled *E.* The function of the tensor with the levator is formed in the first manner (see text).

bundles of the levator muscle (Fig. 51–31); (2) the tendon did not disperse at all but passed into the anterior bundles of the levator muscle as a coherent and unexpectedly thick and single musculotendinous bundle. The second arrangement was found in more than two-thirds of the autopsies.

Levator Veli Palatini

The levator (see Figs. 51–29, 51–30) is a cylindric muscle, the posterior bundles of which arise from the undersurface of the apex of the petrous portion of the temporal bone and anteromedially from the edge of the canal for the passage of the internal carotid artery. The anterior bundles arise from the posteromedial side and from the base of the cartilaginous portion of the eustachian tube.

The levator elevates and shifts the soft palate backward (the muscles of both sides form a sling suspended from the base of the skull like a swing). It also, in a complicated fashion, affects the shape of the eustachian tube—mainly by constricting the opening of the tube. According to Riu and associates (1966), it dilates the tube synergistically with the tensor.

In 1980 Latham, Long, and Latham performed a detailed study of the structure of the velar muscles in a 5 month old infant with a cleft of the secondary palate. They used a special Plexiglas reconstruction method based on serial histologic sections. The three-dimensional reconstruction demonstrated the anterior insertion of the levator, palatopharyngeus, and uvulus muscles and the abnormal (anterior) position of the velar muscles generally. It appeared from this study that the levator muscle was in a position to obstruct the auditory tube during muscle contraction. A bundle of the muscle fibers from the tensor veli palatini did not pass around the pterygoid hamulus but coursed anteriorly to insert on the maxillary tuberosity. These results, in accordance with the studies of Honjo, Harada, and Kumazawa, (1976), Bell-Berti (1976), and Lavorato and Lindholm (1977), provide documentation that the levator muscle is responsible for synchronous lateral wall motion as well as velar displacement during lateral wall motion. Medial movement of the lateral pharyngeal wall, as caused by contraction of this muscle, occurs primarily at the torus tubarius. The electromyographic studies of Bell-Berti (1976) documented that the contribution of the superior and middle constrictors was relatively slight during the production of sounds. The paired levators are the primary elevators of the soft palate (Kuehn, Folkins, and Cutting, 1982).

A study by Boorman and Sommerlad (1985a) was designed to evaluate the significance of the palatal dimples. These dimples are noted on the oral surface of the soft palate of normal patients when they say "aah." The convexities occur at points of maximal excursion of the palate. They are always present in normal subjects without a cleft, and they occur at the junction of the middle and posterior thirds of the soft palate, slightly off the midline. Cleft subjects were found not to have these dimples, but rather grooves running obliquely forward toward the posterior edge of the hard palate coincident with the direction of the cleft muscles. In cadavers the oral palatal dimpling could be reproduced by traction on the levator muscles. As noted in this study, the palatal length of normal subjects is between 30 and 50 mm, with a mean of 40 mm. The dimple position, which is the point of maximal excursion for the levator muscles, was noted primarily at approximately 25 mm from the edge of the hard palate. The levator insertion starts approximately 17 mm from the hard palate in the intermediate 40 per cent of the soft palate. Dissections also showed that the dimples were close to the posterior border of the levators, and were

related to a point where the fibers of the levator and palatopharyngeus muscles intermingled and became inseparable. As noted by Katsuki (1975), it may be important to reconstruct the normal velopharyngeal valving mechanism by retrodisplacing the levator muscles in the proper position. Since the study by Boorman and Sommerlad (1985b) documented that the normal position for the levators is in the intermediate 40 per cent, these data would indicate that surgical retrodisplacement should proceed to that area to achieve normal anatomy. This should be the goal of the surgeon at the time of intravelar veloplasty.

Autopsies in Newborns with Cleft Palate. The levator muscles in all cases investigated were considerably hypoplastic bilaterally. Sometimes they did not exceed one-half the muscle thickness observed in normal newborn children. The thinner the muscle belly, the thicker was the layer of loose connective tissue in its bed.

In most cases the posterior bundles ran posterolaterally toward the bundles of the palatopharyngeus, penetrated the posterior palatine arch to the vicinity of the base of the uvula, and joined them. The medial bundles radiated like a fan into the margin of the cleft. The anterior bundles were either (1) attached by a triangular tendinous area coming laterally from the posterior nasal spine to the posterior edge of the hard palate, while the lateral distinct part of these tendinous bundles arched into the tensor tendon; or (2) directly linked with the compact portion of the tensor tendon (Fig. 51–32).

In the first case (and it usually occurred in the lesser forms of clefts), some anterior bundles of the levator advanced for several millimeters along the cleft margin of the hard palate as a part of the "cleft muscle." Additional views of levator attachments are shown in Figures 51–33 and 51–34.

Palatopharyngeus

The palatopharyngeus (see Fig. 51–29) is generally divided into three parts:

1. *The palatine part.* This component passes from the thyroid cartilage and the adjacent part of the pharyngeal wall through the palatopharyngeal arch to its fan-shaped insertion in the raphe.

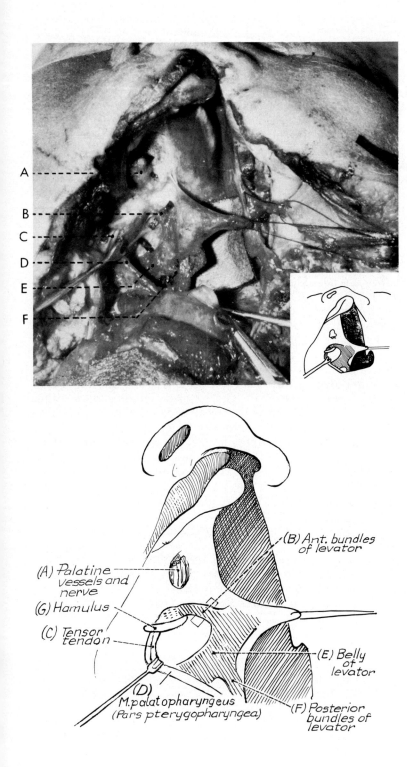

A

B

C

D

E

F

Figure 51–32. Complete cleft on left side (fresh specimen). The belly and insertions of the right levator are only partially dissected. The junction of the tensor and levator muscles is formed in the second manner (see text).

(A) Palatine vessels and nerve

(G) Hamulus

(C) Tensor tendon

(D) M. palatopharyngeus (Pars pterygopharyngea)

(B) Ant. bundles of levator

(E) Belly of levator

(F) Posterior bundles of levator

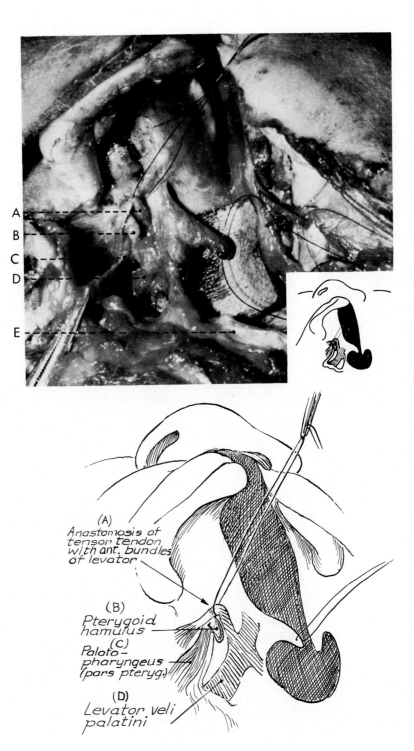

Figure 51–33. Complete cleft on left side (fresh specimen). The suture raises a wide area of the junction of the tensor tendon with the frontal bundles of the right levator. *E,* Palatine portion of the palatopharyngeus freed from its hard palate insertion and turned to the left.

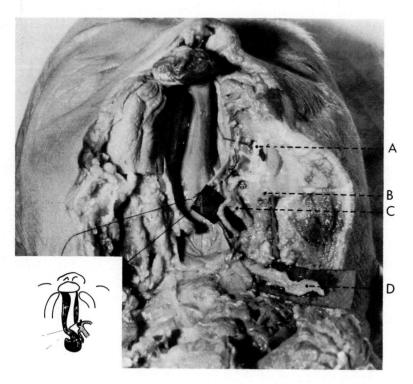

A

B

C

D

Figure 51–34. Complete bilateral cleft (material fixed for several weeks in 10 per cent formalin). On the left side of the specimen, the levator belly is dissected with all of its insertions. The palatine portion of the palatopharyngeus was freed from its hard palate insertion and turned laterally.

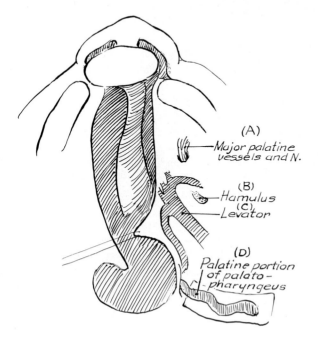

(A)
Major palatine vessels and N.

(B)
Hamulus
(C)
Levator

(D)
Palatine portion of palato-pharyngeus

2. *The pterygopharyngeal part.* This part arises from the posterior and lateral parts of the pharynx and inserts on the hamulus and the palatine aponeurosis, intermingling to a high degree with the pterygopharyngeal part of the superior pharyngeal constrictor.

3. *The salpingopharyngeal part.* This is the weakest portion. Its muscle bundles detach from the previous part and become inserted onto the inferior edge of the cartilage of the eustachian tube orifice.

The function of the palatopharyngeus is to narrow the pharyngonasal isthmus by bringing the palatopharyngeal arches together. The soft palate is drawn posteroinferiorly, as the palatopharyngeal arches stretch and adduct. At the same time the thyroid portion lifts the larynx and pharynx, mainly during deglutition. The tubal portion facilitates dilation of the eustachian tube by stabilizing its cartilage.

Autopsies in Newborns with Cleft Palate. All portions of the palatopharyngeus were relatively well developed. Its fibrous transformation was less significant, in comparison with the tensor and the levator. However, its palatine insertion differed from the normal. Even though the smaller part of its fibers ended in the cleft margin, most of its bundles passed forward along this margin and inserted on the posterior edge of the hard palate (Fig. 51–35) and on the posterior nasal spine. Some fibers finally advanced along the cleft margin, together with bundles from the levator, as a part of the "cleft muscle." In three exceptional cases of wide bilateral total clefts, most of the muscle bundles turned up to the cleft margin of the soft palate (Fig. 51–36). The posterior bundles of the palatopharyngeus, turning to the base of the uvula, passed into the posterior bundles of the levator.

The circular fibers of the palatopharyngeus on the posterior pharyngeal wall were difficult to distinguish from the bundles of the superior constrictor. Thirteen newborns with various types of clefts (50 per cent of the cases) showed condensation and even thickening of the circular fibers of the palatopharyngeus. These bundles were crossed in Passavant's pad, which bulged visibly in the autopsy material. This was not seen in any case of sectioned normal newborns.

The powerful insertion of the pterygoid portion extended from the hamulus across the medial plate of the pterygoid, as far as the lateral portion of the aponeurosis.

Palatoglossus

The palatoglossus (see Fig. 51–29) is a slender muscle, arising from the transverse bundles of the tongue. It passes up into the palatoglossal arch and inserts, fan shaped, into the muscles of the soft palate.

Together with its opposite muscle, it forms the anterior pretonsillar sphincter, which narrows the pharyngo-oral isthmus. It is antagonistic to the levator. The palatoglossus lifts the tongue and propels food.

Autopsies in Newborns with Cleft Palate. In newborns with cleft palate, the palatoglossus passed in a posteroanterior direction in the cleft margin to the posterior edge of the hard palate, where it broadened and flattened as it reached its insertion. It was the most superficial of the soft palate muscles, lying close to the layer of the submucous fat. Its palatal attachment extended in many cases beyond the posterior edge of the hard palate and became inserted more anteriorly, 3 to 5 mm into the oral periosteum of the hard palate (Fig. 51–37).

Uvulae

The uvular muscles (see Fig. 51–29) are a cylindric pair, arising from the palatine aponeurosis and from the posterior nasal spine. They pass nasalward from the other palatine muscles, on either side of the medial sagittal plane, to the top of the uvula, where they end. They lift and bend the uvula backward and shorten it and the entire soft palate longitudinally. Their bundles pierce the stratum of the glands on the nasal side of the velum and thus support their excretion.

The uvular muscle is the most nasal of the soft palate musculature. In Dickson's review (1975) of velopharyngeal anatomy he speculated that the contraction of this muscle could result in humping of the third quadrant of the velum, thus producing what has formally been called the "levator eminence." In 1977 Azzam and Kuehn found that the uvulus was a true paired muscle consisting of two discrete bundles separated by a median septum. The separate bundles coursed posteriorly and converged medially, approximating each other as a cylindrically shaped bundle over the levator sling. The most anterior fibers had no direct attachment to the hard palate. Similar findings were noted in the fetus by Langdon and Klueber (1978).

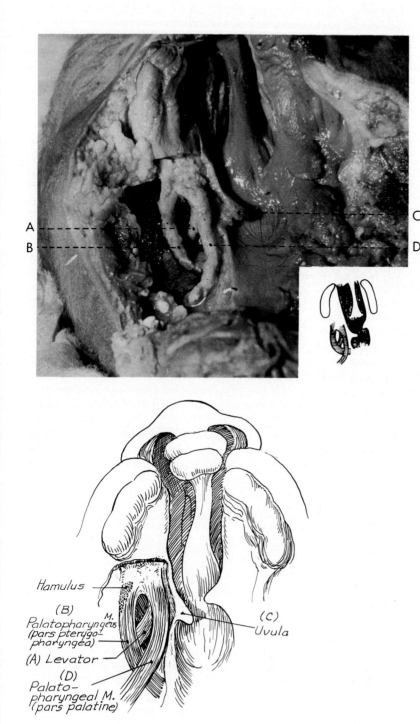

Figure 51–35. Complete bilateral cleft (fresh specimen). On the right can be seen the palatine portion of the palatopharyngeus muscle with its insertion on the posterior edge of the palatine bone, as well as the pterygopharyngeal portion with its insertion on the hamulus continuing to the aponeurosis. Between these the belly of the levator is visible.

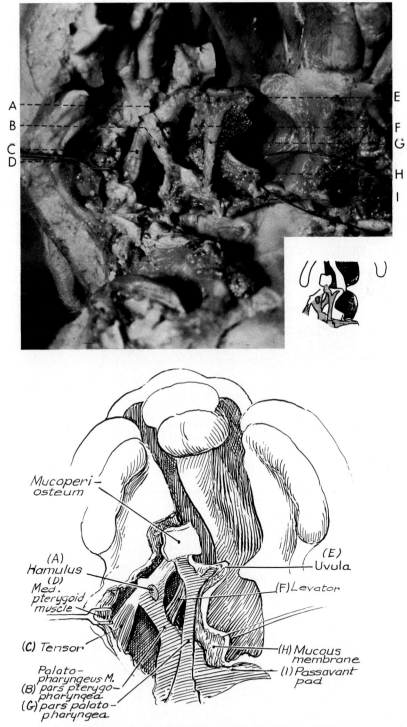

Figure 51–36. Wide complete bilateral cleft (fresh specimen), right side dissected. The greater part of the palatopharyngeus muscle fibers of the palatine portion is inserted into the cleft margin (which is atypical). The remaining muscle fibers are attached to the posterior edge of the palatine bone. On the posterior pharyngeal wall, bulging of the Passavant pad is visible. It is caused by a condensation, thickening, and bulging of the circular fibers of the palatopharyngeus muscle.

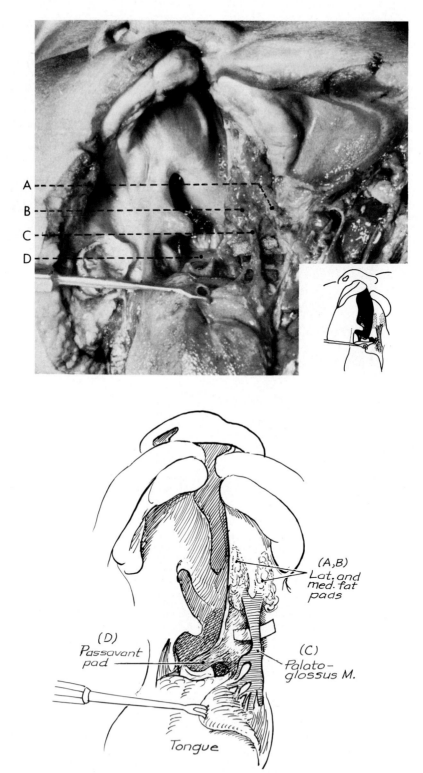

Figure 51–37. Total cleft on left side (fresh specimen). On the left is seen the palatoglossus with its origin in the muscle of the tongue and with its main insertion on the palatine bone. On both sides of the bony insertion, large areas of fat are visible.

The hypothesis that some of the levator eminence is produced by the uvular muscle was substantiated by studies using nasoendoscopy and video fluoroscopy. Patients with hypernasality who were evaluated demonstrated central velar gaps on the nasal surface, thus substantiating the absence of the uvular muscle bulge in that region. Shprintzen and associates (1976) observed small midline gaps in 11 per cent of subjects studied for hypernasal speech.

The nerve supply to the uvular muscle was studied in cadavers (Broomhead, 1951) and fetuses (Broomhead, 1957), and was found to be via the lesser palatine nerve, not via the pharyngeal plexus as are the other intrapalatal muscles. Domenech-Ratto (1977) reached the same conclusion from a developmental study in human embryos. A nerve block of the lesser palatine nerve does not produce any change in speech or change in the nasoendoscopic appearance of the velopharyngeal mechanism during speech (Boorman and Sommerlad, 1985b). These findings suggested that the uvular muscle was not essential for normal speech in the noncleft subject. They provided further evidence that other muscles, i.e., the levators, must also be responsible to some degree for the normal convexity on the nasal surface of the palate during velopharyngeal closure. Piggott, Bensen, and White (1969) suggested that, since the lesser palatine nerve is divided and is distracted during palate repair, long-term atrophy of the uvular muscle should probably be expected after palate repair.

Autopsies in Newborns with Cleft Palate. The muscle passed in the cleft margin, and its bundles intermingled with those of the palatopharyngeus and the levator. The isolation of its fibers was technically difficult.

Superior Pharyngeal Constrictor

The superior constrictor (see Figs. 51–29, 51–30) is a quadrangular muscle surrounding, from behind and laterally, the upper third of the pharyngeal wall. It is the deepest of the pharyngeal constrictors. According to its insertions there are four parts: the pterygopharyngeal, the buccopharyngeal, the mylopharyngeal, and the glossopharyngeal.

In both normal and cleft conditions, a close intermingling of its bundles with those of the pterygopharyngeal part of the palatopharyngeus was typical. This occurred at the point of origin of the muscle in the posterior pharyngeal wall and at the point of its insertion on the pterygoid process.

The upper fibers of the superior constrictor muscle are of considerable importance since they may be responsible for the formation of Passavant's ridge. Data presented by Honjo, Kojima, and Kumazawa (1975) actually suggest that this ridge is of little significance in compensating for velopharyngeal incompetence and that the formation of the ridge is not associated with any degree of closure necessary for the production of specific speech sounds. In 1977 Shprintzen and associates looked at this more closely in patients who demonstrated incompetence resulting from absent lateral pharyngeal wall motion. They were of the opinion that, since velar movement is controlled by levator activity, pharyngeal motion must be controlled by superior constrictor activity and there must be synchronous movement between the two to effect satisfactory speech. The consensus is that Passavant's ridge may be helpful in obtaining normal speech in only about one-third of patients, because the ridge occurs at the proper level for velar closure in only one-third.

Overall Muscle Arrangement in Cleft Palate

The differences between the normal and the cleft arrangement of the muscles of velopharyngeal closure are considerable, yet readily comprehensible. They occur because the muscles extending toward the central line of the soft palate cannot attach themselves to a fixed point in the raphe of the soft palate. They insert, therefore, at various substitute points. These points, however, prevent the muscles from becoming fully functional, so that their development is retarded.

The ability of the muscles in a cleft palate to find suitable substitute insertions depends on the size of the angle formed by each muscle as it proceeds from its origin to the usual insertion point in the absent raphe.

The *palatoglossus* and *palatopharyngeus* muscles, through their palatine portions, find attachment at a very acute angle. Thus, most of their muscle bundles easily bypass the margin of the cleft soft palate and find a reliable substitute insertion, in line with their long axis, on the posterior edge of the hard palate. Some bundles may proceed further forward along the cleft margin of the hard palate like a "cleft muscle." This typical arrangement of the medial bundles of the anterior insertions of the palatine portion of the palatopharyngeus, of the palatoglossus (in most cases), and of the anterior bundles of the levator was described in cleft patients by Veau (1931). It is more clearly seen in operations on older children than in autopsies on stillborn children. The fact is that, in all forms of clefts, the "cleft muscle" becomes thicker in postnatal life, because of the increasing demands made upon the substitute muscular insertion.

The frequency of the substitute insertion of the palatoglossus on the hard palate and the comparatively satisfactory development of the whole muscle in all the author's autopsies of stillborn children were at variance with the experiences of Veau (1931). Veau stated that the palatoglossus in cleft palates is so hypoplastic that in autopsies it cannot be handled at all. The author's findings, on the contrary, seemed to indicate that the functional significance of the pharyngo-oral sphincter in cleft palates is considerable.

The palatoglossus and the palatopharyngeus, especially their palatine portion, are alike in that each of these muscles forms a muscular sling with a thinner compact central part and with fan-shaped ends. The ends of both muscles radiate into mobile organs, i.e., into the soft palate on one side and into the tongue or pharynx on the other, making their origins and insertions variable. In cleft palates, the palatoglossus muscles, because of their main insertion in the posterior margin of the palatine plate, have practically no effect on their respective halves of the soft palate. However, the thickness of their bellies and their firm anchorage in the tongue muscle and on the posterior edge of the hard palate prove their functional importance in lifting the base of the tongue and perhaps the walls of the pharynx.

The *levator,* on the other hand, as it advances to its insertion point in the midline of the palate almost at a right angle, is in a far less favorable situation. It approaches as far as the margin of the cleft. There, however, it fails to secure a sufficiently firm point of insertion and links up, by means of its substitute insertion, with the tendinous bundles of the tensor anteriorly and with the uvulus

and palatopharyngeus posteriorly. This mutual conjugation of all three main muscles of the soft palate is a typical cleft palate arrangement, because of the absence of the usual muscular insertions in the raphe. With little practical effect, this arrangement causes each pair or adjacent muscles joined in this way to form a new functional unit, i.e., a muscular sling, like a double-bellied muscle. Despite this, the levator cannot function adequately, and atrophy follows.

The situation is similar in the case of the *tensor.* Likewise, it has no proper chance to function fully and fails to develop as it should. The absence of a fixed point in the midline, which is necessary for the insertion of the fan-shaped tendon, causes not only an incomplete and atypical growth of the tendon itself, but also a severe hypoplasia of the palatine aponeurosis. Indeed, the very existence of the aponeurosis is due to the extension and penetration of the tensor tendon into it. Thus, the aponeurosis in its lateral area is short. As it approaches the cleft margin, it practically disappears. The pull of the inserted bundles of the circular pharyngeal muscles contributes considerably to the improved development of the lateral parts of the aponeurosis.

In stillborn children (both normal and cleft), the upper end of the lower bundles of the pterygopharyngeal part of the palatopharyngeus passes into the corresponding portion of the superior constrictor. This is in harmony with the genesis of the palatine muscles, which originate in the pharyngeal muscles. The anterior muscles of the soft palate, the tensor and the levator, become more independent and acquire special functions, while the palatopharyngeus retains its original connection with the muscles of the pharynx from a morphologic, functional, and neurologic point of view.

Because of the atypical arrangement of the muscles, certain *bony changes* usually seen in clefts occur. Among these, frequently, is a rather large hamulus, which becomes hypertrophied because of the pull of the muscle bundles attached to it and the greater strain imposed on the pharyngeal sphincter by the cleft.

The pterygopharyngeal part of the palatopharyngeus and the superior constrictors in clefts compensate for the loss of function of the soft palate on the pharyngeal side, although the elevation of the soft palate plays the main part in velopharyngeal closure under normal conditions. This compensatory burden on the above-mentioned sphincter also explains another phenomenon often observed in clefts. In the author's autopsies of stillborn children, he noted a better arrangement of the circular bundles of the palatopharyngeus than in normal individuals, and this forms *Passavant's pad* (see previous discussion under Superior Pharyngeal Constrictor).

In the autopsies, however, the author did not find exostoses on the oral side of the palatine plates as large as in older children at surgery. Apparently these develop only during the first years of life as a result of the excessive strain produced by the atypical insertions of the palatopharyngeus and the palatoglossus when all the functions of swallowing and speech are occurring.

In newborn children the oral mucous membrane can easily be separated from the periosteum, but in older children these layers are firmly attached and are considered from the surgical point of view as one unit—the *mucoperiosteum*. In most autopsies an interposed layer of fat, often quite thick, was noted generally medial to the greater palatine foramen. In this layer, the palatoglossus (and occasionally the palatopharyngeus) extended as far as its insertion within the oral periosteum of the palatine plate. Apparently this fatty tissue tends to disappear postnatally, and the mucous membrane unites firmly with the periosteum as the ends of the muscle bundles move to the posterior edges of the palatine plate.

The *gradation in the development* of these muscles, from the severest form of cleft to the least severe one, was clearly seen in the author's studies. It was most distinctly visible in the belly of the levator, which in equally developed children was almost twice as thick in an isolated soft palate cleft as in a wide, complete bilateral cleft. In a minimal cleft including the posterior edge of the hard palate, the muscle bundles have a better chance to be inserted near the midline and thus to function. This may account for the improved development of the whole muscle, as compared with the case in severe clefts with narrow and widely separated palatine plates. The degree of hypoplasia of the levator was directly proportional to the severity of the palatal cleft.

The levator muscles in clefts illustrate clearly the *effect of a morphologic disorder on function,* from the point of view of both quantity and quality. Indeed, the effect of the activity of these muscles in a cleft palate is almost opposite to that in a normal one. While the muscles of both sides normally join in the raphe to form a sling lifting the palate upward, in patients with cleft palates each muscle pulls its own half of the soft palate in an entirely different direction, i.e., superolaterally, causing a further widening of the cleft. Detaching the cleft insertions and joining the muscles of both halves of the soft palate in the midline must therefore be considered the basic principle of cleft palate surgery (see Chap. 54).

REFERENCES

Azzam, N. A., and Kuehn, D. P.: The morphology of musculus uvulae. Cleft Palate J., *14*:78, 1977.

Bell-Berti, F.: An electromyographic study of velopharyngeal function in speech. J. Speech Hear. Res., *19*:240, 1976.

Boorman, J. G., and Sommerlad, B. C.: Levator palati and palatal dimples: their anatomy, relationship and clinical significance. Br. J. Plast. Surg., *38*:326, 1985a.

Boorman, J. G., and Sommerlad, B. C.: Musculus uvulae and levator palati: their anatomical and functional relationship in velopharyngeal closure. Br. J. Plast. Surg., *38*:333, 1985b.

Broomhead, I. W.: The nerve supply of the muscles of the soft palate. Br. J. Plast. Surg., *4*:1, 1951.

Broomhead, I. W.: The nerve supply of the soft palate. Br. J. Plast. Surg., *10*:81, 1957.

Dickson, D. R.: Anatomy of the normal velopharyngeal mechanism. Clin. Plast. Surg., *2*:235, 1975.

Domenech-Ratto, G.: Development and peripheral innervation of the palatal muscles. Acta Anat., *97*:4, 1977.

Doyle, W. J., Kitajiri, M., and Sando, I.: The anatomy of the auditory tube and paratubal musculature in a one month old cleft palate infant. Cleft Palate J., *20*:218, 1983.

Hairston, L. E., and Sauerland, E. K.: Electromyography of the human palate: discharge patterns of the levator and tensor veli palatini. Electromyogr. Clin. Neurophysiol., *21*:287, 1981.

Honjo, I., Harada, H., and Kumazawa, T.: Role of the levator veli palatini muscle in movement of the lateral pharyngeal wall. Arch. Otorhinolaryngol., *212*:93, 1976.

Honjo, I., Kojima, M., and Kumazawa, T.: Role of Passavant's ridge in cleft palate speech. Arch. Otorhinolaryngol., *211*:203, 1975.

Honjo, I., Okazaki, N., and Kumazawa, T.: Experimental study of the eustachian tube function with regard to its related muscle. Acta Otolaryngol., *87*:84, 1979a.

Honjo, I., Okazaki, N., and Nozoe, T.: Role of the tensor veli palatini muscle in movement of the soft palate. Acta Otolaryngol., *88*:137, 1979b.

Kamerer, D. B.: Electromyographic correlation of tensor tympani and tensor veli palatini muscles in man. Laryngoscope, *88*:651, 1978.

Katsuki, T.: Palatoplasty with muscle sling retention of levator veli palatini and palatopharyngeal speech results and ear disease. Jpn. J. Plast. Reconstr. Surg., *18*:4, 1975.

Keller, J. T., Saunders, M. C., Van Loveren, H., and Shipley, M. T.: Neuroanatomical considerations of palatal muscles: tensor and levator veli palatini. Cleft Palate J., *21*:70, 1984.

Kuehn, D. P., Folkins, J. W., and Cutting, C. B.: Relationships between muscle activity and velar position. Cleft Palate J., *19*:25, 1982.

Langdon, H. L., and Klueber, K.: The longitudinal fibromusclar component of the soft palate in the fifteen-week human foetus: musculus uvulae and palatine raphe. Cleft Palate J., *15*:337, 1978.

Latham, R. A., and Deaton, T. G.: The structural basis of the philtrum and the contour of the vermilion border: a study of the musculature of the upper lip. J. Anat., *121*:151, 1976.

Latham, R. A., Long, R. E., and Latham, E. A.: Cleft palate velopharyngeal musculature in a five-month-old infant: a three dimensional histological reconstruction. Cleft Palate J., *17*:1, 1980.

Lavorato, A. S., and Lindholm, C. E.: Fiberoptic visualization of motion of the eustachian tube. Trans. Am. Acad. Ophthalmol. Otolaryngol., *84*:534, 1977.

Lehman, J. A., Jr., and Artz, J. S.: The minimal cleft lip. Plast. Reconstr. Surg., *58*:306, 1976.

Maher, W. P.: Artery distribution in the prenatal human maxilla. Cleft Palate J., *18*:51, 1981.

Maue-Dickson, W.: Section II. Anatomy and physiology. Cleft Palate J., *14*:270, 1977.

Maue-Dickson, W.: The craniofacial complex in cleft lip and palate: an updated review of anatomy and function. Cleft Palate J., *16*:291, 1979.

Nairn, R. I.: Circumoral musculature: structure and function. Br. Dental J., *138*:49, 1975.

Piggott, R. W., Bensen, J. F., and White, F. D.: Nasendoscopy in the diagnosis of velopharyngeal incompetence. Plast. Reconstr. Surg., *43*:141, 1969.

Riu, R., Flottes, L., Bouche, J., and LeDen, R.: La Physiologie de la trompe d'eustache. Paris, Librairie Arnette, 1966.

Shprintzen, R. J., Lewin, M. L., Rakoff, S. J., Sipott, E. J., and Croft, C.: Diagnosis of small central gaps in the velopharyngeal sphincter. Paper presented at the annual meeting of the ACPA, San Francisco, California, May, 1976. Abstract. Cleft Palate J., *13*:415, 1976.

Shprintzen, R. J., Rakoff, S. J., Skolnick, M. L., and Lavorato, A. S.: Incongruous movements of the velum and lateral pharyngeal walls. Cleft Palate J., *14*:148, 1977.

Veau, V.: Division palatine. Anatomie, Chirurgie, Phonétique. En collaboration avec Mad. Borel. Paris, Masson et Cie, 1931.

Veau, V.: Embryologie du bec-de-lièvre. Scritti in honore del Prof. Donati. Arch. Ital. Chirurg., *54*:845, 1938.

Vogt, T.: Tip rhinoplastic operations using a transverse columellar incision. Aesth. Plast. Surg., *7*:13, 1983.

Zide, B. M.: Nasal anatomy: the muscles and tip sensation. Aesth. Plast. Surg., *9*:193, 1985.

D. Ralph Millard, Jr.

Unilateral Cleft Lip Deformity

The unilateral cleft of the lip and palate, in its asymmetry, is a very complex deformity. Its ideal correction involves alignment of the dental arch, creation of a growing platform for the lip and nose, joining of the separated lip, and correction of the distorted nose. In addition, there must be physiologic division of the oral and nasal cavities by closure of the cleft of the alveolus and hard and soft palate, to make possible normal velopharyngeal closure.

TREATMENT PLAN

As in most architectural constructions, the platform deserves priority (Millard, 1986a). Presurgical orthodontics can achieve alveolar arch alignment, which in turn facilitates clo-

sure of the anterior cleft and construction of the nasal floor. The first stage in the author's treatment of the complete unilateral clefts is carried out by Latham with a method published in 1980.

A split appliance (Fig. 52–1) is secured to the palatal segments with pins in an intraosseous position in the horizontal process of the maxillary bones. A stainless steel bar is placed transversely from one tuberosity to the other, supporting movable metal arms that lie along each alveolar ridge. The transverse bar is required to maintain the retentive angle of the intraosseous pins and to direct the action of the 1-inch long activation screw.

As the deformity to be corrected represents mainly an anteroposterior discrepancy (Fig. 52–2A, B, C), the screw is placed anteroposteriorly in the cleft. The posterior end of the screw is anchored to the appliance, which is

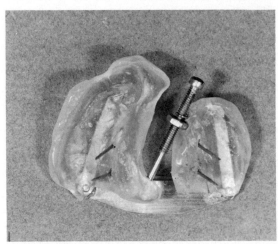

Figure 52–1. The Latham split appliance, which is secured with pins and worked with a screw.

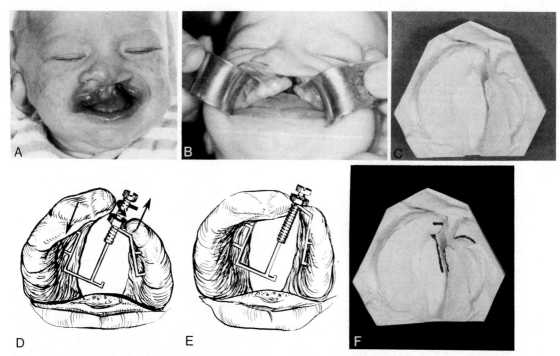

Figure 52–2. *A, B,* Complete cleft of the lip, alveolus, and palate presents outward rotation of the medial maxillary element and a posterior positioning of the lateral maxillary element. *C,* A dental model demonstrates the anteroposterior discrepancy in maxillary alignment. *D,* Diagrammatic positioning of the split appliance and the direction of the forces transmitted through the screw. *E,* Improvement of the maxillary alignment by the appliance. *F,* Gingivoperiosteoplasty. Marking on the dental model to illustrate the mucoperiosteal flaps for two-layer closure of the alveolar and anterior hard palate cleft.

attached to the noncleft segment. A nut is threaded onto the screw and placed at the midpoint. A wire attached to the appliance of the cleft segment makes a loop around the screw in front of the nut. Thus, turning the screw moves the nut forward and pulls the cleft maxillary segment forward (Fig. 52–2D). The other side of the appliance tends to pull back on the projecting premaxillary area of the alveolar ridge (Fig. 52–2E).

The overall effect of the split appliance reduces the width of the cleft, corrects the depression of the cleft alar base, and improves alveolar segment alignment. In seven to ten days alveolar alignment is usually accomplished and gingivoperiosteoplasty is possible. This involves splitting the edges of the cleft alveolus and anterior hard palate so that mucoperiosteal flaps can be elevated and approximated in two layers across the alveolar cleft. Latham has devised alveolar flaps to reconstruct the alveolar ridge (Fig. 52–2F) (Millard, 1980a) and, when all layers have been carefully sutured, a watertight closure across the cleft is achieved without tension.

This technique exposes the alveolar bone on either side of the cleft within the reconstructed mucoperiosteal flap tunnel, which should fill with clot and later with bone and finally attract teeth into the cleft. The one concern is the effect of early alveolar and hard palate closure on subsequent maxillary growth.

After the alveolar and anterior hard palate cleft has been closed in two layers of mucoperiosteum, a symmetric, intact maxillary platform is presented (Fig. 52–3A). To allow this stage of construction to heal without undue tension, the cleft edges of the lip are freshened within the bounds of natural landmarks, joined in a simple adhesion, and left for several months. This technique converts the complete cleft into an incomplete cleft and simplifies definitive construction of the lip (Fig. 52–3B).

When the patient is 4 to 6 months of age the definitive lip construction and partial nasal correction are accomplished (Fig. 52–3C, D, E).

Although the lip adhesion renders the cleft

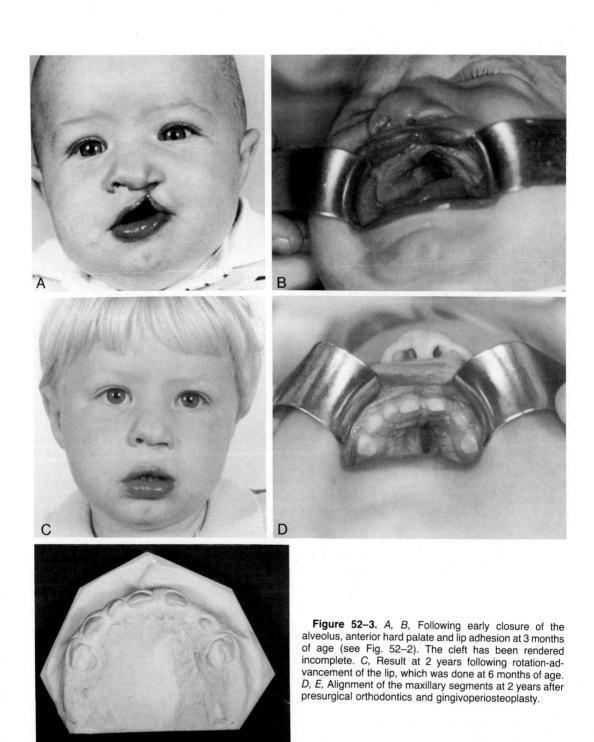

Figure 52–3. *A, B,* Following early closure of the alveolus, anterior hard palate and lip adhesion at 3 months of age (see Fig. 52–2). The cleft has been rendered incomplete. *C,* Result at 2 years following rotation-advancement of the lip, which was done at 6 months of age. *D, E,* Alignment of the maxillary segments at 2 years after presurgical orthodontics and gingivoperiosteoplasty.

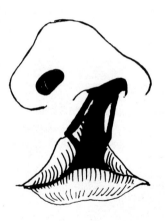 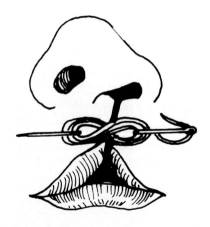

Figure 52–4. Paré pared the cleft edges of the lip, approximated the lip, and fixed it with a straight needle passed through both lip elements and wrapped with a thread in a figure-of-eight.

incomplete, the specific deficiencies of the original deformity are still present. In the author's opinion, the one most important step in the treatment of this entire deformity is construction of the lip and, during this process, the nose. If the definitive lip surgery is poorly planned or executed, the scars are often irreversible and the result severely compromised.

EVOLUTION OF CLEFT LIP SURGERY

The evolution of the unilateral cleft lip closure represents a gradual increase in surgical sophistication. The earliest records of cleft closure date back to 390 A.D. in China and document the cutting and suturing of the cleft lip edges. Ambroise Paré in 1564 was still achieving a straight line freshening of the cleft edges, but he obtained approximation by introducing a long needle through both lip elements wrapped with a thread in

a figure-of-eight (Fig. 52–4). This technique, of course, closed the lip cleft but left a residual notching. Rose (1891) and Thompson (1912) described angled excisions of the short cleft edges to obtain length with closure, and produced a more balanced result (Fig. 52–5). These methods were popular for many years. Numerous varieties of lip operations were devised in an attempt to improve results, but most did not succeed and were not adopted generally. An example was the method of Giraldes (1866) (Fig. 52–6).

Mirault (1844) described a lateral inferior triangular flap to be approximated to a medial paring, which provided increased length to the lip closure. Blair (1930) modified this approach and Brown (1945), his associate, reduced the size of the triangular flap (Fig. 52–7). The result was a nearly straight line scar without a Cupid's bow and with an asymmetric vermilion tubercle. This method was popular through the 1930's and 1940's. In 1949, LeMesurier presented his rendition of the Hagedorn technique described in 1892, which, with a lateral quadrilateral flap intro-

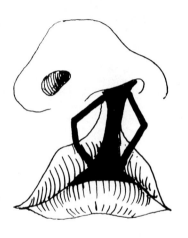 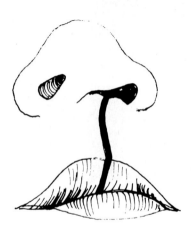

Figure 52–5. Rose and Thompson lengthened the cleft edges by various angled excisions and approximated the lip with sutures.

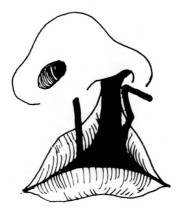
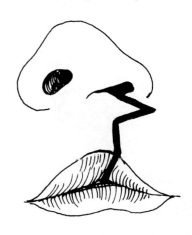

Figure 52–6. Various flap techniques such as that of Giraldes were employed to interrupt the straight line closure, but the unimpressive results prevented adoption of the method.

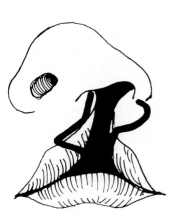
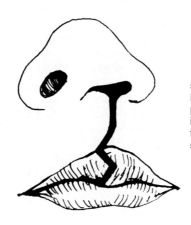

Figure 52–7. A method first described by Mirault, later developed by Blair and modified by Brown, became popular because of the simple markings. The technique, like most of those before it, was essentially a straight line closure.

Figure 52–8. The first method that created a Cupid's bow was described by Hagedorn but popularized by LeMesurier. A quadrilateral flap was transposed across the cleft into a releasing incision in the medial element. By fashioning the width of the distal portion of the flap wider than its base, an artificial Cupid's bow was created. This was an esthetic improvement over previous methods.

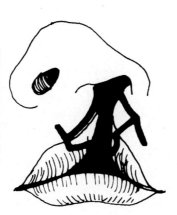
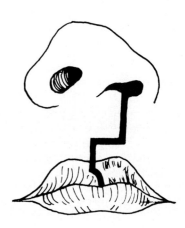

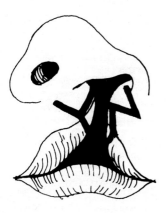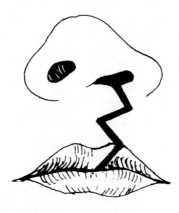

Figure 52–9. Tennison designed a Z-plasty closure of the lip, which preserved the natural Cupid's bow.

duced into a releasing incision in the medial element, created an artificial Cupid's bow (Fig. 52–8). There followed a struggle between the proponents of the Blair-Brown and those of the LeMesurier methods, but the latter found greater application because of the increased sophistication of having created a Cupid's bow for the first time.

Tennison (1952) had been frustrated by the contraction of the straight line scar of the Blair-Brown method in black patients. He designed a Z-plasty, aided with a bent wire, which Marcks, Trevaskis and DaCosta (1953) realized conserved the Cupid's bow and placed it in normal position (Fig. 52–9). In 1952, Cardoso designed a technique similar to the approach that, in fact, was like the one described by Jalaguier in 1880 (1922). The improvement in sophistication of the Tennison method was the preservation and positioning of the natural remnant of the Cupid's bow.

In 1959, Randall did to the Tennison method what Brown had done to the Blair procedure by reducing the size of the inferior triangular flap and defining the mathematics of the method (Fig. 52–10A). The method finally described by Skoog (1969) is also similar to the Randall approach (Fig. 52–10B, C).

Surgical Goal

It is well to outline the ideal goal of cleft lip repair. Approximation of the cleft edges should be achieved without loss of natural landmarks, including any remnant of the Cupid's bow or the philtral dimple. There should be little to no discard of tissue. The Cupid's bow should end in a balanced position. The scar of union should be placed along a natural line. The muscles should be brought together with full-bodied alignment, resulting in eversion of the lip's free border. The alar bases should be balanced and the columella equal on both sides. The definite result should be symmetrically functional and esthetically natural. In 1955 the author presented rotation-advancement as a method to achieve these goals, and this was first published in 1957.

LIP ADHESION

In 1963 the author did his first lip adhesion and for many years transformed a complete cleft into an incomplete one by a preliminary adhesion procedure. When operating outside his home unit and faced with complete clefts that have not had the advantage of presurgical orthodontics or a lip adhesion, the author has become more and more convinced of the value of these actions. While a complete cleft can be closed with a primary rotation-advancement operation, it is technically more difficult and the final result may not be quite as satisfactory. To force the definitive lip scar to mold the maxillae is to place more tension on it than is ideal.

Before adopting presurgical orthodontics to align the maxillary components, the author's adhesion procedure utilized a superiorly based flap of vermilion pared from the cleft edge of the lateral lip segment. This flap was transposed to fill the vestibular lining defect created when the alar base was released from its posterior positioned attachments to the maxilla (Figs. 52–11, 52–12). With preoperative orthodontic alignment of the maxillary segments, it is no longer necessary to release the vestibular lining. Rather, the nasal floor

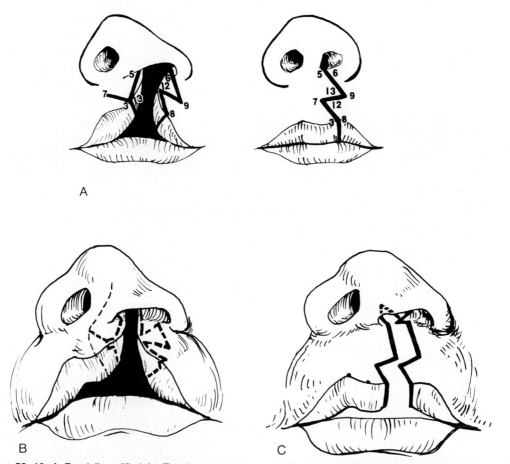

Figure 52–10. *A,* Randall modified the Tennison procedure and with mathematical markings simplified the method. *B,*
C, Skoog later modified his approach by keeping the inferior lateral flap. He moved the upper flap into the nasal vestibule
in a manner similar to the technique of Randall.

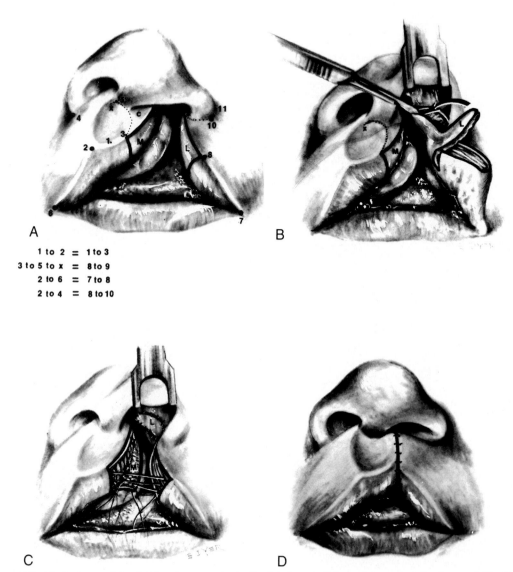

1 to 2 = 1 to 3
3 to 5 to x = 8 to 9
2 to 6 = 7 to 8
2 to 4 = 8 to 10

Figure 52–11. *A,* A complete cleft has been marked with dots for a rotation-advancement lip closure (Millard). The design for an adhesion procedure has been marked in heavy lines to create an L-flap and an M-flap, which also freshen the cleft edges. *B,* The L mucosal flap is incised with its base superior in order that it can be transposed into the incision in the mucosa, which releases the alar base from the retroposed lateral maxillary element. *C,* The M-flap of mucosa provides lining, and 4-0 chromic catgut sutures approximate the muscle across the cleft. *D,* Completed repair.

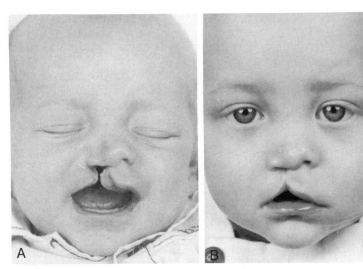

Figure 52–12. *A,* A complete cleft in an infant. *B,* An incomplete cleft after the lip adhesion.

is constructed and the lip adhesion becomes a simple procedure. The edges of the lip cleft are merely incised along the mucocutaneous junction, and the mucosa is turned back to allow approximation in three layers without tension. It is important when preparing the lip for the adhesion that all natural landmarks are noted and preserved. It should be stressed that the adhesion is merely an expedient step toward easing the definite closure and it should serve to create a *bridge* rather than represent *burning bridges.*

CLEFT LIP REPAIR

Whether the cleft deformity is a microform, an incomplete cleft, or a complete cleft with an adhesion, the actions required are similar even if the amount of missing tissue or distortion varies.

First, the difference in the vertical length of the lip from the height of the Cupid's bow on the noncleft side and the cleft side to the base of the columella indicates the lack of Cupid's bow symmetry and the amount of rotation necessary to place normal tissue into normal position. Whatever the discrepancy, correction is possible by rotation and back cut. A controversy continues to exist about the adequate use of rotation in complete clefts. There should be no difficulty if the surgeon understands rotation. Georgiade (1976) has often said he has no problem with complete clefts, but Randall (1986) still maintains that more than a 3 to 4 mm discrepancy

creates a problem for him in using the rotation-advancement technique. He also admits that "about 62 per cent" of his rotation-advancement cases are short, similarly reported by Saunders, Malek, and Karandy in 1986. This emphasizes the importance of understanding the technical details of the rotation technique and creating an advancement to maintain the rotation.

The second measurement involves the vertical height of the lateral lip segment, which must be developed to a length equal to the rotated side in order to match in approximation. This leads to the third measurement that determines the amount of permissible lateral lip paring. Lateral lip paring is used to lengthen the amount of vertical height to join the rotated side. Measurement of the distance from the commissure to the height of the Cupid's bow on the noncleft side should serve as a general guide. If this measurement is marked on the lateral lip element with the latter under the approximate tension to which it will be submitted for cleft closure, the paring should not digress more laterally than this mark. There are instances when it may be necessary to encroach 1 or 2 mm beyond the ideal mark for lateral paring in order to create sufficient vertical height to match the rotation. Within these limits there should be no concern. A difference in vertical height of 1 mm out of an average height of 10 mm total is far more noticeable to the eye than 2 or 3 mm horizontal difference in the distance from commissure to height of Cupid's bow, which measures more than 20 mm with a total horizontal field length of 45 mm from commissure to commissure.

Under general endotracheal anesthesia with the aid of local infiltration of the incision areas, the rotation-advancement markings are made and the exact points of future approximation of the opposite mucocutaneous junctions are stabbed with a needle dipped in methylene blue. A point (1) is placed at the mucocutaneous junction in the middle of the displaced Cupid's bow. A point (2) is placed at the height of the bow on the noncleft side. The distance from 1 to 2 determines the exact distance toward the cleft for point 3 (Fig. 52–13A). It is advisable to mark with dots the normal philtrum column to indicate the ideal matching philtrum column position of the scar of union during cleft closure.

Rotation. The rotation incision starts at point 3, freshening the cleft with a gentle curve in a superior direction to the base of the columella (Fig. 52–13A). This maneuver usually provides at least 4 mm of edge toward matching the 10 mm on the normal side. At the columella base the rotation incision continues two-thirds of the way across, closely hugging the base, which provides another 3 mm of edge (Fig. 52–13B). In rare instances when the normal side is short, this length of rotation may suffice. More commonly it is necessary to increase the rotation with an acute back cut at approximately 90 degrees running parallel but medial to the normal philtrum column. This portion of the incision is best stabbed with a No. 11 scalpel. This provides another 2 to 3 mm of edge on the rotation side (Fig. 52–13C). It is vital that the rotation incision does *not* cross the normal philtrum and lengthen the normal vertical height of the lip. The rotation incision is carried through the muscles to liberate the labial mucosa from the maxilla to achieve total release of the medial lip element. The skin of the rotation edge is elevated no more than 1 to 2 mm from the muscle, and again the mucosa is freed only 1 to 2 mm from the muscle. More radical freeing destroys the coveted philtrum dimple!

A dividend of the rotation is flap *C*, which during the incision is cut free from the lip but is left attached to the side of the columella. It is also freed along the membranous septum to allow columellar advancement (a unilateral forked flap). The attenuated top of flap *C* may be trimmed and rotated around into the upper half of the rotation back cut

(Fig. 52–14A). This maneuver provides extra length at the base of the unilaterally short columella, and also reduces the resulting defect of the back cut, presenting a more ideal rotation gap for the tip of the lip advancement flap. Flap *C* is sutured into position with 6-0 silk to the skin and with 5-0 catgut in the membranous septal mucosa. This completes preparation of the medial side of the cleft, and the height of the arch of the Cupid's bow should be equal on both sides.

Advancement. The advancement flap is marked generally to fit the rotation. The lateral cleft edge should be extended as superiorly as there is usable skin and muscle. The lateral lip element must be pared to equal the length of the rotation side. The limit of paring is set while this element is under the tension it will be subjected to when the lip elements are approximated. If the distance from the commissure to the height of bow on the normal side, 2 to 5, is marked on the cleft side, 7 to 8, paring can extend to point 7 (Fig. 52–14B). Release of the lip from the alar base by a horizontal incision helps to free the advancement flap (Fig. 52–14C). The cleft edge is pared to the mark 7 that indicates bow arch to commissure distance on the normal side. The lateral lip element is freed from its attachments to the maxilla and advanced into the rotation gap to observe the fit. Minor corrections can then be carried out, such as rendering the vertical edge slightly concave to match the convexity of the rotation edge.

Muscle Dissection. The muscle of the lateral lip element deserves careful consideration. It should be freed generously from the skin by careful undermining and also liberated from the mucosa. Usually the tip of the advancement flap is left undissected so that the muscle and skin advance together. If the muscle of the lateral lip element is bunched into a bulge, greater care should be taken in its dissection to allow flattening by stretching, and its bulk can also be reduced by shaving (Fig. 52–14D).

Alar Base Cinch. When the alar base was left attached to the lateral lip element, its flare, of course, was improved during the advancement. This is all that is necessary in microforms and some incomplete clefts. However, in complete clefts and the more severe incomplete clefts it is necessary to advance the alar base ahead of the advancement of the lateral lip element. A technique called

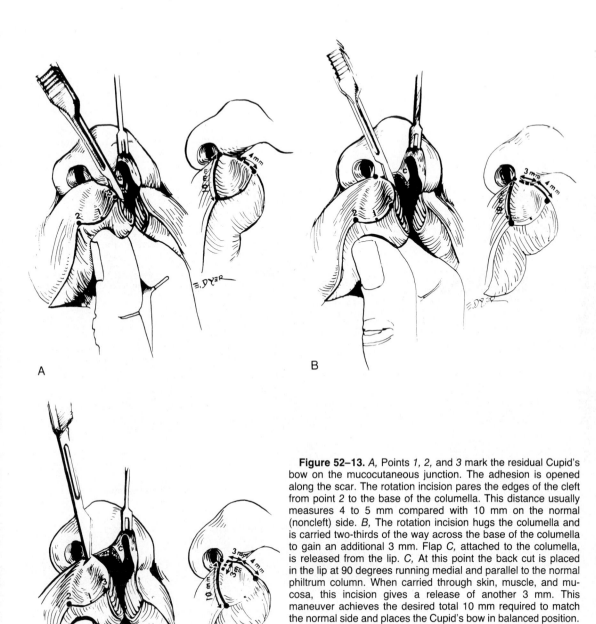

Figure 52–13. *A*, Points *1*, *2*, and *3* mark the residual Cupid's bow on the mucocutaneous junction. The adhesion is opened along the scar. The rotation incision pares the edges of the cleft from point *2* to the base of the columella. This distance usually measures 4 to 5 mm compared with 10 mm on the normal (noncleft) side. *B*, The rotation incision hugs the columella and is carried two-thirds of the way across the base of the columella to gain an additional 3 mm. Flap *C*, attached to the columella, is released from the lip. *C*, At this point the back cut is placed in the lip at 90 degrees running medial and parallel to the normal philtrum column. When carried through skin, muscle, and mucosa, this incision gives a release of another 3 mm. This maneuver achieves the desired total 10 mm required to match the normal side and places the Cupid's bow in balanced position.

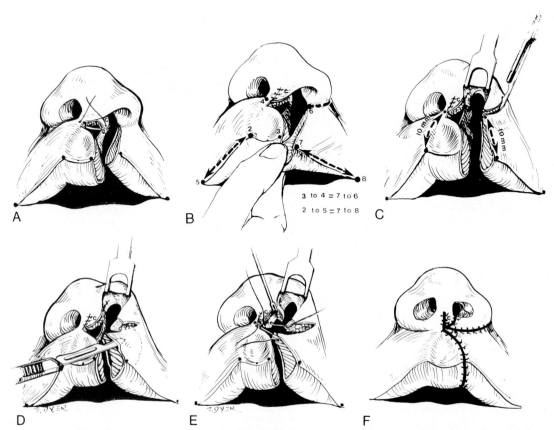

Figure 52–14. *A,* Flap *C* is transposed into the back cut and is sutured to add length to the columella. *B,* The highest point of the lateral lip is marked at point *6* where a transverse incision will free the lip from the flared alar base. As the pared edge of the advancement flap must match the rotation incision (*3* to *4*), point *7* is marked along the free edge so that *6* to *7* = *3* to *4*. The same distance from the height of the Cupid's bow to the commissure on the normal side (*2* to *5*) should be marked on the cleft lip element. With the lateral lip under the tension necessary to close the lip, there is more running room from point *8* for positioning point *7* so that *2* to *5* = *7* to *8*. *C,* Flap *C* has been sutured into the back cut and advanced along a membranous septal incision. The alar base is released from the lip. The height of the lateral lip (10 mm) equals the rotation of 10 mm, thus matching the bow peak to columella base of 10 mm on the noncleft side. *D,* The bunched muscle of the lateral lip element is freed generously from the skin and mucosa so that with muscle approximation across the cleft there is no residual muscle bulge. The tip of the alar base is denuded of epithelium. *E,* The denuded tip of the alar base is sutured to the septum near the anterior nasal spine to cinch the alar flare. The key suture first picks up the muscle in the tip of the advancement flap and then crosses into the back cut of the rotation. *F,* After the alar cinch suture and the key lip suture have been tied, the tissues are in corrected position and require only three-layer closure of the mucosa, muscle, and skin.

the *alar cinch* (Millard, 1976b, 1980b) was developed to facilitate this maneuver. The alar base is freed from the lip by a circumalar incision. The tip of the alar base flap is denuded of epithelium or, if it is too short, a subcutaneous-dermal flap is cut out of the base of the ala, turned out, and used as the tether for the alar base advancement. The alar extension is threaded under flap *C* and sutured to the base of the septum to cinch the alar flare (Fig. 52–14*C, D, E*). The excess skin of the alar base flap is trimmed if necessary and sutured to the side of flap *C* to create a nostril sill in continuity with the columella base.

Suturing. This is the time to place the key suture (Fig. 52–14*E*). A 4-0 chromic catgut suture is used to pick up the muscle of the tip of the advancement flap and then cross over and grasp the muscle in the depth of the rotation back cut. It is important to pick up the medial edge just above the rotation so as not to pull up on the rotation during the tying of the key suture. The muscles are sutured carefully across the cleft using 4-0 chromic catgut, with emphasis on stretching the lateral musculature into normal contour. It is important to free the peripheral orbicularis oris muscles from the mucosa at the edges and approximate the muscles with a suture. This avoids a slight tendency toward retraction at the edge. The skin point of the advancement flap is sutured into the back cut of the rotation with 6-0 silk. The skin edges are trimmed for a perfect fit and sutured with 6-0 silk, making certain that the opposing methylene blue dots in the mucocutaneous junction are in exact apposition (Fig. 52–14*F*).

Further advancement of the alar base can be promoted by 4-0 catgut sutures between the subcutaneous tissue of the alar base and the edge of the upper lip. The posterior mucosa of the lip is closed with 4-0 chromic catgut, and if there is any evidence of tightening, a posterior mucosal interdigitation can be used to lengthen the straight line scar. Moreover, this interdigitation is out of sight.

If there is a discrepancy in the contour of the upper portion of the lateral lip element, more often seen in incomplete clefts, a flap of muscle from the edge of the medial lip element, based superiorly, can be transferred into a tunnel under the depressed skin by transposition. This not only improves the deficiency but interrupts the contracting scar.

A Logan bow is applied to the lip for a few days to reduce tension on the healing scar. An antibiotic ointment is applied regularly on the lip suture line to prevent nasal discharge bathing the stitches.

If all goals have been achieved as planned at this stage, the lip is united and balanced and the nasal deformity has been corrected except for the deviated septum and the slumped alar cartilage. These are treated later.

Warning. If the skin length from alar base to arch of Cupid's bow has been rendered equal on both sides at the end of surgery and the muscles have been well approximated, the final result a year later should be perfectly balanced. Often, during the healing phase, scar contracture of the rotation incision causes an early vertical lift that is disconcerting to parents and surgeon. This contracture often becomes apparent at about one month and may persist for six months or more. By one year the contracture has relaxed and the lip is in balance (Millard, 1976d).

Three random examples of rotation-advancement are presented. One is in an incomplete cleft (Fig. 52–15) and one in a black patient (Fig. 52–16). The nasal correction performed simultaneously with rotation-advancement has rendered the nose reasonably balanced, and only minor surgery will be required later. The Caucasian complete cleft requires more nasal correction at the preschool age of 5 years (Fig. 52–17).

Modifications in Rotation. Adequate rotation has been a problem for a number of surgeons. Saunders, Malek, and Karandy (1986) estimated that 62 per cent of their rotations were short. As their concluding premise was to the effect that technique rather than growth determines the final result, this suggests that they must not understand the method.

Others have used adjuncts to increase the rotation. The most common action has been a small, inferior, triangular interdigitation across the philtrum line in addition to the regular rotation. Skoog (1958) found this necessary and developed his earlier approach based on this (Fig. 52–18). Bernstein (1970) used it, as have several Japanese surgeons, Sasaki (1972) and Onizuka (1966). In principle, and in the author's opinion, this maneuver has never been necessary or justified.

Mohler (1986a) suggested that advancement of the lateral lip into the rotation back

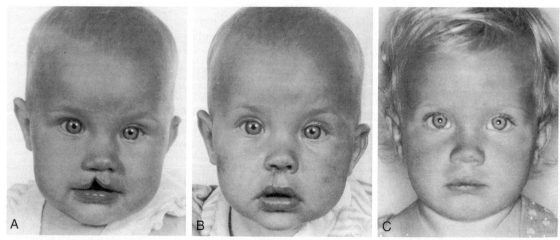

Figure 52–15. *A,* Incomplete cleft lip. *B,* Rotation with small back cut and advancement placed the scar in perfect balance with the normal philtrum. *C,* Result at 1 year.

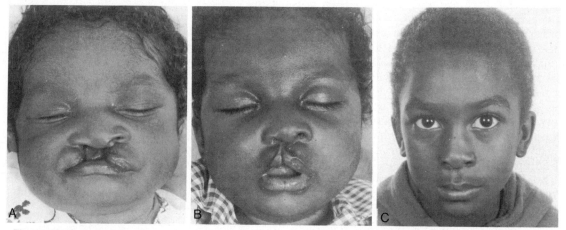

Figure 52–16. *A,* Severe complete cleft lip with nasal deformity. *B,* Early lip adhesion molded the maxillary components. *C,* Result of rotation-advancement at 4½ years with minimal scar balancing the philtrum column. Minimal nasal correction was necessary because of racial nasal characteristics.

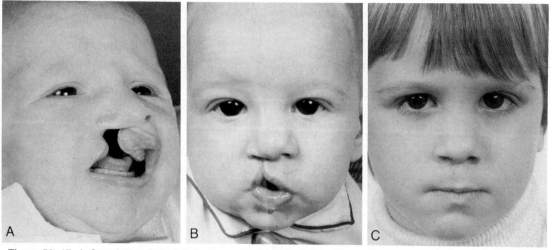

Figure 52–17. *A,* Complete unilateral cleft of lip and palate with deficient lateral lip segment and severe nasal distortion. *B,* Lip adhesion served to render the complete cleft incomplete. *C,* At one year, rotation-advancement procedure achieved positioning of the Cupid's bow in balanced position, with the skin scar symmetric to the opposite philtrum column. Result seen at age 5 years with need for alar cartilage lift indicated.

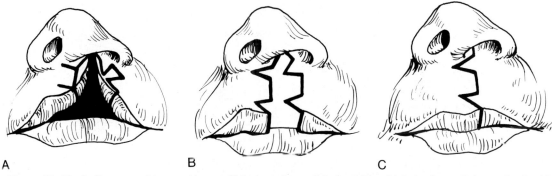

Figure 52–18. *A,* Skoog, unable to achieve sufficient rotation, used an additional inferior flap to balance the Cupid's bow.

cut crosses natural lines. This is partially true in those cases with the philtrum column running toward the floor of the nostril, but not in the more attractive cases with the philtrum column joining its mate inferior to the base of the columella. On the premise that in a large percentage of youths the philtrum columns run toward the nostril floor, Mohler has modified the upper end of the rotation by extending the back cut into the base of the columella, hopefully not including medial crura of the alar cartilages. He used the nasal point of the back cut for approximation to the lip advancement. The back cut in the infant's columella can be closed with flap *C* as in the regular rotation. There is not much extra tissue provided in this technique over the regular rotation and back cut, but direct approximation of the point of the back cut and the lateral lip places the scar in a more lateral position (Fig. 52–19). The real problem is adequate rotation in many cases. If the medial length of the cleft edge is the usual 4 to 5 mm and the columella extension is 3 mm, the incision gives no more than 7 to 8 mm length to the medial cleft edge. The normal vertical lip height usually

measures 10 to 11 mm. The difficulty in getting adequate rotation with this modification was reflected in several of the cases presented by Mohler (1986a). Intraoperative photographs of one patient (Mohler, 1986b) revealed encroachment on the cleft side Cupid's bow to get enough length to lower the Cupid's bow to near-balanced position. This is not justified. If the lip is naturally short on the normal side and the normal column runs into the nostril floor, this modification may be of value if enough rotation can be achieved.

In the author's opinion, this modification offers more difficulties than advantages. As the standard rotation incision may seem slightly asymmetric to the normal column at the time of surgery, it gradually rights itself, as seen in cases presented in this chapter.

EARLY ALAR CARTILAGE LIFT

Before school age (approximately 5 years), correction of the displaced alar cartilage should be considered. In cases of severe alar displacement that would evoke derogatory comments from peers, the alar lift procedure

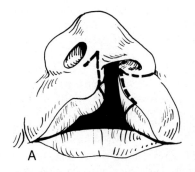 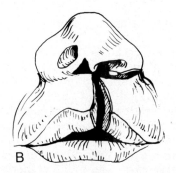 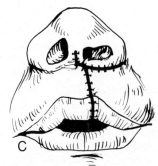

Figure 52–19. *A,* Mohler extended the rotation into the base of the columella and made a back cut. *B,* The point of the back cut is sutured to the lateral lip. *C,* This places the scar more lateral in the upper portion of the lip.

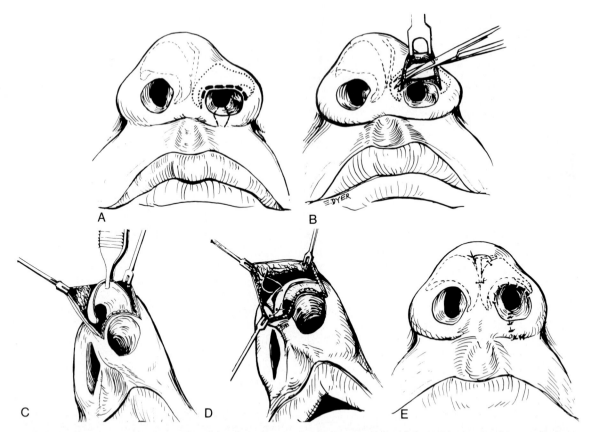

Figure 52–20. *A,* Alar margin (rim) incision provides access to the displaced alar cartilage. *B,* The alar cartilage is freed from the skin and the lining over its medial three-quarters. *C,* The cartilage is lifted free so that it can be rearranged into a more normal position. *D,* The alar cartilage is sutured to the septum with 4-0 Prolene and to the opposite alar cartilage at the tip of the septum to create an alar cartilage contour symmetric with the opposite side. *E,* An onlay cartilage graft from the normal side can be used to bolster the cleft side if indicated. Any other minor nasal revisions, including partial resection of the nostril sill, can be carried out at the same time.

(Millard, 1982) is carried out. Through an alar margin (rim) incision, the alar cartilage is freed from the overlying skin (Fig. 52–20*A,B*). With care the cartilage is dissected free from its slumped position to the lining. The attachments are adherent and the lining is thin; this portion of the procedure is technically demanding. With fine scissors or scalpel the alar cartilage is liberated from the columella and from its peripheral position on the lining. It is also cut free from its attachments along the bridge of the septum, because this is part of the malrotation of the alar cartilage. Thus, the medial three-quarters of the alar cartilage is free, living on its lateral attachment (Fig. 52–20*C*). If the cartilage is attenuated, an extra piece of cartilage from the stronger contralateral alar cartilage may be taken and sutured as an onlay graft for extra strength. The liberated alar cartilage is lifted into normal position and fixed with one or two sutures (4-0 Prolene) to the septum. The key suture is placed between the projected angle of the medial and lateral crus, not only to lift the alar cartilage but also to create symmetry of tip contour. The distal end of the cartilage, which was originally displaced in the columella, is tacked to the opposite alar cartilage at the tip of the septum with a 4-0 catgut suture (Fig. 52–20*D*). This maneuver arches the alar cartilage in its normal position. The lining, which has been freed in order to allow the alar cartilage to be placed into normal position, is advanced into the vestibule by one 4-0 catgut suture, which includes the lining and septal tissue and comes back out through the lining. When tied, this suture lifts the vestibular lining into its natural position. The excess skin and lining along the alar margin are excised to match themselves and the opposite side and are sutured (Fig. 52–20*E*). Three examples of alar cartilage lift are presented: two in children (Figs. 52–21, 52–22); and one augmented with auricular cartilage in childhood and later lifted at age 16 during corrective rhinoplasty, but illustrated at age 21 (Fig. 52–23).

If the slump has been severe, the excess marginal skin can be designed as a triangular flap based on the superior columella (Fig. 52–24A). After the alar cartilage lift, the flap is inserted into a release of the lining from the columella (Fig. 52–24B), which not only allows correction of the alar rim but in fact actually lengthens the upper columella on the shortened cleft side (Fig. 52–24C). This technique, which has been used in secondary deformities (Millard, 1969) and for years in clefts (Millard, 1976c), was described by Thomson in 1985.

During the alar lift procedure, excision of a vestibular skin web or a V-Y advancement improves the nasal airway on the cleft side. Any minor discrepancies of the lip closure can be revised at this time, such as improvement of some part of the lip scar or trimming of excess border vermilion for improved symmetry.

Secondary procedures for the correction of the cleft lip nasal deformity are discussed in Chapter 56.

PRIMARY NASAL SURGERY

Primary correction of the cleft lip nose deformity at the time of lip repair, as described by Salyer (1986), is similar to that practiced by Brown and McDowell during the

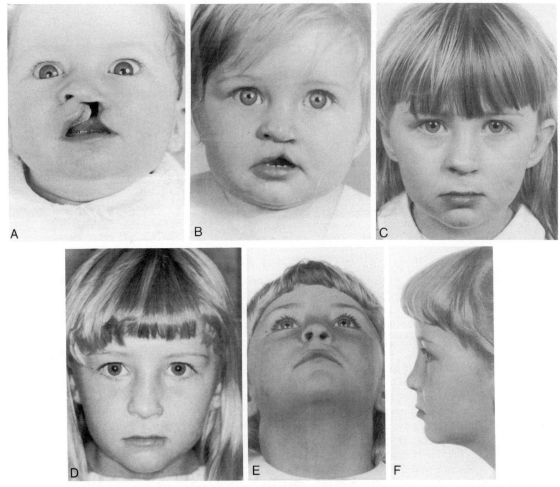

Figure 52–21. *A,* Complete cleft lip with severe nasal distortion. *B,* Complete cleft rendered incomplete with lip adhesion at 2 months. *C,* Rotation-advancement closure of the lip was done at 6 months, and the patient is seen at 5 years with a balanced Cupid's bow. The lip scar is symmetric with the opposite philtrum, but a slump of the alar cartilage is noticeable. *D* to *F,* Alar lift procedure improved the symmetry of the nasal tip contour. Minor correction will be indicated at age 16 years.

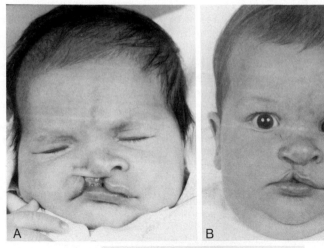

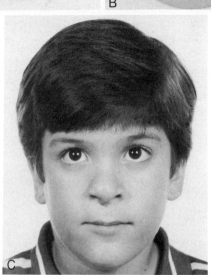

Figure 52–22. *A,* Wide, complete cleft lip with severe nasal distortion. *B,* Lip adhesion was carried out at 6 weeks. *C,* Rotation-advancement was peformed at age 5 months and the alar cartilage lift at age 4 years. The result is illustrated at age 7 years.

1930's and 1940's, with freeing of the skin from the alar cartilage and elevating the cartilage with temporary sutures tied over the external skin. Salyer also released the mucosal attachments laterally. This general approach was used several years ago by the author (Millard, 1976a), who inserted an L-flap into the lateral mucosal release but eventually discontinued its use. Brown and McDowell proved that these actions did not affect growth and that they modestly improved the asymmetric nasal deformity. However, by adulthood more surgery was required for complete correction of the nasal deformity. Probably the same will be true of Salyer's cases. McComb (1986) reviewed Salyer's report and noted that 15 years of personal follow-up will be required for proper evaluation. Incidentally, although this case was not shown in worm's eye view, a residual displacement of the ala is still visible.

Nasal Rotations. A radical method of rotation of the slumped half of the nose through an external incision, splitting the columella and extending over the nasal tip, was developed by Blair and Brown (1930). Others modified this approach, including Sheehan (1925), Joseph (1931), Gillies and Kilner (1932), Young (1949), and Wilkie (1969). It was applied during the primary lip operation in infancy by Berkeley (1959). Recent follow-up of Berkeley's patients revealed reasonable long-term results (Matthews and associates, 1986), but the surgeons who had worked with Berkeley no longer use this approach. In 1982 Dibbell modified this approach through a skin excision with the incision inside the alar rim, rotating the core of the vestibular contents

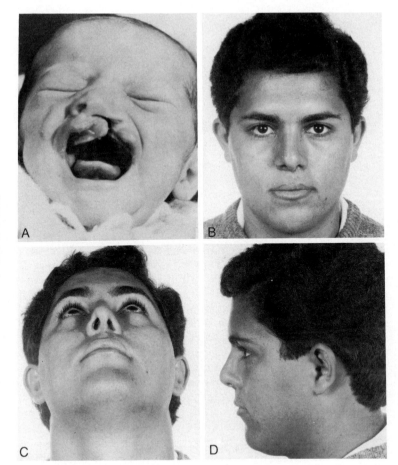

Figure 52–23. *A,* Complete cleft of the lip and palate with a severe nasal deformity treated with rotation-advancement at 3 months of age. An alar cartilage lift was performed during corrective rhinoplasty at age 16 years. *B* to *D,* Result at age 21 years.

clockwise and fixing the rotation with external sutures (Fig. 52–25). This avoids the external scar and gives some improvement but does not solve all nasal problems.

Primary nasal surgery at the time of unilateral or bilateral cleft lip repair is discussed in Chapter 53.

Author's Surgical Timing Plan. If presurgical orthodontics starts in the early weeks, the gingivoperiosteoplasty and lip adhesion can be carried out at two months. The definitive rotation-advancement procedure to repair the lip and nose can be performed at six months, and the remaining

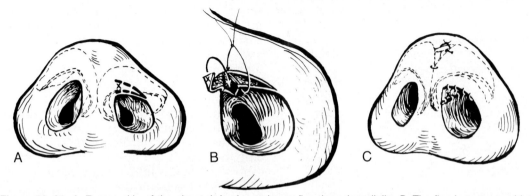

Figure 52–24. *A,* Excess skin of the alar web is elevated as a flap, based medially. *B,* The flap is transposed into a releasing incision high in the vestibular lining to interrupt the circular contracture of the lining and to allow it to be approximated to the alar margin without tension. This tends to improve the symmetry of the alar margin arches. *C,* Flap sutured in place. Additional suturing of the alar cartilages is also illustrated.

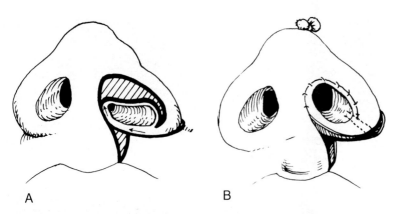

Figure 52–25. *A,* Excision of the dorsal alar skin at the margin and rotation of the vestibular contents clockwise (Dibbell). *B,* The rotation is fixed with external sutures.

A   B

palate cleft closed at 18 months. The tissues can then be allowed to heal and grow. At five years, before school attendance begins, the slumped alar cartilage is lifted into normal position, if indicated, and any minor lip and nose discrepancies are improved. Before the Latham approach of presurgical orthodontics was adopted, bone grafting of the alveolar cleft at eight years was advocated. In the present regimen, however, the interval from five to 16 years is a time for growth to be aided, when indicated, by orthodontic treatment. At 16 years, if indicated, a corrective rhinoplasty and septal correction are carried out with the goal of making the nasal proportions as attractive as possible.

SECONDARY SURGERY

If all goes as expected, the secondary deformities should be minimal. Yet each patient poses a different problem and may react to surgery differently. Maxillary growth can vary. A maxilla developing normally presents a platform with normal facial contour and dental occlusion. Orthodontic manipulation can be used to help achieve this goal. If, in spite of orthodontic treatment, there is lack of maxillary projection and malocclusion, surgery is indicated to correct the deficiencies. The Le Fort I osteotomy with maxillary advancement, mandibular setback, maxillary onlay grafting, and other procedures (see Chaps. 29, 56) are available.

Skin Scars

When the lip scars resulting from the primary lip repair hypertrophy, contract, or spread, time is required for complete healing. This may mean waiting several years. Usu-

ally, when the muscles of the lateral lip element have been liberated and sutured carefully to the muscles of the medial element, there is no tension on the skin closure and the skin scar heals admirably. It is generally true that the scars of infancy tend to heal far better than scars incurred between the ages of 8 and 18 years. After waiting several years, giving the scar a chance to soften and fade, the surgeon should undertake revision (Millard, 1976e). Again the freeing and approximation of the underlying muscles remove the tension from the skin closure with a better prognosis for the appearance of the resulting scar. If only one part of the scar is objectionable, only that part should be revised.

Orbicularis Oris Muscles

When the muscles of the lip elements have not been well positioned and approximated during the primary lip closure, secondary correction is indicated. The most common secondary deformity is the muscle bulge observed in the lateral lip segment. The deformity is more difficult to correct secondarily than during the primary closure. The scar is excised and the skin of the lateral element undermined. The orbicularis oris musculature is also freed from its adherence to the labial mucosa in order that the muscle can be advanced medially and partially flattened. It may be necessary to excise some of the scar from the superior surface of the muscle, not only to shape it but also to convert it from a contracted bulge into a more flattened contour. The muscles of the medial lip edge are freed modestly to preserve the philtrum dimple, and sutured carefully to the lateral muscle edge. An example of a rotation-advancement repair without adequate muscle positioning is shown in Figure 52–26, along with the result after scar revision and alar cartilage lift.

Primary positioning of the orbicularis oris musculature, in which the fibers join across the cleft more or less end-on, is ideal. As noted first by Pennisi, Shadish, and Klabunde (1969), and later by others, the rotation-advancement comes the closest to normal alignment of the lip muscle fibers. Lip closure by the Z-plasty and the rectangular flap tends to correct only the inferior muscle fibers, and the Blair-Brown and straight line closures offer no correction of muscle fiber malalignment. After rotation-advancement positioning of the lip muscle fibers, aided by freeing the lateral muscle bulge and meticulous approximation of near–end-on fiber alignment,

lip function and expression seem to be within normal limits.

COMMON SECONDARY LIP DEFORMITIES

When the technique of rotation and advancement has been used, the most common secondary discrepancy has been failure of adequate rotation. The scar is excised and the rotation is increased by a back cut. Adequate lateral lip edge is created to match the additional rotation edge by lateral paring with the normal limit of height of bow arch to commissure as measured on the noncleft (see Fig. 52–14B). An occasional discrepancy is seen when the distance from the midline

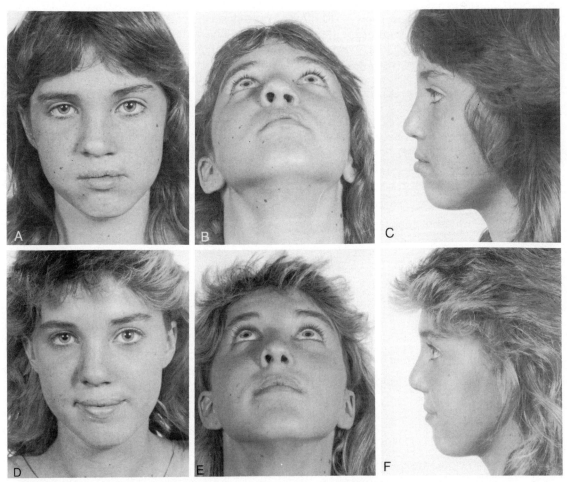

Figure 52–26. *A to C,* Rotation-advancement procedure by another surgeon had achieved balance of the Cupid's bow but had not approximated the orbicularis oris muscle adequately. There were also a residual flare of the alar base and a slumped distortion of the alar cartilage. *D to F,* Through a scar revision the lateral musculature was advanced. The alar cartilage was lifted into a more normal position and the alar web flap technique was used to lengthen the columella. An alar cinch procedure improved the alar base balance.

to the height of the bow arch on the cleft side is longer than on the normal side. In such circumstances the excess can be excised to balance the bow and matched to the lateral element by slight paring if necessary.

If the methods that preserve and place the Cupid's bow in normal position by Z-plasty (Tennison, 1952; Cardoso, 1952; Randall, 1959; and Skoog, 1969) have not achieved balance of the bow, they must be revised to do so. However, in such cases the interdigitation of flaps in disregard for natural skin lines has made definitive scar revision impossible. The irreversibility of this situation leaves minor scar revision as its only exit. Saunders, Malek, and Karandy (1986) reported that 48 per cent of their triangular flap closures were either too short or too long. They also concluded that the errors were inherent in their measurements and technique and not in subsequent growth. Randall (1986) reported that his triangular flap closures were more often too long (vertical dimension) than too short; thus, he undercorrected by 1 mm.

Discard of the normal Cupid's bow and construction of an artificial one by the rectangular flap of Hagedorn-LeMesurier, if a balanced Cupid's bow has not been achieved (Fig. 52–27), calls for redoing the operation to correct the bow (Millard, 1976f). Otherwise, little else can be done for the lip except better

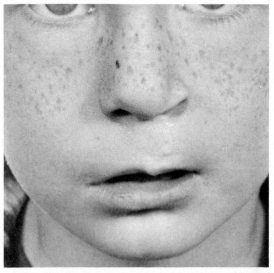

Figure 52–27. The result of the LeMesurier quadrilateral flap in this patient reveals an artificial Cupid's bow with unacceptable asymmetry. Secondary correction involves excision of sufficient skin in the transverse dimension to elevate the long cleft side. Even with improved symmetry the result will still present a scar in an unnatural position.

muscle approximation and skin scar revision when indicated.

After vertical straight line closure, if the residual Cupid's bow is still present but malpositioned, it can be placed correctly by a secondary rotation-advancement.

The straight line closure and the inferior triangular flap of Mirault-Blair-Brown have, more often than not, destroyed the natural landmarks of the Cupid's bow and philtrum dimple. A more radical secondary correction is required. In these cases there is also a discrepancy in the upper and lower lip relationship. The upper lip may be actually too tight or merely relatively tight compared with the loose and often protuberant lower lip.

Special Lip-Switch Flap. A relative tightness of the upper lip in relation to the lower lip is unnatural and ugly. Abbé (1898) first described a lip-switch flap in bilateral clefts. The same general thought had been applied to the tight upper lips secondary to a unilateral cleft. In 1950 Blair and Letterman reported a multitude of lip-switch flaps being used in cleft cases. They invariably inserted the flap into the unilateral scar in an asymmetric position, which relieved the relative tightness of the upper lip but did little else esthetically. In the early 1960's the unilateral positioning of the lip-switch flap dissatisfied the author, who at that time began to ignore the old unilateral scar, to divide the lip in the midline, and to insert the lip-switch flap into the central position (Fig. 52–28). This was published in 1964 and elaborated in *Cleft Craft I* (1976g).

As this approach was practiced, certain facts became evident. A lip-switch flap is certainly performed according to the Robin Hood principle (Millard, 1986b). It also presents "like tissue," and if planned esthetically can be even more "philtrum like." When taken from the center of the lower lip, it usually carries an inherent dimple that imitates the normal philtrum hollow. If fashioned in a shield shape, the flap resembles the normal philtrum. The design also eases the donor closure and reduces the chance of straight line contracture. If the shape of the flap is cut as diagrammed, it also suggests a Cupid's bow (Fig. 52–28). The size of the flap should be the ideal philtrum dimensions and extend the complete vertical height of the lip like a philtrum. Its insertion into the midline of the released upper lip doubly increases its effectiveness on lip tensions. As the upper lip

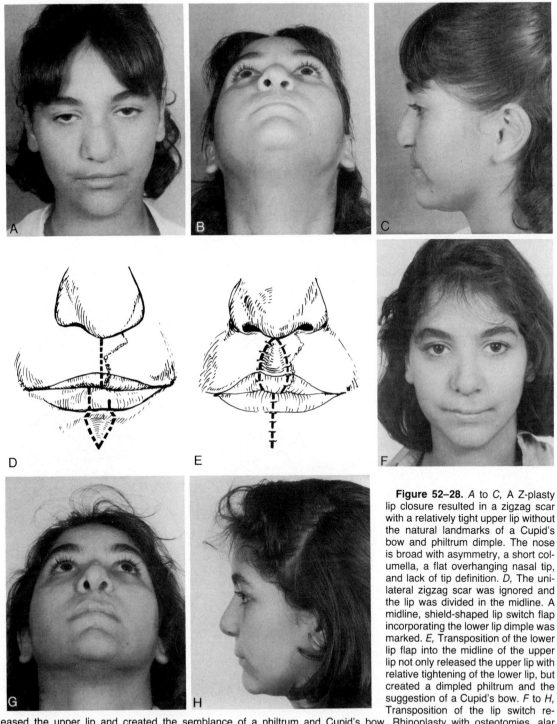

Figure 52–28. *A* to *C,* A Z-plasty lip closure resulted in a zigzag scar with a relatively tight upper lip without the natural landmarks of a Cupid's bow and philtrum dimple. The nose is broad with asymmetry, a short columella, a flat overhanging nasal tip, and lack of tip definition. *D,* The unilateral zigzag scar was ignored and the lip was divided in the midline. A midline, shield-shaped lip switch flap incorporating the lower lip dimple was marked. *E,* Transposition of the lower lip flap into the midline of the upper lip not only released the upper lip with relative tightening of the lower lip, but created a dimpled philtrum and the suggestion of a Cupid's bow. *F* to *H,* Transposition of the lip switch released the upper lip and created the semblance of a philtrum and Cupid's bow. Rhinoplasty with osteotomies, alar cartilage lift, and septal cartilage strut to the columella produced more nasal symmetry and definition. There is still swelling present as these final photos were taken eight days postoperatively.

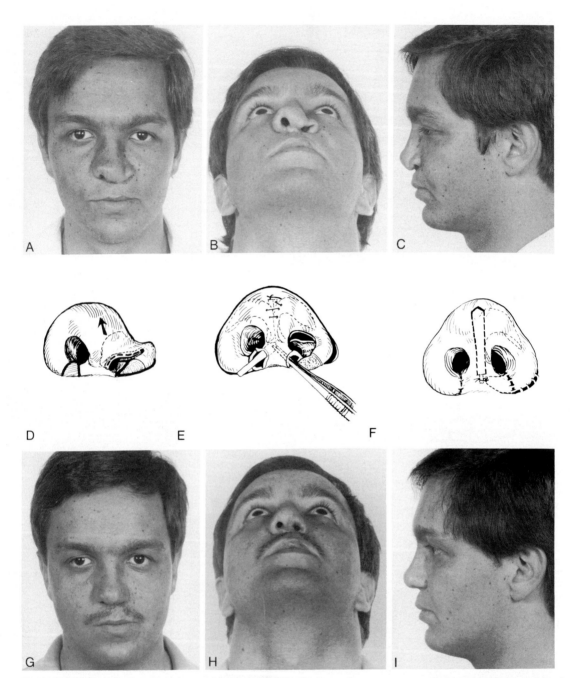

Figure 52–29. *A to C,* Rotation-advancement closure of the lip by another surgeon resulted in a well-balanced lip. A LeFort I advancement osteotomy had improved the maxillary platform. The unusually severe nasal deformity demanded radical action during corrective rhinoplasty. *D,* Alar cartilage lift through the alar margin (rim) incision improved tip contour. Alar base wedge resection on the right and alar cinch procedure on the left have been marked. *E,* Alar cartilage lift has been fixed with Prolene sutures. Left alar base has been denuded for an alar cinch procedure. The septal cartilage obtained during a submucous septal cartilage resection has been fashioned into a strut. *F,* Septal strut inserted into the columella for extra tip support. The alar cinch sutured to the base of the septum corrected the left nostril, while the right alar base was reduced by wedge resection and sutures. *G to I,* Further minor revision, including vertical reduction of the columella width, achieved final improvement.

is relaxed by the width of the new philtrum, the lower lip is being tightened by the same amount, to the mutual benefit of both (Fig. 52–28).

Surgical correction of secondary cleft lip deformities is also discussed in Chapter 56.

CORRECTIVE RHINOPLASTY

If the displaced alar cartilage on the cleft side has been placed into normal position when the child is 5 years old or at any time thereafter, bilateral anterior vestibular incisions allow further correction and reduction of these cartilages as in a standard corrective rhinoplasty. If the alar cartilage is still in a displaced position (Fig. 52–29), inclusion of its correction during the rhinoplasty varies the procedure slightly.

On the normal (noncleft) side, an anterior vestibular incision is made through mucosa and alar cartilages so that all cartilage proximal to the incision can be removed after submucous dissection. On the cleft side an alar marginal (rim) incision gives exposure for freeing the nasal skin from the alar cartilage (Fig. 52–29D). The alar cartilage is freed carefully from the mucosal lining without liberating the thin inferior extension. It is also dissected out of the columella and divided from its unrotated position along the septum. The skin of the dorsum of the nose is freed to give access for lowering the nasal bridge. A membranous septal incision, which is in continuity with the anterior vestibular incision on the normal (noncleft) side, is not connected to the alar margin incision on the cleft side. The anterior septal resection required to shorten a long nose is nonetheless possible. After maintaining an L-shaped cartilage framework along the dorsal and caudal borders of the septum, submucous resection of obstructing cartilage is carried out. The remaining bridge strut is scored on its concave side, and the anterior septal prow is freed from its abnormal dislocation from the anterior nasal spine and reestablished in the midline. The alar cartilage on the cleft side, bolstered by an onlay graft from the resected portion from the normal (noncleft) side, is sutured with 4-0 Prolene to the septum in as near-normal position as possible. The tip of the freed alar cartilage is sutured to the opposite alar cartilage and to the tip of the septum. The vestibular lining is reestablished

with the through and through sutures to the septum, and all lining incisions are sutured. If the alar base is still flared, an alar cinch is carried out on the cleft side and the tether of the alar base is corrected by a suture to the straightened anterior septal prow (Fig. 52–29E). The septal cartilage obtained during the submucous resection can be fashioned into a strut to support the columella and nasal tip (Fig. 52–29F). If a vestibular web persists, it can be excised or reduced with a Z-plasty or a V-Y advancement. Through the vestibular incisions, bilateral osteotomies (lateral) with infracture are performed to realign the nasal bones to the corrected septum. Packing for three days, combined with taping and a splint for seven days, facilitates healing (Fig. 52–29G,H,I).

REFERENCES

Abbé, R.: A new plastic operation for the relief of deformity due to double harelip. Med. Rec., N.Y., 53:477, 1898.

Berkeley, W. T.: The cleft-lip nose. Plast. Reconstr. Surg., 23:567, 1959.

Bernstein, L.: Modified operation for wide unilateral cleft lips. Arch. Otolaryngol., 91:11, 1970.

Blair, V. P., and Brown, J. B.: Mirault operation for single harelip. Surg. Gynecol. Obstet., 51:81, 1930.

Blair, V. P., and Letterman, G. S.: The role of the switched lower lip flap in upper lip restoration. Plast. Reconstr. Surg., 5:1, 1950.

Brown, J. B., and McDowell, F.: Simplified design for repair of single cleft lips. Surg. Gynecol. Obstet., 80:12, 1945.

Cardoso, A. D.: A new technique for harelip. Plast. Reconstr. Surg., 10:92, 1952.

Dibbell, D. G.: Cleft lip nasal reconstruction: correcting the classic unilateral defect. Plast. Reconstr. Surg., 69:264, 1982.

Georgiade, N.: Personal communication, 1976.

Gillies, H. D., and Kilner, T. P.: Operations for the correction of secondary deformities of cleft lip. Lancet, 2:1369, 1932.

Giraldes, J.: Bec-de-lièvre compliqué operation. Bull. Soc. Chir., Paris, 6:407, 1866.

Hagedorn, W.: Die Operation der Hasenscharte mit Zickzarknaht. Zentralbl. Chir., 19:281, 1892.

Jalaguier: À propos de la staphylorrhaphie. Bull. Mem. Soc. Chir. Par., 48:484, 1922.

Joseph, J.: Nasenplastik und Sonstige Gesichtsplastik. Leipzig, Curt Kabitsch, 1931.

Latham, R. A.: Orthopedic advancement of the cleft maxillary segment: a preliminary report. Cleft Palate J., 17:227, 1980.

LeMesurier, A. B.: Method of cutting and suturing lip in complete unilateral cleft lip. Plast. Reconstr. Surg., 4:1, 1949.

Marcks, K. M., Trevaskis, A. E., and DaCosta, A.: Further observation in cleft lip repair. Plast. Reconstr. Surg., 12:392, 1953.

Matthews, D. C., Jacobs, W. E., Mullis, W. F., Walker, A. W., and Chaplin, C. H.: Long-term follow-up of Berkeley primary cleft lip nasal repair. Presented at Am. Assoc. Plast. Surg. meeting, May, 1986.

McComb, H.: Discussion. Primary correction of the unilateral cleft lip nose: a 15-year experience. Plast. Reconstr. Surg., 77:567, 1986.

Millard, D. R., Jr.: A primary camouflage of the unilateral harelip. Trans. 1st Intl. Congr. Plast. Surg., Stockholm, Baltimore, Williams & Wilkins Company, 1957, p. 160.

Millard, D. R., Jr.: Composite lip flaps and grafts in secondary cleft deformities. Br. J. Plast. Surg., 17:22, 1964.

Millard, D. R., Jr.: Secondary corrective rhinoplasty. Plast. Reconstr. Surg., 44:545, 1969.

Millard, D. R., Jr.: Cleft Craft I. Boston, Little, Brown & Company, 1976a, pp. 264, 456, 463.

Millard, D. R., Jr.: Cleft Craft I. Boston, Little, Brown & Company, 1976b, p. 480.

Millard, D. R., Jr.: Cleft Craft I. Boston, Little, Brown & Company, 1976c, p. 483.

Millard, D. R., Jr.: Cleft Craft I. Boston, Little, Brown & Company, 1976d, pp. 520, 581.

Millard, D. R., Jr.: Cleft Craft I. Boston, Little, Brown & Company, 1976e, p. 531.

Millard, D. R., Jr.: Cleft Craft I. Boston, Little, Brown & Company, 1976f, pp. 561, 574.

Millard, D. R., Jr.: Cleft Craft I. Boston, Little, Brown & Company, 1976g, pp. 600–628.

Millard, D. R., Jr.: Cleft Craft III. Boston, Little, Brown & Company, 1980a, p. 289.

Millard, D. R., Jr.: The alar cinch in the flat, flaring nose. Plast. Reconstr. Surg., 65:669, 1980b.

Millard, D. R., Jr.: Earlier correction of the unilateral cleft lip nose. Plast. Reconstr. Surg., 70:64, 1982.

Millard, D. R., Jr.: Principlization of Plastic Surgery. Boston, Little, Brown & Company, 1986a, p. 10.

Millard, D. R., Jr.: Principlization of Plastic Surgery. Boston, Little, Brown & Company, 1986b, p. 292.

Mirault, G.: Deux lettres sur l'opération du bec-de-lièvre. Malgaigne, J. Chir. (Paris), 2:257, 1844.

Mohler, L. R.: Unilateral cleft lip repair. Presented at Am. Assoc. Plast. Surg. meeting, May, 1986a.

Mohler, L. R.: Personal communication, 1986b.

Onizuka, T.: My experience with cleft lip repair: Part I on Millard's method. Jpn. J. Plast. Reconstr. Surg., 9:268, 1966.

Paré, A.: Dix Livres de la Chirurgie. Paris, Jean de Roger, 1564.

Pennisi, V. R., Shadish, W. R., and Klabunde, E. H.: Orbicularis oris muscle in cleft lip repair. Cleft Palate J., 6:141, 1969.

Randall, P.: A triangular flap operation for the primary repair of unilateral clefts of the lip. Plast. Reconstr. Surg., 23:331, 1959.

Randall, P.: Discussion. Growth of the cleft lip following a triangular flap repair. Plast. Reconstr. Surg., 77:238, 1986.

Rose, W.: On Harelip and Cleft Palate. London, H. K. Lewis, 1891.

Salyer, K. E.: Primary correction of the unilateral cleft lip nose: a 15-year experience. Plast. Reconstr. Surg., 77:558, 1986.

Sasaki, M.: Repair of cleft lip. Jpn. J. Oral Surg., 18:148, 1972.

Saunders, D. E., Malek, A., and Karandy, E.: Growth of the cleft lip following a triangular flap repair. Plast. Reconstr. Surg., 77:227, 1986.

Sheehan, J. E.: Plastic Surgery of the Nose. New York, Hoeber, 1925, p. 122.

Skoog, T.: A design for the repair of unilateral cleft lips. Am. J. Surg., 95:223, 1958.

Skoog, T.: Repair of the unilateral cleft lip deformity, maxilla, nose and lip. Scand. J. Plast. Reconstr. Surg., 3:109, 1969.

Tennison, C. W.: The repair of the unilateral cleft lip by the stencil method. Plast. Reconstr. Surg., 9:115, 1952.

Thompson, J. E.: An artistic and mathematically accurate method of repairing the defects in cases of harelip. Surg. Gynecol. Obstet., 14:498, 1912.

Thomson, H. G.: The residual unilateral cleft lip nasal deformity: a three-phase correction technique. Plast. Reconstr. Surg., 76:36, 1985.

Wilkie, T. F.: The "alar shift" revisited. Br. J. Plast. Surg., 22:70, 1969.

Young, F.: The surgical repair of nasal deformities. Plast. Reconstr. Surg., 4:59, 1949.

53

Thomas D. Cronin
Ernest D. Cronin
Pamela Roper
D. Ralph Millard, Jr.
Harold McComb

Bilateral Clefts

A lip that is completely cleft on both sides is usually associated with a complete cleft of the palate, but it may involve only the primary palate, the secondary palate being uncleft. In such cases the premaxilla is unrestrained by attachment to either segment of the maxilla and is projected forward by the growth of the cartilaginous septum (Scott, 1956, 1959a,b). The prolabium, which is variable in size, appears to be attached to the tip of the nose by an almost nonexistent columella. The prolabium in complete clefts demonstrates total absence of orbicularis oris muscle, whereas in incomplete clefts, some muscle fiber may be present (see Chap. 51). Skin appendages may be lacking or deficient in this structure. The alae are flared and stretched out to the maxilla on each side.

The premaxilla may vary in size and development (Figs. 53–1, 53–2). It may contain the four incisor teeth; often only one or two teeth are present, and occasionally a supernumerary or a normal tooth may be encased in a saclike structure protruding from one side of the premaxilla. The prevomerine bone, which is the stem of the premaxilla, is distinguished from the vomer by a suture line 5 to 8 mm posterior to the base of the premaxilla. The site of the suture line is indicated by a bulge or enlargement of the inferior border of the vomer (Fig. 53–1).

The maxillary processes, lacking attachment to the premaxilla and not influenced by the growing septal cartilage, may appear small and retruded. There may be adequate space to accommodate the premaxilla, or the maxillary segments may have collapsed medially, leaving no room for the premaxilla in the alveolar arch (Fig. 53–1D). The premaxilla may be united to the maxilla on one side and cleft on the other or united to the maxilla on both sides, although this usually occurs when the clefts of the lip are incomplete. In fact, there may be any degree or combination of incomplete cleft of the lip or palate, or both.

INCIDENCE

The incidence of bilateral clefts has been variously reported, as shown in Table 53–1.

DIAGNOSIS

Before a plan of treatment is undertaken, an accurate assessment of the degree of deformity should be made. The evaluation should determine (1) whether the cleft is complete or incomplete (Fig. 53–2); (2) the

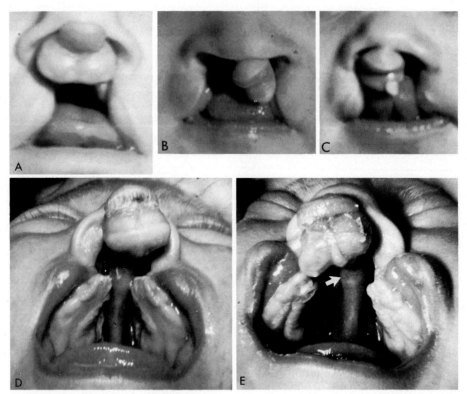

Figure 53–1. Variations in the size and relationships of the premaxilla and prolabium. *A,* Large premaxilla. *B,* Small and rotated premaxilla. *C,* Premaxilla with accessory tooth. *D,* Maxillary segments collapsed behind the protruding premaxilla. *E,* Adequate space between the maxillary segments to accommodate the premaxilla. Arrow points to the vomeropremaxillary suture.

size and position of the premaxilla and prolabium; (3) the length of the columella; (4) in complete clefts, whether the interalveolar space is sufficient to accommodate the premaxilla; and (5) the presence or absence of associated anomalies, such as congenital lower lip pits (Fig. 53–3), indicating an autosomal dominant mode of transmission (Murray, 1860; Van der Woude, 1954). The surgeon should note whether the child is thriving and whether coexisting anomalies are present. If the child has a cleft of the secondary palate, the parents must be cautioned about the almost universal occurrence of middle-ear disease.

TREATMENT

Principles and Objectives

All plans of treatment are predicated on the following: complete correction of the lip and nasal deformity; control of the relationship of the premaxilla and maxillary segments; and closure, or provision for closure, of the anterior palate and subsequently the posterior palate.

In any plan of treatment, the following principles should be observed (Cronin, 1957):

1. The prolabium should be used to form the full vertical length of the lip.

2. The thin prolabial vermilion is turned down for lining.

3. The central vermilion is immediately built up with vermilion-muscle flaps from the lateral lip segments.

4. The vermilion ridge should come from the lateral lip segments.

5. No lateral lip skin should be used below the prolabium.

6. Repositioning of the severely protruding

Table 53–1

Author	Number of Clefts	Percentage of Bilateral Clefts
Ladd (1926)	622	16
Davis (1928)	425	12.94
Veau (1931)	500	9.6
Gabka (1960)	3142	15
Total:	4689	14.33

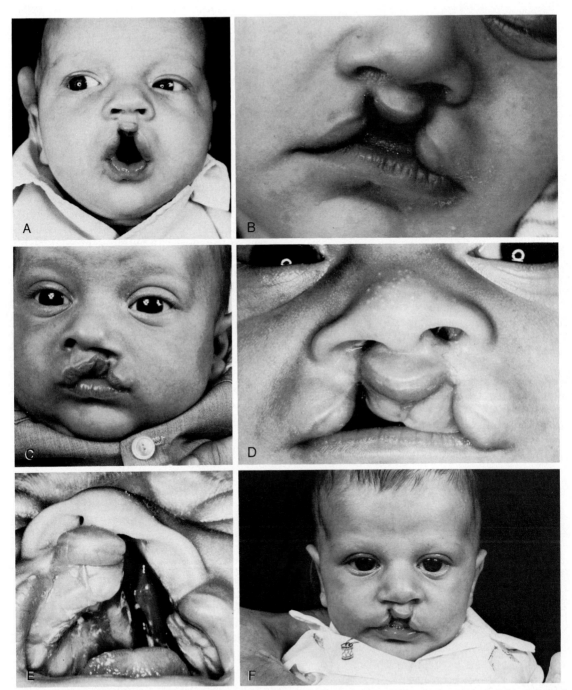

Figure 53–2. *A, B,* Bilateral incomplete cleft lip with small prolabium. *C,* Left unilateral incomplete cleft lip with small Simonart's band and healed cleft on the right. *D,* Bilateral incomplete cleft lip. *E,* Bilateral complete cleft lip with unilateral complete cleft palate. *F,* Bilateral incomplete cleft lip.

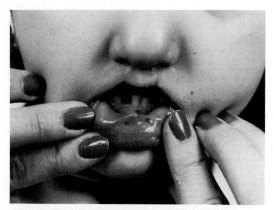

Figure 53–3. Lower lip pits in a patient with bilateral incomplete cleft lip. These findings are indicative of autosomal dominant inherited Van der Woude syndrome.

premaxilla, surgically or nonsurgically, not only permits earlier and better repair of the lip by relieving undue tension but also makes one-stage repair possible unless contraindicated by the method itself.

7. Collapse of the maxillary processes behind the protruding premaxilla requires prevention or expansion with maxillary orthopedics.

8. Bone grafting is indicated to stabilize the premaxilla when it is not united on either side, but is not necessary if one side is fused with the maxilla. It may be required by the orthodontist in order to move a tooth into the cleft or to add contour support of the alar base.

TIMING OF REPAIR

Repair of the lip is generally deferred until an infant weighs approximately 12 to 14 lbs in order to have more tissue with which to work. If the premaxilla protrudes excessively and nonsurgical methods are to be used for its correction, it is important to begin immediately, so that advantage may be taken of the soft pliable condition of the bones and the rapid growth that occurs during the first few months.

USE OF THE PROLABIUM

The prolabium appears to be entirely inadequate for its function of forming the full vertical height of the middle of the lip. The reason for this appearance is that, at its periphery, the prolabium is unattached except at one point. Consequently, there is no

stretching force, and the natural elasticity of the skin causes it to contract. Furthermore, it has no muscle if the cleft is complete (Rees, Swinyard, and Converse, 1962; Fára, 1968); consequently, the prolabium is thinner than the lateral lip segments (see Chap. 51).

Most of the earlier authors, such as Koenig, Maas, Rose, and Thompson (Holdsworth, 1951), and some subsequent ones (Smith, 1950; Barsky, 1950) were deceived by this appearance, and they recommended flaps of skin, muscle, and mucosa from the lateral lip segments to increase the vertical length of the lip. Such a procedure almost always results in a lip that is excessively long in the vertical dimension and excessively tight in the horizontal dimension. Skin has been taken at the expense of the horizontal width, where it can ill be afforded, and used to increase the vertical height where it is not required. Furthermore, the prolabial skin becomes entrapped—like a peninsula, it is almost completely surrounded by scar, so that it bulges, domelike, in the center of the lip as the scar contracts. Worse results ensue when the entire prolabium is used to form the columella, with the lateral lip segments closed in the midline (Adams and Adams, 1953). The prolabium embryologically belongs in the lip, as pointed out by Stark and Ehrmann (1958). Marcks, Trevaskis, and Payne (1957a) demonstrated hair follicles, sebaceous glands, and submucosa of lip tissue. They also noted hair growth on the prolabial skin in some adult males. Current opinion strongly supports the use of the prolabium to form the full vertical height of the lip (Axhausen, 1932; Brown, 1938; Davis, 1940; Vaughn, 1946; Schultz, 1946; Huffman and Lierle, 1949b; Trusler, Bauer, and Tondra, 1955; Cronin, 1957; Bauer, Trusler, and Tondra, 1959; Berkeley, 1961; Skoog, 1965; Manchester, 1970; Millard, 1971a,b).

To achieve a more natural-appearing philtrum, Mulliken (1985) advocated radically narrowing the prolabium to a width of 2 mm. The authors recommend a width of 6 to 8 mm.

MANAGEMENT OF THE PREMAXILLA

According to Scott (1956, 1959a,b) and Baume (1961), the growth of the cartilage of the nasal septum acts as the force for downward and forward growth of the maxilla. Latham (1970) showed that this force is

transmitted by the septopremaxillary ligament coursing from the caudal border of the
nasal septum in a posteroinferior direction to
blend with the premaxillary periosteum and
the interpremaxillary suture (see Chap. 50).
Growth of the septum thus results in a pull
on the premaxilla. Latham (1968) pointed out
that, contrary to earlier views, the septal
cartilage is not important as a growth force
to the maxilla after birth. He demonstrated
that postnatal maxillary growth is due to the
deposition of new bone on the orbital and
posterior free surfaces of the maxilla (the
maxillary tuberosities). The force of this
growing bone against the adjacent soft tissues
(orbital fat, eyeball, temporal muscle) results
in a downward and forward movement of the
maxilla at the maxillary sutures, the latter
acting as sliding planes. Latham and Scott
(1970) postulated that, because this mechanism would supplement the action of the
cartilaginous nasal septum, a basic biologic
principle of "multiple assurance" applies to
facial growth: i.e., there is usually more than
one process involved in the growth mechanism, so that if one does not operate, others
are available.

Latham (1967, 1973) demonstrated overgrowth at the vomeropremaxillary suture in
patients with bilateral cleft lip and palate, as
evidenced by a change in the structure of the
sutural margins to chondroid tissue. The

chondroid tissue is not the force causing the
growth but rather a fill-in, as the cartilaginous septum grows forward, pulling the premaxilla with it by the attachment of the
septopremaxillary ligament.

A diagrammatic representation of the septopremaxillary relationship in the normal
infant and the infant with bilateral cleft is
shown in Figure 53–4. Note that a large part
of the premaxillary protrusion is due to the
abnormally anterior position of the alveolar
process over a period of seven to eight months
of intrauterine life. One can also note the
oblique direction of the vomeropremaxillary
suture (Fig. 53–5).

Control of Protruding Premaxilla.
When the position of the premaxilla is fairly
normal or the protrusion is only moderate,
the lip can be repaired over it with little
tension, although nonsurgical methods may
be employed to further reduce any mild protrusion.

Excessive protrusion is a serious complicating factor, however, in relation to the
planned repair of both the lip and palate.
Attempts to repair the lip over a conspicuously protruding premaxilla may, because of
excessive tension, result either in actual dehiscence of the wound or in spreading of the
scar. The inordinately protruding premaxilla
is in an abnormal relationship to the tip of
the nose. Instead of being located at the base,

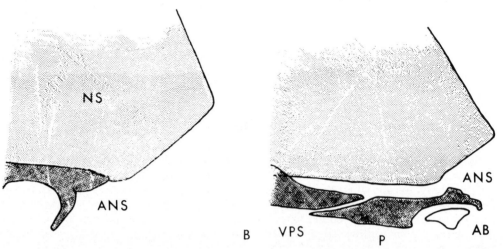

Figure 53–4. *A,* Normal sagittal relationships, drawn from a reconstruction of the nasal septum, basal premaxillary
bone, and alveolar bone at birth. Note that the anterior nasal spine (ANS) lies posterior to the anteroinferior angle of the
nasal septum. *B,* Sagittal relationships in a newborn infant with bilateral cleft lip and palate. The dentoalveolar bone (AB)
protrudes and lies in the same horizontal plane as the basal premaxillary bone, which is also protruding. Note the position
of the anterior nasal spine (ANS), alveolar bone (AB), and vomeropremaxillary suture (VPS). The parts have been
artificially separated to show the inferior septal border. (From Latham, R. A.: Development and structure of the premaxillary
deformity in bilateral cleft lip and palate. Br. J. Plast. Surg., 26:1, 1973, by permission of E. & S. Livingstone.)

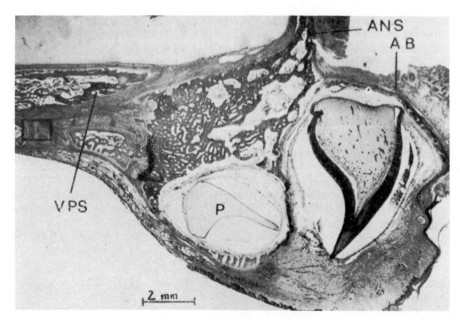

Figure 53–5. Sagittal section through the premaxillary segment of a bilateral cleft. The basal premaxillary bone has an attachment to the nasal septum by the septopremaxillary ligament to the anterior nasal spine (ANS) and in the fibrous septopremaxillary joint generally. Growth is rapid in the vomeropremaxillary suture (VPS); a deciduous incisor tooth lies completely anterior to the nasal septal cartilage. Note the protrusive labial alveolar bone (AB) and the permanent incisor organ (P). (From Latham, R. A.: Development and structure of the premaxillary deformity in bilateral cleft lip and palate. Br. J. Plast. Surg., 26:1, 1973, by permission of E. & S. Livingstone.)

it has grown out to the tip; thus, the shortness of an already too short columella is accentuated.

Listed in order of preference are the methods currently used in dealing with the prominent premaxilla:

1. Traction by external elastic with head cap.
2. Closure of the clefts, one side at a time.
3. Lip adhesion.
4. Intraoral elastic traction devices.
5. Surgical setback of the premaxilla, seldom indicated.

Elastic Traction. Clodius (1964) attributed early use of a head cap and traction to Franco (1561), Levret (1772), and Desault (1791).

As shown in Figure 53–6, an elastic band attached to a head cap by Velcro is worn continuously, except when the infant is being fed, to restrain forward growth and to pull the premaxilla back to some extent while permitting the maxillary segments to grow. Lateral pressure from the elastic may cause collapse of the maxillary segments; therefore, if the segments are in a satisfactory position, an intraoral acrylic plate suffices. A screw plate would be advisable to correct a collapse that was already present (Rutrick, Black, and Jurkiewicz, 1984). Therapeutic results can be expected over a period of weeks or of up to two to three months. If retropositioning of the premaxilla has not been achieved, lip adhesion may be indicated. A disadvantage of the elastic traction procedure is the essential prerequisite of intelligent cooperation from the mother. Moreover, frequent checks are required to ensure a sufficient amount of pressure, but not an excessive amount, which would cause buckling of the septum with lingual tilting of the premaxilla.

Closure of Clefts One Side at a Time. Setback of the premaxilla can be achieved by the pressure of the repaired lip without preliminary orthopedics or surgery. The widest side is usually closed first. When this method of combating the protruding premaxilla is used, the second side usually must be closed under extreme tension, with consequent danger of breakdown of the wound or spreading of the scar. Repair of the second side is performed when the tissues of the first closure are soft, usually two to three months postoperatively. Unless the points for incision of the second side are lightly marked with India ink at the time of the first repair, accurate marking may be difficult owing to distortion of the prolabium by the first operation.

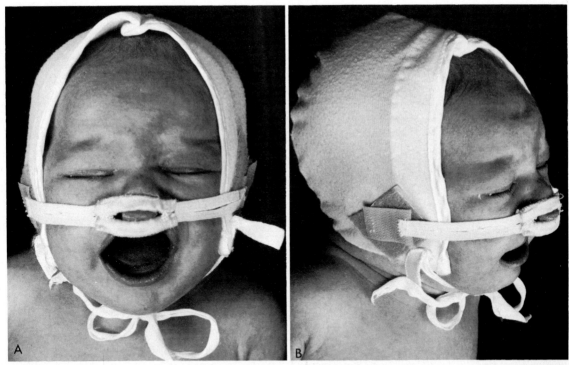

Figure 53–6. Head cap to which ¼ inch elastic is attached by means of Velcro or hooks and eyes. Two or three eyes may be spaced on the cap to allow adjustment of tension. The band is retained in place more easily when split so that one piece lies over the prolabium and one piece below it. A piece of smooth material protects the lip from the rough elastic. The traction is used continuously, except when feeding.

Lip Adhesion. A repaired lip is an efficient means of controlling a protruding premaxilla. An attempt at definitive repair over an excessively protruding premaxilla, however, can result in a spreading hypertrophic scar or actual dehiscence of the repair. A lip adhesion may be indicated when external elastic traction has failed or may be of value as a primary procedure, especially if the external elastic traction cannot be properly supervised. In these circumstances, lip adhesions avoid the possibility of a poor definitive repair because of excessive tension (Fig. 53–7). After the tissues have softened over several months, the definitive repair is performed.

Hamilton, Graham, and Randall (1971) recommended the use of two equal rectangular flaps from the cleft margins, the medial one being based anteriorly and the lateral one posteriorly. Only tissue that would be discarded in the definitive repair is used. Closure is accomplished in three layers: skin, subcutaneous tissue, and mucosa. These authors advised freeing up the lateral segment as needed to avoid undue tension, and they also recommended use of a heavy (3-0 silk or nylon) retention suture if there was much

tension. Spina (1966) performed a fairly elaborate preliminary adhesion while delaying definitive repair for approximately five years. The authors feel this is an inordinate wait for definitive repair.

Intraoral Traction (Fig. 53–8A). Georgiade (1971) placed a pin in the premaxilla anterior to the prevomerine suture line. An acrylic expansion plate with 0.32 spring was positioned and secured with staples into the maxillary segments. Elastic threads were attached from the premaxillary pin to hooks on the acrylic plate. Over two to three weeks the premaxilla was brought into position slowly.

Latham (1973) developed a sophisticated intraoral device with acrylic plates held with a staple over the maxillary segments. A screw controls the expansion of the lateral segments while a pin through the posterior premaxilla is fastened to the acrylic plate with elastic traction. This device can align the premaxillary and lateral segments in a few weeks (Fig. 53–8B). The technique is also discussed in Chapter 57.

Surgical Setback of Premaxilla. This procedure is indicated only when other previous methods, including lip adhesion and

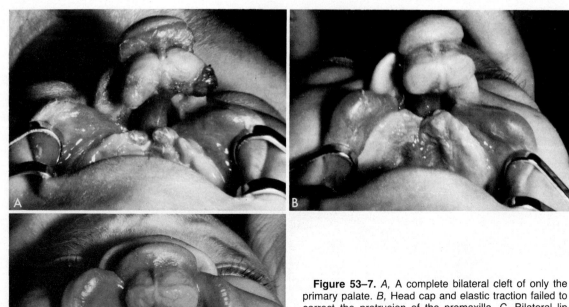

Figure 53–7. *A,* A complete bilateral cleft of only the primary palate. *B,* Head cap and elastic traction failed to correct the protrusion of the premaxilla. *C,* Bilateral lip adhesions achieved retropositioning of the premaxilla in two months. (Courtesy of Dr. R. O. Brauer.)

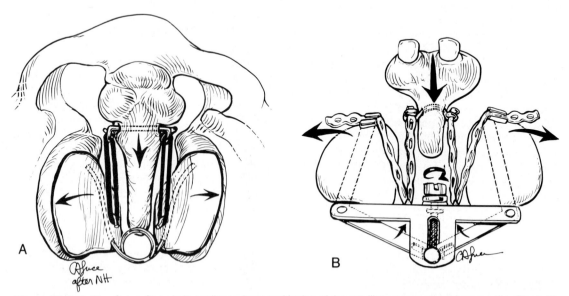

Figure 53–8. *A,* The Quinn-Georgiade appliance for repositioning of the maxillary segments and premaxilla. Stapled in place, the acrylic plates with a spring expand the lateral segments. Traction from elastics, passing from a pin anterior to the prevomerine suture to the acrylic plate, promotes forward movement of the maxillary segments while pulling the premaxilla backward. *B,* The Latham device uses acrylic plates on the lateral segments pinned in place. A screw can be turned to expand the arch. A pin is placed through the premaxilla anterior to the prevomerine suture line. Elastic bands are connected to the premaxilla, looped around a pulley and attached to the anterior part of the acrylic plates.The appliance promotes alignment of the premaxilla and lateral segments.

closure of one side of the lip at a time, have failed to correct a severe protrusion. Surgical setback might also be considered in an older child for whom lip repair has not corrected a severely procumbent premaxilla.

Setback of the premaxilla (Cronin, 1957) may be carried out in the young infant under general endotracheal anesthesia. Strips of cotton sparingly moistened with 5 per cent cocaine are packed into the nose and laid over the inferior border of the vomer for a hemostatic effect.

The surgeon sits at the head of the table with the infant's neck hyperextended and a Lane side mouth gag in place. The suture line of the vomer-prevomerine bone is identified by the bulge or enlargement at this point. The resection of bone should be made from the vomer posterior to the suture line. An incision is made through the mucosa and extended anteriorly over the prevomerine bone (Fig. 53–9).

The thin mucosa is elevated from each side of the septum with care taken to avoid tearing. The amount of protrusion is measured, and 4 to 5 mm less than this amount of vomer is removed as a rectangle. A sharp osteotome or a thin, fine-toothed saw is used to make the anterior cut; if the posterior cut is made first, the other osteotomy is difficult to accomplish, since the vomer is loose. A right-angled knife is used to make a horizontal cut through the septal cartilage from the area of resection toward the tip of the nose. This makes it possible to slide the premaxilla posteriorly without any tilting.

Instead of incising the septal cartilage horizontally, an alternative method (Burston and Kernahan, 1961) is to free the cartilage from the groove in the bone with a septal elevator and slide the premaxilla backward. This method may possibly be less likely to cause any disturbance in the growth of the septal cartilage.

Sectioning through the vomer is preferred because one has a "handle" with which to control the premaxilla. Sectioning through the prevomerine bone deprives one of this handle and makes control and fixation of the premaxilla difficult.

The prolabium is lifted with a hook, and a Kirschner wire (0.035 inch) is drilled through the premaxilla and vomer until the point exits on the cut surface. The drill and excess wire are removed, the two fragments of the vomer are carefully aligned, and the K-wire

is driven into the posterior portion with a mallet. When driven in this way, the wire is tighter than if drilled, and holds the premaxilla firmly in position. The wire should be placed close to the inferior border of the vomer where the thickness of the bone is greatest. The resected piece of vomer is cut into small chips and packed around the junction to promote bony union. The mucosa is sutured with 6-0 silk. The protruding end of the K-wire is removed close to the skin surface so that it lies buried.

TECHNIQUES OF LIP REPAIR

Method 1: Straight Line Closure (Veau III Operation)

Several techniques of lip repair are available. The simplest is essentially a straight line closure and it can produce a satisfactory result (Fig. 53–10). There is some resulting contracture of the scars. However, as they are symmetric, the contracture usually is not noticeable and merely accentuates the formation of the Cupid's bow.

Berkeley (1961) called attention to the importance of not placing point "a" too high as this results in an unduly short columella. He recommended lifting the dome of the ala with a hook to accentuate the presence of the medial crus and placing point "a" well below the tip of the medial crus. Although Berkeley feels that this placement of point "a" results in a columella of normal length, many surgeons believe that in most complete clefts some lengthening will subsequently be necessary. The distance between the two points "a" should be approximately 6 mm. It is advisable that the "a" on each side of the upper part of the prolabium not be farther apart than the two points "b" on the lower prolabium. It is preferable that the vermilion of the lip not be tighter than the upper part of the lip, to avoid reduction of protrusion of the lip.

Point "a'" is located medial to the tip of the base of the ala. Point "c" is placed in the midline of the valley of the Cupid's bow on the vermilion ridge. Point "b" is placed 3 mm lateral to point "c" on the vermilion ridge. When it is certain that the points are in correct position, a 25 gauge needle is dipped in methylene blue and the point of the needle is inserted through the skin. If line "ab" is

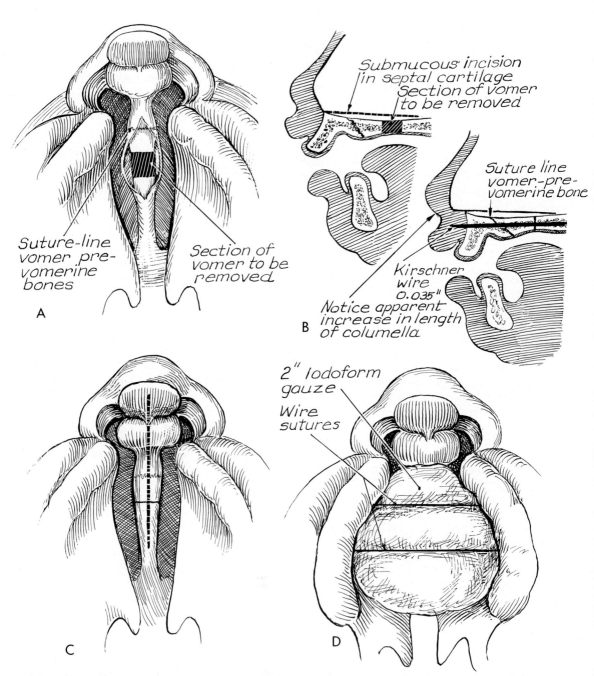

Figure 53–9. Surgical setback of the protruding premaxilla. *A*, Bone is removed from the vomer behind the vomeropremaxillary suture. *B*, Incision of the septal cartilage to allow the premaxilla to slide back. The cartilage may alternatively be freed from the groove in the bone. *C*, The premaxilla has been moved back and the Kirschner wire inserted for fixation. *D*, Complete retrodisplacement has been avoided as further displacement is anticipated. The iodoform packing protects the suture line for five to seven days.

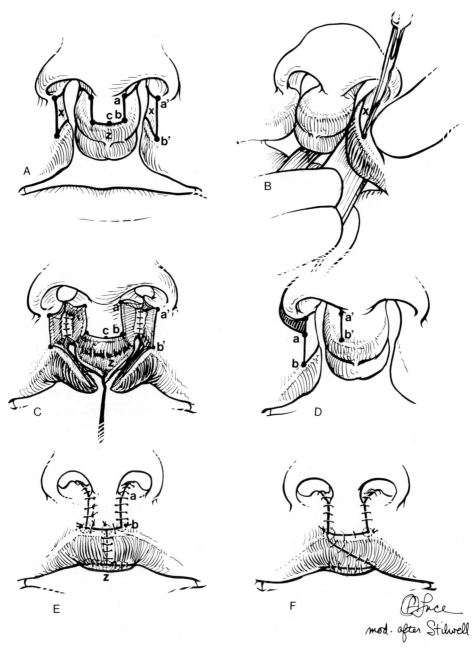

Figure 53–10. Straight line closure (Veau III). *A,* The philtral width should not exceed 6 mm. The vermilion ridge of line "bc" is completely excised. *B,* The incision is made with a No. 15 blade, vertical to the skin and through to the wooden tongue depressor. Flap X should contain sufficient bulk to augment the prolabium and form a small tubercle. *C,* The skin has been removed from the X-flaps, leaving white roll vermilion ridge, vermilion, mucosa, and muscle. Instead of excess skin in the floor of the nose being trimmed, it is retained for future advancement to lengthen the columella. *D,* If the lateral lip is excessive in vertical height, a full-thickness wedge of lip can be removed from the area immediately below the ala (*shaded*). *E,* The preferred closure of the X-flaps in the midline with the Z-flap posteroinferiorly. Note the excess skin protruding as mounds in the nostril floors. *F,* Alternative technique of crosslapping of the X-flaps may be more suitable if the X-flaps are narrow.

Illustration continued on following page

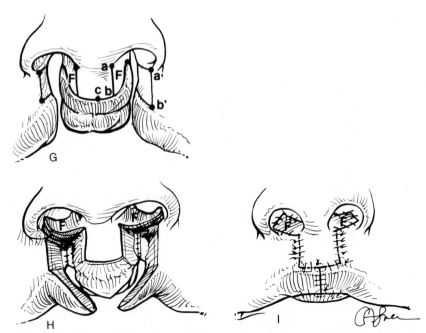

Figure 53–10 *Continued G* to *I*, Development and banking of fork flaps as a modification of straight line closure in a patient with a wide prolabium.

slightly shorter than "a'b'," the prolabium should be stretched with a skin hook during the suturing. Greater differences in length can be corrected by excision of a small wedge from the full thickness of the lip just below each ala (Fig. 53–10*D*). If the prolabium is wide, forked flaps can be developed as in Figure 53–10*G,H* and banked in the nasal floor. If the prolabium is extremely small, the method of Millard (rotation-advancement) (1960b) or that of Wynn (1960) should be used. When incorporated into the lip, the prolabium will enlarge rapidly (see Millard repair). If only one side is to be repaired, the marks "ab" and "a'b'" on the other side are lightly marked by dipping the needle in India ink, thus avoiding later confusion in locating these marks because of distortion of the prolabium resulting from the first repair. The India ink marks should be 0.5 mm out of place so that they can be excised at the next operation.

After the marking is completed, 1 per cent lidocaine (Xylocaine) with epinephrine 1:100,000 is injected sparingly into the buccal sulcus, the base of the ala and columella, the prolabium, and the lip. A 25 to 27 gauge needle is used and the total solution injected should not exceed 1 to 1.5 ml in order not to distort the lip tissues.

Anterior Palate Repair. Before making the lip incisions, the experienced surgeon may choose to repair the anterior palate (Fig. 53–11), particularly if the premaxilla and maxilla are in a fairly acceptable relationship and the clefts are not too wide to prevent suturing the vomer flaps to the edge of the cleft. One or both sides may be repaired. The less experienced surgeon should devote all his attention to achieving an excellent lip repair. However, he should schedule the anterior palate repair before the premaxilla and maxillary segments become opposed by the action of the repaired lip. If the latter occurs, complete repair of the anterior palate is quite difficult owing to the limited access to the area.

If the cleft is complete, it is usually necessary to liberate the base of the ala and the cheek from the maxilla. This is done through an incision in the labiobuccal sulcus, the tissues being freed with scissors superficial to the periosteum just enough so that the lip can be closed without tension. At this time the attachment of the alar cartilages to the margin of the piriform aperture may be severed, including, if necessary, incision of the nasal mucosa. This maneuver facilitates a freer rotation of the alar base.

To control bleeding, the lip is fixed firmly against a wooden tongue depressor as the line "a'b'" is incised completely through the lip with a No. 15 knife blade (see Fig. 53–10*A,B*). The incision is made vertical to the skin

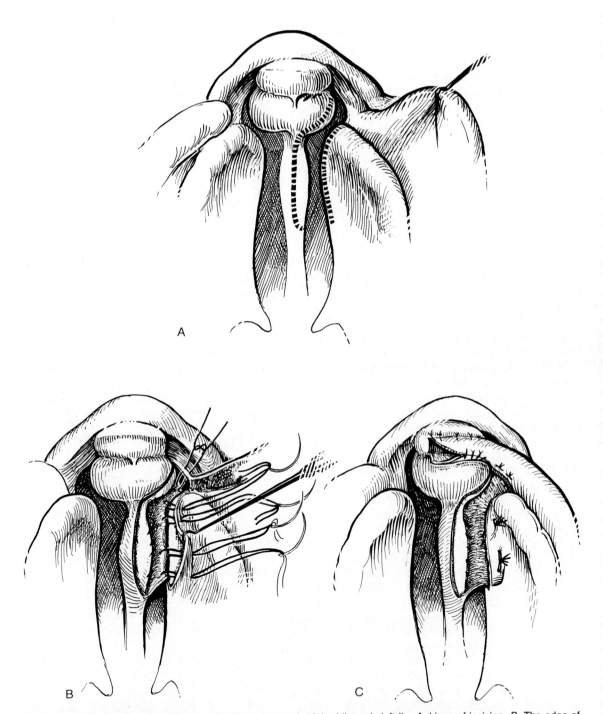

Figure 53–11. Anterior palate repair combined with repair of the bilateral cleft lip. *A,* Lines of incision. *B,* The edge of the vomer flap being advanced under the mucoperiosteum. After the needle is passed through the vomer flap, the other end of the 4-0 catgut suture is threaded through the needle, and the latter is inserted beneath and through the mucoperiosteum. After all sutures have been inserted, they are tied in pairs. *C,* Completed repair of the lip and anterior palate. Alternatively the vomer flap can be sutured laterally to the nasal mucoperiosteum, but this is not as secure as the above method.

surface, care being taken to retain sufficient muscle bulk in flap X to augment the prolabial vermilion with a tubercle in the center. The skin between "a'b'" and the vermilion border is excised, leaving a flap consisting of muscle, vermilion, and mucosa for use in building up the deficient prolabial vermilion. The vermilion ridge is preserved on the muscle vermilion flap.

With finger pressure used again for fixation and hemostasis, line "ab" is incised. If sufficient tissue is available, forked flaps are created lateral to line "ab" to be banked in the nasal floor, otherwise the skin is excised. The remaining vermilion border and mucosal flaps are turned back to be sutured to the mucosa of the respective lateral lip segment as needed.

The vermilion border is incised from "b" on one side to "b" on the other side. This incision should be on the skin side of the vermilion ridge unless the white roll and vermilion ridge are well developed. In the latter case the incision may be made 2 mm on the vermilion side, but if this is done the white roll vermilion ridge should be trimmed off the X-flaps. Flap Z is thus formed and is turned down (see Fig. 53–10C), opening a space into which the X-flaps are fitted (see Fig. 53–10E,F). This maneuver results in deepening of the labial sulcus. Lateral vermilion flaps are preferred, as a uniform color results. The prolabial vermilion border is hinged where it will not show, because it often is not of the same color as the lateral lip vermilion; moreover, there is a tendency for the epithelium to desquamate.

The floor of the nose is formed by continuing "ab" inside the nose, and, if the anterior palate is to be repaired, it continues around on the posterior aspect of the premaxilla and along the midline of the vomer. Likewise, the incision "a'b'" would become continuous with the incision along the edge of the cleft of the anterior palate (Fig. 53–11A).

In making these extensions, as much of the skin on each side of the cleft in the region of the nasal floor as possible is preserved for subsequent use in lengthening the columella (Fig. 53–12). If forked flaps have been made they are turned 90 degrees into the nasal floor and banked (see Fig. 53–10C).

A 4-0 plain catgut or a 4-0 armed Vicryl suture is inserted into the muscle at the base of the right ala. The needle is passed subcutaneously through the base of the columella and out into the cleft on the left, then across the cleft, taking a generous bite in the muscle at the base of the ala, then back through the columella into the cleft on the right. If only one side is being repaired, it may be necessary to pass the suture entirely through the columella and then back over a small bolster, since the subcutaneous tissues are scanty.

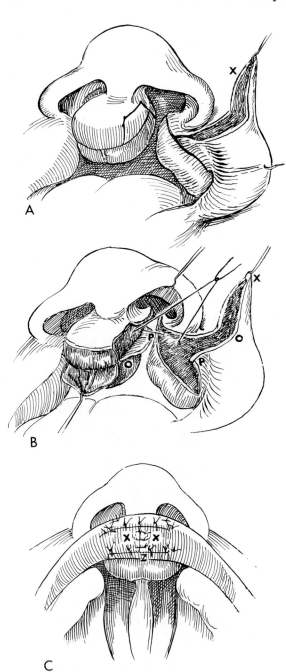

Figure 53–12. *A*, Note the incision in the labial sulcus. The soft tissues are elevated off the periosteum as needed to achieve a relaxed suture line. *B*, Insertion of deep muscle suture. P is approximated to P and O to O. *C*, The final closure.

The ends of the suture are tightened to determine if the alae and columella approximate as desired. If they do not, the suture is removed and reinserted. Before the muscle suture is tied, the skin flaps forming the floor of the nose are sutured with 5-0 plain catgut. Rather than trim the excess skin in the floor, it is "banked" by approximating the raw undersurface together, thus forming an elevated ridge in the floor of the nose (see Fig. 53–10E). Subsequently, this skin can be advanced to lengthen the columella.

The first 6-0 silk suture is placed at the base of the ala and columella. The vermilion ridge is approximated by placing a 6-0 suture about 1 mm from the vermilion ridge; if placed directly upon the ridge or border, the suture may cause sufficient scar to make the vermilion border appear irregular. If the prolabium is short, it is stretched with a skin hook, or if the lateral lip is excessively long, a full-thickness wedge of the lip is removed from below the ala (see Fig. 53–10D), so that the vermilion border of the lateral lip and the prolabial portions can be accurately aligned. Two or three 4-0 plain catgut or 5-0 Vicryl sutures may be used in the muscle on the lateral side and in whatever tissue is available on the prolabial side. The skin is approximated with 6-0 sutures. The thin prolabial vermilion border is augmented with the vermilion-muscle X-flaps (see Fig. 53–10E,F). This maneuver increases the vertical length of the deficient mucosal surface of the prolabium, in effect deepening the labial sulcus. If the lateral vermilion-muscle flaps have been cut to an adequate thickness, a normal-appearing tubercle will result. In any event, the prolabium should be built up enough to avoid a whistle deformity. Figures 53–13 to 53–16 show patients whose lips were repaired by this method.

Others (Millard, 1977; Mulliken, 1985; Black, 1985; Trier, 1985) have advocated more radical elevation of the prolabium and complete dissection and closure of the orbicularis muscle beneath the prolabium. Manchester (1970) does not close the orbicularis muscle because he feels that this results in a closure that is tight and may cause maxillary retrusion (Trusler, Bauer, and Tondra, 1955; Bauer, Trusler, and Tondra, 1959; Brauer, 1974; Spina, Kamakura, and Lapa, 1978; Cronin, 1987). Long-term results of extensive muscle closure have yet to be evaluated.

The arms are splinted with elbows extended to prevent disruption of the repair. These are left in place for two weeks.

Postoperative Care. When the operation is finished, the suture lines are covered lightly with an antibiotic ointment, and a small gauze dressing is taped in place for 24 hours. The authors have not used a Logan's bow for many years. It is certainly not needed when the protruding premaxilla has been repositioned. The next day, exudation from the suture line usually having ceased, the dressing is no longer needed and should be removed, especially since it may become soiled when the infant is fed.

For 10 to 14 days postoperatively the infant is fed through a bulb syringe with a short piece of rubber tubing on the tip. Some skin sutures may be removed on the third postoperative day. Usually all the skin sutures are removed by the fourth day. If there is concern about tension on the lip, the sutures in the floor of the nose and on the vermilion may be left in place a few days longer. After removal of the skin sutures, the scar may be supported by painting the skin with a glue material and applying Steri-Strips for approximately ten days. Bottle and breast feeding is resumed after five days. Packing is removed in five to seven days.

Lengthening the Columella. The shortened columella is practically always associated with complete bilateral clefts. Lengthening of the columella can be done any time after the patient is 2 or 3 years of age. After reviewing their patients, the authors found that the columella was lengthened at an average age of 6 years.

Columellar lengthening is not attempted at the time of initial lip repair. Millard (1988) delays lengthening procedures until school age. He found that very early repair results in downward slippage of the columella and lip over the premaxilla.

The senior author described a method of advancing skin from the floor of the nose and base of the ala into the columella (Cronin, 1958). Converse (1957) used skin from the floor of the nose. Millard (1958, 1971a), Marcks, Trevaskis, and Payne (1957b), and Peskova and Fára (1960) advocated methods that used a forked flap from the prolabium. Brauer and Foerster (1966) employed the V-Y principle in the region of the wide tip.

As described by the senior author, bipedicle flaps are formed, based medially on the col-

Text continued on page 2673

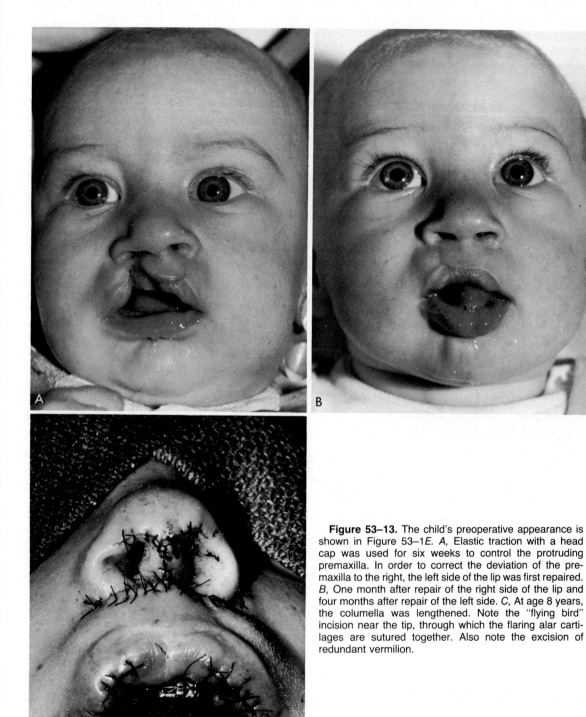

Figure 53–13. The child's preoperative appearance is shown in Figure 53–1E. A, Elastic traction with a head cap was used for six weeks to control the protruding premaxilla. In order to correct the deviation of the premaxilla to the right, the left side of the lip was first repaired. B, One month after repair of the right side of the lip and four months after repair of the left side. C, At age 8 years, the columella was lengthened. Note the "flying bird" incision near the tip, through which the flaring alar cartilages are sutured together. Also note the excision of redundant vermilion.

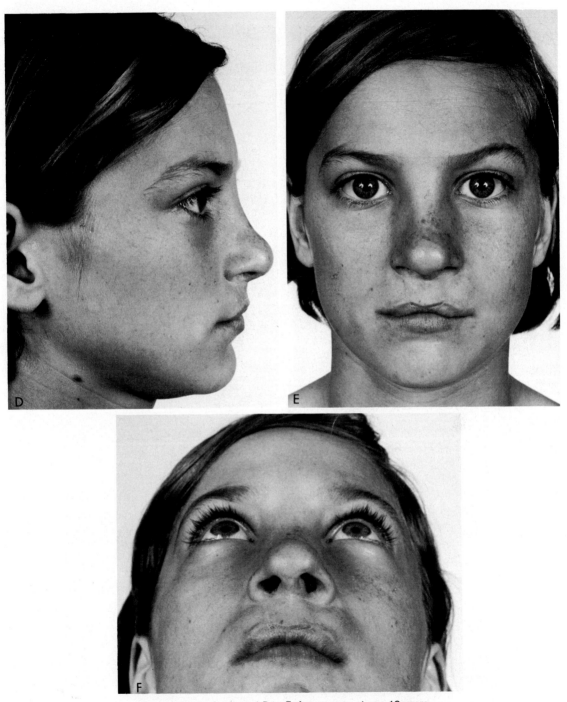

Figure 53–13 *Continued D* to *F,* Appearance at age 12 years.

Illustration continued on following page

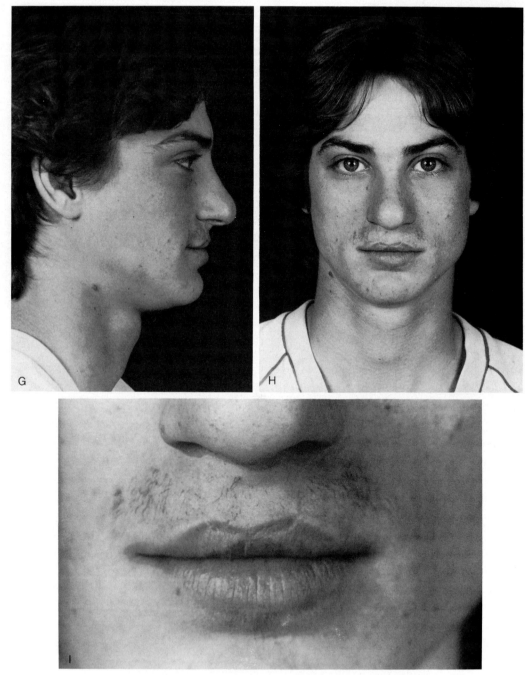

Figure 53–13 *Continued G* to *I,* Appearance at age 21 years.

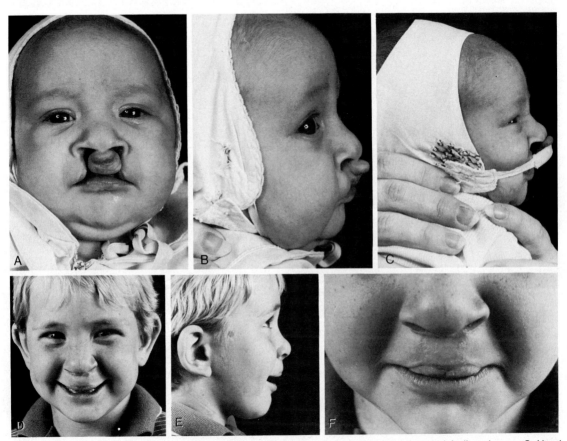

Figure 53–14. *A, B,* Example of a patient with complete bilateral cleft lip repaired using straight line closure, *C,* Head cap with elastic traction on premaxilla worn for two months. *D* to *F,* The patient at 5 years of age, after Veau III lip repair and six months after Cronin columellar lengthening procedure.

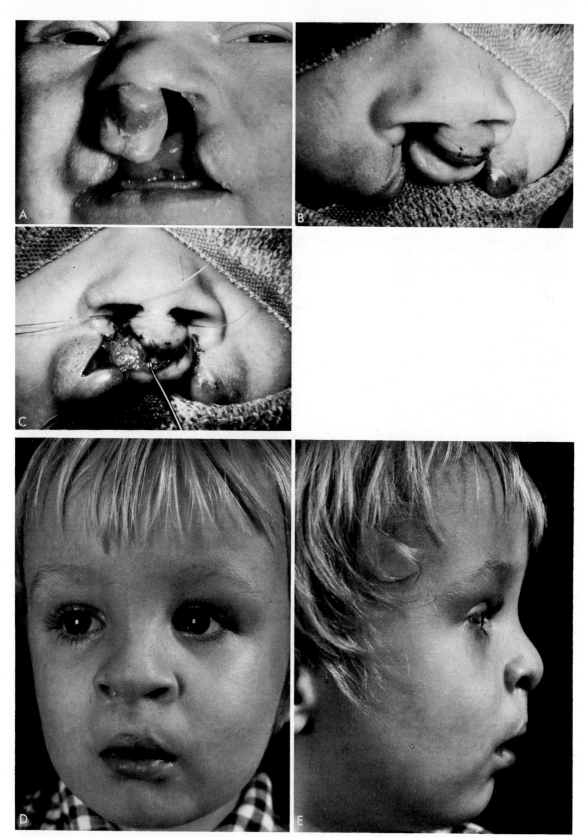

Figure 53–15. *A,* Complete bilateral cleft lip with protruding premaxilla. *B,* Another infant showing lip marking after correction of the protruding premaxilla with elastic traction and a head cap. *C,* The vermilion of the prolabium has been turned down as the Z-flap. The X-flap and lateral lip are ready to be sutured to the prolabium. Deep catgut sutures are being placed to build up the floor of the nose. *D, E,* Appearance at age 3½ years prior to elongation of the columella.

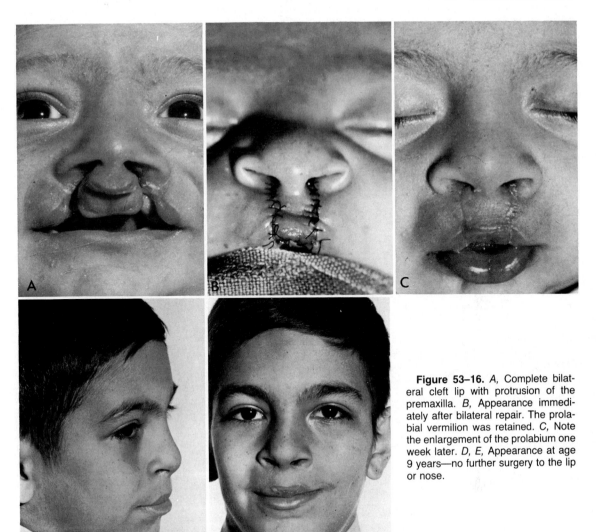

Figure 53–16. *A,* Complete bilateral cleft lip with protrusion of the premaxilla. *B,* Appearance immediately after bilateral repair. The prolabial vermilion was retained. *C,* Note the enlargement of the prolabium one week later. *D, E,* Appearance at age 9 years—no further surgery to the lip or nose.

umella and laterally on the alae (Fig. 53–17). If the flaps diverge, a small triangle of skin is left attached to the lip. The flaps contain sufficient bulk to form the columella and are somewhat thicker laterally, so that the base of the lengthened columella will be pyramidal and therefore more normal in appearance. The medial incision that separates the columella from the septum is continued laterally and posteriorly across the floor of the nose in order to make the flaps progressively wider in the lateral aspect. As the flaps are advanced into the columella, the increased width aids in displacing the base of the columella downward. In this way, a retracted appearance, such as might result with narrow flaps, can be avoided. If the alae are of exces-

sive length, the amount of excess is determined, and a wedge is outlined at the base of the ala (Fig. 53–17C). The wedge includes only one-half of the thickness of the ala. The remaining or inner half is advanced medially to make more skin available to the columella. The incision at the base of the ala is made in the same plane as the surface of the skin of the cheek. Thus, after removal of the half-thickness wedge, the upper cut surface fits down against the lower cut surface.

When the flaps have been freely mobilized, the tip of the nose is lifted forward by a hook. If any tightness remains, the flaps are further undermined laterally. The flaps are sutured together in the midline for a distance sufficient to give the desired increase in length.

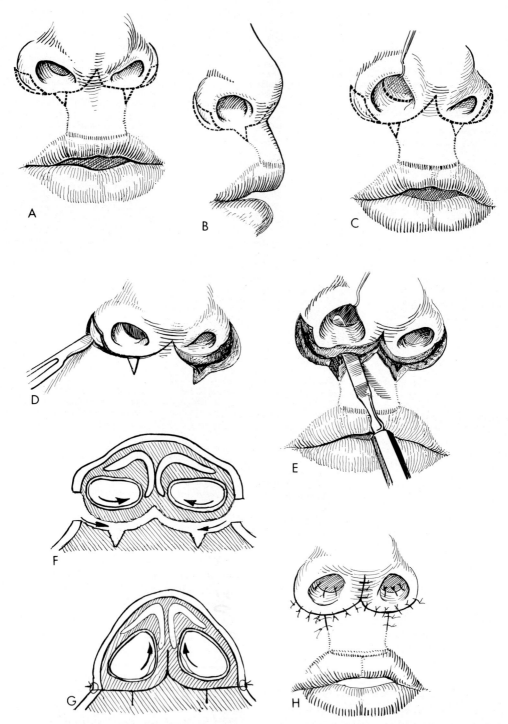

Figure 53–17. Technique of lengthening the short columella associated with bilateral cleft lip (Cronin). *A, B,* External incisions. *C,* The ala is elevated to show the incision separating the columella from the caudad border of the septum and extending across the nasal floor in a posterolateral direction. *D,* The lower incision is made parallel to the surface of the cheek. *E,* The half-thickness wedge of the ala has been removed, and the flap in the floor of the nose has been completely elevated. *F,* Cross section of the nose showing the half-thickness excision of the alae and the manner in which the two cut surfaces of alae fit together when the flaps are advanced into the columella. *G,* Cross section of the lengthened columella. *H,* The completed operation.

The adjacent tissues of the cheek are freed from the maxilla, and a buried, nonabsorbable suture is inserted from side to side in order to draw the tissues medially to conform to the narrowed base of the nose. The columellar-septal incision is sutured with the columella in a more forward position. As the lateral portions of the incisions are closed, the cut edge of skin on the lip side will be visibly in excess because of the medial displacement of the alae. The excess makes possible the revision of old scars of the original cleft lip repair, since a wedge of the desired size can be removed on one side or on both (Fig. 53–17C). In this way, there is no additional scarring of the lip. If the scars do not require revision, the excess length can be used in the closure. The operation can be repeated if necessary.

To avoid subsequent settling of the lengthened columella, it is occasionally advisable to extend the length of the medial crura of the alar cartilages if they are poorly developed.

Ear cartilage is ideal for this purpose. An elliptic piece of cartilage is taken from the posterior surface of the concha of the ear (Fig. 53–18). This is cut into two pieces, which are sutured together, convex surface to convex surface, but the ends are left in a spreading position posteriorly astride the spinous process. The anterior ends are sutured to the medial crura. In rare situations, the alar cartilages are so thin that the tip of the nose is almost devoid of support. In such cases, a longer piece of conchal cartilage is taken, which will reach from the tip of the nose to the maxilla.

In some patients, the lip scars from the original repair may be so inconspicuous that it is undesirable to remove wedges from the lip. Often it is possible to use the excess length on the lip side of the incision. A variation is possible by the use of a Z-plasty, with the ala as one arm and a flap from the floor of the nose as the other (Fig. 53–18C). The ala is shifted medially; the base of the

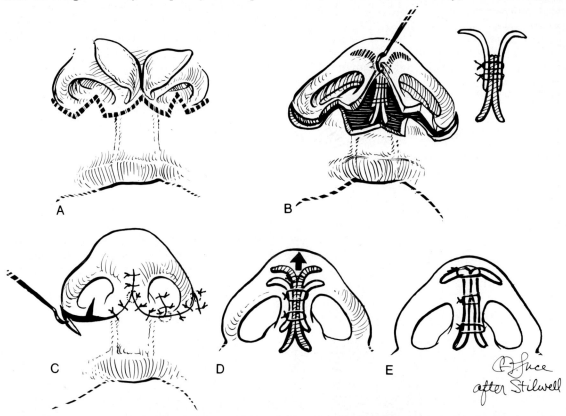

Figure 53–18. Variations of technique in columella lengthening (Cronin). *A,* A Z-plasty, one arm being the ala and the other the floor of the nostril, permits narrowing of the alar base without disturbing the lip, if the scars do not require revision. Sutures may be used to approximate the alar cartilage domes. *B,* Two pieces of ear cartilage sutured back to back to lengthen the medial crura. *C,* Closure of the wound and completion of the Z-plasty. *D,* Use of a longer piece of ear cartilage when the alar cartilages are delicate and more support is required for the tip. *E,* Technique of removal of an elliptic piece of cartilage from the concha of the ear.

nose is narrowed, and the flaring is corrected. The transposed flap from the nasal floor covers the defect that is left laterally and relieves any tendency for lateral spread of the ala. The small triangular flaps have to be sutured into place with great accuracy to avoid conspicuous scars.

Bone Grafting. In complete bilateral clefts the premaxilla is usually unstable. It may be stabilized quite successfully with bone grafts (see Chap. 55) after adequate alignment of the arch by maxillary orthopedics or orthodontics. Studies (Robertson and Jolleys, 1983) have indicated that early bone grafting may inhibit the forward growth of the maxilla, although it is still advocated by some (Rosenstein and associates, 1982).

Late bone grafting can both stabilize the premaxilla and augment the bony base for the support of the nasal ala. The ideal age for bone grafting is approximately 9 to 12 years when the canine roots are approximately one-fourth to one-half formed (El Deeb and associates, 1982). Cancellous bone is packed into the clefts either one side at a time or at one operation. Not only is the ilium a satisfactory source for cancellous bone, but the cranial bone (Wolfe and Berkowitz, 1983) can be used for the same purpose. Pruzansky (1983) argued that, since all these patients will require a fixed bridge, the premaxilla does not need to be stabilized. He did, however, see the advantages of contour augmentation of the alar base.

Method 2: Adaptation of Tennison Unilateral Cleft Lip Repair

This repair results in zigzag scars; however, they are usually not as inconspicuous as in unilateral clefts, especially if the flaps are large. The central part of the vermilion margin protrudes in a more normal manner than is ordinarily achieved with the straight line closure, because of the increased horizontal length of the vermilion, the tissue obtained from the prolabium, and the relative tightness of the lip a few millimeters above the vermilion border. Usually a two-stage procedure is necessary because of the horizontal cuts in the prolabium. Revision, if necessary, may be more difficult because of the zigzag design of the incisions and the resulting scars. For the above reasons, the authors do not prefer this method. Variations of this type of incision have been described by Brauer (1957), Marcks, Trevaskis, and Payne (1957a), Bauer, Trusler, and Tondra (1959), and Berkeley (1961).

The incisions are marked as illustrated in Figures 53–19 and 53–20. At one side of the base of the columella, "a′" is placed, care being taken not to locate it too high, and "b′" is placed at the end of the vermilion ridge, approximately 4 to 6 mm from "a′." The point "c′" is placed about 3 mm from "b′" so that "b′c′" forms a slightly acute angle with the lower vermilion border. It is preferable to make "b′c′" short, since it makes flap "a′b′c′" less conspicuous in the repaired lip and also makes the horizontal length of the lip greater, as points "c′" are thus farther apart. Within the tip of the base of the ala, point "a" is placed with point "d" as high on the lip as the normal thickness extends and where there is still a vermilion ridge. Further up on the vermilion border, point "c" is placed at a distance equal to "b′c′." Point "b" is located so that "a′b′" = "ab," "b′c′" = "bc," and "c′d′" = "cd." Both sides of the lip are marked at this time. Points on the side to be repaired at a later date are marked with India ink,

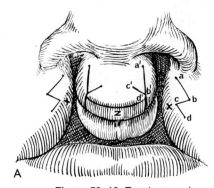 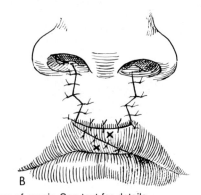

Figure 53–19. Tennison or zigzag type of repair. See text for details.

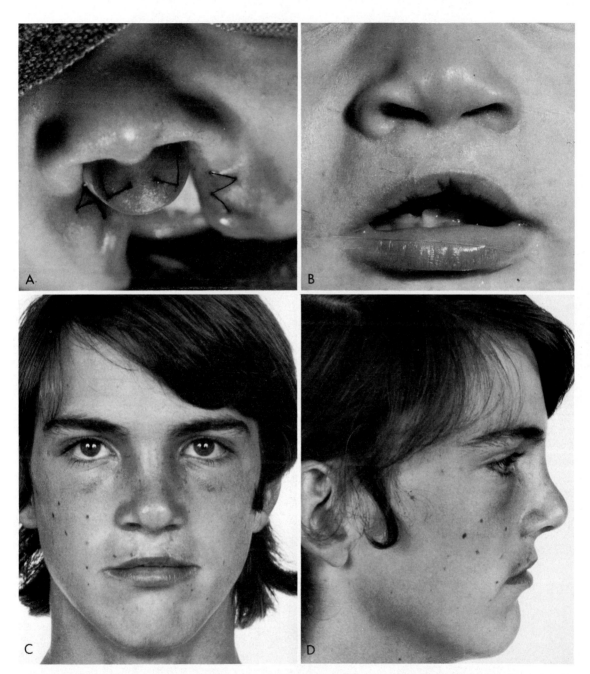

Figure 53–20. Lip repair using the Tennison type of repair. *A,* Both sides of the cleft are marked at the time of repair of the first side, but the points of the second side are marked lightly with India ink to facilitate making the lines of incision at the time of the second stage. *B,* Appearance nine months after two-stage lip repair. *C to G,* Appearance at age 16 years. The lip scars are more noticeable than in the unilateral cleft lip. The columella was elongated by the Cronin method at age 2 years. The dental occlusion and arch have benefited from orthodontic therapy. Rhinoplasty was performed at age 16 years.

Illustration continued on following page

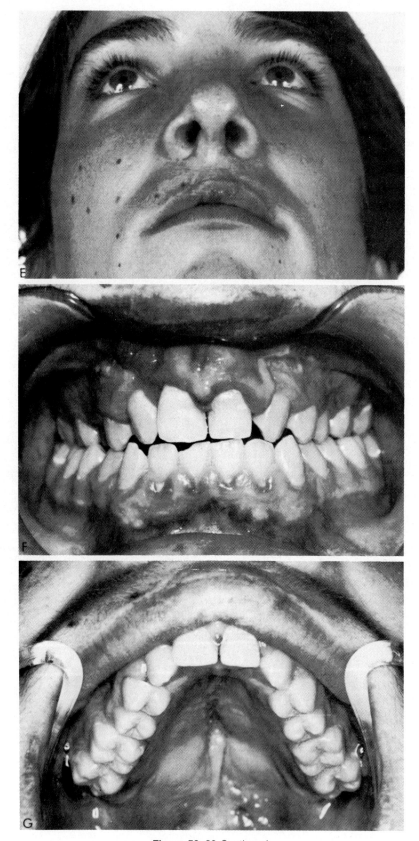

Figure 53–20 *Continued*

0.5 mm out of place, so that they can be excised at the time of repair. This practice simplifies the second stage, since the lines of incision can be drawn between the existing marks. Distortion of the prolabium by the first repair makes accurate marking most difficult if it has not been done previously.

Only one side of the lip is repaired at a time, otherwise the "c'd'" incisions might dangerously impair the circulation to the lower part of the prolabium. The lateral vermilion muscle flap is turned down as flap X, being hinged at "d," and any skin is trimmed away. The incision "a'b'" is made through the prolabial skin and subcutaneous tissue, with the vermilion flap turned laterally to be used as needed to suture to the mucosa of the lateral lip segment. The incision "b'c'" is extended to the underlying premaxilla, across the vermilion border. The vermilion muscle flaps X may be used, as in Figures 53–10E and 53–19B. The floor of the nose is repaired as described in the first method. Figure 53–21 illustrates the application of this method to an incomplete cleft lip. The columella can be lengthened, if necessary, after a few years (see Fig. 53–20).

Method 3

Bauer, Trusler, and Tondra (1959, 1971) strongly opposed any surgery on the protruding premaxilla and preferred to control the protrusion by repairing one side at a time. Skin incisions similar to those of Method 2 (see Fig. 53–19) are used with partial liber-

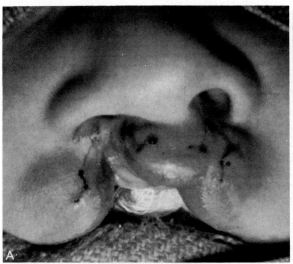
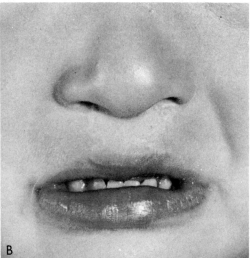
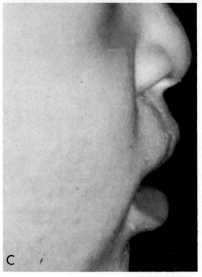

Figure 53–21. An incomplete bilateral cleft repaired by the zigzag method. *A,* Incisions marked. The wider cleft was repaired first. *B, C,* Result two years later.

ation of the prolabium and lining of the latter with lateral mucosal flaps. The technique is illustrated in Figures 53–22 and 53–23.

Technique of First Stage of Lip Repair. The diagram in Figure 53–22A shows the lines of incision. Two points are marked in the floor of the nose on either side of the cleft. Point "a' " is located on the vermilion border of the prolabium at the level of the base of the columella. Point "a" is located inside the vermilion border and slightly above the alar level. Point "b" is chosen on the lateral side where the vermilion border makes a definite change from a horizontal to a more vertical direction as it passes toward the nose. It is also at this point that the diameter of the vermilion portion of the lip begins to decrease in thickness.

Point "c" is located inside the vermilion line at the junction of the lower third and the upper two-thirds of the lip. A line is drawn at right angles to line "bc." Along this line

point "d" is located so that "cd" is slightly less than "bc." The length of "cd" is a negotiable distance and can be adjusted for smooth closure when required. The distance "ad" is transposed to the prolabium for location of point "d'." This is placed just inside the vermilion border. The distance "c'd'," which is equal to "cd," is drawn at a right angle to the line "a'd'." The point "b' " is located on the vermilion border adjacent to "d'." The diagram in Figure 53–22B illustrates the development of flap A after the incisions have been made. Flap A is a mucosal flap containing some of the muscle fibers from the lip. Figure 53–22C shows partial release of the prolabium from the premaxilla and Figure 53–22D illustrates the completed first-stage repair.

The lateral crus of the alar cartilage is rotated medially toward the tip by a series of carefully placed through and through mattress sutures tied over a bolster. This maneu-

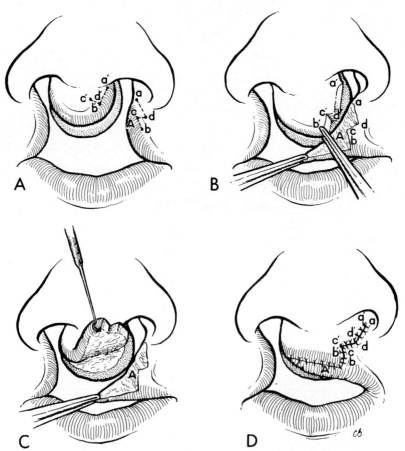

Figure 53–22. Bauer, Trusler, and Tondra method. See text. (From Bauer, T. B., Trusler, H. M., and Tondra, J. M.: Bauer, Trusler, and Tondra's method of cheilorrhaphy in bilateral lip. *In* Grabb, W. C., Rosenstein, S. W., and Bzoch, K. R. (Eds.): Cleft Lip and Palate. Boston, Little, Brown & Company, 1971, p. 311.)

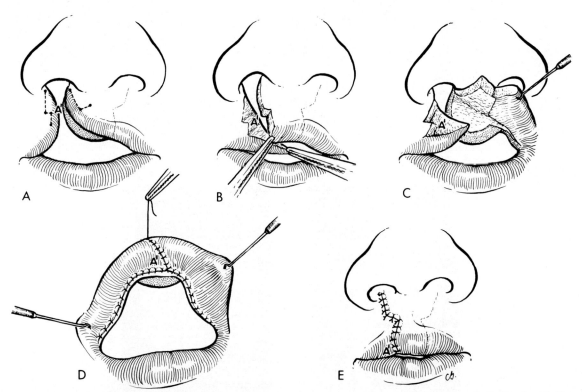

Figure 53–23. Second stage of the Bauer, Trusler, and Tondra method. See text. (From Bauer, T. B., Trusler, H. M., and Tondra, J. M.: Bauer, Trusler, and Tondra's method of cheilorrhaphy in bilateral lip. *In* Grabb, W. C., Rosenstein, S. W., and Bzoch, K. R. (Eds.): Cleft Lip and Palate. Boston, Little, Brown & Company, 1971, p. 311.)

ver increases the length of the columella slightly and rounds out the nostril into a more normal contour.

Technique of Second Stage of Lip Repair. The incisions are designed in the same fashion (Fig. 53–23*A,B*). The mucosal incision is extended around the prolabium and into the superior buccal sulcus on the opposite side (Fig. 53–23*C*). The prolabium is thus completely released from the premaxilla. In designing the skin incision, care should be taken that lines "c'd' " (see Fig. 53–22) do not meet. If this happens, a continuous scar will be established that exerts a pursestring effect on the tissues of the upper portion of the prolabium, producing an unsightly bulge. The mucosal flap A' is brought beneath and behind the lower part of the prolabium and sutured into place. It is attached to the prolabium at a slightly higher level in order to form a sulcus. The vermilion incisions are closed (Fig. 53–23*D*). Figure 53–23*E* illustrates the final appearance.

A patient with cleft lip repaired by this technique is shown in Figure 53–24. As in

Method 2, because of scar placement and the staged nature of the procedure, the authors do not favor this technique.

Method 4A: Millard Repair of Incomplete Bilateral Clefts

Millard (1960b) adapted his rotation-advancement method of unilateral cleft lip repair for use with bilateral cleft lips (Fig. 53–25). In patients with symmetric, incomplete clefts, the columella is usually of adequate length, although the prolabium is characteristically small.

This procedure moves the short prolabium from the normal nose component into the natural philtrum position of the lip and is therefore preferred by the authors. One side of the prolabium is freed from the columella by a curvilinear incision extending almost halfway across the base of the columella (Fig. 53–25*A*). The gap thus produced is filled by the advancement of a large triangular flap from the lateral lip segment. When there is

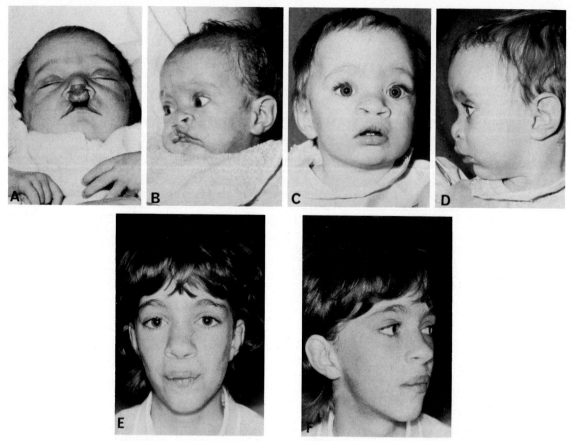

Figure 53–24. Patient repaired by the technique of Bauer, Trusler, and Tondra. *A,* Preoperative view at 2 weeks of age showing severely protruding premaxilla. (From Bauer, T. B., Trusler, H. M., and Tondra, J. M.: Bauer, Trusler, and Tondra's method of cheilorrhaphy in bilateral lip. *In* Grabb, W. C., Rosenstein, S. W., and Bzoch, K. R. (Eds.): Cleft Lip and Palate. Boston, Little, Brown & Company, 1971, p. 311.) *B,* Appearance after repair of the first side at 2 weeks of age. *C, D,* Appearance after repair of the second side; note how the premaxilla has begun to recede under the pressure of the repaired lip. *E, F,* Appearance at 13 years of age. The columella has been elongated by the technique of Cronin.

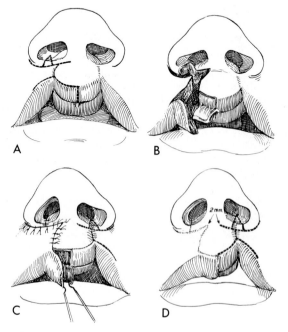

Figure 53–25. Millard rotation-advancement procedure for incomplete bilateral cleft lip. *B,* Incisions have been made. Note that the lateral flap carries the vermilion ridge, or white roll. *C,* The closure of the first side being completed. *D,* Proposed incisions for the second stage.

absent muscle in the prolabium, the lateral flap muscle and mucosa are advanced beneath the prolabium and sutured under it to the midline (Fig. 53–25B). A wedge of skin is removed from the nasal floor as needed. A Cupid's bow is formed, and the deficient prolabium is augmented by advancing a vermilion flap from the lateral portion of the lip. The flap contains the vermilion ridge, muscle, and mucosa unless the white roll is fully present on the prolabium. The prolabial vermilion border is reflected inferiorly from the adjacent half of the prolabium to permit inset of the flap.

When all induration has subsided, the other side is repaired in the same manner. The upper end of the rotation incision should be ended 2 to 3 mm short of the scar on the first side to try to avoid excessive lengthening of the lip in the vertical direction. Figure 53–26 illustrates a patient repaired by this method.

When there is a complete cleft on one side and an incomplete one on the other, the same technique is employed. The complete side is repaired first, since the union on the incomplete side maintains the blood supply of the prolabium. The C-flap described in the Millard (1960b) unilateral lip repair can be used to lengthen the columella on the complete side.

Method 4B: Millard Repair of Complete Bilateral Clefts

Observing that the best scars were obtained with a primary repair in infancy and that entering the lip later to raise forked flaps produced objectionable scarring, Millard (1971a,b) developed a method in which the forked flaps are raised initially and stored for future use while the lip is closed in one stage (Fig. 53–27). A prime requisite of this technique is a fairly large prolabium. If the prolabium is very small, the Veau III or rotation-advancement method should be used, with a resulting enlargement of the prolabium. The

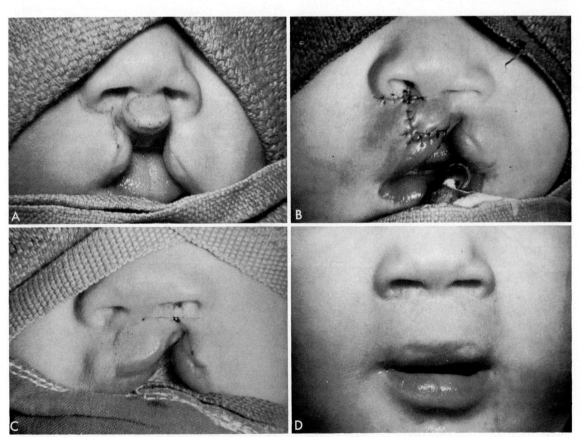

Figure 53–26. Bilateral incomplete cleft lip repair with the rotation-advancement technique. *A,* Markings for rotation-advancement repair of a symmetric, incomplete cleft. *B,* Right side completed. *C,* Markings for the second side three months later. *D,* Appearance one year later.

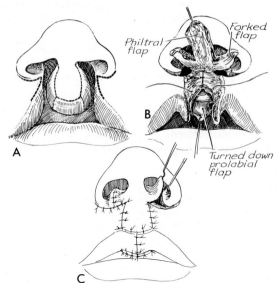

Figure 53–27. Millard two-stage method of lip repair and elongation of the columella. *A,* A shaped philtrum is outlined with a turn-down flap of prolabial vermilion; the lateral prolabial tissues become the forked flaps. Cicumalar marks design the alar base flaps; lateral lip marks show the turn-down of vermilion flaps carrying the white roll of the mucocutaneous junction. *B,* The lateral mucosa and muscle are sutured together behind the prolabium, which has been elevated temporarily. *C,* The lip has been approximated, a slight excess of the vermilion flaps creating a tubercle. The fork flaps are sutured end-on to the alar base flaps, their raw surfaces being approximated to form a mound in the floor of the nose for future columellar lengthening.

lateral vermilion mucosal flaps with the white roll are brought to the midline while the prolabial vermilion is turned downward. Millard also advocated a complete mucosa-muscle to mucosa-muscle suture behind a philtral strip of prolabium. As a second stage, a V-Y advancement of the banked flaps in the floor of the nose is employed to lengthen the columella (Cronin, 1958).

Although a complete muscle to muscle suture beneath the entire prolabium may possibly give improved lip function, the senior author (Cronin) is not at all convinced that the tightness thus produced may not cause retrusion of the face. Past experience, such as that of Adams and Adams (1953), demonstrated the constrictive effect of suturing the lateral lip segments together after advancement of the prolabium to lengthen the columella. Long-term observations will determine whether the present-day complete muscle suture will be any less harmful than in the past. An alternative procedure, favored by the authors, involves less tight muscle to muscle flaps sutured at the vermilion level

without raising the entire prolabium. This has been found to provide satisfactory oral sphincter function (see Figs. 53–10, 53–22).

Although Millard (1971a,b) in his original communication proposed that the columellar lengthening be done one to three months later, he subsequently (1973) advised that in complete clefts this procedure should be delayed until the preschool period (Fig. 53–28). However, he would be willing to proceed within a year for incomplete clefts if lengthening of the columella were necessary. He found that doing the columellar lengthening immediately tended to result in a long vertical dimension to the lip. Repair by this method is illustrated in Figure 53–29.

Method 5: Manchester Method

Manchester (1965, 1970, 1971) advocated a two-stage program for repair of the bilateral lip and palate (Figs. 53–30, 53–31). The first stage consists of a five month presurgical orthopedic program followed by a straight line lip repair preserving most of the prolabium. The prolabial vermilion is elevated and the vermilion ridge is left intact. Caution is taken not to undermine the prolabium itself. The lateral mucosal flaps are brought together beneath the prolabial vermilion to produce a tubercle. The anterior palate is closed at the primary procedure. Pushback palate repair is performed when the infant is 9 months of age.

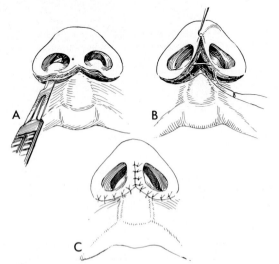

Figure 53–28. Second-stage columellar lengthening. Just before school age, the stored skin flap is advanced in the nostril floor to elongate the columella, in the manner of the Cronin procedure (see Fig. 53–17).

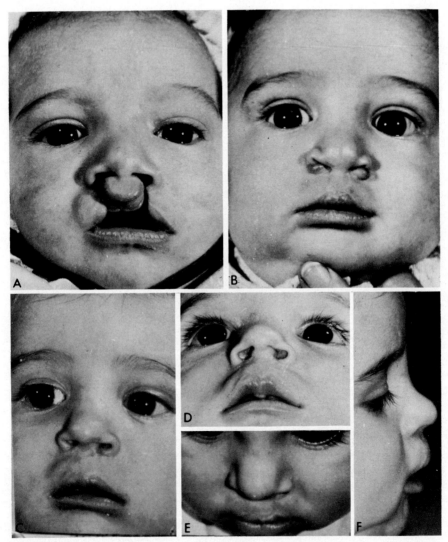

Figure 53–29. Repair by the Millard technique. *A,* Preoperative appearance. *B,* Note the forked flaps "banked" in the floor of the nose after the first stage. *C* to *F,* Three months after the second stage (columellar lengthening). (Note: Millard currently delays the second stage until preschool age.) (From Millard, D. R., Jr.: Closure of bilateral cleft lip and elongation of columella by two operations in infancy. Plast. Reconstr. Surg., *47:*324, 1971. Copyright © 1971, The Williams & Wilkins Company, Baltimore.)

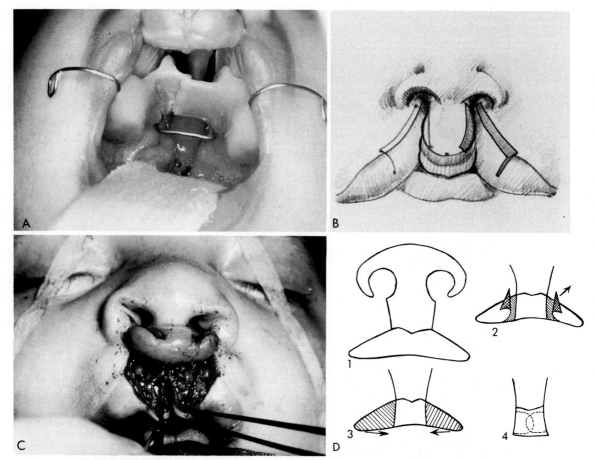

Figure 53–30. Manchester method. *A,* A spring-actuated acrylic plate with sliding leaves to prevent the tongue thrusting on the premaxilla. A head cap with elastic band is used with the plate for five months, at which time surgery is performed. *B,* On one side the points and lines are marked. On the other side, incisions have been made and the mucocutaneous ridges bordering the cleft have been excised. *C,* Mucosal flaps from each lateral lip segment are approximated in the sulcus over the premaxilla. The prolabial vermilion has been trimmed and elevated completely except for a skin attachment in the Cupid's bow area. *D, 1,* The prolabial vermilion spread out. *2, 3,* The lateral wings are deepithelized. *4,* The deepithelized flaps are folded under to produce a tubercle. If not needed, the flaps are simply trimmed. (From Manchester, W. M.: The repair of double cleft lip as part of an integrated program. Plast. Reconstr. Surg., *45*:207, 1970. Copyright © 1970, The Williams & Wilkins Company, Baltimore.)

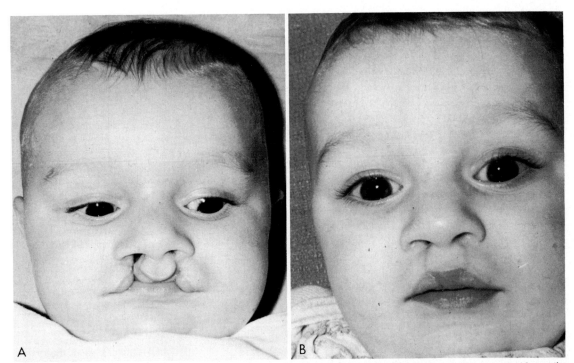

Figure 53–31. Manchester method. *A,* A bilateral cleft, incomplete on the left side. *B,* Appearance at age 10 months. One disadvantage of using the prolabial vermilion in an exposed position is the fact that in some cases there is an appreciable difference in color, compared with that of the lateral segments, as is apparent in this patient. (From Manchester, W. M.: The repair of double cleft lip as part of an integrated program. Plast. Reconstr. Surg., *45*:207, 1970. Copyright © 1970, The Williams & Wilkins Company, Baltimore.)

Method 6: Skoog Method

Skoog (1965) staged the bilateral repairs, the first operation being performed when the infant reaches 3 months of age. He used about one-third of the prolabium for columellar construction. As shown in Figure 53–32, a triangular flap based superiorly at the side of the columella is raised and rotated 90 degrees into a cut across the base of the columella, thereby lengthening the columella by the width of the flap. This flap is similar to one side of the so-called forked flap of Millard (see p. 2684), but it is used in the same manner as in the Marcks, Trevaskis, and Payne (1957b) method for secondary elongation of the columella. Two triangular flaps from the lateral lip element are used to elongate the prolabium, break up a straight scar, and give some degree of protrusion to the lip (Figs. 53–33, 53–34).

Method 7: Wynn Method

In the Wynn procedure (1960), a long, narrow, triangular flap, based superiorly on the lateral lip segment, is inserted into an incision between the columella and the prolabium. The columella is lengthened at the same time that the vertical dimension of the prolabium is increased (Fig. 53–35). The method may have particular merit when the prolabium is unusually small. On the other hand, it tends to make the lip too long in the presence of a large prolabium. The lateral flap sacrifices a minimum of horizontal length in the lower part of the lip where it is needed, unlike many of the older operations (exemplified by Barsky, 1950), which sacrifice horizontal length in the lower part of the lip to gain vertical length (Fig. 53–36). The Wynn operation has the disadvantage of not providing a sufficient augmentation of the thin prolabial vermilion, but the modification of Cronin (Fig. 53–35*D,E*) corrects this deficiency.

The markings in Figure 53–35*C* correspond to the markings placed on the lip. Wynn states that measurement A is made by the compass caliper between point 1, which is made just inside the vermilion mucous membrane at a level with the base of the nasal ala, and point 2, which is placed in the ver-

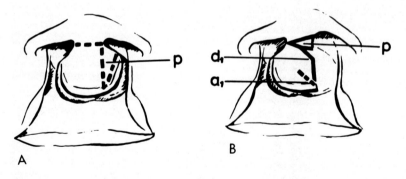

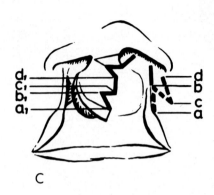

Figure 53–32. Skoog method. *A,* Flap P for elongation of the columella is shown together with the line of incision across the base of the columella. *B,* The P-flap has been transposed through 90 degrees to fill the cut at the base of the columella. An incision is made from a, toward the midline of the prolabium to elongate the border. *C,* Point a is marked on the mucocutaneous ridge where the lip has normal thickness. Point d is placed medial to and sufficiently below the alar base to allow the latter to rise to the correct level when the eversion of the ala is later corrected by rotation of the upper triangular flap ("b–c–d"). The lines "ab" = "bc" = "cd" = "a_1b_1 = b_1c_1 = c_1d_1." (From Skoog, T.: The management of the bilateral cleft of the primary palate. Plast. Reconstr. Surg., *35*:34, 1965. Copyright © 1965, The Williams & Wilkins Company, Baltimore.)

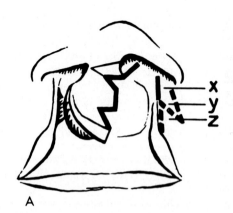

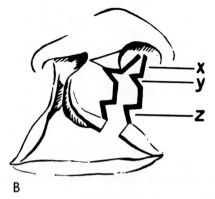

Figure 53–33. *A, B,* Flaps x, y, and z are fitted into the medial side. (From Skoog, T.: The management of the bilateral cleft of the primary palate. Plast. Reconstr. Surg., *35*:34, 1965. Copyright © 1965, The Williams & Wilkins Company, Baltimore.)

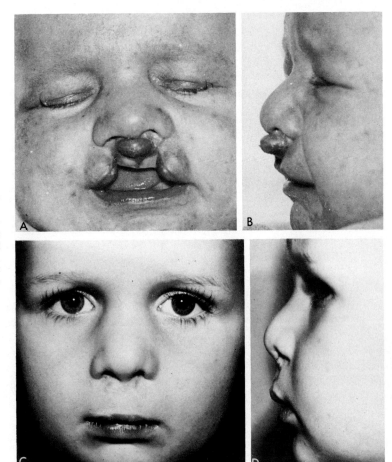

Figure 53–34. Bilateral cleft lip repaired by the Skoog technique. *A, B,* Preoperative appearance. *C, D,* Postoperative views. (From Skoog, T.: The management of the bilateral cleft of the primary palate. Plast. Reconstr. Surg., *35*:34, 1965. Copyright © 1965, The Williams & Wilkins Company, Baltimore.)

milion border where the lip tissue changes to a more horizontal direction with adequate musculature. Measurement B is made by the compass caliper between point 3, which is marked at the upper end of the prolabium just inside the mucocutaneous junction at the level of the base of the columella, and point 4, which is marked at the mucocutaneous junction at the lower end of the prolabium lateral to the midline at about where the Cupid's crest should be. The line from 3 to 4 hugs the vermilion to make a convex curve. The actual length of the line 3 to 4, because of the convexity, will be longer than the straight line measurement taken. This will allow additional lateral flap base usage for lengthening at the columella base. Subtracting the measurement B from A will give the figure that indicates the shortness or deficiency of the central lip tissue. This is called figure C. For example, if A is equivalent to 8 mm and B is equivalent to 5 mm, this would

indicate that there is a 3 mm deficiency in medial or prolabial tissue. In other words, the lateral flap base width will make up the shortness of the medial segment of the lip, as compared with the lateral segment. Then the compass caliper is taken and measured laterally from point 1 to establish point 5, which should be the width of the base of the flap. A line is then drawn from point 5 down to point 2. This gives line D, which completes the lateral flap X outline. Point 6 is made at the junction of the columella with the prolabium just lateral to the midline opposite to the side being operated on. The points 2' and 4' are merely extensions diagonally downward to the mucous membrane.

Subsequently, lengthening of the columella, if necessary, would have to be done according to the technique of Cronin (see Fig. 53–18) or Converse (1957), since the transverse incision across the base of the prolabium precludes use of the forked flap.

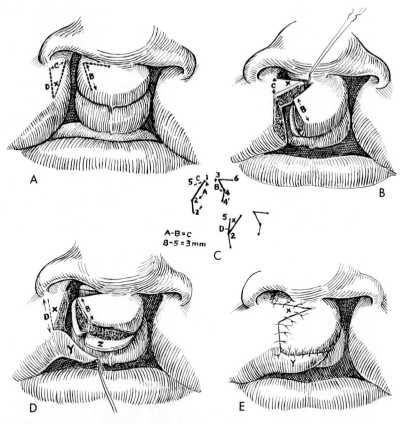

Figure 53–35. Technique of Wynn. *A* to *C,* Markings as recommended by Wynn (see text for details). *D, E,* Modification of Cronin using vermilion-muscle flap Y to augment the thin prolabial vermilion, which Wynn's original operation fails to accomplish.

Method 8: Barsky Technique (1950) (Veau II Operation, 1931)

This method of repair is typical of most of the older procedures and is included mainly for historical coverage (Fig. 53–37). It should never be used, as all too often it results in an unnatural-appearing lip: too long vertically, tight from side to side, and frequently presenting a bulging, unsightly island of prolabial skin in the middle of the lip. There is also a lack of a Cupid's bow effect (Fig. 53–38).

Simon (1970) stated that he abandoned the operation and has had to revise many patients so treated by removal of full-thickness, transverse wedges in an attempt to shorten the lip vertically. A modified Abbé procedure, as described by Peterson, Ellenberg, and Carroll (1966), is often employed to lengthen the vermilion transversely.

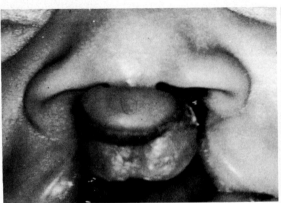

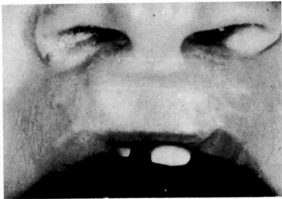

Figure 53–36. Example of a lip repaired by the technique of Wynn. Note that the prolabial vermilion is thinner than the lateral vermilion. For optimal appearance, the columella will require lengthening.

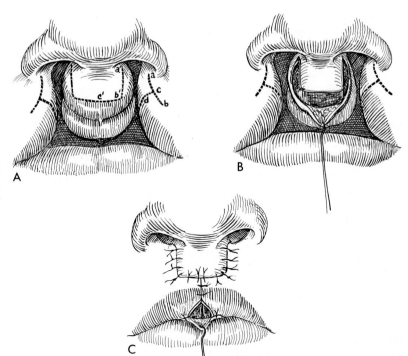

Figure 53–37. Method of Barsky. *A,* Markings are described in the text. *B,* The prolabium incised. *C,* Method of closure after advancement of the lateral flaps.

Method 9: Primary Abbé Flap

The Abbé flap has long been recognized as a secondary treatment for the tight bilateral cleft lip but is not ordinarily considered as a primary procedure. Clarkson (1954) advocated the use of a primary Abbé flap in wide bilateral clefts at 1 month of age. He initially sutured only one side to avoid respiratory obstruction and sutured the other side seven to ten days later; the pedicle was divided at three weeks. Hönig (1964) also recommended the Abbé flap in a young infant. Antia (1973) reported its use in ten patients, most of whom were 1 year of age or older. He advanced the prolabium to elongate the columella and de-

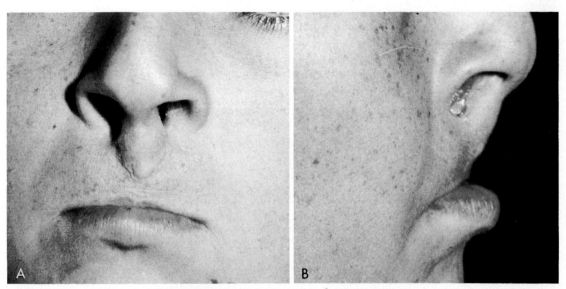

Figure 53–38. Patient repaired by the Barsky method, illustrating the side to side tightness of the lower part of the lip, the excessive vertical length, and the isolated island of prolabial skin in the middle of the lip.

signed an Abbé flap a little over one-half the width of the defect of the upper lip, being careful not to make the flap excessively long. He reported no difficulties with feeding or respiration when the procedure was done in the usual two stages (Fig. 53–39).

Method 10: Method of Mulliken (1985)

Presurgical orthopedic manipulation using an appliance with both sagittal and coronal jackscrews is used for alignment and expansion of the lateral segments and retrusion and rotation of the premaxilla. The first operation is done at 3 to 5 months of age.

Stage I. The prolabial markings are made in a biconcave shape (Fig. 53–40). The Cupid's bow peaks are set no more than 4 to 5 mm apart and the base of the philtral flap is 2 mm at the columellar-labial junction. Fork flaps are delineated. Alar base incisions are marked only on the alar side. The prolabium is elevated as a trefoil (Fig. 53–40). The central vermilion is turned down, and the alar bases are cut free from the lateral lip

segment. The labiogingival sulcus is incised and the lateral lip segments are freed from the maxilla.

The lateral alar cartilages are dissected on the superior and inferior surfaces via intercartilaginous incisions so that the crura can be advanced superiorly.

The muscle bundles are freed from the lateral lip flap extending the subdermal dissection to the melolabial folds. The muscle is freed from the mucosal attachments. The muscle bundles are both cut superiorly to assume a horizontal orientation.

The intercartilaginous incisions are closed first; the lateral crura are advanced superiorly and sutured to overlap the upper lateral cartilages. Next the nostril floor is constructed, the mucosa sutured, and the orbicularis approximated. The alar base flaps are transposed medially and sutured to one another.

The underside of the prolabial flap is incised vertically to unfurl the flap and to give it a more concave surface. The lateral lip vermilion-mucosa flaps are approximated.

The forked flaps are trimmed, rotated 90 degrees, and banked beneath the alar bases.

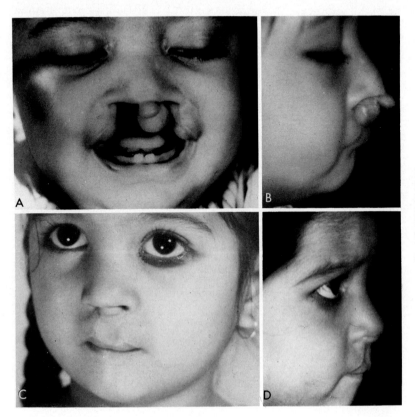

Figure 53–39. Patient repaired by the method of Antia. *A, B,* Preoperative appearance. *C, D,* Appearance after lip repair with a primary Abbé flap. (From Antia, N. H.: Primary Abbé flap in bilateral cleft lip. Br. J. Plast. Surg., *19*:215, 1966, by permission of E. & S. Livingstone.)

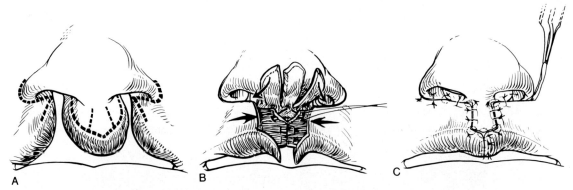

Figure 53–40. Method of Mulliken. Stage 1. *A,* Skin markings. The biconcave prolabial flap should be 2 mm at its base and 4 to 5 mm between the Cupid's bow peaks. *B,* Elevation of the prolabial flaps. The central vermilion-mucosa flap is turned inferiorly to form the anterior sulcus. Approximation of the orbicularis oris layer, placing sutures more laterally in the upper lip. A final suture is inserted into the anterior nasal spine. *C,* Formation of the median tubercle from the lateral vermilion-mucosa flaps; closure after trimming of the lateral lip and forked flaps.

Stage II. At 8 to 9 months of age the alar bases are incised so that they can be transposed medially. The forked flaps are reelevated and the upper incision is extended superiorly through the membranous septum posteriorly to the medial crura and into the intercartilaginous line (Fig. 53–41). A midline nasal tip incision exposes the domes. The medial crura are fully exposed and sutured to one another through the membranous septum incision. The bifid tip is corrected by suturing the domes of the alar cartilages together (Fig. 53–41). The overhanging superior nostril rim is excised and closed.

A custom stent is worn for two to three months. Mulliken (1985) reported that the prolabial measurements at 2 years of age showed a 2.5-fold increase in width at the columella junction and a 2.0-fold increase at the Cupid's bow. A case repaired by this method is illustrated in Figure 53–42.

Method 11: Method of Black (1984, 1985)

Presurgical orthopedics are used to align the segments and premaxilla before lip surgery at 2 to 3 months of age. Short lateral advancement flaps are made; direct apposition is made with a narrow prolabial flap hinged superiorly and retaining the Cupid's bow (Fig. 53–43*A* to *E*), the central vermilion cutaneous margin, and vermilion directly below it. A triangular rotation flap from the prolabial area bilaterally is rotated to each alar base for nasal floor construction. After nasal floor construction, the muscle is realigned and the oral splinter is constructed. The labial sulcus construction (Fig. 53–43*F*) is made with advancement flaps from the lateral prolabium and turnback flaps from the lateral cleft margins. A representative case is illustrated in Figure 53–44.

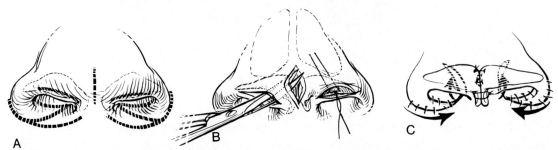

Figure 53–41. Stage 2. *A,* Incisions: nasal tip, nostril rim, alar base, and banked forks. *B,* The inferiorly displaced alar domes are dissected by means of rim and tip incisions. Exposure of the left medial crus via the rim incision. *C,* Apposition of the medial crura and alar domes and transposition of the forked flap into the medial intercartilaginous incision. After medial advancement of the alar bases and suspension of the alar cartilages to the septal–upper lateral cartilage junction.

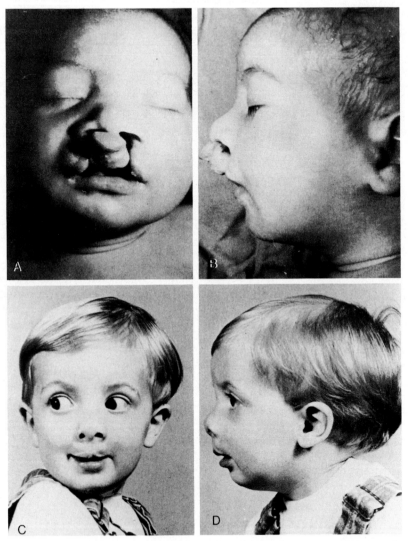

Figure 53–42. *A,* Preoperative photograph of bilateral complete cleft lip after upper arch orthopedics. *B,* Lateral view of the child showing the position of the premaxilla. *C,* The child 3½ years after two-stage lip and nasal correction. *D,* Lateral view to demonstrate the columella.

Figure 53–43. Black technique. *A,* Outline of incisions. *B,* Infranasal view shows a-flaps remaining attached as posterior hinges turn down flaps, and b-flaps remaining attached to the premaxilla. Incisions continue directly posteriorly from the lateral advancement flaps and from the lateral base of the triangular c-flaps along the cleft margins, in preparation for repair of the nasal floors. The prolabium (PL) is elevated with attached vermilion as a superiorly based flap. An acute vermilion-cutaneous angle is relieved by an incision underneath. PM = premaxilla. *C,* The b-flaps are sutured together in the midline of the premaxilla. The a-flaps are ready to be approximated. The muscles have been liberated from their abnormal superior insertion and rotated into better orientation to meet each other and restore orbicularis continuity. *D,* Muscles repaired. At this stage the prolabial flap may be dropped; the c-flaps may be rotated into place; and the skin may be repaired. *E,* Completed skin repair. *F,* The lip and sulcus construction. Note the supporting suture placed at the superior margin of the muscle flaps and labial sulcus lining a-flaps. (From Black, P. W., and Scheflan, M.: Bilateral cleft lip repair: putting it all together. Ann. Plast. Surg., *12:*118, 1984.)

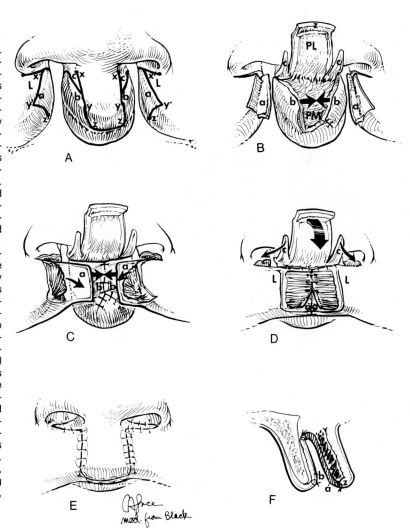

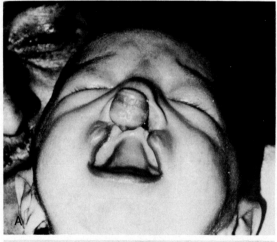

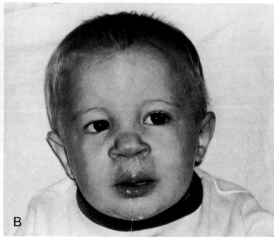

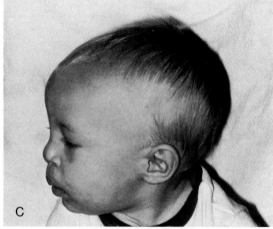

Figure 53–44. Black technique. *A,* Preoperative view. *B, C,* Postoperative appearance.

Method 12: Method of Noordhoff (1986)

Preoperative orthopedics are not routinely used but rubber band traction with tape helps to prevent severe protrusion of the premaxilla. The lip is repaired at 3 months of age.

The Cupid's bow is made 6 to 8 mm in width. The lateral prolabial forked flap varies considerably in width depending on the size of the prolabium. The lateral lip markings are made in a straight line as in Figure 53–45, corresponding to those of the prolabium.

A buccal mucosa flap is made 0.5 to 0.75 cm in width and 1.5 to 2.0 cm in length. The alar cartilage is freed with a minimal amount of dissection by extending the incision from the piriform aperture between the upper and lower lateral cartilage (Fig. 53–45C). The orbicularis mucosa is freed from the alar base to create the orbicular flap (Fig. 53–45D).

The prolabium and forked flaps are freed from the premaxilla.

The prolabial mucosa is thinned of subcutaneous tissue and used to close the lower two-thirds of the premaxilla.

The domes of the lower lateral cartilages are sutured together and to the upper lateral cartilages. The buccal alveolar mucosal flap is sutured into the lower half of the intercartilaginous incision (Fig. 53–45C,D). This maneuver gives more length for nasal floor reconstruction. Additional mucosa can be obtained from the inferior turbinate.

The orbicularis muscle with attached posterior mucosa is approximated with interrupted sutures (Fig. 53–45E). It is important to suture the muscle to the nasal spine so that the lip does not drift inferiorly.

If there is sufficient skin to develop the lateral forked flaps, they are elevated and inserted at the apex of the posterior columella

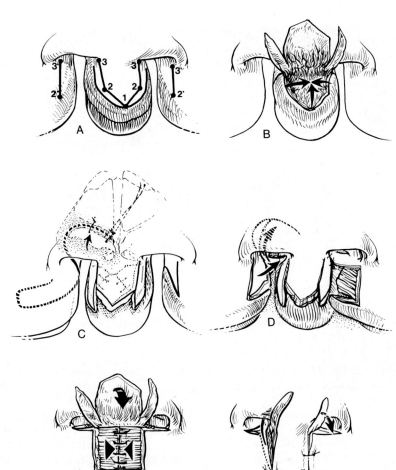

Figure 53–45. The Noordhoff technique. See text for details.

incision behind the prolabial forked flap (Fig. 53–45D).

The orbicularis mucosal flaps are trimmed and sutured, creating the Cupid's bow and tubercle (Fig. 53–45F).

The columella is lengthened at between 1 and 6 years of age by advancing tissue from the nasal floor as described by Cronin (1958). A representative case is illustrated in Figure 53–46.

Complications

Wound Infection. Any contamination of the suture line should be cleaned immediately with cotton applicators and hydrogen peroxide. Repeated, meddlesome cleansing of a clean lip should be avoided. A pustule along the suture line usually indicates an infected buried suture, which should be lifted out as soon as possible with needle-pointed tweezers. Systemic antibiotics are not routinely used.

Wound Disruption or Spreading of Scar. This finding is almost always due to excessive tension, but infection could initiate or complicate the problem. Prevention is best accomplished by reducing the marked disparity between the premaxilla and the maxillary segments before repairing the lip. If the wound does break down, efforts to support it with tapes are in order, but no definitive repair should be attempted until all induration has subsided.

Tilting or Retrusion of Premaxilla. Tilting or retrusion can be avoided by preventing excessive traction by whatever means. The vomer should not be resected in the region of the prevomerine-vomeral suture.

Whistle Deformity. Whistle deformity can be prevented by using lateral muscle ver-

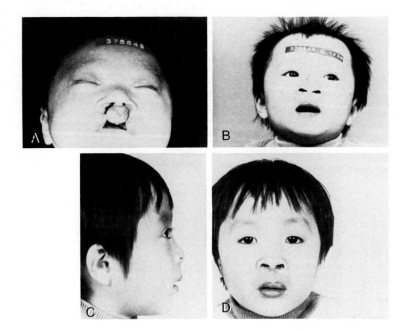

Figure 53–46. The Noordhoff technique. *A,* Preoperative bilateral cleft lip. *B* to *D,* Postoperative views. (From Noordhoff, M. S.: Bilateral cleft lip reconstruction. Plast. Reconstr. Surg., *78*:45, 1986.)

milion flaps to augment the thickness of the prolabium.

Excessively Long Lip. If lateral skin-muscle flaps are not used to increase the length of the lip, the resulting lip will have the proper vertical dimension.

Collapse of Maxillary Segments Behind Premaxilla. Collapsed maxillary segments can be prevented or expanded with an acrylic screw or spring plates.

Summary

Twelve different techniques have been evaluated. Method 1 (Veau III) is probably the simplest and most commonly used. It affords uniformly good results, except in instances of an extremely small prolabium, for which Method 4A (Millard) would be preferable. These are the two methods most frequently used by the authors.

In Method 3, Bauer, Trusler, and Tondra reject surgical setback of the protruding premaxilla and depend on closure of one side of the lip at a time to control protrusion. Their incisions are similar to those of Method 2, but they free up the prolabium and line it with lateral lip mucosa, at the same time building up the prolabial vermilion with a lateral vermilion-muscle flap. Subsequently, they lengthen the columella using the Cronin (1958) method.

Method 4A, the two-stage rotation-advancement of Millard, is the treatment of choice for the incomplete cleft lip with a small prolabium. Method 4B is recommended only for complete clefts with a fairly large prolabium; Millard stores the forked flaps in the nostril floor. When the patient is at preschool age, he advances the flaps to lengthen the columella; thus, the lip is not violated again. Millard also advocates complete muscle to muscle suture, but the senior author is not convinced that this may not have a retrusive effect on maxillary growth.

In Method 5 Manchester advocates a one-stage repair of the lip and anterior palate at 5 months of age after maxillary orthopedics to control the premaxilla and maxillary segments. He uses lateral mucosal flaps to line the prolabial sulcus but feels that muscle to muscle suture would produce a lip that is too tight. Manchester emphasizes construction of a tubercle but retains the prolabial vermilion, which may not always match the color of the lateral vermilion. No special provision is made for lengthening the columella.

In Method 6, Skoog uses a vertical triangular prolabial flap to elongate the columella, and two lateral triangular flaps to interrupt the line of repair and to elongate the lip. The repair is done in two stages.

Method 7 (Wynn's method with Cronin's modification) should be of value when the prolabium is small. If columellar lengthening were required, Cronin's method would be necessary because of the transverse scar across the upper part of the lip, which would preclude the use of a forked flap.

The use of full-thickness lateral skin and muscle flaps (Method 8) is included only to prevent experimentation by the uninformed surgeon. Such repairs generally produce a lip that is excessively long in the vertical dimension and tight from side to side, often with constricted prolabial skin in the center of the lip.

The authors see no need for use of the primary Abbé flap (Method 9) in the infant in view of present-day techniques of repair.

In Method 10, Mulliken advocates a two-stage repair with banked forked flaps and a radical trimming of the prolabium. He makes full muscle closure beneath the prolabium. He performs an intercartilaginous incision and dissects free the lower lateral cartilages. The second stage involves elevation of the banked forked flaps, rerotation of the alar bases, and dissection and suturing of the domes of the lower lateral cartilages.

In Method 11, Black uses straight line closure with elevation of the prolabium and complete muscle closure. He leaves the prolabial vermilion attached to the prolabium. Small forked flaps are used for nasal floor closure. Care is taken to construct the sulcus with turnover flaps from the lateral segments for the labial side and advancement flaps from the prolabium for the premaxillary surface.

In Method 12, Noordhoff uses prolabial and lateral segment forked flaps for nasal floor reconstruction. The straight line repair includes complete muscle closure beneath the prolabium. The prolabial vermilion is constructed from the lateral segments. The premaxilla is partially covered with prolabial vermilion.

CLEFT PALATE REPAIR

If the anterior palate has not been repaired at the time of the lip repair, it should be done before the premaxilla and maxillary segments are forced together by the action of the repaired lip. This is often done within a few weeks or months after the lip repair.

The entire palate should be repaired before the child begins to talk; therefore, the entire palate repair should be done between 12 and 24 months of age.

The authors recommend the pushback procedure as offering the most anatomic repair with a functioning palate of adequate length (see also Chap. 54).

Authors' Technique

The postoperative palatal length can be maintained if the raw surface on the nasal side of the retroposed soft palate is avoided (or lined). The preferred method is that of using the nasal mucosa to cover the raw palatal surface. The rationale is as follows: (1) the mucosa in the floor of the nose is close by and is a normal covering for the purpose; (2) a raw area on soft tissue (nasal surface of the mucoperiosteal flaps) that is subject to contracture during healing is covered, at the expense of a raw area over bone (floor of nose), which cannot contract. Thus, the surgeon can reasonably expect that the retrodisplacement attained at surgery will remain with minimal change (Brauer, 1965).

Technique. To minimize bleeding, the proposed lines of incision of the mucoperiosteum and the margins of the cleft are infiltrated with a solution of lidocaine 1 per cent with 1:100,000 epinephrine. Cocaine 5 per cent pledgets are placed along the nasal floor. The incisions of the mucoperiosteum are made as shown in Figure 53–47. The flaps thus outlined are elevated back to the posterior bony margin. The greater palatine vessels are isolated and teased from the foramen and off the palatal flap for a distance, as well as possible, to prevent tethering of the pushback flap. Unless the palate appears to be exceptionally long, the posteromedial wall of the foramen is removed with an osteotome. After the vessels have been freed by removal of the bony wall of the canal, the elevator is passed laterally and posteriorly, separating the soft tissues from the medial plate of the pterygoid bone. The levator muscles can be identified as they are dissected from the hard palate. The free edge of the soft palate is split open. At this stage, one should estimate the amount of posterior displacement of the soft palate that will be required for normal function. This may range from 1 to 2 cm. A special right-angled knife is inserted through each nostril in turn, and the cutting end is brought into view in the cleft at a point in line with the posterior bony border (Fig. 53–48). The mark on the shaft nearest to the alar margin is noted and the knife is withdrawn a distance

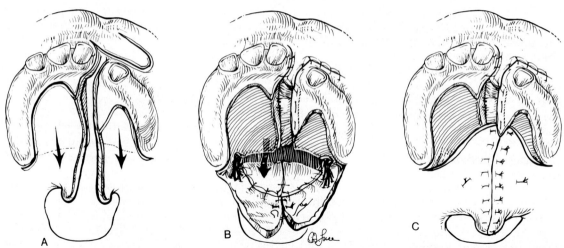

Figure 53–47. *A,* Incisions made when a single cleft is narrow, thus permitting complete repair of the cleft and retropositioning in a single surgical stage. *B,* Elevation of the palatal flaps. Note the lining flaps. *C,* The vomer flap has been advanced beneath the triangular piece of mucoperiosteum that was left for that purpose. The mucosal flaps obtained from the floor of the nose cover the mucoperiosteal flaps. Note how the posterior part of the vomer flap is attached to the edge of the bony palate by a suture through a small drill hole.

equal to the length of the flap desired, approximately 1.5 cm (Fig. 53–48). With the blade firmly pressed against the bony floor of the nose, the knife is moved from side to side several times, producing a transverse cut in the mucosa (Fig. 53–48). Similarly, a Freer septal knife is inserted through each nostril in turn, and drawn back and forth several times on the lateral and medial boundaries of the nasal floor, thus completing the outline of the mucosal flaps with pedicles based on the soft palate.

The levator muscles, aponeurosis, and nasal mucosa are carefully separated from the posterior bony margin, care being taken not to tear the mucosa. A right-angled elevator, or the Robertson tonsil knife, inserted at the posterior bony margin, is used to complete the elevation of each mucosal flap, permitting the flaps to drop into full view in the field of operation. At this stage, if there is any tendency for the palate not to shift back the desired amount, a vertical cut is made behind the posterior bony border of the palate through the thick layer of fascia and mucosa forming the lateral wall of the nasal cavity as it joins the pharynx (Fig. 53–48). The soft palate drops back in a striking manner when this is done.

Beginning anteriorly, the soft palate cleft

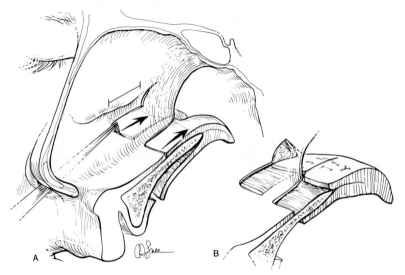

Figure 53–48. Paramedian section of the nose, nasopharynx, and palate. *A,* The starting point of the knife at the posterior border of the palatal bone is shown by the dashed lines. It is withdrawn 1.5 cm (*bracketed line*), as measured by the lines on the shaft, and the transverse cut is made through the mucosa. *B,* The soft palate has been retrodisplaced 1.5 cm and the mucosal flaps cover what would have been a large raw area on the retroposed mucoperiosteal flaps. The residual raw area overlies bone, thus effectively preventing contracture.

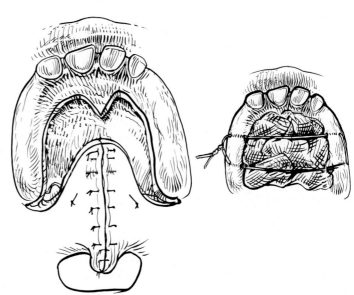

Figure 53–49. Final appearance of the palate in a pushback position. The inset shows the 2 inch iodoform gauze pack used to hold the mucoperiosteal flaps against the bone. The pack is held in place by stainless steel wire of 32 gauge. The wire is threaded on a needle, which is passed through the alveolus as shown. The pack and sutures are removed on the seventh postoperative day.

is sutured, using vertical mattress sutures of 4-0 plain catgut on the nasal side first, and 4-0 vertical mattress sutures of plain catgut or Vicryl on the oral side (see Fig. 53–47). The sutures should include the levator muscle in order to obtain muscle to muscle apposition. After repair of the soft palate, vertical mattress sutures of 4-0 plain catgut or Vicryl are continued on the mucoperiosteal flaps. The vertical mattress sutures produce a ridge or strut of thick mucoperiosteum as the flaps are broadly approximated to each other in the midline. This type of closure is secure and helps to prevent postoperative fistula formation (Fig. 53–49), particularly in midline clefts of the posterior part of the bony and soft palate. The mucoperiosteal flaps are turned downward toward the tongue, exposing the raw nasal surface. The mucosal flaps previously obtained from the floor of the nose are now stretched over the raw surface, the margins being tacked down with interrupted sutures of 4-0 plain catgut.

The soft tissues of the palate are pushed back into the desired position, and if the mucosal flaps have been measured accurately, it will be noted that essentially all of the nasal surface of the posterior bony border

is covered with nasal mucosa. If there is any difficulty in holding the mucoperiosteal flaps in their proper position, a small hole may be drilled through the bone on each side of the cleft, through which anchoring sutures can be inserted.

Brauer (1965) reported an average 12 mm lengthening in the Cronin procedure when evaluating 75 patients with radiopaque tags. Aaronson, Fox, and Cronin (1985) described speech results in 92 patients and found normal resonance in 78 per cent repaired by the Cronin procedure.

Double Reverse Z-Plasty

A procedure (see Chap. 54) involving a double reverse Z-plasty was presented by Furlow (1986) and also reported by Randall and associates (1986). This was designed in an attempt to improve speech results while allowing for adequate maxillary growth after palate repair. The authors think it has the theoretical advantage of less disturbance of maxillary growth. It involves two opposing Z-plasties of the soft palate, one on the oral and one on the nasal surface (see Chap. 54).

A PERSONAL TECHNIQUE

D. Ralph Millard, Jr.

The present treatment regimen of the author for bilateral cleft lip and palate was described in *Cleft Craft III* (Millard, 1980) and has been subsequently modified (Millard, 1986).

Presurgical Orthodontic Therapy

The first step in treatment involves the Latham method of presurgical orthopedics, a technique first described by Georgiade and Latham (1974, 1975). Orthopedic appliances of the pin-retained type are fixed on the maxillas in addition to a restraining chain around the projecting premaxilla (Fig. 53–50). The combination achieves restraint of the premaxilla with expansion and advancement of the maxillas to obtain rapid alignment of the cleft segments in the first month of life (Fig. 53–51). After the segments are in reasonable alignment, the patient is anesthe-

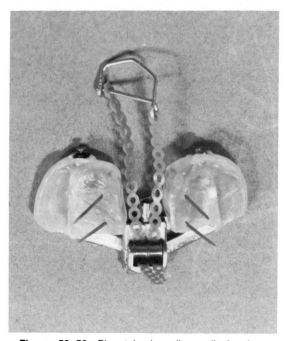

Figure 53–50. Pin-retained appliance (Latham) constructed to be fixed to the maxillas and used to expand and advance these elements. The chain is placed around the premaxilla for restraint.

tized, the appliance is removed, and a bilateral gingivoperiosteoplasty is carried out.

Gingivoperiosteoplasty

The use of the periosteum in the closure reflects the philosophy of Skoog (1967), but the method was specifically designed to reconstruct the alveolar ridge bilaterally (Latham, 1980). After injection of local anesthetic solution along the edges of the alveolar and anterior hard palate cleft, incisions are made in the mucoperiosteum (Fig. 53–52A). The incisions run along the lateral edges of the cleft, curving around the alveolus and extending toward both alar bases. The nasal and oral mucoperiosteum is elevated to present adequate layers for suturing. The incisions are made on each side of the vomer, leaving an intact strip of mucoperiosteum on the undersurface of the septum. The incisions extend around the premaxilla toward the columella. At 90 degrees to the incisions a cut is made on each side of the bulge of the premaxilla, extending down to the point at which the premaxilla and maxilla touch. This maneuver develops two flaps on each side. The flaps are dissected off the bone with the scalpel in a careful manner to avoid injury to the tooth buds. The purpose of this type of careful dissection is to peel the mucoperiosteum out of the cleft in order to expose the bone.

The nasal lining of the lateral edge is elevated from the maxilla in order that it can be advanced medially to aid in closing the nasal floor. The medial nasal flap, dissected from the septal cartilage, is advanced laterally. The two flaps are sutured together on each side to reconstruct the nasal floors (Fig. 53–52B). On both sides the closure extends posteriorly as the lateral and medial nasal flaps are sutured approximately halfway posterior in the hard palate cleft. The oral mucoperiosteal flaps, which have also been liberated from the edges of the cleft, are sutured to each other along the cleft for a two-layer closure. The alveolar closure is achieved anteriorly by interdigitating the alveolar mucoperiosteal flaps as designed (Fig. 53–52B,C). This step produces a tunnel of mucoperiosteum across both clefts with exposed bone at each end and exposed premaxillary bone in the middle.

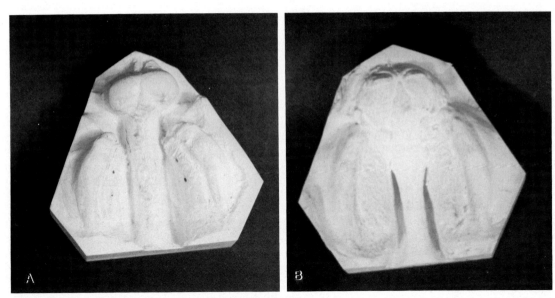

Figure 53–51. Presurgical Orthopedics. *A,* Bilateral cleft with projecting premaxilla and moderately collapsed lateral segments. *B,* Alignment of the three maxillary segments after orthopedic manipulation.

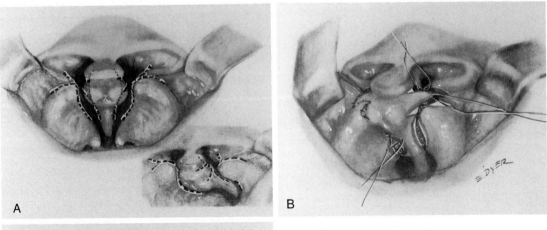

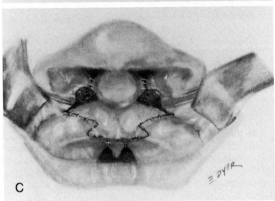

Figure 53–52. Gingivoperiosteoplasty. *A,* Incisions marked along the lateral edges of the anterior hard palate and extended around the alveolus join with the labial mucosa on each side. Corresponding incisions are marked on each side of the vomer extending along the premaxilla toward the base of the columella. An incision at 90 degrees to the horizontal incisions is marked over the bulge of the premaxilla to the point where the premaxilla and lateral maxilla meet. *B,* After dissection of the nasal and oral mucoperiosteal flaps in the area of the anterior hard palate, the two layers are sutured. The two flaps on each side of the alveolus are used for anterior oral closure and are interdigitated across the cleft to reconstruct the alveolar ridge. *C,* Dissection of the lateral mucoperiosteum from the maxilla develops a flap that is advanced medially. Dissection of the mucoperichondrium from the septum produces a flap that is advanced laterally. The two flaps, which are extensions of the anterior hard palate flaps, are sutured to each other to construct the nasal floor.

Lip Adhesion

Extension of the incisions from the alveolar closure are carried into the cleft lip elements to create an adhesion of the lip (Fig. 53–53) (Millard, 1971a). The edges of the prolabium are pared by elevating the mucosa laterally. The inferior vermilion of the prolabium is turned down and may be partially trimmed. The lateral lip edges are pared by turning mucosa and carrying the white roll of the mucocutaneous ridge as flaps. The flaps are transposed over the turndown flap of prolabium vermilion along the inferior border (Fig. 53–54). This maneuver enables closure of the bilateral cleft as a straight line on each side but creates a Cupid's bow along the inferior border. Minimal tension is required in this

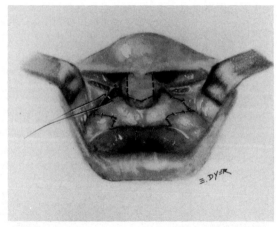

Figure 53–53. After the gingivoperiosteoplasty has been completed, the tunnels are closed off with suturing of the labial mucosa as shown. The incisions for the adhesion extend along the cleft edges of the lip elements.

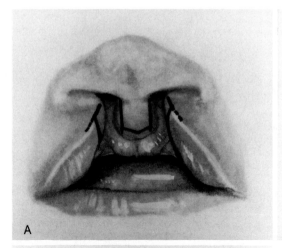

A

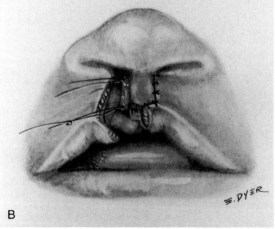

B

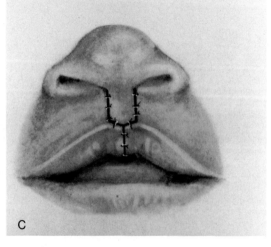

C

Figure 53–54. Lip adhesion. *A,* Design of the incisions when the prolabium is small. The prolabium vermilion is pared from the lateral and inferior edges by turning mucosal flaps posteriorly. The lateral lip elements are incised to match the sides of the prolabium by turning mucosa, which becomes a mucocutaneous flap (*dotted line*). *B,* The mucosa is sutured. The subcutaneous tissue of the prolabium is approximated to the lateral muscle and the skin is closed in a straight line. The lateral mucocutaneous flaps are transposed over the turndown vermilion of the prolabium to create a natural looking Cupid's bow. *C,* The adhesion with small prolabium and short columella should stretch the prolabium sufficiently for a forked flap by two years.

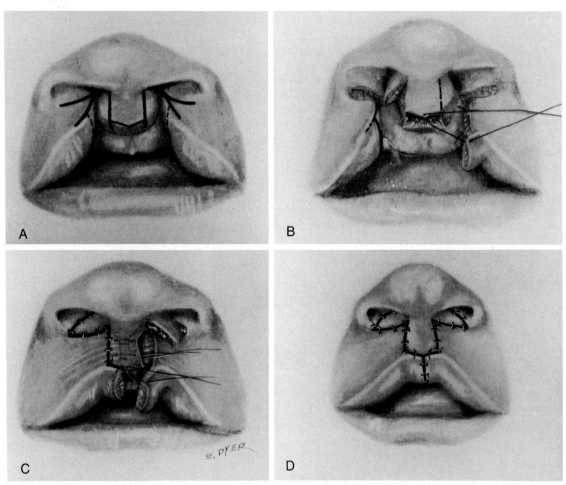

Figure 53–55. *A,* Design of the lip adhesion when the prolabium is wide. Forked flaps are pared off the sides of the prolabium and will be banked in "whisker" position. *B,* All other parings are similar to those of the simple adhesion. *C,* Since the forked flap is banked outside of the actual lip and there will be no need for subsequent lip repair, a definitive lip closure is performed. The lateral muscles are liberated, advanced into the sides of the prolabium, and held with through and through sutures of 4-0 Prolene. The lateral mucocutaneous flaps are transposed along the inferior border of the prolabium. *D,* The forked flaps have been temporarily banked in "whisker" position.

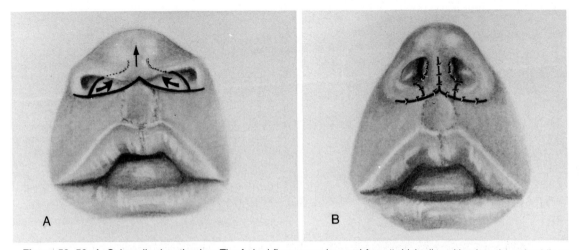

Figure 53–56. *A,* Columellar lengthening. The forked flaps are advanced from "whisker" position into the columella to release the depressed nasal tip. *B,* The soft tissues have been distributed as desired. Revisions should be minor.

type of lip closure as the alveolar segments have already been placed in alignment.

The approach is used when the prolabium is small. Eventually the lateral muscle pull stretches the prolabium until a forked flap is available (Millard, 1977). If the prolabium is wide at the time of lip adhesion, forked flaps can be elevated from the lateral sides and inserted laterally between the alar base and the lip in "whisker" position. The lateral lip segments are advanced and sutured to the reduced prolabium in the definitive bilateral lip closure, the lateral muscles being inserted into the sides of the prolabium (Fig. 53–55).

At approximately 12 to 18 months the remainder of the hard palate cleft and the entire soft palate cleft are closed in three layers.

Columella Lengthening

After the clefts have been closed in the alveolus and hard palate, the bony platform is satisfactory for final correction of the lip and nose. If the forked flaps have been banked primarily, they can be advanced into the columella without disturbing the lip (Fig. 53–56). If not, the prolabium should have spread

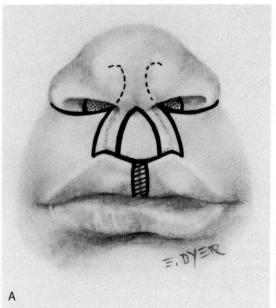

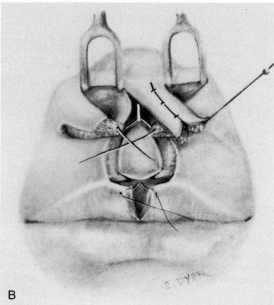

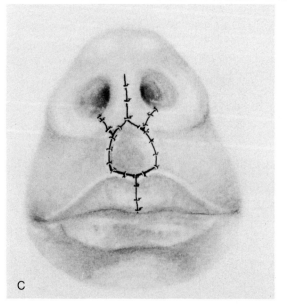

Figure 53–57. *A,* After the prolabium has widened, the forked flap can be taken, including the bilateral lip scars and sufficient prolabium to create a philtrum-shaped centerpiece. *B,* With the aid of a membranous septal incision, the forked flaps can be advanced to release the depressed nasal tip. The alar bases are cinched toward the midline. The lateral lip muscles are liberated and advanced into the sides of the prolabium, and the mucocutaneous flaps are advanced to each other to maintain the Cupid's bow. *C,* A redistribution of soft tissues has been achieved to satisfy nose and lip reconstruction.

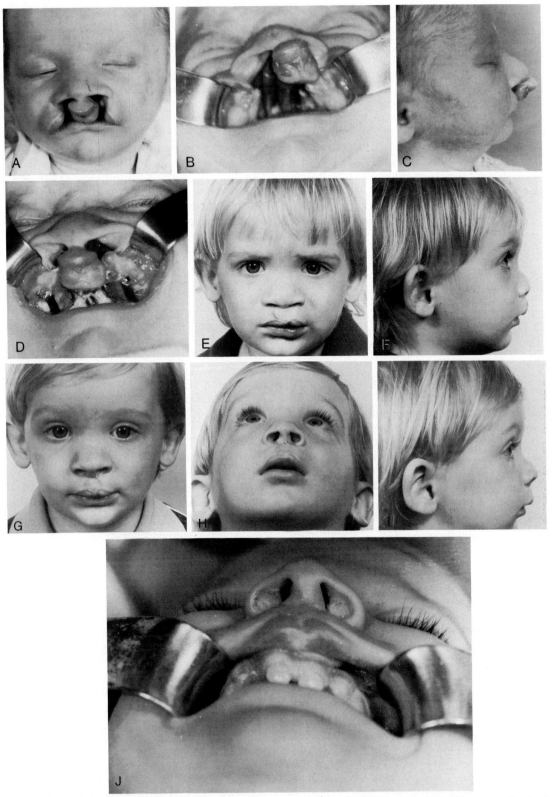

Figure 53–58. *A to C,* Infant with a bilateral cleft of the lip and palate with an asymmetric projecting premaxilla. *D,* The appliance has achieved alignment of the premaxilla with the maxillary segments. *E, F,* After presurgical orthopedics, gingivoperiosteoplasty, and lip adhesion the prolabium has widened but the nose is still flat. *G to I,* Early result after forked flap advancement to release the nasal tip and lengthen the columella. The scars require time to mature but the soft tissues have been redistributed to the benefit of both the lip and the nose. *J,* Note the intact alveolar arch with little evidence of the severe deformity that had been present at birth. Orthodontic therapy will eventually be required for minor dental corrections.

sufficiently to allow a forked flap at approximately 2 years of age. A forked flap is advanced out of the lip in order to release the tethered nasal tip and to lengthen the columella (Millard, 1958, 1986). The lateral lip elements are advanced medially and the muscle is freed and advanced into the sides of the narrowed prolabium. The mucocutaneous ridges and vermilion free border are advanced to create a satisfactory tubercle (Fig. 53–57).

By 2 years of age the alveolus, the hard and soft palate, and the lip have been closed and the columella is lengthened to allow growth to proceed. Little additional surgery is anticipated until adolescent years. A case example with evidence of a small prolabium is illustrated (Fig. 53–58). After presurgical orthopedics the premaxillary and maxillary elements are in alignment (Fig. 53–58*D*). Following the gingivoperiosteoplasty and lip adhesion, the prolabium had stretched sufficiently to supply a forked flap (Fig. 53–58*E,F*). An early result at 2½ years of age demonstrates an elongated columella with release of the nasal tip, lip construction, and an intact alveolar arch (Fig. 53–58*G* to *J*).

PRIMARY REPAIR OF THE CLEFT LIP NOSE

Harold McComb

Sixty years ago, when improved methods of cleft lip repair were being developed, attempts were also made to correct the associated nasal deformity. However, noses that looked good on the operating table usually reverted to the typical cleft lip nasal deformity with additional scarring and stenosis that resulted from this type of early surgery.

This experience with primary repair of the cleft lip nose led to the conclusion that correction of the nasal deformity should be postponed until nasal growth is complete. Consequently, the affected children suffered much embarrassment from their appearance during childhood, and the established deformity is difficult to treat.

Primary repair of the cleft lip nose has been reappraised in recent years. Experience has shown that careful primary surgery does not interfere with subsequent growth of the nose, and several surgeons (Berkeley, 1959, 1971; Skoog, 1969; Wynn, 1972; McComb, 1975a,b, 1985, 1986; Sawhney, 1976; Kernahan, Bauer, and Harris, 1980; Broadbent and Woolf, 1984; Anderl, 1985; Pigott, 1985; Salyer, 1986) have reported the results of primary repair in which the deformity has remained corrected over the long term. It is probable that more harm is done by not repairing the nasal deformity at the time of lip repair.

Documentation is still incomplete and the results of primary nasal repair at the end of the patients' second decade are still to be published. To date the results in only two unselected series of patients have been presented (McComb, 1985, 1986) when the children were 10 years old.

Pathogenesis

At least two factors are involved in the development of cleft lip nasal deformity. First, there is agenesis of tissues in the vicinity of the cleft, arising from deficiencies of mesoderm and ectoderm in the region of the developing primary palate (His, 1901; Stark, 1954; Avery, 1962; Takahashi and Yamazaki, 1963; Brown, 1964; Stenström and Thilander, 1965; Cosman and Crikelair, 1966; Atherton, 1967; Boo-Chai and Tange, 1968; Tulenko, 1968; Brown, 1971; Patten, 1971; Stark and Kaplan, 1973; Noordhoff and Cheng, 1982; Dado and Kernahan, 1986). Second, there is deformity resulting from the mechanical stresses that occur as the cleft widens in utero (Latham, 1969; Kernahan, Dado, and Bauer, 1984; Siegel and associates, 1985).

Shortly after the cleft is established, the premaxillary segment begins to move forward at the sixth week of fetal life, being pulled by the growing nasal septum to which it is attached by the septopremaxillary ligament (Latham, 1969). The alar base region is also retroposed because of lack of forward development of the maxilla (Dado and Kernahan, 1986). Therefore, there is increased widening of the distance between the base of the columella and the alar base. This separation reaches an extreme degree in bilateral clefts, in which the premaxilla is thrust far forward.

When the medial and lateral crura of the alar cartilage are pulled apart, there initially is lowering of the alar arch in a dorsal direction. As this continues, the fascia nasalis connecting the upper border of the alar cartilage to the lower border of the upper lateral cartilage is tightened. The infundibulum between the two cartilages disappears and the alar arch is forced to tilt downward in a caudal direction. The lower edge of the alar cartilage is also displaced dorsally (Huffman and Lierle, 1949a; Stenström and Öberg, 1961).

However, there are other variables. Cleft lip nasal deformity with significant caudal rotation of the alar cartilage is commonly seen in mild clefts where displacement of the cartilage cannot entirely be accounted for by the effects of mechanical tension. The shortening of the columella that occurs in bilateral clefts is due to wide distraction of the alar cartilages. The alar domes are separated and the anterior parts of the medial crura are displaced away from the tip of the nasal septum. The columella is therefore progressively shortened toward its base at the junction of the prolabium.

Anatomy

The extent and nature of the cleft lip nasal deformity have been clarified by nasal dissections in stillborn infants with unilateral and bilateral clefts. The dissections have emphasized the basic role that the alar cartilage plays in the deformity (McComb, 1985, 1986).

THE UNILATERAL CLEFT

In the unilateral cleft there is considerable distortion of the underlying skeletal base. The premaxilla on the side of the cleft is displaced forward and medially toward the noncleft side. It also is often tilted upward into the cleft. When the cleft is complete, the piriform margin is retroposed because of the limited forward growth of the maxilla. The anterior part of the nasal septum is displaced increasingly toward the noncleft side of the nose, from above downward. There is therefore considerable widening of the distance between the anterior nasal spine and the piriform margin in both the coronal and sagittal planes.

The alar cartilage is the centerpoint of the cleft lip nasal deformity. In the normal infant the alar cartilages are situated high in the nasal tip (Fig. 53–59A). On the side of the cleft, in addition to the splayed-out deformity,

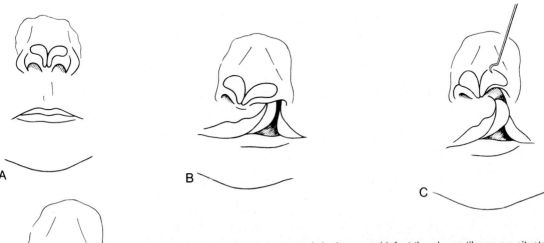

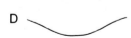

Figure 53–59. Nasal anatomy. *A,* In the normal infant the alar cartilages are situated high in the nasal tip. *B,* In the unilateral cleft the alar cartilage on the cleft side is rotated downward. *C,* Lifting the alar cartilage is an essential step in the correction of the cleft lip nasal deformity. *D,* In the bilateral cleft the alar cartilages are rotated downward. They are pulled apart and displaced out of the nasal tip. The columella is shortened back toward its base.

the alar cartilage is rotated caudally in a downward direction like a bucket handle (Fig. 53–59B). The upper border of the cartilage no longer overlaps the lower border of the upper lateral cartilage, and the infundibulum is opened out.

The alar dome is displaced downward, backward, and laterally. The medial crus moves downward and the lower margin of the lateral crus moves downward and backward.

The caudal rotation of the alar cartilage causes drooping of the nostril rim and lengthening of the half-nose on the side of the cleft. The caudal edge of the lateral crus pushes up an oblique ridge within the vestibule of the nose. In extreme cases, tightness along the caudal margin of the alar cartilage also creates a corresponding oblique groove on the external surface of the nose. The groove may extend to the nostril margin where it produces a concavity in the rim.

Movement of the alar dome and the adjacent portion of the medial crus away from the nasal tip and columella causes shortening of the columella on the side of the cleft. Although the alar cartilage is splayed out across the cleft, its length remains unchanged. The alar base is usually, but not always, lower than on the opposite side.

Caudal rotation of the alar cartilage is of threefold importance in the cleft lip nasal deformity. First, the alar arch must be lifted to shorten the nose on the side of the cleft and to level the nostril rims. Second, elevation of the alar cartilage with the attached nasal lining corrects the oblique fold within the vestibule. Third, when the alar cartilage is lifted at the time of lip repair, the compound curve that produces the typical flare of the cleft lip nostril is avoided (Fig. 53–59C).

THE BILATERAL CLEFT

In the skeletal base of the bilateral cleft lip nose, there is projection of the premaxilla as well as the caudal part of the nasal septum. Both maxillas are shortened in an anteroposterior direction and the margins of the piriform aperture are retroposed in varying degrees. The septum is usually in the midline, but if a Simonart's band is present on one side or if one cleft is incomplete, considerable twisting and deviation of the premaxilla can occur.

Both alar cartilages are rotated caudally and inferiorly, duplicating the deformity that is found in a severe unilateral cleft (Fig. 53–59D). The alar domes are widely separated and the medial crura are stripped away from their positions along the length of the caudal border of the cartilaginous septum. In external appearance, the columella appears to be shortened or nonexistent, and the prolabium often appears to be directly joined to the tip of the nose. The nasal tip is broad and flat without the prominence usually created by the alar domes.

The nostril rims droop, and concave dips may appear in the margins. Oblique ridges are pushed up within the vestibules by the lower borders of the alar cartilages that are in caudal rotation.

The base of the columella lies at the junction of the nasal tissues and the prolabium. This may be the only normal finding in the bilateral cleft deformity. Dissections of the bilateral cleft lip nose suggest that the columella should be reconstructed by reuniting the columellar crura and the alar domes, while simultaneously rebuilding the nasal tip.

The Unilateral Cleft Lip Nose

HISTORICAL ASPECTS

When improved methods of lip repair were being developed 50 to 60 years ago, attempts were also made at correcting the associated nasal deformity. These techniques usually consisted of mobilization of the alar cartilage to allow repositioning and bending of the nostril wall. To achieve this goal, internal incisions were made along the piriform margin, between the upper and lower lateral cartilages, and along the nostril rim. In some cases the nostril was split into layers. External incisions were also used (Blair and Brown, 1930; McIndoe, 1938; Brown and McDowell, 1945, 1950; Steffensen, 1949; Lamont, 1953; Bauer, Trusler, and Glanz, 1953; Brauer, 1953; Gelbke, 1956).

In general the results were unsatisfactory so that Kilner (1958) recommended that nothing should be done to the nose at the time of lip repair. Others (O'Connor, McGregor, and Tolleth, 1963; Marcks and associates, 1964) abandoned the use of external incisions. Millard (1964) simply excised a crescent of tissue from the nostril margin to level the nostril rims at the time of lip repair. Randall (1971) preferred to do nothing to the nose except in cases of severe nasal deformity. He then re-positioned the medial crus of the alar carti-lage through a midcolumellar incision, and also excised any excess skin over the nasal tip.

From time to time it has been suggested that early surgery on infants' noses produces alteration in growth of the nasal cartilage. After their experience with early repair, McIndoe and Rees (1959) stated that "any direct surgical attack upon the alar cartilage at the time of lip repair is likely to increase the deformity by interfering with growth." However, no specific documentation of such interference has been published. On the con-trary, many surgeons (Brown and McDowell, 1945; Lamont, 1953; Berkeley, 1971; Sten-ström, 1975; Ortiz-Monasterio and Olmedo, 1981; Broadbent and Woolf, 1984; Anderl, 1985; Pigott, 1985; McComb, 1985, 1986; Sal-yer, 1986) have observed that there is no alteration in growth of the cartilage after early nasal surgery.

There appear to be three possible reasons for the unsatisfactory results following pri-mary correction of the cleft lip nasal defor-mity. First, little or no attention has been paid to the correction of the caudal rotation of the alar cartilage. This maneuver is essen-tial to elevate the displaced nostril rim, to correct the oblique ridge within the vestibule, and to avoid the flaring nostril margin.

Lifting of the alar cartilage was originally described in secondary cleft lip rhinoplasty (Stenström and Öberg, 1961; Reynolds and Horton, 1965; Stenström, 1966). Skoog (1969) first reported incorporation of an alar lift in primary repair of the cleft lip nose.

It is important that the alar cartilage should be lifted, so that the vault of the vestibule is established and the lining is in position, before the nostril floor is repaired. If the nose is repaired while the alar dome is slumped and retroposed, the transverse cir-cumference of the nasal lining is short. The alar dome is thus displaced in its retroposed position. It follows that the alar cartilage should be lifted at the start of the operation, before the nostril floor is closed. A few lifting sutures inserted at the completion of the lip repair are not sufficient and do not give permanent correction of the alar cartilage, which will be pulled down again by the teth-ered lining.

The second reason for the unsatisfactory results in primary repair of the cleft lip nose is the effect of scarring (Erich, 1953), partic-ularly from incisions made in the nostril lining. Although early surgery does not in-terfere with growth, tissues can nevertheless be displaced and deformed by contraction of scar tissue (Mir y Mir, 1957).

Circumferential scars in the lining of an infant's nose carry a high risk of contraction and stenosis. Some methods of primary repair of the cleft lip nose have been reported (Berkeley, 1959; Wynn, 1972; McComb, 1975a; Kernahan, Bauer, and Harris, 1980; Anderl, 1985) in which no circumferential incisions were made in the nostril lining.

The relatively large changes in the size and shape of the nose that occur during growth spurts, particularly at adolescence, constitute a third reason for unsatisfactory results fol-lowing primary repair.

Unless perfect lifting and repositioning of the alar cartilage have been achieved at the time of primary lip repair, any small discrep-ancy is magnified at subsequent growth spurts. The cleft lip nasal stigma will then reappear in greater or lesser degree.

A number of papers have been published (Berkeley, 1959, 1971; Skoog, 1969; Wynn, 1972; McComb, 1975a,b, 1985, 1986; Sawh-ney, 1976; Kernahan, Bauer, and Harris, 1980; Broadbent and Woolf, 1984; Anderl, 1985; Pigott, 1985; Salyer, 1986) showing that careful, early primary surgery of the unilateral cleft lip nose can correct the defor-mity in the long term without interfering with growth.

SURGICAL PROCEDURE

Presurgical orthopedic procedures (see Chap. 57) are important in preparing a sym-metric bony platform on which primary re-pair of the nose can be based. The maxillary segments are aligned and the displacement of the nasal septum is also reduced. A cleft of the lip and palate is no exception to the rule that displaced tissues should be returned to their normal positions before a defect is re-paired.

Surgical correction essentially consists of a hemirhinoplasty to reposition the displaced alar cartilage (Fig. 53–60). The first step in the repair is to elevate the alar cartilage with its attached vestibular lining to recreate the vault of the vestibule and to obliterate the vestibular ridge. The cartilage should be in its correct position before the nasal floor is

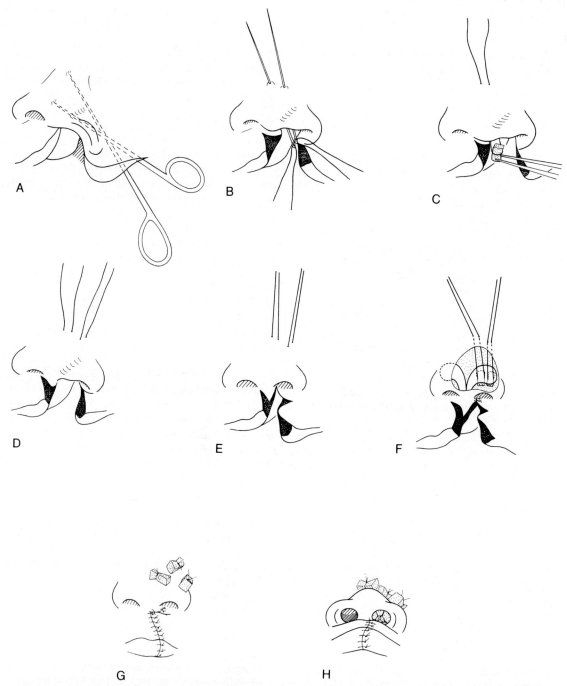

Figure 53–60. Primary repair of the unilateral cleft lip nose consists of a hemirhinoplasty to lift and reposition the displaced alar cartilage. The nose is also shortened on the side of the cleft. *A,* Extensive dissection through the buccal sulcus. *B,* Insertion of elevation suture. *C,* Application of bolster. *D,* The sutures are withdrawn in the region of the nasion. Note the preparation of the lip repair. *E, F,* Traction on the sutures demonstrates the position of the alar cartilage, nostril rim, and vault. *G, H,* Final appearance. Nasal sutures are tied over the bolsters.

closed. This maneuver establishes the circumference and the position of the lining without tethering of the displaced alar cartilage.

The lip and nose are repaired when the child is approximately 3 months old. At an earlier age the technical difficulties are increased and the alar cartilage cannot be controlled as readily.

The following method of primary nasal correction can be combined with any type of lip repair. When the lip incisions are being marked, a flap should be designed that can be turned to augment the nostril sill. In a rotation-advancement repair this is achieved with a C-flap. In other forms of lip repair an alar base flap is used.

No incisions are made in the nostril lining. Dissection is begun with sharp-pointed scissors introduced through the upper buccal sulcus, deep to the base of the nostril (Fig. 53–60A). The alar base is separated from its attachment near the margin of the piriform aperture. Scissor dissection continues over the anterior surface of the alar cartilage and extends to completely undermine the skin of the nose on the cleft side (from the nostril rim below to the nasion above). The undermining continues across the nasal tip over the dome of the opposite alar cartilage and over the lower part of the upper lateral cartilage on the noncleft side. Wide undermining is essential to allow easy lifting of the alar cartilage and the attached nostril lining. It also permits contraction and shortening of the lengthened skin on the cleft side of the nose.

Scissors are also inserted through the upper buccal sulcus in the region of the anterior nasal spine to liberate the medial crus of the alar cartilage in the columella from its attachment to the overlying skin. Dissection continues cephalically over the medial crus through the columella to join the area that has been undermined previously over the nasal tip and along the nostril margin.

Dissection of the lip elements is completed. If the alveolar arch is cleft, a mucosal flap is preserved from the pared margin of the lateral lip element. This is based at the anterior end of the buccal sulcus. It is subsequently turned back to provide the lower layer of a two-layered closure of the alveolar cleft and nostril floor. It is similar to the flap described by Muir (1966). The nostril lining is freed from the lower part of the cartilaginous septum and from the lateral wall of the nose in the region of the piriform aperture. When the dissection is complete, the alar cartilage and the nasal lining can be lifted easily. The alar cartilage can be rotated upward and forward, raising the nostril rim and reestablishing the vault of the vestibule with obliteration of the vestibular fold. The infundibulum is reestablished, and the upper edge of the alar cartilage lies above and superficial to the caudal border of the upper lateral cartilage.

The first sutures that are placed in the repair are long, elevating mattress sutures of 5-0 silk that lift the alar cartilage and establish the correct position of the nostril lining before the nasal floor is closed.

The correct site of the dome is selected by the points of forceps lifting from inside the nasal vestibule. This is also the site of insertion of the first lifting suture. The suture is introduced on straight needles that pass through the mucosa and the alar cartilage in the vicinity of the alar dome (Fig. 53–60B). They are passed subcutaneously upward and slightly medially to emerge in the region of the nasion, toward the noncleft side. A second elevating suture is inserted through the lateral crus of the alar cartilage; it also emerges in the region of the nasion (Fig. 53–60D). Within the nostril the sutures are looped around small bolsters that lift and round out the dome and the lateral wall of the vestibule (Fig. 53–60C). Gentle traction on the sutures lifts the alar cartilage to its correct position (Fig. 53–60E). The nose immediately loses the typical cleft lip appearance. The nostril rim is level with the contralateral side and the vestibular vault is established (Fig. 53–60F).

When the alar cartilage and the nostril lining are in position, the nostril floor is repaired. The nostril sill is augmented with local flaps and muscle union is established beneath the floor of the nose (between the alar base and the columella).

At the completion of the lip repair, the nasal tip and nostril rims are probably not positioned perfectly. It is almost always necessary to remove, replace, and realign the direction of the lifting sutures. Finally, the long sutures are tied over bolsters in the region of the nasion. One or two lateral mattress sutures are inserted through the wall of the nose; one of these is placed in the lateral sulcus at the base of the nostril. The sutures are also tied over bolsters to obliterate the potential dead space (Fig. 53–60G,H).

No attempt is made to realign the cartilaginous septum completely at the time of primary nasal repair. Displacement of the septum is largely corrected by presurgical orthopedic procedures. The incidence of significant septal displacement has been considerably reduced with this type of treatment. Although dissection of the septal cartilage in infancy does not interfere with subsequent growth, fibrosis and scarring around the cartilage can make future secondary correction more difficult.

The nose and lip sutures are removed on the fifth postoperative day. By this time the covering skin has shortened and healed, and the alar cartilage is fixed in its correct position. It is important that the nostril rims should be placed exactly level. Slight overcorrection is also possible. On the other hand, any mild residual droop of the nostril rim is accentuated by later nasal growth.

There has been no interference with growth following this procedure and the position of the nasal tip and the alar cartilages has been maintained (Fig. 53–61).

The Bilateral Cleft Lip Nose

HISTORICAL ASPECTS

The technical difficulties associated with closure of wide, distorted bilateral clefts of the lip have discouraged simultaneous correction of the associated nasal deformity. The usual plan of treatment has been to repair the lip, and to delay release of the nasal tip by reconstruction of the columella until 3 years of age.

Two-staged methods of primary closure (Skoog, 1965; Trauner and Trauner, 1967) have been advocated in which closure of each lip cleft is accompanied by partial lengthening of the columella.

Millard (1967) described a primary forked flap for reconstruction of the columella at the time of lip repair. The central prolabial element that remained was left attached to the premaxilla, which provided its blood supply. It therefore was not possible to join mucomuscular flaps behind the prolabium. A method of "banking" forked flaps was subsequently described (Duffy, 1971; Millard, 1971a). Primary columella reconstruction at the time of lip adhesion was also reported (Randall and Brown, 1973; Randall and Lynch, 1974; Tolhurst, 1985).

Noordhoff (1986) described elevation of the alar cartilages at the time of lip repair in bilateral clefts with subsequent lengthening of the columella. Stenström (1966) reported secondary repair of bilateral cleft lip nasal deformity by means of lifting the alar cartilages after initial lengthening of the columella.

Although it is embryologically part of the lip (Stark and Ehrmann, 1958), the prolabium is generally used as a convenient compromise for reconstruction of the columella. However, nasal dissections in bilateral clefts demonstrate wide separation of the alar cartilages in the region of the nasal tip. This finding suggests that the columella should be lengthened by rearrangement of tissues of the nasal tip—by uniting the medial crura, joining the splayed intercrural angles of the alar cartilages, and excising the excess covering skin. Secondary columella lengthening using tissues from the nasal tip in this way was described by Morel-Fatio and Lalardrie (1966). Broadbent and Woolf (1984) advocated medial advancement of the alar cartilages, combined with excision of the excess skin of the nasal tip, in primary repair of a bilateral cleft lip nasal deformity.

SURGICAL PROCEDURE

Alignment of the bony platform by presurgical orthopedic procedures is the first step in primary correction of the bilateral cleft lip nose (see Chap. 57). The premaxilla is also centralized and any twisting is corrected. When the skeletal displacement is reduced, it is possible to repair both clefts simultaneously. Prolabial tissues that have already been narrowed by migration of a forked flap can be used to reconstruct the philtrum.

Surgical treatment is in two stages. First, the columella is lengthened to release the nasal tip and permit elevation of the alar cartilages (McComb, 1975b). Six weeks later, simultaneous repair of the lip and nose is performed.

In a healthy infant, primary reconstruction of the columella is performed at 6 weeks of age using a forked flap of skin, occasionally with edges of mucosa taken from the sides of the prolabium (Fig. 53–62). The forks are quadrilateral in shape, with pointed tips (Fig. 53–62A). If triangular forked flaps are used, the prolabium becomes globular in shape.

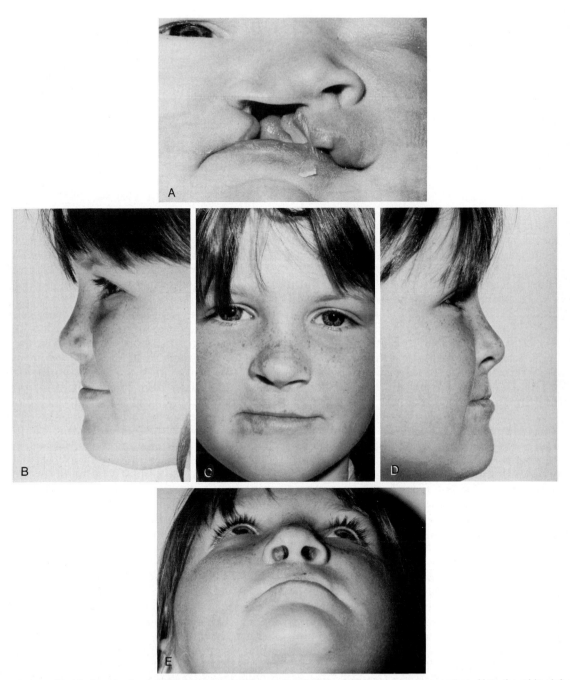

Figure 53–61. Repair of a severe unilateral cleft lip nasal deformity. *A,* Preoperative appearance. Note the wide cleft of the lip with a severe nasal deformity. *B* to *E,* Appearance at 7 years of age. The patient had undergone correction by the technique illustrated in Figure 53–60.

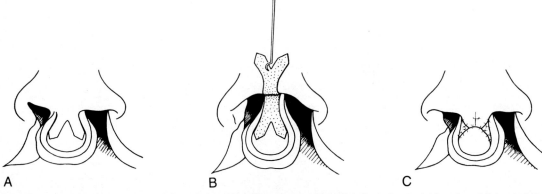

Figure 53–62. Primary reconstruction of the columella using a forked flap from the prolabium in a bilateral cleft. *A,* Outline of forked flaps. *B,* Elevation of the flaps. *C,* Lengthening of the columella and closure.

When the lip is repaired, the columella base is narrow and the nostril sills are tight.

The flaps of the columella are lifted completely out of the prolabium (Fig. 53–62*B*). Their apices are carefully fixed together with a deep suture, which also passes through the tissues in the region of the anterior nasal spine. This maneuver is designed to avoid any later tendency for the columella base to drift into the prolabium. Difficulties have been reported with downward displacement of the columellar base in this way (Randall and Brown, 1973; Randall and Lynch, 1974).

In a 1986 study, 220 Caucasian children were examined to determine the length to which the columella should be constructed (McComb, 1986). Each columella was measured from its base to the level of the intercrural angles of the nostrils. The measurements show that in an infant's nose the columella is 5.0 to 5.5 mm in length, with no difference between males and females. Furthermore, growth of the columella does not start until the child is approximately 18 months old. The lag in nasal development is presumably due to the requirement of maintaining a nasal airway during the period of breast feeding. Accordingly, in the author's patients, the columella is lengthened to 5 mm (Fig. 53–62*C*).

During the phase of columella reconstruction and healing, the elastic strapping across the prolabium that is used in presurgical orthopedic procedures is discontinued. An extension is added to the sucking plate to maintain the premaxilla in its correct position. As soon as the prolabium is healed, pressure from the elastic strapping is resumed.

Simultaneous repair of the lip and nasal deformity is performed six weeks after lengthening of the columella, usually when the child is 3 months old. The lip is repaired with a modified Manchester technique (Fig. 53–63) (Manchester, 1970).

At the initial lip marking, a central prolabial segment, approximately the width of the philtrum, is outlined (Fig. 53–63*A*). Alar base flaps are also marked to augment the nostril sills. The prolabial tissue is carefully dissected and lifted from the premaxilla, proceeding just far enough superiorly to allow the mucomuscular flaps containing the orbicularis muscles to be joined together behind the prolabial philtrum in the midline (Fig. 53–63*C*). The nasal repair essentially consists of correction of the caudal rotation of the alar cartilages, as performed in repair of the unilateral cleft lip nose. The nostril rims are lifted and the vaults of the vestibules are established (without shortage of the lining) before the nostril floors are repaired.

The nasal skin is completely elevated over the sides of the nose and nasal tip, from the nostril rims below to the nasion above. No dissection is performed in the region of the reconstructed columella or the membranous septum, because the remaining central prolabial tissue of the lip now receives its blood supply solely from this area.

The alar cartilages are elevated by one or two long mattress sutures of 5-0 silk on each side (Fig. 53–63*B*). These are passed through the alar cartilages as previously described. They run subcutaneously upward and slightly medially over the nasal skeleton to emerge in the region of the nasion. Gentle

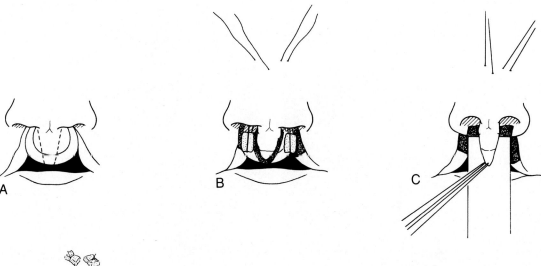

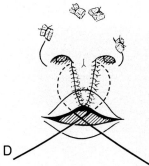

Figure 53–63. Simultaneous repair of the bilateral cleft lip and nasal deformity. *A*, Outline of the prolabial segment. *B*, Elevation of the alar cartilages by mattress sutures on both sides. *C*, Traction on the sutures raises the alar cartilages and nostril rims and establishes the vault of the vestibules. *D*, Position of the elevation sutures, which are tied in bolus fashion. The lip clefts have been repaired. Note the encircling wire that unites the orbicularis musculature behind the prolabium.

traction on the sutures raises the alar cartilage and the nostril rims and also establishes the vaults of the vestibules (Fig. 53–63C). The intercrural angle of each alar cartilage is moved upward, forward, and slightly medially. The cephalic borders of the alar cartilages should lie above and superficial to the caudal borders of the upper lateral cartilages.

The lifting sutures are the first sutures that are placed in the repair. They establish the position of the nasal lining. The alar cartilages are in their correct position before the nostril floors are closed without transverse shortage of lining. The lip repair is completed using alar base flaps to augment the nostril sills.

As in unilateral clefts, it is almost always necessary to remove, replace, and realign the elevating sutures at the completion of the operation. Finally, the ends of the sutures are tied over small bolsters on the skin to maintain the level of the nostril rims and the position of the alar cartilages. One or more lateral mattress sutures are inserted on each side to obliterate the dead space between the dissected layers. One suture is always placed in the lateral groove at the base of each nostril (Fig. 53–63D). The lip musculature is joined behind the prolabium by an encircling wire suture, which is inserted before the repair of the nasal floor is completed. It is also passed through the deep tissues in the region of the anterior nasal spine to prevent downward drag on the columella base.

The mattress sutures are removed on the fifth postoperative day, when the final lip sutures come out. The wire suture is removed on the seventh postoperative day.

Although scars are present across the base of the prolabium, there has been no loss of tissue in the central segment. At completion of the repair, tension across the lip may cause the philtral segment to become pale or dusky blue, depending on the vascular supply. There has been no interference with growth following this procedure (Fig. 53–64). In some patients the nasal tip has remained broad.

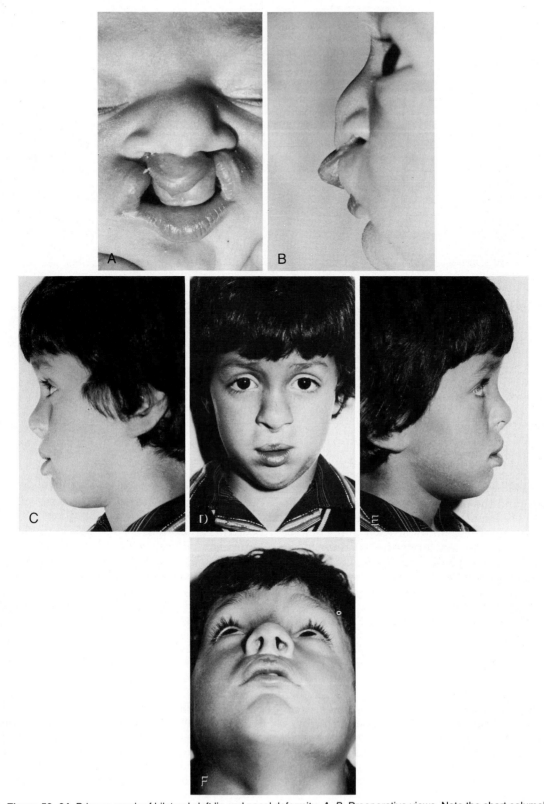

Figure 53–64. Primary repair of bilateral cleft lip and nasal deformity. *A, B,* Preoperative views. Note the short columella and displaced alar cartilages. *C* to *F,* At 7 years of age.

REFERENCES

Aaronson, S. M., Fox, D. R., and Cronin, T. D.: The Cronin push-back palate repair with nasal mucosal flaps: a speech evaluation. Plast. Reconstr. Surg., 75:805, 1985.

Adams, W. M., and Adams, L. H.: The misuse of the prolabium in the repair of bilateral cleft lip. Plast. Reconstr. Surg., 12:225, 1953.

Anderl, H.: Simultaneous repair of lip and nose in the unilateral cleft (a long term report). In Jackson, I. T., and Sommerlad, B. C. (Eds.): Recent Advances in Plastic Surgery. Edinburgh, Churchill Livingstone, 1985, p. 1.

Antia, N. H.: Primary Abbé flap in bilateral cleft lip. Br. J. Plast. Surg., 12:215, 1973.

Atherton, J. D.: A descriptive anatomy of the face in human fetuses with unilateral cleft lip and palate. Cleft Palate J., 4:104, 1967.

Avery, J. K.: The nasal capsule in cleft palate. Anat. Anz. (Suppl.), 109:722, 1962.

Axhausen, G.: Technik und Ergebnisse der Lippenplastik. Stuttgart, Georg Thieme Verlag, 1932.

Barsky, A. J.: Principles and Practice of Plastic Surgery. Baltimore, Williams & Wilkins Company, 1950.

Bauer, T. B., Trusler, H. M., and Glanz, S.: Repair of unilateral cleft lip—advantages of Le Mesurier technique use of mucous membrane flaps in maxillary clefts. Plast. Reconstr. Surg., 11:56, 1953.

Bauer, T. B., Trusler, H. M., and Tondra, J. M.: Changing concepts in the management of bilateral cleft lip deformities. Plast. Reconstr. Surg., 24:321, 1959.

Bauer, T. B., Trusler, H. M., and Tondra, J. M.: Bauer, Trusler, and Tondra's method of cheilorrhaphy in bilateral lip. In Grabb, W. C., Rosenstein, S. W., and Bzoch, K. R. (Eds.): Cleft Lip and Palate: Surgical, Dental, and Speech Aspects. Boston, Little, Brown & Company, 1971.

Baume, L. T.: The postnatal growth activity of the nasal cartilage septum. Helv. Odontol. Acta, 5:9, 1961.

Baxter, H.: A new method of elongating short palate. Canad. Med. Assoc. J., 46:322, 1942.

Berkeley, W. T.: The cleft lip nose. Plast. Reconstr. Surg., 23:567, 1959.

Berkeley, W. T.: The concepts of unilateral repair applied to bilateral clefts of the lip and nose. Plast. Reconstr. Surg., 27:505, 1961.

Berkeley, W. T.: Correction of the unilateral cleft lip nasal deformity. In Grabb, W. C., Rosenstein, S. W., and Bzoch, K. R. (Eds.): Cleft Lip and Palate: Surgical, Dental, and Speech Aspects. Boston, Little, Brown & Company, 1971, p. 227.

Black, P. W.: Bilateral cleft lip. Symposium on cleft lip and cleft palate. Clin. Plast. Surg., 12:627, 1985.

Black, P. W., and Scheflan, M.: Bilateral cleft lip repair: "putting it all together." Ann. Plast. Surg., 12:118, 1984.

Blair, V. P., and Brown, J. B.: Mirault operation for single harelip. Surg. Gynec. Obstet., 51:81, 1930.

Boo-Chai, K., and Tange, I.: The isolated cleft lip nose. Plast. Reconstr. Surg., 41:28, 1968.

Brauer, R. O.: A consideration of the Le Mesurier technique of single harelip repair with a new concept as to its use in incomplete and secondary harelip repairs. Plast. Reconstr. Surg., 11:275, 1953.

Brauer, R. O.: Personal communication, 1957.

Brauer, R. O.: Push-back repair of the cleft palate with nasal mucosal flaps to prevent late contracture; follow-up results of the Cronin procedure. Plast. Reconstr. Surg., 36:529, 1965.

Brauer, R. O.: Repair of the bilateral cleft lip. In Georgiade, N. C., and Hagerty, R. F. (Eds.): Symposium on Management of Cleft Lip and Palate and Associated Deformities. St. Louis, C. V. Mosby Company, 1974.

Brauer, R. O., Cronin, T. D., and Reaves, E. L.: Early maxillary orthopedics, orthodontia and alveolar bone grafting in complete clefts of the palate. Plast. Reconstr. Surg., 29:625, 1962.

Brauer, R. O., and Foerster, D. W.: Another method to lengthen the columella in the double cleft patient. Plast. Reconstr. Surg., 38:27, 1966.

Broadbent, T. R., and Woolf, R. M.: Cleft lip nasal deformity. Ann. Plast. Surg., 12:216, 1984.

Brown, J. B.: Elongation of the partially cleft palate. Am. J. Orthod., 24:878, 1938.

Brown, J. B., and McDowell, F.: Simplified design for repair of single cleft lips. Surg. Gynec. Obstet., 80:12, 1945.

Brown, J. B., and McDowell, F.: Small triangular flap operation for the primary repair of single cleft lips. Plast. Reconstr. Surg., 5:392, 1950.

Brown, R. F.: A reappraisal of the cleft-lip nose with the report of a case. Br. J. Plast. Surg., 17:168, 1964.

Brown, R. F.: The cleft lip nasal deformity in the absence of cleft lip. Transactions of the 5th International Congress of Plastic and Reconstructive Surgery, Melbourne, Australia. Australia, Butterworths, 1971, p. 407.

Burston, W. R., and Kernahan, D. A.: Personal communication, 1961.

Clarkson, P.: Use of the Abbé flap in the primary repair of double cleft lip. Br. J. Plast. Surg., 7:175, 1954.

Clodius, L.: Maxillary orthopedia by means of extraoral forces. In Hotz, R. (Ed.): Early Treatment of Cleft Lip and Palate. International Symposium, April 9–11, 1964, University of Zurich Dental Institute. Berne, Hans Huber, 1964.

Converse, J. M.: Corrective surgery of the nasal tip. Laryngoscope, 67:16, 1957.

Cosman, B., and Crikelair, G. F.: The minimal cleft lip. Plast. Reconstr. Surg., 37:334, 1966.

Cronin, T. D.: Surgery of the double cleft lip and protruding premaxilla. Plast. Reconstr. Surg., 19:389, 1957.

Cronin, T. D.: Lengthening the columella by use of skin from the nasal floor and alae. Plast. Reconstr. Surg., 21:417, 1958.

Cronin, T. D.: Management of the bilateral cleft lip, palate, and nose. In Brent, B. (Ed.): The Artistry of Reconstruction Surgery. St. Louis, MO, C. V. Mosby Company, 1987, pp. 242–252.

Cronin, T. D., Brauer, R. O., and Penoff, J. H.: Maxillary orthopedics, orthodontia and bone grafting. In Cole, R. M. (Ed.): Proceedings of 2nd International Symposium on Early Treatment of Cleft Lip and Palate. Chicago, IL, Northwestern University Cleft Lip and Palate Institute, 1969.

Cronin, T. D., and Penoff, J. H.: Bilateral clefts of the primary palate. Cleft Palate J., 8:349, 1971.

Dado, D. V., and Kernahan, D. A.: Radiographic analysis of the mid face of a stillborn infant with a unilateral cleft lip and palate. Plast. Reconstr. Surg., 78:238, 1986.

Davis, W. B.: Harelip and cleft palate; study of 425 consecutive cases. Ann. Surg., 87:536, 1928.

Davis, W. B.: Methods preferred in cleft lip and cleft palate repair. J. Int. Coll. Surg., 3:116, 1940.

Desault, P. J.: Chorin: sur l'operation d' un bec-de-lièvre double, avec fente; la voute du palais. J. Chir. Paris, 1:97, 1791.

Dorrance, G. M., and Bransfield, J. W.: Cleft palate. Ann. Surg., 117:1, 1943.

Dorrance, G. M., and Bransfield, J. W.: The push-back operation for repair of cleft palate. Plast. Reconstr. Surg., 1:145, 1946.

Duffy, M. M.: Restoration of orbicularis oris muscle continuity in the repair of bilateral cleft lip. Br. J. Plast. Surg., 24:48, 1971.

El Deeb, M., Messer, L. B., Lehnert, M. W., Hebda, T. W., and Waite, D. E.: Canine eruption into grafted bone in maxillary alveolar cleft defects. Cleft Palate J., 19:9, 1982.

Erich, J. B.: A technique for correcting a flap nostril in cases of repaired harelip. Plast. Reconstr. Surg., 12:320, 1953.

Fára, M.: Anatomy and arteriography of cleft lips in stillborn children. Plast. Reconstr. Surg., 42:29, 1968.

Franco, P.: Traité des hernies. Lyon, Thiebaud Payen, 1561, Chap. 118.

Furlow, L. T., Jr.: Cleft palate repair by double opposing Z-plasty. Plast. Reconstr. Surg., 78:724, 1986.

Gabka, J.: Aetiology and statistics of harelips and cleft palate. In Wallace, A. B. (Ed.): Transactions of the International Society of Plastic Surgeons, 2nd Congress, 1959. Edinburgh, E & S Livingstone, 1960.

Gelbke, H.: The nostril problem in unilateral harelips and its surgical management. Plast. Reconstr. Surg., 18:65, 1956.

Georgiade, N. G.: The management of premaxillary and maxillary segments in the newborn cleft palate. Cleft Palate J., 7:411, 1970.

Georgiade, N. G.: Improved technique for one-stage repair of bilateral cleft lip. Plast. Reconstr. Surg., 48:318, 1971.

Georgiade, N. G., and Latham, R. A.: Intraoral traction for positioning the premaxilla in the bilateral cleft lip. In Georgiade, N. G., and Hagerty, R. F. (Eds.): Symposium on Management of Cleft Lip and Palate and Associated Deformities. St. Louis, MO, C. V. Mosby Company, 1974, pp. 123–127.

Georgiade, N. G., and Latham, R. A.: Maxillary arch alignment in the bilateral cleft lip and palate infant, using the pinned coaxial screw appliance. Plast. Reconstr. Surg., 56:52, 1975.

Hamilton, R., Graham, W. P., III, and Randall, P.: Adhesion procedure on cleft lip repair. Cleft Palate J., 8:1, 1971.

His, W.: Beobachtungen zur Geschichte der Nasen-und Gaumenbildung beim menschlichen Embryo. Abhandl. d. math.-phys. Cl. d. k.-sächs Gesellsch. d. Wissensch., Leipzig, 27:1901.

Holdsworth, W. G.: Cleft Lip and Palate. New York, Grune & Stratton, 1951.

Hönig, C. A.: The operative treatment of bilateral complete clefts of the primary and secondary palate in the first year of life. In Hotz, R. (Ed.): Early Treatment of Cleft Lip and Palate. International Symposium, University of Zurich Dental Institute, 1964. Berne, Hans Huber, 1964.

Huffman, W. C., and Lierle, D. M.: Studies on the pathologic anatomy of the unilateral hare-lip nose. Plast. Reconstr. Surg., 4:225, 1949a.

Huffman, W. C., and Lierle, D. M.: The repair of the bilateral cleft lip. Plast. Reconstr. Surg., 4:489, 1949b.

Kahn, S., and Winsten, J.: Surgical approaches to the bilateral cleft lip problem. Br. J. Plast. Surg., 13:13, 1960.

Kernahan, D. A., Bauer, B. S., and Harris, G. D.: Experience with the Tajima procedure in primary and secondary repair in unilateral cleft lip nasal deformity. Plast. Reconstr. Surg., 66:46, 1980.

Kernahan, D. A., Dado, D. V., and Bauer, B. S.: The anatomy of the orbicularis oris muscle in unilateral cleft lip based on a three-dimensional histologic reconstruction. Plast. Reconstr. Surg., 73:875, 1984.

Kilner, T. P.: The management of the patient with cleft lip and/or palate. Am. J. Surg., 95:204, 1958.

Ladd, W. E.: Harelip and cleft palate. Boston Med. Surg. J., 194:1016, 1926.

Lamont, E. S.: Plastic surgery in reconstructing the primary cleft lip and nasal deformity. Am. J. Surg., 86:200, 1953.

Latham, R. A.: Facial growth mechanisms in the human and their role in the formation of the cleft lip and palate deformity. Ph.D. Thesis, University of Liverpool, 1967.

Latham, R. A.: A new concept of the early maxillary growth mechanism. Transactions of the European Orthodontic Society, 1968, pp. 53–63.

Latham, R. A.: The pathogenesis of the skeletal deformity associated with unilateral cleft lip and palate. Cleft Palate J., 6:404, 1969.

Latham, R. A.: Maxillary development and growth: the septopremaxillary ligament. J. Anat., 107:471, 1970.

Latham, R. A.: Development and structure of the premaxillary deformity in bilateral cleft lip and palate. Br. J. Plast. Surg., 26:1, 1973.

Latham, R. A.: Orthopedic advancement of the cleft maxillary segment. A preliminary report. Cleft Palate J., 17:227, 1980.

Latham, R. A., and Scott, J. H.: A newly postulated factor in the early growth of the human middle face and the theory of multiple assurance. Arch. Oral Biol., 15:1097, 1970.

LeMesurier, A. B.: The quadrilateral Mirault flap operation for hare-lip. Plast. Reconstr. Surg., 16:422, 1955.

Levret: Des nouvelles observations sur l'allaitement des enfants. J. Med. Chir. Pharm. Paris, 37:233, 1772.

Manchester, W. M.: The repair of bilateral cleft lip and palate. Br. J. Surg., 52:878, 1965.

Manchester, W. M.: The repair of double cleft lip as part of an integrated program. Plast. Reconstr. Surg., 45:207, 1970.

Manchester, W. M.: A method of primary double cleft lip repair. In Huston, J. T. (Ed.): Transactions of the 5th International Congress of Plastic and Reconstructive Surgery, Melbourne, Australia. Australia, Butterworths, 1971.

Marcks, K. M., Trevaskis, A. E., Berg, E. M., and Puchner, G.: Nasal defects associated with cleft lip deformity. Plast. Reconstr. Surg., 34:176, 1964.

Marcks, K. M., Trevaskis, A. E., and Payne, M. J.: Bilateral cleft lip repair. Plast. Reconstr. Surg., 19:401, 1957a.

Marcks, K. M., Trevaskis, A. E., and Payne, M. J.: Elongation of columella by flap. Plast. Reconstr. Surg., 20:466, 1957b.

McComb, H.: Treatment of the unilateral cleft lip nose. Plast. Reconstr. Surg., 55:596, 1975a.

McComb, H.: Primary repair of the bilateral cleft lip nose. Br. J. Plast. Surg., 28:262, 1975b.

McComb, H.: Primary correction of unilateral cleft lip nasal deformity: a 10-year review. Plast. Reconstr. Surg., 75:791, 1985.

McComb, H.: Primary repair of the bilateral cleft lip nose: a 10-year review. Plast. Reconstr. Surg., 77:701, 1986.

McIndoe, A.: Correction of alar deformity in cleft lip. Lancet, 1:607, 1938.

McIndoe, A., and Rees, T. D.: Synchronous repair of secondary deformities in cleft lip and nose. Plast. Reconstr. Surg., 24:150, 1959.

Millard, D. R., Jr.: Columella lengthening by a forked flap. Plast. Reconstr. Surg., 22:454, 1958.

Millard, D. R., Jr.: A primary compromise for bilateral cleft lip. Surg. Gynecol. Obstet., 111:557, 1960a.

Millard, D. R., Jr.: Adaptation of the rotation-advancement principle in bilateral cleft lip. In Wallace, A. B. (Ed.): Transactions of the International Society of Plastic Surgeons, 2nd Congress, 1959. Edinburgh, E & S Livingstone, 1960b, p. 50.

Millard, D. R., Jr.: The unilateral cleft lip nose. Plast. Reconstr. Surg., 34:169, 1964.

Millard, D. R., Jr.: Bilateral cleft lip and primary forked flap: a preliminary report. Plast. Reconstr. Surg., 39:59, 1967.

Millard, D. R., Jr.: Closure of bilateral cleft lip and elongation of columella by two operations in infancy. Plast. Reconstr. Surg., 47:324, 1971a.

Millard, D. R., Jr.: Complete bilateral cleft lip; primary lip and nose correction. In Huston, J. T. (Ed.): Transactions of the 5th International Congress of Plastic and Reconstructive Surgery, Melbourne, Australia. Australia, Butterworths, 1971b, p. 185.

Millard, D. R., Jr.: Personal communication, 1973.

Millard, D. R., Jr.: Cleft Craft II. Boston, Little, Brown & Company, 1977, pp. 313–374, 384–388.

Millard, D. R., Jr.: Cleft Craft III. Boston, Little, Brown & Company, 1980, pp. 292–296.

Millard, D. R., Jr.: Principlization of Plastic Surgery. Boston, Little, Brown & Company, 1986, pp. 287, 298, 359–363.

Millard, D. R., Jr.: Personal communication, 1988.

Mir y Mir, L.: Nasal deformity and single cleft lip. In Skoog, T. (Ed.): Transactions of the International Society of Plastic Surgeons, First Congress, Stockholm and Uppsala, 1955. Baltimore, Williams & Wilkins Company, 1957, p. 171.

Morel-Fatio, D., and Lalardrie, J. P.: External nasal approach in the correction of major morphologic sequelae of the cleft lip nose. Plast. Reconstr. Surg., 38:116, 1966.

Muir, I. F. K.: Repair of the cleft alveolus. Br. J. Plast. Surg., 19:30, 1966.

Mulliken, J. B.: Principles and techniques of bilateral cleft lip repair. Plast. Reconstr. Surg., 75:477, 1985.

Murray, J. J.: Undescribed malformation of the lower lip occurring in four members of one family. Br. For. Med.-Chir. Rev., 26:502, 1860.

Noordhoff, M. S.: Bilateral cleft lip reconstruction. Plast. Reconstr. Surg., 78:45, 1986.

Noordhoff, M. S., and Cheng, W-S.: Median facial dysgenesis in cleft lip and palate. Ann. Plast. Surg., 8:83, 1982.

O'Connor, G. B., McGregor, M. W., and Tolleth, H.: The nasal problem in cleft lips. Surg. Gynec. Obstet., 116:503, 1963.

Ortiz-Monasterio, F., and Olmedo, A.: Corrective rhinoplasty before puberty: a long-term follow-up. Plast. Reconstr. Surg., 68:381, 1981.

Patten, B. M.: Embryology of the palate and the maxillofacial region. In Grabb, W. C., Rosenstein, S. W., and Bzoch, K. R. (Eds.): Cleft Lip and Palate: Surgical, Dental, and Speech Aspects. Boston, Little, Brown & Company, 1971.

Peskova, A., and Fára, M.: Lengthening of the columella in bilateral cleft. Acta. Chir. Plast., 2:18, 1960.

Peterson, R. A., Ellenberg, A. H., and Carroll, D. B.: Vermilion flap reconstruction of bilateral cleft lip deformities (a modification of the Abbé procedure). Plast. Reconstr. Surg., 38:111, 1966.

Pigott, R. W.: "Alar leapfrog." A technique for repositioning the total alar cartilage at primary cleft lip repair. Clin. Plast. Surg., 12:643, 1985.

Pruzansky, S.: Discussion. The use of cranial bone grafts in the closure of alveolar and anterior palatal clefts. Plast. Reconstr. Surg., 72:669, 1983.

Randall, P.: In Grabb, W. C., Rosenstein, S. W., and Bzoch, K. R. (Eds.): Cleft Lip and Palate: Surgical, Dental, and Speech Aspects. Boston, Little, Brown & Company, 1971, p. 204.

Randall, P., and Brown, A.: Primary reconstruction of the columella in bilateral clefts of the lip. Abstracts of the 2nd International Congress on Cleft Palate. Copenhagen, 1973, p. 251.

Randall, P., LaRossa, D., Solomon, M., and Cohen, M.: Experience with the Furlow double reversing Z-plasty for cleft palate repair. Plast. Reconstr. Surg., 77:569, 1986.

Randall, P., and Lynch, D. J.: Primary reconstruction of the columella in bilateral prepalatal clefts. Presented to the American Association of Plastic & Reconstructive Surgeons, Seattle, May, 1974.

Rees, T. D., Swinyard, C. A., and Converse, J. M.: The prolabium in the bilateral cleft lip. An electromyographic and biopsy study. Plast. Reconstr. Surg., 30:651, 1962.

Reynolds, J. R., and Horton, C. E.: An alar lift procedure in cleft lip rhinoplasty. Plast. Reconstr. Surg., 35:377, 1965.

Robertson, N. R. E., and Jolleys, A.: An 11-year follow-up of the effects of early bone grafting in infants born with complete clefts of the lip and palate. Br. J. Plast. Surg., 36:438, 1983.

Rosenstein, S. W., Monroe, C. W., Kernahan, D. A., Jacobson, B. N., Griffith, B. H., and Bauer, B. S.: The case for early bone grafting in cleft lip and cleft palate. Plast. Reconstr. Surg., 70:297, 1982.

Rutrick, R., Black, P. W., and Jurkiewicz, M. J.: Bilateral cleft lip and palate: presurgical treatment. Ann. Plast. Surg., 12:105, 1984.

Salyer, K. E.: Primary correction of the unilateral cleft lip nose: a 15-year experience. Plast. Reconstr. Surg., 77:558, 1986.

Sawhney, C. P.: Nasal deformity in unilateral cleft lip. Cleft Palate J., 13:291, 1976.

Schultz, L. W.: Bilateral cleft lips. Plast. Reconstr. Surg., 1:338, 1946.

Scott, J. H.: Growth at facial sutures. Am. J. Orthod., 42:381, 1956.

Scott, J. H.: The growth of the nasal cavities. Acta Otolaryngol., 50:215, 1959a.

Scott, J. H.: Further studies on the growth of the human face. Proc. R. Soc. Med., 52:263, 1959b.

Siegel, M. I., Mooney, M. P., Kimes, K. R., and Gest, T. R.: Traction, prenatal development, and the labioseptopremaxillary region. Plast. Reconstr. Surg., 76:25, 1985.

Simon, B. E.: Personal communication, 1970.

Skoog, T.: The management of the bilateral cleft of the primary palate (lip and alveolus). Part 1: General considerations and soft tissue repair. Plast. Reconstr. Surg., 35:34, 1965.

Skoog, T.: The use of periosteum and Surgicel for bone restoration in congenital clefts of the maxilla. Scand. J. Plast. Reconstr. Surg., 1:113, 1967.

Skoog, T.: Repair of unilateral cleft lip deformity: maxilla, nose and lip. Scand. J. Plast. Reconstr. Surg., 3:109, 1969.

Smith, F.: Plastic and Reconstructive Surgery. Philadelphia, W. B. Saunders Company, 1950.

Spina, V.: Cirugia del labio leporino bilateral. In Transactions of the Third International Congress of Plastic Surgery, Washington, DC, 1963. Amsterdam, Excerpta Medica Foundation, p. 314.

Spina, V.: The advantages of two stages in repair of bilateral cleft lip. Cleft Palate J., 3:56, 1966.

Spina, V., Kamakura, L., and Lapa, F.: Surgical management of bilateral cleft lip. Ann. Plast. Surg., 1:497, 1978.

Stark, R. B.: The pathogenesis of harelip and cleft palate. Plast. Reconstr. Surg., 13:20, 1954.

Stark, R. B., and Ehrmann, N. A.: The development of the center of the face with particular reference to surgical correction of bilateral cleft lip. Plast. Reconstr. Surg., 21:177, 1958.

Stark, R. B., and Kaplan, J. M.: Development of the cleft lip nose. Plast. Reconstr. Surg., 51:413, 1973.

Steffensen, W. H.: A method for repair of the unilateral cleft lip. Plast. Reconstr. Surg., 4:144, 1949.

Stenström, S. J.: The alar cartilage and the nasal deformity in unilateral cleft lip. Plast. Reconstr. Surg., 38:223, 1966.

Stenström, S. J.: Follow-up clinic: the alar cartilage and nasal deformity in unilateral cleft lip. Plast. Reconstr. Surg., 55:359, 1975.

Stenström, S. J., and Öberg, T. R. H.: The nasal deformity in unilateral cleft lip. Plast. Reconstr. Surg., 28:295, 1961.

Stenström, S. J., and Thilander, B. L.: Cleft lip nasal deformity in the absence of cleft lip. Plast. Reconstr. Surg., 35:160, 1965.

Takahashi, R., and Yamazaki, Y.: Studies on the external nose in cases of cleft lip and their application to plastic surgery. Transactions of the Third International Congress of Plastic Surgery, Washington, DC, 1963. Amsterdam, Excerpta Medica Foundation, p. 336.

Tolhurst, D. E.: Primary columella lengthening and lip adhesion. Br. J. Plast. Surg., 38:89, 1985.

Trauner, R., and Trauner, M.: Results of cleft lip operations. Plast. Reconstr. Surg., 40:209, 1967.

Trier, W. C.: Repair of bilateral cleft lip: Millard's technique. Clin. Plast. Surg. 12:605, 1985.

Trusler, H. M., Bauer, T. B., and Tondra, J. M.: The cleft lip–cleft palate problem. Plast. Reconstr. Surg., 16:174, 1955.

Tulenko, J.: Cleft lip nasal deformity in the absence of cleft lip: case report. Plast. Reconstr. Surg., 41:35, 1968.

Van der Woude, A.: Fistula labii inferioris congenita and its association with cleft lip and palate. Am. J. Hum. Genet., 6:244, 1954.

Vaughn, H. S.: Importance of premaxilla and philtrum in bilateral cleft lip. Plast. Reconstr. Surg., 1:240, 1946.

Veau, V.: Division Palatine, Anatomie, Chirurgie, Phonétique. Paris, Masson et Cie, 1931.

Wilde, N. J.: Repositioning of the premaxilla and its fixation. Br. J. Plast. Surg., 13:28, 1960.

Wolfe, S. A., and Berkowitz, S.: The use of cranial bone grafts in the closure of alveolar and anterior bilateral clefts. Plast. Reconstr. Surg., 72:659, 1983.

Wynn, S. K.: Lateral flap cleft surgery technique. Plast. Reconstr. Surg., 26:509, 1960.

Wynn, S. K.: Primary nostril reconstruction in complete cleft lips. The round nostril technique. Plast. Reconstr. Surg., 49:56, 1972.

54

Peter Randall
Don LaRossa

Cleft Palate

HISTORICAL ASPECTS

Unlike cleft lip, the surgical correction of a cleft palate eluded surgeons for centuries. Indeed, an unnamed Chinese surgeon repaired a cleft lip in the fourth century A.D. The result must have been reasonably successful since his patient, Wei Yang-Chi, became Governor General of six Chinese provinces (Boo-Chai, 1966). In thirteenth century Europe, Jehan Yupperman, a Flemish surgeon, was the first to describe in detail the repair of cleft lips, but he made no mention of clefts of the palate (Rogers, 1964, 1971). However, it was as late as the sixteenth century that Franco (1561) noted that "those who have cleft palates are more difficult to cure." He described the hypernasal speech characteristic of patients with unrepaired clefts and observed that it could be corrected if plugged with cotton or even "better a plate of silver or lead" (Barsky, 1964). Franco was, in all likelihood, drawing from the centuries-old experience with obturating palatal clefts introduced into Western medicine by Arabic and Eastern traditions. The use of dental prostheses is evidenced by the discovery of one dating from about 2500 B.C. in the old empire of Egypt (Rogers, 1971). Undoubtedly, these methods resulted in the evolution of intraoral prostheses fabricated later in Western medicine. Paré (1564) first used the term "obturateur" to describe the plates of gold or silver he used to occlude palatal clefts (Paget, 1899). However, Lusitanius probably described the use of gold plates held in place by a sponge four years before (Lusitanius, 1566; Rogers, 1971). Most writings of this era are concerned with repair of palatal defects resulting from gunshot wounds or syphilis. Only Franco in this group of sixteenth century surgeons elaborated on congenital clefts of the palate. Indeed, the commonly held belief that palatal malformations were syphilitic in origin may have retarded the development of surgical procedures to repair clefts. In the eighteenth century, obturators became quite sophisticated. Devices with movable wings and sponge padding were described. In 1757, Bourdet reported the attachment of obturators to the teeth by means of clasps (Bourdet, 1757; Rogers, 1971).

The nineteenth century witnessed the successful surgical closure of clefts of the soft palate by von Graefe in 1816 and Roux in 1819 (Francis, 1963; von Graefe, 1817, 1820). The details of Roux's operation from the patient's perspective are clearly described by his first patient, John Stephenson, a Canadian medical student, in his graduation thesis (Francis, 1963; Rogers, 1971). Shortly thereafter, in 1826, Dieffenbach (1828, 1845) recommended separating the hard palate mucosa from the bone as a means of closing the hard palate. He even employed lateral osteotomies in 1828 to aid in the closure (Peer, 1959, 1964). Von Langenbeck (1859, 1861) extended these concepts and emphasized the need to create subperiosteal undermining and mucoperiosteal flaps in his bipedicle flap procedure. His concepts represented a major contribution in that the incidence of wound disruption was reduced.

The importance of relaxing incisions to reduce tension on the repair was described in the writings of Pancoast (1843), Warren (1828, 1843a,b), and Fergusson (1845) in the United States.

Refinements of these basic principles of repair and greater attention to the details of anatomy and function mark the history of palate surgery from the beginning of the 20th century to the present. Veau (1931) converted the bipedicle flaps of von Langenbeck to single pedicle flaps based on the greater palatine vessels (Converse, 1962). In addition, he emphasized the need for palatal lengthening. Wardill (1937) and Kilner (1937) modified Veau's procedure and ushered in an era of numerous techniques aimed at achieving increased palatal length. Concern about the eventual contraction of the raw surfaces left by palatal lengthening led to the description of a variety of procedures by numerous authors in the decades that followed. Dorrance and Bransfield (1946) described the use of a skin graft to prevent contracture. Cronin (1957) used nasal flaps to line the nasal surface. Kaplan (1975a) described buccal mucosal flaps, while Millard (1966) used flaps of hard palate mucoperiosteum based on the greater palatine vessels in the form of a sandwich to fill the gap between the hard and soft palate. The latter procedure was later abandoned after it was realized that the scar-

ring left on the hard palate would result in significant skeletal deformities.

In the 1960's, the muscular anatomy of the palate became the focus of attention. Although Veau (1931) had described the abnormal musculature of the palate earlier in the century, Kriens (1970, 1975) spearheaded the interest in muscular reconstruction of the disoriented levator and tensor palatini muscles. His procedure, the intra-velar-veloplasty, involved releasing the anterior muscular attachments from the posterior edge of the palatal shelves and suturing them across the midline during palatal repair. Although not all surgeons have followed Kriens' advice with an extensive muscular dissection, most have recognized the need to detach the muscles from the hard palate and thereby achieve some lengthening of the soft palate, restoration of the levator sling, and improved muscular function. This interest in muscular reconstruction resulted in the development of a double reversing Z-plasty palatoplasty (Furlow, 1980, 1986).

After the principles of repair had become defined and established, questions about the appropriate timing for cleft palate repair and the potential effects on skeletal growth began to be addressed.

It was abundantly clear that the palate was an important organ of speech and that the earlier that surgical closure could be achieved, the better were the speech results. However, wide undermining and the development of mucoperiosteal flaps, particularly in the pushback procedures that were popular from the 1930's onward, had the potential for impairing facial skeletal growth (see Chap. 49). Surgeons gravitated into one of the two schools, depending on their philosophic beliefs.

Warren (1828) noted that wide clefts of the hard palate could be narrowed by first closing the soft palate. Schweckendiek (1955, 1962) repopularized this approach for treating wide clefts, leaving the hard palate unrepaired to allow for maxillary growth before closing the hard palate. A number of centers have adhered to this philosophy, delaying hard palate closure until the ages of 5 to 9 years, to allow the maxilla to achieve most of its lateral growth (Schweckendiek, 1955; Hotz, 1964; Dingman and Grabb, 1971; Perko, 1979). The hard palate cleft is obturated in the interval.

The other school advocates closure of the hard and soft palate simultaneously, emphasizing the beneficial effects on speech as opposed to the potential adverse effects on facial skeletal growth (Fara and Brousilova, 1969; Cosman and Falk, 1980; Bardach, Morris, and Olin, 1984; Witzel, Salyer, and Ross, 1984).

The latest chapter in the history of cleft palate surgery concerns the management of the bony cleft of the alveolus. A more thorough review of the historical aspects of maxillary orthopedics and bone grafting can be found in Chapter 55. In brief, it was not until the early twentieth century that reports of bone grafting of the alveolus began to appear. Lexer (1908) and Drachter (1914) described the first attempts, while Schmid in 1944 is reported to have performed the first bone graft using costal bone (Schultz, 1964). During the 1950's and 1960's primary and secondary bone grafting was performed by numerous surgeons using tibial, costal, and iliac bone (Nordin and Johanson, 1955; Nordin, 1957; Schrudde and Stellmach, 1958, 1959; Stellmach, 1959; Johanson and Ohlsson, 1961; Schuchardt and Pfeifer, 1962, 1966). Skoog (1965) reported the use of maxillary periosteum in a technique called the "boneless bone graft."

Early bone grafting met with enthusiasm but it was only temporary. Reports of the detrimental effects of bone grafting on maxillary growth began to appear (Pruzansky, 1964; Kling, 1964; Ortiz-Monasterio and associates, 1966; Rehrmann, Koberg, and Koch, 1970; Jolleys and Robertson, 1972). These workers suggested that early bone grafting interfered with maxillary growth and caused malocclusion, and that the technique should therefore be abandoned. However, other investigators had not experienced the same poor results. They carefully followed patients treated with early bone grafting in infancy and during the period of mixed dentition, and demonstrated a beneficial outcome (Nylen, 1966; Nylen and associates, 1974; Abyholm, Bergland, and Semb, 1981; Rosenstein and associates, 1982; Bergland and associates, 1986; Bergland, Semb, and Abyholm, 1986).

Coupled with bone grafting were investigations into the management of the malaligned alveolar segments. Burston (1960, 1965) and McNeil (1954) were advocates of early maxillary orthopedics. Numerous reports of the use of fixed and nonfixed prostheses in infancy followed (Nordin, 1960; Conway and Goulian, 1963; Georgiade, Pickrell, and Quinn, 1964; Horton and associates,

1964; Georgiade, 1970; Brauer and Cronin, 1964; Rosenstein and associates, 1972).

A historical review of cleft palate management emphasizes the complex and multifaceted nature of the problem. Solutions have emanated from careful, long-term observation of patients and the imaginative application of principles and techniques from many disciplines.

GENERAL CONSIDERATIONS

A child born today with a cleft palate, with or without a prepalatal cleft, should receive comprehensive care. Surgical care is much more than simply obtaining closure of the hard and soft palate cleft at the appropriate age. Clefts can adversely affect every function of the face except that of sight. A cleft palate can be associated with malnutrition, malocclusion, deficiencies in maxillary and malar bone growth, eustachian tube malfunction, reduced air conduction in the middle ear, deafness, and nasorespiratory obstruction. As such, there can be problems in speaking, alimentation, hearing, nasal breathing, taste, and smell as well as in normal facial appearance and expression. Priorities in timing are critical. For example, a postoperative soft palate incompetence producing speech distortion usually should be corrected before a malocclusion, even though the time might be best for orthodontic care. Often, these two problems can be treated simultaneously. However, if there is an articulation problem that is due to an anterior malocclusion, it makes little sense to insist on speech training before the malocclusion is corrected. Similarly, it appears that the best time to reconstruct the alveolar defect with gingival mucosal flaps and bone grafts is when the adjacent permanent teeth are erupting, i.e., at approximately 9 to 11 years of age (Abyholm, Bergland, and Semb, 1981; Bergland and associates, 1986; Bergland, Semb, and Abyholm, 1986). Satisfactory results are currently being obtained by bone grafting at an earlier age if the defect is wide (Mayro, 1986). This surgical step must be coordinated with the plans of the orthodontist and the speech pathologist.

The plastic surgeon responsible for the care of these children not only should be aware of these manifestations but also should have at least a rudimentary knowledge of the disciplines of dentistry, speech pathology, pediatrics, genetics, and otolaryngology. In this way, the surgeon can collaborate effectively with these specialists and with others who may also be involved.

ANATOMY

The *palate* is limited anteriorly by the *incisive foramen/papilla* and extends posteriorly through the structures of the hard palate, the soft palate, and the uvula (Fig. 54–1). The structures anterior to the incisive foramen include the alveolus, the upper lip, and the nasal tip. These are collectively referred to as the *prepalatal structures* or the *primary palate,* the incisive foramen being the point of separation. Those posterior to the incisive foramen are called either the *palate* or the *secondary palate.* The terms *prepalatal* and *palatal* structures are preferred because they are explicit. It is somewhat confusing to refer to the *lip structures* as the *primary palatal structures* and to the *palate structures* as *secondary palatal* structures. "Secondary" implies something less important than "primary," whereas there seems to be nothing less important about the palatal structures as opposed to the prepalatal structures.

The maxillas are paired and join each other in the midline in the normal palate. They meet at the incisive foramen anteriorly and

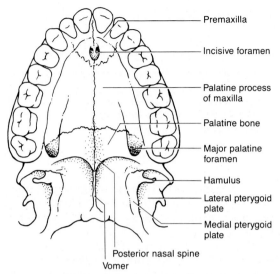

Figure 54–2. The normal bony topography of the palate. The locations of the major palatine foramen, the incisive foramen, and the hamulus are important surgical landmarks. (After Millard, D. R., Jr.: Cleft Craft. Vol. III. Boston, Little, Brown & Company, 1980, p. 19.)

extend posteriorly to the two palatal bones (Fig. 54–2). Superiorly, they form the bony groove that holds the nasal cartilaginous septum anteriorly and the vomer posteriorly. The *premaxilla* is situated centrally and anterior to the incisive foramen. It includes the nasal spine and the four incisor teeth. The palatine bones define the posterior edge of the hard palate, including the *major* and *minor palatine foramina* on either side, which contain the major vascular supply to the palate as well as a sensory nerve supply as part of the middle division of the trigeminal nerve. Blood vessels and sensory nerves also pass through the incisive foramen.

The palatine bone articulates with the *medial plate* of the *sphenopterygoid* bone, from which projects the *pterygoid hamulus.* The hamulus acts as a pulley for the tensor palatini muscle.

The muscles of the palate (Fig. 54–3) are paired and divided into those used primarily for speaking and those used primarily for swallowing. However, there is some overlap for both of these functions, i.e., *the levator palatini muscles are the most important and most active muscles for achieving velopharyngeal closure* for speech, but they are usually assisted by some contraction of the superior pharyngeal constrictor muscles and the palatopharyngeus muscles (see also Chap. 51).

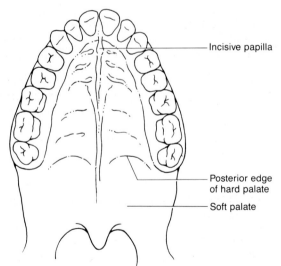

Figure 54–1. The normal surface topography of the palate. Although the mucosa of the hard palate is thick, it is easy to identify the major palatal vessels and the posterior nasal spine.

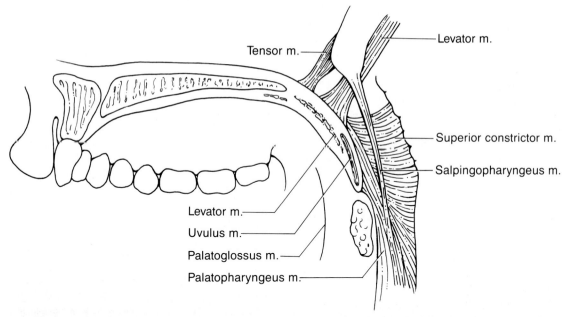

Figure 54–3. Sagittal view of a normal adult palate showing the relationships of the levator, the uvulus, and the palatoglossus muscles within and beyond the palate. The adjacent superior pharyngeal constrictor muscle is also shown. (After Millard, D. R., Jr.: Cleft Craft, Vol. III. Boston, Little, Brown & Company, 1980, opposite p. 36.)

In swallowing, the tensor palatini muscles contract, and while there is some contraction in the levator palatini to achieve velopharyngeal closure, there is even more activity in the superior pharyngeal constrictors than is seen during speech. In gagging, the forceful contraction of both the levator palatini and the superior pharyngeal constrictors can produce an observable bulge or ridge in the posterior pharynx above the arch of the atlas, *Passavant's ridge* or *pad*.

During normal speech, velopharyngeal closure is achieved primarily by the contraction of the levator palatini muscles and, to a lesser extent, the superior pharyngeal constrictor and the palatopharyngeus muscles (Fig. 54–4). In fact, the *musculus uvulae*, while contracting, causes thickening in the central portion of the soft palate, thus contributing to velopharyngeal closure by adding thickness at the site of maximal levator contraction. This site is known as the *levator eminence* and, as seen on radiographs of the normal palate, it rises to a position above the plane of the nostril floor. During yawning, the palatal musculature contracts but with little movement of the palate. The eustachian tube orifices are also opened and equalization of middle ear pressure is achieved.

It used to be thought that the musculus uvulae had little function in speech, swallowing, or anything else. However, Croft and associates (1978) described velopharyngeal incompetence in several patients with either isolated absence or noncontractibility of the musculus uvulae. This defect is visible radiographically by using the basilar view or by

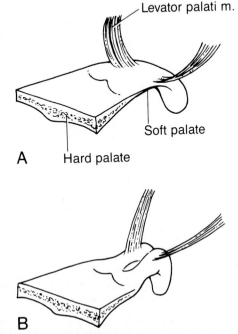

Figure 54–4. The levator muscle is the most important muscle for velopharyngeal closure. Note that the pull is approximately 45 degrees superiorly and posteriorly. *A*, At rest. *B*, Following contraction.

nasendoscopy, which shows a notch or groove in the levator eminence instead of a bulge.

The *levator palatini muscles* take their origin from the undersurface of the temporal bone and the medial lamina of the cartilaginous auditory tube, and insert into the palatine aponeurosis in the midportion of the soft palate. The nerve supply is by way of the pharyngeal plexus and, as a pair, they act as a sling to pull the middle and posterior portions of the soft palate upward and backward into intimate contact with the adenoid tissue (Fig. 54–4). This must be a rapid, easy motion and must be as effortless as a blink if it is to function properly. The levator palatini muscles have their blood supply and innervation entering laterally so that the medial portion can be dissected free and repositioned in the soft palate repair without interference with function.

The *palatopharyngeus muscles* extend laterally, downward, and posteriorly in the posterior edge of the soft palate and into the posterior tonsillar pillar (Fig. 54–5). They contract synergistically with the levator palatini muscles and help to pull the palate posteriorly, although they are not strong muscles. Their innervation from the pharyn-

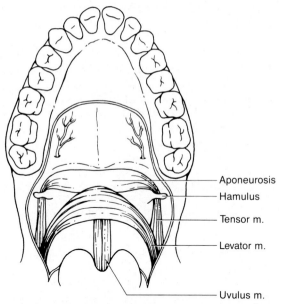

Figure 54–6. Normal musculature of the soft palate. Note the transverse orientation of the levator muscle in the middle portion of the soft palate. (After Millard, D. R., Jr.: Cleft Craft. Vol. III. Boston, Little, Brown & Company, 1980, following p. 37.)

geal plexus enters the muscles somewhat medial to the central portion so that their inferior and lateral portions can be used in a type of pharyngoplasty described by Orticochea (1968, 1983).

The *tensor palatini muscles* (Fig. 54–6) take their origin lateral to the levator from the base of the medial pterygoid plate, the spina angularis of the sphenoid, and the lateral wall of the cartilaginous auditory canal. Each courses around the pterygoid hamulus and inserts mainly into the anterior midline aponeurosis of the soft palate with a small attachment to the palatal bone laterally. They serve to tighten the anterior palate so that the tongue has a firm surface against which it can oppose to force a bolus of food into the pharynx. As swallowing muscles, they are innervated by the trigeminal nerve.

The *palatoglossus muscles* pass from the posterior soft palate into the anterior tonsillar pillar and then into the tongue, and elevate the midportion of the tongue, as in swallowing.

The *superior pharyngeal* constrictor muscles can contract in several ways. Superiorly, the lateral walls of the pharynx can be moved medially to contribute to velopharyngeal closure with little or no posterior pharyngeal wall motion. Additionally, the posterior wall

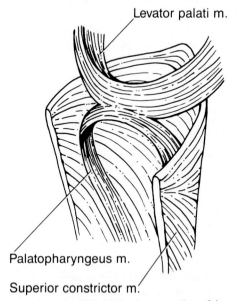

Figure 54–5. Braithwaites's demonstration of how the levator sling and the palatopharyngeus muscles supplement each other in moving the soft palate posteriorly while the superior pharyngeal constrictor muscles narrow the pharynx by moving the lateral walls medially, causing the posterior wall to bulge forward. (After Braithwaite F.: *In* Gibson, T. (Ed.): Modern Trends in Plastic Surgery. Washington, Butterworths, 1964.)

musculature can be contracted to move the posterior pharyngeal wall forward. In some forms of palatal incompetence, this is seen as a shelflike projection, previously noted as "Passavant's ridge" or "pad." It is typically seen in children with unrepaired clefts of the palate or repaired clefts that are too short. The level of maximal anterior movement of the posterior wall, although above the arch of the atlas, is inferiorly located and is usually at a lower level than is seen in normal velopharyngeal closure. This motion, however, is useful in providing valving against a prosthetic obturator when this technique is used for achieving velopharyngeal competence.

Skolnick and associates (1975) noted that the level of maximal lateral pharyngeal wall excursion can vary greatly in normal individuals, both in position and in the amount of movement. In the normal, the excursion is high and is located just below the level of the adenoid pad. In the normal palate, medial movement of the lateral pharyngeal walls is not great; in an incompetent palate, it can increase considerably to compensate for reduced soft palate motion. Hence, excessive movement in the lateral pharyngeal walls may well indicate less than normal activity in the soft palate.

From this description of the anatomy and the functional movement of the soft palate, it can be seen that the adenoid pad is an integral part of velopharyngeal closure, and increased excursion of the soft palate is needed as the adenoid tissue atrophies in early adolescence. Conversely, the palatine tonsils have virtually no role in velopharyngeal closure, although in the hypertrophied state they occasionally intrude into the velopharyngeal port and interfere with velopharyngeal closure. *Tonsillectomy,* when indicated, should have little effect on palatal function unless it is followed by excessive scarring (Shprintzen, 1985). In children with a repaired or submucosal cleft, *adenoidectomy* can produce a disastrous amount of velopharyngeal incompetence. This result is particularly likely if the palate is barely achieving velopharyngeal closure against hypertrophied adenoids, so that the adenoidectomy suddenly deepens the nasopharynx beyond the ability of the soft palate to achieve closure. In the normal individual, as the adenoids atrophy, the palatal excursion increases to compensate and maintain velopharyngeal

competence. A child is occasionally seen with an adequately repaired cleft palate without incompetence who becomes incompetent when the adenoids atrophy. Presumably this palate achieved satisfactory closure against the hypotrophied adenoids but with maximal excursion. As the adenoids involute, additional compensatory excursion is not possible (Subtelny and Baker, 1956; Mason and Warren, 1980).

In the child with a cleft palate, the cleft in the hard and the soft palate can vary greatly in extent and in width. At times, the defect is a narrow slit and at other times it has a horseshoe-shaped configuration as though the entire tongue can fit into the cleft as during early gestation. Under these conditions, the amount of tissue in the soft palate and the palatal shelves is usually deficient. Some cleft palates, before surgery, appear to have considerable scarring along the edge of the soft palate and the uvula is pulled anteriorly into an abnormal position. On examination it should be noted whether the uvula touches the pharynx behind the adenoid pad, whether it touches the posterior or anterior half of the adenoids, or whether, if it is so short, it does not reach the adenoid pad at all (Types I, II, III, or IV). These findings may be predictive of the functional result.

Perhaps the most important anatomic distortion seen in the child with a cleft is the *disorientation* of the *levator palatini muscles* (Fig. 54–7). In the normal patient, the muscles come together in the midline with a transverse orientation (see Fig. 54–6). Their insertion is located at approximately the middle third of the soft palate. However, in the child with a cleft, instead of being transversely oriented, the bundles are much more longitudinally oriented. Instead of being inserted into the palatal aponeurosis that is easily moved, they insert into the posterior edge of the palatine bone close to the cleft margin and also along the bony cleft itself (Veau, 1931; Fara and Dvorak, 1970; Kriens, 1970, 1975; Dickson and Dickson, 1972; Latham, Long, and Latham, 1980). In this position, the bulk of the levator muscle bundle in the palate is directed diagonally forward and medially (see also Chap. 51).

In a *submucous cleft palate,* in addition to the obvious bifid uvula, the abnormal orientation of the levator muscle may be easily seen as a converging diagonal ridge on each side, a finding accentuated on gagging. The

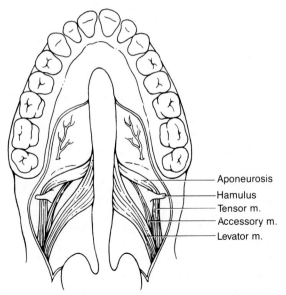

Figure 54–7. The musculature as seen in most palatal clefts. The levator muscles are oriented more longitudinally, and insert on the posterior edge of the palatal bone and along the bony cleft margins. (After Millard, D. R., Jr.: Cleft Craft. Vol. III. Boston, Little, Brown & Company, 1980, following p. 37.)

mucosa between the two abnormally positioned muscles usually is thin and is referred to as the *zona pellucida.* Under these conditions, there is also a cleft in the posterior portion of the bony palate so that, instead of being able to palpate a small tubercle in this area (the posterior nasal spine), one actually can feel a notch in the posterior edge of the bony palate. Thus, a submucous cleft palate can include a cleft uvula, displaced levator muscles, a zona pellucida, and a cleft in the posterior edge of the hard palate. The anteroposterior dimension of the palate can also be diminished, and velopharyngeal incompetence is frequent.

An interesting variation occurs in the attachment of the *vomer* to the maxilla. In clefts of only the hard and soft palate, the vomer is usually seen in the midline and is not attached to either maxilla. However, if a cleft of the hard and soft palate is also associated with a unilateral *prepalatal* cleft, the vomer usually has nearly a right-angled deviation in its inferior portion and articulates with the entire length of the maxilla on the non-cleft side. There are occasional exceptions, but this seems to point to a different mechanism of hard palate clefting in these two frequently seen clefts. The vomer configura-

tion in bilateral clefts is usually midline and it is not attached to the maxilla on either side. The deviation seen in the septum in the unilateral cleft improves with surgical closure of the cleft and with growth, but often is still present in older patients, producing a significant degree of nasorespiratory obstruction on the cleft side. In the patient with an unoperated hard palate cleft, the palatal shelves are often more vertically oriented than in the normal or postoperative patient.

CLASSIFICATION

The classification (Fig. 54–8) of various types of clefts is described in Chapter 45. Clefts of the palate can be described as being one-third, two-thirds, and three-thirds clefts of the soft palate and one-third, two-thirds, and three-thirds clefts of the hard palate extending up to the incisive foramen (Ker-

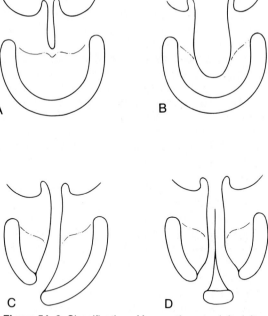

Figure 54–8. Classification of frequently seen clefts (after Veau). *A,* A cleft of the soft palate only. One can usually palpate a notch in the posterior hard palate and there is generally a submucosal extension into the hard palate. *B,* A complete palatal cleft extending anteriorly to the incisive foramen. This cleft may be narrow but often has a wide horseshoe-shaped defect. *C,* A unilateral palatal and prepalatal cleft. Note that the vomer is attached to the maxilla on the noncleft side. *D,* Bilateral complete cleft of the palate and prepalate. The premaxilla without any restraining force from the lip can protrude markedly and is stabilized only by the vomer. (After Veau, V.: Division Palatine. Paris, Masson et Cie, 1931.)

nahan and Stark, 1958; Tessier, 1976; Watson, 1980b). The bifid uvula is a cleft of the uvula or a rudimentary soft palate cleft. It can be either partial or complete. The incidence of bifid uvula is surprisingly high, approximately 2 per cent of the normal American population as reported by Meskin, Gorlin, and Isaacson (1964). Most individuals with a simple bifid uvula *do not have any speech problems* and do not require surgery. However, an appreciable percentage of "cleft uvulae" are also associated with a reduction in the anteroposterior dimension of the entire soft palate and with palatal incompetence, or may be associated with a submucosal cleft palate (Randall, Bakes, and Kennedy, 1960; Calnan, 1971; Trier, 1983).

Family medicine doctors, pediatricians, plastic surgeons, and those in otolaryngology should be aware of these possible problems and, on seeing a bifid uvula, should look very carefully for a submucosal cleft. Additional evidence of palatal incompetence is regurgitation of oral contents into the nose and/or hypernasal speech. The diagnosis of a submucosal cleft with a bifid uvula is often overlooked until the child has developed "cleft palate–type speech," or until the adenoids are removed (perhaps because the child "talks through his nose"), and his speech is made much worse.

FEEDING

The most immediate problem facing parents of a newborn with a cleft is that of feeding, yet the problem and its solution are not difficult. The child usually accomplishes all the mouthing and sucking motions necessary to feed, but as long as the palate is open it is impossible to build up a negative pressure (except in minimal clefts). As a result, the child works to the point of exhaustion and finally falls asleep only to wake up about two hours later still hungry. The deception is that the sleep is usually due to *fatigue* and *not a full stomach.* Lack of weight gain and failure to thrive quickly follow, and the exasperated physician and parents often seek hospitalization and gavage feeding, neither of which is usually necessary or advisable.

The answer is simply to deliver the milk into the mouth without the infant needing to suck it out of the bottle. One solution is to make large crosscuts in a soft nipple or to use cuticle scissors to cut a larger hole in the nipple so that the milk literally drips out upon compression.

A plastic squeeze bottle can also be used. The so-called "cleft palate nipples" with a rubber flange to obturate the cleft rarely if ever prove satisfactory. The child should take a full feeding in about 30 minutes; if it takes longer, the child probably is working too hard to eat.

The child is usually held at a 45 degree angle so that less milk escapes into the nasal passages. The ability to swallow is not usually impaired. The child with a cleft palate can be expected to swallow more than the usual amount of air, and requires more than the usual amount of "burping." The test is whether the child sleeps longer than two or three hours between feedings and shows a healthy weight gain. The usual formulas, dietary increases, and vitamins are used. Direct breast feeding has not usually been successful; however, a breast pump may permit a motivated mother to provide breast milk for her infant (Grabb, 1971; Pashayan and McNab, 1979; Styer and Freeh, 1981; Balluff, 1986).

It is advisable to have a trained "outreach" person from a cleft palate team meet with the parents soon after birth, discuss the problem, answer questions, and review some of the relevant literature on the subject.

Another point the authors believe to be important is to have the mother take over as many feedings as possible. Those that she cannot do should be carried out if possible by a different nurse each time. In this way the mother soon masters the little details noted above, becomes the real expert in feeding her child, and realizes that she is the most important person in keeping the child alive. The importance of early "bonding," particularly when the child has a facial deformity, cannot be overstressed. Often, however, the oldest and most experienced nurse in the nursery literally "takes over" the feeding "problem" and willingly relieves the anxious mother of this additional burden. This separates the mother and child at a critical time in a basic need and function, and should be avoided if at all possible.

SPEECH

The most important objective in cleft palate repair is to achieve *normal speech* (see Chap.

58). This is speech that not only is articulated well with normal resonance, but is also produced with a fairly normal amount of effort and consistency. Speech that may simply have a hypernasal quality, even though it may be well understood, still calls attention to itself, and leads to stigmatization, teasing, and cruel jokes. The child or adult is often reluctant to recite in class or to speak in public.

At times, a child or adult with a cleft palate is able to speak distinctly and with near-normal resonance, but only with considerable effort and concentration. When such a person is tired or is speaking rapidly, voice quality usually deteriorates. If much effort is needed for proper speech production, it can lead to straining, hoarseness, and even the development of vocal cord nodules. Speech ideally should be well articulated, and produced with normal resonance and without the need for excessive effort and concentration.

Speech is a highly complex learned function that even though under voluntary control, is so automatically produced that it should not be necessary to think about how to speak properly. A video recording of the normal soft palate shows an extremely mobile, rapid, delicate action with a bouncing quality that reminds one of the ease and speed of an eyelid blink. Unless the surgeon can reconstruct a palatal sphincter that can achieve this type of mobility and competence, it probably will not produce *normal, relaxed, conversational speech,* even though it may be able to achieve *velopharyngeal closure* (soft palate to posterior pharyngeal wall). Velopharyngeal closure (i.e., "v. p. closure") is needed to build up intraoral pressure for *all the consonant sounds* in the English language *except* the *nasal consonants* "m," "n," and "ng" (as in "ring"). The *nasal consonants* are pronounced with the lips closed and the air stream directed through the nose. An adequate nasal airway is needed for their proper production.

All the other consonants are divided into two groups—those produced by a small explosion, called "plosives" or "stop plosives," such as "b," "p," and "t," and those produced by the sound of friction, called "continuants," such as "s," "sh," and "z." The two groups are further subdivided depending on whether or not the vocal cords are used, i.e., "voiced" or "unvoiced," and they also differ depending on the site of stoppage for the "stop plosives" and the site of constriction in the "continuants."

For example, the "p" as in "pig" differs only from the "b" as in "big" in the use of the vocal cords on the "b" sound. Both are "bilabial stop plosives." The "p" is unvoiced and the "b" is voiced. The unvoiced continuants are called "sibilants," such as the "s" and "sh" sound. Voiced continuants are called "fricatives," as in "v" and "z." The only difference between "Sue" and "zoo" is the use of the vocal cords on "z," both consonants being "lingual dental continuants." In general, it takes more control of the air stream to produce a continuant such as "s" or "sh" accurately than to produce a plosive such as "b" or "k." Even with a partially incompetent soft palate, a child can often say "big" or "pig" well but is unable to say "Sue" or "zoo." Alternatively, the child may muster the extra effort with an incompetent palate to force velopharyngeal closure and say "Sue" in isolation while being tested, yet may be unable to say it accurately in relaxed conversational speech or in rapid speech when fatigued. Similarly, a distortion of the incisor teeth can interfere with the production of the "s" and "sh" sounds but not with the production of "w," as in "when" or "way."

Vowels in the English language require a slight amount of nasal resonance and usually need complete velopharyngeal closure for proper production.

Lacking closure (*velopharyngeal incompetence–v.p.i.*) the amount of air which passes into the nose increases, thus adding the resonance of the nasal passages and paranasal sinuses in the production of the sound with a resulting *hypernasal quality.* This is the typical "nasality" of the cleft palate type speech. Obstruction of the nasal airway, on the other hand, produced either by occlusion of the velopharyngeal valve, such as with hypertrophied adenoids or severe obstruction by a deviated septum, or by severe congestion from a cold or an allergic rhinitis, produces *hyponasality* or denasalized speech. Normal nasal resonance is not completely denasalized. The adult with large nasal passages and additional paranasal air spaces normally has more resonance than the child.

Usually a professional singer or speaker carefully increases the amount of resonance to make the voice "carry" or "project," but not to the extent of sounding "hypernasal." The velopharyngeal port, therefore, does not function in a simple open or closed position but requires delicate control for normal speech production.

A number of languages, particularly those of the Orientals, use nasalized vowels. However, they use the nasalized sounds in a controlled way, since the sounds are present in some words and not in others. The listener is even more critical of incorrect nasal resonance than is the average English-speaking listener. Some words, in fact, have an entirely different meaning depending on whether the vowels are intentionally nasalized or denasalized.

A third area of speech distortion is called *nasal escape,* which is the sound of air leaking inappropriately into the nose. It is entirely different from misarticulation or hypernasality, and consists of a "sniffing" or "snorting" sound caused by air leakage or "escaping" into the nose on a sound when the entire air stream should be directed through the mouth. The leakage may be through a fistula in the hard or soft palate or through an incompetent soft palate.

These distortions—*misarticulation, hyper-* or *hyponasality,* and *nasal escape*—interfere with the understandability or the *intelligibility* of the individual words or sentences. These are the four most important aspects of speech production that are studied in determining whether a child with a cleft is speaking correctly.

Another measure of speech proficiency concerns the child's ability to combine articulation sounds, such as the "s" and the "l" as in "slow" or the "s" and the "m" as in "small." To pronounce "small" the palatal port must first be closed, then opened and closed again. This maneuver must be performed quickly as in the words "simple" and "sample," which can be used to test the speed and agility of the repaired palate. Young children with normal palates gradually learn these skills, and the speech pathologist attempts to determine whether cleft palate children are developing sounds and words that are appropriate for their age and stage of development and also whether this can be done with consistency (Weatherley-White, Stark, and De Haan, 1965; Spriestersbach and Sherman, 1968; Van Demark, Morris, and Vandehaar, 1979; Brookshire, Lynch, and Fox, 1980; Trost, 1981; McWilliams, Morris, and Shelton, 1984).

A trained speech *pathologist* with a particular interest in the problems of cleft palate is a key member of the cleft palate team. Often school speech therapists do not have the insight to diagnose or treat these problems, although, with competent guidance, they can be of great help for speech training. The plastic surgeon who treats children with clefts should also be familiar with the details of speech production as well as with the *function* and *malfunction* of the speech mechanism. The plastic surgeon who examines the child with a cleft should listen to the speech of the patient and be able to assess the speech and the possible need for further therapy or surgery. He should have the skills and insight to understand what the speech pathologist might advise. The speech pathologist is needed for critical evaluation, diagnosis, and therapy management, but the surgeon must be able to understand the implications.

DENTAL OCCLUSION

Any cleft that does not involve the alveolus (i.e., a cleft of the palate only) should not disturb the anterior alveolar arch. Operative scarring in the region of the palatal shelves can cause midpalatal transverse constriction and an "hourglass" distortion of the maxillary arch, but the anterior dentition should be intact. Mandibular defects as seen in the Robin sequence can be associated with a number of problems of malocclusion, and although usually associated with a cleft of the palate, they are not directly due to the cleft.

A cleft involving the alveolus is a cleft of the prepalatal area and not a palatal cleft. Because of the proximity to the palate and the effect of palatal surgery on alveolar structures as well as the importance of the latter to speech, these structures will be briefly discussed. Clefting is thought to result from mesenchymal deficiencies (Stark, 1954). The deficiency is manifest in the alveolar area as a reduction in maxillary and premaxillary size and position. There usually is a vertical deficiency of bone in the region of the canine or premolar tooth (Jordan, Kraus, and Neptune, 1966). Adults who have had no surgery can have deficiencies, particularly in the area of vertical growth, but the facial profile, particularly the angle of convexity, usually approaches normal. Ortiz-Monasterio and associates (1966), who have studied unoperated adult patients with clefts, often are misquoted as saying that the unoperated adults have "normal facial growth." Actually, *none* has had normal facial growth or normal occlusion and all have had some deficiencies, except in this angle of convexity.

For two generations, Schweckendiek (1955, 1962; Schweckendiek and Doz, 1978) has intentionally delayed closure of the hard palate until the patient is 11 to 12 years of age to allow for facial growth unimpaired by surgical scar. The cases have been studied critically and were indeed found to have satisfactory facial growth but, unfortunately, poor speech (Morris, 1976; Bardach, Morris, and Olin, 1984). Part of the poor speech was attributed to the technique of soft palate closure (done at 6 months of age), but part was thought also to be due to the delay in hard palate closure. The improved results in facial growth have led many surgeons to plan early soft palate closure for speech production, to obturate the hard palate cleft with a dental plate, and to delay hard palate closure so as to allow maxillary growth. However, Cosman and Falk (1980) have documented significantly poorer speech in these patients in spite of "adequate" prosthetic obturation, and have advised against this delay. The authors of this chapter have found the same results in patients in whom hard palate closure was delayed, and, further, did not consider that it significantly improved the eventual occlusion in the permanent dentition (Morris, 1976; Henningsen, 1983; Bardach, Morris, and Olin, 1984; Witzel, Salyer, and Ross, 1984).

One must compare the priorities for improved speech production with better facial growth. Palatal surgery has been blamed for restriction of palatal growth, particularly when associated with extensive hard palate surgery, but Bardach and Mooney (1984) reported that in beagles any surgical closure of an artificially produced *cleft lip* causes a persistent compression force on the alveolus. Premaxillary structures often are flared anteriorly (labially) in the unrepaired unilateral prepalatal cleft, and extremely so in the unrepaired total bilateral prepalatal cleft. This is a condition seen only when the constricting forces of the intact lip are lost, as in the cleft lip deformity. In the uncleft child, there is a balance between the normal pressure of the intact lip on the labial side of the teeth and the pressure of the tongue on the lingual side. After a cleft lip repair, the force from the external structures is increased and the tongue may be retropositioned. In addition, these structures, particularly the lateral maxillary structures, often are deficient in bulk and virtually always are deficient at the cleft margin in vertical height. This deficiency is seen even in incomplete clefts. The abnormal compression of the lip, the inherent deficiency in bony bulk, and the added constriction of scar from surgery in this area early in life are factors that can interfere with normal bone growth and occlusion.

A wide variety of surgical procedures have also been advocated for hard palate closure, extending from the simple vomer flap closure to the raising of mucoperiosteal flaps from the maxilla for early alveolar reconstruction or hard palate closure, to an extreme recommendation in which Brophy (1923) placed wires transversely from one maxilla to the other in the buccal sulcus, achieving closure by twisting the wires until the cleft edges were approximated. Surgery today is less traumatic than in the past, but any surgical incision leaves residual scar and should be suspected of interfering with bone growth, until it is proved otherwise.

TIMING OF TREATMENT

The speech pathologist, recognizing that vocalization starts at birth, would prefer to have the speech mechanism intact as soon as possible. The orthodontist would like to have a minimal amount of surgical scarring in the palatal area until facial growth has been completed. Without an intact speech mechanism, the child with a cleft palate usually either substitutes a consonant he can produce for one that he cannot produce, or simply omits the sound he cannot make. A *glottal stop* is a stop plosive made by using the glottis instead of the tongue or the lips. It is similar to a gutteral "g." The older child with an unrepaired cleft palate usually can say "mama," since the "m" is a nasal consonant, although the "a" will have a hypernasal resonance. This is not very noticeable in the child with small nasal passages, rudimentary paranasal sinuses, and a high-pitched voice. "Dada," however, either is not attempted or is produced as a glottal "gaga," substituting the glottal "g" for "d," or as "aa-aa," simply omitting the "d" sound altogether. When *patterns of substitution and omission* become established in the mind and speech pattern of the older child, they are very difficult to change through speech therapy.

Infantile speech normally omits some sounds, such as the "s" in the final position, so that "bus" becomes "bu." The more complicated combination of consonant sounds, called "blends," such as the "str" in "strong," are not completely pronounced. A speech pathologist's expertise is essential to differentiate what is pathologic and what is within the normal range development.

In comparing these two problems, i.e., established misarticulation versus dental crossbites, the trade-off is not satisfactory. Established misarticulation is difficult to treat through speech therapy and can interfere drastically with development such as schooling and social activities. A simple crossbite usually is not difficult to treat orthodontically and interferes little with these activities. A major maxillary underdevelopment, on the other hand, which produces a severe crossbite and malocclusion, may be beyond orthodontic treatment and may require orthognathic surgery.

Rationale for Early Soft Palate Closure

The first three activities of the newborn infant, aside from moving arms and legs, are to take a deep breath, to utter a lusty cry, and shortly thereafter to start swallowing. To be accomplished normally, all three functions involve use of the soft palate, and each requires a rather complex sequence of muscular activity. The action of sucking and swallowing while intermittently breathing through the nose must require extremely complex neurologic control and programming.

Two of the functions, swallowing and respiratory movement, are normally active in the intrauterine period. What happens in the child with a cleft? At the time of birth, it is not unusual to see Passavant's ridge or an abnormal anterior bulging of the posterior pharyngeal wall, findings that may indicate incorrect compensatory programming as a neonate.

Another concern regarding this neurologic control may have significant bearing on the newborn with a palatal cleft. The neurologic control of the extraocular muscles in a child with true strabismus indicates that the usual system is sensitive to the effects of abnormal experience only during a limited time early in life when it is immature and plastic (Greenwald and Parks, 1983). Failure to correct the impairment at an early age may prevent the usual system from functioning normally. In some individuals, compensatory systems develop and the normal system may never be recalled into the control system. The compensatory mechanisms may allow for depth perception and tracking, but they are not comparable with the normal process. A songbird, isolated from sound during a critical time in development, never sings (Konishi, 1965). However, in the infant with a palatal cleft, involving similarly complex muscular functions that are used and needed well before sight develops, one wonders whether a similar pattern of neurologic control and development is taking place. If the soft palate "program" is not put to proper use early in life, perhaps it too will be bypassed, and substitute actions and controls will take its place. This reasoning would argue for early closure of the soft palate.

The question in cleft palate closure is how early is "early," and the answer at present is not known. In most series in which speech is compared with surgery performed at two different ages, the speech is better in the younger age group (Grabb, 1971; Evans and Renfrew, 1974). It had been traditional to close the palate cleft at 18 to 24 months of age. Today most soft palate clefts are repaired at 12 to 18 months. The authors would prefer to repair the soft palate cleft at 3 to 9 months, but as yet there are few hard data to confirm the benefits of early closure. Dorf and Curtin (1982), noting that persistent misarticulation is a difficult speech problem to care for in the older child, found this to be present in 86 per cent of children whose soft palates were closed between 12 and 24 months of age, and in only 10 per cent of children whose cleft palates were closed before 12 months of age (p <0.0001).

In the authors' patients, 48 per cent of the overall cleft population eventually required a secondary operation (usually a posterior pharyngeal flap) for velopharyngeal incompetence. This is a high percentage but it reflects a very critical evaluation of the speech results rather than an inferior surgical technique. In 17 patients whose soft palates were closed between 3 and 7 months of age and who could be evaluated carefully, the need for a pharyngeal flap was decreased to 13 per cent (p <0.001) (Randall and associates, 1983). There are many studies that do not provide hard data but suggest advantages in early soft palate closure. Kaplan (1981) reported that early repair was associated with an earlier onset of language, fewer speech errors, less middle ear disease, less parental tension, and a more rapid inclusion of the child into the family unit. The cleft of the palate had been closed at the same time as the cleft of the lip repair at age 3 to 6 months. Davies (1966) combined the palate repair with the lip repair in newborns (age 7 to 28 days). However, he now feels that this represents a great deal of surgery in the infant and should be reserved for those rare occasions when one probably would never see the child again after the first operation. Malek, Psaume, and Genton (1985) believed that closing the soft palate helps to position the tongue forward against the alveolus; they closed the soft palate in patients 3 months of age, and the lip and hard palate clefts three to four months later. The authors believe that patients who have had any difficulty maintaining an airway, such as those with the Robin sequence or the Treacher Collins syndrome, and those who are not thriving and doing well *should not be considered candidates for early soft palate closure.* These clefts should be repaired at 12 to 18 months of age.

In 1960, Stark suggested that a posterior pharyngeal flap adds little morbidity to the initial operation and, if done at the time of the soft palate closure ("primary posterior pharyngeal flap"), the child has the best opportunity for achieving velopharyngeal competence (Stark and Dehaan, 1960; Stark and Frileck, 1971). Others have argued that only 15 to 25 per cent of children with clefts ever require secondary pharyngoplasty. One would thus be adding the flap for 75 to 85 per cent of children who would not need it. Grabb (1975) set up a prospective double-blind randomized series to study this problem, and came to believe that those who had had primary posterior pharyngeal flaps were doing so much better than their counterparts without the flap that he discontinued the study. The authors have felt that a primary posterior pharyngeal flap was indicated if the primary surgery was delayed until 3 to 4 years of age, if the soft palate was particularly short or had little soft tissue, such as in the horseshoe-shaped defect, or if little levator muscle is found. Since 48 per cent of the clefts that were closed at 12 to 18 months of age in the authors' series eventually needed a secondary pharyngoplasty, the authors reasoned that by *not* doing a primary posterior pharyngeal flap in the 12 to 18 month age group, roughly half of the patients would have palatal incompetence persisting until the time that their faulty speech confirmed the diagnosis. This would be 2 to 5 years of age under the usual conditions. Such a long delay in providing an adequate speech mechanism could be extremely detrimental to speech in this group of children. This is the authors' reason for *considering* a primary posterior pharyngeal flap in those patients closed at the "late" age of 12 to 18 months.

Two additional points should be made concerning *primary* posterior pharyngeal flaps. First, the flaps performed at an early age need not and should not be very wide. They should be constructed by utilizing approximately one-half to two-thirds of the posterior pharyngeal wall. If they are too wide, there is a significant risk of nasorespiratory obstruction and sleep apnea. Second, and for the same reasons, a primary posterior pharyngeal flap is *not* advised in any patients whose soft palate is closed at 3 to 6 months of age. The authors have done six of these at the early age, and three had to be taken down because of severe sleep apnea (Barot, Cohen, and LaRossa, 1986). The primary posterior pharyngeal flap is also contraindicated in patients who have had any difficulty maintaining an airway, such as those with the Robin sequence or the Treacher Collins syndrome, and those who are not thriving (Randall and associates, 1983).

Early Orthodontic Therapy

McNeil (1954) and later Burston (1960) initiated the enthusiasm for early manipulation of the alveolar and maxillary segments with the purpose of improving dental arch alignment in the infant (*presurgical orthodontics*). The technique has since been improved and many have been encouraged by the results. At present, some surgeons virtually always use presurgical orthodontics, some use it occasionally, particularly in wide clefts, and some do not use it at all or have discontinued using it (Jolleys and Robertson, 1972; Hotz and associates, 1978).

There is no question that the bony segments can be moved easily and quickly, giving rise to the term "presurgical orthopedics."

Better arch alignment can be achieved in the newborn to facilitate lip closure. This is particularly helpful in the wide unilateral and in the bilateral cleft. A more permanent prosthesis with metal pins (see Chap. 57) that achieve fixation in the maxilla is preferred by others (Georgiade, 1970; Latham, Kusy, and Georgiade, 1976; Hagerty and Hagerty, 1985).

Perhaps the most critical evaluation is measured by the long-term results of early orthodontic therapy (either presurgical or postsurgical) on the deciduous teeth and the *eventual occlusion in the permanent dentition.* While it is easy to see a difference and a change as a result of early orthodontic (or orthopedic) therapy in the infant, Huddart (1979, 1984), in a well-controlled series, showed that these early efforts had virtually *no effect* on the eventual occlusion in the *permanent dentition.* Although the authors' studies are not as well controlled, the impression has been the same. At present, the authors rarely use orthodontic or orthopedic appliances before the eruption of the permanent dentition. Much of the improvement in the alignment of the alveolar segments before lip surgery can also be achieved with a lip adhesion operation, which is a more natural and a more gentle way of achieving the same goal (Randall, 1965).

In the severe bilateral cleft, some surgeons prefer to expand the maxillary segments early in life and to move the premaxilla back into the maxillary arch (see Chap. 53) (Latham, Kusy, and Georgiade, 1976). Repositioning of the premaxilla in a dorsal direction should be approached with the knowledge that, in the bilateral cleft, the most *deficient* growth over the next dozen years is likely to be in the anterior-posterior direction so that eventually, in the adolescent and adult with a bilateral cleft, one is likely to be struggling with *retrusion* of the middle third of the face and a Class III malocclusion, rather than the *protruding premaxilla* seen in the newborn.

For these reasons, the authors have been treating the premaxilla in a different way, leaving it in the anterior position and "locked out" of the maxillary arch. The maxillary segments are collapsed behind the premaxilla during early life. With the eruption of the permanent dentition, the maxillary arches are expanded; the premaxilla is appropriately positioned into the arch; and the alveolar

clefts are grafted with autogenous cancellous bone and closed with gingival flaps (see Chap. 55). A study of 24 children with bilateral clefts who reached the age of 18 to 21 years showed a satisfactory profile with minimal midface retrusion (Mayro, LaRossa, and Randall, 1985). Only two of these patients had, or needed, orthognathic surgery. This plan is not without its problems, and some of the children, at 5 to 8 years of age, have an abnormally prominent premaxilla that is disfiguring. In these patients, the authors believe that a compromise must be made and earlier expansion is carried out. Some of the patients have also had a marked overbite with the upper incisor teeth positioned over the lower incisor teeth. At the time of bone grafting, patients with this problem require an osteotomy to reposition the premaxilla more superiorly.

Bone Grafting

Bone grafting of the alveolus has long been a concern in both unilateral and bilateral clefts with alveolar involvement. It seems that with a deficiency of bone it is helpful to fill the gap at an early age and to provide a "keystone" in the deficient arch (see Chap. 55). After this concept was eagerly adopted by many with bone grafting in the first year of life, Pruzansky and Aduss (1964) pointed out that there was no good evidence to show that this was worthwhile. Studies also appeared showing that early bone grafting tended to restrain rather than supplement maxillary growth, and the technique was largely abandoned (Kling, 1964, 1966; Johanson, 1966; Rehrmann, Koberg, and Koch, 1970; Jolleys and Robertson, 1972). At the present time, Nylen and associates (1974), Rosenstein and associates (1982), and Nordin and associates (1983) have continued to bone graft the alveolar segments at an early age and have had impressive data showing satisfactory facial growth, good arch formation, and well-reconstructed alveolar ridges.

Bone grafts in the alveolar cleft not only tend to stabilize the adjacent bony segments, particularly in the complete bilateral cleft, but also provide a matrix into which the adjacent permanent teeth can erupt. Without the bony matrix, the teeth usually angle away from the alveolar ridge and erupt in a diagonal direction. In addition, with full eruption of the permanent teeth, the teeth adjacent to the cleft on either side have little bone on the cleft side of the tooth root extending to the apex of the tooth. Frequently, the teeth are deformed, the roots being angled away from the cleft. This represents an unstable situation, and the teeth adjacent to the cleft may be lost or abandoned in early life.

The authors are enthusiastic about the protocol of the Norwegian team Abyholm, Borchgrevink, Bergland, and Semb (Abyholm, Bergland, and Semb, 1981; Bergland, Semb, and Abyholm, 1986; Bergland and associates, 1986). Cancellous bone is packed into the cleft at 9 to 11 years of age when the adjacent permanent teeth are erupting. Coverage is achieved with flaps of gingival mucosa. This tends to augment the deficient alveolus, to stabilize the "floating premaxilla" in the bilateral clefts, to provide a matrix into which adjacent teeth can erupt, and to provide thick bony support along the entire tooth root to stabilize the teeth adjacent to the cleft. In the past, badly displaced teeth were often removed; today, many permanent teeth can be saved. Mucosal coverage in this area, in the past, was achieved with a flap of buccal mucosa. This tissue is readily available and easily transferred, but it does not provide ideal gingival mucosa; the teeth also do not erupt as well through this tissue. Flaps of gingival mucosa are far more satisfactory for alveolar reconstruction. They can be elevated widely, undermined, and shifted with little difficulty. Nonabsorbable or slowly absorbable sutures are needed, because these tissues heal much more slowly than other mucosal flaps. A completely watertight closure over the bone graft is not absolutely necessary.

Bonded orthodontic appliances are often left in place during the bone grafting operation to ensure the best positioning of the adjacent teeth and to stabilize movable segments while the bone graft is becoming vascularized. A postoperative retainer plate can be used for the same purpose, although fitting a retainer over edematous mucosal flaps is somewhat difficult. Replacement of teeth is best achieved by bonding them in a semipermanent fashion to the adjacent teeth. These so-called "Maryland bridges" are effective but they require that the adjacent teeth be sound and stable. A bonded bridge is not strong enough to stabilize a movable premaxilla in the complete bilateral cleft. In this situation the stress of a limited dental bridge bonded to adjacent teeth with an unstable premaxilla is too great. If the premaxilla is unstable and prosthetic replacement of teeth is needed, an anterior plate or shell containing the missing teeth is required or the alveolar arches must be stabilized first with a bone graft. If bone grafting is done before orthodontic bonding, orthodontic therapy should be begun about three months after bone grafting (Bergland, Semb, and Abyholm, 1986).

A two-layer mucosal closure of alveolar and hard palate fistulas usually leaves an appreciable amount of "dead space" between the nasal and oral closure. There is often a disappointingly high incidence of fistula recurrence. When the dead space is filled with bone or other similar material (such as hydroxyapatite), few fistulas recur (Schultz, 1986). One disadvantage of hydroxyapatite compared with cancellous bone is that it solidifies like cement; consequently, it is virtually impossible to move adjacent teeth into it and teeth cannot erupt through it.

OTOLOGY

In the past, most patients with clefts of the soft palate had chronic middle ear infections, extensive scarring, and significant permanent hearing loss. Masters, Bingham, and Robinson (1960) reported a 45 per cent incidence of a 40 decibel *permanent* loss of hearing in one or both ears in teenagers. Stool and Randall (1967) and Paradise and Bluestone (Paradise and Bluestone, 1969; Bluestone, 1971; Bluestone, Wittel, and Paradise, 1972) reported almost constant middle ear effusion in infants with palatal clefts. The effusion is not the usual serous otitis fluid seen intermittently in younger children, but is a thick, tenacious, inspissated material apparently associated with incompetent eustachian tube function. Indeed, Schultz (1986) in 1970 produced surgical clefts in the soft palate in rabbits, and within weeks he consistently found pieces of grass in the middle ear. The attachment of the levator palatini muscles and the tensor palatini muscles to the cartilaginous portion of the eustachian tubes appears to be critical for normal eustachian tube function. When these muscles do not function normally (as in the unrepaired cleft), the eustachian tube orifice can be incompetent. There is evidence that palatal repair at least partly reestablishes eustachian tube competence (Bluestone and Stool, 1983).

Early examination of the ears by a qualified otolaryngologist, with prompt evacuation of middle ear fluid and insertion of ventilating tubes or grommets in the tympanic incision, has become routine. This approach, plus the vigilance of the otolaryngologist and the concerned parent aiming to treat middle ear infection early in the process, rather than late, has reduced the incidence of permanent hearing loss, cholesteatoma, tympanic membrane scarring, perforation, and atrophy. Since hearing is so critical for speech production, improved hearing is extremely valuable (Spriestersbach and associates, 1962; McWilliams, Morris, and Shelton, 1984).

SURGICAL TECHNIQUE

The child must be in good health and free from acute respiratory tract infections. With a cleft open into the nose there usually is mucopurulent material in the nasopharynx, but this should not interfere with surgery.

The foot pad of the operating table is put at the head of the table about halfway onto the head rest, so that the child can be placed with the head on the foot pad for intubation, and then moved slightly to the head of the table with the foot pad under the shoulders after intubation. In this way the head can be extended adequately by dropping the head rest, allowing satisfactory vision for the surgeon sitting or standing at the head of the table.

General anesthesia is used with an oral endotracheal tube, which is taped to the midline of the chin; an intravenous line and cardiac monitors are employed. It is helpful to use the anesthesiologist's laryngoscope to inject the operative area with small amounts of lidocaine 1 per cent and epinephrine 1/100,000 before the surgeon prepares the skin and drapes the patient. In this way at least seven to ten minutes elapse before the surgical incisions are made. A Dingman mouth gag (Dingman and Grabb, 1962) is used for maximal exposure.

Perioperative antibiotics may help to reduce postoperative fever and to facilitate more rapid resumption of oral intake and a shortened hospital stay (Jolleys and Savage, 1963; McClelland and Patterson, 1963; Duffy, 1966; LaRossa, Vaniver, and Randall, 1986).

Double Reversing Z-Plasty

In recent years the authors have preferred the "double reversing Z-plasty" technique (Fig. 54–9) described by Furlow (Furlow, 1980, 1986; Randall and associates, 1986) for cleft palate repair.

The "double Z" operation consists of two Z-plasties, one on the oral mucosa of the soft palate and the other in the reverse orientation on the nasal mucosa of the soft palate. The levator muscle is included in the posteriorly based mucosal flap of the Z-plasty so that the levator muscle on one side is included in the posteriorly based *oral* mucosal flap and the levator muscle from the opposite side is included in the posteriorly based *nasal* mucosal flap. The hard palate cleft is closed by a vomer flap in one or two layers. Because the palatal shelves are displaced upward, it is possible to raise small mucoperiosteal flaps from the oral mucosa at the edges of the cleft in the hard palate and to achieve a two-layer closure in the hard palate. This leaves dead space but has not caused a problem. The advantages of this operation are that it lengthens the soft palate within the substance of the soft palate, making it unnecessary to raise large mucoperiosteal flaps from the hard palate, with possible retardation of midfacial growth. In addition, the Furlow operation reorients the malposition of the levator muscles; allows approximation of the muscles in an overlapped position; reduces the amount of dissection around the muscles; and avoids a straight midline incision in the soft palate, which has the potential of contracting and shortening the length of the palate. It can be used with a primary posterior pharyngeal flap if desired and it can also be used as a secondary operation if lengthening and reorientation of the levator muscles are desired.

As noted by Furlow (1980, 1986), it is probably easiest for the right-handed surgeon to place the posteriorly based oral mucomuscular flap on the patient's left side. The length and the limit of the Z-plasty vary *inversely* with the width of the cleft: usually one would expect that the wider the void, the larger the required flap should be, but the reverse is true. The reason is that one is sacrificing width to gain length in a Z-plasty, and if the cleft is wide there simply is not much width to use. Furlow does not agree with this and uses a large flap even in a wide cleft, but he

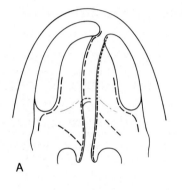

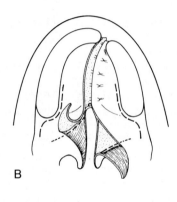

Figure 54–9. The Furlow "double Z-plasty" operation. The levator muscle is included in the posteriorly based flap of the *oral* mucosal Z-plasty, and the levator from the other side is included in the posteriorly based *nasal* mucosal flap. The Z-plasty in the nasal mucosa is the reverse of the one in the oral mucosa. *A,* The incisions. *B,* The anterior palate is closed with a vomer flap (see Fig. 54–10). *C,* The nasal mucosal closure. Note that the levator muscle has been re-oriented in a transverse direction. *D,* Suturing completed. By achieving lengthening within the soft palate, large mucoperiosteal flaps from the hard palate are avoided. In addition, the orientation of the levator muscles is improved and they are closed in an overlapped position.

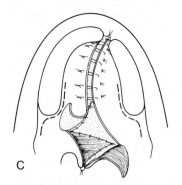

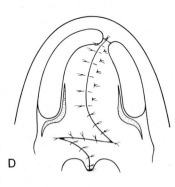

notes that at times it does not reach the lateral apex of the recipient incision. Regardless of the size of the mucosal flaps, the full amount of the underlying levator muscle can be used, which is usually larger than the size of the mucosal flaps. The incision for the anteriorly based oral mucosal flap of the Z-plasty is not made at the classical 60 degree angle with the cleft margin, but more at an 80 degree angle. The levator muscle from the opposite side thus has less tendency to be bound down to the posterior edge of the hard palate and lies more in the transverse position.

Furlow (1986) does not recommend lateral relaxing incisions, but the authors do not hesitate to use them if the closure appears to be tight. The cleft margins are *incised* longitudinally and the margins of the uvula are *excised* so as to provide a broader approximation of the cleft at this level. The oral mucosa and submucosa of the soft palate are thick, and the dissection is taken down to the levator muscle by making the incision for the anteriorly based mucosal flap first. In this way the location of the levator muscle can be ascertained. The dissection is continued between the oral mucosa and the levator muscle

on the patient's right side, progressing anteriorly to the posterior edge of the bony palate. The dissection is continued anteriorly along the cleft margin to the alveolus or the anterior extent of the cleft by using a small dental elevator to lift the mucoperiosteum off the hard palate for a short distance laterally. Similar elevation is carried out on the left side, extending from front to back and continuing on the oral side of the levator muscle. The elevator is used to lift the nasal mucosa off the hard palate so that the plane of dissection between the levator muscle on the left side and the nasal mucosa can be clearly defined. The levator muscle is separated from its attachment to the palatal bone. A toothed bayonet forceps is useful to grasp the tip of the posteriorly based oral mucomuscular flap in a gentle manner, and the dissection is carried out carefully between the muscle and the thin nasal mucosa. The levator muscle is bluntly dissected from the adjacent tissue so as not to injure its nerve or vascular supply. The posteriorly based oral mucomuscular flap is completely dissected so that it can be shifted easily into the transverse position.

The anteriorly based nasal mucosal flap can then be developed with ease by cutting from posterior to anterior with a pair of scissors. The lateral extent of the cut is located close to the eustachian tube. The anteriorly based nasal mucosal flap is the one most likely to be in short supply when the nasal mucosa is being sutured; additional length can be obtained by placing its distal tip close to the base of the uvula.

The posteriorly based nasal mucomuscular flap is dissected. The right levator muscle is detached from its bony attachment and is released by cutting the nasal mucosa, leaving an anterior edge for suturing and again extending laterally close to the eustachian tube.

A wide-based flap of nasal mucosa is elevated from the vomer with the base oriented superiorly, and is used for hard palate closure. In bilateral clefts vomer flaps are obtained from each side of the vomer. This maneuver completely avoids the need for large mucoperiosteal flaps from the hard palate and should minimize late growth disturbances of the maxilla.

If closure of the mucomuscular flaps seems excessively tight, lateral relaxing incisions can be employed. These are started in the oral mucosa at a point anterior to the anterior tonsillar pillar at the lateral edge of the soft palate, and they extend anteriorly to a position just lateral to the posterior maxillary tubercle. They pass around the maxillary tubercle and anteriorly through the mucoperiosteum of the hard palate between the major palatine vessels and the gingiva. Scissors are used to open the space lateral to the soft palate musculature (space of Ernst) and to liberate the tissues of the soft palate. The pterygoid hamulus can be fractured medially if desired (with a greenstick fracture), and this apparently can be done with impunity so far as the function of the tensor palatini muscles is concerned. There appears to have been no interference with eustachian tube function in a group of patients in whom this was done on one side and not on the other (Noone and associates, 1973). The mucoperiosteum can be elevated laterally from the hard palate, dissecting around the palatine foramen and stretching the major palatine vessels for a short distance out of the foramen if necessary. Jackson (1986) noted that the mucosa stretches rather quickly even during the time of the operation; after closure of the palate cleft, he also closes the relaxing incisions sequentially until they are completely closed.

The palatal incisions are closed with one layer of sutures on the nasal mucosa and another on the oral mucosa. A 4-0 chromic catgut suture is used on the mucomuscular flaps, and either 4-0 or 5-0 chromic on the uvula and vomer flaps. A single suture is also placed approximating the anterior edge at the midportion of the two muscular flaps to each other, so as to minimize any dead space in this area.

The vomer is closed with mattress sutures, achieving a good deal of overlap with the opposite oral mucoperiosteal flap, and the edges of the hard palate mucoperiosteal flaps are approximated with mattress sutures (Fig. 54–10).

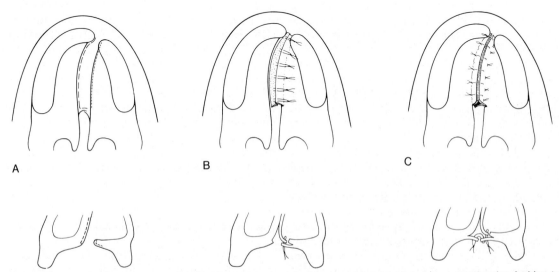

Figure 54–10. Vomer flap. *A*, Elevation of the vomer flap. *B*, The vomer flap is sutured in an overlapping fashion to the opposite oral mucosal flap. *C*, Completed two-layer closure. Upper inset—oral view. Lower inset—coronal view.

If the mucomuscular flaps of the Z-plasties or the mucosal flaps of the Z-plasty are too short to reach the desired positions laterally, they can be sutured just short of the apex of the incisions, and the incisions can be closed in a "Y" rather than a "V" configuration. On the nasal side a raw area is left laterally if closure was difficult, since the oral flaps provide ample coverage.

It should be noted that a primary posterior pharyngeal flap can also be inserted at the time of the soft palate closure. Lining flaps of mucosa can be raised from the mucosa posterior to the Z-plasty and based at the free edge of the soft palate. Usually a superiorly based posterior pharyngeal flap is preferred, with lining flaps from the nasal mucosa. The posterior pharyngeal flap is not wide (about one-half to two-thirds of the posterior pharyngeal wall) and primary closure of the donor site is achieved.

The most likely area for an oronasal fistula is at the junction of the hard and soft palate closure. However, this has occurred in only three of the authors' first 112 patients. When soft palate closure is done at the same time as the cleft lip repair, the hard palate cleft is left open and closed three to six months later. This is done to reduce the amount of surgery in the infant, and also to keep from occluding the nasal airway completely. Infants are usually obligatory nose breathers, so that an adequate nasal airway is essential postoperatively. In addition, by closing the cleft of the lip and the cleft in the soft palate simultaneously, a dramatic narrowing of the hard palate cleft occurs. In fact, if the second step of closure of the hard palate cleft is unduly delayed, the cleft can become so narrow as to make it almost impossible to achieve a two-layer closure.

At the end of the operation a large (No. 18 to 22 French) nasopharyngeal airway is placed and taped securely in place. A heavy 2-0 silk suture is placed deeply in the tongue, tied as a loop, and taped loosely to the cheek. Tension by hand on the tongue suture may be needed to help maintain an adequate airway postoperatively, particularly if the child has a borderline airway. This must be done by holding the stitch manually, since taping it under tension is not reliable.

The ears are always inspected by an otolaryngologist either immediately before or after the palate repair. Most of the time serositis is encountered; myringotomies are performed; and the fluid is aspirated and ventilating tubes are placed in the myringotomy incisions. Antibiotic drops are placed in the ears.

Intravelar Veloplasty

Kriens (1970, 1975) clearly emphasized the abnormal orientation of the levator palatini muscles, and the need to detach them from their insertion on the posterior edge of the palatal bone and reorient the muscles in the transverse direction (see Chap. 51). Kriens sutured the muscles end to end, but they usually are long enough for an overlap of the muscles to be achieved and a tighter levator sling obtained.

Before the Furlow operation this was the authors' preferred method of soft palate closure. However, the muscles have to be dissected completely free from both the oral and the nasal mucosa, which could increase fibrosis. A three-layer closure is used with the same suture material as previously noted.

If added length is needed in the nasal mucosal closure (as when a lengthening procedure is done on the hard palate), the authors prefer to use a large Z-plasty in the nasal mucosa of the soft palate, as described by Stark (1963). Cronin (1957, 1971) also described an ingenious method of obtaining nasal mucosa flaps from the hard palate for lining of the soft palate.

If the intravelar veloplasty is not done, it is important at least to cut the levator muscles from their attachment to the posterior edge of the hard palate and to suture them in the midline, otherwise the levator muscles add virtually nothing to soft palate excursion. In the authors' series additional improvement in speech was achieved by reorienting the muscle as in the intravelar veloplasty (Brown, Cohen, and Randall, 1983; Dreyer and Trier, 1984). Further improvement has been obtained by using the Furlow technique and also by operating in patients 3 to 9 months of age instead of 12 to 18 months (Dorf and Curtin, 1982; Randall and associates, 1983).

von Langenbeck Operation

The von Langenbeck (1859, 1861) operation is an established procedure that includes the

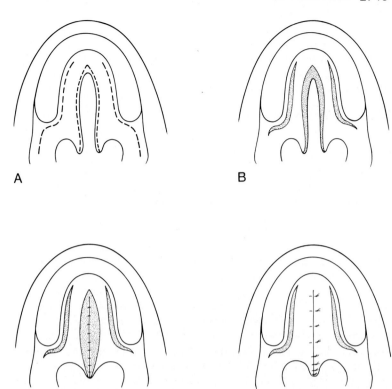

A

B

C

D

Figure 54–11. The von Langenbeck operation. *A,* Tho incisions. *B,* The mucosa of the hard palate is elevated between the bone and periosteum. The major palatal vessels are identified and stretched out of their canals. *C,* The nasal mucosa is closed and the muscles sutured side to side after being detached from their insertion. *D,* The oral closure.

elevation of large mucoperiosteal flaps from the hard palate (Fig. 54–11). It is a side to side approximation of the cleft margins of both the hard and soft palate, with detachment of the levator muscles from their bony insertions and the use of long relaxing incisions laterally. It does not include a lengthening maneuver.

The edges of the cleft are incised from the alveolus to the base of the uvula, the sides of which are excised. Relaxing incisions are made from the anterior tonsillar pillar at the lateral edge of the soft palate to a point lateral to the posterior maxillary tubercle. The incision passes around the tubercle, anterior between the major palatine vessels and the gingiva, up to approximately the level of the premolar teeth.

The incision is carried through the periosteum, and the mucoperiosteum is lifted widely off the bone with a blunt elevator. Lateral relaxing incisions are opened widely in both the soft and hard palate areas. Scissors are used bluntly posteriorly, and the dissection is carried along the posterior edge of the hard palate and around the major palatine vessels. The hamulus process may be fractured.

The hard palate mucoperiosteum is also elevated widely between the cleft margins from the lateral relaxing incisions. A vomer flap can be elevated to provide a two-layer hard palate closure.

The dissection is carried around the major palatine vessels. With an elevator on either side of the vessels they are firmly but gently stretched out of the canal. If this does not achieve sufficient length to allow approximation of the hard palate mucoperiosteal flaps without tension, additional lengthening can be achieved by cutting between the vessels and the mucoperiosteal flap. The vessels course along the nasal side of this flap and can be dissected away safely from it for 6 to 10 mm if necessary (Edgerton, 1962).

The levator muscle is detached completely from its bony attachment. A finger is placed in the lateral relaxing incision and the soft palate musculature is pressed toward the midline until suturing can be accomplished without tension.

Closure is achieved in three layers in the soft palate, using 4-0 or 5-0 chromic catgut sutures. End-on mattress sutures are preferred on the oral mucosa, particularly in the hard palate, to prevent inversion of the mucosal edges, which can lead to fistula formation. As previously mentioned, a two-layer closure can be achieved in the hard palate by elevating a vomer flap based superiorly and suturing this past the oral mucosal closure, using through and through sutures through the mucoperiosteal flaps.

Wardill-Kilner-Veau Operation

Most palate repairs that fail to achieve velopharyngeal competence do so either because there is insufficient motion in the soft palate or the entire repaired palate is not long enough. To increase the anteroposterior length of the palate at the time of primary palatoplasty, various mucoperiosteal flap maneuvers in the hard palate have been recommended. The Wardill-Kilner operation (Fig. 54–12) is somewhat similar to that developed by Veau (Veau, 1931; Wardill, 1937; Kilner, 1937). A V-Y lengthening operation is done in the tissues of the mucoperiosteum of the hard palate. The rigid mucoperiosteum probably maintains the length that is achieved, although a similar amount of lengthening must be obtained in the nasal

mucosa of the soft palate. The authors prefer a large nasal mucosa Z-plasty as described by Stark (1963), although the Cronin flaps (1971) from the mucosa of the nasal floor can also be used.

The V-Y lengthening procedure invariably leaves bare membranous bone exposed in the area from which the flaps were taken. These areas usually granulate quickly and epithelize promptly within two to three weeks. However, they remain as areas of fibrous scar and probably are the most likely cause of distortions in maxillary growth and dental occlusion (Kremenak, Huffman, and Olin, 1967; Bardach and Salyer, 1987). Lateral and anterior crossbites with maxillary collapse, in the authors' experience, are more frequently seen in the von Langenbeck operation and most often seen in the Wardill-Kilner operation. They are infrequent when hard palate repair is achieved with a vomer flap in a one- or two-layer closure by simply elevating the mucoperiosteum adjacent to the cleft.

Perko (1979) attempted to minimize this contraction by elevating the hard palate mucosal flaps between the mucosa and the periosteum. This probably does reduce scar contraction, as the bare area will now be covered

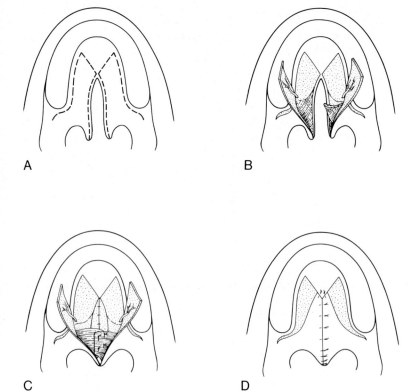

Figure 54–12. The Wardill-Kilner operation. *A,* A V-Y lengthening gains length but leaves an exposed area of bone that granulates and epithelizes. *B,* The levator muscles are detached, reoriented, and sutured either end-on or in an overlapped position. *C,* Nasal closure and muscle approximation. *D,* Oral closure.

A

B

C

D

by periosteum, but the dissection in this plane must be done sharply and is difficult. It also deprives the flaps of their major blood supply.

Innumerable other approaches to gain length in the palate have been suggested. Flaps of buccal mucosa based posterior to the maxillary tubercle can be used for both oral and nasal mucosal supplementation (Kaplan, 1975a). However, the mucosa is loose and lacks stiffness. There once was enthusiasm for a unilateral or bilateral island flap of hard palate mucoperiosteal tissue taken from the anterior hard palate, based on a long segment of the palatine vessels and repositioned transversely behind the hard palate at its junction with the soft palate on the oral side, the nasal side, or both sides (Millard, 1966). However, this maneuver left such a large area of denuded bone anteriorly that severe bone growth disruption and malocclusion usually resulted.

PROSTHETIC OBTURATION

During the 1930's and 1940's the results of palatal surgery, particularly in the United States, were often poor. It was not unusual to see teenagers who had had multiple operations on their palates and ended up with scarred, immobile soft palates, multiple fistulas and distorted maxillae, dental malocclusion, and impaired speech. The orthodontists and prosthodontists of that era achieved heroic improvement with these cleft palate cripples. This led to a feeling that perhaps every cleft or at least every wide cleft should be treated with a dental prosthesis obturating the anterior cleft, and using a bulb extension beyond the soft palate and into the pharynx so that the superior pharyngeal constrictor could valve against it (see Chap. 72).

Even the best speech results with the obturated palates were usually not nearly as good as the best speech results following surgery. Furthermore, such a prosthesis puts great stress on the remaining teeth, which are already subject to increased dental caries and less than the usual amount of bone support. Today, "primary" prosthetic closure of even wide clefts probably has no place if state of the art surgery and anesthesia are available. On the other hand, some patients are extremely poor surgical risks or almost impossible to intubate (such as those with severe Treacher Collins syndrome or the Robin sequence), and a primary prosthesis can be a satisfactory alternative. Finally, if poor surgery has been followed by scarring, fistulas, and extremely poor tissue with which to work, a dental appliance with a speech bulb remains a satisfactory salvage maneuver (Mazaheri, 1962; Shelton and associates, 1968; Blakeley, 1969; Adisman, 1971).

POSTOPERATIVE CARE

Patients are observed carefully in the anesthetic recovery room for at least an hour. Infants under 12 months of age are kept for an additional hour at minimum. If there is concern about the airway or the child's general condition, the patient is transferred to the intensive care unit, but this is not usually required. The fingertip pulse oxygen monitor is a helpful guide to the postoperative aeration.

Mothers are encouraged to hold their children, because these patients are usually irritable for 24 to 48 hours and sedation can depress the respiratory center severely. Meperidine hydrochloride (Demerol) is used sparingly for sedation (0.75 mg/kg) or codeine is given (0.5 mg/kg). Patients are watched carefully to check for an adequate airway, oxygenation, color, respiration, secretions, and bleeding. Suction can be used in the anterior mouth or through the nasopharyngeal tube. Intravenous fluids are given to keep the children well hydrated; full liquids are offered by mouth, usually the afternoon of surgery, by way of a rubber-tipped syringe or from a cup. Usually the intravenous line and the tongue suture can be removed 24 to 48 hours after surgery. *A bottle with a nipple is not used,* as undue negative pressure on the suture line can conceivably produce disruption. Arm cuffs (elbow splints) are used continuously except when the child is bathed and are maintained for three weeks. Soft baby food or junior foods by way of a spoon, syringe, or cup are usually started on the third day after surgery. Feedings are followed by water to clear food particles. Patients are usually discharged two to four days after surgery on a soft diet. This diet and routine are continued for three weeks, after which the arm cuffs are removed and a normal diet and feeding techniques are resumed.

After discharge, patients are seen in the office at ten days, or sooner if there is any concern about their condition. They are seen again at three weeks, at which time they can usually return to normal feedings and care. Mothers are encouraged to talk with their children and to encourage any kind of verbal expression. Within three to six months of complete closure of the palate, the mothers are also asked to encourage sucking and blowing games such as sucking through straws, blowing bubbles through a straw using soap bubble pipes, and using whistles or mouth organs. This should be done several times a day to stimulate velopharyngeal closure. If the hard palate cleft has been left open, the children are seen two months after surgery. If healing is satisfactory with narrowing of the hard palate cleft, they are scheduled for hard palate–vomer flap closure in two to three months. Children are usually seen by the plastic surgeon again in six months, and by 18 to 24 months of age they are examined by the whole cleft palate team. The otolaryngologist usually sees the children at monthly or three-monthly intervals.

When the patient is seen in the cleft palate clinic, the parents are asked how the child is progressing, what verbalization he or she is producing, what words can be produced easily, and with which ones there is difficulty. They are asked about the child's ability to blow bubbles, to whistle, and to drink through a straw. They are questioned as to whether there is any leakage of food or liquid into the nose, particularly chocolate milk, chocolate ice cream, or chocolate pudding. They are also asked whether there have been any continuing ear problems.

Even in patients of 6 to 12 months of age, some evaluation can usually be made as to how the speech is progressing—whether the child can produce a "b," "t," "d," or "s" sound, and whether or not there is an abnormal hypernasal quality. Almost any sample of relaxed conversational speech is of great value in assessing palatal function.

After this evaluation has been made, the palate is inspected with a tongue blade and light. The general appearance is noted and any evidence of fistula or breakdown is sought. If the child is old enough he is asked to say "kah, kah, kah." The excursion of the soft palate is noted and the movement of the velum straight back or more to one side than the other is recorded. In addition, an attempt is made to determine the amount of lateral and posterior pharyngeal wall motion. A slight amount of lateral pharyngeal wall movement is usually seen; an *excess* of movement may indicate a *decreased* amount of palatal movement, with a compensatory attempt at closure by using the superior pharyngeal constrictor muscles. Occasionally, even an anterior bulge of the posterior pharyngeal wall can be seen (Passavant's ridge), additional evidence of inadequate soft palate movement. After verbalization, a quick attempt is made to elicit a gag reflex and to see if further palatal and pharyngeal movement is possible.

A metal mirror held under the nostril is used while the child pronounces words with sibilant sounds to determine whether there is fogging and an abnormal escape of air through the nose. The mirror can also be used with nasal consonants to see if the nasal airway is adequate or obstructed.

Patients are usually seen in the cleft palate clinic by the plastic surgeon, the speech pathologist, the pedodontist and/or orthodontist, the pediatrician, and the otolaryngologist. Screening hearing tests and tympanography are carried out, and in the authors' clinic a physical anthropologist also examines the child.

If the child is doing well in all respects, particularly in regard to speech, nothing further is recommended except continued speech stimulation at home, good dental hygiene, and careful observation for ear infections. The parents are urged to treat the child as normally as they would a child without a cleft, and not to provide undue protection or limitations of activity. A return visit is usually scheduled within one year. If the child's speech is not progressing satisfactorily, definitive steps are taken (see Chap. 58), or the child is seen within a three to six month period for further evaluation.

COMPLICATIONS

Bleeding

One of the major complications of cleft palate surgery is bleeding. It does little good to inject the palate with a vasoconstrictor and to start operating immediately. One should wait at least seven minutes after completing the injection for full effectiveness. It is also helpful to have a little head tilt to the table.

Under these conditions the field should be dry with little need for suction.

If there is much bleeding during the operation, the surgeon can simply stop, place a moist gauze on the field, and hold pressure for three to four minutes. In the worst of bleeding, if pressure is held seven to ten minutes and the gauze sponge removed, the surgeon usually has five to ten seconds of a dry field and opportunity to pick up a bleeding point with a hemostat or even a suture ligature. Bleeding at the end of the operation must be controlled because it is bound to become worse as the child awakens and the epinephrine disappears. The area can be reinjected; suture ligatures can be used; cauterization with a disposable suction cautery is useful, or packing with a hemostatic agent or simply Vaseline gauze soaked in balsam of Peru or Whitehead's varnish. Packing can be sutured over a bleeding spot and removed three to four days later.

Airway Maintenance

The airway is a major concern in the postoperative cleft palate patient. A No. 18 or 20 French nasopharyngeal airway tube is excellent for maintaining an airway in the infant and young child. It is secured with tape or a suture *through the alar base* and is left in for 12 to 48 hours or longer. A tongue stitch looped and loosely taped to the cheek represents another precautionary measure.

Dehiscence

Dehiscence or breakdown is fortunately rare. If it is due to an injury such as falling down with a spoon in the mouth in the first two to three weeks, it can be repaired immediately. If it is a gradual breakdown with more than the usual amount of inflammation, resuturing probably will not hold and can be detrimental by adding more trauma and more foreign material to the area. Under these conditions, it is better to let the infection subside and to allow the tissues to soften before repair is attempted. It often takes four to six months before the tissues are in satisfactory condition. A slight dehiscence of the uvula is frequently seen and is probably of no consequence.

Oronasal Fistula

A persistent oronasal fistula is bothersome. If tiny it may cause little if any trouble. Larger fistulas leak fluid and air and can distort articulation. Leakage from the nose is embarrassing. Impacted food particles in a crevice or fistula can produce malodorous breath. Small fistulas in the alveolus or prealveolar area often are almost asymptomatic.

The repair of a fistula, except when tiny, can be difficult. Repeat surgery should not be attempted until the area is thoroughly healed and inflammation has completely subsided. Furthermore, the healing process is often accompanied by diminution in the size of the fistula. It occasionally closes completely. Persistent fistulas represent a problem in which a large operation is needed for a small defect.

A soft palate fistula can frequently be excised and the defect closed in two to three layers. In the hard palate, however, this is much more difficult, as the tissue is not elastic and a sizable adjacent flap is often needed. The flaps must be freed up sufficiently to fall into place or they are likely to fail (see Chap. 56).

In the alveolus and anterior hard palate, a simple two-layer closure normally leaves a dead space between the nasal and oral closure. Secondary breakdown is frequently seen. On the other hand, the insertion of autogenous bone taken from the ilium, cranium, or rib and placed between the layers of closure (nasal and oral mucosa) has been found to be very successful (see Chap. 55). If the area has completed growth, if the alveolus does not have to be moved orthodontically, and if the permanent dentition is fully erupted, hydroxyapatite as a block or as granules is a good substitute. However, hydroxyapatite has no flexibility or "give" as does autogenous bone. In large alveolar and hard palate defects, hydroxyapatite can be placed posteriorly and autogenous bone can be used anteriorly. Gingival mucosal flaps provide the best coverage in the alveolar area.

REFERENCES

Abyholm, F. E., Bergland, O., and Semb, G.: Secondary bone grafting of alveolar clefts. Scand. J. Plast. Reconstr. Surg., *15*:127, 1981.

Adisman, I. K.: Cleft palate prosthetics. *In* Grabb, W. C., Rosenstein, S. W., and Bzoch, K. R. (Eds.): Cleft

Lip and Palate: Surgical, Dental, and Speech Aspects. Boston, Little, Brown & Company, 1971.

Bäckdahl, M., and Nordin, K. E.: Bone defect in cleft palate. Acta Chir. Scand., *122*:131, 1961.

Bäckdahl, M., Nordin, K. E., Nylén, B., and Strömbeck, J. O.: Bone grafting to the maxillary defect in cleft lip and palate by the method of Bäckdahl and Nordin. Transactions of the Third International Congress of Plastic Surgery. Amsterdam, Excerpta Medica, 1964, p. 193.

Balluff, M. A.: Nutritional needs of an infant or child with a cleft lip or palate. Ear, Nose, Throat J., *65*:311, 1986.

Barclay, T. L., and Kernahan, D. A.: Plastic Surgery. London, Butterworth, 1986.

Bardach, J., Bakowska, J., McDermott-Murray, J., Mooney, M. P., and Dusdieker, L. B.: Lip pressure changes following lip repair in infants with unilateral clefts of the lip and palate. Plast. Reconstr. Surg., *74*:476, 1984.

Bardach, J., and Mooney, M. D.: The relationship between lip pressure following lip repair and craniofacial growth: an experimental study in beagles. Plast. Reconstr. Surg., *73*:544, 1984.

Bardach, J., Morris, H. L., and Olin, W. H.: Late results of primary veloplasty: the Marburg project. Plast. Reconstr. Surg., *73*:207, 1984.

Bardach, J., and Salyer, K.: Surgical Techniques in Cleft Lip and Palate. Chicago, Year Book Medical Publishers, 1987.

Barot, L. R., Cohen, M. A., and LaRossa, D.: Case reports: surgical indications and techniques for posterior pharyngeal flap revisions. Ann. Plast. Surg., *16*:527, 1986.

Barsky, A. J.: Pierre Franco, father of cleft lip surgery: his life and times. Br. J. Plast. Surg., *17*:335, 1964.

Bergland, O., Semb, G., and Abyholm, F. E.: Elimination of the residual alveolar cleft by secondary bone grafting and subsequent orthodontic treatment. Cleft Palate J., *23*:175, 1986.

Bergland, O., Semb, G., Abyholm, F., Borchgrevink, H., and Eskeland, G.: Secondary bone grafting and orthodontic treatment in patients with bilateral complete clefts of the lip and palate. Ann. Plast. Surg., *17*:460, 1986.

Blakeley, R. W.: The rationale for a temporary speech prosthesis in palatal insufficiency. Br. J. Disord. Commun., *4*:134, 1969.

Bluestone, C. D.: Eustachian tube obstruction in the infant with cleft palate. Ann. Otol. Rhinol. Laryngol., Suppl. 2:1, 1971.

Bluestone, C. D., and Stool, S. E. (Eds.): Pediatric Otolaryngology. Vol. II. Philadelphia, W. B. Saunders Company, 1983.

Bluestone, C. D., Wittel, R. A., and Paradise, J. L.: Roentgenographic evaluation of eustachian tube function in infants with cleft and normal palates. Cleft Palate J., *9*:93, 1972.

Boo-Chai, K.: An ancient Chinese text on a cleft lip. Plast. Reconstr. Surg., *38*:89, 1966.

Bourdet, B.: Recherches et Observations sur Toutes les Parties de l'Art du Dentiste. Paris, J. T. Herissant, 1757.

Boyne, P. J., and Sands, N. R.: Secondary bone grafting of residual alveolar and palatal clefts. J. Oral Surg., *30*:87, 1972.

Brauer, R. O., and Cronin, T. D.: Maxillary orthopedics and anterior palate repair with bone grafting. Cleft Palate J., *1*:31, 1964.

Brescia, N. J.: Anatomy of the lip and palate. In Grabb, W. C., Rosenstein, S. W., and Bzoch, K. R. (Eds.), Cleft

Lip and Palate: Surgical, Dental, and Speech Aspects. Boston, Little, Brown & Company, 1971.

Brookshire, B. L., Lynch, J. L., and Fox, D. R.: A Parent-Child Cleft Palate Curriculum: Developing Speech and Language. Tigard, OR, CC Publications, 1980.

Broomhead, I. W.: The nerve supply of the muscles of the soft palate. Br. J. Plast. Surg., *4*:1, 1951.

Brophy, T. W.: Cleft Lip and Palate. Philadelphia, P. Blakiston Company, 1923.

Brown, A. S., Cohen, M. A., and Randall, P.: Levator muscle reconstruction: does it make a difference? Plast. Reconstr. Surg., *72*:1, 1983.

Burston, W. R.: The pre-surgical orthopaedic correction of the maxillary deformity in clefts of both primary and secondary palate. In Transactions of the International Society of Plastic Surgeons. Second Congress. Edinburgh, E. & S. Livingstone, 1960, p. 28.

Burston, W. R.: The early orthodontic treatment of alveolar clefts. Proc. R. Soc. Med., *58*:767, 1965.

Bzoch, K. R. (Ed.): Communicative Disorders Related to Cleft Lip and Palate. Boston, Little, Brown & Company, 1979.

Calnan, J. S.: Congenital large pharynx. A new syndrome with a report on 41 personal cases. Br. J. Plast. Surg., *24*:263, 1971.

Converse, J. M.: Victor Veau (1871–1949): the contributions of a pioneer. Plast. Reconstr. Surg., *30*:225, 1962.

Converse, J. M. (Ed.): Reconstructive Plastic Surgery. 2nd Ed. Vol. IV. Philadelphia, W. B. Saunders Company, 1977.

Conway, H., and Goulian, D., Jr.: Experiences with maxillary orthopedics. Ann. Surg., *158*:431, 1963.

Cosman, B., and Falk, A. S.: Delayed hard palate repair and speech deficiencies: a cautionary report. Cleft Palate J., *17*:27, 1980.

Croft, C. B., Shprintzen, R. J., Daniller, A., and Lewin, M. L.: The occult submucous cleft and the musculus uvulae. Cleft Palate J., *15*:150, 1978.

Cronin, T. D.: Method of preventing raw areas on the nasal surface of soft palate in push-back surgery. Plast. Reconstr. Surg., *20*:474, 1957.

Cronin, T. D.: Pushback palatorrhaphy with nasal mucosal flaps. In Grabb, W. C., Rosenstein, S. W., and Bzoch, K. R. (Eds.): Cleft Lip and Palate: Surgical, Dental, and Speech Aspects. Boston, Little, Brown & Company, 1971.

Davies, D.: The one-stage repair of unilateral cleft lip and palate: a preliminary report. Plast. Reconstr. Surg., *38*:129, 1966.

Desai, S. N.: Early cleft palate repair completed before the age of 16 weeks: observations on a personal series of 100 children. Br. J. Plast. Surg., *36*:300, 1983.

Dickson, D. R., and Dickson, W. M.: Velopharyngeal anatomy. J. Speech Hear. Res., *15*:372, 1972.

Dieffenbach, J. F.: Beiträge zur Gaumennath. Lit. Ann. Heilk., *10*:322, 1828.

Dieffenbach, J. F.: Die Operative Chirurgie. Vol. I. Leipzig, F. S. Brockhaus, 1845.

Dingman, R. O., and Grabb, W. C.: A new mouth gag. Plast. Reconstr. Surg., *29*:208, 1962.

Dingman, R. O., and Grabb, W. C.: A rational program for surgical management of bilateral cleft lip and cleft palate. Plast. Reconstr. Surg., *47*:239, 1971.

Dorf, D. S., and Curtin, J. W.: Early cleft palate repair and speech outcome. Plast. Reconstr. Surg., *70*:74, 1982.

Dorrance, G. M.: The Operative Story of Cleft Palate. Philadelphia, W. B. Saunders Company, 1933.

Dorrance, G. M., and Bransfield, J. W.: The pushback operation for repair of cleft palate. Plast. Reconstr. Surg., *1*:145, 1946.

Drachter, R.: Operation for cleft palate. Dtsch. Z. Chir., *131*:1, 1914.

Dreyer, T. M., and Trier, W. C.: A comparison of palatoplasty techniques. Cleft Palate J., *21*:251, 1984.

Duffy, M. M.: Fever following palatoplasty: an evaluation based on "fever volume." Plast. Reconstr. Surg., *38*:32, 1966.

Dunn, F. S.: Results of the vomer flap technic used in surgery of the cleft palate during the past eleven years. Am. J. Surg., *92*:825, 1956.

Edgerton, M. T.: Surgical lengthening of the cleft palate by dissection of the neurovascular bundle. Plast. Reconstr. Surg., *29*:551, 1962.

Evans, D., and Renfrew, C.: The timing of primary cleft palate repair. Scand. J. Plast. Reconstr. Surg., *8*:153, 1974.

Fara, M., and Brousilova, M.: Experiences with early closure of velum and later closure of hard palate. Plast. Reconstr. Surg., *44*:134, 1969.

Fara, M., and Dvorak, J.: Abnormal anatomy of the muscles of the palatopharyngeal closure in cleft palates. Plast. Reconstr. Surg., *46*:488, 1970.

Fergusson, W.: Observations on cleft palate and on staphylorraphy. Med. Times & Gaz., Lond., *2*:256, 1845.

Fergusson, W.: Cleft palate. Med. Times & Gaz., Lond., *4*:433, 1852.

Fergusson, W.: Observations on hare lip and cleft palate. Br. Med. J., *1*:403, 1874.

Francis, W. W.: Repair of cleft palate by Philibert Roux in 1819: a translation of John Stephenson's De Velosynthesi. J. Hist. Med., *18*:217, 1963.

Franco, P.: Petit Traité Contenant une des Parties Principales de Chirurgie. Lyon, Antoine Vincent, 1556.

Franco, P.: Traité des Hernies. Lyon, Thibauld Payan, 1561.

Friede, H., and Johanson, B.: Adolescent facial morphology of early bone-grafted cleft lip and palate patients. Scand. J. Plast. Reconstr. Surg., *16*:41, 1982.

Friede, H., Lilja, J., and Johanson, B.: Cleft lip and palate treatment with delayed closure of the hard palate. Scand. J. Plast. Reconstr. Surg., *14*:49, 1980.

Furlow, L. T., Jr.: Double reversing Z-plasty for cleft palate. *In* Millard, D. R., Jr. (Ed.): Cleft Craft. Vol. III: Alveolar and Palatal Deformities. Boston, Little, Brown & Company, 1980, p. 519.

Furlow, L. T., Jr.: Cleft palate repair by double opposing Z-plasty. Plast. Reconstr. Surg., *78*:724, 1986.

Georgiade, N. G.: The management of premaxillary and maxillary segments in the newborn cleft palate patient. Cleft Palate J., 7:411, 1970.

Georgiade, N. G., Pickrell, K. L., and Quinn, G. W.: Varying concepts in bone grafting of alveolar palatal defects. Cleft Palate J., *1*:43, 1964.

Gorlin, R. J., Pindborg, J. J., and Cohen, M. M., Jr.: Syndromes of the Head and Neck. New York, McGraw-Hill Book Company, 1976.

Grabb, W. C.: General aspects of cleft palate surgery. *In* Grabb, W. C., Rosenstein, S. W., and Bzoch, K. R. (Eds.): Cleft Lip and Palate: Surgical, Dental, and Speech Aspects. Boston, Little, Brown & Company, 1971.

Grabb, W. C.: Personal communication, 1975.

Grabb, W. C., and Smith, J. W.: Plastic Surgery. A Concise Guide to Clinical Practice. Boston, Little, Brown & Company, 1971.

Gray, H.: Anatomy of the Human Body. 28th Ed. Goss, C. M. (Ed.). Philadelphia, Lea & Febiger, 1966.

Greenwald, M. J., and Parks, M. J.: Amblopia. *In* Duane, T. E. (Ed.): Clinical Ophthalmology. Vol. I. Philadelphia, Harper & Row, 1983.

Hagerty, R. F., and Hagerty, H. F.: Towards an optimal resolution of the cleft lip and palate defect. Presented at the Fifth International Congress on Cleft Palate and Related Craniofacial Disorders. Monte Carlo, 1985.

Henningsen, G.: Speech results in delayed hard palate closure. Presented at the First International Meeting of the Craniofacial Society of Great Britain. Birmingham, England, July 16, 1983.

Horton, C. E., Crawford, H., Adamson, J., Buxton, S., Cooper, R., and Kanter, J.: The prevention of maxillary collapse in congenital lip and palate cases. Cleft Palate J., *1*:25, 1964.

Hotz, M. M., Gnoinski, W. M., Nussbaumer, H., and Kistler, E.: Early maxillary orthopedics in CLP cases: guidelines for surgery. Cleft Palate J., *15*:405, 1978.

Hotz, R. (Ed.): Early Treatment of Cleft Lip and Palate, International Symposium, April 9-11, 1964, University of Zurich. Bern, Huber, 1964.

Huddart, A. G.: Presurgical changes in unilateral cleft palate subjects. Cleft Palate J., *16*:147, 1979.

Huddart, A. G.: Late findings in dental occlusion in unilateral clefts with presurgical treatment. Presented at the Third International Symposium on the Early Treatments of Cleft Lip and Palate. Zurich, Switzerland, Sept. 1984.

Jackson, I.: Personal communication, 1986.

Johanson, B.: Discussion of paper by R. Stellmach: Modern procedures in uni- and bilateral clefts of the lip, alveolus, and hard palate, with respect to primary osteoplasty. *In* Schuchardt, K. (Ed.): Treatment of Patients with Clefts of Lips, Alveolus, and Palate. Second Hamburg International Symposium, 1964. Stuttgart, Georg Thieme Verlag, 1966.

Johanson, B., and Ohlsson, A.: Bone grafting and dental orthopaedics in primary and secondary cases of cleft lip and palate. Acta Chir. Scand., *122*:112, 1961.

Jolleys, A., and Robertson, N. R.: A study of the effects of early bone grafting on complete clefts of the lip and palate—five year study. Br. J. Plast. Surg., *25*:229, 1972.

Jolleys, A., and Savage, J. P.: Healing defects in cleft palate surgery—the role of infection. Br. J. Plast. Surg., *16*:134, 1963.

Jordan, R. E., Kraus, B. S., and Neptune, C. M.: Dental abnormalities associated with cleft lip and/or palate. Cleft Palate J., *3*:22, 1966.

Kaplan, E. N.: Soft palate repair by levator muscle reconstruction and a buccal mucosal flap. Plast. Reconstr. Surg., *56*:129, 1975a.

Kaplan, E. N.: The occult submucous cleft palate. Cleft Palate J., *12*:356, 1975b.

Kaplan, E. N.: Cleft palate repair at 3 months? Ann. Plast. Surg., 7:179, 1981.

Karl, H. W., Swedlow, D. B., Lee, K. W., and Downes, J. J.: Epinephrine-halothane interactions in children. Anesthesiology, *58*:142, 1983.

Kernahan, D. A., and Stark, R. B.: A new classification for cleft lip and cleft palate. Plast. Reconstr. Surg., *22*:435, 1958.

Kernahan, D. A., and Bauer, B. S.: Cleft palate. *In* Georgiade, N. G., Georgiade, G. S., Riefkohl, R., and Barwick, W. J. (Eds.): Essentials of Plastic, Maxillofacial, and Reconstructive Surgery. Baltimore, Williams & Wilkins Company, 1987.

Kilner, T. P.: Cleft lip and palate repair technique. St. Thomas Hosp. Rep., 2:127, 1937.

Kling, A.: Evaluation of results in references to the bite. *In* Hotz, R. (Ed.): Early Treatment of Cleft Lip and Palate. International Symposium, April 9-11, 1964, University of Zurich. Bern, Huber, 1964, pp. 193–197.

Kling, A.: Procedures and limits of orthodontic treatment. *In* Schuchardt, K. (Ed.): Treatment of Patients with Clefts of Lip, Alveolus, and Palate. Second Hamburg International Symposium, 1964. Stuttgart, Georg Thieme Verlag, 1966, pp. 123–124.

Konishi, M.: Effects of deafening on song development in American robins and black-headed grosbeaks. Z. Tierpsychol., 22:584, 1965.

Kremenak, C. R., Huffman, W. C., and Olin, W. H.: Growth of maxillae in dogs after palatal surgery. Cleft Palate J., 4:6, 1967.

Kriens, O. B.: Fundamental anatomic findings for an intravelar veloplasty. Cleft Palate J., 7:27, 1970.

Kriens, O. B.: Anatomy of the velopharyngeal area in cleft palate. Clin. Plast. Surg., 2:261, 1975.

Krogman, W. M., Jain, R. B., and Oka, S. W.: Craniofacial growth in different cleft types from one month to ten years. Cleft Palate J., 19:206, 1982.

LaRossa, D., and Randall, P.: The unilateral cleft lip. *In* Georgiade, N. G., Georgiade, G. S., Riefkohl, R., and Barwick, W. J. (Eds.): Essentials in Plastic, Maxillofacial, and Reconstructive Surgery. Baltimore, Williams & Wilkins Company, 1987.

LaRossa, D., Vaniver, K., and Randall, P.: The Effect of Preoperative Antibiotics on Post-operative Morbidity in Patients with Cleft Lip and Palate. A Retrospective Study. Presented at the American Cleft Palate Association Meeting, New York, 1986.

Latham, R. A., Kusy, R. P., and Georgiade, N. G.: An extraorally activated expansion appliance for cleft palate infants. Cleft Palate J., 13:253, 1976.

Latham, R. A., Long, R. E., and Latham, E. A.: Cleft palate velopharyngeal musculature in a five-month-old infant: a three-dimensional histological reconstruction. Cleft Palate J., 17:1, 1980.

Lexer, E.: Die Verwendung der freien Knochenplastik nebst Versuchen über Gelenkversteifung und Gelenktransplantation. Langenbecks Arch. Klin. Chir., 86:939, 1908.

Lusitanius, A.: Curationum Medicinalium . . . Tomus Seconde, Continens Centurias Tres, Quintam Videlcet. Venetiis, Apud Vincentium Valgrislum, 1566. Curatio 14, p. 39.

Malek, R., Psaume, J., and Genton, N.: New timing and new sequence for operative interventions on cleft palate patients. Presented at the Fifth International Congress on Cleft Palate and Related Craniofacial Anomalies. Monte Carlo, 1985.

Mason, R. M., and Warren, D. W.: Adenoid involution and developing hypernasality in cleft palate. J. Speech Hear. Disord., 45:469, 1980.

Masters, F. W., Bingham, H. G., and Robinson, D. W.: The prevention and treatment of hearing loss in the cleft palate child. Plast. Reconstr. Surg., 25:503, 1960.

Mayro, R.: Personal communication, 1986.

Mayro, R., LaRossa, D., and Randall, P.: The "locked out" premaxilla in bilateral clefts—an 18 year follow-up study. Presented at the Fifth International Congress on Cleft Palate and Related Craniofacial Anomalies. Monte Carlo, 1985.

Mazaheri, M.: Indications and contraindications for prosthetic speech appliances in cleft palate. Plast. Reconstr. Surg., 30:663, 1962.

McClelland, R. M. A., and Patterson, T. J. S.: The influence of penicillin on the complication rate after repair of clefts of the lip and palate. Br. J. Plast. Surg., 16:144, 1963.

McNeil, C. K.: Oral and Facial Deformity. London, Sir Isaac Pitman & Sons, 1954.

McWilliams, B. J., Morris, H. L., and Shelton, R. L. (Eds.): Cleft Palate Speech. Philadelphia, B. C. Decker; St. Louis, C. V. Mosby, 1984.

Melnick, M., Bixler, D., and Shields, E. D. (Eds.): Etiology of Cleft Lip and Cleft Palate. New York, A. R. Liss, 1980.

Meskin, L. H., Gorlin, R. J., and Isaacson, R. J.: Abnormal morphology of the soft palate: I. The prevalence of cleft uvula. Cleft Palate J., 1:342, 1964.

Millard, D. R., Jr.: A new use of the island flap in wide palate clefts. Plast. Reconstr. Surg., 38:330, 1966.

Millard, D. R., Jr.: Cleft Craft. Vols. I, II, III. Boston, Little, Brown & Company, 1976, 1977, 1980.

Morris, H. L. (Ed.): The Bratislava Project: Some Results of Cleft Palate Surgery. Iowa City, University of Iowa Press, 1976.

Musgrave, R. H., and Bremner, J. C.: Complications of cleft palate surgery. Plast. Reconstr. Surg., 26:180, 1960.

Noone, R. B., Randall, P., Stool, S. E., Hamilton, R., and Winchester, R. A.: The effect on middle ear disease of fracture of the pterygoid hamulus during palatoplasty. Cleft Palate J., 10:23, 1973.

Nordin, K. E.: Bone grafting to the alveolar process clefts following orthodontic treatment of secondary cleft palate deformity. *In* Skoog, T., and Ivy, R. H. (Eds.): Transactions of the International Society of Plastic Surgery. First Congress. Baltimore, Williams & Wilkins Company, 1957, p. 228.

Nordin, K. E.: Early jaw orthopaedics in the cleft palate program with a new orthopaedic–surgical procedure. Transactions of the European Orthodontic Society, 1960, p. 150.

Nordin, K. E., and Johanson, B.: Freie Knochentransplantation bei Defekten im Alveolarkamm nach kieferothopädischer. Einstellung der Maxilla bei Lippen-Kiefer-Gaumenspalten. *In* Schuchardt, K., and Wassmund, M. (Eds.): Fortschritte der Kiefer- und Gesichts-Chirurgie. Vol. I. Stuttgart, Georg Thieme Verlag, 1955, pp. 168–171.

Nordin, K. E., Larson, O., Nylen, B., and Eklund, G.: Early bone grafting in complete cleft lip and palate cases following maxillofacial orthopedics. I. The method and skeletal development from seven to thirteen years of age. Scand. J. Plast. Reconstr. Surg., 17:33, 1983.

Nylen, B.: Surgery of the alveolar cleft. Plast. Reconstr. Surg., 37:42, 1966.

Nylen, B., Korlof, B., Arnander, C., Leanderson, R., Barr, B., and Nordin, K. E.: Primary, early bone grafting in complete clefts of the lip and palate. A follow-up study of 53 cases. Scand. J. Plast. Reconstr. Surg., 8:79, 1974.

Orticochea, M.: Construction of a dynamic muscle sphincter in cleft palates. Plast. Reconstr. Surg., 41:323, 1968.

Orticochea, M.: A review of 236 cleft palate patients treated with dynamic muscle sphincter. Plast. Reconstr. Surg., 71:180, 1983.

Ortiz-Monasterio, F., Serrano, A., Barrera, G., Rodriguez-Hoffman, H., and Vinageras, E.: A study of untreated adult cleft palate patients. Plast. Reconstr. Surg., 38:36, 1966.

Paget, S.: Ambroise Paré and His Times: 1510–1590. New York, G. P. Putnam's Sons, 1899.

Pancoast, J.: On staphylorrhaphy. Am. J. Med. Sci., 6:66, 1843.

Paradise, J. L., and Bluestone, C. D.: The universality of otitis media in fifty infants with cleft palate. Pediatrics, 44:35, 1969.

Paré, A.: Die Livres de la Chirurgie. Paris, Jean le Royer, 1564, p. 211.

Parks, M. M.: Ocular Motility and Strabismus. Vol. I. New York, Harper & Row, 1975.

Pashayan, H. M., and McNab, M.: Singlefeed method of feeding infants born with cleft palate with or without cleft lip. Am. J. Dis. Child., 133:145, 1979.

Peer, L.: Cleft palate deformity and the bone-flap method of repair. Surg. Clin. North Am., 39:313, 1959.

Peer, L. A., Walker, J. C., and Meiger, R.: The Dieffenbach bone-flap method of cleft palate repair. Plast. Reconstr. Surg., 34:472, 1964.

Perko, M. A.: Two-stage closure of cleft palate. J. Maxillofac. Surg., 7:76, 1979.

Piaget, J.: Play, Dreams and Imitations in Childhood, Part I. Translated by C. Gettegno and F. M. Hodgson. New York, Norton, 1962.

Pruzansky, S.: Pre-surgical orthopedics and bone grafting for infants with cleft and palate: a dissertation. Cleft Palate J., 1:164, 1964.

Pruzansky, S., and Aduss, H.: Arch form and the deciduous occlusion in complete unilateral clefts. Cleft Palate J., 1:411, 1964.

Randall, P.: A triangular flap operation for the primary repair of unilateral clefts of the lip. Plast. Reconstr. Surg., 23:331, 1951.

Randall, P.: A lip adhesion operation in cleft lip surgery. Plast. Reconstr. Surg., 35:371, 1965.

Randall, P.: Secondary surgery. In Edwards, M., and Watson, A. C. H. (Eds.): Advances in the Management of Cleft Palate. Edinburgh, Churchill Livingstone, 1980a.

Randall, P.: The Cleft Palate. In Barron, J. N., and Saan, M. N. (Eds.): Operative Plastic and Reconstructive Surgery. London, Churchill Livingstone, 1980b.

Randall, P., Bakes, F. P., and Kennedy, C.: Cleft palate–type speech in the absence of cleft palate. Plast. Reconstr. Surg., 25:484, 1960.

Randall, P., LaRossa, D., Fakhraee, S. M., and Cohen, M. A.: Cleft palate closure at three to nine months of age: a preliminary report. Plast. Reconstr. Surg. 71:624, 1983.

Randall, P., LaRossa, D., Solomon, M., and Cohen, M.: Experience with the Furlow double reversing Z-plasty for cleft palate repair. Plast. Reconstr. Surg., 77:569, 1986.

Randall, P., Whitaker, L. A., and LaRossa, D.: The importance of muscle reconstruction in primary and secondary cleft lip repair. Plast. Reconstr. Surg., 54:316, 1974.

Rehrmann, A. H., Koberg, W. R., and Koch, H.: Long-term postoperative results of primary and secondary bone grafting in complete clefts of the lip and palate. Cleft Palate J., 7:206, 1970.

Riski, J. E., and DeLong, E.: Articulation development in children with cleft lip palate. Cleft Palate J., 21:57, 1984.

Rogers, B. O.: Harelip repair in Colonial America: a review of 18th century and earlier surgical techniques. Plast. Reconstr. Surg., 34:142, 1964.

Rogers, B. O.: History of cleft lip and palate treatment. In Grabb, W. C., Rosenstein, S. W., and Bzoch, K. R.: Cleft Lip and Palate: Surgical, Dental, and Speech Aspects. Boston, Little, Brown & Company, 1971, pp. 142–169.

Rosenstein, S. W., Jacobson, B. N., Monroe, C., Griffith, B. H., and McKinney, P.: A series of cleft lip and palate children five years after undergoing orthopedic and bone grafting procedures. Angle Orthod., 42:1, 1972.

Rosenstein, S. W., Monroe, C. W., Kernahan, D. A., and Jacobson, B. N.: The case for early bone grafting in cleft lip and cleft palate. Plast. Reconstr. Surg., 70:297, 1982.

Rune, B., Sarnas, K. V., Selvik, G., and Jacobsson, S.: Movement of maxillary segments after expansion and/or secondary bone grafting in cleft lip and palate. A roentgen stereophotogrammetric study with the aid of metallic implants. Am J. Orthod., 77:643, 1980.

Schrudde, J., and Stellmach, R.: Die primäre Osteoplastik des Defekte des Kieferbogens bei Lippen-Kiefer-Gaumenspalten am Saugling. Zentralbl. Chir., 83:849, 1958.

Schrudde, J., and Stellmach, R.: Primäre Osteoplastik und Kieferbogenformung bei Lippen-Kiefer-Gaumenspalten. Fortschr. Kiefer-und Gesichts-Chir., 5:247, 1959.

Schuchardt, K., and Pfeifer, G.: Primary and secondary operations for cleft palate. J. Int. Coll. Surg., 38:237, 1962.

Schuchardt, K., and Pfeifer, G.: Erfahrungen über primäre Knochen Transplantationen bei Lippen-Kiefer-Gaumenspalten. Langenbecks Arch. Klin. Chir., 295:881, 1966.

Schultz, R. C.: A survey of European and Scandinavian bone grafting procedures for cleft palate deformities. Cleft Palate J., 1:188, 1964.

Schultz, R. C.: Personal communication, 1986.

Schweckendiek, H.: Zur zweiphasigen Gaumenspalten Operation bei primäre Velum Verschluss. In Schuchardt, K., and Wassmund, M. (Eds.): Fortschritte der Kiefer- und Gesichts-Chirurgie. Vol. I. Stuttgart, Georg Thieme Verlag, 1955, pp. 73–76.

Schweckendiek, W.: Die Ergebnisse der Kieferbildung und die Sprache nach der primären Veloplastik. Arch. Ohr. Nas. Kehlkopfheilk., 180:541, 1962.

Schweckendiek, W., and Doz, P.: Primary veloplasty: long-term results without maxillary deformity—a 25 year report. Cleft Palate J., 15:268, 1978.

Shelton, R. L., Lindquist, A. F., Chisum, L., Arndt, W. B., Youngstrom, K. A., and Stick, S. L.: Effect of prosthetic speech bulb reduction on articulation. Cleft Palate J., 5:195, 1968.

Shprintzen, R.: Personal communication, 1985.

Skolnick, M. L., Shprintzen, R. J., McCall, G. N., and Rakoff, S.: Patterns of velopharyngeal closure in subjects with repaired cleft palate and normal speech: a multiview videofluoroscopic analysis. Cleft Palate J., 12:369, 1975.

Skoog, T.: The use of periosteal flaps in the repair of clefts of the primary palate. Cleft Palate J., 2:332, 1965.

Spriestersbach, D. C., Lierle, D. M., Moll, K. L., and Prather, W. F.: Hearing loss in children with cleft palates. Plast. Reconstr. Surg., 30:336, 1962.

Spriestersbach, D. C., and Sherman, D. (Eds.): Cleft

Palate and Communication. New York & London, Academic Press, 1968.

Stark, D. B.: Nasal lining in partial cleft palate repair. Plast. Reconstr. Surg., *32*:75, 1963.

Stark, R. B.: The pathogenesis of harelip and cleft palate. Plast. Reconstr. Surg., *13*:20, 1954.

Stark, R. B.: Cleft palate. *In* Plastic Surgery. New York, Hoeber Med. Div., Harper & Row, 1962.

Stark, R. B., and DeHaan, C. R.: The addition of a pharyngeal flap to primary palatoplasty. Plast. Reconstr. Surg., *26*:378, 1960.

Stark, R. B., and Frileck, S.: Primary pharyngeal flap and palatorrhaphy. *In* Grabb, W. C., Rosenstein, S. W., and Bzoch, K. R. (Eds.): Cleft Lip and Palate: Surgical, Dental, and Speech Aspects. Boston, Little, Brown & Company, 1971.

Stellmach, R.: Primäre Knochenplastik bei Lippen-Kiefer-Gaumenspalten am Saugling unter besonderer Berücksichtigung der Transplantations Deckung. Langenbecks Arch. Klin. Chir., *292*:865, 1959.

Stool, S. E., and Randall, P.: Unexpected ear disease in infants with cleft palate. Cleft Palate J., *4*:99, 1967.

Styer, G. W., and Freeh, K.: Feeding infants with cleft lip and/or palate. J.O.G.N. Nurs., *10*:329, 1981.

Subtelny, J. D., and Baker, H. K.: The significance of adenoid tissue in velopharyngeal function. Plast. Reconstr. Surg., *17*:235, 1956.

Tessier, P.: Anatomical classification of facial, craniofacial, and latero-facial clefts. J. Maxillofac. Surg., *4*:69, 1976.

Tessier, P.: Autogenous bone grafts taken from calvarium for facial and cranial applications. Clin. Plast. Surg., *9*:531, 1982.

Trier, W. C.: Velopharyngeal incompetency in the absence of overt cleft palate: anatomic and surgical considerations. Cleft Palate J., *20*:209, 1983.

Trier, W. C.: Surgery for congenital cleft palate. *In* Habal, M. B., Moran, W. D., Lewin, M. L., Parsons, R. W., and Woods, J. E. (Eds.): Advances in Plastic and Reconstructive Surgery. Vol. II. Chicago, Year Book Medical Publishers, 1986.

Trost, J. E.: Articulatory additions to the classical description of the speech of persons with cleft palate. Cleft Palate J., *18*:193, 1981.

Van Demark, D. R., Morris, H. L., and Vandeharr, C.: Patterns of articulation abilities in speakers with cleft palate. Cleft Palate J., *16*:230, 1979.

Veau, V.: Division Palatine, Anatomie, Chirurgie, Phonetique. Paris, Masson et Cie, 1931.

von Graefe, C. F.: Kurze Nachrichten und Auszuge. J. Pract. Arznek. Wundarzk., *44*:116, 1817.

von Graefe, C. F.: Die Gaumennath, ein neuentdecktes Mittel gegen angeborene Fehler der Sprache. J. Chir. Augenh., *1*:1, 1820.

von Langenbeck, B.: Beitrage zur Osteoplastik. Deutsche Klin., *2*:471, 1859.

von Langenbeck, B.: Operation der angebornen totalen Spaltung des harten Gaumens nach einer neuer Methode. Gösch. Deutsche Klin., *3*:231, 1861.

Wardill, W. E. M.: Techniques of operation for cleft palate. Br. J. Surg., *25*:117, 1937.

Warren, J. C.: On an operation for the cure of natural fissures of the soft palate. Am. J. Med. Sci., *3*:1, 1828.

Warren, J. M.: Operations for fissures of the soft and hard palate (palatoplastie). N. Engl. Q. J. Med. Surg., *1*:538, 1843a.

Warren, J. M.: Operations for fissures of the soft and hard palate. Am. J. Med. Sci., *(N.S.)6*:257, 1843b.

Watson, A. C. H.: Primary surgery in cleft palates. *In* Edwards, M., and Watson A. C. H. (Eds.): Advances in the Management of Cleft Palate. Edinburgh, Churchill Livingstone, 1980a.

Watson, A. C. H.: Classification of cleft palate. *In* Edwards, M., and Watson, A. C. H. (Eds.): Advances in the Management of Cleft Palate. Edinburgh, Churchill Livingstone, 1980b.

Weatherley-White, R. C., Stark, R. B., and De Haan, C. R.: The objective measurement of nasality in cleft palate patients. Plast. Reconstr. Surg., *35*:588, 1965.

Weinburger, B. W.: An Introduction to the History of Dentistry. Vol. I. St. Louis, C. V. Mosby Company, 1948, pp. 117, 248, 390.

Witzel, M. A., Salyer, K. E., and Ross, R. B.: Delayed hard palate closure: the philosophy revisited. Cleft Palate J., *21*:263, 1984.

Wolfe, S. A., and Berkowitz, S.: The use of cranial bone grafts in closure of alveolar and anterior palate clefts. Plast. Reconstr. Surg., *72*:659, 1983.

55

S. Anthony Wolfe
G. Wesley Price
James M. Stuzin
Samuel Berkowitz

Alveolar and Anterior Palatal Clefts

The word alveolus is the diminutive of the Latin "alveus," meaning trough, and it thus designates a small trough that contains the tooth buds. The maxillary alveolar ridge separates the palate from the lip, and clefts of the primary palate (from the anterior surface of the lip to the incisive foramen), by definition, have a cleft of the alveolus as well. In the most common clefts of the primary palate, the alveolar portion of the cleft is located between the lateral incisor, if present, and the canine. This corresponds to a No. 4 cleft in the Tessier classification (Tessier, 1976). The cleft may also pass between the central incisor and the lateral incisor, corresponding to a No. 3 cleft (see Chap. 59). Rarer forms of clefts may pass between the central incisor (No. 0 cleft), or more distally on the maxillary arch (Nos. 5 and 6 clefts).

A complete cleft of the alveolus passes superiorly into the nasal cavity and posteriorly into the anterior palate, with continuity of the alveolar, nasal, and palatal mucoperiosteum.

DENTAL CONSIDERATIONS

The affected dental lamina (the embryonic tooth layer) may give rise to variations in the number as well as the position and form of the involved teeth. If the lateral incisor bud is involved, it may develop into two perfectly formed teeth on either side of the cleft. More often, a malformed or completely missing lateral incisor may result. The malpositioned lateral incisor usually erupts palatally in the line of the cleft. Additional partially malformed teeth may be present and can be located only by periapical radiographs. Tooth eruptions in both the deciduous and permanent dentition are delayed (Bailit, Doykos, and Swanson, 1968). The incidence of supernumerary lateral incisors in the deciduous dentition varies between 5 and 30 per cent, although there are instances when they may be present in the permanent dentition. Absent permanent lateral incisors are reported in 10 to 40 per cent of patients (Millhon and Stafne, 1941; Bohn, 1963; Olin, 1964; Fishman, 1970; Ranta, 1971a,b, 1972). The central incisor and second bicuspid on the cleft side are often small or have deformed crowns, and have areas of poor enamel formation.

CLOSURE OF ALVEOLAR CLEFTS

Plastic surgeons have focused their attention on the closure of clefts of the lip and more posterior portions of the palate, and many patients in whom results are excellent from the point of view of appearance, speech, and dental occlusion have been left with persistent clefts of the alveolus. Moreover, the late surgical closure of alveolar defects is difficult. Kilner, acclaimed by many who saw him operate as one of the most proficient of cleft palate surgeons, is reported to have stated that closure of clefts of the anterior palate was the most trying procedure in cleft palate surgery (Millard, 1972).

Why should one attempt to close an alveolar cleft? If there is a satisfactory lip repair, albeit with a slight deficiency of alar base support on the cleft side; if there is adequate speech; and if prosthetic dentistry, when necessary, can provide a bridge to span the gap created by the missing tooth, why should the surgeon attempt the technically difficult closure of a small defect in an older patient? Or, if he is to try to close the alveolar defect with or without preliminary neonatal maxillary orthopedics at the time of the primary lip closure, he must be concerned about interference with subsequent midfacial development. This controversial area of neonatal maxillary orthopedics is discussed in Chapter 57.

This chapter attempts to provide reasons why alveolar clefts *should* be closed, and why bony continuity of the maxillary alveolar arch is a worthwhile surgical goal. There are still considerable differences of opinion as to the optimal time for closure of alveolar defects, with or without concomitant bone grafting.

Rationale

Reasons for closing alveolar clefts are listed below.

1. *To provide stability of the maxillary arch.* This is of particular importance in bilateral clefts, in which the premaxilla may be quite mobile. If a maxillary advancement becomes necessary at a later date, it is much easier to advance the maxilla in one piece by a standard Le Fort I osteotomy than to have to deal with three separate osseous segments. The premaxilla will also be assured of sufficient blood supply.

2. *To close oronasal fistulas and anterior palatal clefts.* These openings are irritating to patients, since food and drink can often pass into the nasal cavity. Closure can be

accomplished without bone grafting, but the success rate is greater when a bone graft is used. Bone grafts are also used to construct a piriform rim that is symmetric with the normal side, providing a better platform for the alar base, improving nasal symmetry, and preventing the inferior turbinate's prolapsing into the cleft (Millard, 1980).

3. *To provide better periodontal support for teeth bordering the cleft.* Bone grafting before the eruption of the permanent dentition, it is hoped, will create a bony matrix through which the teeth can erupt, improving the orthodontic result, providing greater longevity for the teeth on the borders of the cleft, and possibly avoiding the need for any permanent fixed prosthodontic appliances (Bergland, Semb, and Abyholm, 1986).

Since there is a wide difference between the therapeutic approaches used in the management of alveolar clefts by various cleft palate teams (Witsenburg, 1985), it will be of value to examine first the evolution of this surgery over the past century.

Historical Evolution

In the last century and in the early part of this century, the treatment of clefts was primarily in the hands of surgeons (Veau, 1931; Dorrance, 1933). Numerous procedures were described for closure of the palatal cleft and lengthening of the soft palate. When the palatal cleft was too large for surgical closure, the prosthodontist was called upon to fabricate an obturator. In the adult, the obturator was also used to replace missing teeth, to seal the alveolar and palatal fistulas, and to provide lip support to improve facial esthetics (Harkins, 1960). If speech was hypernasal, a posterior extension (speech bulb) was added to divert air flow through the mouth in order to improve speech tone.

After World War II, a multidisciplinary approach to the treatment of cleft palate children began to appear. Clinics were established at Lancaster, Pennsylvania, and the Universities of Illinois and Iowa, to name a few. Orthodontists Pruzansky (1964), Slaughter and Brodie (1949), and Graber (1954), using lateral cephaloroentgenographics and cast analyses of children who had undergone various types of cleft palate repair, decried what was being done. They showed long-term results with evidence of extensive midfacial deformity and severe speech disorder.

These studies condemned early surgery and associated extensive mucoperiosteal undermining, which left wide areas of denuded bone with secondary scar formation and major distortions of the maxillary arch. Such reports influenced many surgeons to accept the postponement of palatal surgery until patients were 5 years of age or older, when most palatal growth was completed.

With the advent of orthodontic methods to correct arch alignment, the residual alveolar cleft received more attention. Clinical problems relating to the alveolar cleft include instability of the maxillary segments, a tendency to relapse after orthodontic treatment, the need for fixed and elaborate bridgework, nasal asymmetry, and persistent oronasal fistulas. Axhausen, in 1952, wrote that surgical closure of the alveolar cleft was "the final problem in the repair of complete clefts at present." His idea of surgical restoration of arch integrity and restoration of the alveolar cleft as a potential tooth-bearing segment was the beginning of the osteoplastic era in alveolar cleft surgery (Koberg, 1973).

Although Lexer in 1908 attempted to bone graft an alveolar cleft, Drachter (1914) is given credit for the first successful bone graft, using tibial bone and periosteum. Beck and Jesser (1921) described using a mucoperiosteal flap from the inferior turbinate to close a cleft of the primary palate. In 1931, Veau attempted closure of an anterior alveolar cleft using vomerine and mucoperiosteal flaps with tibial bone grafts (one-layer closure), but failed. Campbell (1926) was one of the first to recognize the importance of a two-layer mucoperiosteal closure of the anterior palate.

Schmid and associates (1954, 1955, 1960, 1963, 1964, 1974) deserves credit for directing the attention of contemporary cleft surgeons to bone grafting of alveolar clefts. Extrapolating from bone grafting techniques used in reconstruction of jaw defects resulting from war injuries, Schmid performed successful bone grafting of the alveolar cleft, using the iliac crest as donor. In 1955, Johanson and Nordin reported bone grafting alveolar clefts primarily (at the time of lip closure), using tibial or iliac bone grafts in a three-stage procedure. They achieved closure of the lip, palate, and alveolus by 1 year of age. Burian (1957) also described a buccal flap to provide additional mucoperiosteum for a two-layer closure.

Schrudde and Stellmach introduced the concept of primary osteoplasty of the alveolar cleft in 1958. Their aim was to stabilize the mobile premaxilla by obtaining soft tissue closure of the lip and bony continuity of the alveolus in infants with bilateral clefts. Early success with primary bone grafting was similarly reported by Schuchardt and Pfeifer (1960), using two full-thickness rib grafts placed within the alveolus at the time of lip closure. Steinhardt (1966) advocated a two-layer closure of alveolar clefts using vomerine and alveolar mucoperiosteal flaps with bone grafts.

The early reports of successful primary bone grafting caused rapid acceptance of the procedure. The proposed advantages of primary bone grafting were the prevention of maxillary collapse and the possibility of more normal craniofacial development. It was also felt that bone grafting might indeed "stimulate" maxillary growth (McNeil, 1954; Burston, 1965; Metz and Gunther, 1967). By the end of the 1950s, most major European centers were performing early closure of alveolar clefts with primary bone grafting (Nordin and Johanson, 1955; Schrudde and Stellmach, 1958; Schuchardt and Pfeifer, 1960; Steinhardt, 1966), and many American groups soon followed suit (Brauer and Cronin, 1964; Georgiade, Pickrell, and Quinn, 1964; Monroe and associates, 1968).

In the early 1960's, concern began to manifest itself about the effect of subperiosteal undermining and bone grafting on maxillary growth. The possibility of harm arising from the orthopedic alignment of infant maxillary arches was also considered. Although Ritter (1959) and Gabka (1964) were among the first to raise these concerns about the impairment of maxillary growth, Pruzansky (1964) is remembered as the most outspoken critic of these procedures. He challenged the view that presurgical orthopedic treatment and primary bone grafting were necessary or beneficial, and presented a longitudinal study of 1000 children to show that the results achieved by early orthopedic management could be arrived at spontaneously in untreated patients. Pruzansky believed that preschool orthodontic arch alignment was appropriate, but that before that time there was neither need nor place for maxillary orthopedics. He recommended that bone grafting should be delayed until after eruption of the permanent dentition, and, in support of this view, cited a 1959 report by Ortiz-Monasterio, Rebeil, and Valderrama on untreated adult cleft lip and palate patients who all demonstrated satisfactory arch development.

Johanson (1964) was disturbed by the effect of primary bone grafting on maxillary growth, and later reported that he had stopped primary bone grafting, waiting until eruption of the permanent dentition. In a long-term follow-up of their patients who had been treated by primary bone grafting, Friede and Johanson (1982) documented severe maxillary retrusion and poor maxillary development in the vertical dimension in both bilateral and unilateral cleft patients. They reported that 40 per cent of the bilateral and 50 per cent of the unilateral cases treated with primary bone grafting eventually required a Le Fort I maxillary advancement. In 1968, Pickrell, Quinn, and Massengill reported 25 patients who had been bone grafted primarily. They showed absence of growth of the bone graft, continued collapse of the maxillary arch without orthodontic support, and failure of tooth eruption through the bone grafts. Kling, at the 1964 Hamburg International Symposium, described a series of poor results in patients treated by primary bone grafting, and showed an 88 per cent increase in the incidence of maxillary retrusion. In the late 1960's, other groups reported that they had abandoned primary bone grafting (Hollman, 1964; Perko, 1966; Mazaheri, Harding, and Nanda, 1967; Rehrmann, Koberg, and Koch, 1970).

By the early 1970's, there were numerous reports showing that primary bone grafting tended to inhibit midfacial growth, with resultant Class III malocclusion. Several centers, however, continued to report satisfactory results with primary bone grafting and to advocate its use (Schrudde and Trauner, 1972; Nylen and associates, 1974; Schmid and associates, 1974; Rosenstein and associates, 1982). Rosenstein and associates are one of the few groups still performing primary bone grafting in the United States.

It is not clear why primary or early bone grafting inhibits subsequent midfacial growth. Dixon and Sarnat (1982) suggested that inhibition of bone growth is brought on by any surgery that affects the blood supply to developing bone. Stenström and Thilander (1967a,b) demonstrated experimentally that bone grafting in surgically created clefts resulted in inhibition of facial development. Engdahl (1972) showed experimentally that cortical bone grafts, but not particulate marrow grafts, caused severe growth retardation. Lynch and Peil (1966) and Ross (1970) suggested that maxillary growth inhibition was mainly the result of subperiosteal dissection in an infant, with subsequent scar formation. It is possible that the groups who continued to advocate primary bone grafting were much more vigorous in the subsequent orthodontic treatment of their patients, with a resultant lower incidence of maxillary retrusion. However, there is also no evidence that orthodontic treatment can effectively prevent skeletal (i.e., basal bone, and not dentoalveolar) maxillary retrusion.

As an alternative to primary bone grafting, Skoog (1967b) developed the periosteoplasty, or "boneless bone graft" technique, in which periosteal continuity was established between maxillary segments by the transfer of local periosteal flaps from the anterior maxillary wall (Skoog, 1965, 1967a,b). This procedure, which takes advantage of the propensity of periosteum to form bone in young children, leads to the formation of new bone within the alveolar cleft in spite of the fact that no bone graft is used. In a longitudinal follow-up (Hellquist and Ponten, 1979), 47 per cent of patients had satisfactory bone formation after infant periosteoplasty, as compared with 80 per cent with good bone formation when the periosteoplasty was delayed (but performed before the age of 7 years). No adverse effects on facial growth were seen in either group. Despite these findings, periosteoplasty has not become a widely accepted procedure, although the concept is attractive. Millard and Latham are currently evaluating gingivoplasty-periosteoplasty performed at the time of lip closure, following presurgical neonatal maxillary orthopedics (see Chap. 52).

ORTHODONTIC CONSIDERATIONS

In complete clefts of the lip and palate, the palatal segments at birth are laterally displaced as a result of the aberrant muscle pull of the cleft orbicularis oris muscle, coupled with protrusion of the tongue. This action is reversed when the lip is repaired, causing the palatal segments to move together (molding), thereby reducing the cleft space. Aduss and

Pruzansky (1967) demonstrated three potential arch relationships that could result within a few months after lip repair: (1) the palatal segments approximate, (2) the larger segment overlaps the smaller segment, and (3) the segments move together but do not make contact (owing to premature contact of the inferior turbinate with the nasal septum).

Berkowitz (1985) reported serial growth changes from birth to 6 years of age in 36 complete unilateral cleft lip and palate patients and 29 complete bilateral cleft lip and palate patients when cleft palate closure was performed between 12 to 24 months using conservative surgical techniques. He demonstrated that molding action is completed within the first three months after the lip is repaired, additional cleft space closure being due to appositional bone growth. This study also showed that appositional bone growth in the palatal segments is most rapid during the first year; thereafter its rate of growth slowly decreases.

At age 3 years, the size of the palate appeared to be within normal size as judged by the dental occlusion. Dental crossbite of the deciduous cuspid due to mesioangular rotation of the lesser segment was the most common finding in both the unilateral and the bilateral cleft lip and palate patients. By the age of 3 years the premaxilla made contact with the lateral segments and the anterior cleft space was obliterated in 25 of the 29 bilateral cases. Periapical radiographs of the cleft area showed a space between the bony anterior ends of the palatal segments. Dental crossbite correction was generally initiated between 3 and 4 years of age and completed within three months. The new arch form was retained by fixed palatal archwires. In some patients a second stage of palatal expansion was required, depending on growth of the maxilla relative to the mandibular arch.

SECONDARY BONE GRAFTING

The possibility of interference with midfacial growth has been the reason for delaying bone grafting procedures until later in childhood, although the optimal age for secondary bone grafting remains under debate.

Many centers now favor secondary bone grafting during the period of mixed dentition, generally between the ages of 7 and 11 years (Boyne and Sands, 1976; Waite and Kersten, 1980; Abyholm, Bergland, and Semb, 1981; El Deeb and associates, 1982). The sagittal and transverse growth of the anterior maxilla is largely completed by age 8 years (Bjork and Skieller, 1974) and most subsequent maxillary growth is in the vertical dimension, occurring mainly by the addition of alveolar bone (see Chap. 47). It is thought that the eruption of the permanent dentition stimulates the formation of alveolar bone and provides an impetus for vertical maxillary growth (Steedle and Proffit, 1985). By use of bone grafts to achieve closure of the alveolar arch and later orthodontically guiding the permanent teeth into the former cleft site, alveolar bone is generated by the erupting teeth. Vertical maxillary height is also maintained (Bergland, Semb, and Abyholm, 1986).

Waite and Kersten (1980) indicated that the permanent teeth that erupt into the dental arch adjacent to a nongrafted cleft are often deficient in bony and periodontal support, thus affecting tooth longevity. Secondary bone grafting before tooth eruption can often provide such support. The lateral incisor generally erupts at 7 or 8 years of age and the canine at 11 to 12 years of age (McDonald, 1974). Many centers advocate bone grafting between the ages of 9 and 11 years when the canine root is one-fourth to one-half formed (Boyne and Sands, 1972, 1976; Abyholm, Bergland, and Semb, 1981; El Deeb and associates, 1982; Bergland, Semb, and Abyholm, 1986). Their rationale has been that no adverse effect on midfacial growth has been noted with bone grafting at this age, and that grafting at this time has led to satisfactory canine migration and eruption through the bone graft. The question remains to be answered about grafting at ages 5 to 6 years, performed to provide support for the erupting lateral incisor. While the effects of surgery on maxillary growth at this age are uncertain, one must consider the high incidence of abnormalities in lateral incisor formation.

It is probably best to individualize the age at which bone grafting is performed. When the maxillary segments are in satisfactory alignment with a small cleft space, surgery can proceed in unilateral clefts between 5 and 6 years of age, and in bilateral clefts after the permanent central incisors have erupted and the arch has been properly aligned orthodontically. Since the latter correction involves the movement of bony segments rather than simple movement of teeth, orthodontic correction would be difficult if not impossible if it was attempted after bone grafting. These segments need to be stabilized with fixed retention immediately after bone grafting. In most cases the permanent central incisors in bilateral clefts need to be utilized to upright the premaxilla, in order to align it with the lateral palatal segments. One of the main advantages of performing a bone graft at this relatively early age is to permit the normal eruption of the permanent lateral incisors through the bone grafted site. In unilateral cases this approach appears to allow more room for the erupting central incisors as well. It must be stressed, however, that the bone grafted segments frequently fail to maintain the corrected arch form even after lengthy fixed stabilization (six to 12 months). It still needs to be determined whether performing alveolar surgery at this earlier age leads to a greater incidence of anterior crossbites than in a series of patients in whom the grafting was performed between 9 and 10 years of age. Any abnormally formed deciduous tooth or severely malpositioned tooth found in the line of the cleft is extracted at the time of surgery, in order to permit proper "pocket" construction for the bone graft.

In bilateral cases when an anterior cleft space of 5 mm or more exists, bone grafting is postponed until the premaxillary central and lateral incisors have erupted, in order that the premaxilla can be retropositioned orthodontically. In these cases a 5 mm soft tissue gap space usually represents a bony gap space of 10 to 13 mm, a size too large for successful bone grafting.

Finally, bone grafting during adolescence has been advocated, since maxillary growth is then completed and the occlusion is stable (Matthews and associates, 1970). The principal disadvantage of grafting after formation of the permanent dentition is that periodontal and alveolar support for fissural teeth is not improved. Crestal height uniformly reverts to preoperative levels (Turvey and associates, 1984). Patients grafted after canine eruption also show a lower rate of successful orthodontic closure, a finding necessitating an increased need for prosthodontics (Bergland, Semb, and Abyholm, 1986).

FLAP DESIGN

The gingiva along the margins of teeth is a specialized structure consisting of keratinized squamous epithelium; it is termed *attached gingiva*. The attached gingiva provides a protective covering over the tooth root and is attached to the teeth via the fibers of the periodontal membrane. The gingiva formed by the alveolar mucosa is nonkeratinized epithelium; it is more mobile than attached gingiva and lacks attachments to the teeth.

An evaluation of mucobuccal versus mucogingival incisions (Troxell, Fonseca, and Osbon, 1982; Hinrichs and associates, 1984; Witsenburg, 1985; El Deeb and associates, 1986; Bergland, Semb, and Abyholm, 1986) shows the superiority of using flaps of attached gingiva in providing periodontal support for the erupting canines. These flaps, which are developed pericoronally along the tooth margin, provide a greater width of attached gingiva, especially at the mesiofacial surface of the erupting canine. Flaps of buccal mucosa may actually impede canine eruption and increase the need for surgical exposure. If buccal mucosal flaps are used to cover bone grafts through which teeth are to erupt, they should be replaced by split palatal grafts before tooth eruption occurs.

BONE GRAFTING

Most bone grafting techniques utilize particulate cancellous bone to promote the formation of new bone. Autogenous cancellous bone has been shown to be an active osteogenic substance that can produce rapid healing in osseous defects (Boyne, 1970). It incorporates rapidly into alveolar bone and responds to the migration and orthodontic movement of teeth. In cancellous bone grafts, viable cells are transplanted and, under ideal conditions, early revascularization is noted within one week and full revascularization within three weeks (Albrektsson, 1980). Cortical bone requires the relatively slow ingrowth of vessels through established vascular networks, a process known as *creeping substitution;* the graft is slowly replaced by host tissue before full incorporation.

For successful bone grafting of alveolar defects, certain conditions must be satisfied. A watertight repair of the palatal cleft and the nasal lining, and a secure closure of the soft tissues across the anterior alveolus are essential. Bone grafts with a predominance of cancellous particles are more rapidly vascularized. In general, small particle grafts are quicker to revascularize than larger ones (Fonseca and associates, 1980), but extremely small bone particles may not be "recognized" as bone and may undergo complete resorption (Burwell and Gowland, 1961). Atraumatic surgical technique, avoidance of heat generation during the harvesting of the graft, and storage of the bone particles in a saline-soaked sponge to avoid desiccation are important in maintaining cell viability before transplantation.

The use of allogenic material such as lyophilized bone or hydroxyapatite are mentioned only to be condemned. Lyophilized bone has much less osteogenic potential than autologous bone and is only slowly and incompletely revascularized (Frost, Fonseca, and Burkes, 1982). Similar findings are seen with the use of hydroxyapatite, vascularization and bone ingrowth being seen only at the periphery of the implant material (Finn, Bell, and Brammer, 1980). Both materials are inert and do not fulfill the requirements of alveolar bone, providing an adequate substrate for tooth migration and arch restoration.

Sources of Bone Grafts

Most of the reports on primary or early bone grafting of alveolar clefts described the use of autogenous rib, which has a high ratio of cortical to cancellous bone (Robertson and Jolleys, 1968; Pickrell, Quinn, and Massengill, 1968; Hogeman, Jacobsson, and Sarnas, 1972). Some authors later showed dissatisfaction with rib grafting perhaps for this reason, though it is still used by Rosenstein and associates (1982) in primary grafting.

Johanson and associates (1974) used the tibia, where a large amount of purely cancellous bone is available. A small trapdoor of tibia covered by a proximally based periosteal flap is elevated, cancellous bone is removed with a curette, and the cortical trapdoor is replaced and maintained with a single wire.

In older patients, iliac bone has been most frequently used since it is a rich source of purely cancellous bone. Unfortunately, one cannot expect to find large amounts of cancellous iliac bone in children under the age of 9 to 10 years, since the apophysis of the iliac crest in younger patients is still largely cartilaginous. To harvest cancellous bone from the ilium, a small incision is made below the iliac crest, the medial lip of the crest is reflected, and cancellous bone is removed from the medial portion of the ilium. The medial lip of the crest is wired in place to maintain the contour of the crest and to minimize postoperative discomfort.

In 1970, Shehadi described the use of calvarial bone dust harvested with a neurosurgical perforator to reconstruct skull defects. In 1978 the authors began using bone harvested from the skull for the reconstruction of alveolar defects, and published the method in 1983 (Wolfe and Berkowitz).

The calvaria is an excellent donor source for bone grafts for alveolar clefts, since it is in an adjacent area, the bone can be rapidly harvested, there is virtually no pain postoperatively, and the technique does not leave a visible scar (Wolfe and Berkowitz, 1983; Kawamoto and Zwiebel, 1985). If one harvests the graft by the method to be described, it will not be a purely cancellous graft. One should try to have as high a percentage of diploic bone as possible, but some cortical bone shavings will inevitably be present. An incision is made over the parietal region, where the skull is thickest (see Chap. 18), and a number of superficial perforations are made with a neurosurgical perforator to remove and discard most of the cortical bone of the outer table. When brisk bleeding is encountered from the diploic bone, the surgeon uses a hand-driven Hudson brace or the neurosurgical perforator at a very slow speed, with constant irrigation (an important point so that viable bone cells are not injured during harvesting). The diploic bone is removed down to the inner table, and hemostasis is obtained with bone wax. Five to six perforations provide sufficient bone for closure of an alveolar cleft (5 to 10 ml).

The cranium is used as the bone graft donor source in approximately 90 per cent of patients. In older patients with large clefts, in patients with large bilateral clefts, and in patients in whom there has been a failure with cranial bone, iliac bone is preferred. It is favored in these situations because of its higher percentage of cancellous bone and slightly more substantial consistency. It may be that the smaller particle size of bone harvested with a drill is a negative factor, and that if diploic bone were taken with a curette (a possibly dangerous maneuver), cranial bone would perform as well as iliac bone. In general, cancellous iliac grafts can be expected to perform better than cranial bone, harvested as described above, in difficult clinical situations.

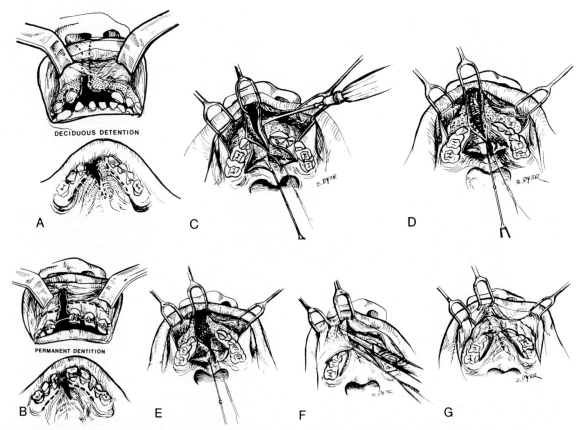

Figure 55–1. Technique to close an alveolar cleft. *A,* In the deciduous dentition, incisions are used to strip the gingiva from its lowest dental attachment (pericoronal incision). *B,* In the permanent dentition, the incisions are made higher to preserve this attachment. *C, D,* Dissection of the anterior maxilla and the cleft is carried out and, when required, incisions can be made on the palatal surface to facilitate closure of the anterior palatal cleft. *E,* After dissection and closure of the nasal lining, the bone graft is packed into the deficient area. *F,* An undercutting of the superiorly based flap from the surface of the upper lip is performed to allow tension-free closure over the bone graft. *G,* Completed repair.

SURGICAL TECHNIQUE

After preliminary injection with an epinephrine-saline solution, a superiorly based mucogingival triangular flap is elevated, extending as far as possible into the depths of the alveolar cleft (Fig. 55–1). Deciduous teeth along the edges of the cleft, if present, are removed. A pericoronal incision is used along *deciduous* teeth, and over *permanent* teeth an incision is made 3 to 4 mm above the gingivodental junction. An incision is made along the edges of the cleft, midway between the palate and the nasal floor. Superiorly based flaps are developed for nasal lining, and inferiorly based flaps are reflected caudally for closure of the palate. This maneuver is easy on the lateral side of the cleft; on the medial side, the raising of the mucoperiosteum from

the vomer is much more tedious. The dissection should extend posteriorly well beyond the extent of the palatal cleft, which in some patients is as far back as the hard palate–soft palate junction. The nasal lining is closed with fine catgut or Vicryl sutures tied on the nasal side. The palatal closure is accomplished with larger sutures tied on the palatal side.

Bilateral alveolar clefts can usually be repaired in one surgical stage, although this is technically more demanding than a unilateral closure (Fig. 55–2). An adequate blood supply to the premaxilla must be maintained through the labial mucoperiosteum. If needed, posteriorly based palatal flaps can be raised to allow better exposure for closure of the nasal lining from the palatal side and for a tension-free palatal repair.

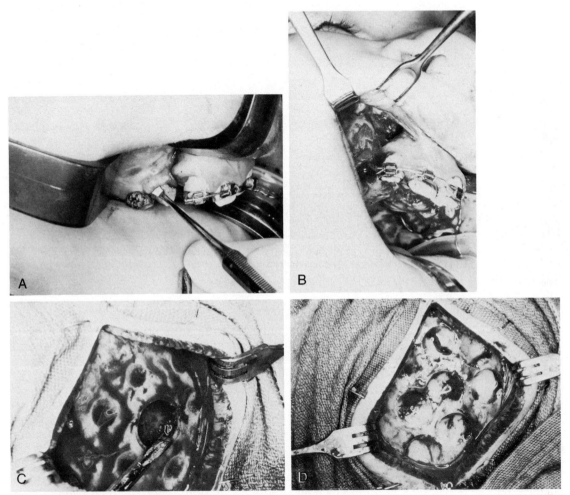

Figure 55–2. Cranial bone grafting of a bilateral cleft at age 6 years. *A,* A pericoronal incision is used; the deciduous tooth along the cleft margin will be removed. *B,* After closure of the nasal lining. *C,* An incision in the parieto-occipital region of the nondominant side is used. A number of superficial perforations through the outer table are made until bleeding bone is encountered. The outer table bone is discarded and diploic bone is harvested. *D,* Bone wax is used for hemostasis.

Illustration continued on following page

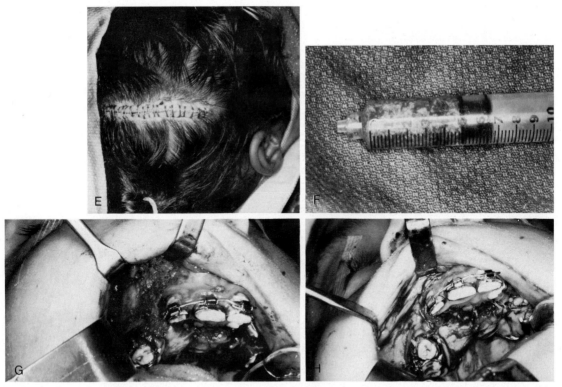

Figure 55–2 *Continued E*, The scalp is closed in two layers. *F*, The diploic bone is compressed in a syringe. *G*, The bone graft is packed into the alveolar defect. *H*, The anterior closure is performed after undermining the superiorly based flap from the lip.

After the nasal lining and the palatal cleft have been closed, the bone graft, either iliac or cranial, is packed into the entire extent of the cleft, thus providing bone for the nasal floor and palate. Bone is also used to constitute a piriform rim and is packed into the alveolar defect as inferiorly as possible. Any remaining bone is placed as an onlay over the upper portion of the piriform rim to augment the maxilla and provide support for the alar base of the nose. The previously developed triangular flap is then brought down for anterior closure. It may be necessary to extend the flap into the lip or lengthen the incision into the buccal sulcus with a back cut. The flap can then be transferred over the bone graft to provide anterior alveolar closure without tension (Fig. 55–3). When there has been a poor lip repair, reopening the lip facilitates closure of large alveolar clefts (Fig. 55–4). Patients are given antibiotics (penicillin, if they are not allergic to this agent) before and during the procedure, and this is continued for one week postoperatively. Clear liquids are given by mouth for the first two days and the patients are advanced to a soft diet, on which they remain for three weeks.

RESULTS

Incorporation of Bone Grafts. Approximately 90 per cent of the authors' patients have undergone successful closure of alveolar defects with the use of cranial bone (Fig. 55–5) (Wolfe and Berkowitz, 1983). This rate is similar to that reported by Kawamoto and Zwiebel (1985) but below that of Johanson and associates (1974), who reported success in 96 per cent of patients with tibial bone grafts.

Other series have reported success rates of 97 per cent after use of iliac bone grafts (Troxell, Fonseca, and Osbon, 1982; Hall and Posnick, 1983; Bergland, Semb, and Abyholm, 1986). Jackson and associates (1982) reported an 84 per cent initial success rate using iliac bone grafts and a 95 per cent success rate of alveolar cleft closure following secondary operations.

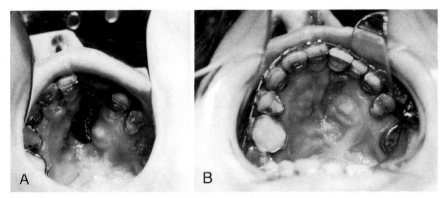

Figure 55–3. Closure of the anterior palatal fistula is crucial to the success of the bone graft. In large clefts, anterior palatal flaps must be developed to allow closure without tension over the bone graft. *A,* Preoperative view. Note the alveolar cleft and the associated palatal fistula. *B,* Following repair and bone grafting.

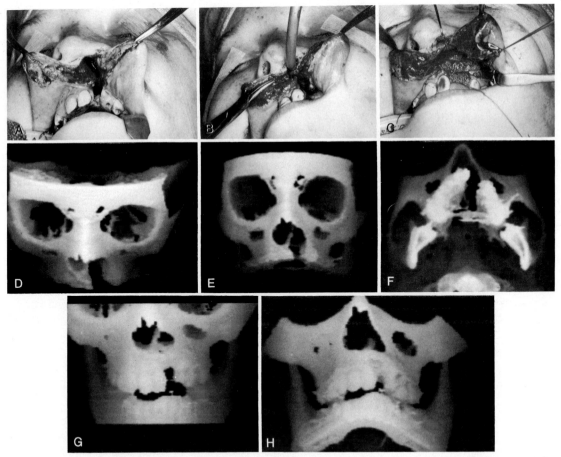

Figure 55–4. When there has been a poor lip repair, reopening the lip facilitates closure of large alveolar clefts. *A,* The reopened lip, giving a clear view of a large alveolar cleft. *B,* The nasal lining is closed over a catheter to establish an adequate nasal passage. *C,* After closure of the anterior palatal cleft, the bone graft is packed into the defect. Posteriorly, it extends along the entire length of the maxillary cleft; superiorly it reconstitutes a piriform rim, and inferiorly it is extended as low as possible. *D–H,* Pre- and postoperative three-dimensional CT scans of the same patient (one year postoperatively). This is a large cleft, and it can be clearly seen on the preoperative views that the bony cleft extends through almost the entire hard palate.

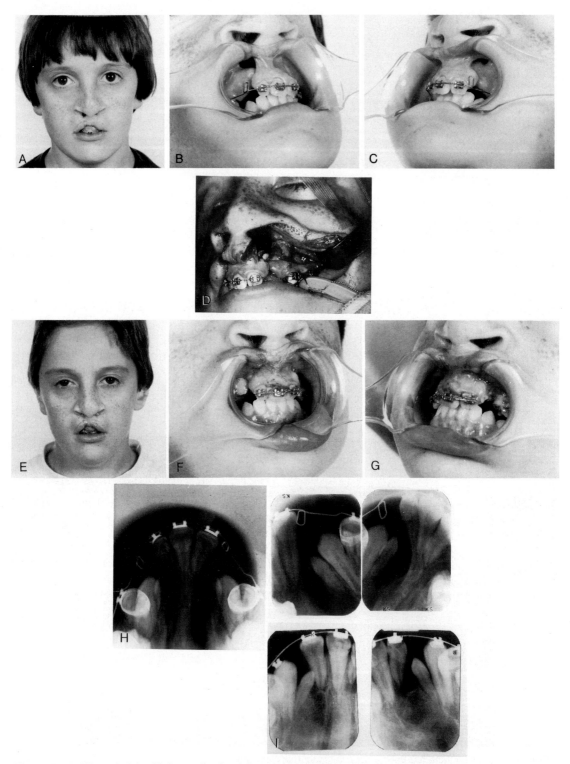

Figure 55–5. Bilateral cleft with large alveolar defects and a mobile premaxilla. Preliminary orthodontic therapy has brought the maxillary segments into satisfactory alignment. *A,* Preoperative appearance of the patient. *B, C,* The alveolar clefts. There is little labial sulcus over the premaxilla. *D,* Closure of defects of this magnitude probably would not be possible without reopening the lip. *E,* Postoperative appearance at one month. *F, G,* The alveolar defects one month postoperatively. *H, I,* Preoperative and four-month postoperative radiographs showing satisfactory bone formation (iliac donor site). This patient will almost certainly need an Abbé flap reconstruction of the upper lip, with the prolabial skin used to reconstruct the columella.

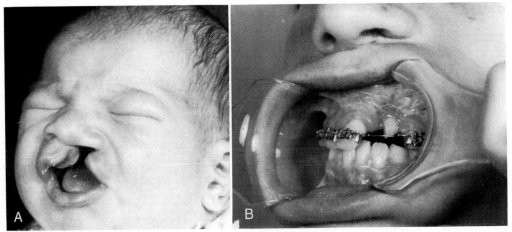

Figure 55–6. *A,* An infant with a unilateral complete cleft. Cranial bone grafting of the alveolar defect was performed at age 6 years. *B,* At age 10, a tooth is seen erupting through the bone graft.

Eruption of Canine. El Deeb and associates in 1982 showed that in 27 per cent of patients the canines at the alveolar cleft erupted spontaneously after alveolar bone grafting (Figs. 55–6, 55–7), while the remaining 73 per cent underwent surgical uncovering to allow canine eruption. Fifty-six per cent of patients also required orthodontic guidance following canine eruption.

Similar findings were noted by Hinrichs and associates (1984); 56 per cent of canines required surgical exposure and 44 per cent of patients required orthodontic assistance to allow eruption into functional occlusion. These data compare with the reports of Bergland, Semb, and Abyholm (1986) in which only 15 per cent of patients required surgical exposure of the canine to allow eruption into

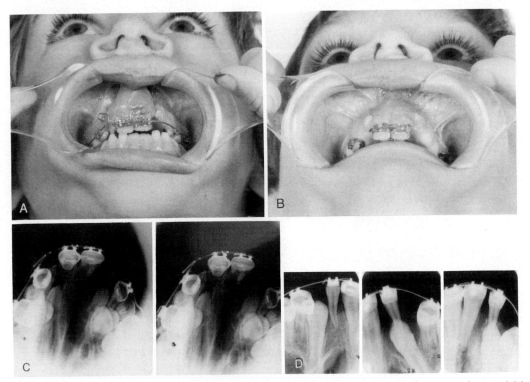

Figure 55–7. A patient with bilateral alveolar clefts. *A,* Preoperative occlusal view. *B,* One year after cranial bone grafting. The lateral incisors are erupting spontaneously through the bone graft. *C,* Preoperative occlusal radiographs. *D,* Postoperative periapical radiographs of the same patient.

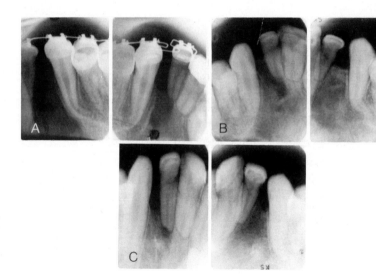

Figure 55–8. *A,* Preoperative, *B,* one-year postoperative, and *C,* four-year postoperative radiographs after cranial bone grafting of bilateral alveolar clefts. Note that a small apical cyst has formed above one lateral incisor and that there has been slight regression of crestal height.

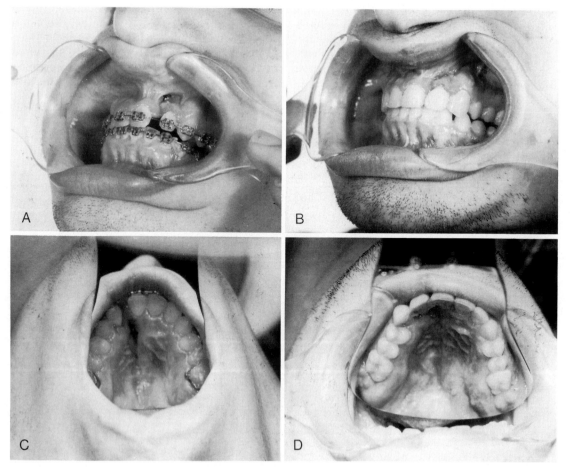

Figure 55–9. An 18 year old patient who underwent bone grafting of an alveolar cleft and closure of an oronasal fistula. The lateral incisor is present and is located distal to the cleft. *A,* Preoperative view. *B,* In the postoperative view, the size of the lateral incisor has been increased by dental bonding. *C,* Preoperative palatal view. *D,* Postoperative palatal view.

the cleft site. In the series by Turvey and associates (1984), only 5 per cent required surgical exposure. Overall, satisfactory canine eruption is seen after alveolar bone grafting performed during the period of mixed dentition.

Closure of Cleft Space. According to Bergland, Semb, and Abyholm (1986), in patients grafted before canine eruption, the success rate of closure of the cleft space was 90 per cent, only 10 per cent of the patients requiring prosthodontic devices. In patients who underwent late secondary bone grafting during the period of permanent dentition, the success rate fell to 72 per cent, 28 per cent of the patients requiring prosthodontic closure of the cleft space.

COMPLICATIONS

Minor postoperative complications occur occasionally. Failure rates with this procedure in the authors' hands remain approximately 10 per cent and are almost always due to problems with soft tissue closure (either inadequate closure of the palatal cleft, or separation of the anterior suture line due to excessive tension). Bilateral alveolar cleft repairs have had a higher complication rate, perhaps owing to the difficulty in developing adequate flaps from the posterior surface of the premaxilla (Fig. 55–8). If the soft tissue closure is successful, the bone graft usually is also successful.

Minor bone graft exposure should be managed conservatively with a soft diet and antibiotic therapy. Healing of small areas of exposed bone usually proceeds uneventfully with only a minor loss of graft material (Fig. 55–9) (Witsenburg, 1985).

REFERENCES

Abyholm, F., Bergland, O., and Semb, G.: Secondary bone grafting of alveolar clefts. Scand. J. Plast. Reconstr. Surg., 15:127, 1981.

Aduss, H., and Pruzansky, S.: The nasal cavity in complete cleft lip and palate. Arch. Otolaryngol., 85:53, 1967.

Albrektsson, T.: Repair of bone grafts. A vital microscopic and histological investigation in the rabbit. Scand. J. Plast. Reconstr. Surg., 14:1, 1980.

Axhausen, G.: Technik und Ergebnisse der Spaltplastiken. Munchen, Hanser, 1952.

Bailit, H. L., Doykos, J. D., III, and Swanson, L.: Dental development in children with cleft palate. J. Dent. Res., 47:664, 1968.

Beck, J. C., and Jesser, J. J.: Plastic surgery of the face. Dental Items Interest, 43:359, 1921.

Bergland, O., Semb, G., and Abyholm, F. E.: Elimination of the residual alveolar cleft by secondary bone grafting and subsequent orthodontic treatment. Cleft Palate J., 23:175, 1986.

Berkowitz, S.: Cleft lip and palate research: an updated state of the art. Section III. Orofacial growth and dentistry. Cleft Palate J., 14:288, 1977.

Berkowitz, S.: State of the art in cleft palate orofacial growth and dentistry. Am. J. Orthod., 74:564, 1978.

Berkowitz, S.: Timing in cleft palate closure: age should not be the sole determinant. J. Craniofac. Genet. Dev. Biol. [Suppl.], 1:69, 1985.

Bjork, A., and Skieller, V.: Growth in width of the maxilla studied by the implant method. Scand. J. Plast. Reconstr. Surg., 8:26, 1974.

Bohn, A.: Dental anomalies in harelip and cleft palate. Acta Odont. Scand., 21:Suppl. 38, 1963.

Boyne, P. J.: Autogenous cancellous bone and marrow transplants. Clin. Orthop., 73:199, 1970.

Boyne, P. J., and Sands, N. R.: Secondary bone grafts of residual alveolar and palatal clefts. J. Oral Surg., 30:87, 1972.

Boyne, P. J., and Sands, N. R.: Combined orthodontic-surgical management of residual palato-alveolar cleft defects. Am. J. Orthod., 70:20, 1976.

Brauer, R. O., and Cronin, T. D.: Maxillary orthopedics and anterior palatal repair with bone grafting. Cleft Palate J., 1:31, 1964.

Burian, F.: On the disturbances of growth of the upper jaw in operated cleft lip and palate. In Skoog, T., and Ivy, R. H. (Eds.): Transactions of the International Society of Plastic Surgeons, First Congress. Baltimore, Williams & Wilkins Company, 1957, pp. 224–227.

Burston, W. R.: The early orthodontic treatment of alveolar clefts. Proc. R. Soc. Med., 58:767, 1965.

Burwell, R., and Gowland, G.: Studies in the transplantation of bone. Assessment of antigenicity. Serological studies. J. Bone Joint Surg., 43B:814, 1961.

Campbell, A.: The closure of congenital clefts of the hard palate. Br. J. Surg., 13:715, 1926.

Dixon, A. D., and Sarnat, B. G.: Factors and Mechanisms Influencing Bone Growth. Progress in Clinical and Biological Research. Vol. 101. New York, Alan R. Liss, 1982.

Dorrance, G. M.: The Operative Story of Cleft Palate. Philadelphia, W. B. Saunders Company, 1933.

Drachter, R.: Die Gaumenspalte und ihren operative Behandlung. Dtsch. Z. Chir., 131:1, 1914.

El Deeb, M. E., Hinrichs, J. E., Waite, D. E., Bandt, C. L., and Bevis, R.: Repair of alveolar cleft defects with autogenous bone grafting: periodontal evaluation. Cleft Palate J., 23:126, 1986.

El Deeb, M., Messer, L. B., Lehnert, M. W., Hebda, T. W., and Waite, D. E.: Canine eruption into grafted bone in maxillary alveolar defects. Cleft Palate J., 19:9, 1982.

Engdahl, E.: Bone regeneration in maxillary defects. An experimental investigation on the significance of the periosteum and various media on bone formation and maxillary growth. Scand. J. Plast. Reconstr. Surg., 8:1, 1972.

Finn, R. A., Bell, W. H., and Brammer, J. A.: Interpositional "grafting" with autogenous bone and coralline hydroxyapatite. J. Maxillofac. Surg., 8:217, 1980.

Fishman, L. S.: Factors related to tooth number, eruption time, and tooth position in cleft palate individuals. J. Dent. Child., 37:303, 1970.

Fonseca, R. J., Clark, P. J., Burkes, E. J., Jr., and Baker, R. D.: Revascularization and healing of onlay particulate autologous bone grafts in primates. J. Oral Surg., *38*:572, 1980.

Friede, H., and Johanson, B.: Adolescent facial morphology of early bone-grafted cleft lip and palate patients. Scand. J. Plast. Reconstr. Surg., *16*:41, 1982.

Frost, D. E., Fonseca, R. J., and Burkes, E. J.: Healing of interpositional allogeneic lyophilized bone grafts following total maxillary osteotomy. J. Oral Maxillofac. Surg., *40*:776, 1982.

Gabka, J.: Hasenscharten und Wolfsrachen. Entstehung und Behandlung. Berlin, Gruyter, 1964.

Georgiade, N. C., Pickrell, K. L., and Quinn, G. W.: Varying concepts in bone grafting of alveolar palatal defects. Cleft Palate J., *1*:43, 1964.

Graber, T. M.: Acephalometric analysis of the developmental pattern and facial morphology in cleft palate. Angle Orthod., *19*:91, 1949.

Graber, T. M.: The fundamentals of occlusion. J. Am. Dent. Assoc., *48*:177, 1954.

Hall, H. D., and Posnick, J. C.: Early results of secondary bone grafts in 106 alveolar clefts. J. Oral Maxillofac. Surg., *41*:289, 1983.

Harkins, C. S.: Principles of Cleft Palate Prosthesis. New York, Columbia University Press, 1960.

Harvold, E.: Observations on the development of the upper jaw by harelip and cleft palate. Odontol. Tidskr., *55*:289, 1947.

Harvold, E.: Prinsippene for den kjeveontopediske behandling av overkjaven med ensidig total ganespalte. Nor. Tannlaegeforen Tid., *59*:395, 1949.

Hellquist, R., and Ponten, B.: The influence of infant periosteoplasty on facial growth and dental occlusion from five to eight years of age in cases of complete unilateral cleft lip and palate. Scand. J. Plast. Reconstr. Surg., *13*:305, 1979.

Hellquist, R., and Skoog, T.: The influence of primary periosteoplasty on maxillary growth and deciduous occlusion in cases of complete unilateral cleft lip and palate. Scand. J. Plast. Reconstr. Surg., *10*:197, 1976.

Hinrichs, J. E., El Deeb, M. E., Waite, D. E., Bevis, R. R., and Bandt, C. L.: Periodontal evaluation of canines erupted through grafted alveolar cleft defects. J. Oral Maxillofac. Surg., *42*:717, 1984.

Hogeman, K. E., Jacobsson, S., and Sarnas, K. V.: Secondary bone grafting in cleft palate: a follow up of 145 patients. Cleft Palate J., *9*:39, 1972.

Hollman, K.: Bemerkungen zum Osteoplastik bei Lippen-Kiefer-Gaumenspalten. Ost. Z. Stomatol., *61*:388, 1964.

Jackson, I. T., Vandervord, J. G., McLennan, J. G., Christie, F. B., and McGregor, J. C.: Bone grafting of the secondary cleft lip and palate deformity. Br. J. Plast. Surg., *35*:345, 1982.

Johanson, B.: Secondary osteoplastic completion of maxilla and palate. *In* Schuchardt, K. (Ed.): Treatment of Patients with Clefts of Lip, Alveolus and Palate. Topic 10. Second Hamburg International Symposium, 1964. Stuttgart, Georg Thieme Verlag, 1966.

Johanson, B., and Nordin, K. E.: Freie knochen Transplantation bei Defekten in Alveolarkamm nach Kiefer orthopadischer Einstellung der Maxilla bei Lippen-Kiefer-Gaumenspalten. Fortschr. Kiefer-Gesichtschir., *1*:168, 1955.

Johanson, B., Ohlsson, A., Friede, H., and Ahlgren, J.: A follow-up study of cleft lip and palate patients treated with orthodontics, secondary bone grafting,

and prosthetic rehabilitation. Scand. J. Plast. Reconstr. Surg., *8*:121, 1974.

Kawamoto, H. K., and Zwiebel, P.: Cranial bone grafts in alveolar cleft. *In* Caronni, E. (Ed.): Craniofacial Surgery. Boston, Little, Brown & Company, 1985.

Kling, A.: Evaluation of results in reference to the bite. *In* Schuchardt, K. (Ed.): Treatment of Patients with Clefts of Lip, Alveolus and Palate. Second Hamburg International Symposium, 1964. Stuttgart, Georg Thieme Verlag, 1966.

Koberg, W. R.: Present view on bone grafting in cleft palate. J. Maxillofac. Surg., *1*:185, 1973.

Lexer, E.: Die Verwendung der freien Knochenplastik nebst Versuchen über Gelenkversteifung und Gelenktransplantation. Arch. Klin. Chir., *86*:939, 1908.

Lynch, J. B., Brelsford, H., Lewis, S., and Blocker, T.: Maxillary bone grafts in cleft lip–cleft palate reconstruction. Texas J. Med., *61*:172, 1965.

Lynch, J. B., and Peil, R.: Retarded maxillary growth in experimental cleft palate. Mechanical binding of scar tissue in puppies. Am. Surg., 32:507, 1966.

Matthews, D., Broomhead, I., Grossmann, W., and Goldin, H.: Early and late bone grafting in cases of cleft lip and palate. Br. J. Plast. Surg., 23:115, 1970.

Mazaheri, M., Harding, R. L., and Nanda, S.: The effect of surgery on maxillary growth and cleft width. Plast. Reconstr. Surg., *40*:22, 1967.

McDonald, R. E.: Dentistry for the Child and Adolescent. St. Louis, C. V. Mosby Company, 1974, p. 70.

McNeil, C. K.: Oral and Facial Deformity. London, Pitman, 1954.

Metz, H., and Gunther, H.: Indications and techniques of secondary osteoplastic procedures in clefts of the alveolus and palate. Panminerva Med., *9*:400, 1967.

Millard, D. R., Jr.: Personal communication, 1972.

Millard, D. R., Jr.: Cleft Craft III. Alveolar and Palatal Deformities. Boston, Little, Brown & Company, 1980.

Millhon, J. A., and Stafne, E. C.: Incidence of supernumerary and congenitally missing lateral incisor teeth in eighty-one cases of harelip and cleft palate. Am. J. Orthod. (Oral Surg.), 27:599, 1941.

Monroe, C. W., Griffith, B. H., Rosenstein, S. W., et al.: The correction and preservation of arch form in complete clefts of the palate and alveolar ridge. Plast. Reconstr. Surg., *41*:108, 1968.

Nordin, K., and Johanson, B.: Freie Knochentransplantation bei Defekten im Alveolarkamm nach Kieferortopadischer Einstellung der Maxilla bei Lippen-Kiefer-Gaumenspalten. *In* Schuchardt, K., and Wassmund, M. (Eds.): Fortschritte der Kiefer- und Gesichts-Chirurgie. Vol. I. Stuttgart, Georg Thieme Verlag, 1955, pp. 168–71.

Nylen, B., Körlof, B., Arnander, C., Leanderson, R., Barr, B., and Nordin, K. E.: Primary, early bone grafting in complete clefts of the lip and palate. Scand. J. Plast. Reconstr. Surg., *8*:79, 1974.

Olin, W. H.: Dental anomalies in cleft lip and palate patients. Angle Orthod., *34*:119, 1964.

Ortiz-Monasterio, F., Rebeil, A. S., Valderrama, M., and Cruz, R.: Cephalometric measurements on adult patients with nonoperated clefts. Plast. Reconstr. Surg., *24*:53, 1959.

Perko, M.: Gleichzeitige Osteotomie des Zwischenkiefers, Restspaltenverschluss und Zwischenkieferversteifung durch sekundäre Osteoplastik bei Spätfällen von beidseitigen Lippen-Kiefer-Gaumenspalten. Dtsch. Zahn Mund Kieferheilk., *47*:1, 1966.

Pickrell, K., Quinn, G., and Massengill, R.: Primary bone

grafting of the maxilla in clefts of the lip and palate: a four year study. Plast. Reconstr. Surg., 41:438, 1968.

Pruzansky, S.: Pre-surgical orthopedics and bone grafting for infants with cleft lip and palate: a dissent. Cleft Palate J., 1:164, 1964.

Pruzansky, S.: Discussion of the use of cranial bone grafts in the closure of alveolar and anterior palatal clefts by Wolfe, S. A., and Berkowitz, S. Plast. Reconstr. Surg., 72:669, 1983.

Ranta, R.: The effect of congenital cleft lip, alveolar process and palate on the tooth germ of the lateral incisor and on its position in relation to the cleft. Suom. Hammaslaak. Toim., 67:295, 1971a.

Ranta, R.: On the development of central incisors and canines situated adjacent to the cleft in unilateral total cleft cases. Suom. Hammaslaak Toim., 67:345, 1971b.

Ranta, R.: The development of the permanent teeth in children with complete cleft lip and palate. Proc. Finn. Dent. Soc., 68:Suppl. III, 1972.

Rehrmann, A. H., Koberg, W., and Koch, H.: Long-term postoperative results of primary and secondary bone grafting in complete clefts of lip and palate. Cleft Palate J., 7:206, 1970.

Ritter, R.: Beuterlung des Zwischenkiefers bei Spaltkindern von Seiten des Kieferchirurgien des Orthopaeden und des Prosthetikers. Fortschr. Kiefer-Gesichtschir., 5:243, 1959.

Robertson, N. R., and Jolleys, A.: Effects of early bone grafting in complete clefts of lip and palate. Plast. Reconstr. Surg., 42:414, 1968.

Rosenstein, S.: Orthodontic and bone grafting procedures in a cleft lip and palate series. An interim cephalometric evaluation. Angle Orthod., 45:227, 1975.

Rosenstein, S. W., Monroe, C. W., Kernahan, D. A., Jacobson, B. N., Griffith, B., and Bauer, B.: The case for early bone grafting in cleft lip and cleft palate. Plast. Reconstr. Surg., 70:297, 1982.

Ross, R. B.: The clinical implications of facial growth in cleft lip and palate. Cleft Palate J., 7:37, 1970.

Ross, R. B.: The management of dental arch deformity in cleft lip and palate. Clin. Plast. Surg., 2:325, 1975.

Schmid, E.: Die aufbauende Kieferkammplastik. Ost. J. Stomatol, 51:582, 1954.

Schmid, E.: Die Annaherung der Kieferstumpfe bei Lippen-Kiefer-Gaumenspalten: ihre schädlichen Folgen und Vermeidung. Fortschr. Kiefer-Gesichtschir., 1:37, 1955.

Schmid, E.: Die Osteoplastik bei Lippen-Kiefer-Gaumenspalten. Langenbecks Arch. Klin. Chir., 295:868, 1960.

Schmid, E.: Bone grafting as an aid to the formation of normal alveolar and dental arch. In Hotz, R. (Ed.): Early Treatment of Cleft Lip and Palate. Bern, Huber, 1964.

Schmid, E., and Widmaier, W.: La greffe osseuse simultanée a la fermeture du bec-de-lièvre. Ann. Chir. Plast., 8:23, 1963.

Schmid, E., Widmaier, W., Reichert, H., and Stein, K.: The development of the cleft upper jaw following primary osteoplasty and orthodontic treatment. J. Maxillofac. Surg., 2:92, 1974.

Schrudde, J., and Stellmach, R.: Die primäre Osteoplastik der Defekte des Kieferbogens bei Lippen-Kiefer-Gaumenspalten am Säugling. Zentralbl. Chir., 83:849, 1958.

Schrudde, J., and Stellmach, R.: Primäre Osteoplastik und Kieferbogen Formung bei Lippen-Kiefer-Gaumenspalten. Fortschr. Kiefer-Gesichtschir., 5:247, 1959.

Schrudde, J., and Trauner, M.: Über das Schicksal der freien Rippenknochentransplantate nach der primaren Osteoplastik der Kieferspaltz die Lippen-Kiefer-Gaumenspalten. Transact d. III Tag. d. Verein. d. Dtsch. Plast. Chir. Pilgram, Hoffnungsthal, 1972.

Schuchardt, K., and Pfeifer, G.: Erfahrungen über primare Knochentransplantationen bei Lippen-Kiefer-Gaumenspalten. Langenbecks Arch. Klin. Chir., 295:881, 1960.

Shehadi, S. I.: Skull reconstruction with bone dust. Br. J. Plast. Surg., 23:227, 1970.

Skoog, T.: The management of the bilateral cleft of the primary palate (lip and alveolus). Part II. Bone Grafting. Plast. Reconstr. Surg., 35:140, 1965.

Skoog, T.: Diskussion zum Vortrag von R. Stellmach: Modern procedures in uni- and bilateral clefts of lip, alveolus and hard palate with respect to primary osteoplasty. In Schuchardt, K. (Ed.): Treatment of Patients with Clefts of Lip, Alveolus and Palate. Second Hamburg International Symposium, 1964. Stuttgart, Georg Thieme Verlag, 1966.

Skoog, T.: Repair of the cleft maxilla using periosteal flaps. Panminerva Med., 9:405, 1967a.

Skoog, T.: The use of periosteum and Surgicel for bone restoration in congenital clefts of the maxilla. A clinical report and experimental investigation. Scand. J. Plast. Reconstr. Surg., 1:113, 1967b.

Slaughter, W. B., and Brodie, A. G.: Facial clefts and their surgical management in view of recent research. Plast. Reconstr. Surg., 4:311, 1949.

Steedle, J. R., and Proffit, W. R.: The pattern and control of eruptive tooth movements. Am. J. Orthod., 87:56, 1985.

Steinhardt, G.: Diskussion zum Vortrag von R. Stellmach: Modern procedures in uni- and bilateral clefts of the lip, alveolus and hard palate, with respect to primary osteoplasty. In Schuchardt, K. (Ed.): Treatment of Patients with Clefts of Lip, Alveolus and Palate. Second Hamburg International Symposium, 1964. Stuttgart, Georg Thieme Verlag, 1966.

Steinhardt, G. Der operative Verschluss die Lippen-Kiefer-Gaumenspalten mittels Pichler-Vomer-Lappen und Alveolar Lappen. In Schuchardt, K., Steinhardt, G., and Schwenzen, N. (Eds.): Fortschr. der Kiefer-und Gesichts-Chirurgie. Vol. 16–17. Stuttgart, Georg Thieme Verlag, 1973, pp. 80–83.

Stenström, S. J., and Thilander, B. L.: Facial skeleton growth after bone grafting to surgically created premaxillary suture defects: an experimental study on the guinea pig. Plast. Reconstr. Surg., 40:1, 1967a.

Stenström, S. J., and Thilander, B. L.: The growth retarding effect of bone grafting to the defect after extirpation of the premaxillary suture in guinea pigs. Panminerva Med., 9:406, 1967b.

Tessier, P.: Anatomical classification of facial, craniofacial and latero-facial clefts. J. Maxillofac. Surg., 4:69, 1976.

Troutman, K. C.: Maxillary arch control in infants with unilateral clefts of the lip and palate. Am. J. Orthod., 66:198, 1974.

Troxell, J. B., Fonseca, R. J., and Osbon, D. B.: A retrospective study of alveolar cleft grafting. J. Oral Maxillofac. Surg., 40:721, 1982.

Turvey, T. A., Vig, K., Moriarty, J., and Hoke, J.: Delayed bone grafting in the cleft maxilla and palate: a retrospective multidisciplinary analysis. Am. J. Orthod., 86:244, 1984.

Veau, V.: Division Palatine: Anatomie, Chirurgie, Phonetique. Paris, Masson et Cie., 1931.

Waite, D. E., and Kersten, R. B.: Residual alveolar and palatal clefts. *In* Bell, W. H., Proffit, W. R., and White, R. P. (Eds.): Surgical Correction of Dentofacial Deformities. Philadelphia, W. B. Saunders Company, 1980, pp. 1329–1367.

Witsenburg, B.: The reconstruction of anterior residual bone defects in patients with cleft lip, alveolus and palate. J. Maxillofac. Surg., *13*:197, 1985.

Wolfe, S. A., and Berkowitz, S.: The use of cranial bone grafts in the closure of alveolar and anterior palatal clefts. Plast. Reconstr. Surg., *72*:659, 1983.

56

Ian T. Jackson
Michael C. Fasching

Secondary Deformities of Cleft Lip, Nose, and Cleft Palate

Secondary deformities can exist after repair of cleft lip or cleft lip and palate and can affect some or all of the previously cleft regions. There may be lip distortion, nasal deformity, and maxillary hypoplasia; the alveolus may be partly edentulous; and there may be malocclusion, fistula, and palatal dysfunction. The degree of the deformities is usually related to several variables: the severity of the original defect, the method of repair and subsequent healing, the inherent and familial patterns of the patient's craniofacial growth, the effectiveness of orthodontic therapy, and the adequacy of prosthetic rehabilitation. The evolution of sophisticated lip repairs (e.g., LeMesurier, 1949; Tennison, 1952; Millard, 1955; Skoog, 1958; Manches-ter, 1965; Trauner and Trauner, 1967) ensures satisfactory results for the majority of cleft patients. The stigmas of the cleft are usually located in other areas (e.g., the nose), although management of the lip continues to be a surgical challenge in bilateral cleft repair in Caucasians.

Brown and McDowell (1941) advised patients with secondary cleft deformities to adopt a livelihood in which they would not appear in the public eye and to develop a retiring personality. This statement is an admission of defeat and is no longer acceptable to either the surgeon or the patient.

The correction of secondary cleft deformities is difficult and requires the efforts of a multidisciplinary team, including a speech pathologist, an orthodontist, a prosthodontist, an otologist, a psychologist, a medical social worker, and a plastic surgeon, who frequently heads the team. Even with the expertise of such a team, there may be residual problems. Bardach and associates (1984) reported that only 16 per cent of patients had completed treatment to the satisfaction of all specialists in their clinic, and totally acceptable results were achieved in fewer than 50 per cent of patients in any one area of special interest.

Correction of the complex interrelated secondary deformities of the lip, the nose, and the alveolus requires a careful and systematic evaluation of the deformity, an integrated treatment plan, and high quality surgical technique. As is the case for primary cleft, secondary deformities are interconnected, and isolated operations on the nose, the lip, or the alveolus (except when the initial defect was fairly minimal) often give less than optimal results.

Table 56–1. Evaluation of Secondary Cleft Defects

I. The foundation of the lip and nose
  A. Evaluate the alveolar defect
  B. Determine the position of the maxilla
  C. Identify missing or malpositioned dental units
II. Lip
  A. Assess the total amount of lip tissue
  B. Evaluate the freedom of the buccal aspect of the lip from the anterior aspect of the alveolar process Does the upper lip pout?
  C. Evaluate the vermilion mucosa for equal bulk along the entire margin
  D. Cupid's bow
    1. Determine if all components are present
    2. Determine the position of components
  E. Philtral structures
    1. Assess the length of philtral ridges
    2. Evaluate the direction of ridges as well as the location and direction of lip scars
    3. Assess the width of the philtral column
  F. Check the alignment of the circumoral muscles
III. Nose
  A. From the front
    1. Locate the lower lateral cartilages
    2. Locate the alar bases: to each other, to the eyes, and to the structures of the Cupid's bow
    3. Determine the size and shape of the alae
    4. Locate the upper lateral cartilages
    5. Determine the width of the bony pyramid
  B. From *both* profiles
    1. Determine the nasolabial angle
    2. Assess the length and direction of the septum
    3. Evaluate the visibility of the columella
    4. Assess the length of the columella and the relative position of the nasal tip
  C. From below
    1. Determine the size, shape, and direction of nostrils
    2. Assess the length of both sides of the columella and the direction of the columella
    3. Evaluate deviation of the caudal septum
    4. Evaluate the vestibules for the presence of a web or distorted lateral border of the lower lateral cartilages
    5. Evaluate the alae for size, shape, and position
  D. From above
    1. Assess the straightness of the septum
    2. Determine the size, shape, and position of the upper and lower lateral cartilages
    3. Assess the size, shape, and position of the alae

From Wilson, L. F.: Correction of residual deformities of the lip and nose in repaired clefts of the primary palate (lip and alveolus). Clin. Plast. Surg. *12:*719, 1985.

SECONDARY DEFORMITIES OF UNILATERAL CLEFT

Brown and McDowell (1941) stated the requirements for satisfactory repair of the cleft lip and the associated nasal deformity, and Steffensen (1953) expanded this list: (1) accurate skin, muscle, and mucosal union with adequate lip lengthening; (2) rotation of the deflected lateral portion of the orbicularis oris muscle into a horizontal position with its medial component; (3) measures to obtain symmetric alar bases and nostril floors; (4) a nasal tip with an adequate columellar-labial angle and sufficient columellar length; (5) a symmetric vermilion border with a Cupid's bow; (6) a slight eversion, or pouting, of the central portion of the lip; and (7) a minimal scar, which, as it contracts, does not interfere with the achievement of the other objectives. Unfortunately, this list ignores the effect of the nasal septum and the maxillary deformity on the production of lip and nose distortion, and thus this simplistic approach needs to be amended.

A format for evaluating secondary cleft

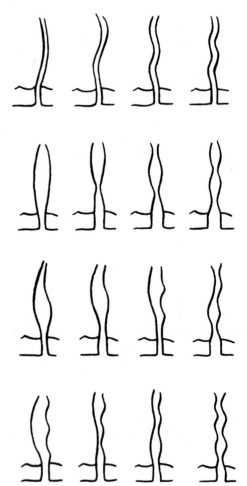

Figure 56–1. Various designs of "wave-line" repair for revision of an old lip scar. (After Pfeifer. From Millard, D. R., Jr.: Cleft Craft. Vol. I. Boston, Little, Brown & Company, 1976.)

defects is presented in Table 56–1. For assessment of the secondary cleft deformity, whether unilateral or bilateral, the deformed nose must be placed in a normal position. This is done by gently pulling on the nasal rim with a hook until symmetry or correct nasal tip position is achieved. In this way, *true lip shortness* and other subtle features, such as the force required to achieve this nasal symmetry, can be determined.

Lip Deformities

Residual lip deformities after primary repair may be esthetic or functional and include scars, skin shortage or excess (vertical and transverse), orbicularis oris muscle malposition or diastasis, lip landmark abnormalities, vermilion deficiencies or deformities, mucosal contracture, and buccal sulcus obliteration.

Lip Scars. Lip scars are unavoidable. In patients between 8 and 18 years of age, surgery often results in an exaggerated healing reaction, with increased periods of scar erythema and hypertrophy (Millard, 1976). The first scar is often the best, and repeated revision is contraindicated. This approach, however, is not always practical, since significant deformity causes distress and should be corrected. Bone grafting at the time of canine eruption requires surgery when the patient is between 8 and 10 years of age; if necessary, lip revision can be done at this time.

Revision techniques include Z- or W-plasty or "wave-line" excisions (Fig. 56–1) (Pfeifer, 1973), which may improve the scars but leave zigzag incisions across normal anatomic contours. This may be an acceptable result, particularly after correction of wide, obvious scars. During revision, the scar can be deepithelized and buried to add projection to the philtral ridge in a "vest-over-pants" fashion (Fig. 56–2) (Stal and Spira, 1984). The buried dermal scar may absorb the tension of closure in addition to providing philtral bulk. This can be done only when the scar lies over the philtral column. A narrow conchal cartilage graft placed vertically in the lip can also form a philtral column. Dermabrasion may be used on lip scars, but this must be done with care because of the possibility of color changes.

A scar revision designed to correct the specific deformity as it affects the skin, the muscle, and the mucosa is logical. The lip dynamics are corrected, and with uncomplicated healing the scar should be satisfactory. Removal of sutures at three to four days postoperatively eliminates crosshatching, and tape reinforcement for a few weeks certainly does no harm. Mild chromic catgut (6-0)

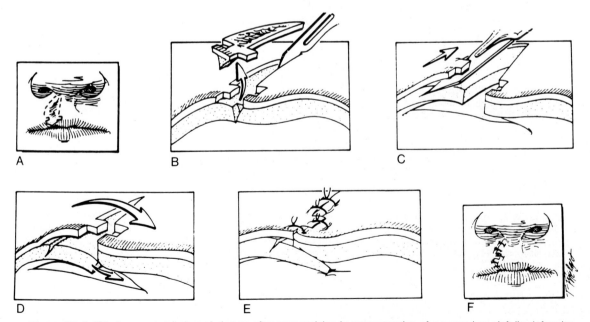

Figure 56–2. "Vest-over-pants" dermal closure after scar revision in reconstruction of a secondary cleft lip deformity. (From Stal, S., and Spira, M.: Secondary reconstructive procedures for patients with clefts. *In* Serafin, D., and Georgiade, N. G. (Eds.): Pediatric Plastic Surgery. St. Louis, MO, C. V. Mosby Company, 1984.)

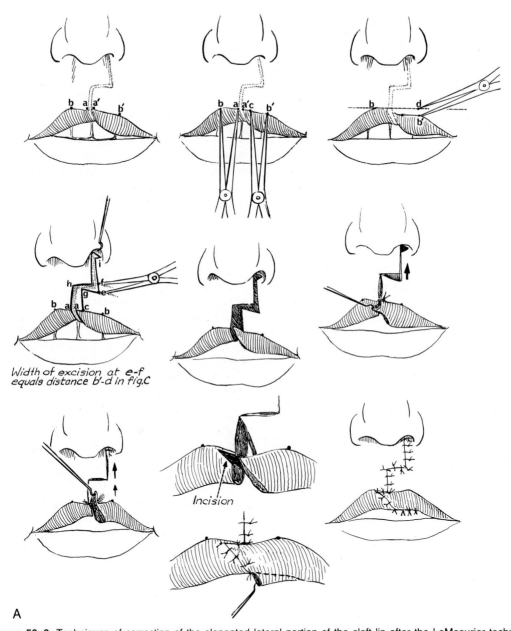

Figure 56–3. Techniques of correction of the elongated lateral portion of the cleft lip after the LeMesurier technique. *A*, Excision of the previous scar, with the focus on removing an adequate amount of tissue in the horizontal limb of the incision. (From Converse, J. M.: Correction of the drooping lateral portion of the cleft lip following LeMesurier repair. Plast. Reconstr. Surg., *55*:501, 1975. Copyright 1975, The Williams & Wilkins Company, Baltimore.)

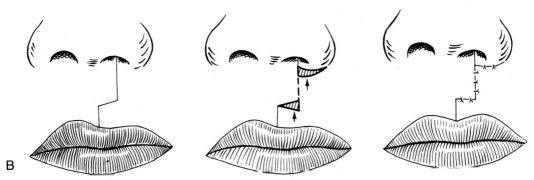

B

Figure 56–3 *Continued B,* Reduction of the height of the quadrilateral flap by horizontal excisions. (From Millard, D. R., Jr.: Cleft Craft. Vol. I. Boston, Little, Brown & Company, 1976.)

suture material is usually dissolved by four to five days, and its use prevents suture marks without the necessity of suture removal (Jackson, 1984).

Long Lip (Vertical Excess). The length of the lip is largely related to the primary repair technique. An excessively long lip is unusual, particularly if the method of assessing lip length described above is used. However, some flap repairs (LeMesurier, 1949; Tennison, 1952; Randall, 1959) can produce this deformity. This condition is corrected by a full-thickness horizontal excision from the superior portion of the lip below the nostril sill. Tessier and Tulasne (1984) described the resection of a thick infranasal wedge of full-thickness lip tissue, 8 to 12 mm wide, from one nasolabial fold to the other. If there is a transverse scar in the philtral area, it can be excised in a triangular horizontal fashion for additional lip shortening (Fig. 56–3) (Converse, 1975). More inferiorly situated resec-

tions are not recommended, since these may cause further anatomic distortion.

A long lip can occur as a result of the rotation-advancement lip repair owing to excessive rotation (Millard, 1974; Bardach and Salyer, 1987a); this becomes apparent only with growth and development of the face. This situation is rare. The scar should be excised; the lesser lip segment is derotated and de-advanced, with repair of the incision that crossed into the normal side. The lateral segment edge is adjusted to match the medial edge. Much more common after the rotation-advancement repair is relative lengthening of the lip lateral to the repair with cranial displacement of the alar base attributable to insertion of the C-flap under the alar base. The C-flap should be excised and the alar base advanced inferiorly. Usually the lip is elevated; rarely is total correction of the alar base position achieved. If increased total height is the only deformity, a transverse

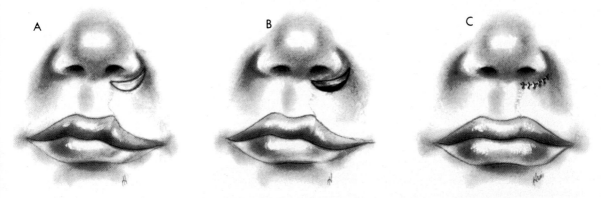

Figure 56–4. Correction of the long lesser segment that may occur with the rotation-advancement repair. *A,* Design of excision for shortening of the long lip on the cleft side. *B,* Excision of the subalar base crescent. *C,* The alar base is brought down and the lip is brought up. (From Bardach, J., and Salyer, K. E.: Surgical Techniques in Cleft Lip and Palate. Chicago, Year Book Medical Publishers, 1987.)

crescentic excision is the preferred but not the universal method of treatment (Fig. 56–4).

Short Lip (Vertical Deficiency). It has been stated that vertical scar contracture along the suture line subsequent to primary lip repair is the most common cause of a short lip (Bardach and Salyer, 1987a). This explanation is too simplistic and is not borne out in practice. The components of a short lip are found in each layer: the static elements of scar contracture in the skin, the muscle, and the mucosa and the dynamic one of the uncorrected, abnormal muscle function. Clinical assessment is critical, and a total secondary lip repair is frequently necessary. As stated above, *the length of the lip can be gauged only with the nasal tip in its correct anatomic position.* The skin and the mucosa are examined, and the lines of tension are looked for, especially in relation to the frenulum.

Muscle function is assessed by observing the patient's pursing of the lips. The vermilion-cutaneous junction is carefully inspected. The transverse dimensions of the lip are measured. In the unilateral cleft lip, vertical shortness is likely to result from straight-line or slightly curved repairs (Rose, 1891; Thompson, 1912). The rotation-advancement method has been criticized for producing reduction of the vertical height of the lip, especially in wide clefts (Millard, 1968). Frequently, this is a temporary condition, and within six months resolution of the scar allows the Cupid's bow to settle into a normal position. Usually permanent shortness is due to technical errors: inadequate rotation; failure to extend the incision across the base of the columella; failure to use a back cut; and inadequate dissection, repositioning, and lengthening of the muscular layer. Treatment consists of scar excision and rerotation of the

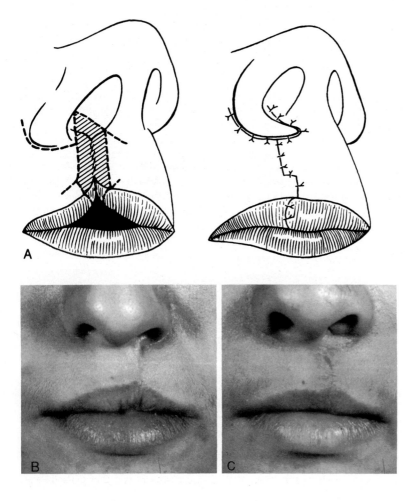

Figure 56–5. Correction of the short lip after a rotation-advancement primary repair. *A,* Alar advancement technique. (After Grignon. From Millard, D. R., Jr.: Cleft Craft. Vol. I. Boston, Little, Brown & Company, 1976.) *B,* Straight-line closure has partially obliterated the Cupid's bow and produced a short lip. *C,* Early postoperative result after scar excision and alar advancement.

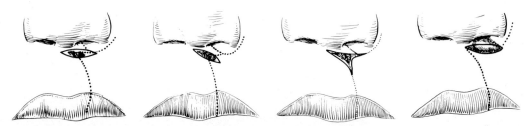

Figure 56–6. Various excision designs for lengthening and adjusting secondary deformities resulting from the rotation-advancement repair. (After Onizuka. From Millard, D. R., Jr.: Cleft Craft. Vol. I. Boston, Little, Brown & Company, 1976.)

flap with a back cut to increase the downward rotation of the medial segment; the lateral segment is adjusted accordingly, and the muscle is lengthened by interdigitation of the cut ends (Fig. 56–5).

For major discrepancies of the lateral and medial elements with an intact philtrum, a rotation-advancement revision is recommended, ignoring any previous quadrilateral flap or triangular flap repairs (Hogan and Converse, 1971). If the deformity is minor, excision of the scar and a Z-plasty placed close to the nasal sill in the shadow of the nostril can be adequate (Fig. 56–6). These methods are not particularly recommended, since the most accurate and satisfactory tech-nique (with minimal additional scarring) is a rotation-advancement of the upper vertical scar (Fig. 56–7). If there is a lower vertical scar, additional lengthening can be achieved by a Rose-Thompson scar excision (Fig. 56–8).

Transpositions have also been described by Ginestet (1977) (Fig. 56–9), Merville (1962) (Fig. 56–10), and Trauner (1956) (Fig. 56–11) for repair of previous straight-line closures. The Hagedorn-LeMesurier technique is suitable for straight-line closures in which a portion of the Cupid's bow has been destroyed, but again the rotation-advancement revision is preferred. The LeMesurier revision is not recommended in young children, as use of the

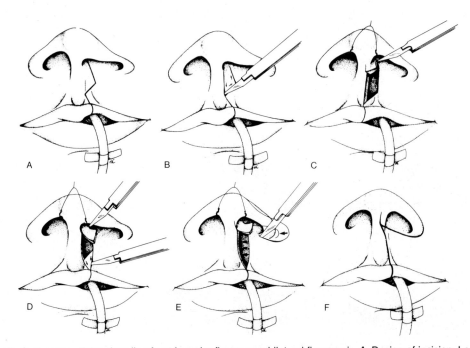

Figure 56–7. Revision of the short lip after triangular flap or quadrilateral flap repair. *A,* Design of incision. Lengthening of the short lip. *B* to *D,* Rose-Thompson excision and lengthening of the lower portion of the lip. *E, F,* Rotation-advancement of the upper vertical scar. (From Wilson, L. F.: Correction of residual defects of the lip and nose in repaired clefts of the primary palate (lip and alveolus). Clin. Plast. Surg., *12*:719, 1985.)

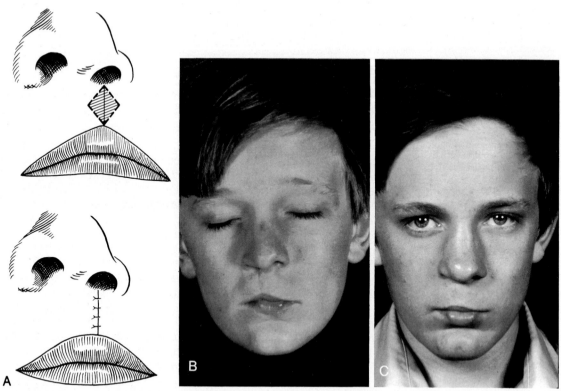

Figure 56–8. *A,* Rose-Thompson excision and closure to lengthen the short lip. (From Millard, D. R., Jr.: Cleft Craft. Vol. I. Boston, Little, Brown & Company, 1976.) *B,* Short lip with peaking of the vermilion and notching of the border. *C,* Postoperative result after diamond-shaped excision of scar and reconstruction of the orbicularis oris muscle.

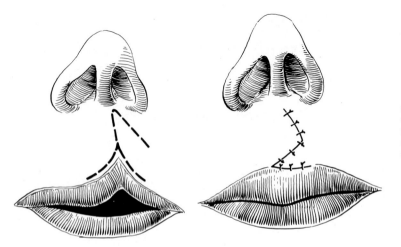

Figure 56–9. Lengthening of the short lip by transposition of an inferiorly based oblique flap. (After Ginestet. From Millard, D. R., Jr.: Cleft Craft. Vol. I. Boston, Little, Brown & Company, 1976.)

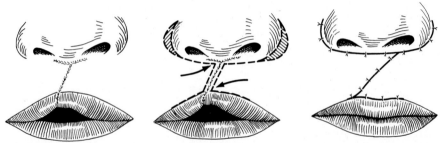

Figure 56–10. Lengthening of the lip by advancement flaps and circumalar crescent excisions. (After Merville. From Millard, D. R., Jr.: Cleft Craft. Vol. I. Boston, Little, Brown & Company, 1976.)

quadrangular flap may result in asymmetric growth, which may cause secondary deformities (Fig. 56–12) (Bardach and Salyer, 1987a).

Tight Lip (Horizontal Deficiency). In the normal situation, the upper lip is full, pouts, and protrudes slightly in front of the lower lip. Sacrifice of excessive soft tissue during the primary repair produces an indrawn upper lip, which is stretched across the teeth, with the upper lip lying behind the somewhat redundant lower lip. This situation is accen-

tuated in the presence of maxillary retrusion (Fig. 56–13).

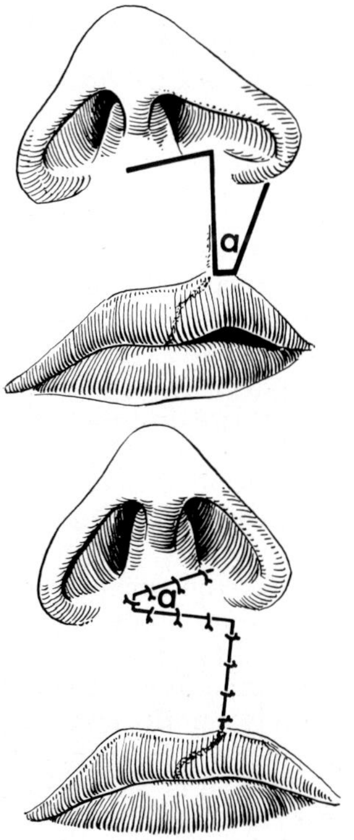

Any of the standard primary lip operations can result in a tight upper lip in relation to the protuberant lower lip, especially the straight-line and Blair-Brown triangular flap repairs (Millard, 1977). It is important to determine whether the tightness is actual or whether it is due to maxillary retrusion and can be corrected by an advancement osteotomy.

Correction of marked horizontal deficiencies with gross lip disproportion may require an Abbé flap. The cross lip flap (see Chap. 38) was initially described by Sabbatini (1838) and was subsequently modified by Stein (1848), Buck (1864), Estlander (1872), and Abbé (1898). The flap is basically a composite transfer of skin, muscle, and mucosa based on a pedicle containing the inferior labial vessels (Figs. 56–14 to 56–16). The 180 degree transposition of the lower lip flap and its insertion into the upper lip is facilitated by minimizing the bulk of the pedicle. This may be reduced to the mucosa surrounding the labial wall (Gillies and Millard, 1957; McGregor, 1963; Lehman, 1978; Jackson and Soutar, 1980). The flap is divided and inset under local anesthesia after ten days. Maintenance of the lip flap on the mucosal pedicle alone after inadvertent division of the labial artery was described (Millard and McLaughlin, 1979). If this occurs, it is prudent to replace the flap in the lower lip and to transfer it later. Free composite grafts from the lower lip to the upper lip (1 cm or less in width) with at most superficial skin necrosis were reported by Flanagin (1956).

Reinnervation may occur in Abbé flaps in one year or less (DePalma, Leavitt, and Hardy, 1958; Smith, 1960, 1961; Thompson and Pollard, 1961; Isaksson and associates, 1962). However, clinical evidence of muscular

Figure 56–11. Lengthening of the short lip by a superiorly based transposition flap. (After Trauner. From Millard, D. R., Jr.: Cleft Craft. Vol. I. Boston, Little, Brown & Company, 1976.)

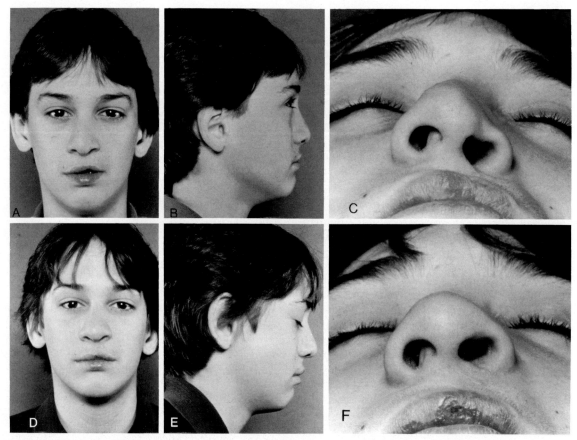

Figure 56–12. Short lip and asymmetric growth of the lip after the LeMesurier repair. *A to C,* Preoperative appearance. *D to F,* Postoperative appearance after orbicularis oris reconstruction, rotation-advancement of the upper part of the lip, and Rose-Thompson excision of the lower part to lengthen the lip.

activity in large Abbé flaps is minimal or absent, particularly if the flap is square. A triangular flap has the advantage of closer apposition to the upper lip orbicularis oris muscle superiorly. The flap should *always be placed in the midline* of the upper lip, regardless of the type or location of the previous repair. In this position, it recreates the philtrum, the Cupid's bow, and the philtral tubercle.

McGregor (1963), an advocate of unilateral insertion, added a modified Gillies' Cupid's bow operation (Fig. 56–17) by excising a wedge of skin and muscle from the flap rather than just skin. This technique should not be used.

Placement of the flap in the upper lip midline was encouraged by the superior results achieved in bilateral clefts (Peet and Patterson, 1963; Millard, 1964b). The results can be most satisfactory, despite the thin island

of residual skin between the midline flap and the scar of the primary repair (Fig. 56–18) (Onizuka, 1966; Schuh, Crikelair, and Cosman, 1970; Hogan and Converse, 1971).

As stated above, the central insertion reproduces the central fullness or pout of the upper lip. There is a resemblance to a Cupid's bow when the Abbé flap is taken from the center of the lower lip. Its design is such that it simulates the normal philtrum. The width of the adult philtrum ranges from 0.8 to 1.2 cm at the vermilion border and from 0.6 to 0.9 cm at the columellar base. Clifford and Pool (1959) reported that the maximal length of the normal adult philtrum is 1.7 cm. These dimensions should be remembered when planning the flap—it is *not* square and should *not* be overlong.

Various modifications of the flap have been described. In the "shelving muscle flap" (Hogan and Converse, 1971) the suture lines are

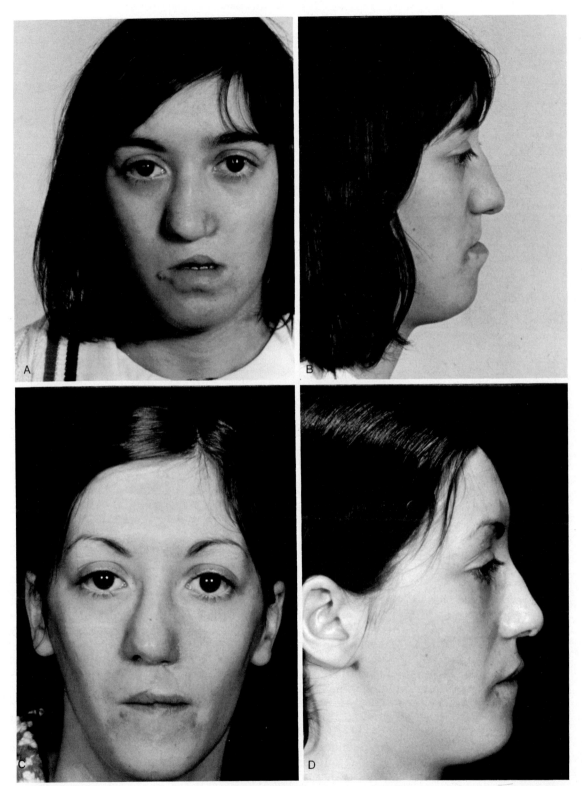

Figure 56–13. Correction of a tight lip. *A, B,* Preoperative appearance. Oversacrifice of upper lip tissue resulted in a reversed lip deformity, which is accentuated by maxillary retrusion. *C, D,* Postoperative appearance after Abbé flap and Le Fort I advancement osteotomy. The Abbé flap could not be placed in the midline.

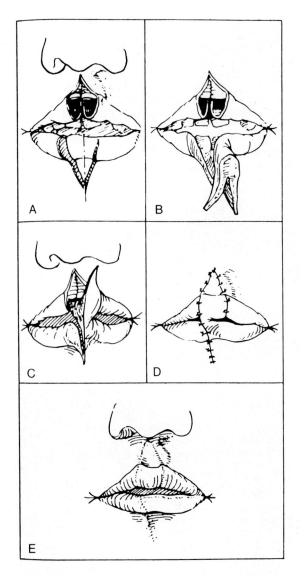

Figure 56–14. Operative technique for a sandwich Abbé flap. *A,* Dissection of the orbicularis oris muscle. *B,* Elevation of the Abbé flap. *C,* Transfer of the lower lip flap and insertion into the upper lip. *D,* Sutures hold the flap in position. *E,* The flap is divided after ten days. (From Jackson, I. T., and Soutar, D. S.: The sandwich Abbé flap in secondary cleft lip deformity. Plast. Reconstr. Surg., *66*:38, 1980.)

staggered at the base of the columella to decrease scar formation and the tourniquet effect (see Fig. 56–16). Lehman (1978) described a dynamic Abbé flap, which produces a better functioning lip. The technique consists of dissection and repair of the orbicularis oris muscle across the midline before the inset of the flap. The Abbé flap is then split in the coronal plane and enveloped around the orbicularis repair. The sandwich Abbé flap of Jackson and Soutar (1980) also includes orbicularis oris muscle repair, but flap bulk is decreased by raising the flap as skin and mucosa without the lower lip orbicularis oris muscle. For revision of bulky, immobile, curtain-like Abbé flaps, the scars are excised, the fibrous center of the flap is removed, and the orbicularis oris is repaired through the flap. The skin and mucosa are sutured into their proper relationships.

The routine use of Abbé flaps for the repair of deficient upper lip tissue has been questioned. Repair of defects of upper lip contour and position is intimately dependent on correction of the following elements: (1) the maxilla, which is often retruded; (2) the alveolus, which is deficient through the nasal floor defects; (3) the columella, which is particularly short in bilateral clefts; and (4) the lower lip, which tends to compensate to achieve lip seal. Tessier and Tulasne (1984) quoted Pichler: "first the bone, then the soft

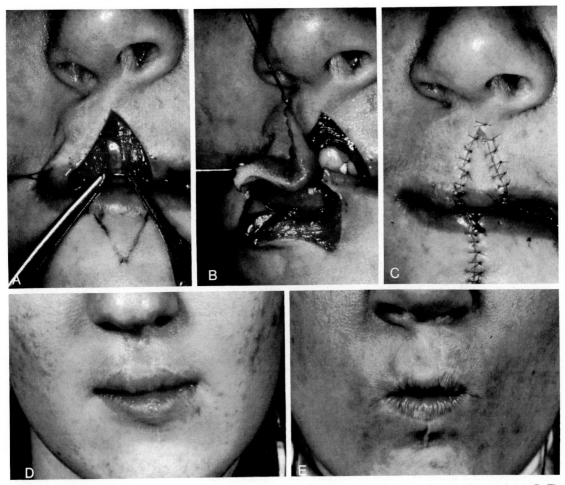

Figure 56–15. Sandwich Abbé flap (see Fig. 56–14). *A,* Orbicularis oris muscle of upper lip is dissected out. *B,* The skin-mucosal Abbé flap is elevated. *C,* Flap is sutured in position. *D, E,* Postoperative result to show good muscle function in the area of the flap.

tissue." In most cases, maxillary advancement restores the upper lip profile more satisfactorily than does an Abbé flap. Reconstruction of the hypoplastic maxilla and alveolus are addressed below. However, in some patients, the soft tissue deficiency is excessive. In these cases, the tight (horizontally deficient) lip, by exerting pressure on an advanced maxilla and alveolus, can cause lingual version of the anterior maxillary teeth. The experienced surgeon tends to use Abbé flaps rarely. After careful assessment, any maxillary deficiency or retrusion is corrected by osteotomy or onlay bone grafting. The lip is revised with orbicularis oris reconstruction at the same time or later. The Abbé flap skin is of a different texture and color

from that of the upper lip; moreover, hair is scanty and grows in a different direction from upper lip hair. The lower lip scar may become hypertrophic and obvious. The Abbé flap procedure should be avoided if at all possible.

A generalized flattening of the repaired cleft lip on the cleft side may have several causes. There may be hypoplasia of the edges of the lip cleft, which should be corrected by the orbicularis oris reconstruction (Veau, 1931; Stark, DeHaan, and Washio, 1964; Stark and Kaplan, 1973). Mobilization of the orbicularis oris muscle from the alar base area may leave a residual soft tissue deficit. Measures to fill this void include dermal fat grafts (Cosman and Crikelair, 1965), muscle and scar flaps (Ragnell, 1946), or interdigi-

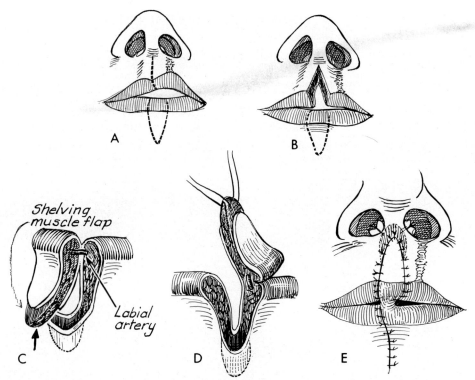

Figure 56–16. Abbé shelving muscle flap. *A,* The design of the flap is made on the lower lip. The new philtrum is trapezoid in shape with a somewhat rounded tip. The measurements of width fall within 0.9 and 1.2 cm for the vermilion, or basal, portion and between 0.6 and 0.9 cm for the subnasal, or distal, portion. *B,* A full-thickness incision is made in the center of the upper lip. In determining where the center lies, allowance must be made for distortion caused by the repaired cleft. *C,* The flap is prepared by applying the principle of the muscle shelf. The shelf fits snugly under the columella, producing an elevation of the columella and facilitating skin-to-skin approximation in the repair of the subnasal area. *D,* The vascular supply. The flap is rotated on a small vascular pedicle, which includes a mucosal bridge. *E,* The shelving muscle flap is drawn under the columella by mattress sutures, which are tied over a small cotton ball within the nostril. The mucosal and muscle layers of the upper and lower lip are closed with 4-0 chromic catgut and the skin with 5-0 nylon sutures. The flap is divided in ten days. (From Hogan, V. M., and Converse, J. M.: Secondary deformities of unilateral cleft lip and nose. *In* Grabb, W. C., Rosenstein, S. E., and Bzoch, K. R. (Eds.): Cleft Lip and Palate. Boston, Little, Brown & Company, 1971.)

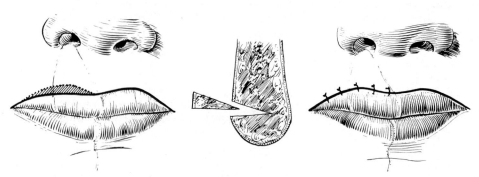

Figure 56–17. Method of simulating half of the Cupid's bow after an asymmetric Abbé flap by resection of skin, subcutaneous tissue, and muscle wedge. (After McGregor. From Millard, D. R., Jr.: Cleft Craft. Vol. I. Boston, Little, Brown & Company, 1976.)

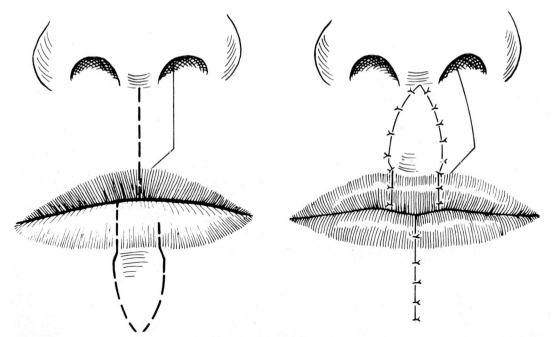

Figure 56–18. Correction of a tight lip after Blair-Brown triangular flap closure. The placement of the Abbé flap is in the midline of the upper lip, disregarding the previous lip repair scar. (From Millard, D. R., Jr.: Cleft Craft. Vol. I. Boston, Little, Brown & Company, 1976.)

tation of a portion of the contralateral muscle (Millard, 1974). Actually the flattening is largely due to maxillary hypoplasia with a deficient bony platform at the piriform aperture. Improvement in the skeletal support of the lip, as well as the alar base, corrects the flattened upper lip appearance and also improves nasal symmetry. In addition to the above attempts to improve soft tissue deficiency, cartilage grafts have been placed beneath the alar base. Cancellous bone grafts are used to fill larger bony defects, particularly when tooth roots are unsupported. The placement of cancellous bone grafts to augment the hypoplastic maxilla at the piriform aperture is often done concurrently with alveolar bone grafting. Absorbable cellulose gauze (Surgicel) mixed with blood beneath the periosteum of the piriform aperture improves support for the alar base during the primary repair. This is useful as an alternative to cancellous bone grafts in incomplete clefts (Jackson and Mustardé, 1988).

Orbicularis Oris Abnormalities. In recent years, the importance of muscle reconstruction in the primary correction of the cleft lip has been emphasized. In secondary cleft lip repair, abnormalities of muscle function resulting from muscle deficiency, malposi-

tion, discontinuity, or diastasis may be noted and should be corrected.

One of the first signs of inadequate muscle continuity across a lip repair may be a widened scar resulting from lateral tension on the skin suture line. In addition, there is thinning of the lip under the repair with relative thickness of the adjacent lip (Schafer and Goldwasser, 1984). An inadequate muscle repair without interdigitation will result in a short, or vertically deficient, lip (Kernahan and Bauer, 1983). Lip lengthening can be obtained by adequate muscle repair (Jackson, 1973). In bilateral clefts, orbicularis oris union in the midline effectively lengthens the lip (Oneal, Greer, and Nobel, 1974).

Inadequate muscle reconstruction results in a lip that functions improperly in speech, facial expression, whistling, and mastication. Without integrity of the circumoral muscular ring, attempts to whistle result in a lateral bunching of the muscle, accentuating the tissue deficiency in the region of the repair (Fig. 56–19).

The muscles that move the lip and the nose are integrally related. Aberrant orientation of muscle fibers and muscle action abnormalities in the cleft tend to displace the alar base laterally and widen the nostril sill on the

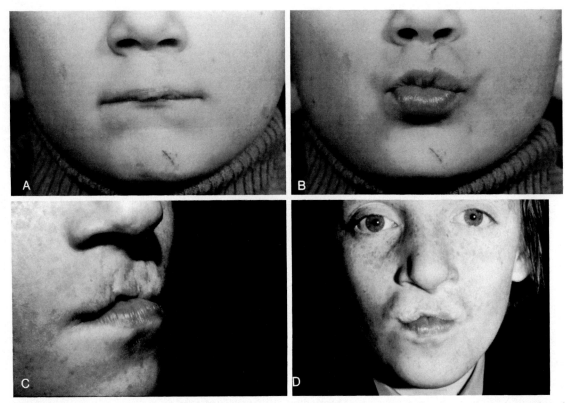

Figure 56–19. Functional deformities after lip repair as a result of inadequate orbicularis oris muscle reconstruction. *A, B,* Left-sided unilateral cleft. *C, D,* Bilateral cleft.

affected side. Borchgrevink (1970) attributed original nasal deformities, in part, to the unopposed muscle action on the ala laterally and the septum medially. If this is uncorrected in the primary repair, the nasal deformity persists. Delaire (1975) and Delaire and Prechious (1987) pointed out that the orbicularis oris and paranasal muscles are important for the normal development of the upper jaw. Recent data suggested that reconstruction of the paranasal and perioral muscles is a decisive factor in shaping the midfacial bones and the upper jaw (Joos, 1987). This principle applies to secondary as well as primary repairs, but the potential to modify facial growth decreases considerably after the age of 8 to 10 years, since the sutures of the skull begin to close and growth areas become less active.

In the presence of a cleft, the insertions of the paranasal and oral muscle groups are abnormal, with the muscle fibers paralleling the cleft margin (Fig. 56–20). Fara (1968) described the location and orientation of the

orbicularis oris muscles in stillborn children with clefts and found 70 to 80 degrees of upward displacement of muscle fibers in the lateral lip segments of bilateral clefts. In the unilateral cleft, muscle fibers run parallel to the lateral margin, inserting into the alar base region (Fig. 56–20*A*). An important feature to note is the narrowing of the muscle as it sweeps cephalad to its insertion.

Kernahan (1978) mapped the orientation of the orbicularis oris in clefts by electric stimulation and advised the use of this technique for accurate muscle repair. As opposed to Fara's (1968) findings, he showed that the orbicularis fibers appeared to insert into the dermis and mucosa of the cleft margins, not the alar base. In the normal lip, the perioral musculature decussates in the upper lip midline, terminating in the skin lateral to the philtral columns on the contralateral side (Latham and Deaton, 1976; Briedis and Jackson, 1981). Kernahan's findings were interpreted by Briedis and Jackson as indicating that only a small superficial portion of the

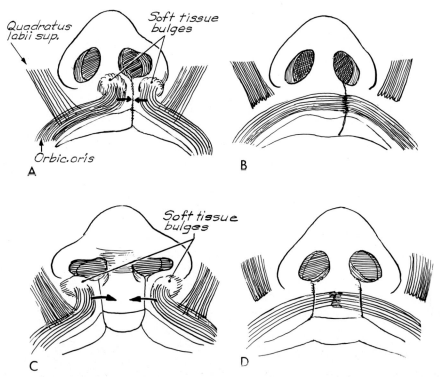

Figure 56–20. Orbicularis oris abnormalities. *A,* The orbicularis oris fibers are misdirected in the unilateral cleft lip, forming two orbicularis bulges, one on each side of the cleft. *B,* After division of the fibers of the quadratus labii superioris muscle, the orbicularis oris muscle is redirected and sutured. *C,* A similar misdirection is found in the bilateral complete cleft. *D,* The fibers of the orbicularis oris are redirected and introduced into the prolabial segment in which muscle is sparse or absent.

orbicularis oris muscle inserts into the dermis and mucosa of the cleft margins, with the remainder paralleling the cleft.

Numerous techniques for approximating and aligning the orbicularis oris muscle during primary or secondary repair have been proposed (Randall, 1959; Fara, 1968; Millard, 1968; Climo, 1969; Borchgrevink, 1970; Jackson, 1973; Randall, Whitaker, and LaRossa, 1974; Delaire, 1975; Kernahan, 1978; Schendel and Delaire, 1981; Kernahan and Bauer, 1983; Tajima, 1983; Schafer and Goldwasser, 1984; Tessier and Tulasne, 1984). All these investigators noted that the muscle anatomy of the mouth and nasal area is extremely complex and that an exact restoration is impossible, especially in previously repaired lips. In some cases of secondary cleft lip deformity, older repairs with inadequate dissection may have been used primarily, and the orbicularis oris may lie lateral and parallel to the cleft margins as in the nonoperated cleft. Each case is unique, but all short (previously repaired) lips should be com-

pletely incised, with excision of all scar. The dissection displays the horizontal, oblique, and incisal bundles of the orbicularis oris muscle. In small children, the insertions of the orbicularis are difficult to identify, but wide mobilization ensures availability of all three bundles. Elevation of the alar base enables mobilization of the lateral nasal muscles, which are the principal lip elevators. In older children and in adults the quadratus labii superioris muscle can be identified by entering the deep portion of the orbicularis oris. The lateral mucosal muscles are rotated medially and downward to be inserted into the base of the septum and columella; the orbicularis is sutured medially in the midline of the lip. The upper or oblique fibers of the orbicularis should be anchored to the periosteum of the nasal spine, and the lower internal fibers of the orbicularis are directed into the pouting tubercle of the lip (Schafer and Goldwasser, 1984). Dissection and positioning of the muscle fibers in a horizontal direction with interdigitation and lengthening are es-

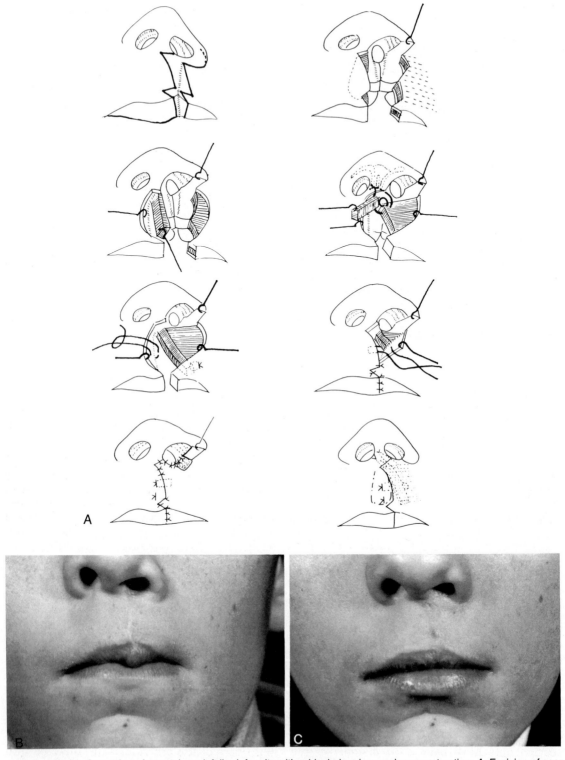

Figure 56–21. Correction of secondary cleft lip deformity with orbicularis oris muscle reconstruction. *A,* Excision of scar and repositioning of orbicularis oris muscle. (From Onizuka, T., Akagawa, T., and Tokunaga, S.: A new method to create a philtrum in secondary cleft lip repairs. Plast. Reconstr. Surg., *62:*842, 1978.) *B,* Preoperative appearance. *C,* Postoperative appearance.

sential. Three separate-layer closures (mucosa, muscle, and skin) are recommended (Fig. 56–21).

When previous repair of the orbicularis oris has broken down or a diastasis is present, a Z-plasty incorporating the scarred medial and lateral muscular segment edges (Kernahan and Bauer, 1983) results in a secure closure and an increase in lip length. When a satisfactory lip scar without the need of revision is present with muscular incompetence, a mucosal approach is advised, but this is rarely indicated. Kapetansky (1971) described an approach through the free vermilion border, leaving a horizontal scar.

Lip Landmark Abnormalities. The characteristic feature of the upper lip is the central dimple and the philtral columns. The two most common lip landmark abnormalities occurring after primary repair are loss of philtral definition and obliteration of the Cupid's bow (Rohrich and Tebbetts, 1987).

The philtrum plays a key role in the appearance of the upper lip. In unilateral clefts, preservation of the philtral columns and the central dimple was emphasized by Veau (1931, 1937–1938). The major portion of the philtrum is present in the medial (noncleft) segment of the unilateral cleft lip (Cardoso, 1952). The techniques of Tennison (1952), Millard (1955), and Randall (1959) were designed to preserve these structures. The LeMesurier repair (1949) and the majority of previous techniques transgress the philtral structure. Patients with bilateral clefts lack philtral structures and require production of a philtrum-like structure. Simultaneous construction of a philtral dimple and central muscle approximation is difficult to achieve at the initial repair. The philtral dimple is composed of centrally located, dense subcutaneous tissue bordered by loose subcuta-

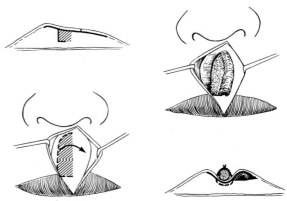

Figure 56–23. Roll-over muscle flap from central philtrum to reconstitute philtral columns and central dimple. (After Onizuka. From Millard, D. R., Jr.: Cleft Craft. Vol. I. Boston, LIttle, Brown & Company, 1976.)

neous connective tissue, producing the philtral ridges laterally (Monie and Cacciatore, 1962). Fibers of the contralateral orbicularis oris are inserted into the dermis lateral to each philtral ridge, augmenting this contour (Latham and Deaton, 1976; Briedis and Jackson, 1981).

Reconstruction of Philtrum and Cupid's Bow. Millard (1971) modified the primary bilateral cleft lip repair with a deep suture from the dermis to the premaxillary periosteum to create an illusion of a dimple. If significant upper lip tissue deficiency exists, a secondary repair using a centrally placed Abbé flap may effect a philtral dimple in addition to providing lip tissue.

Subcutaneous rotation flaps harvested in the midline and pivoted on inferior pedicles horizontally at the vermilion-cutaneous border produced a central dimple and upswing of the upper lip (Fig. 56–22) (O'Connor and McGregor, 1958). A roll-over flap of muscle tissue from the central philtrum was used to provide a philtral column and dimple (Fig. 56–23) (Onizuka, Akagawa, and Tokunaga, 1978). Chondrocutaneous composite grafts and subcutaneous auricular cartilage grafts (Fig. 56–24) were transplanted to reconstruct the philtrum and philtral columns, respectively (Schmid, 1964; Neuner, 1967).

The components of the free border of the upper lip flow in a double upward arch with a central downward curve to form the Cupid's bow. The mucocutaneous junction creates a ridge of tissue, the "white roll," distinctly separating the vermilion from the lip skin. Asymmetry of Cupid's bow is common and

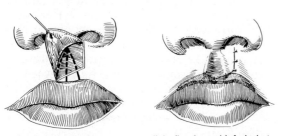

Figure 56–22. Cutaneous pedicle flap based inferiorly to form a philtral ridge. (After O'Connor and McGregor. From Millard, D. R., Jr.: Cleft Craft. Vol. I. Boston, Little, Brown & Company, 1976.)

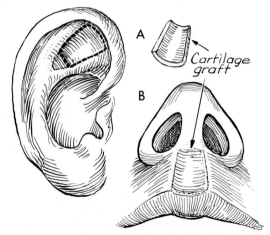

Figure 56–24. Subcutaneous auricular cartilage graft *(A)* for reconstruction of the philtrum *(B)*. (After Neuner.)

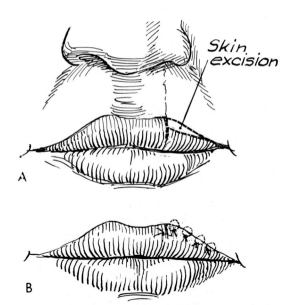

Figure 56–26. Repair of a deficiency of the vermilion border of the upper lip. *A,* To avoid flattening of the lip, a portion of the lip dermis is left and the vermilion is advanced over it. *B,* Approximation is by half-buried mattress sutures with the knots on the vermilion side. (After Stark. Modified from Converse, 1964.)

results from poor alignment of the lip and the vermilion during the initial lip repair. Cupid's bow deformity may include (1) shortness (horizontal deficiency) because of repeated scar revisions and wide excisions, (2) flatness due to excessive tension, (3) notching as a result of poor approximation, and (4) distortion caused by unbalanced flaps or retraction of scar (Tessier and Tulasne, 1984). When misalignment is minor, correction of the vermilion-cutaneous junction defect can be accomplished with a small localized Z-plasty, secondary white roll flap, or white roll free graft (Millard, 1976). Stal and Spira (1984) have reported injections of artificial collagen (Zyderm) into the dermis as an alternative to surgical reconstruction of the white roll. This is only a temporary solution.

Gillies and Kilner (1932) reconstructed the Cupid's bow by advancing the vermilion bor-

der of the lip as double peaks after full-thickness skin excision (Fig. 56–25). However, this gives an artificial appearance and is avoided if possible. By deepithelizing rather than excising the lip skin, Stark (1968) attempted to retain the pout of the vermilion border with flap advancement (Fig. 56–26). In unilateral deformities with absence of the Cupid's bow peak on the cleft side, a unilateral Gillies' procedure was advocated by Millard (1976). Preservation of the white roll–cutaneous junction by excision of skin above the white roll may result in a more natural appearance by maintaining the white roll highlights (Millard, 1976). McGregor (1963) modified the classic Cupid's bow operation by excising a wedge of skin and muscle down to mucosa before advancing the vermilion in unilateral clefts with previously placed Abbé flaps as noted above. Incisions horizontally oriented at or above the vermilion-cutaneous junction compromise a majority of these techniques. Major discrepancies may necessitate complete take-down and repair of the lip or, in the case of severe tissue deficiency, an Abbé flap.

Vermilion Deficiency or Deformity. The most common secondary deformity of the vermilion in unilateral cleft lips is deficiency of

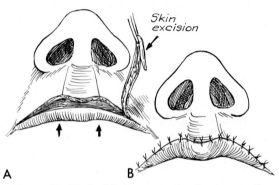

Figure 56–25. Cupid's bow reconstruction by vermilion advancement. *A,* Full-thickness skin excision. *B,* Vermilion advancement. (After Gillies and Kilner.)

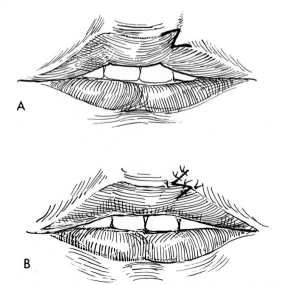

Figure 56–27. A step deformity of the upper lip *(A)* corrected by a Z-plasty *(B)*.

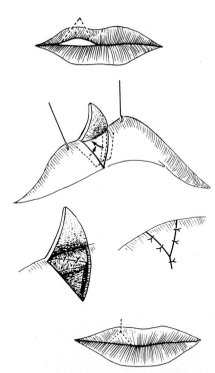

Figure 56–29. Whistle deformity. V-Y advancement with additional subcutaneous flaps to reconstruct deficiency of the vermilion margin. (From Millard, D. R., Jr.: Cleft Craft. Vol. I. Boston, Little, Brown & Company, 1976.)

the Cupid's bow. This may be vertical in orientation, with a notching deformity of the vermilion, a mismatch of the vermilion margins, or an attenuated or absent vermilion ridge. In bilateral cleft lips, the classic "whistle deformity" or central notching defect is common.

The reconstructive procedures used in unilateral vermilion defect revisions can also be applied to bilateral deformities. These techniques involve Z-plasties, V-Y advancements, transposition flaps, free grafts, and cross lip flaps. Minor misalignment of the vermilion border or notching can be corrected with a Z-plasty (Fig. 56–27), V-Y advancement (Figs. 56–28, 56–29), or advancement of lip mucosa. Transposition or advancement of mucosa re-

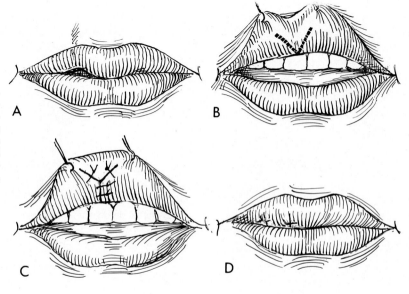

Figure 56–28. Whistle deformity. Minor deficiency of tissue *(A)* may be corrected by a V-Y advancement of the vermilion tissue *(B to D)*. Undermining must extend for at least 0.75 cm in all directions; closure is by interrupted 4-0 chromic catgut sutures.

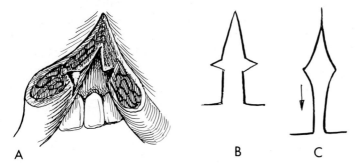

Figure 56–30. Technique of lengthening the mucosal aspect of the upper lip. *A,* The incised area is spread to form an inverted V; short lateral incisions are made into the mucosa and muscle on each side of the wound. *B,* Vertical and lateral incisions, oral aspect. *C,* Stretching out the lateral incisions lengthens the mucosal margins of the wound for straight-line suturing. (After Erich.)

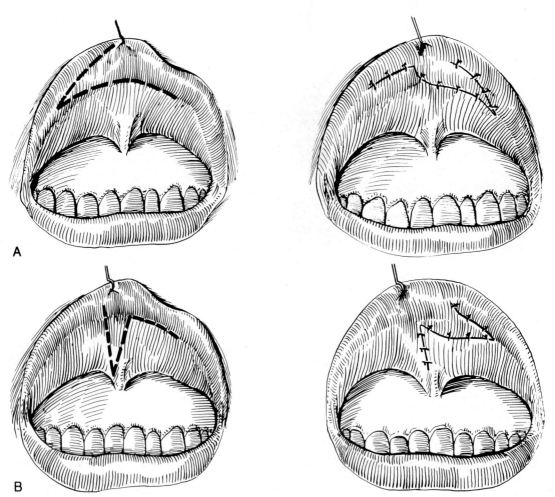

Figure 56–31. Inner lip transposition flaps to correct lip deficiency. *A,* Horizontal transposition flap, 180 degrees. *B,* Vertical transposition flap, 90 degrees. (After Ginestet. From Millard, D. R., Jr.: Cleft Craft. Vol. I. Boston, Little, Brown & Company, 1976.)

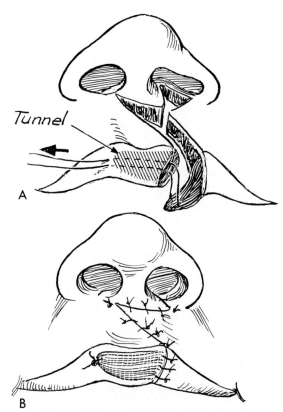

Figure 56–32. Modification of the Millard operation to prevent notching of the vermilion border. *A,* A tunnel is prepared in the medial portion of the vermilion border. A mattress guide-suture is used to introduce the denuded flap into the tunnel. *B,* Operation completed. (After Guerrero-Santos and associates.)

quires care not to place "wet" mucosa in the "dry" mucosal area. Erich (1953) lengthened the mucosal aspect of the lip by a vertical closure of horizontal incisions (Fig. 56–30). Ginestet (1976) was able to compensate for vertical vermilion deficiency by developing large inner lip mucosal flaps turned 180 degrees or 90 degrees (Fig. 56–31).

Secondary vermilion notching can be minimized by denuding a flap of the excess lateral vermilion tissue; the flap is then tunneled into the medial segment of the vermilion border (Fig. 56–32) (Guerrero-Santos and associates, 1971).

Whistle deformities are relatively common, particularly after bilateral cleft lip repairs. When they involve the visible mucosa and vermilion alone, a variety of corrective techniques have been utilized. For small defects, a V-flap based in the vermilion-cutaneous border is advanced toward its base and closed

in a V-Y fashion (Fig. 56–33). In larger defects, the entire labial sulcus is released by two large buccal mucosal flaps and rotated and advanced inferiorly toward the free border and the vermilion-cutaneous junction (Hogan and Converse, 1971). This technique results in a vertical scar in the wet mucosa with overall lengthening of the central vermilion (Fig. 56–34). The correction is frequently insufficient, and any significant scarring in the labial sulcus from previous procedures limits the effectiveness of this technique.

A double V-Y advancement from the lateral vermilion toward the midline was described by Robinson, Ketchum, and Masters (1970) (Fig. 56–35). Kapetansky (1971) used double pendulum (island) flaps of lateral vermilion, mobilized with the underlying orbicularis oris muscle; the flaps are moved from the lateral vermilion medially into the midline (Fig. 56–36; see also Fig. 56–95). Further inferior medial rotation of these flaps by Juri, Juri, and de Antueno (1976) was used to define and elevate a central tubercle (Fig. 56–37). These techniques work well if the flaps in the wet mucosa are designed correctly. Correction of midline notching or a whistle defect with the above methods requires inclusion of adequate vermilion bulk. Conservation of "excess" vermilion during the primary repair is crucial. When there is a significant whistle deformity, lip function is carefully evaluated to ascertain whether orbicularis oris reconstruction was performed during the initial repair. Until the orbicularis oris muscle is reconstructed, all methods of correcting the whistle deformity will have suboptimal results.

Correction of large tissue defects in the vermilion may require transfer of tissue from the lower lip or the tongue. A tongue flap can be used to resurface the lip in this situation or for complications of transposition flap loss (Guerrero-Santos, 1969). Free composite tissue grafts from the lower lip for defects smaller than 1 cm were described by Flanagin (1956). Neither technique is advocated: the first entails color and texture differences between tongue and vermilion and a ten day interposition of the tongue between the teeth; the composite graft technique is tenuous, and only a limited amount can be transferred.

Contour and color match often are improved by using a centrally based flap of exposed vermilion in cross lip flaps. Kawa-

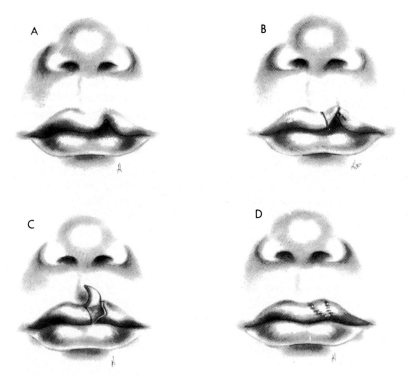

Figure 56–33. Transposition of a superiorly based mucosal flap to correct notching of the upper lip. *A,* Whistle deformity. *B,* Design of unequal Z-plasty. *C,* Elevation of the flap, which is transposed to correct vermilion deficiency. Z-plasty is performed simultaneously. *D,* Appearance after closure. (From Bardach, J., and Salyer, K. E.: Surgical Techniques in Cleft Lip and Palate. Chicago, Year Book Medical Publishers, 1987.)

Figure 56–34. Whistle deformity. *A,* Diagram of the whistle deformity. *B,* The upper lip is elevated, and an outline is drawn of the extent of the whistle deformity. The upper buccal sulcus incision should be about 0.5 cm from the depth of the sulcus so that there is an adequate cuff to permit suture of the flaps after they have been advanced. The length of the original incision is determined by the width of the whistle deformity; it should extend laterally beyond the confines of the whistle deformity so that the full length of the incision line equals three times the width of the whistle deformity. *C,* Advancement of the flaps in a V-Y manner is facilitated by placing a hook at the apex of the incised mucosa and starting the suture of the flaps at this point. One should be careful not to advance too much tissue, since it is relatively easy to overcorrect the deformity. *D,* Operation completed.

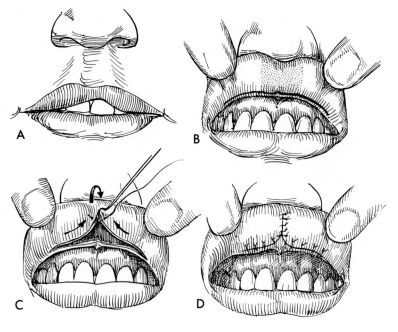

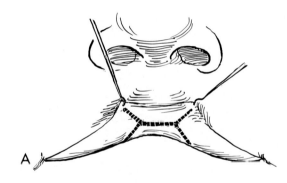

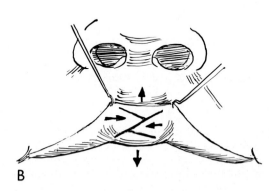

Figure 56–35. Double lateral V-Y advancement to correct notching of the vermilion border. *A,* Outline of the V-Y flaps. *B,* The direction of the advancement of the flaps. (After Robinson, Ketchum, and Masters.)

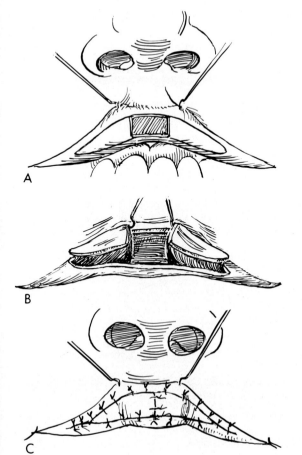

Figure 56–36. Double "pendulum" flaps (island flaps with an orbicularis muscle pedicle) to correct notching of the vermilion border. *A,* Two lateral island flaps are designed. *B,* The island flaps before being advanced centrally. *C,* Operation completed. (After Kapetansky.)

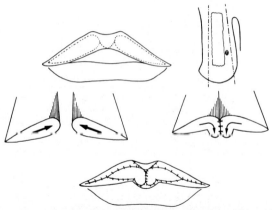

Figure 56–37. Over-rotation of pendulum flaps in the midline to form a central lip tubercle. (From Juri, J., Juri, C., and de Antueno, J.: A modification of the Kapetansky technique for repair of whistling deformities of the upper lip. Plast. Reconstr. Surg., 57:70, 1976.)

moto (1979), using a modification of Gillies and Millard's (1957) technique, provided a cross lip flap of mucosa from the inner surface of the lower lip. The pedicle is divided in five to seven days, and tailoring of the remaining lower lip has the added benefit of reducing the bulk of the frequently protuberant lower lip (Fig. 56–38).

Deficient Buccal Sulcus. A shallow buccal sulcus is unusual in unilateral cases but commonly occurs in the prolabial area in bilateral clefts. An inadequate primary surgical technique with failure to provide a deep sulcus is the usual cause. The presence of a sulcus not only aids the orthodontist and the prosthodontist in performing corrective procedures but also enhances lip function.

The raw area resulting from construction of a sulcus can be covered by split-thickness skin, oral mucosal, or palatine mucoperiosteal grafts or local rotation flaps. A variable amount of contraction and loss of depth of the newly created sulcus occurs regardless of what technique is used, but it is particularly apparent after graft techniques. Maintaining buccal sulcus depth generally requires an appliance, and thus sulcoplasty is best delayed until the child is 4 to 6 years of age and can cooperate. The use of local flaps is usually unsatisfactory because of their bulk and lack of adhesion to the underlying alveolus.

Adhesions of the buccal sulcus may be released with widely undermined, laterally based mucosal advancement flaps (Fig. 56–

39) (O'Connor and associates, 1972). Horton and associates (1970) combined Z-plasty and V-Y advancement flap techniques, including supplemental mucosal grafting of the sulcus when necessary (Fig. 56–40). Horton and associates' (1970) technique can give satisfactory results when there is proper indication. The technique of O'Connor and associates

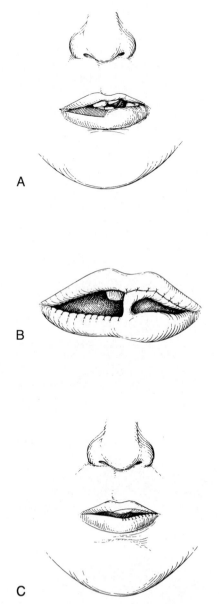

A

B

C

Figure 56–38. Cross lip mucosal flap from the inner surface of the lower lip. *A,* Incision and design of flap. *B,* Flap in place prior to division of the pedicle. *C,* Final result. (From Kawamoto, H. K.: Correction of major defects of the vermilion with a cross-lip vermilion flap. Plast. Reconstr. Surg., 64:315, 1979.)

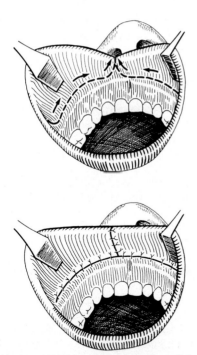

Figure 56–39. Wide undermining and medial advancement of mucosa. V-Y advancement releases buccal sulcus adhesions and lengthens the lip in area of repair. (After O'Connor, McGregor, and Tolleth. From Millard, D. R., Jr.: Cleft Craft. Vol. I. Boston, Little, Brown & Company, 1976.)

to provide support and stabilization of the graft; it was then replaced by a retainer for six months. In this way, a sulcus with proper depth can be maintained. Premature discontinuation of use of the appliance or the retainer almost always results in a shallow sulcus. Esser (1917) and Gillies and Kilner (1932) used split-thickness skin grafts, but Cosman and Crikelair (1966) favored oral mucosal grafts, which seemed to undergo less contraction. The authors prefer split-thickness skin grafts.

In patients with alveolar clefts and fistulas, or poor lip repairs, concomitant sulcoplasty may be performed with lip revision, gingivoplasty, and bone grafting. This is achieved by gingival and mucosal shifting procedures as indicated by the local conditions.

Cleft Lip Nasal Deformity

An enhanced understanding of the total anatomic deformity of the primary cleft and the consequent refinement of surgical techniques has led to a significant improvement in results of primary and secondary repair of the lip. It is probably fair to say that the situation with regard to the nasal deformity is less satisfactory. The greatest corrective challenge lies in management of the nose. According to Trier (1984), there are two reasons: First, the abnormality of the cleft lip and palate has been studied to a greater degree than the nasal deformity, with resulting improvement in surgical design and results. Second, the lip line and shadow beneath

(1972) often deforms the lip and is not recommended. Bardach and Salyer (1987a) detached the lip from the alveolar ridge and created a triangular gap of proper depth (Fig. 56–41). A thin skin graft was held in position by using a dental splint formed preoperatively from an impression. The appliance was wired to the teeth and retained for one month

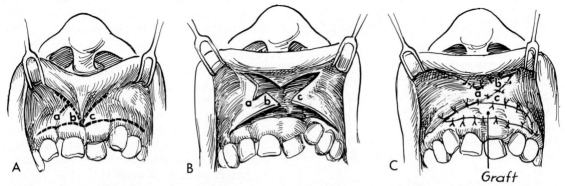

Figure 56–40. Secondary correction of upper sulcus adhesions. *A,* Short central segment of the upper lip; incisions shown are for a V-Z advancement. *B,* V-Z advancement. Note that the central portion of the vermilion border is increased in size. All flaps are undermined widely. *C,* The V-flap has been advanced to fill out the vermilion border. The Z-flaps avoid a straight scar. A mucous membrane graft has been sutured to the denuded alveolar process. (Adapted from Horton, C. E., Adamson, J. E., Mladick, R. A., and Taddeo, R. J.: The upper lip sulcus in cleft lips. Plast. Reconstr. Surg., *45:*31, 1970. Copyright 1970, The Williams & Wilkins Company, Baltimore.)

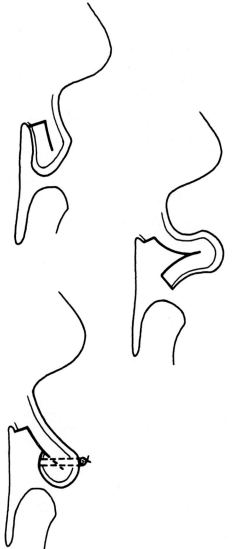

Figure 56–41. Lengthening of lip mucosa with insertion of a split-thickness skin graft into the superior raw area intraorally. (After Johnson. From Millard, D. R., Jr.: Cleft Craft. Vol. II. Boston, Little, Brown & Company, 1977.)

the nose deemphasize the lip, whereas the nose is always more obvious. The actual reason is that the total interrelated lip, nose, maxilla, and palate deformity has been poorly analyzed and understood, and consequently treatment objectives have not been realized.

PATHOLOGIC ANATOMY

While the cleft lip nasal deformity is usually characteristic, its severity varies with each case and is directly related to the extent of the lip deformity and particularly the alveolar cleft. "Formes frustes" of the cleft lip nose can occur with a normal lip (Brown, 1964; Stenström and Thilander, 1965; Boo-Chai and Tange, 1968). It is now well accepted that these are often associated with high orbicularis defects and deficiencies of the underlying nostril sill, the nasal spine, and the maxilla.

Components of the nasal deformity include defects of the lower lateral cartilage on the cleft side, the nasal septum, the columella, the nasal tip, and the entire nasal pyramid. The maxillary cleft and hypoplasia and malpositioning of the maxillary segments also contribute significantly to the asymmetry. The anatomic and functional deformity of the orbicularis muscle also contributes to the nasal deformity.

The etiology of the unilateral cleft nasal deformity is still a subject of considerable debate. Studies of the development of the facial area, specifically the medial and lateral nasal processes, suggest an intrinsic defect or a deficiency of growth and development of the nasal structures. Failure of neural crest cells to migrate results in absence of mesodermal penetration of the soft tissues in the cleft region and is a plausible cause (Veau, 1937–1938; Stark, 1968; Stark and Kaplan, 1973; Johnston, Hassell, and Brown, 1975). The growth disturbance can result from an inherited tendency (Fogh-Andersen, 1942) or from an environmental influence (Fraser, 1963, 1971; Patton, 1968, 1971). The degree of severity is related to the embryologic period in which the disturbance occurs, with misdirection during an earlier period causing even greater deformity. Noting that cartilage provides support for the soft tissues of the face and early embryonic development, Avery (1961) demonstrated marked differences in the nasal cartilaginous capsules of five embryos with clefts when compared with those of unaffected embryos. The cartilage in the embryos with clefts was deficient and malformed and showed delayed growth. In addition, there were abnormalities of the vomer and contiguous maxillary bones. Millicovsky, Ambrose, and Johnston (1982) demonstrated a lack of epithelial activity in the nasal pit area of the medial nasal prominence of cleft-prone strains versus cleft-resistant strains of mice. The "isolated cleft lip-nose" concept seems to argue for an intrinsic tissue abnormality, a hypothesis supported only by Brown

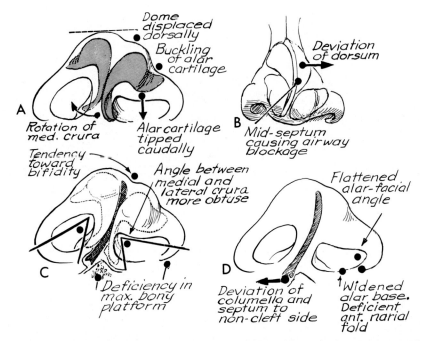

Figure 56–42. Deformities of the nasal tip in the cleft lip nose. *A*, Deviation of the nasal tip. *B*, Deviation of the nasal dorsum. The alar cartilage is tipped caudally. *C*, The angle between the medial and lateral crura is more obtuse, and the dome is displaced dorsally. Note the buckling of the lateral crus and the deficiency of the maxillary bone platform. *D*, The columella and caudal septum are deviated to the noncleft side. The septum on the convex side causes varying degrees of obstruction and also causes the tendency to bifidity.

(1964). Boo-Chai and Tange (1968) and Stenström and Thilander (1965) reported abnormal canine and supernumerary teeth in these patients and, because of this finding, believe that the cleft lip nasal deformity is an expression of lip and palate diathesis. These researchers failed to examine the orbicularis muscle and the underlying maxilla.

Most investigators believe that cleft lip nasal deformities result from tissue deficiency of the cleft lip, a deficiency of the maxilla, or abnormal muscular pull on the nasal structures (Figs. 56–42, 56–43). They have emphasized the role of tissue deficiencies "extrinsic" to the nasal tissues. Characteristic anatomic abnormalities of the unilateral cleft lip nasal deformity were described by Blair (1925), Gillies and Kilner (1932), McIndoe (1938), Huffman and Lierle (1949), Stenström and Oberg (1961), Converse, Hogan, and Barton (1977), and Bardach and Salyer (1987a). Huffman and Lierle (1949) based their description of the "typical" cleft lip nasal deformity on information obtained from photographs of and dental impressions taken from a large number of patients. Their descriptions remain fairly accurate and are as follows:

1. The tip of the nose is deflected toward the noncleft side.
2. The dome on the cleft side is retrodisplaced.
3. The angle between the medial and lateral crura on the cleft side is excessively obtuse.
4. The ala buckles inward on the cleft side.
5. The alar-facial groove on the cleft side is absent.
6. The alar-facial attachment is at an obtuse angle.
7. There is real or apparent bony deficiency of the maxilla on the cleft side.
8. The circumference of the naris is greater on the cleft side.
9. The naris on the cleft side is retrodisplaced.
10. The columella is shorter in the anteroposterior dimension on the cleft side.
11. The medial crus is displaced on the cleft side.
12. The columella is positioned obliquely, with the dorsal ends slanted toward the noncleft side.

Not all deformities are present in each patient, nor are they present to the same degree.

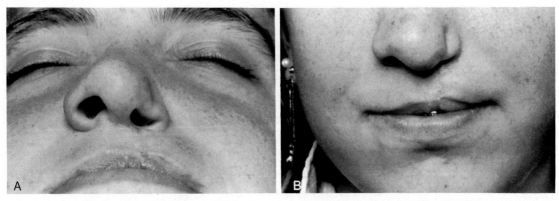

Figure 56–43. Secondary cleft lip nose. A, B, Typical appearance (see Fig. 56–42).

Bardach and Salyer (1987b) emphasized the individuality of the cleft lip nasal deformity; their description of the cleft lip nose included, in addition to the above, nasolabial fistula, absence of the nasal floor, hypertrophy of the inferior turbinate on the cleft side, and displacement of the noncleft maxillary segment. That the alar crease continues unopposed across the alar cartilage, often to the alar rim, was observed by Millard (1976). Berkeley (1959), Brown and McDowell (1941), and Uchida (1971) described what was referred to as a vestibular web—a characteristic linear contracture of the interior nostril from its apex to the piriform aperture along the upper border of the alar cartilage. This defect is due to the anteroposterior shortness of the maxilla (i.e., piriform aperture on the cleft side). There is general agreement on these observations, although Broadbent and Woolf (1984) stated that the columella is not short and that it simply extends laterally to a dipped area on the rim of the nostril. It is true that the columella is not short, but it appears so owing to malpositioning because of the absence of the nasal spine on the cleft side.

Maxillary hypoplasia as a component of the cleft nasal deformity was recognized by Gillies and Kilner (1932) and McIndoe (1938). A deficient piriform aperture and its adverse effect on the alar base have been emphasized by Fomon, Bell, and Syracuse (1956), Farrior (1962), Longacre and associates (1966), Hogan and Converse (1971), Ortiz-Monasterio and Olmedo (1981), Jackson (1984), and Anderl (1985). Bone grafts, cartilage grafts, and other materials placed on the piriform aperture have significantly improved the nasal contour by providing elevation of the alar

base. Berkeley (1969) attributed the cleft lip nasal deformity to incomplete rotation of the alar cartilage; Onizuka (1972) believed that nostril asymmetry was due in part to absence of the alar base fullness on the affected side. The nasal deformity has been attributed to hypoplasia of the lateral crus of the alar cartilage by Spira, Hardy, and Gerow (1970), Schwenzer (1973), and Sawney (1976). A normal alar cartilage distorted by mechanical forces was theorized by Blair (1925), Gillies and Kilner (1932), McIndoe (1938), and Huffman and Lierle (1949). Dissections of stillborn infants with unilateral and bilateral clefts (McComb, 1984, 1985) revealed that the cleft nostril was larger than that of the unaffected side, but the alar cartilages were symmetric when lifted into their correct positions. Cadaver dissections demonstrated that the unilateral cleft lip nasal deformity resulted from abnormal muscular tension on nasal structures, especially the alar base. Loss of orbicularis oris muscle continuity was also suggested as a cause of the nasal deformity (Stenström and Oberg, 1961; Skoog, 1969; Sawney, 1976).

Converse, Hogan, and Barton (1977) considered the pathologic anatomic features under three categories: the nasal tip (alar cartilages and columella), the lateral bony platform (piriform aperture), and the midline supporting structures (cartilaginous septum and anterior nasal spine). Hogan and Converse (1971) represented the unilateral cleft nasal deformity as a "tilted tripod" resting on a hypoplastic maxilla to explain the characteristic bending and deformity of the nasal cartilages (Fig. 56–44). The tripod of the two alae and the septum supports the nasal soft tissue. When one of the bony platforms (hy-

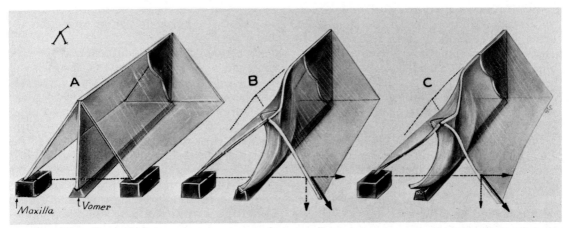

Figure 56–44. The tilted tripod. *A,* Schematic representation of the nose illustrating the basic tripod nature of the nasal structure. The tripod consists of the dorsal portion of the septum and nasal bones, and the two alar arms. *B,* The tilting effect resulting from maxillary hypoplasia with secondary deformity of the septum and cleft ala. *C,* More dramatic illustration of the convex deformity of the septum and the vertical bending of the septum posterior to the junction of the membranous and cartilaginous portions of the septum. Restriction of the caudal border of the septum in its anterior thrust causes it to bend toward the normal nostril. If there is a more severe deformity of the vomer, the septum is displaced into the normal nostril. (From Hogan, V. M., and Converse, J. M.: Secondary deformities of unilateral cleft lip and nose. *In* Grabb, W. C., Rosenstein, S. E., and Bzoch, K. R. (Eds.): Cleft Lip and Palate. Boston, Little Brown & Company, 1971.)

poplastic maxilla) is deficient, the tripod collapses on the ipsilateral ala and deflects the septum into the contralateral normal naris. With marked hypoplasia, the septum is lifted out of the vomerine groove and encroaches on the opposite nostril, as occurs in 70 to 80 per cent of unilateral cleft lip noses.

In addition to the extrinsic deficiencies theory, intrinsic hypoplasia of the involved soft tissue and cartilage has been postulated. Using anthropometric techniques, Lindsay and Farkas (1971) noted abnormalities of the noncleft side of the face in patients with clefts, as compared with normal controls. Whether cleft lip nasal deformity is caused by malpositioning of normal structures due to an extrinsic mechanism or a secondary inherent deficiency of nasal development, or both, a significant amount of secondary deformity can be prevented by a primary lip repair that also includes nasal correction. It is important to recognize that failure to reconstruct the nasal floor in the primary cleft repair leaves the nose attached directly to the lip through the intact orbicularis and to the palate through the lateral mucoperiosteum of the alveolar cleft. Thus, although the lip defect may improve with time, the primary nasal deformity will *never* improve. This is a basic tenet of cleft development! The small constricted nostril resulting from oversacrifice of the lip or nose elements is dif-

ficult to correct and should not be produced initially. The rotation-advancement repair of Millard (Gillies and Millard, 1957) preserves tissue, repositions the alar base, lengthens the columella, restores lip muscle continuity, reconstructs the nostril sill and floor (if the primary palate is repaired), adds tissue for vestibular lining, and generally offers the greatest opportunity for nasal correction.

SURGICAL CORRECTION

In both primary and secondary procedures, functional and esthetic problems must be addressed. Nasal symmetry with improved nasolabial and nasofacial relationships and minimal evidence of surgical intervention fulfill the esthetic requirements. Functional objectives include a patent airway, proper position of the maxilla to provide Class I interdental occlusion, and the achievement of normal speech.

Timing of Surgery

Repair of nasal deformities in unilateral cleft lip patients may be done at the time of primary lip repair, in the preschool years (age 4 to 6 years), during puberty (age 10 to 12 years), or as an adult. There is now less credence given to the concept of disturbance of nasal growth by surgery.

Simultaneous Primary Lip and Alveolar Repair. The optimal time to attempt correction of a cleft lip nasal deformity remains controversial. The possibility of simultaneous primary lip and nose repairs interfering with nasal and maxillary growth as a result of postoperative scarring was raised by Blair (1925), Veau (1931), Gillies and Kilner (1932), Peet and Patterson (1963), Marcks and associates (1964), and Matthews (1968). Direct surgical attack on the nasal tip or alar cartilages of the unilateral cleft lip nasal deformity in infancy presupposes the technical ability to work with small and fragile cartilages and the capacity to predict the outcome of developing structures. Operating on the adult nose, in the opinion of these investigators, offers the advantage of producing a definitive result. However, it sentences the individual to years of ridicule and unhappiness. This concept cannot be accepted.

Correction at the primary lip repair was advised by McIndoe (1938), Brown and McDowell (1941), Huffman and Lierle (1949), Berkeley (1959, 1969), and O'Connor, McGregor, and Tolleth (1968). They argued that the future nasal configuration would be more satisfactory if the cartilages were in their correct position during the growth period. There is no evidence to support this hypothesis. Over the last two decades, more radical correction of the nasal deformity at the time of lip repair has been described by Berkeley (1959), Skoog (1969), Pigott and Millard (1971), Wynn (1972), Broadbent and Woolf (1984), Anderl (1985), McComb (1985), Salyer (1986), and Bardach and Salyer (1987b). The subject is discussed in detail in Chapter 53.

Preschool Age. Social pressures at age 4 to 6 years heighten the patient's awareness of residual cleft lip nasal deformity, and consequently demands for correction intensify. Millard (1982) believed that the alar cartilages are adequately developed and can be manipulated at this age. Bardach and Salyer (1987b) delayed secondary correction until the patient was 8 to 12 years old for three reasons: (1) to allow completion of orthodontic correction of the skeletal base; (2) to allow as much growth and development of the lower lateral cartilages as possible and thus to have a stronger, more stable support for the reconstructed nasal tip; and (3) to allow bone grafting of the hypoplastic maxillary segment on the cleft side, which when performed in patients aged 8 to 9 years results in a more symmetric alar base, improving conditions for successful nasal deformity correction at a later age.

Converse, Hogan, and Barton (1977) recommended only closure of the anterior cleft nasal floor, repositioning of the flaring ala, and bone grafting of the hypoplastic piriform aperture. They preferred to delay secondary rhinoplasty until nasal growth had been completed. This occurs in females by age 16 and in males by age 18 years (Hajnisova, 1967). Growth activity in the septal cartilage of septoplasty patients from 6 to 35 years of age was studied by Vetter, Pirsig, and Heinze (1983). Study after incorporation of a labeled sulfate in septal specimens indicated that the highest growth activity was in the suprapremaxillary and anterior border of the septal cartilage between the ages of 6 and 10 years. Thus, they recommended no septal resection or revision before age 20. The vomer is essential for general nasal growth and downward and forward growth of the maxilla until 7 to 8 years of age (Reidy, 1968). Patients who underwent resection of the vomer during palatal closure at 1 year of age were found to have marked maxillary retrusion. The effect of septal resection on nasal growth has also been studied in rabbits by Sarnat (1967), who found that resection of the cartilaginous nasal septum resulted in severe arrest of growth, whereas dislocation caused little growth disturbance. On the other hand, no significant reduction in facial growth was noted after early resection of septal cartilage in chimpanzees (Siegel and Sadler, 1981; Siegel, 1983).

Rhinoplasty performed before puberty has not been fraught with growth disturbances or poor long-term results (Ortiz-Monasterio and Olmedo, 1981; Salyer, 1986). Ortiz-Monasterio and Olmedo (1981) performed "complete rhinoplasties" in 44 patients between the ages of 8 and 12 years; three-fourths of the nasal deformities were associated with unilateral or bilateral cleft lip or cleft palate. Lateral and medial osteotomies, extensive alar dissection, and septoplasty were performed in the majority of patients. There were no obvious growth problems during a five year follow-up.

Most authorities agree that early correction (during the preschool years) of the unilateral cleft lip nose is indicated. A rational approach is rotation-advancement lip repair with primary closure of the cleft nostril floor and repositioning of the alar base. Onlay bone grafts (Converse, Hogan, and Barton, 1977) or surgical augmentation of the hypoplastic piriform aperture to elevate the cleft alar platform should represent the extent of the primary procedure. Secondary correction of residual nasal deformity by limited septoplasty, reconstruction of the nasal tip and alar cartilages, and cartilage grafts as described below is also appropriate during the preschool years.

Puberty/Adolescence. According to the studies of Hajnisova (1967), nasal growth is complete in females by age 16 and in males by age 18 years. As noted above, rhinoplasty can be performed at earlier ages without upsetting nasal and facial growth (Ortiz-Monasterio and Olmedo, 1981; Millard, 1982). Delay of definitive rhinoplasty until the patient is 14 years of age or older is desirable. According to Bardach and Salyer (1987a), by this age the canine teeth have erupted and bone grafting has been performed, thus providing bony support for the nasal base with augmentation of the hypoplastic maxilla. Osteotomies of the maxilla and correction of skeletal or occlusal abnormalities should precede definitive rhinoplasty, as advancement of the maxilla may alter the nasal contour significantly. Although it has been advised to wait for one year after maxillary osteotomy before doing the rhinoplasty (Bardach and Salyer, 1987b), it is quite reasonable to correct nasal deformity after six months. Although correction of a deformity of the lower third of the nose can and should be performed at the time of other surgery, such as closure of an alveolar cleft and alveolar bone grafting, definitive rhinoplasty should be delayed until after surgical advancement, expansion, or repositioning of the maxilla. Schendel and Delaire (1981) combined lip and nose revision with orthognathic surgery, since the latter results in significant profile alteration.

Definitive rhinoplasty may include septal resection, osteotomies, cartilage or bone grafting, and extensive dissection of the upper and lower lateral cartilages. Salyer (1986) summarized the principles of correction of the cleft lip nasal deformity as follows: (1) the more severe the deformity, the earlier and more radical the secondary procedure should be; (2) correction of the nasal deformity is designed to improve form and function and to alleviate psychologic stress; (3) correction of nasal deformities includes the skeletal base, the septum, the tip, and the alae; (4)

bone grafting and cartilage augmentation may be indicated; (5) definitive rhinoplasty is performed when the patient is 14 years of age or older; and (6) severe asymmetry of the skeletal base is a contraindication to definitive rhinoplasty. The authors, however, would advocate much earlier correction for a severe deformity.

Corrective Surgery Techniques

No single procedure developed to date has given sufficiently satisfactory results to provide a surgical standard for cleft lip nasal deformity correction. Familiarity with the wide range of repairs is necessary to choose the appropriate technique for each patient (Musgrave, 1961; Converse, Hogan, and Barton, 1977). The historical evolution of unilateral cleft nasal deformity correction has been chronicled by Millard (1976) and reviewed by Denecke and Meyer (1967), Spira, Hardy, and Gerow (1970), Converse, Hogan, and Barton (1977), Trier (1984), and Rohrich and Tebbetts (1987).

To restore nasal symmetry, the alar cartilages must be modified by repositioning, suspension, alteration in size, or augmentation with grafts. Reduction of the bulk of the unaffected larger-appearing naris may be required. Nasal tip deformity may also result from septal deflection, which in turn is adversely affected by defective maxillary development.

The various techniques for correction of the unilateral cleft lip nasal deformity have been listed by Rohrich and Tebbetts (1987) (Fig. 56–45): (1) external approach, (2) alar cartilage mobilization and suspension, (3) alar cartilage incision and repositioning, and (4) graft augmentation. Additional techniques include orthognathic procedures, bone grafting, vestibular web revisions, and nostril hood modifications.

Rotation of Cleft Lip Lobule and External Incisions. In 1925, Blair noted that the width of the nostril on the cleft side was almost always increased. In addition, the alar base remained in association with the hypoplastic maxilla. He initially carried out superior and medial rotation of the alar base to correct the abnormal orientation of the nares, and he advanced the downwardly displaced medial crura by a midcolumellar incision that extended under the alar base (Fig. 56–45A). This procedure elevated the dome and nar-

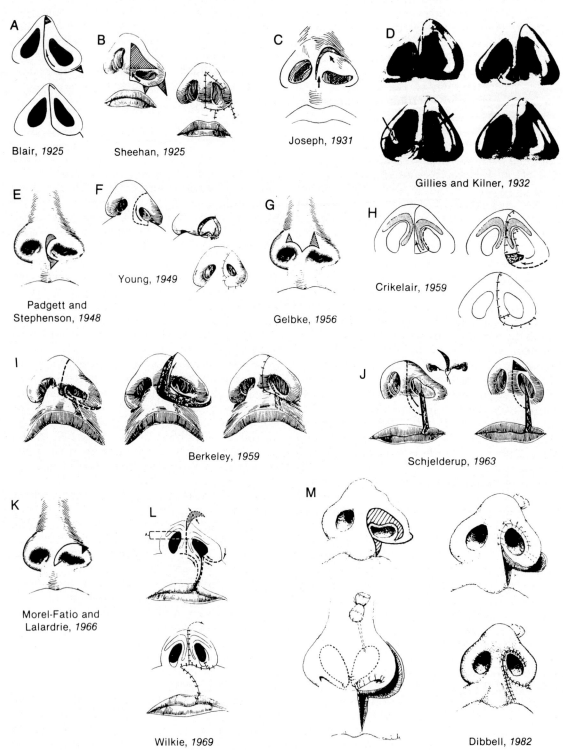

Blair, *1925*

Sheehan, *1925*

Joseph, *1931*

Gillies and Kilner, *1932*

Padgett and
Stephenson, *1948*

Young, *1949*

Gelbke, *1956*

Crikelair, *1959*

Berkeley, *1959*

Schjelderup, *1963*

Morel-Fatio and
Lalardrie, *1966*

Wilkie, *1969*

Dibbell, *1982*

Figure 56–45. Selection of methods for correction of the unilateral cleft lip nasal deformity using a columellar incision and nasal tip skin resection.

rowed the alar base but left the caudal dislocation of the alar margin to be corrected by a wedge excision. Rerotation of the ala was further espoused by Blair and Brown (1931), and this began a trend toward rotation of the alar lobule as a complex unit. Modifications of Blair's technique of excision and rotation-advancement were described by Sheehan (1936) (Fig. 56–45B), Padgett and Stephenson (1948) (Fig. 56 45E), Gelbke (1956) Fig. 56–45G), Farrior (1962), Schjelderup (1963) (Fig. 56–45J), Morel-Fatio and Lalardrie (1966) (Fig. 56–45K), and Pitanguy (1963). This operation resulted in external scarring and fortunately has been abandoned in most centers.

A semilunar excision of dorsal skin to correct the downward displacement of the ala was described by Joseph (1931). This technique brought the dome of the alar cartilage into a more normal position but was not a definitive correction of the problem (Fig. 56–45C). Crikelair, Ju, and Symonds (1959) stated that external skin excisions were justifiable in patients with marked abnormalities (Fig. 56–45H). In all these procedures, medial advancement of the alar base is usually done as a separate procedure.

Gillies and Kilner (1932) extended Blair's procedure by lengthening the midcolumellar incisions upward over the cleft side of the dome (Fig. 56–45D) as in Joseph's (1931) incision technique. This was illustrated incorrectly in their initial publication, the incision being extended over the tip of the nose on the normal side. Later it was corrected by Wilkie (1969), who noted that Joseph's dorsal

incision was part of the rotation-advancement of the alar columella. A separate rim incision corrected downward displacement of the ala (Fig. 56–45L).

Berkeley (1959) described a more extensive rotation upward and medially of the entire half of the nose on the cleft side (Fig. 56–45I). Wilkie (1969) and Velazquez and Ortiz-Monasterio (1974) advocated the same technique. Correction of the flaring alar base, downward displacement of the alar dome, and inferior medial displacement of the medial crus results from the extensive mobilization of the lobule complex. These techniques have been abandoned by most surgeons treating cleft patients because of unacceptable scarring.

Instead of rotating the nostril floor into the columella, Hugo and Tumbusch (1971) and Neuner (1967) incorporated lip skin and scar to lengthen the columella on the cleft side (Fig. 56–46).

Dibbell (1982) described excision of excess alar rim skin, mobilization of the alar cartilage from the skin, and rotation of the nostril peripherally rather than rotation of half of the columella (see Fig. 56–45M). The disadvantage of this method is the introduction of a fresh lip scar.

Controversy continues as to the location of the incisions through which the alar cartilages are dissected, exposed, and repositioned. Routine intranasal incisions provide adequate exposure of the lateral and medial crura. Although this approach is not as satisfactory as that afforded by the external

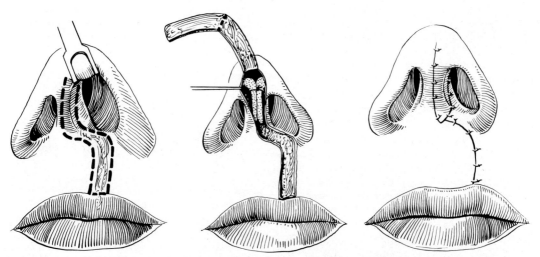

Figure 56–46. Use of lip scar and columellar skin to provide unilateral lengthening of columella. (After Hugo and Tumbusch. From Millard, D. R., Jr.: Cleft Craft. Vol. I. Boston, Little, Brown & Company, 1976.)

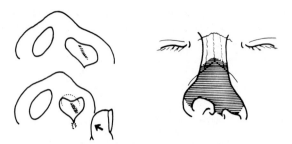

Figure 56–47. Degloving of lower nose to expose and correct lower lateral cartilage deformity. (From Tajima, S., and Maruyama, M.: Reverse U incision for secondary repair of cleft lip nose. Plast. Reconstr. Surg., 60:256, 1977.)

incision, it is adequate for surgeons trained in esthetic rhinoplasty. In unilateral and bilateral secondary cleft lip nasal deformities, through a combination of rim and upper labial sulcus incisions, Black (1982) was able to deglove the lower nasal skeleton and enhance exposure. "C-flap" extensions as described by Tajima (1983) are an additional means of simultaneous exposure and skin tailoring (Fig. 56–47). Often secondary revisions of the lip and nose defects are combined.

Proponents of the external incision cite the following advantages: (1) wide exposure, (2) increased alar mobilization, (3) possibly enhanced long-term stability, and (4) superior correction of severe deformities. The major disadvantage of some external incisions is the presence of a scar on the nasal tip. Converse, Hogan, and Barton (1977) have used dermabrasion for midline nasal scars two to three months after healing to produce relatively inconspicuous scars. External incisions were advocated by Crikelair, Ju, and Symonds (1959) in the following situations: (1) severe deformities as a result of cleft deficiency or previous repairs, (2) thick alar skin, and (3) previous unsuccessful intranasal procedures.

External nasal incisions, excluding those for skin excision or alar lobule rotation, are generally designed to provide exposure of the medial crura and dome area (Fig. 56–48). Erich (1953) advocated a "flying wing" incision at the nasal tip (Fig. 56–48a); it is especially prone to cause scarring and pincushioning in the tip area. DeKleine (1955) and O'Connor, McGregor, and Tolleth (1968) described a midcolumellar incision. Figi (1952) recommended a combination of the flying wing and midcolumellar incisions (Fig.

56–48b). The original Gillies and Kilner (1932) incision extended the columellar incision into the cleft floor (Fig. 56–48d). Salyer (1986) used an incision described by Berkeley (1969) without extension into the nostril or over the nasal tip (Fig. 56–49).

Intranasal rim incisions connected across the columella at different levels have been advocated by several investigators (Rethi, 1934; Spira, Hardy, and Gerow, 1970). These are not advised, since placement of the incision at the columellar base and development of a columellar flap produces a less noticeable scar and allows excellent access to alar cartilage (Potter, 1954; McIndoe and Rees, 1959; Uchida, 1971; Schwenzer, 1973; Bardach and Salyer, 1987b). *This is the only acceptable external approach*, since it is also used when indicated in esthetic rhinoplasty. A midline incision along the nasal dorsum to the nasal tip has been described by Converse, Hogan, and Barton (1977) but should not be used.

Alar Cartilage Mobilization and Suspension. Long-term maintenance of cleft lip nasal deformity correction requires accurate

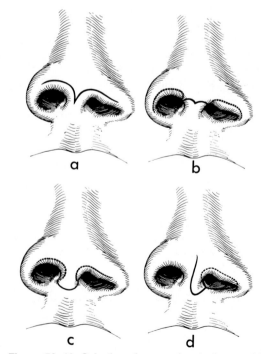

Figure 56–48. Selection of approaches to the nasal tip (see text for details). a, After Erich. b, After Figi. c, After Potter. d, After Gillies. (From Spira, M., Hardy, S. B., and Gerow, F. J.: Correction of nasal deformities accompanying unilateral cleft lip. Cleft Palate J., 7:112, 1970.)

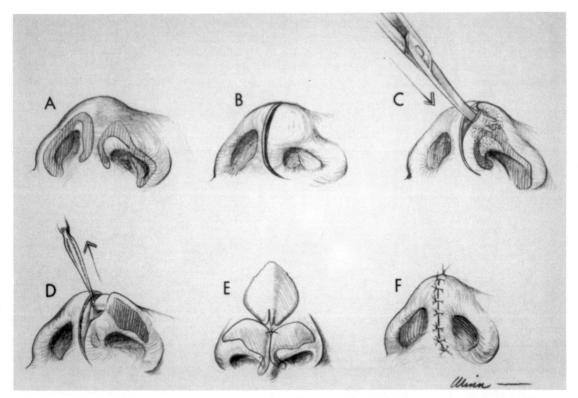

Figure 56–49. Method of exposing and correcting lower lateral cartilage deformity. *A,* The deformed and displaced lower lateral cartilage on the cleft side. *B,* The incision starts along the nasal sill and extends up to the midline of the columella and over the nasal dome to create access to the domes and lower lateral cartilage. *C,* Dissection of the skin from the lateral crus of the lower lateral cartilage. The skin is also dissected over the entire nasal tip. *D,* Elevation of the lower lateral cartilage on the cleft side to the level of the dome on the opposite side. Dissection was carried between the medial crura, exposing the septum. *E,* The lower lateral cartilage on the cleft side has been elevated and matched to the cartilage on the noncleft side by advancing it superiorly and cephalad, correcting the slumped or drooped tip. *F,* Closure of the external incision using interrupted 6-0 nylon sutures or, preferably, pull-out Prolene of 4-0 or 5-0. (After Berkeley. From Bardach, J., and Salyer, K. E.: Surgical Techniques in Cleft Lip and Palate. Chicago, Year Book Medical Publishers, 1987.)

placement of the nasal supporting structures (i.e., alar cartilages). Sufficient surgical exposure for dissection of the alar cartilage from the vestibular and external skin is essential for correction of the alar deformity, and this can be achieved through intranasal incisions. The various types of intranasal incisions have been described by Gillies and Kilner (1932), Steffensen (1949), deKleine (1955), Millard (1964a), Schwenzer (1973), Sawney (1976), Nishimura and Ogino (1977), Tajima and Maruyama (1977), and Broadbent and Woolf (1984). Adequate exposure of the dome area and the medial and lateral crura can be obtained, although not as completely as through an external incision. Converse, Hogan, and Barton (1977) argued that soft tissue redraping is less stable via intranasal incisions versus external incisions; however, scarring cannot be avoided and the claim of

superior long-term results is debatable. Nevertheless, in severe nasal deformity, especially after multiple previous procedures, and in bilateral cases the external approach is recommended.

Regardless of whether intranasal or external incisions are used, maintenance of the cleft alar components in their proper anatomic position after dissection and mobilization is crucial. The likelihood of success is limited in the presence of marked deformity or attenuation of the cleft alar cartilages, inadequate soft tissue mobilization, disruption of delicate structures during dissection, or significant preexisting scarring (Rohrich and Tebbetts, 1987).

Complete exposure of the deformed alar cartilage, delivery of the lateral crus, and suturing of the domes are important components in the nasal correction of Potter (1954)

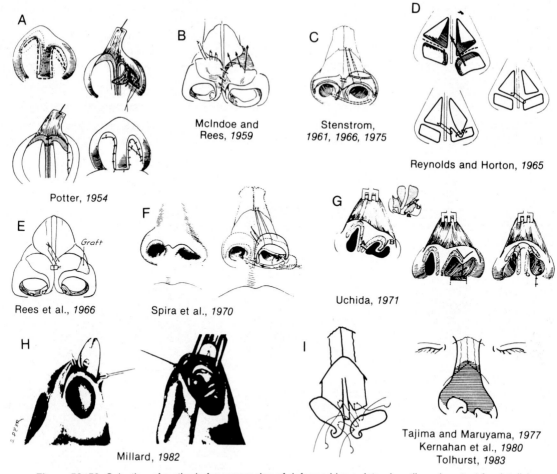

A

Potter, 1954

B

McIndoe and
Rees, 1959

C

Stenstrom,
1961, 1966, 1975

D

Reynolds and Horton, 1965

E

Rees et al., 1966

F

Graft

Spira et al., 1970

G

Uchida, 1971

H

Millard, 1982

I

Tajima and Maruyama, 1977
Kernahan et al., 1980
Tolhurst, 1983

Figure 56–50. Selection of methods for suspension of deformed lower lateral cartilage (see text for details).

(Fig. 56–50). The columellar flap was raised, exposing both lateral crura, in his technique (Fig. 56–50A). Gelbke (1956) sutured the alae at their maximal height through a transverse flying wing incision, but this resulted in pronounced nasal tip scarring. McIndoe and Rees (1959) described a procedure that involved exposing both alar cartilages and securing the alar domes to each other and to the septal angle. The lateral cartilages and crura were secured by sutures to the septum and by mattress sutures through the skin, respectively (Fig. 56–50B). A raw defect in the lateral vestibule either was closed with a composite graft of cartilage and skin or was left to epithelize. Stenström (1966, 1975) and Spira, Hardy, and Gerow (1970) described similar medial rotations of the lateral crus, with suspension sutures to the ipsilateral nasal dome at the caudal edge of the nasal

bones. Spira, Hardy, and Gerow (1970) excised the noncleft lateral crus to fill the lateral vestibular defect on the cleft side. A suture from the alar base passing through the nasal spine and caudal septum provided maintenance of nostril sill width (Fig. 56–50F). A Z-plasty to narrow the alar base with a buried suture anchoring the alar base to the septum was advocated by Stenström (1975) (Fig. 56–50C). Rees, Guy, and Converse (1966) dissected the entire lateral crus on the cleft side from the nasal skin and mucosa and weakened the cartilage by scoring to establish a contour similar to that of the noncleft dome (Fig. 56–50E). Sutures to the contralateral upper lateral cartilage and medial crura maintained the corrected height of the dome. The lateral vestibular defect was closed with a skin graft or composite chondrocutaneous graft. Suspension of the cleft

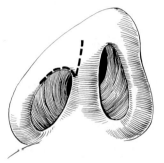 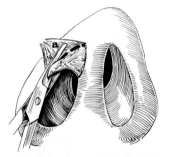 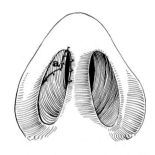

Figure 56–51. Correction of alar-columellar web by modified Z-plasty technique (see Fig. 56–54). (After Straith. From Millard, D. R., Jr.: Cleft Craft. Vol. I. Boston, Little, Brown & Company, 1976.)

lateral alar crus to both ipsilateral and contralateral upper lateral cartilages was described by Reynolds and Horton (1965) (Fig. 56–50D). Elevating and suspending the cleft alar cartilage are facilitated by excision of a portion of the alar cartilage (cephalic edge).

When the alar cartilages are repositioned a shortage of skin may become apparent, particularly in the alar web and vestibular area. Differences of opinion regarding preservation or excision of the alar-columellar web tissue are apparent in the various approaches recommended. Alar-columellar web correction by Z-plasty was performed as early as 1946 by Straith (Fig. 56–51). Excision of alar cartilage from the web area and preservation of skin and lining were reported by Musgrave and Dupertuis (1960), Millard (1964a), and Salyer (1986). Ariyan and Krizek (1978) excised vestibular skin with underlying cartilage and external skin. Tajima and Maruyama (1977) described a reverse U–incision with suture suspension of the repositioned alar cartilages (Fig. 56–50I). The principle of conversion of external skin to nasal lining to correct alar-columellar web has been reported by Isshiki, Sawada, and Tamura (1980), Ogino and Ishida (1980), and Millard (1982). The outcome of Tajima and Maruyama's (1977) technique is an excellent nasal contour with minimal external scar and correction of the alar-columellar web. On the nostril on the cleft side a reverse U–incision begins in the membranous septum, curving forward slightly over the nostril rim parallel to the dome of the cartilage and reentering the nose to end just lateral to the fold in the nasal vestibule; a chondromucocutaneous flap of alar cartilage is raised and widely undermined. Additional undermining over the contralateral alar cartilage and upper lateral cartilage frees the entire nasal skin for re-

draping. The deformed alar cartilage flap is properly positioned and sutured to the contralateral alar cartilage of the noncleft side and the lateral cartilages of both sides by rotating the reverse U–flap medially and superiorly. Kernahan, Bauer, and Harris (1980) and Tolhurst (1983) reported success with minor and severe cleft lip nasal deformities repaired primarily or secondarily with this technique. Nakajima, Yoshimura, and Kami (1986) modified the technique by adding a Z-plasty in the lateral nasal vestibule (Fig. 56–52). Additional means to prevent tightness of the vestibular area include various external and internal Z-plasties (Trauner, 1956; Stenström and Oberg, 1961; O'Connor, McGregor, and Tolleth, 1965; Rees, Guy, and Converse, 1966; Matthews, 1968), skin grafts (Rees, Guy, and Converse, 1966), or composite grafts

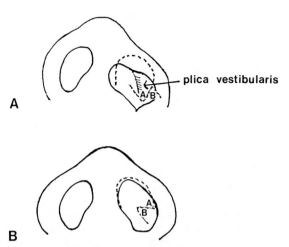

Figure 56–52. Correction of intranasal web by rotation flap and Z-plasty. *A,* Design of the reverse U–incision. *B,* Operation completed. (From Makajima, T., Yoshimura, Y., and Kami, T.: Refinement of the "reverse U" incision for the repair of cleft lip nose deformity. Br. J. Plast. Surg., 39:345, 1986.)

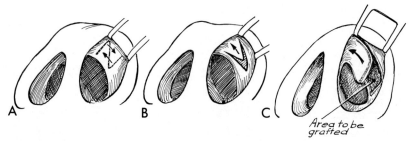

Figure 56–53. Techniques for correction of a web in the lateral vestibule. *A,* Z-plasty. *B,* V-Y advancement. *C,* Medial advancement (arrow) of a medially based flap of vestibular skin and alar cartilage in a unilateral cleft lip and nose deformity. A full-thickness skin graft is placed in the resulting lateral defect. (After Rees, Guy, and Converse.)

(Figs. 56–53, 56–54). Millard's (1982) rotation-advancement flap may have an "L-flap" available for filling in this area.

Long-term correction of the secondary cleft lip nasal deformity depends on an adequate dissection of the alar components, the structural integrity of the dissected elements, and maintenance of proper position by suture and eventual adherence and growth. Suspension sutures secured to bolsters over the nasal skin or rubber stent catheter can secure the nostril; through and through sutures are an alternative means of support.

Spira, Hardy, and Gerow (1970) emphasized overcorrection, since septal displacement and settling of the alar cartilage tend to occur. Deformity or attenuation of the cartilages may necessitate augmentation with grafts or incision and splitting of the cartilages.

Incision and Relocation of Alar Cartilage. In 1938, Humby proposed incision and transposition of the upper portion of the unaffected lateral crus across the midline to augment the lateral crus of the cleft side (Fig. 56–55C). Multiple techniques of incising or splitting portions of the alar cartilages and subsequent relocation followed (Figs. 56–55, 56–56).

Kazanjian (1939) described elevation of the medial crura of both alar cartilages as medially based flaps; these are sutured together vertically after division from the lateral crus (Fig. 56–56). Excision of alar base wedges and semilunar excision of skin from the alar web area also modified nostril width and projection.

Brown and McDowell (1941) divided the cleft lateral crus and repositioned it across the midline over its own medial crus and dome; it was suspended to the contralateral dome through an intranasal incision (Fig. 56–

55A). Using an external incision, Barsky (1950) relocated and suspended the cephalic border of the lateral crus on the cleft side to the dorsum of the septum (Fig. 56–55D). Erich (1953) divided the medial crus on the cleft side through an external incision and suspended the dome area to the contralateral dome (Fig. 56–55B). Whitlow and Constable (1973) used a Figi-type external incision and described a technique of crossed bilateral alar winged flaps suspended through the skin by pull-out bolster sutures (Fig. 56–55E).

The hinged cartilage flaps of Humby (1938), Barsky (1950), and Whitlow and Constable (1973) depend on preservation of cartilage integrity to maintain the elevation and the

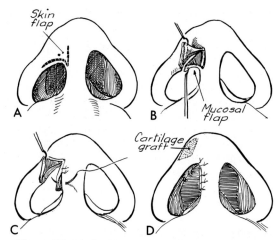

Figure 56–54. Straith technique for the removal of the web of tissue that veils the apex of the naris, with insertion of a cartilage graft. *A,* Outline of the incision. *B,* A skin flap is raised, exposing the cartilage. *C,* The exposed alar cartilage is excised, and the remaining mucosal flap is incised, rotated anteromedially, trimmed, and sutured to the columella. The skin flap is rotated into the vestibule and sutured to the lateral wall. *D,* Cartilage may be added to increase the projection of the dome of the alar cartilage. (After Straith.)

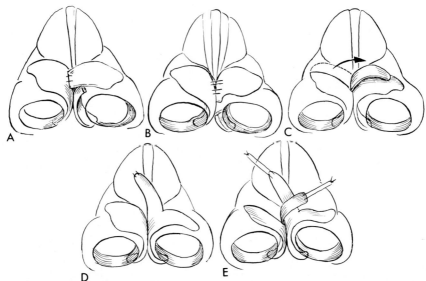

Figure 56–55. Relocation of the alar cartilages (see text for details). *A,* After Brown-McDowell. *B,* After Erich. *C,* After Humby. *D,* After Barsky. *E,* After Whitlow-Constable.

position of the remaining alar cartilage. Prerequisites are a strong, well-developed cartilaginous component that can withstand the stresses necessary to move attached soft tissue. Since the cartilage of the alar dome is frequently thin and fragile, construction of a durable tip may not be possible without the addition of a cartilage graft.

Graft Augmentation. If adequate and symmetric nasal projection is not obtained by suspension and repositioning of the alar cartilages, it can be achieved by cartilage graft augmentation of the cleft ala (Fig. 56–57). Lamont (1945) harvested the cephalic margin of the uninvolved ala to augment the cleft alar dome (Fig. 56–57*A*). Fomon, Bell, and Syracuse (1956) placed ear cartilage grafts over the lateral crus in the columella and the anterior nasal spine (Fig. 56–57*B*). A sutured multitiered cartilage graft was advocated by Musgrave and Dupertuis (1960) (Fig. 56–57*C*). A columellar strut graft of septal cartilage was proposed by Millard (1964b) to increase nasal tip projection (Fig. 56–57*E*). Gorney and Falces (1973) used a "gull-wing" conchal graft (Fig. 56–57*F*). This was formed by suturing conchal grafts together with their convexities apposing one another. Dibbell (1976) shaped costal cartilage into a "bowie knife" strut for placement in a pocket created in the columella and the membranous septum (Fig. 56–57*H*). Support of the nasal tip by positioning the strut with the concave portion

turned cephalically provided a graceful slope for the nasal dorsum and supratip area.

Augmentation of the columella and the tip can be achieved satisfactorily by the "Minerva's helmet" or lily conchal cartilage graft (Fig. 56–57*G*) (Tessier and associates, 1969; Pollet, 1972). A C-shaped costal cartilage graft can be used for tip projection. It is inserted through an incision in the columellar rim, which extends into the floor of the nose. The graft provides support for the depressed ala and augments the nasal sill in addition to its effect on the nasal tip. It is placed

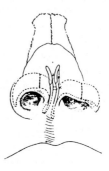

Kazanjian, *1939*

Figure 56–56. Kazanjian's technique for modification of nasal tip deformity. (From Kazanjian, V. H.: Secondary deformities in cleft palate patients. Ann. Surg., *109*:442, 1939.)

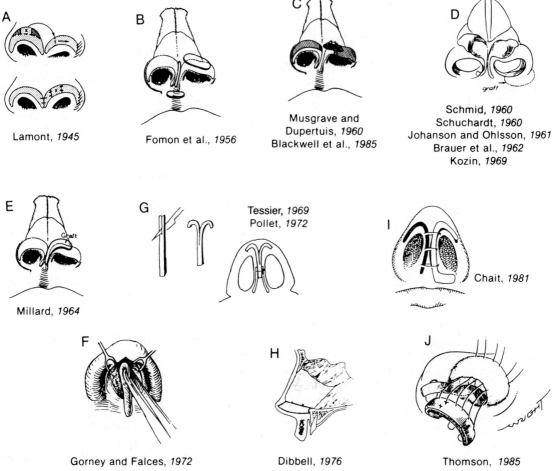

A

Lamont, *1945*

B

Fomon et al., *1956*

C

Musgrave and
Dupertuis, *1960*
Blackwell et al., *1985*

D

Schmid, *1960*
Schuchardt, *1960*
Johanson and Ohlsson, *1961*
Brauer et al., *1962*
Kozin, *1969*

E

Millard, *1964*

G

Tessier, *1969*
Pollet, *1972*

I

Chait, *1981*

F

Gorney and Falces, *1972*

H

Dibbell, *1976*

J

Thomson, *1985*

Figure 56–57. Correction of nasal tip deformity using a selection of cartilage grafts (see text for details).

superficial to the alar cartilage and is secured to the medial crura of both alar cartilages (Fig. 56–57*I*) (Chait, 1981). Thomson (1985) described an incision of the alar rim to produce a medially based flap (Fig. 56–57*J*). Interposition of the alar rim flap resulted in lengthening of the columella. The nasal tip and perialar sulcus are augmented with a conchal cartilage graft.

The long-term maintenance of the graft dimension and position in adults and adolescents has been reasonably well documented by Millard (1976), Sheen and Sheen (1978), and Ortiz-Monasterio and Olmedo (1981). The long-term fate of grafts used at the time of primary procedures has not been well studied with respect to longitudinal growth. Cartilaginous columellar grafts must be sufficiently rigid to produce projection and shaping of the

soft tissues. Subsequently, they may cause distortion or displacement of the nasal tip owing to warping. They should be cut carefully as balanced cross sections (Gibson and Davis, 1958). Alloplastic support for the columella (e.g., silicone) should not be used because of the frequent occurrence of erosion through the skin (Millard, 1976). This complication may also occur with costal cartilage grafts (Rohrich and Tebbetts, 1987).

Grafts of cartilage on bone have also been used to elevate and support the displaced alar base and nostril sill (Fig. 56–57*D*) (Schmid, 1960; Schuchardt, 1960; Johanson and Ohlsson, 1961; Brauer, Cronin, and Reaves, 1962; Farrior, 1962; Longacre and associates, 1966; Hugo and Tumbusch, 1971; Schwenzer, 1973). Dermal fat grafts (Cosman and Crikelair, 1965), Proplast (Jackson, 1984), and Surgicel

(Skoog, 1967; Jackson, Pellett, and Smith, 1983) have also been used to augment the hypoplastic maxilla and overlying alar base. Foreign body implants (e.g., Proplast and hydroxyapatite) are used only when an extremely watertight closure of the mucosa is obtained and hematoma can be avoided. In some severe nasal deformities, it may be necessary to insert cartilage or bone grafts to establish a new nasal dorsum and to obtain satisfactory tip projection.

Ancillary Procedures. Despite adequate primary cleft lip nasal repairs, several characteristic deformities, such as the cleft nostril vestibular web, may remain. A number of supplemental soft tissue procedures have been designed and are occasionally required. To correct the apical overhang of the cleft nostril hood, Ombrédanne (1921), Blair (1925), and Millard (1964a) used a nostril rim excision. As mentioned above, Gillies and Kilner (1932) excised nasal lining and cleft alar cartilage from the free margin to allow rolling of the external skin into the resultant vestibular lining defect. This technique did not work and is no longer used. Simultaneous elongation of the columella and correction of nostril overhang was accomplished by Straith (1946) and Elsahy (1974) by Z-plasty of the alar hood (see Figs. 56–51, 56–54). Deepithelization of the overhanging rim and advancement of the tissue beneath an external skin flap through external and internal rim incisions were described by Pitanguy and Franco (1967) and Meyer (1973), respectively.

Tension of the lining in the lateral aspect of the cleft nasal vestibule, tented over a portion of the lateral crus, has been termed by Berkeley (1959, 1969) the vestibular web. This deformity is attributed to the reduction of the anteroposterior dimensions of the lateral wall of the piriform aperture resulting from maxillary hypoplasia. This can be corrected during the primary repair by elongation of the periosteum of the aperture. Repositioning of the alar base can result in visibility of the fold from a basal view and occlusion of the vestibular portion of the airway in severe cases. Secondary correction includes a V-Y chondromucosal advancement flap based medially as described by Potter (1954) and Stenström (1966) or a Z-plasty of the web as described by O'Connor, McGregor, and Tolleth (1965) and Matthews (1968). Uchida (1971) incorporated a double Z-plasty along the longitudinal axis of the web for

correction. A full-thickness composite graft can be used to close the defect resulting from medial advancement of a medially based flap of vestibular skin and alar cartilage (Rees, Guy, and Converse, 1966). The Gillies and Kilner (1932) repair incorporated a transposition flap from the nostril sill. Redistribution of the vestibular lining may be necessary with any one of the above techniques, despite adequate repositioning of the cleft alar cartilage after undermining and suture suspension. Correction of the excessively narrow nostril sill by a transposed flap taken lateral to the alar base was described by Joseph in 1931 (Fig. 56–58).

In contrast to the situation in noncleft noses, nasal bone infracture is frequently insufficient to establish symmetry in the cleft nose (Salyer, 1986). In the cleft lip nasal deformity, outfracturing may be necessary to mobilize the nasal bones and to place them in symmetric positions. When the nasal tip lacks definition and the nasal dorsum is flat and cannot be corrected by infracture, dorsal grafting is performed with septal cartilage, conchal cartilage, or a calvarial graft. A split-thickness calvarial graft of the required contour and dimensions can be taken from the temporoparietal area and inserted through a small vertical glabellar incision; wiring or lag screwing at the glabellar area results in a cantilever type of dorsal graft, which can accurately project the tip and establish a satisfactory nasal dorsum (Jackson, Pellett, and Smith, 1983). A chondro-osseous rib graft can also be used, but the fine control of the nasal tip position is lacking.

Deviation of the caudal end of the nasal septum toward the noncleft side is an almost constant feature of the unilateral cleft lip nasal deformity. This should be repositioned at the time of the primary repair. Limited

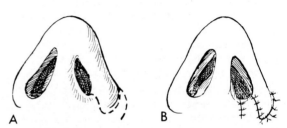

Figure 56–58. Correction of the narrow nostril floor. *A,* Design of flap taken from the area lateral to the ala. *B,* The flap has been transposed into the floor of the vestibule. (After Joseph.)

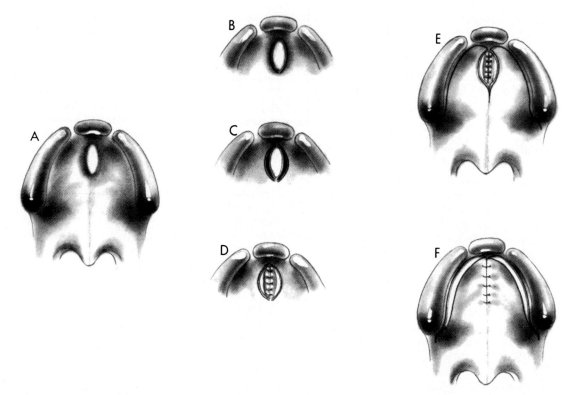

Figure 56–59. Two-layer correction of anterior midline fistula by reconstruction of nasal layer and approximation of bilateral Veau flaps. *A,* Fistula at midline in the anterior palate. *B,* Incisions surrounding the fistula. *C,* Undermining of the turn-over mucoperiosteal flaps. *D,* Turn-over flaps sutured at midline. *E,* Design of two mucoperiosteal flaps on the palate to close the fistula, creating a second layer. *F,* After transposition of both mucoperiosteal flaps, the fistula is closed at midline. An area of bare bone may remain exposed lateral to the mucoperiosteal flaps. (From Bardach, J., and Salyer, K. E.: Surgical Techniques in Cleft Lip and Palate. Chicago, Year Book Medical Publishers, 1987.)

septoplasty can be accomplished at a preschool age during correction of the secondary nasal deformity. When correction of the nasal deformity requires osteotomies, septoplasty, or partial turbinectomy, septal surgery is best delayed until adolescence.

Palatal Fistula

The most common defect in the hard palate after repair is a fistula (Stal and Spira, 1984). It may be located anterior or posterior to the alveolar ridge. Fistulas occur more frequently after palatoplasty for complete clefts of the primary and secondary palates (CL/P) than after that for an isolated secondary palate cleft (CP). Because the alveolar cleft has not been primarily repaired, there is a residual cleft rather than a fistula. True fistulas are caused by infection, hematoma formation between the oral and nasal layers, excess tension on the repair, flap necrosis, inadequate

attachment of the oral to the nasal layer, and a technically insecure anterior closure.

FISTULA CLOSURE

Fistulas are generally small and become obvious within a few weeks of the primary repair; occasionally fistulas may result from orthodontic expansion of the dental arches (in reality, an enlargement of a preexisting fistula). Large defects that affect speech or allow escape of fluid and food particles through the nose should be closed early. When the fistula is small and of no functional significance, closure can be delayed for several years, if performed at all. Oronasal fistulas anterior to the alveolar arch are generally closed at the time of secondary lip surgery or alveolar bone grafting (see Chap. 55). The local blood supply is usually sufficiently robust to allow safe mobilization of local tissue despite the presence of scarring. The hard palate mucoperiosteum rapidly regenerates over denuded areas. Successful closure of palatal defects is almost always possible without resorting to distant flaps.

Closure of defects between the oral cavity and the nasal or maxillary sinus cavities should always be two layered. This is achieved by turning medial and lateral flaps from the cleft margins to form the nasal floor and rotating one or two Veau flaps medially with a buccal or preferably a gingival flap for oral closure (Jackson, Pellett, and Smith, 1983). Many patients have reduction of nasal escape of fluid and food and less nasality after this procedure (Jackson, Jackson, and Christie, 1976). Although infrequently necessary, the use of an obturator is an alternative solution in defects that cannot be closed by local tissue because of size or because of patient preference.

Anterior or Alveolar Palatal Fistula. Oronasal or anterior alveolar palatal fistulas are generally repaired when secondary lip revision is undertaken or are repaired in conjunction with bone grafting of the alveolar cleft (see Chap. 55). Apart from the alveolar bone defect and its dental implications, an oronasal fistula may allow regurgitation of food into the nose, nasal crusting caused by chronic irritation, and oronasal air escape with resulting hypernasality. It is usually the larger fistulas that cause speech problems (Stal and Spira, 1984).

When the alveolar fistula is closed, the alveolar defect should be bone grafted. Jackson (1972a), Lehman (1978), and Jackson and associates (1981, 1982b) showed that large fistulas in the alveolar region and anterior palate could always be closed by means of bone grafts covered with mucoperiosteal or mucosal flaps. Autogenous cancellous bone grafts placed between the two-layer closure obliterate dead space, prevent hematoma formation, and provide stability to the soft tissue repair. A higher risk of unsuccessful closure of the oronasal communication has been demonstrated by Obwegeser and Perko (1968), Perko (1969), Petrovic (1971), Johanson and associates (1974), and Turvey and associates (1984) when bone grafts are omitted. The optimal age for repair, the donor source of bone grafts, and grafting of alveolar clefts in the maxilla are discussed below and in Chapter 55.

In nasolabial and oronasal fistulas, an incision is made around the fistula to create flaps for nasal closure (Figs. 56–59, 56–60).

Any hypertrophic mucosa is resected; failure to do this will impede healing. One or two mucoperiosteal flaps are elevated from the palate and are approximated to achieve oral closure. Larger fistulas or those extending into the buccal sulcus necessitate gingival flaps for closure (Fig. 56–61). In large defects, especially bilateral ones, buccal flaps may be necessary to achieve secure closure. The alveolar cleft and the space between the flaps are packed with autogenous cancellous bone graft. Particular care must be taken with the buccal flap to suture its base high in the buccal sulcus; otherwise, the buccal sulcus is obliterated, making it extremely difficult to fit a prosthesis or a removable bridge (Fig. 56–62). If possible, gingival flaps are used. However, in the case of large fistulas, only buccal mucosa provides a flap of sufficient size to ensure secure closure.

Posterior Palatal Fistula. Palatal fistulas located posterior to the alveolus may vary in size from 2 mm to greater than 10 mm. Frequently there have been prior attempts at closure, resulting in considerable mucoperiosteal scarring. In the majority of cases closure can be obtained by using local palatal flaps. In rare cases, distant flaps are indicated. The use of an obturator is an alternative solution in defects that cannot be closed by local tissue because of size, previous unsuccessful surgical procedures, or patient request (Converse, Hogan, and Barton, 1977). Dentures with an attached obturator can be worn to occlude the larger fistulas if elected by the patient. The authors believe that all fistulas can be closed by one of the techniques described in this chapter.

CLOSURE TECHNIQUES

When designing a mucoperiosteal flap for fistula closure, the flap must be made significantly larger than the defect, and the design must allow sufficient mobility of the flap to cover the defect without tension. Mucoperiosteum is stiff, especially when scarred by previous procedures, and does not adapt to transposition or suturing particularly well. Any defect that remains after palatal flap transposition heals quickly.

A narrow fistula typically follows the line of the palatal cleft. For an anterior fistula, an incision is made along the medial edges of the fistula so that lateral and medial flaps can be raised and sutured to form the nasal

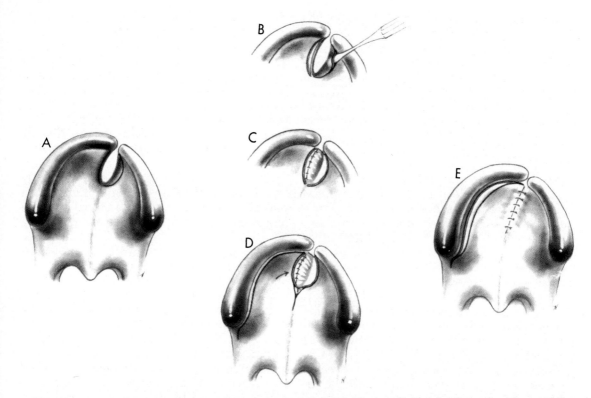

Figure 56–60. Two-layer reconstruction of a typical unilateral cleft fistula or residual cleft with repair of the nasal floor and medial advancement of a single Veau flap. *A,* Design of the incisions surrounding the fistula in the anterior portion of the palate to create turn-over flaps for the inner layer. Note that the lateral flap is larger than the medial flap. The suture line is close to the margin of the fistula to avoid overlapping of the suture lines of the inner and outer layers. *B,* Undermining of the flaps. *C,* Both flaps sutured together. *D,* Design of the mucoperiosteal flap that is raised and transposed toward the fistula to create the second layer. *E,* After transposition of the mucoperiosteal flaps, complete closure of the oral layer is achieved with some exposure of bare bone lateral to the flap. (Reproduced from Bardach, J., and Salyer, K. E.: Surgical Techniques in Cleft Lip and Palate. Chicago, Year Book Medical Publishers, 1987.)

floor. A flap of uninvolved palatal mucoperiosteum on the noncleft side can be elevated entirely and rotated to achieve oral closure (Fig. 56–63). When the defect is longitudinal, a modification of the von Langenbeck procedure (see Chap. 54) with two flaps can provide satisfactory oral reconstruction (Figs. 56–64, 56–65). Bone grafting of the hard palate with a wedge of bone placed between the two layers has been described by Stal and Spira (1984). However, this is unnecessary, since there is little or no dead space. When the fistula is wide and long, total reoperation in the area of the hard palate is indicated to achieve secure closure. *The rule is always to use large palatal flaps; closure with small flaps is almost always doomed to failure.*

A lateral defect of the hard palate is closed by using a lining turn-over flap hinged on the edge of the defect (Fig. 56–66) and a covering flap of mucoperiosteum elevated and mobilized along the alveolar process of the uninvolved side. The palatine vessels exiting from the greater palatine foramen must be preserved to ensure vascularity of the flaps. The use of these flaps with incisions in close proximity to the dentition should be limited to patients in the secondary dentition stage, as the resulting scar may have an adverse effect on dental development. If possible, all flaps should be taken from the midline to avoid encroachment on the alveolar ridge.

A round fistula is closed by raising a hinged semicircular flap on one side of the fistula. This is sutured to the nasal mucosa around the remainder of the fistula to provide the nasal layer. A transposition flap from the opposite side is used for the oral coverage (Fig. 56–67).

Large fistulas in the anterior aspect of the hard palate may result from excision of the premaxilla in bilateral cleft repair or from breakdown or loss of the anterior flaps in a four-flap repair. Two-layer closures in this

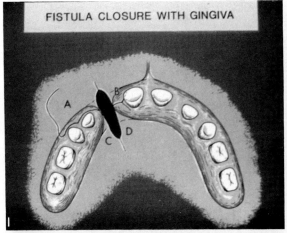

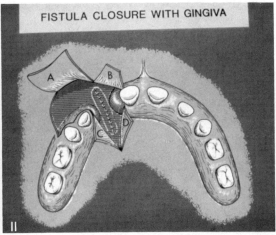

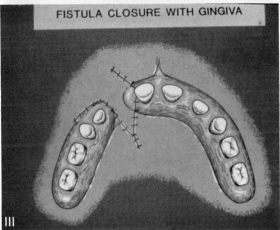

Figure 56–61. Gingival flaps used in addition to palatal flaps in repair of an alveolar fistula. (From Jackson, I. T.: Cleft lip and palate. *In* Mustardé, J. C., and Jackson, I. T. (Eds.): Plastic Surgery in Infancy and Childhood. 3rd Ed. Edinburgh, Churchill Livingstone, 1988.)

defect may be performed by using a vestibular flap from the buccal sulcus for nasal lining; it is transposed through a subperiosteal tunnel along the floor of the nose and secured with its raw surface downward (Fig. 56–68). Closure of the oral side is obtained with Veau mucoperiosteal flaps. It is almost always possible to form a nasal layer by using standard bilateral flaps from the edge of the fistula and to employ a combination of gingival or buccal flaps (unilateral or bilateral) and Veau flaps for the oral layer.

Closure of large palatal defects with a tongue flap was initially described by Guerrero-Santos and Altamirano (1966) (see Chap. 71). This type of procedure is indicated in patients with previous unsuccessful attempts at closure, heavily scarred palatal tissue, and a persistent large palatal defect. This technique can also be employed in young children (Jackson, 1972b; Posnick and Getz, 1987) but should be used only when no other method is

feasible. The palatal mucoperiosteum is mobilized and hinged on the edge of the defect and is sutured to provide nasal closure. An anteriorly based tongue flap of the appropriate dimensions is elevated from the dorsum of the tongue. It is raised with some underlying muscle to provide bulk and to ensure vascularity. After the flap is sutured to the edge of the cleft, additional nonabsorbable sutures are placed around the teeth to provide stability (Fig. 56–69). Intermaxillary fixation (Steinhauser, 1988) additionally ensures the security of the flap insertion. Airway problems may be seen after a previous pharyngoplasty, and it is advisable to continue intubation in these patients for one to two days (Jackson and Mustardé, 1988). After two weeks, the flap is divided and inset and the remaining donor site is closed. A posteriorly based flap can be used for closure of posterior fistulas, although this is a more hazardous procedure. A radial forearm free flap anasto-

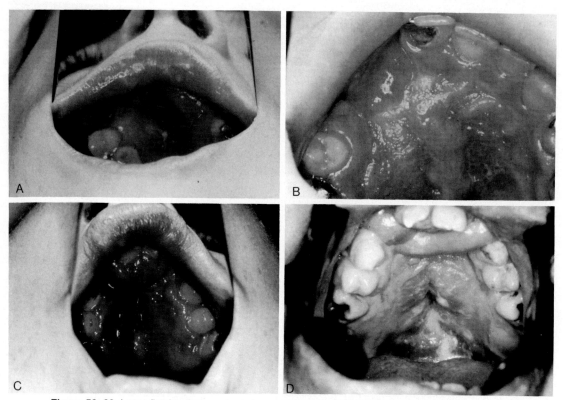

Figure 56–62. Large fistulas that required closure using buccal flaps. *A* to *D,* Postoperative results.

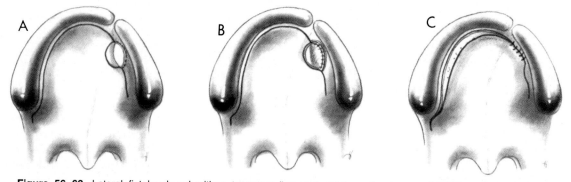

Figure 56–63. Lateral fistula closed with a turn-over flap and rotation of a large palatal flap. *A,* Design of the mucoperiosteal flap for the inner and outer layers. *B,* Turn-over flap sutured in place. *C,* Large mucoperiosteal flap transposed toward the defect and sutured in place. (From Bardach, J., and Salyer, K. E.: Surgical Techniques in Cleft Lip and Palate. Chicago, Year Book Medical Publishers, 1987.)

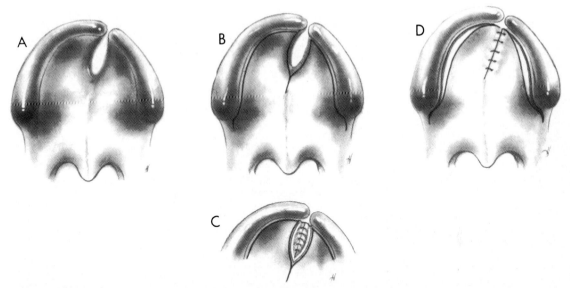

Figure 56–64. Closure of an anterior fistula in a unilateral cleft by upturned flaps for nasal lining and bilateral Veau flaps for oral closure. *A,* Fistula in the anterior palate. *B,* Design of incisions for two-layer closure. *C,* Closure of the inner layer. *D,* Mucoperiosteal flaps transposed toward the fistula and sutured together, creating the second layer. (From Bardach, J., and Salyer, K. E.: Surgical Techniques in Cleft Lip and Palate. Chicago, Year Book Medical Publishers, 1987.)

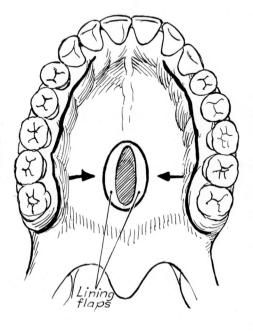

Figure 56–65. Closure of a defect in the posterior portion of the hard palate. Outline of the turn-over hinged flaps for lining and the von Langenbeck flaps for covering. (From Kazanjian, V. H., and Converse, J. M.: Surgical Treatment of Facial Injuries. 3rd Ed. Baltimore, Williams & Wilkins Company, 1974.)

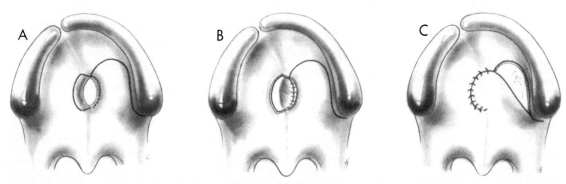

Figure 56–66. Defect closed by a turn-over flap and a lateral transposition flap. The flap for oral lining must be long enough to rotate and close comfortably in the midline. *A,* Incisions around the fistula are designed to create one turn-over flap to be sutured to the margin of the fistula, while a mucoperiosteal flap is transposed to close the defect as an outer layer. *B,* Turn-over flap sutured in place. *C,* Mucoperiosteal flap sutured in place. Some bare bone remains exposed lateral to the transposition flap. (From Bardach, J., and Salyer, K. E.: Surgical Techniques in Cleft Lip and Palate. Chicago, Year Book Medical Publishers, 1987.)

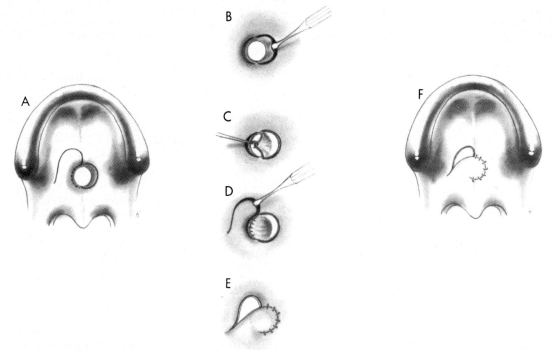

Figure 56–67. Round defect at junction of the hard and soft palates. Closure by a turn-over flap and a local transposition flap. The transposition flap must be large enough and long enough for oral closure. *A,* Design of the turn-over flap to create the inner layer and design of the transposition flap to create the outer layer. *B, C,* Undermining of the mucoperiosteal flap on the margin of the fistula and turning of it over with mucosa toward the nasal cavity. *D,* Turn-over flap sutured in place. *E, F,* Mucoperiosteal flap transposed toward the defect and sutured in place, leaving an area of exposed bone. (From Bardach, J., and Salyer, K. E.: Surgical Techniques in Cleft Lip and Palate. Chicago, Year Book Medical Publishers, 1987.)

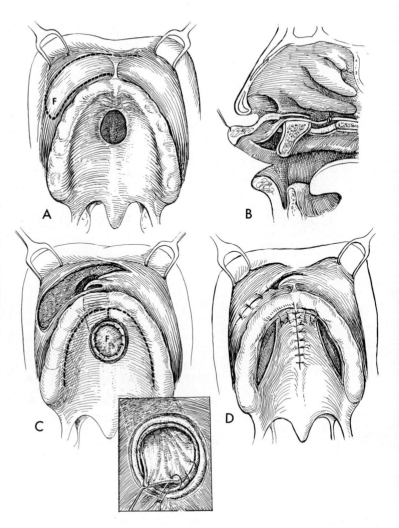

Figure 56–68. Vestibular flap for closure of a palatal defect. *A,* Design of the vestibular flap. *B, C,* Introduction of the vestibular flap through a subperiosteal tunnel along the floor of the nose. Suture of the vestibular flap *(F)* raw surface downward to the edges of the defect. *D,* Closure of the mobilized Veau-type mucoperiosteal palatal flaps. (From Kazanjian, V. H., and Converse, J. M.: Surgical Treatment of Facial Injuries. 3rd Ed. Baltimore, Williams & Wilkins Company, 1974.)

mosed to the facial vessels can be used to provide oral closure of large anterior fistulas after unsuccessful closure using local tissue (MacLeod, 1988). The magnitude of the procedure and the introduction of skin that is often hair bearing into the palate restrict this technique to use in a few selected cases.

Oronasal fistulas in the soft palate may be small and do not require early correction if speech is satisfactory. If bone grafting is performed during the stage of mixed dentition, these fistulas can be closed then. Moderate-sized and large fistulas of the soft palate may be repaired by relaxing incisions and a two-layer closure. Frequently, a total palatal reconstruction is necessary to obtain adequate velopharyngeal function. Large fistulas in association with a short palate may necessitate a concomitant pharyngeal flap procedure. In patients functionally crippled by the fistula

and repeatedly unsuccessful procedures, a properly fitting prosthetic device to replace lost and missing teeth and to function as an obturator may be the only satisfactory solution. This situation should rarely if ever arise where sophisticated services are available.

Deformities of Maxilla

In a complete primary unilateral cleft of the primary and secondary palates, there is frequently a significant bony defect in the maxilla. A varying degree of hypoplasia of the lesser maxillary segment is almost always present. Occasionally the contralateral side may also show hypoplasia but to a lesser degree.

The most significant skeletal changes in patients with clefts are maxillary retrusion

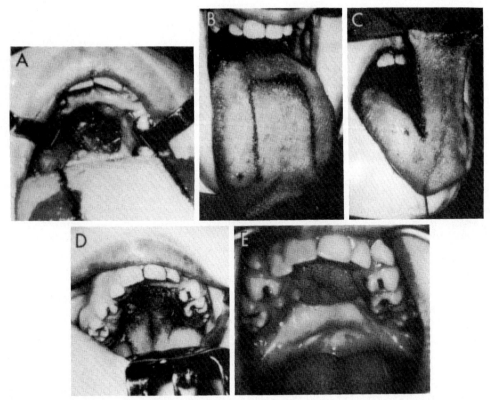

Figure 56–69. Use of an anteriorly based tongue flap to close a large anterior fistula. *A,* Nasal layer closed by local upturned flaps. *B,* Design of the flap. *C,* Elevation of the large anteriorly based tongue flap. *D,* Pedicle of tongue flap is divided in ten days under local anesthesia (the flap is sutured to the palate under general anesthesia). *E,* Postoperative result. (From Jackson, I. T.: Cleft lip and palate. *In* Kelly, V. C. (Ed.): Practice of Pediatrics. Philadelphia, J. B. Lippincott Company, 1985.)

and collapse of the maxillary segment (Mapes and associates, 1974). The alveolar cleft in the disrupted dental arch frequently accentuates facial disfigurement because the anterior maxillary teeth may be malpositioned, malformed, or congenitally absent.

After the initial lip and palate repair, later bone grafting of the alveolar cleft and augmentation of the skeletal hypoplasia may be required to establish a foundation for soft tissue reconstruction and to achieve optimal esthetic and functional results.

ALVEOLAR CLEFTS

A residual anterior palatal or alveolar defect associated with an oronasal fistula has many sequelae (Waite and Kersten, 1980): (1) malposition of one or more teeth in the anterior maxillary region; (2) insufficient periodontal bone support for teeth adjacent to the bony cleft and subsequent loss of these

teeth; (3) caries and periodontal inflammation as a consequence of poor oral hygiene caused by tooth malposition; (4) irregular tooth shape; (5) oronasal air escape, adversely affecting speech; (6) facial asymmetry resulting from lack of bony support for the alar base; and (7) nasal crusting caused by oronasal communication. In addition, there is a deficient bony base for denture retention (Drachter, 1914; Obwegeser and Perko, 1968; Reichert, 1969). A relapse after orthodontic expansion of the collapsed maxillary segments was reported by Johanson and associates (1974) and Boyne and Sands (1976). Insufficient bone in the alveolar cleft area to enable orthodontic manipulation of the teeth into optimal position and occlusion often necessitates extensive prosthetic treatment (Boyne and Sands, 1972, 1976; Abyholm, Bergland, and Semb, 1981; Jackson and associates, 1982b). The altered anatomic features of an oronasal fistula produce nasal airway obstruction owing to hypertrophy of the inferior turbinate and septal displacement (Matthews and associates, 1970; Jackson and associates, 1982b). The lip repair result may be less than optimal because of the lack of support from the alveolus and the teeth (Pickrell, Quinn, and Massengill, 1968; Petrovic, 1971).

From the above observations, there appear to be multiple reasons for reconstruction of the residual alveolar cleft, but in the past the methods and timing have varied. Attention to closure of the alveolar cleft began with von Langenbeck's (1861) palatal closure. Aggressive, traumatic surgical techniques for closure followed and often resulted in severe maxillary collapse. As cephalometric studies became available, evaluation of craniofacial growth became more accurate. Cephalometric studies showed that traumatic surgery caused a long-term inhibition of subsequent growth of the maxillary complex (Graber, 1949; Slaughter and Brodie, 1949).

Harvold (1947, 1949) and Böhn (1963a) collaborated in developing a combined orthodontic and prosthodontic approach to alignment of the maxillary segments and alveolar arch with less surgical manipulation. By repositioning the maxillary segments and the misaligned teeth, they preserved the maxillary dental arch, except for a short bridge across the alveolar cleft gap. The latter was amenable to surgical closure. Ramstad (1973) thought that this management method was superior to the surgical mutilation of the maxilla seen previously, since there was less inhibition of growth.

Despite improvements in orthodontic treatment, the shortcomings mentioned above remain. Orthodontic positioning of maxillary segments and alignment of the alveolar arches and teeth before and after surgical procedures remain an essential part of the approach to bony management of the cleft (Jackson and associates, 1982b; Hall and Posnick, 1983; Enemark, Krantz-Simonsen, and Schramm, 1985; Bergland, Semb, and Abyholm, 1986; Bardach and Salyer, 1987f). Postoperatively dental plates, conventional orthodontic appliances, and retention bands are used for varying lengths of time, depending on the incisor position and stability, the types or degree of malocclusion, or the stage of dentition. Consideration of orthodontic space closure versus prosthetic reconstruction of arch continuity must include the following

variables: (1) the presence or absence of usable fissural teeth, (2) the type of cleft, (3) intermaxillary relationships, (4) aplasia of the teeth beyond the cleft area, and (5) the width of the cleft space (Bergland, Semb, and Abyholm, 1986a).

BONE GRAFTING

The advantages of bone grafting include stabilization of the arch in both unilateral and bilateral clefts with the potential for eruption of the teeth into solid bone. These teeth can be manipulated by the orthodontist and are less prone to periodontal disease or loss resulting from inadequate bony support. Boyne and Sands (1972, 1976) first reported that a cancellous bone graft, inserted into the alveolar cleft, was capable of responding physiologically to orthodontic movement or teeth migration. The relative maxillary stability also allows fixation of a prosthesis. A two-layer repair of the fistula is less prone to break down with incorporation of a bone graft (Jackson, 1972a; Widmaier, 1973; Rintala, 1980; Henderson and Jackson, 1975; Jackson and associates, 1982b). A relatively normal maxillary arch also adds bony support for a more satisfactory lip and nose correction.

Timing of Bone Grafting

There is still dispute about when bone grafting and closure of the alveolar cleft should be performed. To standardize terminology, the following scheme should be employed: (1) primary or delayed primary bone grafting, 0 to 2 years of age; (2) early secondary bone grafting, 2 to 5 years of age; (3) secondary bone grafting, 6 to 12 years of age; and (4) delayed (late secondary) bone grafting, adolescence to adulthood. (Koberg, 1973; Boyne and Sands, 1976).

Interference with maxillary growth has been the concern of surgeons and has been a partial basis for the variety of timing regimens for osteoplasty procedures. It is well known that surgery during the first few months of life as well as repeated aggressive operative procedures has an adverse effect on maxillary development. The interference with facial growth resulting from surgical manipulation of the alveolus and maxilla was described by Ortiz-Monasterio and associates (1966); untreated adults with cleft palates had normal anteroposterior and transverse maxillary growth, in contrast with the re-truded maxilla found in cleft palate patients who had undergone repair. A knowledge of maxillary growth led to more intelligent planning of osteoplasty procedures at earlier ages in general. Maxillary growth and in-crease in width take place mainly in the midpalatal section, with the greater growth and width increase occurring posteriorly, es-pecially when compared with growth in the anterior dimensions. As the palatal skeletal cleft is usually close to the median suture in the primary palate, early cleft repair may interfere with this growth site (Böhn, 1963b). Bjørk and Skieller (1974) showed that the increase in width in the anterior maxilla is minimal after age 6 to 7 years; accordingly, surgical interference with the primary palate after the age of 7 to 8 years would have little effect on growth. If growth is affected after that time, dental alveolar expansion can eas-ily compensate (Abyholm, Bergland, and Semb, 1981).

Maxillary height increases as a result of appositional growth of the occlusal margin of the alveolar process and interaction with su-tural growth in the nasal floor. Eruption of the canine on the cleft side through grafted cancellous bone has been demonstrated by Abyholm, Bergland, and Semb (1981) to stim-ulate an increase in the height of the hypo-plastic alveolar cleft area. Growth of the maxilla in length takes place at the trans-verse palatine suture and by appositional growth in the region of the maxillary tuber-osity (Bjørk and Skieller, 1977). According to Friede (1977, 1978), the vomeropremaxillary and vomeromaxillary sutures may play a role in adolescent facial growth. Bone grafting of the alveolar cleft is unlikely to cause any significant inhibition of growth in this area. Lip repair and resulting lip pressure may also be important factors in retardation of maxillary growth (Bardach and Eisbach, 1977).

Primary Bone Grafting. Bone grafting of the alveolar cleft at the time of the primary repair was first described by Schmid (1955) and Nordin and Johanson (1955). Schmid (1955) implanted small iliac bone-cartilage grafts between the edges of the alveolar cleft prior to surgical closure. Nordin and Johan-son (1955) transplanted iliac crest into the alveolar cleft as a single, wedge-shaped por-tion of bone. Other surgeons followed with enthusiasm (Stellmach, 1959; Rehrmann,

1964; Lynch, Lewis, and Blocker, 1966; Schu-chardt, 1966; Matthews and associates, 1970). These surgeons considered the bone graft an orthodontic appliance and consequently used a solid block of iliac crest or rib to wedge open the alveolar margins (Schuchardt, 1964). After 1964, because of reports of poor results after primary and early secondary osteoplasty, primary bone grafting was per-formed in relatively few institutions. Long-term follow-up from early studies revealed an incidence of anterior dental collapse and crossbite equivalent to that with conventional repairs. Kling (1964, 1966) found a striking increase in the incidence of lateral crossbite (88 per cent) and mandibular pseudoprog-nathism (58 per cent). Jolleys and Robertson (1972) found that primary or early secondary bone grafting impaired maxillary growth. Long-term results in a large group of patients who underwent primary and early secondary bone grafting of the cleft alveolus confirmed the significant deficiencies of maxillary growth (Rehrmann, Koberg, and Koch, 1970; Friede and Johanson, 1974).

Primary bone grafting is being reevalu-ated, as it appears to offer several advan-tages. There is some question about whether the operative technique rather than the in-sertion of a bone graft arrests maxillary de-velopment. Moss (1962) hypothesized that the graft may be introduced to support the nasal bone and nostril floor with the purpose of allowing tooth eruption. If some degree of collapse is considered normal and acceptable after cleft repair, tooth eruption in the correct anatomic area with superior nose formation as a result of primary bone grafting may allow the technique to be deemed satisfactory (Boyne and Sands, 1972; Boyne, 1974).

Early Secondary Bone Grafting. Graft-ing at an older age (after eruption of the majority of the deciduous teeth) was preferred by Johanson and Ohlsson (1961), Longacre (1970), and Koch (1982). Rosenstein and as-sociates (1982) placed a portion of rib graft high in the cleft with minimal subperiosteal dissection in 4 month old patients, who have demonstrated excellent facial growth and tooth development on long-term follow-up. Orthodontic therapy is used, as with all sec-ondary and delayed bone grafting, to expand and reposition the arches by slow movement with a removable appliance or rapidly with a fixed-screw appliance.

Secondary Bone Grafting. Secondary osteoplasty is performed in patients between the ages of 6 and 12 years (the period of mixed dentition). The exact timing of grafting is determined by the position of the canine tooth (Boyne and Sands, 1972, 1976; Abyholm, Bergland, and Semb, 1981; Ames, Ryan, and Maki, 1981; Eskeland and associates, 1985; Bergland, Semb, and Abyholm, 1986a; Bardach and Salyer, 1987g). The optimal time is when the root of the permanent canine has formed by approximately one-fourth to two-thirds of its length. As it begins to upright and align itself to erupt, the bone graft is placed in position and is covered with a gingival flap. This maneuver allows the tooth to erupt into solid bone, thus enabling the orthodontist to begin positioning the tooth (see Chap. 55).

Sagittal and transverse growth of the anterior maxilla has virtually ceased by 8 to 9 years of age (Sillman, 1964; Bjørk and Skieller, 1974). Vertical growth of the maxilla occurs mainly as deposition of additional alveolar bone at the alveolar crest (Bjørk and Skieller, 1976). After a peripubertal growth spurt, vertical maxillary growth continues at a slow rate throughout life (Ainamo and Jalari, 1976; Steedle and Proffit, 1985). The continuous eruption of teeth is thought to be the agent that stimulates bone growth. The bone graft is rapidly transformed into functional alveolar bone, which responds to eruption of the canine and produces bone volume sufficient for vertical height (Bjørk and Skieller, 1976; Bergland, Semb, and Abyholm, 1986a). These same processes of graft incorporation and response would be of greater dental benefit at age 5 to 6 years if it were not for the possibility of arresting transverse maxillary growth. Secondary osteoplasty affects transverse growth of the maxilla to a small extent; however, it has a positive interaction with the developing permanent canine. Grafting before eruption of the permanent canine teeth generally results in more stability with better crestal bone support (Turvey and associates, 1984). Bone grafting at too early an age has resulted in palatal eruption of the ipsilateral permanent canine (Geiger and Wunderlich, 1982).

Late Secondary Bone Grafting. Older patients may still benefit from bone grafting, even though all teeth have erupted. As in the younger patient, it may be carried out in association with lip revision and repositioning of the alar base and lower lateral carti-

lage. The anterior fistula may necessitate a buccal flap closure (Jackson, 1972a) if it is too large for gingival flap closure. If an unerupted canine is present and the fistula is not excessively large, a gingival flap is preferable as tooth eruption into the bone grafted alveolar cleft may still occur (Abyholm, Bergland, and Semb, 1981).

Techniques in Bone Grafting

Periosteal Closure for Primary Palate. Initially, Skoog (1965) described the use of a periosteal flap from the anterior aspect of the maxilla to close the primary palate and to form bone in that area. He categorically stated that there was no resultant maxillary hypoplasia on the side from which the flap was taken. On follow-up, his orthodontist noted that 46 per cent of the patients formed bone in the alveolar cleft area with this technique, and, in many cases, teeth erupted into the cleft area. However, the resulting crossbite and collapse of the maxillary segments were scarcely improved from those occurring in conventionally treated patients (Hellquist, Svärdström, and Ponten, 1983). It is significant that there was tooth eruption through the reconstructed alveolus and that the maxillary donor site showed no residual adverse changes.

Periosteum can also be taken as a free graft (e.g., from the tibia), with resulting bone formation (Ritsila and associates, 1972). Stricker and associates (1977) have placed a large portion of periosteum from the buccal area into the end of the hard palate without oral coverage. They stated that bone formation was achieved, but follow-up was limited. Other surgeons also recommended the use of periosteum (Santoni-Rugiu, 1966; O'Brien, 1970; Schultz, 1984). It is now rarely used in the primary or early repair.

Supplementary Prosthodontic and Orthodontic Treatment. The multidisciplinary team management of clefts is essential to achieve reconstruction of a relatively normal maxillary skeleton, stabilization of the maxilla, and a satisfactory occlusion. Most surgeons favor orthodontic therapy before secondary bone grafting to expand the transverse deficiency of the constricted dentoalveolar region and to relocate the maxillary segments. Hall and Posnick (1983) noted that closure of the mucoperiosteum was easier after presurgical orthodontic expansion.

Movement of a malpositioned central incisor into a more normal position with preoperative orthodontic treatment also allows for closure of the mucosa around the tooth, precluding development of pockets of trapped food and debris between the rotated crown and the incision. Any malocclusion existing in the deciduous dentition is left untreated. Anterior crossbites and severe rotations are corrected after eruption of the permanent incisors (Bergland, Semb, and Abyholm, 1986a).

Patients undergoing bone grafting in the permanent dentition stage can have orthodontic treatment resumed after three months. Studies by Albrektsson (1979) showed that cancellous bone grafts are fully revascularized after three weeks, but transformation of the graft into a normal trabecular pattern is not completed before three months. Turvey and associates (1984) advocated less delay and initiated orthodontic movement at two to three weeks postoperatively. Teeth located posterior to the cleft are therefore free to migrate forward and facilitate space closure. Patients in whom the space is closed orthodontically complete treatment by approximately age 15 years, similarly to the noncleft patient with a malocclusion. Cleft patients generally require retention for longer periods of time when compared with noncleft patients. If orthodontic closure of a space is not achieved, insertion of a permanent bridge is performed when the patient is approximately 18 years of age. Alveolar bone grafting carried out before canine eruption resulted in orthodontic closure of the space in 90 per cent of patients, compared with closure in 72 per cent of patients bone grafted in the period of permanent dentition (Bergland, Semb, and Abyholm, 1986a). Segmental repositioning by orthodontic means is inhibited after alveolar bone grafting, but significant changes in the dental arch can still be accomplished with orthodontic treatment (Abyholm, Bergland, and Semb, 1981). It is now possible to replace missing teeth in bone grafted patients by using the techniques of osseointegration (Brånemark and associates, 1969, 1977; Jackson and Mustardé, 1988) (see Chap. 72).

Donor Sites for Bone Grafts. There is little dispute that bone grafting increases successful closure of a fistula, allows response to tooth eruption, and promotes vertical growth and stability of the maxilla. Opinions vary as to the optimal bone graft donor site. The ribs and iliac crest are the two most common donor sites. Cancellous bone from the iliac crest is generally considered the best material for bone grafting of alveolar and maxillary clefts. In most patients, unless block bone is required, Jackson and associates (1982b) enter the posterior ilium through the cartilaginous bony crest or the inner table via a 1 cm skin incision and use a curette to harvest the bone. Bardach and Salyer (1987g) developed a segment of ilium, including the crest, which is pedicled medially on the periosteum to provide access to the large amounts of cancellous bone contained between the inner and outer tables (Fig. 56–70). Closure of the pedicled segment is thought to avoid deformity of the iliac crest area, although a large skin incision is required and there is pain and prolonged discomfort for the patients. It is not recommended.

Rib grafts, one or more in number, can be harvested through a single incision. Usually only two ribs are harvested sequentially to avoid a flail chest, although three in succession may be removed without significant difficulty. The ribs are split and can be easily bent and contoured to the desired shape. For alveolopalatal reconstruction, rib bone is inadequate (Schmid and associates, 1974; Boyne and Sands, 1976; Abyholm, Bergland, and Semb, 1981). As described by Mowlem (1941) and confirmed by Albrektsson (1979), cortical bone is revascularized by a slow process of restoring flow through existing vessels or cannaliculi. As rib is mostly cortical, the arguments against the use of rib bone for alveolar clefts reflect this phenomenon. In addition, teeth have greater difficulty in erupting into a rib grafted area (Robertson and Jolleys, 1983). The greater resorption of grafted rib bone is a result of delayed revascularization and is an additional factor militating against its use (Schmid, 1966).

Alternative donor sites include the calvaria (Jackson, Pellett, and Smith, 1983; Wolfe and Berkowitz, 1983), the tibia (Jackson and associates, 1981), and the trochanter (Spiessl, 1973). The advantages of calvarial bone grafts include a shorter harvesting time, a camouflaged scar, a large donor area, and location of the donor site in the field of the primary operation. Cranial bone is thought to undergo less resorption than bone from other sites. The main disadvantage of calvarial grafts is that it is difficult to harvest long, contoured strips similar to split rib grafts or to obtain sufficient cancellous bone for the

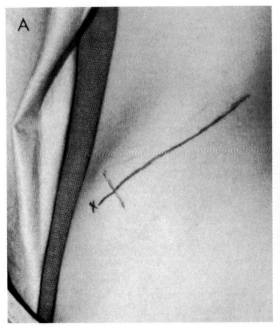
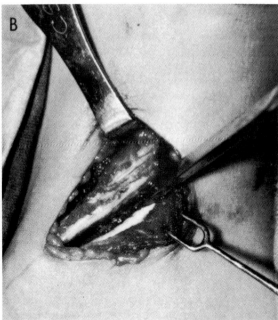

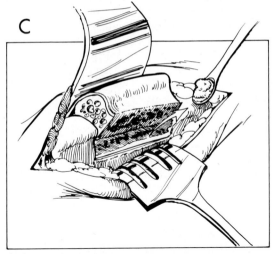

Figure 56–70. Method of taking block iliac crest graft by osteotomy of iliac crest and curettage of cancellous bone. *A, B,* Split incision through the iliac crest facilitates harvesting of cancellous bone without dissecting the muscles or lifting the segment of iliac crest. *C,* Cancellous bone is obtained after a segment of the iliac crest is elevated, leaving its attachment to the periosteum on the inner side. (From Bardach, J., and Salyer, K. E.: Surgical Techniques in Cleft Lip and Palate. Chicago, Year Book Medical Publishers, 1987.)

alveolar defect. Tibial and trochanteric donor sites are used infrequently. If cancellous bone becomes exposed, only a small amount may be lost with subsequent granulation and successful healing. This may happen with ribs but is less likely; cranial bone will always have to be removed in toto.

Materials such as hydroxyapatite have not been used, as autogenous cancellous bone grafts or rib grafts are superior to alloplastic materials (Bardach and Salyer, 1987g). The authors have had successful results with alloplastic materials, but mucosal closure must be absolutely watertight.

Surgical Technique in Secondary Bone Grafting. Revision of the lip defect with muscle repair is often required concomitantly with bone grafting. Examination of the cleft area usually reveals that the lip is in continuity with the mucosa of the alveolus and the nose. The lip is opened completely after the points of the commissure and the Cupid's bow have been measured and marked and after the proposed repair, generally a rotation-advancement type, has been designed. Opening the lip gives excellent exposure of the fistula and the alveolar cleft. The technique is referred to as "recreation of the primary cleft" (Jackson, 1972a).

An incision is made along the edges of the fistula in the buccal sulcus and on the anterior aspect of the alveolus at the level of the alveolar ridge. Palatal subperiosteal dissection, beginning in the mouth and working toward the floor of the nose, allows lateral and medial flaps to be raised adjacent to the fistula. All hypertrophic mucosa at the cleft edge is excised to allow accurate suturing and healing, both prerequisites for successful bone grafting. The flaps are sutured together to form a nasal floor at the same level as on the noncleft side. Care must be taken not to injure any unerupted teeth. The bony lamellae covering the tooth roots adjacent to the cleft should not be traumatized (Fig. 56–71).

Depending on the size of the palatal defect, one or two Veau flaps are elevated and mobilized widely enough to allow closure at the midline. Since the flaps are elevated from a concavity and approximated across the midline, sufficient length is frequently gained to close the lateral secondary defects. The bony defect is now seen to be a wedge-shaped cavity delineated by the nasal repair superiorly, the palatal repair inferiorly, and the edges of the alveolar cleft laterally and medially. The palatoalveolar defect is packed with cancellous iliac bone, and a portion is also placed as an onlay graft beneath the alar base, the nasal sill, and the spine to augment these areas. The anterior opening is closed by suturing the gingival edges together. Direct suturing of the anterior area is not usually possible, and it is often necessary to elevate a superiorly based gingival mucoperiosteal flap from the lesser segment. Some care should be taken to design flaps to cover the marginal portion of the graft with gingiva. Steedle and Proffit (1985) emphasized an interaction between gingiva and alveolar bone, leading to tooth eruption through the alveolar bone graft. Flaps lacking gingiva tend to impede tooth eruption. The gingival flap is transposed medially, inferiorly, and posteriorly to achieve secure closure. The lip is closed with dissection and suturing of the orbicularis oris muscle, followed by reconstruction with lengthening of its edges by interdigitation of

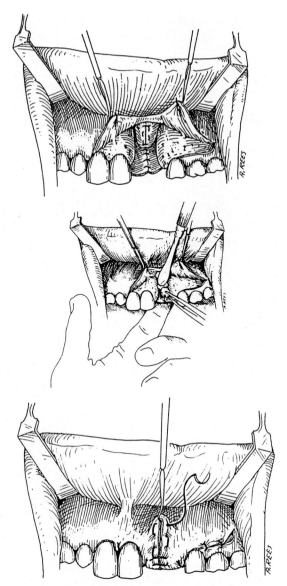

Figure 56–71. Closure of an alveolar fistula with bone grafting. *Top,* Reconstruction of nasal layer from upturned flaps. *Middle,* Bone grafting of alveolar defect. *Bottom,* Closure of gingiva. (From Hall, H. D., and Posnick, J. C.: Early results of secondary bone grafts in 106 alveolar clefts. J. Oral Maxillofac. Surg., 41:289, 1983.)

flaps. The lower lateral cartilage on the cleft side is approached through intranasal incisions and is repositioned to achieve nasal tip symmetry.

Complications. Exposure of the bone graft resulting from dehiscence, flap necrosis, or infection is rare. A foul smell or unpleasant taste may be the first indication of exposure, which can frequently be treated by conservative debridement; the underlying vascularized bone usually heals rapidly. Total flap failure with extensive graft exposure is rare; debridement may be required with repeat grafting after six to nine months. Bone resorption tends to occur after exposure or infection. Often a greater amount of bone graft than is necessary to fill the defect is placed to allow for any subsequent resorption.

External tooth root resorption appears to result from placing osseous tissue adjacent to the cementum of teeth (Boyne and Sands, 1972; Boyne, 1974). Cautious stripping of periosteum avoids exposure of cementum and prevents this complication, especially when the lateral incisor on the cleft side is present. A recurrent oronasal fistula, retention of the permanent canine, and loss of adjacent teeth are other possible complications.

Consolidation of the cancellous bone grafts was found at one year in 90 per cent of patients (Johanson and associates, 1974). After three years, approximately 100 per cent of surviving bone grafts had become incorporated into the alveolar bone. At the present time, a satisfactory result should be obtained in more than 80 per cent of patients, with complete failures occurring in less than 5 per cent.

Surgical Technique in Delayed (Late Secondary) Bone Grafting. The technique is similar to that described for grafting during the period of mixed dentition. Elevation of the flaps is technically easier, as unerupted teeth are unusual. When a wide anterior alveolar ridge defect is present, coverage with gingiva may not be possible. In this instance, a buccal flap (Jackson, 1972b) can be used to cover the defect (Figs. 56–72 to 56–74). The buccal flap is raised on the lip at the apex of the buccal sulcus. The flap is 1 to 2 cm in width and sufficiently long to be transposed into the alveolar ridge area; it is elevated from the highest portion of the lip. The rotation point must be close to the alveolar defect to facilitate complete flap closure (Figs. 56–72, 56–73). The base of the flap remains high in the sulcus to maintain adequate depth for insertion of the prosthesis or the dentures, and the remainder is draped over the bone graft to form a covering for the alveolus. The flap defect can be closed directly without difficulty. The disadvantages of this flap include the inability of teeth to erupt through the heterotopic tissue and the mobility of the

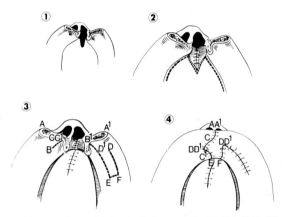

Figure 56–72. Method of closure of anterior cleft with buccal mucosal flap in secondary bone grafting procedures (see Fig. 56–73). (From Jackson, I. T.: Cleft lip and palate. *In* Mustardé, J. C., and Jackson, I. T.: Plastic Surgery of Infancy and Childhood. 3rd Ed. Edinburgh, Churchill Livingstone, 1988.)

buccal mucosa overlying the bone graft, thus making prosthetic rehabilitation difficult. In some cases, it is desirable to excise the buccal flap at a later date and to replace it with a gingival or palatal mucoperiosteal graft.

MAXILLARY RETRUSION

Maxillary retrusion is a frequent sequela to secondary cleft deformity (Converse, Hogan, and Barton, 1977). It is usually manifest with the profile deformity of pseudoprognathism, but occasionally there may be true mandibular protrusion and rarely an isolated mandibular retrusion. The nasomaxillary hypoplasia may be further affected by surgery, since nonoperated clefts do not demonstrate this growth pattern (Slaughter and Brodie, 1949; Kazanjian, 1951; Ortiz-Monasterio and associates, 1959, 1966).

Congenital maxillary hypoplasia and inhibition of growth after cleft lip and palate repair may result in maxillary retrusion. Onlay bone grafts or Le Fort I or II osteotomies may be required (see also Chap. 29).

ONLAY BONE GRAFTS

Onlay grafts may be inserted through a buccal sulcus incision, or they may be applied at the time of a maxillary osteotomy. These are used to augment the anterior surface of the maxilla, around the piriform aperture and in the nostril sill area. No osseous fixation is generally required, as the soft tissue and the

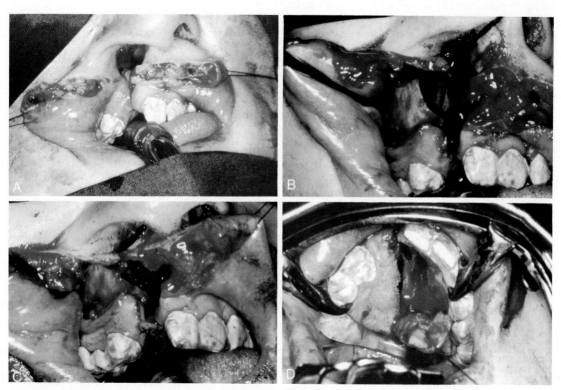

Figure 56–73. Closure of left anterior fistula with bone grafting and buccal flap. *A*, Primary defect recreated. *B*, Lateral and medial flaps elevated for nasal floor closure. *C*, Nasal floor closure. *D*, Raising of the unilateral Veau flap.

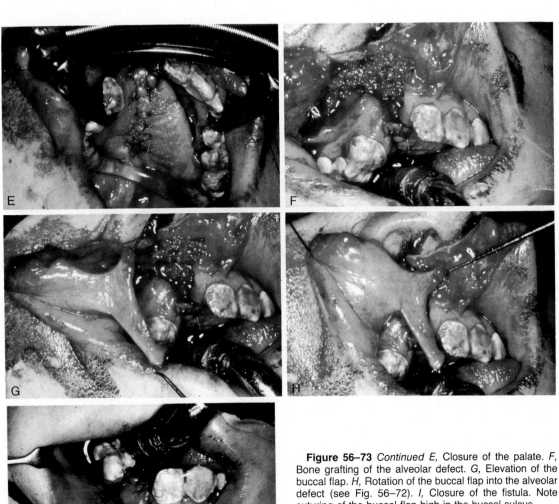

Figure 56–73 *Continued E,* Closure of the palate. *F,* Bone grafting of the alveolar defect. *G,* Elevation of the buccal flap. *H,* Rotation of the buccal flap into the alveolar defect (see Fig. 56–72). *I,* Closure of the fistula. Note suturing of the buccal flap high in the buccal sulcus.

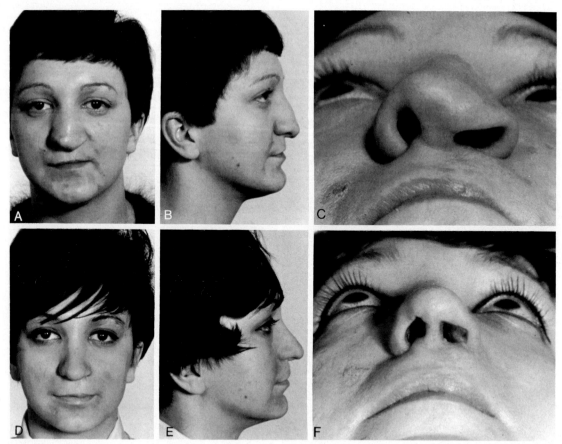

Figure 56–74. Delayed bone grafting technique of Figure 56–72. *A* to *C*, Preoperative appearance of a patient with secondary unilateral cleft deformity. *D* to *F*, Postoperative appearance after fistula closure, lip revision, and bone grafting with repositioning of the lower lateral cartilage of the nose.

periosteum secure the graft. Jackson and associates (1982a, b) carried out augmentation of this area with cancellous iliac bone during lip revision or secondary bone grafting of the alveolus. The extent of bone resorption is unpredictable, but subperiosteal placement decreases resorption (Salyer, 1986). Salyer preferred to overcorrect by 20 to 30 per cent when using rib graft for facial contouring. There is a contemporary shift to augmentation with calvarial grafts secured with lag screws.

OSTEOTOMIES

There are four main assessment techniques for planning of osteotomies. First, the clinical examination must include the lip, the nose, the facial proportions, and the facial profile (see Chapter 29 for details of the preoperative evaluation). In patients with any evidence of velopharyngeal incompetence or nasal emissions, palatal function is assessed by videofluoroscopy and nasal endoscopy. Second, cephalograms document the skeletal pathologic changes, allow facial growth to be monitored, and assess relapse after osteotomy (see Chap. 29). Third, dental impressions are obtained; dental models mounted on an articulator allow the determination of presurgical orthodontic manipulation required to provide satisfactory occlusion. Anteroposterior, vertical, and segmental shifts are calculated, and an occlusal splint is prefabricated to guide intraoperative occlusion. These dental models are useful for later assessment of postosteotomy relapse and growth and the need for postsurgical orthodontic treatment (see Chap. 29). Fourth, life-sized photographs allow detailed studies of facial symmetry and discussion of preoperative planning with the patient (see Chap. 29).

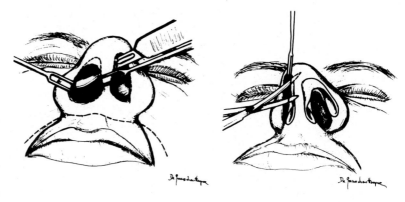

Figure 56–75. Degloving of the face through nasal and buccal sulcus incisions for Le Fort II osteotomy for simultaneous correction of maxillary and nasal deformity. (From Kinnebrew, M. C., Zide, M. F., and Kent, J. N.: Modified Le Fort II procedure for simultaneous correction of maxillary and nasal deformities. J. Oral Maxillofac. Surg., *41*:295, 1983.)

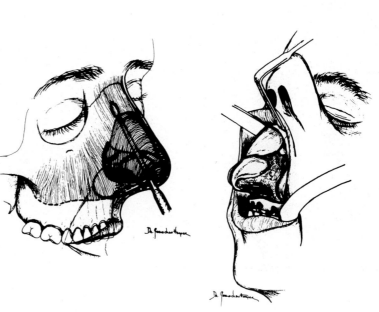

Bardach and Salyer (1987a) listed four indications for maxillary osteotomies in secondary cleft lip and palate deformities: maxillary retrusion, alveolar collapse, premaxillary malpositioning, and esthetic contouring. The management of a unilateral deformity and the associated bony cleft can be accomplished in three ways. For small or intermediate-sized fistulas, closure and bone grafting may be performed simultaneously with the osteotomy. For larger fistulas, it may be safer and may preserve vascular integrity better to do the osteotomy first and to perform fistula closure and bone grafting later. In bilateral cleft deformities and unilateral deformities in which the lesser segment is vertically deficient, the fistula is closed and the alveolar cleft is bone grafted before osteotomy. In the latter group, the upper arch is expanded and the maxillary segment is brought into the correct position before bone grafting. After surgery the arch form is retained by a splint for six months until the maxillary advancement osteotomy is performed.

Esthetic and functional correction of the lip and the lower nose is occasionally performed simultaneously with the osteotomy. Schendel and Delaire (1981) combined lip and nose correction with Le Fort I osteotomy in patients with unilateral cleft deformity. Kinnebrew, Zide, and Kent (1983) entirely degloved the midface in association with a Le Fort II osteotomy and correction of the maxillary and nasal deformities (Fig. 56–75). It is important in all cases to consider the vascular supply of any maxillary segments to be moved and to make sure that this is not interrupted in obtaining exposure for the osteotomy or nasal reconstruction (Henderson and Jackson, 1975). Only nasal tip surgery

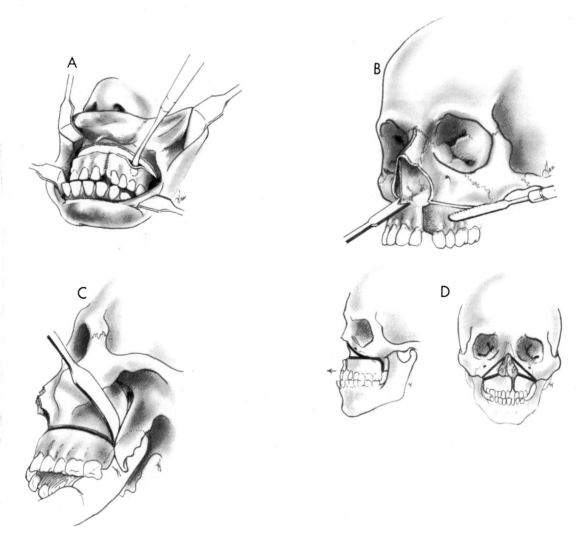

Figure 56–76. Method of performing Le Fort I maxillary osteotomy in the unilateral cleft patient. *A,* Transbuccal incision. The periosteum has been dissected to facilitate Le Fort I osteotomy. *B,* Two-pronged nasal osteotome separates the nasal septum from the maxilla. Le Fort osteotomy is performed with a side-cutting oscillating saw. The osteotomy is carried from the maxillary tuberosity on one side through the posterior wall of the maxilla and the medial and anterior walls at the desired level. This is also performed on the opposite side. *C,* After separation of the maxillary tuberosity from the pterygoid plate (with the left index finger placed intraorally), the right hand guides the modified Dautery-Salyer osteotome between the pterygoid plate and maxillary tuberosity. The maxillary segment is then downfractured. *D,* Anterior and lateral views of variations of the Le Fort I osteotomy. The lower is the standard level of the Le Fort I osteotomy. The higher is the modified Le Fort 1½ osteotomy. This osteotomy is used when there is substantial paranasal hypoplasia and more than a Le Fort I maxillary advancement is indicated. (From Bardach, J., and Salyer, K. E.: Surgical Techniques in Cleft Lip and Palate. Chicago, Year Book Medical Publishers, 1987.)

should be performed at the time of osteotomy, although on occasion a dorsal strut of bone or cartilage graft may be inserted. To achieve an optimal nasal effect, an esthetic rhinoplasty requires a separate procedure with a different objective from an osteotomy procedure.

Osteotomies are generally postponed until adolescence (15 to 16 years of age in girls and 16 to 17 years in boys). Delaying surgery allows for completion of mandibular growth; earlier surgery interferes with maxillary growth. Freihofer (1973) found 70 per cent of 100 patients undergoing osteotomy before 16 years of age had unacceptable results. In contrast, patients operated on at age 16 or 17 years demonstrated much better results, with unacceptable outcomes occurring in only 27 per cent. Earlier intervention, especially in girls, has been recommended by Braun and Sotereanos (1980, 1981), and they reported no inhibition of maxillary growth.

Maxillary advancement procedures for cleft lip and palate differ from those performed for other pathologic conditions, whether traumatic or congenital (see Chap. 29). There are usually skeletal asymmetry and post-tuberosity scarring; the latter impedes forward movement of the osteotomized segment. Because of frequent occurrence of asymmetry, segmental osteotomies with independent forward or lateral movement may be required.

Le Fort I Osteotomy. The Le Fort I advancement osteotomy for maxillary retrusion associated with cleft lip and palate was popularized by Obwegeser (1969) but was described by Axhausen (1932). To effect simultaneous repair of the anterior fistula and maxillary advancement, the incisions and mucoperiosteal elevation of the alveolus and palate are performed as previously described for alveolar bone grafting (see Fig. 56–71). A single Veau flap is raised on the greater segment *only* if the fistula is large (to preserve the blood supply to the maxilla). Cleft lip revision may also be included in the incision to gain exposure of the alveolus and the maxilla. The buccal mucoperiosteum is elevated through two vertical incisions using a tunneling technique to minimize vascular compromise of the maxillary segments. The tunnel is created from the edge of the cleft to the pterygomaxillary fissure (Fig. 56–76). The nasal mucoperiosteum is raised from the floor of the nose and piriform aperture areas. Using a side-cutting bur, or preferably a reciprocating saw, the maxilla is cut at the desired horizontal level from piriform aperture to the pterygomaxillary fissure.

A similar cut is made anteroposteriorly along the lateral wall of the piriform aperture. Mobilization of the segments may require a vertical osteotomy with a curved osteotome at the pterygomaxillary junction to separate the maxillary tuberosity and the pterygoid plate. Advancement of the maxilla to the preplanned position may require the use of the Rowe maxillary disimpaction forceps, the use of the Tessier maxillary mobilizer, or division of retrotuberosity scar tissue. For patients with substantial paranasal hypoplasia, the horizontal osteotomy is placed at a correspondingly higher level.

The nasal and oral layer repairs are per-

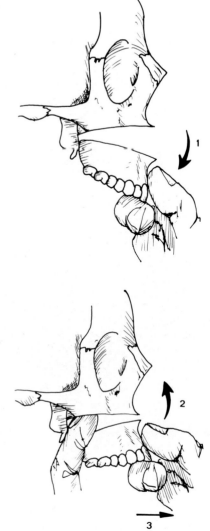

Figure 56–77. Gentle manipulation of the Le Fort I maxillary segment using finger pressure. (From Schendel, S. A., and Delaire, J.: Functional musculoskeletal correction of secondary unilateral cleft lip deformities: combined lip-nose correction and Le Fort I osteotomy. J. Maxillofac. Surg., 9:108, 1981.)

formed before placement of the segments into the interdental splint with transalveolar wires. Intermaxillary fixation is established, and the maxilla is stabilized with wires to the piriform aperture, inferior orbital rims, or zygomatic arch. Stabilization with miniplates is now commonly used (see Chap. 29), and this newer technique may allow the intermaxillary fixation to be removed at the end of the procedure (Drommer and Luhr,

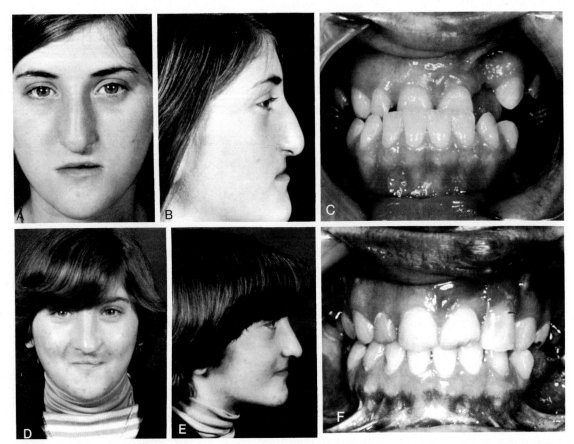

Figure 56–78. Le Fort I osteotomy (see Figs. 56–76, 56–77). *A* to *C,* Typical unilateral cleft deformity with retrusion of the maxilla. *D* to *F,* Postoperative result after Le Fort I advancement osteotomy of the maxilla with lip revision and closure and bone grafting of the anterior fistula.

Figure 56–79. Osteotomies and bone graft sites in the Le Fort II procedure. *A,* Frontal view of the Le Fort II osteotomy for maxillary advancement in unilateral cleft lip, alveolus, and palate. A horizontal osteotomy is carried through the frontonasal suture bilaterally and continues posteriorly to the nasolacrimal groove on each side and inferiorly over the infraorbital rims. The osteotomy is carried inferomedially to the infraorbital nerve and reaches the groove anterior to the pterygoid plates (shown best in the lateral view). The osteotomy turns outward, laterally, above the roots of the teeth and the maxillary tuberosity. *B,* Postosteotomy view after separation of the segments with maxillary advancement and insertion of the bone grafts (shown in white). Bone grafts are placed in the frontonasal junction between the maxillary segments, in the alveolar cleft, and on the nose. *C,* Lateral view showing the hypoplastic maxilla and the osteotomies for Le Fort II maxillary advancement. The osteotomy is carried from the frontonasal junction into the medial orbital wall behind the nasolacrimal groove, across the infraorbital rim and medial to the infraorbital nerve, posterior and below the zygoma along the maxillary tuberosity, and down between the maxillary tuberosity and pterygoid plates. *D,* Oblique view of the Le Fort II osteotomy showing the line of osteotomy. *E,* Maxillary advancement following Le Fort II osteotomy with bone grafts wired into the created gaps. Note that no bone graft is inserted in the space between the maxillary tuberosity and pterygoid plates. *F,* Same view with bone grafts inserted in the gaps after Le Fort II procedure for maxillary advancement and bone grafting on the nose and in the alveolar defect. (From Bardach, J., and Salyer, K. E.: Surgical Techniques in Cleft Lip and Palate. Chicago, Year Book Medical Publishers, 1987.)

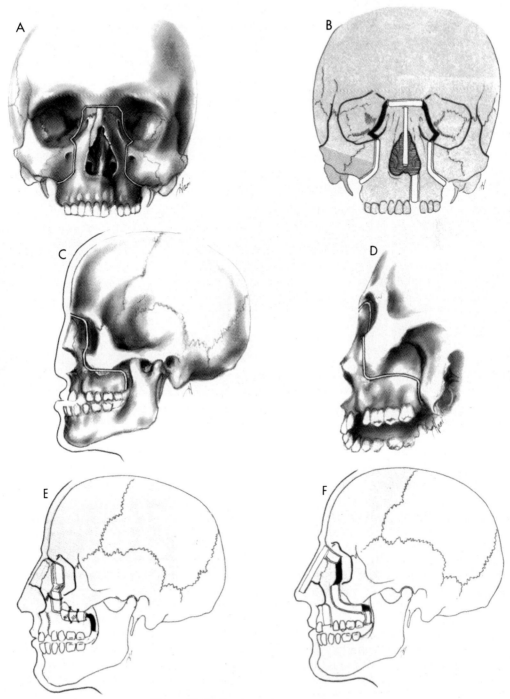

Figure 56–79 *See legend on opposite page*

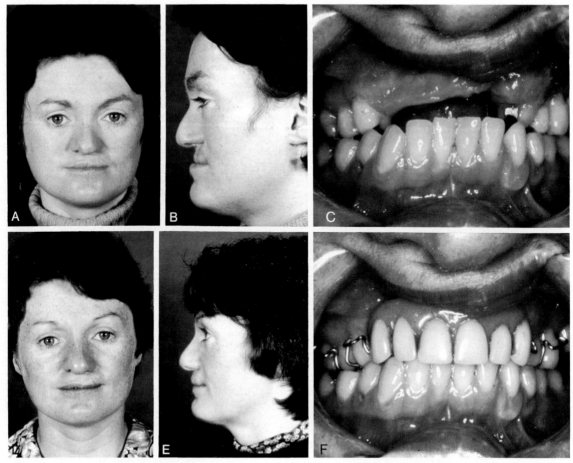

Figure 56–80. Le Fort II osteotomy (see Fig. 56–79). *A* to *C*, Preoperative appearance. *D* to *F*, Postoperative appearance after Le Fort II advancement, lip revision, and closure and bone grafting of the anterior fistula.

1981; Salyer, 1986; Jackson and Mustardé, 1988).

The cleft is grafted in the usual way with cancellous bone. Onlay grafts to the alar base and anterior surface of the maxilla are inserted before closure of the buccal sulcus and alveolar cleft incisions. Bone grafting of the retrotuberosity area is not necessary for maintenance of the anteroposterior position of the segment, especially if plate and screw fixation is used.

A Le Fort I osteotomy undertaken six months after fistula closure and bone grafting may be complicated by adherent nasal mucoperiosteum, which may be difficult to dissect in the area of previous repair. Downfracturing of the Le Fort maxillary segment (see Chap. 29) must be gently performed to avoid fracturing the previously placed alveolar bone graft (Figs. 56–77, 56–78). If the latter

occurs, the management is the same as that of a two-part maxilla, and fixation is identical to that described above.

If wires have been used, intermaxillary fixation is retained for six weeks. If there is any question about stability, fixation is reestablished for two weeks. When miniplate and screw fixation is employed, intermaxillary fixation is usually used only for intraoperative positioning of the segments.

Le Fort II Osteotomy. With additional hypoplasia situated cephalad to the maxilla, a high Le Fort I osteotomy and onlay bone grafting are performed. Severe paranasal hypoplasia extending to the infraorbital rims necessitates a Le Fort II osteotomy as described by Henderson and Jackson (1973), but it should be understood that this is not a common occurrence (Figs. 56–79, 56–80) (see Chap. 29).

Exposure is gained through a bicoronal incision or bilateral paranasal incisions. The former is a more extensive procedure, possibly entailing medial canthal disruption; the latter results in potentially visible external scars.

The medial orbital floor, the infraorbital rim, the medial orbital wall, and the lacrimal sac are exposed in a subperiosteal plane. The medial canthal tendons are left undisturbed. An osteotomy is made with a side cutting bur down the medial orbital wall behind the lacrimal groove. It is extended medially to the infraorbital nerve area through the orbital floor, over the anterior maxilla, and caudally as far as possible. The Aufricht retractor is inserted from one paranasal incision to the other to retract the dorsal nasal skin, and the osteotomies are connected at the nasal dorsum using a reciprocating saw. Any unconnected areas are cut with a fine osteotome; exposure for the osteotomies is improved with the bicoronal approach. Through a posterior buccal sulcus incision the osteotomy cuts are located and are extended across the maxillary tuberosities to the pterygomaxillary fissures. The maxillary tuberosities are separated from the pterygoid plates with a curved osteotome. To complete the osteotomy, a curved osteotome is placed in the transverse cut across the nasofrontal junction and is driven posteriorly and inferiorly to separate the vomer from the anterior skull base. Mobilization of the maxilla is achieved as in the Le Fort I procedure (see Chap. 29).

Management of the fistula, bone grafting of the cleft, fixation, and postoperative management differ little from those described above for the Le Fort I osteotomy. The infraorbital rim defects are accurately bone grafted through the paranasal incisions. The anterior osteotomy sites are filled with inlay and onlay bone grafts using the buccal sulcus approach. Split cranial bone grafts are readily available when a coronal approach is used (Jackson, Pellett, and Smith, 1983). Wire or multiple screws and miniplates placed from the frontal bone to the nasal skeleton provide secure fixation of the central maxilla to the skull. If nasal height is lacking, a split cranial bone graft can be placed beneath the dorsal nasal skin and secured with two screws or wire to provide a cantilever type of dorsal graft.

Segmental Osteotomies. In patients with unilateral cleft lip and palate with the sec-

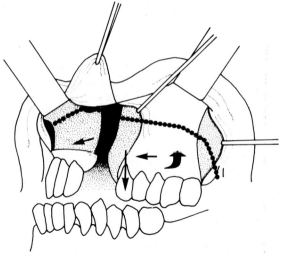

Figure 56–81. Asymmetric Le Fort I maxillary osteotomy. (From Tideman, H., Stoelinga, P., and Gallia, L.: Le Fort I advancement with segmental palatal osteotomies in patients with cleft palates. J. Oral Surg., 38:196, 1980.)

ondary deformities of maxillary hypoplasia, collapse of the lesser maxillary segment, or anterior fistula, it is often difficult to correct the malpositioned segment with orthodontic therapy. Unilateral open bite, crossbite, and total unilateral collapse of the maxillary arch are seen to various degrees. The larger segment is frequently stable and has normal proportions and occlusal relationships. On the cleft side the maxilla lacks the necessary skeletal support and may be adversely influenced by scar tissue from previous palatal surgery. Such unilateral deformities may necessitate segmental osteotomies (Braun and Sotereanos, 1980; Tideman, Stoelinga, and Gallia, 1980). The elimination of crossbite, stabilization of the maxillary arch, and improvement of the alar base and soft tissue relationships with the maxilla are the objectives of a maxillary segmental osteotomy. Whenever possible, orthodontic care is initiated presurgically for arch alignment and palatal expansion.

A unilateral Le Fort I or rarely Le Fort II osteotomy can be performed, depending on the preoperative evaluation. Through a buccal sulcus incision, the mucoperiosteum is elevated to expose the maxilla bilaterally. A Le Fort osteotomy is designed to ensure preservation of intact palatal mucosa to maintain skeletal vascularity (Fig. 56–81). The osteotomized maxilla is placed into proper occlusion with a prefabricated occlusal splint, and intermaxillary fixation is applied. Maxillary osseosynthesis with wires or plates is established when the alignment and position of the dental arch corresponds to the preplanned position in the dental splint. Cancellous iliac bone grafts are used to fill the osteotomy sites and alveolar cleft and are placed over the maxilla and under the alar base. Closure of the alveolar fistula and fixation are as previously described.

Mandibular Osteotomies. Mandibular osteotomies may be indicated in patients with mandibular prognathism, or in patients whose maxillary retrusion is so severe (1.5 to 2 cm) that stability would be unlikely if the required maxillary advancement were performed. In the latter situation, a two-jaw procedure is much less likely to result in relapse. Apart from this indication, a mandibular osteotomy should not be used in patients with pseudoprognathism (Jackson, 1984). When a bimaxillary procedure is carried out, an intermediate interdental splint (see Chap. 29) is essential to obtain the correct, planned position of the maxilla; a definitive splint is then used on completion of the mandibular osteotomy to obtain the final occlusion. The mandible is usually retrodisplaced by the sagittal split technique (Obwegeser, 1957) or rarely by a subcondylar vertical osteotomy. These procedures are described in detail in Chapter 29.

Velopharyngeal Incompetence After Osteotomy. Velopharyngeal incompetence may occur in cleft patients after maxillary advancement and should be discussed with the patient preoperatively (see Chap. 29). Noncleft patients without preoperative nasal emission rarely develop velopharyngeal incompetence because the normal palate can compensate for large forward movements, even those in excess of 10 mm (Schwarz and Gruner, 1976; McCarthy, Coccaro, and Schwartz, 1979; Schendel and associates, 1979). The repaired palate, however, is scarred, and in some cases there is poorly reconstructed palatal musculature; thus, it is less adaptable to maxillary advancement. If velopharyngeal incompetence is present preoperatively, it may be increased postoperatively (Bralley and Schoeny, 1977; Witzel and Munro, 1977; Mason, Turvey, and Warren, 1980). This phenomenon has been reported in approximately 10 per cent of patients postoperatively in one series (Jackson, 1978). If hypernasality develops after maxillary ad-

vancement, a minimum of six months should elapse before a pharyngoplasty is performed. The delay is necessary so that the velopharyngeal function may improve through adaptation. Moreover, premature creation of a pharyngeal flap after maxillary advancement could contribute to postoperative maxillary relapse. For the latter reason, a midline pharyngeal flap that becomes tight during or after advancement should be divided or lengthened. If the pharyngeal flap is transected and velopharyngeal incompetence persists, it is the authors' custom to perform a sphincter pharyngoplasty after six months. It has never been necessary to rearrange a sphincter pharyngoplasty performed before an osteotomy.

SECONDARY DEFORMITIES OF BILATERAL CLEFT

Many of the considerations and techniques for secondary correction of the unilateral cleft lip deformity apply also to bilateral clefts. The results of primary bilateral cleft lip repair are often unsatisfactory and secondary revision is frequently necessary. The secondary deformities may involve the lip, the nose, the alveolus, or the skeleton. The prominent premaxilla with associated alveolar clefts and oronasal fistulas presents specific problems.

Lip Deformities

The most common lip deformities include the following: (1) a V-shaped whistle deformity in the midportion of the lip due to a deficiency of vermilion, lack of muscle reconstruction, and mucosal scarring; (2) a short prolabium; (3) a wide prolabium; (4) asymmetric vermilion; (5) an immobile prolabium; (6) inadequate orbicularis oris repair; (7) deficient gingivobuccal sulcus; (8) a tight upper lip; and (9) an excessively long upper lip.

In most revisions, the lip scar is completely reopened, and the prolabium is narrowed to 15 mm. The resulting lateral fork flaps can be used for columellar lengthening or can be "banked" for later use. Since simultaneous lengthening requires separation of the prolabium from the base of the columella, it is wiser to delay columellar surgery until a later date. The flaps are banked; the orbicularis oris muscle is dissected out and sutured in the midline. If the mucosa of the prolabium is deficient, resulting in a whistle deformity, triangular island flaps of vermilion based on the orbicularis oris muscle and advanced from the lateral lip segments in a V-Y fashion (Kapetansky, 1971) give the most satisfactory correction. In bilateral cases, the nasal deformities are generally corrected after or at the time of columellar lengthening.

Lip Scars. Secondary scar revisions and small irregularities or misalignment of the white roll can be corrected by the same techniques used in management of the unilateral deformities. It is important to visualize the normal position and direction of the bilateral philtral columns and to attempt to place the scars along these anatomic lines, thus avoiding abrupt interruptions of any natural features that may remain.

Tension across the initial suture line is probably responsible for the undesirable scar (Millard, 1977). Secondary scar revisions may be performed on one side at a time to avoid the production of further tension, but this is rarely necessary. The scar tissue can be buried or banked to lengthen the columella or to create a philtral ridge (Millard, 1977; Stal and Spira, 1984). However, the philtral augmentation is rarely maintained.

Upper lip scars may inhibit hair growth, which in the clean-shaven male is a visible

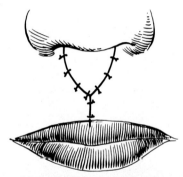

Figure 56–83. Resulting Y-configuration of the scar in the philtrum after excision of previous scars as in Figure 56–82. (After Erich. From Millard, D. R., Jr.: Cleft Craft. Vol.II. Boston, Little, Brown & Company, 1977.)

stigma of a cleft lip repair, especially when the prolabium is excessively wide. Successful rehabilitation of bilateral cleft lips with a philtrum of correct width can be judged by the acceptability of the moustache growth in males. Abbé flaps and temporal island flaps have been described to bring hair-bearing tissue to the upper lip from the lower lip and scalp, respectively (Millard, 1977; Stal and Spira, 1984). Total resurfacing of the upper lip with a full-thickness skin graft in severely scarred bilateral cleft lips was reported by Broadbent (1957). Dermabrasion has been of only limited success. It is exceedingly rare to be forced into using any of these drastic measures.

Long Lip (Vertical Excess). The long upper lip deformity in bilateral clefts is usually the result of the introduction of composite flaps (from the lateral lip elements) between the prolabium and vermilion. These inferiorly positioned flaps are triangular (Mirault-Rose-Blair-Braun) or quadrilateral (Hagedorn-LeMesurier) and are joined end to end. Lengthening can also occur when lateral lip element flaps are joined above the prolabium or when extreme lengthening is accomplished with Z-plasty–type procedures. Incorrect placement of previously inserted Abbé flaps may also produce this deformity. The resultant upper lip appears excessively long and curtain-like, with a short columella and depressed nasal tip.

Erich (1953) reduced the vertical length of the lip by excision of the bilateral scars and reduction of the prolabium (Fig. 56–82), but an unnatural Y-configuration in the philtrum resulted (Fig. 56–83). Vaughan (1940) (Fig. 56–84) and Ragnell (1946) used similar but

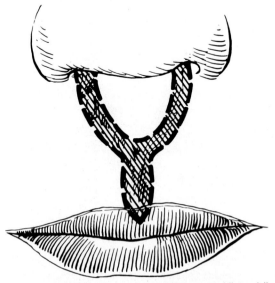

Figure 56–82. Revision of a previous poor bilateral lip repair using excision of the old scars with reduction of vertical lip length and reduction of prolabial size (see Fig. 56–83). (After Erich. From Millard, D. R., Jr.: Cleft Craft. Vol. II. Boston, Little, Brown & Company, 1977.)

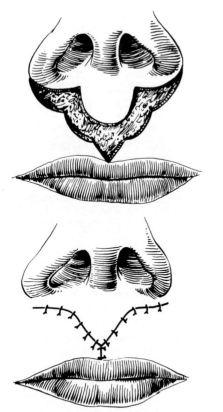

Figure 56–84. Shortening of a long bilateral lip by resection of scars and tissue from the inferior prolabium and the nasolabial junction. "Winged" scar results. (After Vaughan. From Millard, D. R., Jr.: Cleft Craft. Vol. II. Boston, Little, Brown & Company, 1977.)

more radical patterns to reduce the vertical length of the lip. Ragnell's (1946) design produced scars that fell within natural landmarks and appears to be the most satisfactory of the three techniques (Fig. 56–85).

Peterson, Ellenberg, and Carroll (1966) liberated the prolabium, shortened the lateral lip segments by wedge excisions along the nasolabial line, and transferred a central Abbé flap of only vermilion and muscle from the lower lip into the defect beneath the prolabium (Fig. 56–86). A repositioning of scars, compatible with the design of a philtrum, shortened the vertical length of the upper lip and reduced the relative excess of the lower lip. When the lateral lip elements lie beneath the prolabium, the flaps are returned to their vertical positions along the prolabium from whence they were initially taken (Millard, 1977). Four months later the delayed flaps can be advanced into the columella as fork flaps to achieve lengthening. Alternatively, the prolabium can be advanced into the columella and a central Abbé flap transferred from the lower lip into the upper lip defect to reconstruct the philtrum.

If all other aspects of the nose and lip repair are satisfactory, vertical excess of the upper lip can be corrected by a transverse full-thickness excision at the nasolabial junction (Fig. 56–87). When the lip is long but the columella is short or retracted, lip shortening

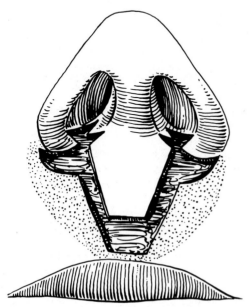
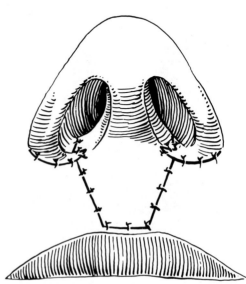

Figure 56–85. Shortening of a long bilateral cleft lip, including scar excision and medial advancement of the alar bases. Note the areas of undermining. The scars fall in natural landmarks. (After Ragnell. From Millard, D. R., Jr.: Cleft Craft. Vol. II. Boston, Little, Brown & Company, 1977.)

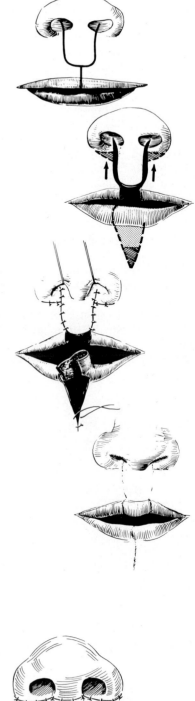

Figure 56–86. Shortening of a long bilateral cleft lip with an increase in the transverse width and reconstruction of the mucosa with a mucomuscular lip switch flap. (After Peterson, Ellenburg, and Carroll. From Millard, D. R., Jr.: Cleft Craft. Vol. II. Boston, Little, Brown & Company, 1977.)

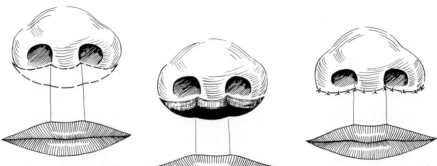

Figure 56–87. Transverse wedge excision at the nasolabial junction to achieve shortening of excess vertical lip length. (From Millard, D. R., Jr.: Cleft Craft. Vol. II. Boston, Little, Brown & Company, 1977.)

and columellar lengthening by a modification of Cronin's (1958) technique is possible.

Short Lip (Vertical Deficiency). When the upper lip is short (vertical deficiency), there is unacceptable incisor show. A short prolabium results when the initially short prolabial segment cannot be stretched to match the lateral lip segments.

For minor deformities with adequate lip width, scar excision or Z-plasty techniques may suffice. Total reoperation and readjustment of the skin and vermilion are likewise acceptable for moderate deformity if adequate tissue is available (Fig. 56–88). Lengthening of the lip without available local tissue in some deformities may necessitate an Abbé flap.

In minor lip shortening Muir and Bodenham (1966) placed a full-thickness ear lobe graft at the vermilion-cutaneous junction in the midline to simulate the central portion of the Cupid's bow (Fig. 56–89). Fork flaps can be used to lengthen both lip and columella (Figs. 56–90, 56–91) (Millard, 1977) but should be avoided because of the frequently poor columellar reconstruction. Lateral advancement flaps as in the LeMesurier or the Ginestet method (Fig. 56–92) achieve vertical length at the price of unnatural scarring and horizontal tightness and should not be used. Bardach and Salyer (1987d) lengthened the short upper lip, corrected the whistle deformity, and narrowed the alar base with a V-Y technique (Fig. 56–93). A gull-wing incision was developed through all lip layers, with wedges of skin being removed from the nostril sill bilaterally. Downward traction at the midline pulled the lip inferiorly, lengthening the midportion and approximating the lateral segments. Cheek advancement flaps can be advanced beneath the alae to increase length as described by Barron (1977) (Fig. 56–94). Although skin lengthening is important, the most effective method of total lip lengthening and of ensuring that the repair is permanent is orbicularis oris reconstruction with interdigitation of the muscle (Figs. 56–95, 56–96).

Tight Lip (Horizontal Deficiency). A tight upper lip can result from excessive tissue excision or from use of the prolabium to lengthen the columella at the primary oper-

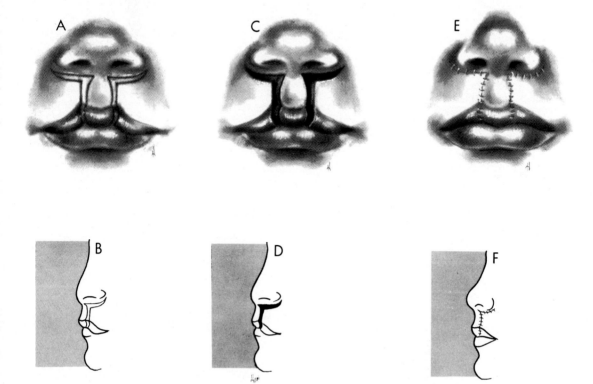

Figure 56–88. Total reconstruction of a previous lip repair by excision of scars and bilateral advancement to reduce the length of the lateral lip segments. *A, B,* Design for incisions. *C, D,* Excision of scars and excision at the alar bases. Incisions are carried through all three layers. *E, F,* Completed operation. (From Bardach, J., and Salyer, K. E.: Surgical Techniques in Cleft Lip and Palate. Chicago, Year Book Medical Publishers, 1987.)

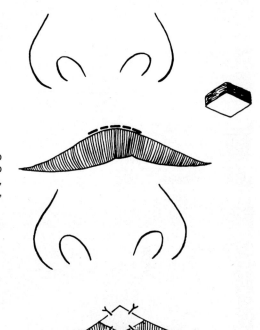

Figure 56–89. Full-thickness skin (ear lobe) graft inserted into the center of the lip just above the mucocutaneous junction to recreate the Cupid's bow. (After Muir and Bodenham. From Millard, D. R., Jr.: Cleft Craft. Vol. II. Boston, Little, Brown & Company, 1977.)

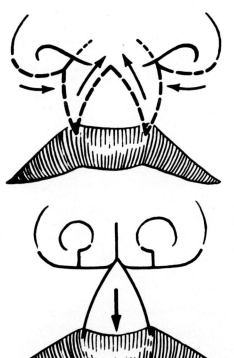

Figure 56–90. Design of fork flaps for lengthening of the columella primarily or as a secondary procedure. (From Millard, D. R., Jr.: Cleft Craft. Vol. II. Boston, Little, Brown & Company, 1977.)

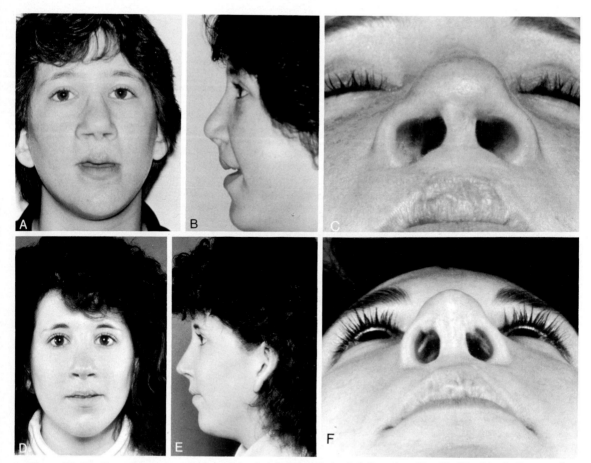

Figure 56–91. Correction of a secondary bilateral cleft deformity by fork flaps (see Fig. 56–90). *A* to *C*, Preoperative appearance. (From Jackson, I. T.: Cleft lip and palate. *In* Mustardé, J. C., and Jackson, I. T. (Eds.): Plastic Surgery in Infancy and Childhood. 3rd Ed. Edinburgh, Churchill Livingstone, 1988.) *D* to *F*, Postoperative appearance after lip revision, closure and bone grafting of anterior fistulas, fork flaps for reconstruction of the columella, and a small cartilage graft to the nasal tip.

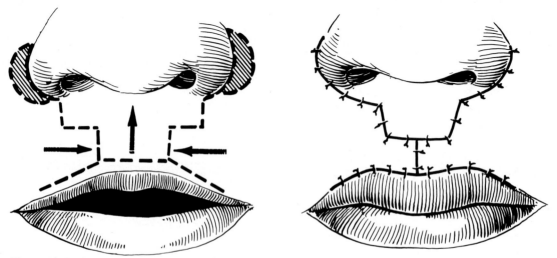

Figure 56–92. Lateral advancement flaps for lengthening of the short bilateral cleft lip. Unnatural scarring and horizontal lip tightening result. (After Ginestet. From Millard, D. R., Jr.: Cleft Craft. Vol. II. Boston, Little, Brown & Company, 1977.)

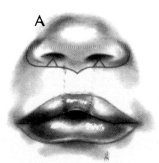 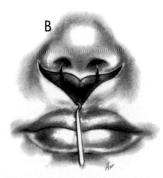 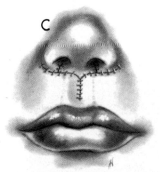

Figure 56–93. Lengthening of the short bilateral lip with a V-Y procedure. *A,* The design of the incisions enables lengthening of the midportion of the lip and narrowing of the alar bases. *B,* Incisions are carried through all lip layers, and a hook is inserted at the midline to pull the lip inferiorly, lengthening the midportion and approximating the lateral lip elements. *C,* Completed procedure. (From Bardach, J., and Salyer, K. E.: Surgical Techniques in Cleft Lip and Palate. Chicago, Year Book Medical Publishers, 1987.)

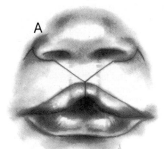 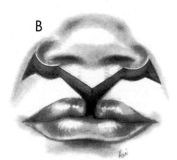 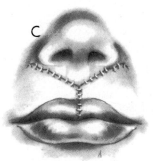

Figure 56–94. Correction of the short midportion of the upper lip after bilateral cleft lip repair and simultaneous narrowing of the alar bases. *A,* Design of incisions. *B,* Incisions are carried through all layers. *C,* The lateral portions slide inferiorly and medially, resulting in adequate lengthening. The alar bases are narrowed at the same time. (From Bardach, J., and Salyer, K. E.: Surgical Techniques in Cleft Lip and Palate. Chicago, Year Book Medical Publishers, 1987.)

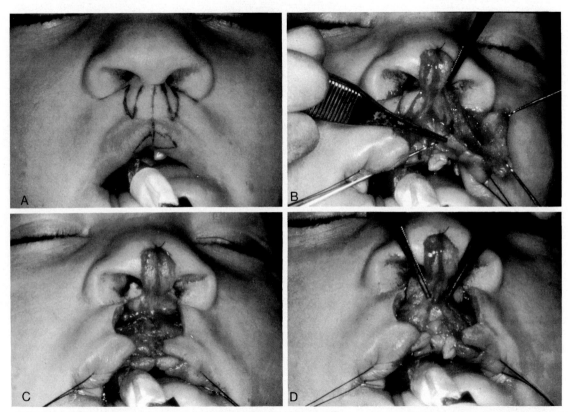

Figure 56–95. Fork flaps and orbicularis oris reconstruction in secondary revision of bilateral cleft lip. *A,* The design of the lip repair is outlined. Note the Kapetansky pendulum flaps drawn on the mucosal aspect of the lip. *B,* Muscle is being mobilized together with the Kapetansky pendulum flaps. *C,* The orbicularis oris muscle is being dissected in the lateral segments. *D,* The fork flaps are stored in the nostril sill area. (From Jackson, I. T.: Cleft lip and palate. *In* Mustardé, J. C., and Jackson, I. T. (Eds.): Plastic Surgery in Infancy and Childhood. 3rd Ed. Edinburgh, Churchill Livingstone, 1988.)

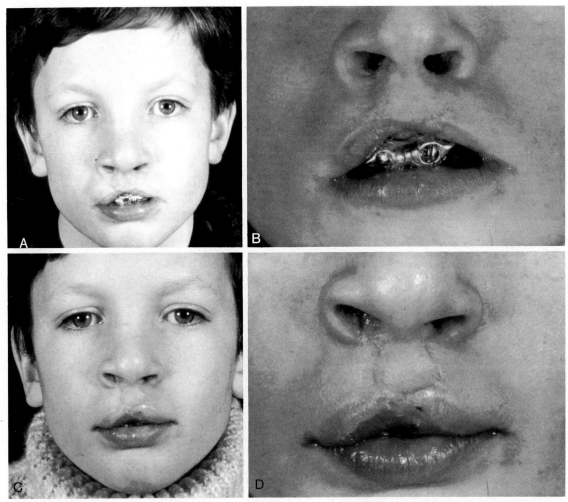

Figure 56–96. Orbicularis oris reconstruction (see Fig. 56–95). *A, B*, Secondary bilateral cleft lip deformity showing thinness of the prolabial segment and a whistle deformity due to lack of orbicularis oris reconstruction. *C, D*, Postoperative appearance after complete revision of the lip with reconstruction of the orbicularis oris muscle. (*B, D*, From Jackson, I. T.: Cleft lip and palate. *In* Mustardé, J. C., and Jackson, I. T.: (Eds.): Plastic Surgery in Infancy and Childhood, 3rd Ed. Edinburgh, Churchill Livingstone, 1988.)

ation. The resulting deformity is classic in profile: the upper lip is tight and the lower lip is slack and protuberant. An assessment of midfacial growth in the anteroposterior dimension should be made, as skeletal surgery in addition to soft tissue repair may be necessary. Most surgeons recommend an Abbé flap to correct the deformity. When a small prolabium is incorporated in the previous lip repair, midline insertion of the Abbé flap may result in four suture lines in the philtral area. Millard (1976) recommended advancement of the prolabium into the columella to avoid this problem. Design of the Abbé flap, as noted above, must include nor-

mal philtral measurements to prevent a large, unesthetic transfer in the upper lip and a tight lower lip. W-shaped or V-shaped flaps are transposed as indicated, and the pedicle is divided in ten days. Several modifications of the Abbé flap have been described. If the upper lip defect is excessively large to be closed with a philtrum-sized Abbé flap, perialar crescentic flaps as described by Webster (1955) allow cheek skin to be advanced and reduce the width of the defect (Fig. 56–97). Good muscle function can be achieved by advancing the upper lip orbicularis into the midline and covering it with a sandwich Abbé flap (Jackson and Soutar, 1980). The indica-

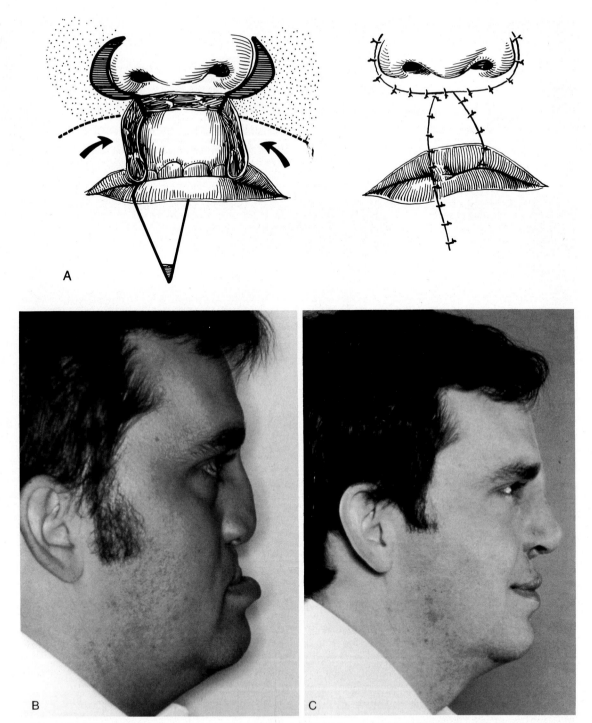

Figure 56–97. Perialar crescent excisions for large lip defect closure. *A,* Perialar advancement flaps used to narrow the upper lip defect after excision of the central scarred area. An Abbé flap is used to reconstruct the upper lip. (*A,* After Webster. From Millard, D. R., Jr.: Cleft Craft. Vol. II. Boston, Little, Brown & Company, 1977.) *B,* Bilateral cleft lip and palate deformity with considerable jaw discrepancy. *C,* Postoperative appearance after bimaxillary osteotomy, closure of the anterior fistula with bone grafting, Abbé flap procedure, and cranial bone grafting to the nose. (*B, C,* From Jackson, I. T.: Cleft lip and palate. *In* Mustardé, J. C., and Jackson, I. T. (Eds.): Plastic Surgery in Infancy and Childhood. 3rd Ed. Edinburgh, Churchill Livingstone, 1988.)

tion to use an Abbé flap is rare. Most lip defects can be rehabilitated with satisfactory muscle repair and, if necessary, advancement of pendulum flaps; rarely a bucket handle mucosal flap can be transferred from the lower lip.

Orbicularis Oris Deformity. In the patient with bilateral cleft lip, the absence of orbicularis oris muscle in the prolabial segment and the surgeon's failure to identify and join the fibers of the muscle from the lateral lip elements at the primary repair result in a characteristic lateral bulge above the vermilion of the upper lip. This distortion can ruin the appearance of an otherwise satisfactory bilateral cleft lip repair and is accentuated by the patient's attempts at facial animation. Schultz (1946), Glover and Necomb (1961), Manchester (1965), Duffy (1971), and Millard (1964b, 1971) have described techniques for primary bilateral cleft repair that provide midline muscle union. Secondary lip correction including union of the orbicularis oris muscle in the midline has been recommended by the same investigators as well as by Jackson (1973), Oneal, Greer, and Nobel (1974), Skoog (1974), and Puckett, Reinisch, and Werner (1980). A modifying influence of an intact orbicularis oris and paranasal musculature on facial bone development before age 8 years has been reported by Joos (1987). His findings suggest that reconstruction of these muscles can prevent or at least reduce secondary skeletal changes to an extent that orthodontic treatment can successfully manage skeletal hypoplasia. The action of the intact lip and the orbicularis oris muscle after primary repair provides a natural orthodontic force to mold the premaxilla.

Correction of the muscle deformity involves separation of the orbicularis oris from its vertical attachment to the alar base and development of a distinct horizontal muscle flap extending laterally as far as the nasolabial folds if necessary. A thin edge of scar is maintained in the medial border of the muscles to allow secure muscle interdigitation, with resulting lengthening in the midline beneath the prolabial skin. As mentioned above, in older children and adults, the shortened fibers of the quadratus labii superioris muscle entering the deep portion of the orbicularis might require partial division to bring the muscles into a satisfactory horizontal position at the midline (Fig. 56–98). With the union of the muscles in the midline, the transverse vectors of lateral muscle pull from each side are replaced by a vector tending to lengthen the prolabium (Duffy, 1971). The problabium has no muscle fibers and remains immobile without muscle union. Contrary to the opinion of most investigators, Bardach and Salyer (1987d) stated that adequate lip function can be obtained by insertion of the orbicularis oris muscle into the edges of the deep layer of the prolabium. This technique is thought to create a midline depression resembling the concavity of the normal philtrum. This technique should be used only if junction of the muscles in the midline is not possible.

Philtral Abnormalities. If correctly designed, a Cupid's bow and philtral dimple can be constructed during the primary repair (Millard, 1971). The philtral dimple is constructed by placing a deep suture from the dermis to the premaxillary periosteum; in addition, the prolabium is trimmed to normal philtral dimensions. It is necessary to overcorrect the philtrum, since it stretches after repair; it is unlikely that the deep suture is of much long-term value. Secondary bilateral cleft deformities involving the philtrum are

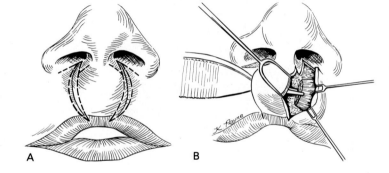

Figure 56–98. Reconstruction of orbicularis oris muscles in bilateral cleft. *A,* Design of incision. *B,* Incision to allow midline muscle union. (From Puckett, C. L., Reinisch, J. F., and Werner, R. S.: Late correction of orbicularis discontinuity in bilateral cleft lip deformity. Cleft Palate J., *17*:34, 1980.)

A   B

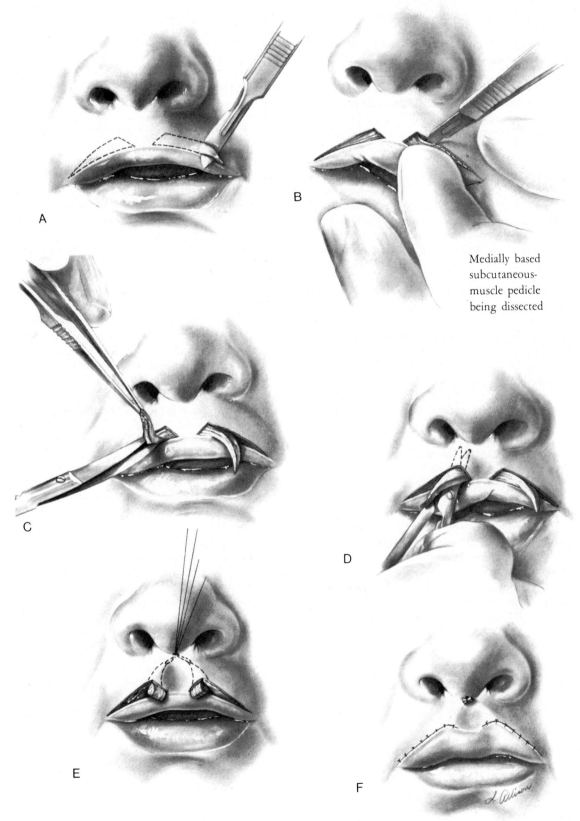

A

B

Medially based
subcutaneous-
muscle pedicle
being dissected

C

D

E

F

Figure 56–99. *See legend on opposite page*

generally amenable to many of the procedures mentioned above for treatment of the unilateral cleft lip deformity. When an extreme upper lip tissue defect is present, secondary reconstruction may require an Abbé flap. In the absence of the need for tissue augmentation, less extensive procedures for philtral reconstruction are sufficient.

Neuner (1967) transposed inferiorly based subcutaneous (bilateral) flaps from the midline to a lateral horizontal position to create a philtral hollow and elevate the lateral vermilion. In addition to performing O'Connor, McGregor, and Tolleth's (1965) procedure, he advanced the vermilion bilaterally in a V-Y fashion to accentuate lip eversion and construct a central tubercle of the Cupid's bow. Onizuka and associates (1978) rolled a midline flap of muscle to enhance the deficient philtral ridge in unilateral clefts. Millard (1977) reported a modification that included two rolls of tissue to elevate the philtral ridges on either side (Fig. 56–99). The best results are frequently obtained by inserting a conchal cartilage graft, especially in scarred lips.

Vermilion Deficiency. The most common vermilion deficiency is the whistle deformity. Correction may require either a bilateral V-Y advancement (Robinson, Ketchum, and Masters, 1970) or bilateral vermilion island flaps based on the orbicularis oris muscle (Kapetansky, 1971). The latter is the most logical and satisfactory technique for the correction of this deformity. Any of the techniques described above for correction of unilateral cleft lip deformities are also suitable for bilateral cleft lip deformities.

Additional techniques for repair include Arons' (1971) double transposition flaps. Small bilateral inverted V-flaps of mucosa and scar on either side of the whistle deformity are based inferiorly. The central segment is elevated as a superiorly based flap and advanced into a roll. The lateral V-flaps are crossed horizontally beneath the rolled central flaps (Fig. 56–100). For minor whistle deformities, Johnson (1972) unrolled the central upper lip and advanced the posterior

mucosa by releasing the lip in the buccal sulcus. A bolster stay suture maintained the proper position of the upper lip vermilion. Secondary healing of the raw mucosal defect in the alveolar area was required. Vermilion flaps from the lower lip were used by Lexer (1931) to augment the free border of the upper lip (Fig. 56–101). Tschopp (1973) devised a fleur-de-lys lip flap, which was a modification of the Lexer technique. After two weeks, these flaps were divided and inset. Cross lip flaps of vermilion, described initially by Gillies and Millard (1957) and subsequently by Kawamoto (1979), are best employed when the lateral vermilion is narrow and tissue for medial advancement is inadequate. The technique of elevation and delayed placement of the flaps has been described above with discussion of Abbé flaps. Tongue flaps (Fig. 56–102) (Guerrero-Santos, 1969) and Abbé flaps are alternative choices. In general, the majority of whistle deformities are automatically corrected by orbicularis oris muscle reconstruction.

Buccal Sulcus Abnormalities. In many bilateral clefts the prolabium is so closely attached to the premaxilla that the gingivobuccal sulcus is absent. Creation of a sulcus is an indispensable step in lip reconstruction. An adequate sulcus enhances the function of the lip and is essential for retention of orthodontic appliances and prostheses. Primary bilateral lip repairs that fail to elevate the prolabium from the premaxilla always necessitate secondary reconstruction of the upper sulcus. Schultz (1946) popularized separation of the prolabium and the premaxilla by lining the posterior aspect of the prolabium with lateral flaps. The premaxilla was allowed to epithelize secondarily as in the primary repair of Bauer, Trusler, and Tondra (1959) and Manchester (1965). The procedure for lining of the premaxilla was provided by Tondra, Bauer, and Trusler (1966).

Numerous techniques for reconstruction of the buccal sulcus have been discussed above under Secondary Deformities of Unilateral Cleft. Flap reconstruction of the buccal sulcus with epithelization of the premaxillary donor

---

Figure 56–99. Formation of philtral columns using deepithelized medially based upper lip flaps with simultaneous construction of the Cupid's bow. *A,* Deepithelizing the skin but preserving the mucocutaneous ridge. *B,* Medially based subcutaneous muscle pedicle being dissected. *C,* Elevation of flaps. *D,* Philtral column tunnel dissected. *E,* Flaps being pulled into tunnels to produce the Cupid's bow, philtral columns, and dimple. *F,* After closure. (From Millard, D. R., Jr.: Cleft Craft. Vol. II. Boston, Little, Brown & Company, 1977.)

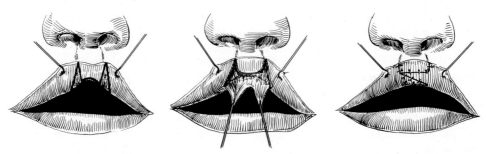

Figure 56–100. Augmentation of central upper lip vermilion by double transposition flaps. (After Arons. From Millard, D. R., Jr.: Cleft Craft. Vol. II. Boston, Little, Brown & Company, 1977.)

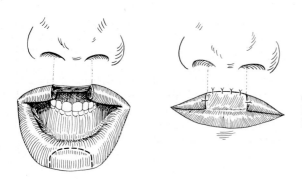

Figure 56–101. Augmentation of the upper lip mucosa using a mucosal-submucosal cross lip flap. (After Lexer. From Millard, D. R., Jr.: Cleft Craft. Vol. II. Boston, Little, Brown & Company, 1977.)

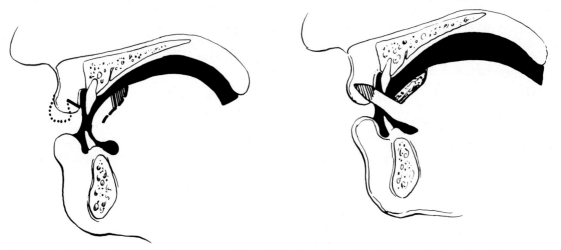

Figure 56–102. Use of a tongue flap to augment the deficient upper lip. (After Guerrero-Santos. From Millard, D. R., Jr.: Cleft Craft. Vol. II. Boston, Little, Brown & Company, 1977.)

site was reported by Falcone (1966) (Fig. 56–103). A flap consisting of prolabium, sulcus, and premaxillary mucosa was produced via an anterior premaxillary incision, and the flap was elevated from the premaxilla at the periosteal level. The flap was advanced into the depths of the new sulcus to line the labial side of the sulcus. The exposed periosteum of the premaxilla was left to reepithelize. Cosman and Crikelair (1966) described application of a full-thickness free mucosal graft to the labial sulcus after dissection of the prolabium from the premaxilla.

Cleft Lip Nasal Deformity

The bilateral cleft nasal deformity is characteristic and varied only in degree. It is usually symmetric, although the protruding and rotated premaxilla may cause asymmetry, as is seen with a complete cleft on one side and an incomplete cleft on the other. Trier (1985) advocated a preliminary lip adhesion in this circumstance to achieve symmetric repair of the cleft and to establish greater symmetry of the nasal deformity for later correction. As compared with secondary repair of the unilateral cleft lip nasal deformity, secondary reconstruction in the bilateral deformity is easier to some extent because of the initial symmetry.

PATHOLOGIC ANATOMY

The following characteristic factors may be present before the primary lip repair and may remain as residual deformities (Fig. 56–104): (1) the columella is short with encroachment of lip tissue; (2) the medial crura of the alar cartilages are displaced inferiorly with lowering of the alar domes; (3) the alar domes are laterally displaced with a bifid appearance to the nasal tip, and the dome angle between the medial and lateral crura is obtuse, resulting in a flattened appearance; (4) lateral displacement of the alar bases on the hypoplastic maxilla results in a flattened alar-facial angle and a widened nostril sill; (5) prominent vestibular skin webs and buckling of the lateral crura produce a collapsed nostril contour; and (6) the caudal septum and the underdeveloped anterior nasal spine are displaced inferiorly or laterally, depending on the degree and asymmetry of the cleft.

Stenström and Oberg (1961) hypothesized that lateral traction on the alar bases and lowering of the alae resulted in the characteristic nasal deformity. Pruzansky (1971) attributed the bilateral cleft lip nasal deformity to an overgrowth or an excess of mesoderm at the vomeropremaxillary suture because of lack of restraint by the nonunited orbicularis oris muscle. Potter (1968) and McComb (1975) ascribed the majority of secondary bilateral cleft nasal deformities to incorporation of the prolabium into the lip repair. McComb (1986) consequently advocated advancing fork flaps into the columella at six weeks postoperatively to prevent the nasal deformity (see Chap. 53). Millard (1982) discontinued primary columellar lengthening because of concerns about the security of the lip closure and the vascularity of the prolabium remaining in the lip. At the present

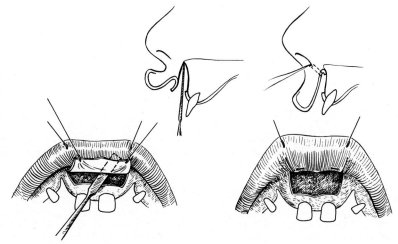

Figure 56–103. Lengthening of the buccal mucosa of the upper lip by advancement of the premaxillary gingiva. Spontaneous reepithelization of the premaxillary defect occurs. (After Falcone. From Millard, D. R., Jr.: Cleft Craft. Vol. II. Boston, Little, Brown & Company, 1977.)

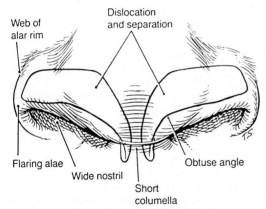

Figure 56–104. Characteristic components of the nasal deformity in the bilateral cleft. (From Rohrich, R. J., and Tebbetts, J. B.: Cleft lip II: secondary cleft lip/nasal/alveolar deformities. Selected Readings in Plastic Surgery, Vol. 4, No. 22, 1987.)

time, most surgeons make only provisions for later columellar lengthening at the time of the initial lip closure.

After measuring the columellas of normal persons and of patients who had undergone bilateral cleft lip repair, Lindsay and Farkas (1971) concluded that in many cases the columellar shortening noted in infancy was more apparent than real. They advised avoiding dissection and displacement of the columella at the initial lip repair, thus allowing columellar growth to continue and reducing the need for secondary revisions. Pigott and Millard (1971) pointed out that the normal infant's nose has less projection and is broader than the adult's nose. The outer angle of the nostrils in the Caucasian infant lies at approximately 90 degrees and decreases to 45 degrees in the adult (Fig. 56–105). The ratio of columellar height to nasal projection above the columella is less than 1:2 in the infant,

but nearly 1:1 in the adult. These observations of nasal projection are important when assessing the infant's nose, either primarily or secondarily.

At the time of primary bilateral cleft lip repair, most surgeons (Bardach and Salyer, 1987e; Millard, 1977) reconstruct the nasal floor and sill, position the alar bases symmetrically, and preserve skin by banking flaps in the nasal floor to later reconstruct the columella (see Chap. 53). Several factors must be considered: the optimal source of available tissue, the site of banking, and the method and timing of transfer (Rohrich and Tebbitts, 1987).

SURGICAL CORRECTION

The columella is the first area to address. Transposition of local tissue from the lip or the nose and the use of composite grafts are the main tissue delivery techniques. Cronin and Upton (1978) reviewed the available procedures according to the source of skin to be transposed to the columella (e.g., the lip, the nose, and distant sites).

Upper lip tissue in the form of a V-Y advancement from the prolabium to lengthen the columella (Fig. 56–106) was first described by Gensoul (1833). Either part of or the entire prolabium can be advanced, depending on the nasolabial relationships. Gillies and Kilner (1932), McIndoe and Rees (1959), and Potter (1954) likewise adopted and used this technique. Lexer (1931) modified the Gensoul V-Y advancement by adding incisions in the nasal floor, which, after advancement of the prolabium into the columella, allowed narrowing of the nostril sill. A midline approximation of the medial crura was also performed. Blair and Letterman

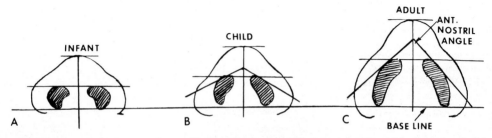

Figure 56–105. The nostril changes shape with age. The angle that the caudal portion of the lateral wall of the nostril makes with the septal plane is called the anterior nostril angle (ANA). The angle is approximately 90 degrees in the infant *(A),* approximately 60 degrees in the child *(B),* and approximately 45 degrees in the adult *(C).* (Redrawn from Pigott, R. W., and Millard, D. R.: Correction of the bilateral cleft lip nasal deformity. *In* Grabb, W. C., Rosenstein, S. W., and Bzoch, K. R. (Eds.): Cleft Lip and Palate. Boston, Little, Brown & Company, 1971.)

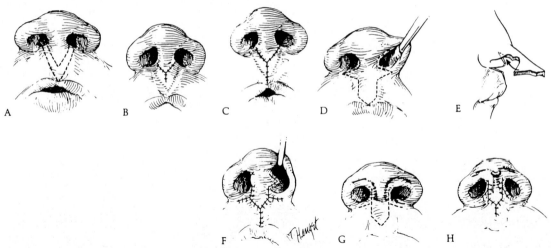

Figure 56–106. Various methods of lengthening the columella based on the V-Y principle. *A* to *C,* Lengthening of the columella with simple upward V-Y advancement of either part of the prolabium *(B)* or the entire prolabium *(C)* (after Gensoul, Lexer, and Joseph). *D* to *F,* Lateral wings taken from a long upper lip (after Brown and McDowell and Blair). Mobilization of the flap and cut-back site *(E)* into the membranous septum. After closure *(F).* *G, H,* Lexer modified the Gensoul V-Y advancement by adding incisions in the nasal floor. Advancement of the central prolabium to lengthen the columella is followed by mobilization of the nasal floor and midline approximation of the medial crura and lower lateral cartilages *(H).* (From Cronin, T. D., and Upton, J.: Lengthening of the short columella associated with bilateral cleft lip. Ann. Plast. Surg., *1*:75, 1978.)

(1950) advanced the prolabium as a "trefoil" with lateral wings harvested from the long upper lip (Fig. 56–107A). The lateral extensions were placed in relaxing incisions in the membranous septum to provide length to the nose and to reduce the overall lip length. As a secondary procedure to the trefoil technique, Blair and Letterman (1950) used a V-Y design in the nasal tip to achieve additional advancement and tip refinement (Fig. 56–107B). Erich and Kragh (1959) designed a similar stellate flap with lateral extensions involving the prolabium to lengthen the columella and shorten the upper lip. The specific indication was deformities that occurred after primary repairs, including transfer of lateral lip elements beneath the prolabium. Closure of the lip unfortunately resulted in T-shaped vertical scar. Brown and McDowell (1941) reduced the lateral wings of the trefoil pattern by reducing the amount of vertical lip shortening. These techniques were criticized by Peskova and Fara (1960); the amount of columellar lengthening was slight, and a third vertical scar was added.

Advancement of the entire prolabium into the columella was first described by Dupuytren (1833). This was accompanied by excision of the premaxilla and direct closure of the lip. Von Deilen (1952), Musgrave (1961), Converse (1964), Converse, Hogan, and Du-

puis (1970), Malik (1974), and Millard (1974) advocated advancement of the prolabium into the columella combined with an Abbé flap to reconstruct the prolabium (Fig. 56–108). This technique is appropriate for the secondary lip deformity caused by overexcision of the prolabium at the primary procedure, with a resulting tight upper lip, short columella, and maxillary hypoplasia. Converse, Hogan, and Barton (1977) also recommended insertion of a cantilevered iliac bone graft to maintain nasal tip projection.

Secondary bilateral fork flap columellar lengthening was described by Millard (1955) and subsequently by Peskova and Fara (1960), Burian (1967), Stark and Kaplan (1973), and Wray (1976). Peskova and Fara (1960) modified Millard's (1955) design by including lateral wings to fill the cutback incisions in the membranous septum. In secondary lip deformities with adequate width vertical "forks" of scar or excess prolabium are elevated and advanced, with the columella undermined to the nasal tip. Millard (1974) described a two-stage fork flap procedure in which the flaps are banked in the nostril sills at the primary lip repair and advanced into the columella secondarily (Figs. 56–109, 56–110). A criticism of the fork flap technique is the presence of multiple, vertical scars in the columella, which

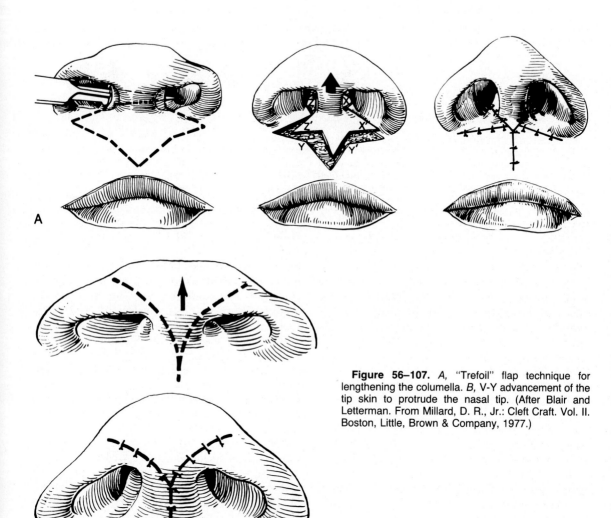

A

B

Figure 56–107. *A,* "Trefoil" flap technique for lengthening the columella. *B,* V-Y advancement of the tip skin to protrude the nasal tip. (After Blair and Letterman. From Millard, D. R., Jr.: Cleft Craft. Vol. II. Boston, Little, Brown & Company, 1977.)

Figure 56–108. Advancement of the prolabium into the columella with augmentation of the upper lip using an Abbé flap. *A,* Defect left in the central portion of the upper lip after the Gensoul V-Y advancement and outline of the Abbé flap. *B,* Transfer of the lower lip flap. *C,* Division of the flap after two weeks. (From Cronin, T. D., and Upton, J.: Lengthening of the short columella associated with bilateral cleft lip. Ann. Plast. Surg., *1:*75, 1978.)

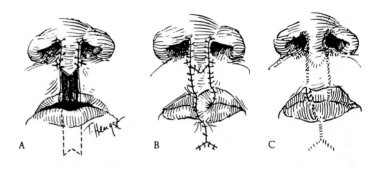

rarely gives a favorable esthetic result. In addition, there may be problems with the vascularity of the flap tips. The use of bilateral vertical flaps from the upper lip with rotation of the columellar base as a secondary procedure has been described by Marcks, Trevaskis, and Payne (1957) and Trauner and Trauner (1967). The latter based two philtral flaps superiorly, rotated them 90 degrees, and sutured them in the midline to create a new columellar base. Marcks, Trevaskis, and Payne (1957) transposed (crisscrossed) similarly designed flaps one over the other (Fig. 56–111).

Skoog (1965) and Wynn (1960) crisscrossed vertical flaps across the midline for lengthening of the columella during the primary repair. Trauner (1956), as part of an initial repair, developed vertical superiorly based flaps from the lateral lip segments to create a new columellar base. This technique gives only minimal lengthening and is now rarely if ever used.

In bilateral cleft lips after adequate muscle and mucosa repair with satisfactory scars, little tissue is available to lengthen the columella without using lip tissue. Columellar lengthening with tissue from the nasal floor was described by Carter (1919), Kazanjian

(1939), Barsky (1950), and Converse (1957) (Fig. 56–112). Wide nasal floor flaps were elevated as bilateral unipedicle flaps based on the columella and were sutured together to provide columellar advancement. The defects in the nostril floors were closed by medial advancement of the alar bases. Cronin (1958) described a refinement of the technique using bilateral, bipedicled flaps that included columellar base, nostril floor, and alar base; the technique simultaneously corrected the alar flaring, the wide nostril floor, and the short columella (Fig. 56–113). If adequate columellar lengthening is not obtained by the first advancement, the procedure can be repeated many months later. Gorney and Rosenberg (1979) modified Cronin's (1958) technique by rotating skin and mucoperiosteum upward and placing a cartilage strut graft for support. The nasal dorsum and tip were used for columellar lengthening, and this procedure was combined with a prolabial V-Y advancement by Blair and Letterman (1950) (Fig. 56–114). Brauer and Foerster (1966) recommended the method to avoid encircling the prolabium with scar (Fig. 56–115). The modified Gillies and Millard (1957) gull-wing technique included external and vestibular incisions along the alae and the

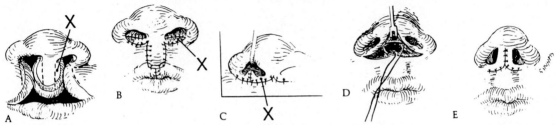

Figure 56–109. Storage of fork flaps after bilateral cleft lip repair or revision with advancement of the nasal tip and lengthening of the columella. *A,* Incisions for the upper lip repair. X denotes the flap to be banked. *B,* Flaps trimmed from the prolabium are banked across the nasal floor (after Duffy). *C,* Flaps positioned as "praying hands" (after Millard). *D, E,* At a second stage, the tissues preserved in the floor of the nose are advanced to lengthen the columella (after Cronin). (From Cronin, T. D., and Upton, J.: Lengthening of the short columella associated with bilateral cleft lip. Ann. Plast. Surg., *1:*75, 1978.)

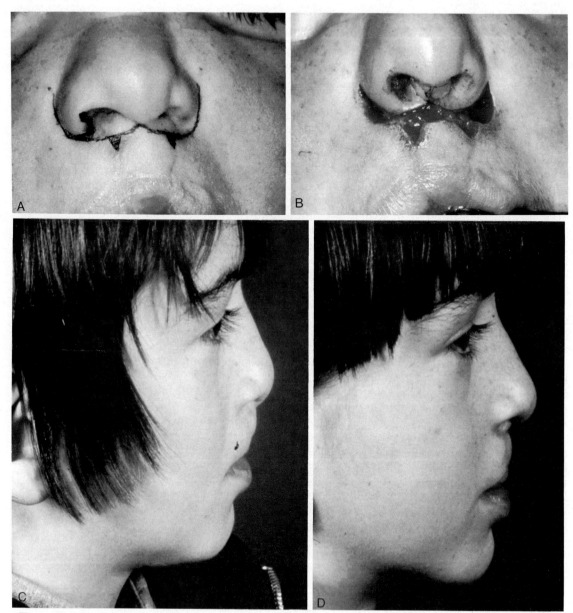

Figure 56–110. Columellar lengthening by bucket handle flaps (see Fig. 56–113). *A,* Cronin rotation design. *B,* Advancement of bucket handle flaps with lengthening of the columella. *C,* Preoperative appearance. *D,* Postoperative appearance after Cronin flap rotation.

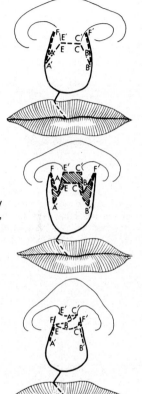

Figure 56–111. Lengthening of the columella using crisscrossed fork flaps, either vertically or transversely in the columella. (After Marcks, Trevaskis, and Payne. From Millard, D. R., Jr.; Cleft Craft. Vol. II. Boston, Little, Brown & Company, 1977.)

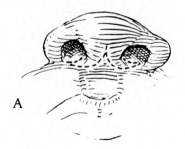

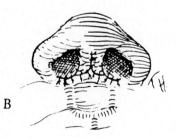

A

B

Figure 56–112. Lengthening of the columella using flaps from the nostril sill region. *A,* Bilateral flaps raised from the nasal floor and advanced. *B,* After closure. (From Cronin, T. D., and Upton, J.; Lengthening of the short columella associated with bilateral cleft lip. Ann. Plast. Surg., *1*:75, 1978.)

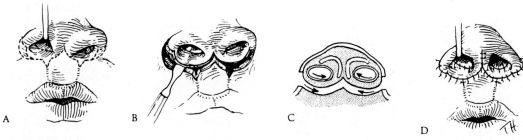

Figure 56–113. Bilateral Cronin advancement flaps for columellar lengthening (see Figure 56–110). *A,* Incisions produce the bipedicle flaps and half-thickness alar wedge excisions and V-excisions in scars of the upper lip. *B,* The flap in the vestibular floor is undermined down to the nasal spine medially. *C,* Cross section of flaps. Arrows indicate the direction of rotation toward the nasal tip. *D,* After advancement and closure. (From Cronin, T. D., and Upton, J.: Lengthening of the short columella associated with bilateral cleft lip. Ann. Plast. Surg., *1*:75, 1978.)

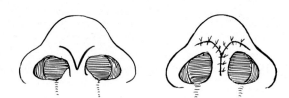

Figure 56–114. V-Y advancement of the tip for columella augmentation. (After Blair and Letterman.)

Figure 56–115. Bilateral alar wing flaps to lengthen the columella. (Gillies and Millard technique; after Brauer and Foerster.)

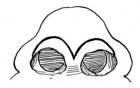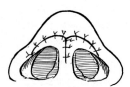

nasal tip to raise essentially a columellar-alar margin flap resembling the fluked tail of a whale (Fig. 56–116). Suturing the flaps together raised and narrowed the nasal tip. This procedure lengthened the columella but often produced a hanging columella effect that usually improved with time but often required secondary revision by excising a portion of the membranous septum. Ecker (1981) further modified the nasal tip V-Y advancement. These techniques have merit when minimal lip is available for columellar lengthening. The nostril floors are narrowed, and the alar bases are brought into better position. As with all external approaches to the nose, scarring may detract from the esthetic result.

Modifications and rearrangements of the columella and nasal dome have been recommended to lengthen the columella; these include the diamond-shaped skin excision of Blair and Letterman (1950) at the junction of the nasal tip and columella, which on closure also narrowed the tip. Inverted V-Y patterns advancing the nasal dorsum into the columella were described by Ombrédanne and Ombrédanne (1928), Dieffenbach (1952), Morel-Fatio and Lalardrie (1966), and Edgerton, Lewis, and McKnelly (1967). Ombrédanne and Ombrédanne's (1928) incisions across the alar-columellar area detract significantly from the esthetic result.

Straith (1946) and Straith, Straith, and Lawson (1957) obtained apparent columellar lengthening by the use of Z-plasties in the nostril apex, but there was a fair amount of noticeable external scarring. However, no true lengthening was obtained by this procedure.

The use of distant tissue to augment the columella was first described by König (1902), Dupertuis (1946), and Musgrave (1961), who transplanted composite grafts of ear lobule to the columellar base (Fig. 56–117). Helical rim was transplanted by Brown and Cannon (1946) and Meade (1959). Pegram (1954) elongated the columella by means of a graft from the alar base, the latter being resected for correction of flaring nostrils. Composite grafts have been useful to gain additional length of the columella in patients with otherwise satisfactory relationships of lip, nasal tip, and alae.

The optimal columellar lengthening procedure should be selected according to the particular nasolabial deformity. If the nasal floor tissue is deficient and especially if resection of lip scar tissue is indicated, the Millard (1968) fork flap technique or the Gensoul (1833) V-Y advancement flap is suitable for lengthening the columella. Satisfactory lip scars and a deficient nostril floor suggest the advisability of either the Brauer and Foerster (1966) procedure (flaps from the nasoalar margins) or an ear lobule graft. Advancement of the prolabium into the columella for lengthening combined with an Abbé flap for upper lip reconstruction is indicated by a deficient upper lip that is unable to yield donor tissue. Cronin's (1958) nostril sill advancement requires adequate upper lip and nasal floor tissue; in addition, the flaring alar bases and wide nostrils are corrected. Converse, Hogan, and Barton (1977) described a technique for correction of the flaring nostrils, exclusive of the columella (Fig. 56–118). A continuous incision from the lateral portion of the alar base is extended circumferentially into the floor of the nasal vestibule. A wedge-shaped flap is created in the nostril sill area, and the incision is extended medially, and then inferiorly on the upper aspect of the philtral ridge. The alae is freed at its base and is transposed with the nasal floor wedge. The flaps are sutured in the new position, with the residual lateral defect being closed by the V-Y technique.

Secondary revision of the nasal deformity, which fortunately is usually symmetric, should be performed during the preschool years. Salyer (1986) performed a Cronin (1958) type of secondary revision in patients

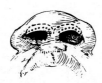

Figure 56–116. Alar margin flaps based medially and inferiorly on the columella like a fluked tail of a whale are sutured in the midline to gain columellar length and tip protrusion. *Left,* Outline of incisions in the skin *(dashed lines)* and in the vestibule *(dotted lines)* (after Brauer). *Center,* Elevation of flaps. *Right,* Closure in midline. (From Cronin, T. D., and Upton, J.: Lengthening of the short columella associated with bilateral cleft lip. Ann. Plast. Surg., *1:*75, 1978.)

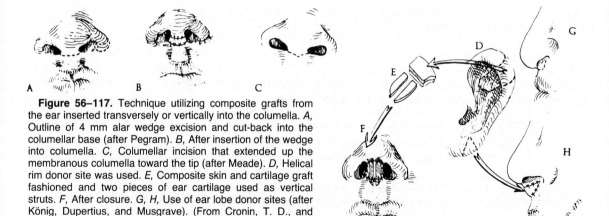

Figure 56–117. Technique utilizing composite grafts from the ear inserted transversely or vertically into the columella. *A,* Outline of 4 mm alar wedge excision and cut-back into the columellar base (after Pegram). *B,* After insertion of the wedge into columella. *C,* Columellar incision that extended up the membranous columella toward the tip (after Meade). *D,* Helical rim donor site was used. *E,* Composite skin and cartilage graft fashioned and two pieces of ear cartilage used as vertical struts. *F,* After closure. *G, H,* Use of ear lobe donor sites (after König, Dupertius, and Musgrave). (From Cronin, T. D., and Upton, J.: Lengthening of the short columella associated with bilateral cleft lip. Ann. Plast. Surg., *1*:75, 1978.)

2 to 3 years of age to increase the amount of nasal soft tissue. The fragile alar cartilages must remain attached to mucosa or skin, and at this age they can make surgical manipulation difficult. Improvement of midface skeletal support and contour by correction of a hypoplastic maxilla generally increases nasal projection. Advancement and suture of the orbicularis oris muscle beneath the prolabium relaxes and augments the midportion of the upper lip in secondary as well as primary repairs.

The most satisfactory method of bilateral cleft nasal correction is the midline prolabial flap (Fig. 56–119). The vertical incisions continue upward on both sides of the prolabium and around and inside the alar rim. The lip, the columella, and the nasal skin are widely dissected to expose the lower lateral cartilage. Soft tissue is excised from between and over the cartilages. The alar cartilages are dissected from the mucosa until they are based on the medial crura. The cartilages are scored at the projected site of the dome, and they are sutured together with 5-0 nylon; if necessary the nasal tip is augmented with a conchal cartilage graft. The lip tissue is advanced into the columella, and the incisions are closed. The procedure achieves nasal tip projection, columellar lengthening, transverse tightening of the upper part of the lip, and lengthening of the central lip (Fig. 56–120).

Deformities of Bilateral Cleft Palate

Bilateral complete clefts of the primary and secondary palates are the most severe malformations among the common cleft anomalies. Particular features characterizing complete bilateral clefts include the following: (1) a frequent incidence of oronasal fistulas after primary palatal repair, (2) a greater deficiency of bony and soft tissue, (3) a protruded premaxilla from the midline, and (4) persistent mobility of the premaxilla (Bergland and associates, 1986). Palatal fistulas in bilateral clefts, although they may occur more frequently, are treated similarly to those accompanying unilateral cleft palate deformities (see above under Palatal Fistula). Increased cleft widths and greater scarring from mobilization of the mucoperiosteum may be encountered in repair of the bilateral cleft pal-

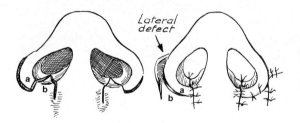

Figure 56–118. Correction of the wide flaring nostrils. *A,* Flap *b* is raised from the floor of the nasal vestibule. An incision frees the alar base. *B,* The alar base flap is rotated and the resulting defect is repaired by the transposition of flap *b* and a V-Y closure.

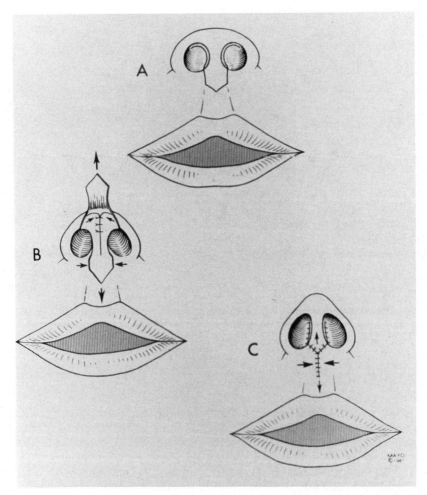

Figure 56–119. Central lip flap for columellar lengthening. *A,* Design of the incisions. Note the position of incisions on the columella and inside the alar rims. *B,* Lip-columellar flap elevated to expose the lower lateral cartilages. The latter are dissected out and placed in correct position. *C,* Flap replaced in an advanced position and the lip sutured. (From Jackson, I. T.: Cleft lip and palate. *In* Mustardé, J. C., and Jackson, I. T. (Eds.): Plastic Surgery in Infancy and Childhood. 3rd Ed. Edinburgh, Churchill Livingstone, 1988.)

ate as compared with correction of the unilateral cleft. Wide mobilization and secure two-layer closure with bone grafting of the anterior palate area are the guiding principles.

ALVEOLAR CLEFTS AND PREMAXILLARY PROTRUSION

The growth pattern of the premaxilla in bilateral clefts differs significantly from that of the normal premaxilla. Excessive anterior growth of the premaxilla occurs in utero owing to lack of restraint by the lateral nasal

processes, especially if the clefts are complete (see Chap. 48). A protrusive maxilla at birth is the result. The position of the premaxilla in bilateral cleft lip and palate is further reflected by the excessive bony deposition at the vomeropremaxillary junction according to Pruzansky (1971), Latham (1977), and Friede and Morgan (1976). Of all the features of the complete bilateral cleft, the excessive and asymmetric projection of the premaxilla, freed from attachment to the lateral segments, presents the dominating challenge. It can prevent lip closure, except with undue tension. Repositioning of the premaxilla has

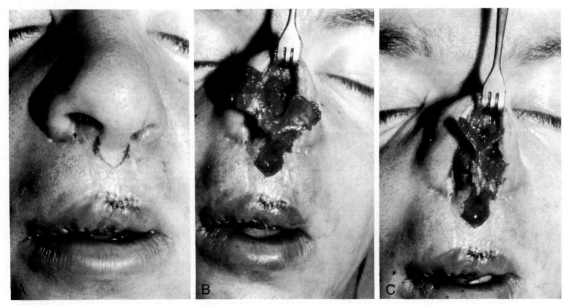

Figure 56–120. Columellar lengthening by a midline flap (see Fig. 56–119). *A,* Design of flap. *B,* Lower lateral cartilages being dissected out. *C,* Suturing of the lower lateral cartilages in the midline.

been attempted with compression bands, head caps, and strapping. The mobility of the premaxilla and the rapid growth of the infant often allow rapid posterior movement, which may result in collapse of the lateral segments, a phenomenon that limits further posterior movement of the premaxilla. Brauer, Cronin, and Reaves (1962) found that the elastic band technique of applying continuous pressure to the projecting premaxilla with a removable dental appliance can achieve alignment of the arch within three weeks, allowing definitive lip repair. Millard (1976) had a similar experience but noted that in Kilner's cases approximately 90 per cent of these attempts resulted in collapse of the lateral segments and trapping of the premaxilla in an anterior position. Skeletal traction applied through interosseous K-wires, expansion screws (Harkins 1958), or coaxial cable devices (Georgiade and Latham, 1975) have also been used to correct the protruding premaxilla.

Excision of the premaxilla results in severe maxillary retrusion and absence of the maxillary incisors, and it is no longer practiced.

Premaxillary set-back had many advocates (Huffman and Lierle, 1949; Cronin, 1957, 1964; Monroe, 1965) and is currently performed in patients aged 5 to 6 years old by Bardach and Salyer (1987c) if orthodontic treatment begun at 3 to 4 years of age has been unsuccessful. In Bardach and Salyer's

(1987c) experience elimination of the vomeropremaxillary suture with proper orthodontic care does not adversely affect anteroposterior facial growth and development. Bergland and associates (1986b) and Vargervik (1983) reported severe maxillary retrusion with surgical set-back of the premaxilla. In a followup study of patients with bilateral clefts Vargervik (1983) reported that the protuberant premaxilla's growth rate from age 4 years to adulthood is only one-half of that in noncleft controls. At age 12 years, the premaxilla is nearly in line with the remaining alveolar arch because of a decelerated growth rate. Ortiz-Monasterio and associates (1966) reported a relatively normal growth of the cleft skeleton in nonoperated clefts and supported the above observations.

Direct surgical manipulation of the premaxilla has been supplanted for the most part by orthodontic therapy and secondary bone grafting (Jackson, 1972a; Hotz and Gnoinski, 1976; Abyholm, Bergland, and Semb, 1981; Bergland, Semb, and Abyholm, 1986a; Bergland and associates, 1986b). Burston (1958) and McNeil (1964) introduced neonatal maxillary orthodontic treatment that aligns the collapsed lateral segments and the protruding maxilla. They used removable appliances to expand the lateral segments and mold the premaxilla into the alveolar arch. The appliances were fitted during the

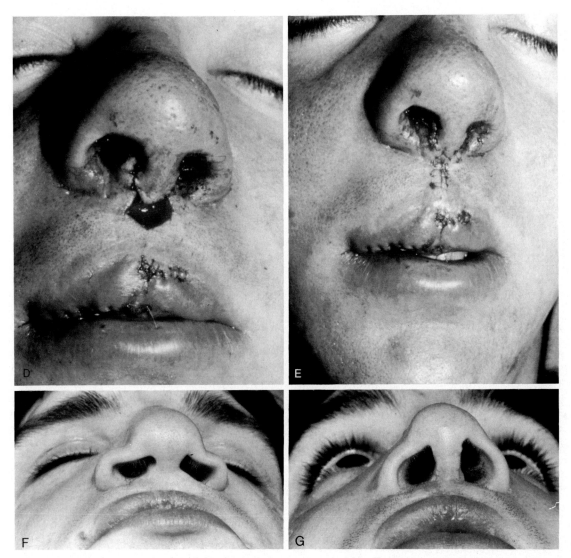

Figure 56–120 *Continued D,* Columellar flap returned to new position. *E,* Closure of the columella and lip. *F,* Preoperative appearance. *G,* Postoperative result. (*A to E,* from Jackson, I. T.: Cleft lip and palate. *In* Mustardé, J. C., and Jackson, I. T. (Eds.): Plastic Surgery in Infancy and Childhood. 3rd Ed. Edinburgh, Churchill Livingstone, 1988.)

first week of life unless other complicating congenital or medical problems existed. The main objective of neonatal orthodontic therapy is to adjust the alveolar arch into reasonable alignment and allow definitive lip closure without undue tension. Long-term follow-up of patients with clefts treated with neonatal maxillary orthodontic techniques reveals little beneficial effect on malocclusion at age 10 years, especially if the patients were bone grafted primarily (Jolleys and Robertson, 1972). This treatment is not now generally considered an essential component of

rehabilitation. However, in wide clefts satisfactory segment alignment can make for technically easier lip repair (Vig and Turvey, 1985). It does not, however, obviate the need for or extent of later orthodontic treatment.

Initiation of orthodontic treatment when all deciduous teeth have erupted (approximately 3 years of age) is recommended by Coccaro (1969) and Coccaro and Valauri (1977) (see also Chap. 57). The advantages of early treatment are believed to be in the areas of function, esthetics, speech, and improved anatomic relationships (Coccaro,

1984). However, orthodontic therapy in the deciduous phase does not necessarily prevent the development of malocclusion or crossbite (Derischsweiler, 1964; Pruzansky and Aduss, 1967). It is probably of little value apart from correcting a reversed incisor relationship or preparing the maxillary arch for bone grafting.

Primary or early bone grafting in bilateral cleft lip and palate has the same advantages as in the unilateral situation (namely, promotion of tooth eruption and closure of alveolar clefts), but has the same disadvantage (i.e., growth inhibition). A specific indication for bone grafting in the bilateral cleft is persistent premaxillary mobility. Before bone grafting, stabilization of the premaxilla can be achieved by insertion of a bridge appliance extending from canine to canine with prosthetic replacement of any missing teeth.

As in unilateral cleft repair, secondary bone grafting is the preferred technique to avoid growth interruption and to enhance tooth development and stability (see Chap. 55). Presurgical orthodontic treatment to align the maxillary segments and premaxilla is begun during the period of mixed dentition, especially the stage of canine eruption. Alveolar bone grafting allows the natural teeth to erupt into the cleft area.

Alveolar bone grafting in bilateral clefts is similar to that performed in unilateral clefts. However, the procedure is technically more difficult. Because medial and lateral flaps must be used to reconstruct the nasal floor, the lateral aspect of the fistula is a donor site, and on the medial aspect large bilateral flaps are taken from the premaxilla and the septal stalk. Bilateral buccal mucosal flaps may be necessary to obtain a secure oral lining closure in large defects, since there may not be sufficient gingiva. If possible, however, gingival flaps are preferred. Postoperative stabilization of the maxilla with a splint for three months is essential to maintain the premaxilla in position until the bone grafts have healed. The goal of later orthodontic treatment is to make final adjustments of the dental occlusion; this can usually be accomplished within six to eight months (Vig and Turvey, 1985).

OSTEOTOMIES

Prominence of the premaxilla in bilateral cleft lip and palate patients is present throughout childhood but gradually disappears as the growth rate of the mandible and lateral maxillary segments exceeds that of the premaxilla by a factor of almost two after age 4 years (Narula and Ross, 1970; Friede and Pruzansky, 1972; Vargervik, 1983). In the young adult with bilateral cleft lip and palate, retrusion of the midface is a more common finding than premaxillary protrusion.

Comparison of the craniofacial morphologic features of unilateral and bilateral clefts in adults by Dahl (1970) showed only a few differences. Maxillary length was greater in bilateral clefts compared with unilateral clefts, a finding demonstrating absence of growth retardation of the maxillary complex in the bilateral deformity. Surgical advancement of the maxilla by Le Fort I osteotomies was rarely necessary in bilateral clefts in Vargervik's (1983) experience, provided a satisfactory lip and palate repair, secondary bone grafting, and pre- and postsurgical orthodontic therapy were carried out. The presence of one or more of the following factors may indicate osteotomies: inherent tissue deficiencies, a premaxillary excision or set-back procedure, aggressive early surgery, inadequate orthodontic therapy, and early bone grafting. These patients may develop maxillary hypoplasia necessitating osteotomies or onlay bone grafts. Many bilateral clefts also are observed in families showing midface hypoplasia or retrusion without clefts. In these patients, maxillary advancement is often necessary. This finding underlines the importance of examining the facial features of family members.

Osteotomies in bilateral cleft lip and palate patients should generally be preceded by bone grafting of the alveolary clefts and fistula closure to stabilize the premaxilla before advancement. Osteotomies are carried out as described above for the unilateral cleft lip and palate deformity.

REFERENCES

Abbé, R.: A new plastic operation for the relief of deformity due to double harelip. Med. Rec. Ann., *53*:477, 1898.

Abyholm, F. E., Bergland, O., and Semb, G.: Secondary bone grafting of alveolar clefts. Scand. J. Plast. Reconstr. Surg., *15*:127, 1981.

Ainamo, J., and Jalari, A.: Eruptive movements of teeth in human adults. *In* Poole, D. F. G., and Stade, M. U.

(Eds.): The Eruption and Occlusion of Teeth. London, Butterworth, 1976.

Albrektsson, T.: Healing of bone grafts: in vivo studies of tissue reactions at osteografting of bone in the rabbit tibia. Thesis, University of Göteborg, 1979.

Ames, J. R., Ryan, D. E., and Maki, K. A.: The autogenous particulate cancellous bone marrow graft in alveolar clefts: a report of forty-one cases. Oral Surg. Oral Med. Oral Pathol., *51*:588, 1981.

Anderl, H.: Simultaneous repair of lip and nose in the unilateral cleft (a long-term report). *In* Jackson, I. T., and Sommerlad, B. (Eds.): Recent Advances in Plastic Surgery. Vol. 3. Edinburgh, Churchill Livingstone, 1985, p. 1.

Ariyan, S., and Krizek, T. J.: A simplified technique for correction of the cleft lip nasal deformity. Ann. Plast. Surg., *1*:568, 1978.

Arons, M. S.: Another method for secondary correction of whistling deformities in bilateral cleft lips. Plast. Reconstr. Surg., *47*:389, 1971.

Avery, J. K.: The nasal capsule in cleft palate. Anat. Anz., *109*:722, 1961.

Axhausen, G.: Technik und Ergebnisse der Lippenplastik. Leipzig, Thieme, 1932.

Bardach, J., and Eisbach, K. J.: The influence of primary unilateral cleft lip repair on facial growth. Cleft Palate J., *14*:88, 1977.

Bardach, J., Morris, H., Olin, W., McDermott-Murray, J., Mooney, M., and Bardach, E.: Late results of multidisciplinary management of unilateral cleft lip and palate. Ann. Plast. Surg., *12*:235, 1984.

Bardach, J., and Salyer, K. E.: Correction of secondary unilateral cleft lip deformities. *In* Bardach, J., and Salyer, K. E.: Surgical Techniques in Cleft Lip and Palate. Chicago, Year Book Medical Publishers, 1987a.

Bardach, J., and Salyer, K. E.: Correction of nasal deformity associated with unilateral cleft lip. *In* Bardach, J., and Salyer, K. E.: Surgical Techniques in Cleft Lip and Palate. Chicago, Year Book Medical Publishers, 1987b.

Bardach, J., and Salyer, K. E.: Bilateral cleft lip repair. *In* Bardach, J., and Salyer, K. E.: Surgical Techniques in Cleft Lip and Palate. Chicago, Year Book Medical Publishers, 1987c.

Bardach, J., and Salyer, K. E.: Correction of bilateral cleft lip deformities. *In* Bardach, J., and Salyer, K. E.: Surgical Techniques in Cleft Lip and Palate. Chicago, Year Book Medical Publishers, 1987d.

Bardach, J., and Salyer, K. E.: Correction of the nasal deformity associated with bilateral cleft lip. *In* Bardach, J., and Salyer, K. E.: Surgical Techniques in Cleft Lip and Palate. Chicago, Year Book Medical Publishers, 1987e.

Bardach, J., and Salyer, K. E.: Cleft palate repair. *In* Bardach, J., and Salyer, K. E.: Surgical Techniques in Cleft Lip and Palate. Chicago, Year Book Medical Publishers, 1987f.

Bardach, J., and Salyer, K. E.: Correction of the skeletal defects in secondary cleft lip and palate deformities. *In* Bardach, J., and Salyer, K. E.: Surgical Techniques in Cleft Lip and Palate. Chicago, Year Book Medical Publishers, 1987g.

Barron, J. N. Cited by Millard, D. R., Jr.: Cleft Craft. Vol. II. Bilateral and Rare Deformities. Boston, Little, Brown & Company, 1977, p. 633.

Barsky, A. J.: Principles and Practice of Plastic Surgery. Baltimore, Williams & Wilkins Company, 1950, p. 243.

Bauer, T. B., Trusler, H. M., and Tondra, J. M.: Changing concepts in the management of bilateral cleft lip deformities. Plast. Reconstr. Surg., *24*:321, 1959.

Bergland, O., Semb, G., and Abyholm, F. E.: Elimination of the residual alveolar cleft by secondary bone grafting and subsequent orthodontic treatment. Cleft Palate J., *23*:175, 1986a.

Bergland, O., Semb, G., Abyholm, F., Borchgrevink, H., and Eskeland, G.: Secondary bone grafting and orthodontic treatment in patients with bilateral complete clefts of the lip and palate. Ann. Plast. Surg., *17*:460, 1986b.

Berkeley, W. T.: The cleft lip nose. Plast. Reconstr. Surg., *23*:567, 1959.

Berkeley, W. T.: Correction of secondary cleft lip nasal deformities. Plast. Reconstr. Surg., *44*:234, 1969.

Bjørk, A., and Skieller, V.: Growth in width of the maxilla studied by the implant method. Scand. J. Plast. Reconstr. Surg., *8*:26, 1974.

Bjørk, A., and Skieller, V.: Postnatal growth and development of the maxillary complex. *In* McNamara, J. A., Jr. (Ed.): Factors Affecting the Growth of the Midface. Ann Arbor, University of Michigan, 1976.

Bjørk, A., and Skieller, V.: Growth of the maxilla in three dimensions as revealed radiographically by the implant method. Br. J. Orthodont., *4*:53, 1977.

Black, D. W.: The cleft lip nose deformity—a definitive repair. Presented at the Annual Meeting of the American Association of Plastic Surgeons, Colorado Springs, 1982.

Blackwell, S. J., Parry, S. W., Roberg, B. C., and Huang, T. T.: Onlay cartilage graft of the alar lateral crus for cleft lip nasal deformities. Plast. Reconstr. Surg., *76*:394, 1985.

Blair, V. P.: Nasal deformities associated with congenital cleft of the lip. J.A.M.A., *84*:185, 1925.

Blair, V. P., and Brown, J. B.: Nasal abnormalities, fancied and real; the reaction of the patient; their attempted correction. Surg. Gynecol. Obstet., *53*:797, 1931.

Blair, V. P., and Letterman, G. S.: The role of the switched lower flap in upper lip reconstructions. Plast. Reconstr. Surg., *5*:1, 1950.

Böhn, A.: Dental anomalies in harelip and cleft palate. Acta Odontol. Scand., *21* (Suppl. 138):1, 1963a.

Böhn, A.: The course of the premaxillary and maxillary vessels and nerves in cleft jaw. Acta Odontol. Scand., *21*:436, 1963b.

Boo-Chai, K., and Tange, I.: The isolated cleft lip nose. Plast. Reconstr. Surg., *41*:28, 1968.

Borchgrevink, H. H. C.: The rotation-advancement operation of Millard as applied to secondary cleft lip deformities. Cleft Palate J., *7*:161, 1970.

Boyne, P. J.: Use of marrow-cancellous bone in maxillary, alveolar and palatal clefts. J. Dent. Res., *53*:821, 1974.

Boyne, P. J., and Sands, N. R.: Secondary bone grafting of residual alveolar and palatal clefts. J. Oral Surg., *30*:87, 1972.

Boyne, P. J., and Sands, N. R.: Combined orthodontic-surgical management of residual palato-alveolar cleft defects. Am. J. Orthodont., *70*:20, 1976.

Bralley, R. C., and Schoeny, Z. G.: Effects of maxillary advancement on speech of a submucosal cleft palate patient. Cleft Palate J., *14*:98, 1977.

Brånemark, P. I., Adell, R., Breine, U., Hansson, B. O., Lindstrom, J., and Ohlsson, A.: Intraosseous anchorage of dental prostheses: experimental studies. Scand. J. Plast. Reconstr. Surg., *3*:81, 1969.

Brånemark, P. I., Hansson, B. O., Adell, R., Breine, U.,

Lindstrom, J., et al.: Osseointegrated implants in the treatment of the edentulous jaw: experience from a 10-year period. Scand. J. Plast. Reconstr. Surg., *16* (Suppl.):1, 1977.

Brauer, R. O., Cronin, T. D., and Reaves, E. L.: Early maxillary orthopedics, orthodontia and alveolar bone grafting in complete clefts of the palate. Plast. Reconstr. Surg., *29*:625, 1962.

Brauer, R. O., and Foerster, D. W.: Another method to lengthen the columella in the double cleft patient. Plast. Reconstr. Surg., *38*:27, 1966.

Braun, T. W., and Sotereanos, G. C.: Orthognathic and secondary cleft reconstruction of adolescent patients with cleft palate. J. Oral Surg., *38*:425, 1980.

Braun, T. W., and Sotereanos, G. C.: Orthognathic surgical reconstruction of cleft palate deformities in adolescents. J. Oral Surg., *39*:255, 1981.

Briedis, J., and Jackson, I. T.: The anatomy of the philtrum: observations made on dissections in the normal lip. Br. J. Plast. Surg., *34*:128, 1981.

Broadbent, T. R.: The badly scarred bilateral cleft lip: total resurfacing. Plast. Reconstr. Surg., *20*:485, 1957.

Broadbent, T. R., and Woolf, R. M.: Cleft lip nasal deformity. Ann. Plast. Surg., *12*:216, 1984.

Brown, J. B., and Cannon, B.: Composite free grafts of skin and cartilage from the ear. Surg. Gynecol. Obstet., *82*:253, 1946.

Brown, J. B., and McDowell, F.: Secondary repair of cleft lips and their nasal deformities. Ann. Surg., *114*:101, 1941.

Brown, R. F.: A reappraisal of the cleft lip nose with the report of a case. Br. J. Plast. Surg., *17*:168, 1964.

Buck, G.: Case report of series of plastic procedures for restoration of right upper lip and adjacent parts of the cheek and nose. Trans. Med. Soc. N.Y., 1864, p. 173.

Burian, F.: Chir rozstepu vty a patra. Cited by Denecke, H. J., and Meyer, R. (Eds.): Plastic Surgery of the Head and Neck. Vol. I: Corrective and Reconstructive Rhinoplasty. New York, Springer-Verlag, 1967.

Burston, W. R.: The early treatment of cleft palate conditions. Dent. Pract. (Bristol), *9*:41, 1958.

Cardoso, A. D.: A new technique for harelip. Plast. Reconstr. Surg., *10*:92, 1952.

Carter, W. W. Cited by Davis, J. S.: Plastic Surgery, Its Principles and Practice. Philadelphia, Blakiston, 1919, p. 492.

Chait, L. A.: The "C" costal cartilage graft in reconstruction of the unilateral cleft lip nose. Br. J. Plast. Surg., *34*:169, 1981.

Clifford, R. H., and Pool, R., Jr.: The analysis of the anatomy and geometry of the unilateral cleft lip. Plast. Reconstr. Surg., *24*:311, 1959.

Climo, M. S.: Diastasis of the orbicularis oris muscle in repaired unilateral clefts of the lip. Cleft Palate J., *6*:316, 1969.

Coccaro, P. J.: Orthodontics in cleft palate children: a continuing process. Cleft Palate J., *6*:495, 1969.

Coccaro, P. J.: Orthodontic treatment in craniofacial anomalies. *In* Serafin, D., and Georgiade, N. G. (Eds.): Pediatric Plastic Surgery. St. Louis, MO, C. V. Mosby Company, 1984.

Coccaro, P. J., and Valauri, A. J.: Orthodontics in cleft lip and palate children. *In* Converse, J. M. (Ed.): Reconstructive Plastic Surgery. 2nd Ed. Philadelphia, W. B. Saunders Company, 1977.

Converse, J. M.: Corrective surgery of the nasal tip. Laryngoscope, *67*:16, 1957.

Converse, J. M.: Reconstructive Plastic Surgery. Philadelphia, W. B. Saunders Company, 1964.

Converse, J. M.: Correction of the drooping lateral portion of the cleft lip following the LeMesurier repair. Plast. Reconstr. Surg., *55*:507, 1975.

Converse, J. M., Hogan, V. M., and Barton, F. E.: Secondary deformities of cleft lip, cleft lip and nose, and cleft palate. *In* Converse, J. M. (Ed.): Reconstructive Plastic Surgery. 2nd Ed. Philadelphia, W. B. Saunders Company, 1977.

Converse, J. M., Hogan, V. M., and Dupuis, C. C.: Combined nose-lip repair in bilateral complete cleft lip deformities. Plast. Reconstr. Surg., *45*:109, 1970.

Cosman, B., and Crikelair, G. F.: The reconstruction of the unilateral cleft lip nasal deformity. Cleft Palate J., *2*:95, 1965.

Cosman, B., and Crikelair, G. F.: Release of the prolabium in the bilateral cleft lip. Cleft Palate J., *3*:122, 1966.

Crikelair, G. F., Ju, D. M. C., and Symonds, F. C.: A method for alar plasty in cleft lip nasal deformities. Plast. Reconstr. Surg., *24*:588, 1959.

Cronin, T. D.: Surgery of the double cleft lip and protruding premaxilla. Plast. Reconstr. Surg., *19*:389, 1957.

Cronin, T. D.: Lengthening columella by use of skin from nasal floor and alae. Plast. Reconstr. Surg., *21*:417, 1958.

Cronin, T. D.: The bilateral cleft lip with bilateral cleft of the primary palate. *In* Converse, J. M. (Ed.): Reconstructive Plastic Surgery. Philadelphia, W. B. Saunders Company, 1964.

Cronin, T. D., and Upton, J.: Lengthening of the short columella associated with bilateral cleft lip. Ann. Plast. Surg., *1*:75, 1978.

Dahl, E.: Craniofacial morphology in congenital clefts of the lip and palate. An x-ray cephalometric study of young adult males. Acta Odontol. Scand., *28* (Suppl. 57):11, 1970.

De Kleine, E. H.: Nasal tip reconstruction through external incisions. Plast. Reconstr. Surg., *15*:502, 1955.

Delaire, J.: La cheilo rhinoplastie primaire pour fente labio maxillaire congenitale unilaterale. Essai de schematisation d'une technique. Rev. Stomatol., *76*:193, 1975.

Delaire, J., and Prechious, B.: Balanced facial growth: a schematic interpretation. Oral Surg. Oral Med. Oral Pathol., *63*:637, 1987.

Denecke, H. J., and Meyer, R. (Eds.): Plastic Surgery of the Head and Neck. Vol. I: Corrective and Reconstructive Rhinoplasty. New York, Springer-Verlag, 1967.

DePalma, A. T., Leavitt, L. A., and Hardy, S. B.: Electromyography in full thickness flaps rotated between upper and lower lips. Plast. Reconstr. Surg., *21*:449, 1958.

Derichsweiler, H.: Early orthodontic treatment of cleft palate patients as related to the prevention of jaw anomalies. *In* Hotz, R. (Ed.): Early Treatment of Cleft Lip and Palate. Proceedings of an International Symposium, University of Zürich Dental Institute, April 1964. Bern, Hans Huber, 1964, p. 132.

Dibbell, D. G.: A cartilaginous columellar strut in cleft lip rhinoplasties. Br. J. Plast. Surg., *29*:247, 1976.

Dibbell, D. G.: Cleft lip nasal reconstruction: correcting the classic unilateral defect. Plast. Reconstr. Surg., *69*:264, 1982.

Dieffenbach, J. F.: Technik und Ergebnisse der Spaltplastiken. München, Hauser, 1952.

Drachter, R.: Die Gaumenspalte und deren operative Behandlung. Dtsch. Z. Chir., *131*:1, 1914.

Drommer, R., and Luhr, H. G.: Chirurgische Massnahmen bei erwachsenen Spaltpatienten mit extremen Gesichtsdeformierungen und nach Resektion des Zwischenkiefers im Säuglingsalter. Dtsch. Zahnärtzl. Z., 36:191, 1981.

Duffy, M. M.: Restoration of orbicularis oris muscle continuity in the repair of bilateral cleft lip. Br. J. Plast. Surg., 47:321, 1971.

Dupertuis, S. M.: Free ear lobe grafts of skin and fat. Plast. Reconstr. Surg., 1:135, 1946.

Dupuytren, G. (par L. Marx): Observation sur une restauration du nez. J. Hebd. Med. Chir. Practique, 12:29, 1833.

Ecker, H. A.: A direct approach to the more severely deformed cleft lip nose. Plast. Reconstr. Surg., 67:369, 1981.

Edgerton, M. T., Lewis, C. M., and McKnelly, L. O.: Lengthening of the short nasal columella by skin flaps from the nasal tip and dorsum. Plast. Reconstr. Surg., 40:343, 1967.

Elsahy, N. I.: A new method for correction of cleft lip nasal deformities. Cleft Palate J., 11:214, 1974.

Enemark, H., Krantz-Simonsen, E., and Schramm, J. E.: Secondary bone grafting in unilateral cleft lip palate patients: medications and treatment procedures. Int. J. Oral Surg., 14:2, 1985.

Erich, J. B.: A technique for correcting a flat nostril in cases of repaired harelip. Plast. Reconstr. Surg., 12:320, 1953.

Erich, J. B., and Kragh, L. V.: Technique for lengthening the columella in cases of repaired bilateral harelip. Minn. Med., 42:1592, 1959.

Esser, J. F. S.: Studies in plastic surgery of the face: plastic operations about the mouth. The epidermal inlay. Ann. Surg., 65:297, 1917.

Eskeland, C., Bergland, O., Borchgrevink, H., et al.: Management of the cleft alveolar arch. In Jackson, I. T., and Sommerlad, B. (Eds.): Recent Advances in Plastic Surgery. Edinburgh, Churchill Livingstone, 1985.

Estlander, J. A.: Eine Methode aus der einen Lippe Substanzverluste der anderen zu ersetzen. Arch. Klin. Chir., 14:622, 1872.

Falcone, A. E.: Release of the adherent prolabium and deepening of the labial sulcus in the secondary repair of bilateral cleft lips. Plast. Reconstr. Surg., 38:42, 1966.

Fara, M.: Anatomy and arteriography of cleft lips in stillborn children. Plast. Reconstr. Surg., 42:29, 1968.

Farrior, R. T.: The problem of the unilateral cleft lip nose. Laryngoscope, 72:289, 1962.

Figi, F. A.: The repair of secondary cleft lip and nasal deformity. J. Int. Coll. Surg., 17:297, 1952.

Flanagin, W. S.: Free composite grafts from lower to upper lip. Plast. Reconstr. Surg., 17:376, 1956.

Fogh-Andersen, P.: Inheritance of Harelip and Cleft Palate. Copenhagen, Nyt Nordisk Forlag Arnold Busck, 1942.

Fomon, S., Bell, J. W., and Syracuse, V. R.: Harelip-nose revision. Arch. Otolaryngol., 64:14, 1956.

Fraser, F. C.: Hereditary disorders of the nose and mouth. In Proceedings of the Second International Congress on Human Genetics, 1963, p. 1852.

Fraser, F. C.: Etiology of cleft lip and palate. In Grabb, W. C., Rosenstein, S. W., and Bzoch, K. R. (Eds.): Cleft Lip and Palate. Boston, Little, Brown & Company, 1971.

Freihofer, H. P. M., Jr.: Results after midface osteotomies. J. Maxillofac. Surg., 1:30, 1973.

Friede, H.: Studies of facial morphology and growth in bilateral cleft lip and palate. Thesis, University of Göteborg, 1977.

Friede, H.: The vomero-premaxillary suture—a neglected growth site in midfacial development of unilateral cleft lip and palate patients. Cleft Palate J., 15:398, 1978.

Friede, H., and Johanson, B.: A follow-up study of cleft children treated with primary bone grafting. I. Orthodontic aspects. Scand. J. Plast. Reconstr. Surg., 8:88, 1974.

Friede, H., and Morgan, P.: Growth of the vomero-premaxillary suture in children with bilateral cleft lip and palate. Scand. J. Plast. Reconstr. Surg., 10:45, 1976.

Friede, H., and Pruzansky, S.: Longitudinal study of growth in bilateral cleft lip and palate, from infancy to adolescence. Plast. Reconstr. Surg., 49:392, 1972.

Geiger, S. A., and Wunderlich, E.: Die Position des Eckzahnes bei Spaltpatienten nach früher sekundärer Plastik. Presented at the Sixth Congress of the European Association for Maxillofacial Surgery, Hamburg, 1982.

Gelbke, H.: The nostril problem in unilateral harelips and its surgical management. Plast. Reconstr. Surg., 18:65, 1956.

Gensoul, M.: Reduction of a thickened columella and advancing the point of the nose. J. Hebd. Med. Chir. Practique, 12:29, 1833.

Georgiade, N. G., and Latham, R. A.: Maxillary arch alignment in the bilateral cleft lip and palate infant, using pinned coaxial screw appliance. Plast. Reconstr. Surg., 56:52, 1975.

Gibson, T., and Davis, W. B.: The distortion of autogenous cartilage grafts: its causes and prevention. Br. J. Plast. Surg., 10:257, 1958.

Gillies, H., and Kilner, T. P.: Harelip: operations for the correction of secondary deformities. Lancet, 2:1369, 1932.

Gillies, H., and Millard, D. R., Jr.: The Principles and Art of Plastic Surgery. Boston, Little, Brown & Company, 1957.

Ginestet, J. G. Cited by Millard, D. R., Jr.: Cleft Craft. Vol. I: The Unilateral Deformity. Boston, Little, Brown & Company, 1976.

Ginestet, J. G. Cited by Millard, D. R., Jr.: Cleft Craft. Vol. II: Bilateral and Rare Deformities. Boston, Little, Brown & Company, 1977.

Glover, D. M., and Necomb, M. R.: Bilateral cleft lip repair and the floating premaxilla. Plast. Reconstr. Surg., 28:365, 1961.

Gorney, M., and Falces, E.: Repair of post cleft nasal deformities with gullwing cartilage graft. In Johanson, B. (Ed.): Abstracts of the Second International Congress on Cleft Palate, Copenhagen, 1973.

Gorney, M., and Rosenberg, H. L.: Centripetal rotation-advancement for cleft lip nasal deformities. Ann. Plast. Surg., 2:374, 1979.

Graber, T. M.: An appraisal of the developmental deformities in cleft palate and cleft lip individuals. Quarterly Bulletin of Northwestern University Medical School, 23:153, 1949.

Guerrero-Santos, J.: Use of a tongue flap in secondary correction of cleft lips. Plast. Reconstr. Surg., 44:368, 1969.

Guerrero-Santos, J., and Altamirano, J. T.: The use of lingual flaps in repair of fistulas of the hard palate. Plast. Reconstr. Surg., 38:123, 1966.

Guerrero-Santos, J., Ramirez, M., Castaneda, A., and Torres, A.: Crossed-denuded flap as a complement to the Millard technique in correction of cleft lip. Plast. Reconstr. Surg., *48*:506, 1971.

Hajnisova, M.: Growth of the nose and mouth in children of 6 to 18 years of age. *In* Sanvenero-Rosselli, G., and Boggio-Robutti, G. (Eds.): Transactions of the Fourth International Congress of Plastic and Reconstructive Surgery. Amsterdam, Excerpta Medica, 1967.

Hall, H. D., and Posnick, J. C.: Early results of secondary bone grafts in 106 alveolar clefts. J. Oral Maxillofac. Surg., *41*:289, 1983.

Harkins, C. S.: Retropositioning of the premaxilla with the aid of an expansion prosthesis. Plast. Reconstr. Surg., *22*:67, 1958.

Harvold, E.: Observations on the development of the upper jaw by harelip and cleft palate. Odontol. Tidskr., *55*:289, 1947.

Harvold, E.: Prinsippene fer den kjeveortopediske behandling av overklieven med ensidig total ganespalte. Nor. Tannbegeforen Tid., *59*:395, 1949.

Hellquist, R., Svärdström, K., and Ponten, B.: A longitudinal study of delayed periosteoplasty to the cleft alveolus. Cleft Palate J., *20*:277, 1983.

Henderson, D., and Jackson, I. T.: Nasomaxillary hypoplasia—the Le Fort II osteotomy. Br. J. Oral Surg., *11*:77, 1973.

Henderson, D., and Jackson, I. T.: Combined cleft lip revision, anterior fistula closure, and maxillary osteotomy: a one-stage procedure. Br. J. Oral Surg., *13*:33, 1975.

Herbert, D. C.: Closure of a palatal fistula using a mucoperiosteal island flap. Br. J. Plast. Surg., *27*:332, 1974.

Hogan, V. M., and Converse, J. M.: Secondary deformities of unilateral cleft lip and nose. *In* Grabb, W. C., Rosenstein, S. E., and Bzoch, K. R. (Eds.): Cleft Lip and Palate. Boston, Little, Brown & Company, 1971.

Horton, C. E., Adamson, J. E., Mladick, R. A., and Taddeo, R. J.: The upper lip sulcus in cleft lips. Plast. Reconstr. Surg., *45*:31, 1970.

Hotz, M., and Gnoinski, W.: Comprehensive care of cleft lip and palate children at Zürich University: a preliminary report. Am. J. Orthodont., *70*:481, 1976.

Huffman, W. C., and Lierle, D. M.: Studies on the pathologic anatomy of the unilateral harelip nose. Plast. Reconstr. Surg., *4*:225, 1949.

Hugo, N. E., and Tumbusch, W. T.: Repair of unilateral cleft lip nasal deformities. Cleft Palate J., *8*:257, 1971.

Humby, G.: The nostril in secondary harelip. Lancet, *1*:1275, 1938.

Isaksson, I., Johanson, B., Petersen, I., and Sellden, U.: Electromyographic study of the Abbé and fan flaps. Acta Chir. Scand., *123*:343, 1962.

Isshiki, N., Sawada, M., and Tamura, N.: Correction of alar deformity in cleft lip by marginal incision. Ann. Plast. Surg., *5*:58, 1980.

Jackson, I. T.: Closure of secondary palatal fistulae with intraoral tissue and bone grafting. Br. J. Plast. Surg., *25*:93, 1972a.

Jackson, I. T.: Use of tongue flaps to resurface lip defects and close palatal fistulae in children. Plast. Reconstr. Surg., *49*:537, 1972b.

Jackson, I. T.: The importance of orbicularis oris in cleft lip repair. *In* Johanson, B. (ed.): Abstracts of the Second International Congress on Cleft Palate, Copenhagen, 1973.

Jackson, I. T.: Clefts and jaw deformities. *In* Whitaker, L. A., and Randall, P. (Eds.): Symposium on Reconstruction of Jaw Deformity. St. Louis, MO, C. V. Mosby Company, 1978.

Jackson, I. T.: Suture removal in babies following cleft lip repair (letter). Chir. Plast., *7*:297, 1984.

Jackson, I. T., and Mustardé, J. C.: Cleft lip and palate. *In* Mustardé, J. C., and Jackson, I. T.: Plastic Surgery in Infancy and Childhood. Edinburgh, Churchill Livingstone, 1988.

Jackson, I. T., Munro, I. R., Salyer, K. E., and Whitaker, L. A. (eds.): Atlas of Craniomaxillofacial Surgery. St. Louis, MO, C. V. Mosby Company, 1982a.

Jackson, I. T., Pellett, C., and Smith, J. M.: The skull as a bone graft donor site. Ann. Plast. Surg., *11*:527, 1983.

Jackson, I. T., Schecker, L. R., Vandervord, J. G., and McLennan, J. G.: Bone marrow grafting in the secondary closure of alveolar-palatal defects in children. Br. J. Plast. Surg., *34*:422, 1981.

Jackson, I. T., and Soutar, D. S.: The sandwich Abbé flap in secondary cleft lip deformity. Plast. Reconstr. Surg., *66*:38, 1980.

Jackson, I. T., Vandevord, J. G., McLennan, J. G., Christie, F. B., and McGregor, J. C.: Bone grafting of the secondary cleft lip and palate deformity. Br. J. Plast. Surg., *35*:345, 1982b.

Jackson, M. S., Jackson, I. T., and Christie, F. B.: Improvement in speech following closure of anterior palatal fistulas with bone grafts. Br. J. Plast. Surg., *29*:295, 1976.

Johanson, B., and Ohlsson, A.: Bone grafting and dental orthopedics in primary and secondary cases of cleft lip and palate. Acta Chir. Scand., *122*:112, 1961.

Johanson, B., Ohlsson, A., Friede, H., and Ahlgren, J.: A follow-up study of cleft lip and palate patients treated with orthodontics, secondary bone grafting, and prosthetic rehabilitation. Scand. J. Plast. Reconstr. Surg., *8*:121, 1974.

Johnson, H. A.: A simple method for the repair of minor postoperative cleft lip "whistling" deformity. Br. J. Plast. Surg., *25*:152, 1972.

Johnston, M. C., Hassell, J. R., and Brown, K. S.: The embryology of cleft lip and palate. Clin. Plast. Surg., *2*:195, 1975.

Jolleys, A., and Robertson, R. E.: A study of the effects of early bone grafting in complete clefts of the lip and palate: five-year study. Br. J. Plast. Surg., *25*:229, 1972.

Joos, U.: The importance of muscular reconstruction in the treatment of cleft lip and palate. Scand. J. Plast. Reconstr. Surg., *21*:109, 1987.

Joseph, J.: Nasalplastik und sonstige Gesichtsplastik nebst Mammaplastik. Leipzig, Curt Kabitzsch, 1931.

Juri, J., Juri, C., and de Antueno, J.: A modification of the Kapetansky technique for repair of whistling deformities of the upper lip. Plast. Reconstr. Surg., *57*:70, 1976.

Kapetansky, K. I.: Double pendulum flaps for whistling deformities in bilateral cleft lips. Plast. Reconstr. Surg., *47*:321, 1971.

Kawamoto, H. K., Jr.: Correction of major defects of the vermilion with a cross-lip vermilion flap. Plast. Reconstr. Surg., *64*:315, 1979.

Kazanjian, V. H.: Secondary deformities in cleft palate patients. Ann. Surg., *109*:442, 1939.

Kazanjian, V. H.: Collective review: secondary deformities of cleft palate. Plast. Reconstr. Surg., *8*:477, 1951.

Kazanjian, V. H., and Converse, J. M.: Surgical Treatment of Facial Injuries. 3rd Ed. Baltimore, Williams & Wilkins Company, 1974.

Kernahan, D. A.: Muscle repair in unilateral cleft lip, based on findings of electrical stimulation. Ann. Plast. Surg., *1*:48, 1978.

Kernahan, D. A., and Bauer, B. S.: Functional cleft lip repair: a sequential, layered closure with orbicularis muscle realignment. Plast. Reconstr. Surg., *72*:459, 1983.

Kernahan, D. A., Bauer, B. S., and Harris, G. D.: Experience with the Tajima procedure in primary and secondary repair in unilateral cleft lip nasal deformity. Plast. Reconstr. Surg., *66*:46, 1980.

Kinnebrew, M. C., Zide, M. F., and Kent, J. N.: Modified Le Fort II procedure for simultaneous correction of maxillary and nasal deformities. J. Oral Maxillofac. Surg., *41*:295, 1983.

Kling, A.: Procedures and limitations of orthodontic treatment. *In* Schuchardt, K. (Ed.): Treatment of Patients with Clefts of Lips, Alveolus, and Palate. Stuttgart, Georg Thieme Verlag, 1966.

Kling, J.: Evaluation of results with reference to the bite. *In* Hotz, R. (Ed.): Early Treatment of Cleft Lip and Palate. Proceedings of an International Symposium, University of Zürich Dental Institute, April 1964. Bern, Hans Huber, 1964, p. 193.

Koberg, W. R.: Present view on bone grafting in cleft palate: a review of the literature. J. Maxillofac. Surg., *1*:185, 1973.

Koch, J.: 15 jährige Erfahrungen mit der primären Knochentransplantation beim Verschluss der Kiefer- und Gaumenspalte im 4. Lebensjahr. *In* Pfeifer, G. (Ed.): Lippen-Kiefer-Gaumenspalten. Stuttgart, Georg Thieme Verlag, 1982, p. 112.

König, F.: Zur Deckung von Defekten der Nasenflugel. Berl. Klin. Wochenschr., *39*:137, 1902.

Kozin, I. A.: Surgical treatment of deformations of the upper lip and nose after plasty of the lip in adults with unilateral hare lip. Acta Chir. Plast. (Praha), *11*:283, 1969.

Lamont, E. S.: Reparative surgery of cleft lip and nasal deformities. Surg. Gynecol. Obstet., *80*:422, 1945.

Latham, R. A. Cited by Millard, D. R., Jr.: Cleft Craft. Vol. II: Bilateral and Rare Deformities. Boston, Little, Brown & Company, 1977, p. 226.

Latham, R. A., and Deaton, T. G.: The structural basis of the philtrum and contour of the vermilion border: a study of the musculature of the upper lip. J. Anat., *121*:151, 1976.

Lehman, J. A., Jr.: The dynamic Abbé flap. Ann. Plast. Surg., *3*:401, 1978.

LeMesurier, A. B.: A method of cutting and suturing the lip in the treatment of complete unilateral clefts. Plast. Reconstr. Surg., *4*:1, 1949.

Lexer, E.: Die gesamte Wiederherstellungschirurgie. Leipzig, Barth, 1931.

Lindsay, L. G., and Farkas, W. K.: The columella in cleft lip and palate anomaly. *In* Hueston, J. T. (Ed.): Transactions of the Fifth International Congress of Plastic and Reconstructive Surgery. Melbourne, Butterworth, 1971, p. 373.

Longacre, J. J.: Cleft Palate Deformation: Correction and Prevention. Springfield, IL, Charles C Thomas, 1970.

Longacre, J. J., Halak, D. B., Munick, L. H., Johnson, H. A., and Chunekamral, D.: A new approach to the correction of the nasal deformity following cleft lip repair. Plast. Reconstr. Surg., *38*:555, 1966.

Lynch, J. B., Lewis, S. R., and Blocker, T. G.: Maxillary bone grafts in cleft palate patients. Plast. Reconstr. Surg., *37*:31, 1966.

MacLeod, A.: Personal communication. Cited by Jackson, I. T., and Mustardé, J. C.: Cleft lip and palate. *In* Mustardé, J. C., and Jackson, I. T.: Plastic Surgery in Infancy and Childhood. 3rd Ed. Edinburgh, Churchill Livingstone, 1988, p. 37.

Malik, R.: Nasal deformities and their treatment in secondary repair of cleft lip patients. Scand. J. Plast. Reconstr. Surg., *8*:136, 1974.

Manchester, W. M.: The repair of bilateral cleft lip and palate. Br. J. Surg., *52*:878, 1965.

Mapes, A. H., Mazaheri, M., Harding, R. L., Meier, J. A., and Canter, H. E.: A longitudinal analysis of the maxillary growth increments of cleft lip and palate patients. Cleft Palate J., *11*:450, 1974.

Marcks, K. M., Trevaskis, A. E., Berg, E. M., and Puchner, G.: Nasal defects associated with cleft lip deformity. Plast. Reconstr. Surg., *34*:176, 1964.

Marcks, K. M., Trevaskis, A. E., and Payne, M. J.: Elongation of columella by flap transfer and Z plasty. Plast. Reconstr. Surg., *20*:466, 1957.

Mason, R., Turvey, T. A., and Warren, D. W.: Speech considerations with maxillary advancement procedures. J. Oral Surg., *38*:752, 1980.

Matthews, D.: The nose tip. Br. J. Plast. Surg., *21*:153, 1968.

Matthews, D., Broomhead, I., Grossmann, W., and Goldin, H.: Early and late bone grafting in cases of cleft lip and palate. Br. J. Plast. Surg., *23*:115, 1970.

McCarthy, J. G., Coccaro, P. J., and Schwartz, M. D.: Velopharyngeal function following maxillary advancement. Plast. Reconstr. Surg., *64*:180, 1979.

McComb, H.: Primary repair of the bilateral cleft lip nose. Br. J. Plast. Surg., *55*:596, 1975.

McComb, H.: Cleft lip nasal deformity. *In* Serafin, D., and Georgiade, N. G. (Eds.): Pediatric Plastic Surgery. St. Louis, MO, C. V. Mosby Company, 1984.

McComb, H.: Primary correction of unilateral cleft lip nasal deformity. A 10-year review. Plast. Reconstr. Surg., *75*:791, 1985.

McComb, H.: Primary repair of the bilateral cleft lip nose: A 10-year review. Plast. Reconstr. Surg., *77*:701, 1986.

McGregor, I. A.: The Abbé flap—its use in single and double lip clefts. Br. J. Plast. Surg., *16*:46, 1963.

McIndoe, A. H.: Correction of the alar deformity in cleft lip. Lancet, *1*:607, 1938.

McIndoe, A. H., and Rees, T. D.: Synchronous repair of secondary deformities in cleft lip and nose. Plast. Reconstr. Surg., *24*:150, 1959.

McNeil, C. K.: Orthopedic principles in the treatment of lip and palate clefts. *In* Hotz, R. (Ed.): Early Treatment of Cleft Lip and Palate. Proceedings of an International Symposium, University of Zürich Dental Institute, April 1964. Bern, Hans Huber, 1964.

Meade, R. J.: Composite ear grafts for construction of columella. Plast. Reconstr. Surg., *23*:134, 1959.

Merville, L. C.: L'asymetrie narinaire au bec-de-lièvre unilateral: correction chirurgicae secondaire. Rev. Stomatol., 392, 1962.

Meyer, R.: Infolding technique for correction of the nares in macrorhinia and harelip nose. Personal communication to Millard, 1973.

Millard, D. R., Jr.: A primary camouflage in the unilateral harelip. *In* Skoog, T. (Ed.): Transactions of the International Congress of Plastic Surgery. Baltimore, Williams & Wilkins Company, 1955.

Millard, D. R., Jr.: The unilateral cleft lip nose. Plast. Reconstr. Surg., *34*:169, 1964a.

Millard, D. R., Jr.: Composite lip flaps and grafts in secondary cleft deformities. Br. J. Plast. Surg., *17*:22, 1964b.

Millard, D. R., Jr.: Extensions of the rotation-advancement principle for wide unilateral cleft lips. Plast. Reconstr. Surg., *42*:535, 1968.

Millard, D. R., Jr.: Closure of bilateral cleft lip and elongation of columella by two operations in infancy. Plast. Reconstr. Surg., *37*:324, 1971.

Millard, D. R., Jr.: Further adjuncts in rotation and advancement. *In* Georgiade, N. G. (Ed.): Symposium on Management of Cleft Lip and Palate and Associated Deformities. St. Louis, MO, C. V. Mosby Company, 1974.

Millard, D. R., Jr.: Cleft Craft. Vol. I: The Unilateral Deformity. Boston, Little, Brown & Company, 1976.

Millard, D. R., Jr.: Cleft Craft. Vol. II: Bilateral and Rare Deformities. Boston, Little, Brown & Company, 1977.

Millard, D. R., Jr.: Earlier correction of the unilateral cleft lip nose. Plast. Reconstr. Surg., *70*:64, 1982.

Millard, D. R., Jr., and McLaughlin, C. A.: Abbé flap on a mucosal pedicle. Ann. Plast. Surg., *3*:544, 1979.

Millicovsky, G., Ambrose, L. J., and Johnston, M. C.: Developmental alterations associated with spontaneous cleft lip and palate in CL/Fr mice. Am. J. Anat., *164*:29, 1982.

Monie, I. W., and Cacciatore, A.: The development of the philtrum. Plast. Reconstr. Surg., *30*:313, 1962.

Monroe, C. W.: Recession of the premaxilla in bilateral cleft lip and palate: a follow-up study. Plast. Reconstr. Surg., *35*:512, 1965.

Morel-Fatio, D., and Lalardrie, J.: External nasal approach in the correction of major morphologic sequelae of the cleft lip nose. Plast. Reconstr. Surg., *38*:116, 1966.

Moss, M. L.: The functional matrix. *In* Kraus, B. S., and Riedel, R. A. (Eds.): Vistas in Orthodontics. Philadelphia, Lea & Febiger, 1962, p. 85.

Mowlem, R.: Bone (iliac) and cartilage transplants to ear and nose: their use and behavior. Br. J. Surg., *29*:182, 1941.

Muir, I. F. K., and Bodenham, D. C.: Secondary repair of cleft lip and palate deformities. *In* Gibson, T. (ed.): Modern Trends in Plastic Surgery. London, Butterworth, 1966, p. 226.

Musgrave, R. H.: Surgery of nasal deformities associated with cleft lip. Plast. Reconstr. Surg., *28*:261, 1961.

Musgrave, R. H., and Dupertuis, S. M.: Revision of the unilateral cleft lip nostril. Plast. Reconstr. Surg., *25*:223, 1960.

Nakajima, T., Yoshimura, Y., and Kami, T.: Refinement of the "reverse-U" incision for the repair of cleft lip nose deformity. Br. J. Plast. Surg., *39*:345, 1986.

Narula, J. K., and Ross, R. B.: Facial growth in children with complete bilateral cleft lip and palate. Cleft Palate J., *7*:239, 1970.

Neuner, O.: Secondary correction of cleft lip and palate. *In* Sanvenero-Rosselli, G., and Boggio-Robutti, G. (Eds.): Transactions of the Fourth International Congress of Plastic and Reconstructive Surgery. Amsterdam, Excerpta Medica, 1967.

Nishimura, Y., and Ogino, Y.: The use of two V-flaps for secondary correction of the cleft lip nose. Plast. Reconstr. Surg., *60*:390, 1977.

Nordin, K. E., and Johanson, B.: Frei Knochen-Transplantation bei Defekten in Alveolarkam nach Kiefer-ortopadischer Enstellung der Maxilla bei Lippen-Kiefer-Gaumenspalten. Stuttgart, Georg Thieme Verlag, 1955.

O'Brien, B. M.: The maxillary periosteal flap in primary palate surgery. Austr. N.Z. J. Surg., *40*:65, 1970.

Obwegeser, H. L.: Surgical correction of mandibular prognathism and retrognathia with consideration of genioplasty. Oral Surg. Oral Med. Oral Pathol., *10*:67, 1957.

Obwegeser, H. L.: Surgical correction of small or retro-displaced maxillae: the "dish face" deformity. Plast. Reconstr. Surg., *43*:351, 1969.

Obwegeser, H. L., and Perko, M.: Die Rekonstruktion des Knochendefektes bei Lippen-Kiefer-Gaumenspalten-Patienten. Dtsch. Zahn. Mund. Kieferheilkd., *50*:203, 1968.

O'Connor, G. B., and McGregor, M. W.: Surgical formation of the philtrum and the cutaneous upsweep. Am. J. Surg., *95*:227, 1958.

O'Connor, G. B., McGregor, M. W., Murphy, S., and Tolleth, H.: Advancement of soft tissues to correct mild midfacial retrusion. Plast. Reconstr. Surg., *52*:42, 1972.

O'Connor, G. B., McGregor, M. W., and Tolleth, H.: The management of nasal deformities associated with cleft lips. Pac. Med. Surg., *73*:279, 1965.

O'Connor, G. B., McGregor, M. W., and Tolleth, H.: The nasal problem in cleft lips. Surg. Gynecol. Obstet., *116*:503, 1968.

Ogino, Y., and Ishida, H.: Secondary repair of the cleft lip nose. Ann. Plast. Surg., *4*:469, 1980.

Ombrédanne, L.: Reconstruction of nostril in single harelip. Presse Med., *29*:703, 1921.

Ombrédanne, L., and Ombrédanne, M.: Le nez aplati des opérés du bec-de-lièvre bilateral complèt. Ann. Mal. Orielle Larynx, *47*:1090, 1928.

Oneal, R. M., Greer, D. M., Jr., and Nobel, G. L.: Secondary correction of bilateral cleft deformities with Millard's midline muscular closure. Plast. Reconstr. Surg., *54*:45, 1974.

Onizuka, T.: Experiences with cleft lip repair. I. On Millard's method. Keisei Geka, *9*:168, 1966.

Onizuka, T.: Repair of columella base deformity in unilateral cleft lip. Br. J. Plast. Surg., *25*:33, 1972.

Onizuka, T., Akagawa, T., and Tokunaga, S.: A new method to create a philtrum in secondary cleft lip repairs. Plast. Reconstr. Surg., *62*:842, 1978.

Ortiz-Monasterio, F., and Olmedo, A.: Corrective rhinoplasty before puberty: a long-term follow-up. Plast. Reconstr. Surg., *68*:381, 1981.

Ortiz-Monasterio, F., Rebeil, A. S., Valderrama, M., and Cruz, R.: Cephalometric measurements on adult patients with non-operated cleft palates. Plast. Reconstr. Surg., *24*:53, 1959.

Ortiz-Monasterio, F., Serrano, R., Barrera, P., Rodriques-Hoffman, H., and Vinageras, E.: A study of untreated adult cleft palate patients. Plast. Reconstr. Surg., *38*:36, 1966.

Padgett, E. L., and Stephenson, K. L.: Plastic and Reconstructive Surgery. Springfield, IL, Charles C Thomas, 1948, p. 382.

Patton, B. M.: Human Embryology. 3rd Ed. New York, McGraw-Hill Book Company, 1968, p. 345.

Patton, B. M.: Embryology of the palate and the maxillary region. *In* Grabb, W. C., Rosenstein, S. W., and Bzoch, K. R. (Eds.): Cleft Lip and Palate. Boston, Little, Brown & Company, 1971.

Peet, E. W., and Patterson, T. J. S.: The Essentials of Plastic Surgery. Oxford, Blackwell Scientific Publications, 1963, p. 324.

Pegram, M.: Repair of congenital short columella. Plast. Reconstr. Surg., 14:305, 1954.

Perko, M.: Die chirurgische Spaltkorrekture von Zahn- und Kieferstellungs-anomalien bei Spaltpatienten. Schweiz. Monatsschr. Zahnheilkd., 79:19, 1969.

Peskova, H., and Fara, M.: Lengthening of the columella in bilateral cleft. Acta Chir. Plast. (Praha), 2:18, 1960.

Peterson, R. A., Ellenberg, A. H., and Carroll, D. B.: Vermilion flap reconstruction of bilateral cleft lip deformities (a modification of the Abbé procedure). Plast. Reconstr. Surg., 38:109, 1966.

Petrovic, S.: Unsere Erfahrungen mit sekundaren Knochenplastiken bei der Therapie der Spaltendeformationen des Oberkiefers und des Gebisses. Dtsch. Zahn. Mund. Kieferheilkd., 57:230, 1971.

Pfeifer, G.: The wave-line procedure for primary cleft lip. In Johanson, B. (Ed.): Abstracts of the Second International Congress on Cleft Palate, Copenhagen, 1973, p. 190.

Pickrell, K., Quinn, G., and Massengill, R.: Primary bone grafting of the maxilla in clefts of the lip and palate. A four-year study. Plast. Reconstr. Surg., 41:438, 1968.

Pigott, R. W., and Millard, D. R., Jr.: Correction of the bilateral cleft lip nasal deformity. In Grabb, W. C., Rosenstein, S. W., and Bzoch, K. R. (Eds.): Cleft Lip and Palate. Boston, Little, Brown & Company, 1971, p. 325.

Pitanguy, I.: Rhino-cheilo-plastie a ciel ouvert dans les sequelles du bec-de-lièvre. Ann. Chir. Plast., 8:47, 1963.

Pitanguy, I., and Franco, T.: Nonoperated facial fissures in adults. Plast. Reconstr. Surg., 39:569, 1967.

Pollet, J.: Three autogenous struts for nasal tip support. Plast. Reconstr. Surg., 49:527, 1972.

Posnick, J. C., and Getz, S. B., Jr.: Surgical closure of end-stage palatal fistulas using anteriorly based dorsal tongue flaps. J. Oral Maxillofac. Surg., 45:907, 1987.

Potter, J.: Some nasal tip deformities due to alar cartilage abnormalities. Plast. Reconstr. Surg., 13:358, 1954.

Potter, J.: The nasal tip in bilateral harelip. Br. J. Plast. Surg., 21:173, 1968.

Pruzansky, S.: The growth of the premaxillary-vomerine complex in complete bilateral cleft lip and palate. Tandlaegebladet, 75:1167, 1971.

Pruzansky, S., and Aduss, H.: Prevalence of arch collapse and malocclusion in complete unilateral cleft lip and palate. Trans. Eur. Orthodont. Soc., 1:16, 1967.

Puckett, C. L., Reinisch, J. F., and Werner, R. S.: Late correction of orbicularis discontinuity in bilateral cleft lip deformities. Cleft Palate J., 17:34, 1980.

Ragnell, A.: Treatment of secondary deformity in case of harelip. Med. Presse, 216:281, 1946.

Ramstad, T.: Post-orthodontic retention and post-orthodontic occlusion in adult complete unilateral and bilateral cleft subjects. Cleft Palate J., 10:34, 1973.

Randall, P.: A triangular flap operation for primary repair of unilateral clefts of the lip. Plast. Reconstr. Surg., 23:331, 1959.

Randall, P., Whitaker, L., and LaRossa, D.: The importance of muscle reconstruction in primary and secondary lip repair. Plast. Reconstr. Surg., 54:316, 1974.

Rees, T. D., Guy, C. L., and Converse, J. M.: Repair of the cleft lip nose: addendum to the synchronous technique with full-thickness skin grafting of the nasal vestibule. Plast. Reconstr. Surg., 37:47, 1966.

Rehrmann, A.: Bone grafting in cleft palate repair. In Gibson, T. (Ed.): Modern Trends in Plastic Surgery. London, Butterworth, 1964, p. 50.

Rehrmann, A. H., Koberg, W. R., and Koch, H.: Long-term postoperative results of primary and secondary bone grafting in complete clefts of lip and palate. Cleft Palate J., 7:206, 1970.

Reichert, H.: Chirurgie der Lippen-Kiefer-Gaumenspalte heute. Dtsch. Stomatol., 19:325, 1969.

Reidy, J. P.: The nasal septum. Ann. R. Coll. Surg. Engl., 43:141, 1968.

Rethi, A.: Raccourcissement du nez trop long. Rev. Chir. Plast., 2:85, 1934.

Reynolds, J. R., and Horton, C. E.: An alar lift in cleft lip rhinoplasty. Plast. Reconstr. Surg., 35:377, 1965.

Rintala, A. E.: Surgical closure of palatal fistula. Scand. J. Plast. Reconstr. Surg., 14:235, 1980.

Ritsila, V., Alhopuro, S., Gylling, U., and Rintala, A.: The use of free periosteum for bone formation in congenital clefts of the maxilla. Scand. J. Plast. Reconstr. Surg., 6:57, 1972.

Robertson, N. R. E., and Jolleys, A.: An 11-year follow-up of the effects of early bone grafting in infants born with complete clefts of the lip and palate. Br. J. Plast. Surg., 36:438, 1983.

Robinson, D. W., Ketchum, L. D., and Masters, F. W.: Double V-Y procedure for whistling deformity in repaired cleft lips. Plast. Reconstr. Surg., 46:241, 1970.

Rohrich, R. J., and Tebbetts, J. B.: Cleft lip II: secondary cleft lip/nasal/alveolar defects. Selected Readings in Plastic Surgery, Vol. 4, No. 22, 1987.

Rose, W.: Harelip and Cleft Palate. London, H. K. Lewis & Co., 1891.

Rosenstein, S. W., Monroe, C. W., Kernahan, D. A., Jacobson, B. N., Griffith, B. H., and Bauer, B. S.: The case of early bone grafting in cleft lip and cleft palate. Plast. Reconstr. Surg., 70:297, 1982.

Sabbatini, P.: Cenno storico dell'origine e progressi della descrizione di queste operazioni sopra un solo individuo. Bella, Arti, 1838.

Salyer, K. E.: Primary correction of the unilateral cleft lip nose: 15-year experience. Plast. Reconstr. Surg., 77:558, 1986.

Santoni-Rugiu, P.: La'ricostruzione dell'orcata alveolare con leimbi perisotie nella labiognato palatoschisi complete. Bol. Soc. Med.-Chir., 34:1, 1966.

Sarnat, B. G.: Differential effect of surgical trauma to the nasal bones and septum upon rabbit snout growth. In Sanvenero-Rosselli, G., and Boggio-Robutti, G. (Eds.): Transactions of the Fourth International Congress of Plastic and Reconstructive Surgery. Amsterdam, Excerpta Medica, 1967.

Sawney, C. P.: Nasal deformity in unilateral cleft lip. Cleft Palate J., 13:291, 1976.

Schafer, M. E., and Goldwasser, M. S.: On the importance of muscle repair in secondary cleft lip deformity. Clin. Plast. Surg., 11:761, 1984.

Schendel, S. A., and Delaire, J.: Functional musculoskeletal correction of secondary unilateral cleft lip deformities: combined lip-nose correction and Le Fort I osteotomy. J. Maxillofac. Surg., 9:108, 1981.

Schendel, S. A., Oeschlaeger, M., Wolford, L. M., and Epker, B. N.: Velopharyngeal anatomy and maxillary advancement. J. Maxillofac. Surg., 7:116, 1979.

Schjelderup, H.: Correction tardive des déformations nasales importantes dans le bec-de-lièvre unilatéral. Acta Chir. Plast. (Prague), 12:427, 1963.

Schmid, E.: Die Annäherung der Kieferstumpfe bei Lippen-Kiefer-Gaumenspalten, ihre schädlichen Folgen und Vermeilung. *In* Schuchardt, K., and Wassmund, M. (Eds.): Fortschritte der Kiefer- und Gesichtschirurgie. Vol. 1. Stuttgart, Georg Thieme Verlag, 1955, p. 37.

Schmid, E.: Die Osteoplastik bei Lippen-Kiefer-Gaumenspalten. Arch. Klin. Chir., *295*:868, 1960.

Schmid, E.: The use of auricular cartilage and composite grafts in reconstruction of the upper lip, with special reference to construction of the philtrum. *In* Broadbent, T. R. (Ed.): Transactions of the Third International Congress of Plastic Surgery. Amsterdam, Excerpta Medica, 1964, p. 306.

Schmid, E.: Discussion of Johanson, B.: Secondary osteoplastic completion of maxilla and palate. *In* Schuchardt, K. (Ed.): Treatment of Patients with Clefts of Lip, Alveolus, and Palate. Stuttgart, Georg Thieme Verlag, 1966.

Schmid, E., Widmaier, W., Reichert, H., and Stein, K.: The development of the cleft upper jaw following primary osteoplasty and orthodontic treatment (a report of 87 cases). J. Maxillofac. Surg., *2*:92, 1974.

Schuchardt, K.: Die Entwicklung der Lippen-Kiefer-Gaumenspalten-Chirurgie. Arch. Klin. Chir., *295*:850, 1960.

Schuchardt, K.: Primary bone grafting in clefts of lip, alveolus, and palate. *In* Gibson, T. (ed.): Modern Trends in Plastic Surgery. London, Butterworth, 1964.

Schuh, F. D., Crikelair, G. F., and Cosman, B.: A critical appraisal of the Abbé flap in secondary cleft deformity. Plast. Reconstr. Surg., *23*:142, 1970.

Schultz, L. W.: Bilateral cleft lips. Plast. Reconstr. Surg., *1*:338, 1946.

Schultz, R. C.: Free periosteal graft repair of maxillary clefts in adolescents. Plast. Reconstr. Surg., *73*:556, 1984.

Schwarz, C., and Gruner, E.: Logopaedic findings following advancement of the maxilla. J. Maxillofac. Surg., *4*:40, 1976.

Schwenzer, N.: Correction of noses associated with clefts of lip and palate. J. Maxillofac. Surg., *1*:91, 1973.

Sheehan, J.: Plastic Surgery of the Nose. New York, Paul B. Hoeber, 1936, p. 115.

Sheen, J. H., and Sheen, A. P.: Aesthetic Rhinoplasty. St. Louis, MO, C. V. Mosby Company, 1978.

Siegel, M. I.: Discussion of "Growth activity in human septal cartilage: age-dependent incorporation of labeled sulfate in different anatomic locations" by U. Vetter, W. Pirsig, and E. Heinze. Plast. Reconstr. Surg., *71*:171, 1983.

Siegel, M. I., and Sadler, D.: Nasal septum resection and craniofacial growth in a chimpanzee animal model: implications for cleft palate surgery. Plast. Reconstr. Surg., *68*:849, 1981.

Sillman, M. A.: Dimensional changes of the dental arches: longitudinal study from birth to 25 years. Am. J. Orthod., *50*:824, 1964.

Skoog, T.: A design for the repair of unilateral cleft lip. Am. J. Surg., *95*:223, 1958.

Skoog, T.: The management of the bilateral cleft of the primary palate (lip and alveolus). Part I. General considerations and soft tissue repair. Plast. Reconstr. Surg., *35*:34, 1965.

Skoog, T.: The use of periosteum and surgical bone reconstruction in congenital clefts of the mandible. Scand. J. Plast. Reconstr. Surg., *1*:113, 1967.

Skoog, T.: Repair of unilateral cleft lip deformity: maxilla, nose, and lip. Scand. J. Plast. Reconstr. Surg., *3*:109, 1969.

Skoog, T.: Plastic Surgery: New Methods and Refinements. Stockholm, Almqvist & Wiksell, 1974, p. 134.

Slaughter, W. B., and Brodie, A. G.: Facial clefts and their management in view of recent research. Plast. Reconstr. Surg., *4*:311, 1949.

Smith, J. W.: The anatomic and physiologic acclimatization of tissue transplanted by the lip switch technique. Plast. Reconstr. Surg., *26*:40, 1960.

Smith, J. W.: Clinical experiences with the vermilion bordered lip flap. Plast. Reconstr. Surg., *27*:527, 1961.

Spiessl, B.: Verschiebeosteotomie und Spongiosatransplantation bei extremer Deformierung des kieferbogens bei Spaltpatienten. Fortschr. Kiefer. Gesichtschir., *16/17*:332, 1973.

Spira, M., Hardy, S. B., and Gerow, F. J.: Correction of nasal deformities accompanying unilateral cleft lip. Cleft Palate J., 7:112, 1970.

Stal, S., and Spira, M.: Secondary reconstructive procedures for patients with clefts. *In* Serafin, D., and Georgiade, N. G. (Eds.): Pediatric Plastic Surgery. Vol. 1. St. Louis, MO, C. V. Mosby Company, 1984, p. 352.

Stark, R. B.: Cleft Palate. New York, Hoeber Medical Division, Harper & Row, 1968, p. 139.

Stark, R. B., DeHaan, C. R., and Washio, H.: Forked flap columellar advance. Cleft Palate J., *1*:116, 1964.

Stark, R. B., and Kaplan, J. M.: Development of the cleft lip nose. Plast. Reconstr. Surg., *51*:413, 1973.

Steedle, J. R., and Proffit, W. R.: The pattern and control of eruptive tooth movements. Am. J. Orthod., *87*:56, 1985.

Steffensen, W. H.: Further experience with the rectangular flap operation for cleft lip repair. Plast. Reconstr. Surg., *11*:49, 1953.

Stein, S. A. V.: Laebedannelse (cheiloplasty) udfort paa en ny methode. Hospitalsmeddelelser, *1*:212, 1848.

Steinhauser, E.: Personal communication. Cited by Jackson, I. T., and Mustardé, J. C.: Cleft lip and palate. *In* Mustardé, J. C., and Jackson, I. T.: Plastic Surgery in Infancy and Childhood. 3rd Ed. Edinburgh, Churchill Livingstone, 1988, p. 37.

Stellmach, R.: Primäre Knochenplastik bei Lippen-Kiefer-Gaumenspalten am Säugling unter besonderer Berücksichtigung der Transplantations Deckung. Langenbecks Arch. Klin. Chir., *292*:865, 1959.

Stenström, S. J.: The alar cartilage and the nasal deformity in unilateral cleft lip. Plast. Reconstr. Surg., *38*:223, 1966.

Stenström, S. J.: Alar cartilage and nasal deformity in unilateral cleft lip (follow-up clinic). Plast. Reconstr. Surg., *55*:359, 1975.

Stenström, S. J., and Oberg, T. R. H.: The nasal deformity in unilateral cleft lip. Plast. Reconstr. Surg., *28*:295, 1961.

Stenström, S. J., and Thilander, B. L.: Cleft lip nasal deformity in the absence of cleft lip. Plast. Reconstr. Surg., *35*:160, 1965.

Straith, C. L.: Elongation of the nasal columella. Plast. Reconstr. Surg., *1*:79, 1946.

Straith, C. L., Straith, R. E., and Lawson, J. M.: Reconstruction of the harelip nose. Plast. Reconstr. Surg., *20*:455, 1957.

Stricker, M., Chancolle, A. R., Flet, F., Molka, G., and Montoya, A.: La greffe périostée dans la réparation de la fente totale du palais primaire. Ann. Chir. Plast., *22*:117, 1977.

Tajima, S.: The importance of the musculus nasalis and the cure of the cleft margin flap in repair of the complete unilateral cleft lip. J. Maxillofac. Surg., *11*:64, 1983.

Tajima, S., and Maruyama, M.: Reverse-U incision for secondary repair of cleft lip nose. Plast. Reconstr. Surg., *60*:256, 1977.

Tennison, C. W.: The repair of unilateral cleft lip by the stencil method. Plast. Reconstr. Surg., *9*:115, 1952.

Tessier, P., Delbet, J. P., Pastoriza, F., and Aiaich, R.: Séquelles labiales et nasales du bec-de-lièvre complet, chez l'adolescent. Relations avec les malformations et déformations du maxillaire. Ann. Chir. Plast., *14*:312, 1969.

Tessier, P., and Tulasne, J. F.: Secondary repair of cleft lip deformity. Clin. Plast. Surg., *11*:747, 1984.

Thompson, J. E.: An artistically and mathematically accurate method of repairing the defect in cases of harelip. Surg. Gynecol. Obstet., *14*:498, 1912.

Thompson, N., and Pollard, A. C.: Motor function in Abbé flaps. Br. J. Plast. Surg., *14*:66, 1961.

Thomson, H. G.: The residual unilateral cleft lip nasal deformity: a three-phase correction technique. Plast. Reconstr. Surg., *76*:36, 1985.

Tideman, H., Stoelinga, P., and Gallia, L.: Le Fort I advancement with segmental palatal osteotomies in patients with cleft palates. J. Oral Surg., *38*:196, 1980.

Tolhurst, D. E.: Secondary correction of the unilateral cleft lip nose deformity. Br. J. Plast. Surg., *36*:449, 1983.

Tondra, J. M., Bauer, T. B., and Trusler, H. M.: The management of the bilateral cleft lip deformity. Acta Chir. Plast., *8*:173, 1966.

Trauner, R.: Operationen bei Lippen-Kiefer-Gaumen-spalten in Chirurgische Operationslehre von B. Breitner. Vol. 1. Vienna, Urban and Schwarzenberg, 1956.

Trauner, R., and Trauner, M.: Results of cleft lip operations. Plast. Reconstr. Surg., *40*:209, 1967.

Trier, W. C.: Cleft lip nasal deformity. *In* Serafin, D., and Georgiade, N. G. (Eds.): Pediatric Plastic Surgery. St. Louis, MO, C. V. Mosby Company, 1984.

Trier, W. C.: Repair of unilateral cleft lip: the rotation advancement operation. Clin. Plast. Surg., *12*:573, 1985.

Tschopp, H. M.: Die Sekundärbehandlung voroperierter doppelseitiger Lippenspalten mittels eines Muskel-Mukosa-Läppchens von der Unterlippe. Fortschr. Kiefer. Gesichtschir., *16/17*:230, 1973.

Turvey, A. T., Vig, K., Moriarty, J., and Hoke, J.: Delayed bone grafting in the cleft maxilla and palate: a retrospective multidisciplinary analysis. Am. J. Orthod., *86*:244, 1984.

Uchida, J. I.: A new approach to the correction of cleft lip nasal deformities. Plast. Reconstr. Surg., *47*:454, 1971.

Vargervik, K.: Growth characteristics of the premaxilla and orthodontic treatment principles in bilateral cleft lip and palate. Cleft Palate J., *20*:289, 1983.

Vaughan, H. S.: Congenital Cleft Lip, Cleft Palate and Associated Nasal Deformities. Philadelphia, Lea & Febiger, 1940.

Veau, V.: Division Palatine—Anatomie, Chirurgie, Phonetique. Paris, Masson et Cie, 1931.

Veau, V.: Hasenscharten menschlicher Keimlinge auf der Stufe. A. Anat. Entwicklungsgesch., *108*:459, 1937–1938.

Velazquez, J. M., and Ortiz-Monasterio, F.: Primary simultaneous correction of the lip and nose in the unilateral cleft lip. Plast. Reconstr. Surg., *54*:558, 1974.

Vetter, U., Pirsig, W., and Heinze, E.: Growth activity in human septal cartilage: age-dependent incorporation of labeled sulfate in different anatomic locations. Plast. Reconstr. Surg., *71*:167, 1983.

Vig, K. W. H., and Turvey, T. A.: Orthodontic-surgical interaction in the management of cleft lip and palate. Clin. Plast. Surg., *12*:735, 1985.

Von Deilen, A. W.: Some aspects in the secondary repair of cleft lip, palate and nasal deformities, with case report. Plast. Reconstr. Surg., *10*:460, 1952.

von Langenbeck, B.: Die Uranoplastik mittels Ablösung des mucosperiostalen Gaumenüberzüges. Arch. Klin. Chir., *2*:205, 1861.

Waite, D. E., and Kersten, R. B.: Residual alveolar and palatal clefts. *In* Bell, W. H., Proffit, W. R., and White, R. P. (Eds.): Surgical Correction of Dentofacial Deformities. Vol. 2. Philadelphia, W. B. Saunders Company, 1980.

Webster, J. P.: Crescentic peri-alar cheek excision for upper lip flap advancement with short history of upper lip repair. Plast. Reconstr. Surg., *16*:434, 1955.

Whitlow, D. R., and Constable, J. D.: Crossed alar wing procedure for correction of late deformity in the unilateral cleft lip nose. Plast. Reconstr. Surg., *52*:38, 1973.

Widmaier, W.: Beitrag zum Verschluss schwieriger Rest-perforationen am Gaumen nit Insellappen und Lyodura. Fortschr. Kiefer. Gesichtschir., *16/17*:299, 1973.

Wilkie, T. F.: The "alar shift" revisited. Br. J. Plast. Surg., *33*:70, 1969.

Wilson, L. F.: Correction of residual deformities of the lip and nose in repaired clefts of the primary palate (lip and alveolus). Clin. Plast. Surg., *12*:719, 1985.

Witzel, M. A., and Munro, I. R.: Velopharyngeal insufficiency after maxillary advancement. Cleft Palate J., *14*:176, 1977.

Wolfe, S. A., and Berkowitz, S.: The use of cranial bone grafts in the closure of alveolar and anterior palatal clefts. Plast. Reconstr. Surg., *72*:659, 1983.

Wray, R. C., Jr.: Secondary correction of nasal abnormalities associated with cleft lip. J. Oral Surg., *34*:113, 1976.

Wynn, S. K.: Lateral flap cleft lip surgery technique. Plast. Reconstr. Surg., *26*:509, 1960.

Wynn, S. K.: Primary nostril reconstruction in complete cleft lips. Plast. Reconstr. Surg., *49*:56, 1972.

Young, F.: The surgical repair of nasal deformities. Plast. Reconstr. Surg., *4*:59, 1949.

57

Barry H. Grayson
Peter J. Coccaro
Augustus J. Valauri

Orthodontics in Cleft Lip and Palate Children

Many professional disciplines are involved in the rehabilitation of the patient with a cleft lip and palate. A large number of them, of necessity, render their services only periodically from birth through adulthood. The orthodontist, however, is one whose services are essential throughout the child's formative years. His knowledge of the growth and development of the jaw and dentition should be considered in planning any treatment designed to counter the adverse impact that the cleft has on the maxilla and developing dentition. The areas of interest to the orthodontist are (1) the skeletal structures (maxilla, mandible, and cranium), (2) the dentoalveolar structures (teeth and alveolar processes), and (3) the relationship of the dentoalveolar structures to the skeletal structures and overlying soft tissue.

In noncleft individuals most of the ordinary malocclusion problems involve only the dentoalveolar structures, while associated skeletal involvement, which requires treatment, occurs in only a minority of patients. Although most of the orthodontist's work is associated with correcting dental irregularities, he can bring specialized skills to the treatment of the cleft lip and palate patient who presents a unique combination of skeletal and dental abnormalities, problems that lend themselves to guidance and complete orthodontic therapy.

HISTORY

Clefts of the lip and palate have probably afflicted the human race since prehistoric times. Archeologic evidence of this malformation, however, is remarkably sparse. The first cleft palate repair in the United States was performed by Stevens in 1827. One of the earliest employed intraoral appliances was the obturator. Fauchard (1786) made valuable contributions and innovations in cleft palate prosthodontics, particularly in the area of obturators.

Two men stand out for their early contributions to the orthodontic and prosthodontic treatment of these deformities. Kingsley, who shares with others the claim to be the "father of orthodontia," wrote his classic textbook *A Treatise on Oral Deformities* in 1880. This book featured the orthodontic appliances of the period, including jack screws, retainers, and arches with ligatures. Case published "A practical treatise on the techniques and principles of dental orthopaedia and prosthetic correction of the cleft palate" in 1921. The appliances described were all of the fixed type.

A considerable amount of cleft palate research, particularly longitudinal growth studies, has been conducted by orthodontists. Cleft palate orthodontics is no longer confined to the local movement of individual teeth; it also involves early treatment for the movement of the distorted maxillary palatal segments into a more normal spatial relationship. The orthodontist is also involved in the planning of orthognathic surgical procedures in the cleft palate patient (see Chap. 56).

THE MAXILLA

It is generally accepted that the maxilla in cleft lip and palate children is deficient in the vertical and anteroposterior dimensions (Graber, 1950; Ross and Johnston, 1972; Grayson and associates, 1987) (see Chap. 50). This finding may vary with the type and severity of the cleft. Clinical and radiographic observations indicate that there are morphologic differences in the character of the palatal defect from one patient to another both within specific cleft palate categories and between the different types of clefts.

The cleft appears to be present more often in the dentoalveolar area where the developing lateral incisor tooth would normally be located (between the maxillary central incisor and the cuspid). In all types of cleft palate, except in the lip and alveolar group (or primary palate), the defect involves the premaxilla, the palatal processes of the maxilla, and the horizontal processes of the palatine bone. The disruption in the continuity of the bony palate contributes toward the abnormality observed in muscle attachments and function.

At birth the configuration of the unilateral cleft alveolar segments may vary. The medial wall of the lesser or cleft segment may be retropositioned and/or laterally displaced (Fig. 57–1A). The incisal portion of the greater or noncleft segment may be displaced anteriorly and laterally by the pull of the orbicularis oris musculature in the incomplete lip. The cleft alveoli often turn upward along their cleft margins (Fig. 57–1B).

The nasal deformity is often related to the magnitude of the underlying dentoalveolar skeletal deformity (Fig. 57–2). The alar base on the cleft side is retropositioned and reveals the deficient forward projection or lateral displacement of the cleft alveolar process and anterior wall of the maxilla. The bilateral cleft alveolar segments in the newborn may be displaced to varying degrees medially or laterally (Fig. 57–3A). The premaxilla is usually everted and superiorly displaced. The presence of Simonart's bands or incomplete clefting of the soft tissue may result in an asymmetric displacement of the cleft skeletal components. The medial wall of the bilateral cleft segments are, like the unilateral cleft, superiorly displaced (Fig. 57–3B).

In early childhood or adolescence the affected palatal segment may be rotated medially, while the larger noncleft segment may be rotated upward and outward in the area of the dentoalveolar process adjacent to the cleft. This results in an overlapping of the palatal segments, with the smaller palatal segment locked in behind the larger noncleft segment (see Fig. 57–1). In bilateral clefts the premaxilla may be advanced or turned in and upward (Fig. 57–3A,C). In both situations, however, the lateral palatal segments are usually rotated medially toward each other (Fig. 57–3B,D). The specific history of surgery and lack of orthodontic follow-up is often associated with this type of secondary dentoalveolar deformity.

Since variations are noted in all clefts, each patient must be analyzed on an individual basis. In each patient the orthodontic approach must employ treatment procedures designed to bring the deformed dental arch within normal limits. Achievement of this goal often involves uncovering the true status of the cleft and the magnitude of the congenital maxillary deformity. The anatomic defect in each cleft lip and palate patient should be adequately defined as early as possible. The defect usually includes bony and soft tissue structures that may be deficient or displaced. Coupe and Subtelny (1962) demonstrated a deficiency of hard palate tissue in all types of clefts involving the hard palate. The deficiency was greatest in bilateral clefts, while unilateral clefts had the least. Although this is not true in all cases, it would appear that treatment procedures (surgical and/or orthodontic) in some cases are much more effective in producing a satisfactory result, whereas in others the reverse is true. This difference may reflect the degree of tissue deficiency with which the clinician must work and the difference in the spatial relationship of the parts to be treated. Such features as the width of the cleft, the extent of the cleft, and the spatial relationships of contiguous anatomic structures are important skeletal considerations that should be evaluated before ortho-

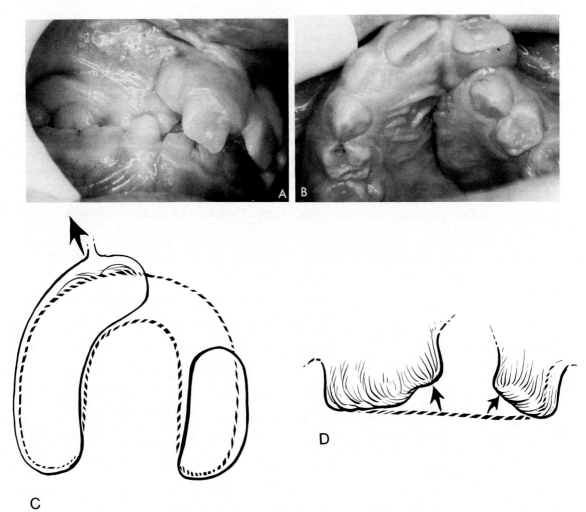

Figure 57–1. Intraoral views of a unilateral cleft lip and palate. *A,* Lateral view showing rotation of the maxillary noncleft palatal segment and the constricted palatal segment with accompanying crossbite. *B,* Palatal view showing the impacted palatal segment behind the rotated noncleft palatal segment. *C,* Dental casts of a newborn with unilateral cleft lip and palate. Occlusal view showing lateral displacement and retroposition of the cleft segment. The noncleft segment may be laterally displaced by muscle pull in the incisal region. *D,* Frontal view showing vertical displacement of the medial wall of the alveolar clefts.

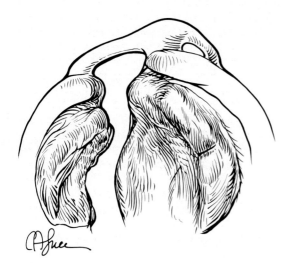

Figure 57–2. Malposition of the underlying dentoalveolar skeletal structures contributes to the retropositioning of the alar base on the cleft side. Efforts may be made to reposition the alveolar structures using molding plates or other orthopedic appliances to enhance the support of the lip and nose before definitive repair.

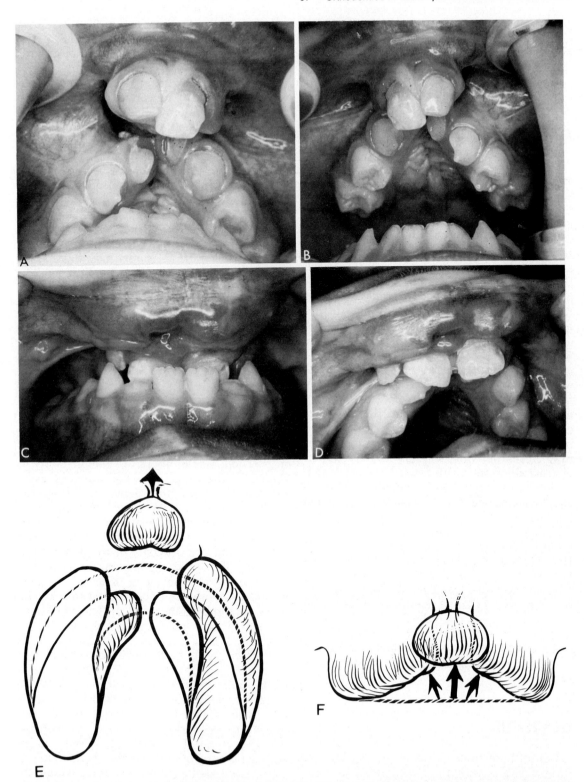

Figure 57–3. Occlusal and palatal views of patients with bilateral cleft. *A, B,* The premaxilla is procumbent and anterior to the medially collapsed palatal segments. *C, D,* A similar defect in another child showing the premaxilla relatively retropositioned but still situated anteriorly; the palatal segments are collapsed medially. Note the differences in malocclusion between the two patients. *E,* The premaxilla is usually everted and superiorly displaced. The presence of Simonart's bands in incomplete clefting of the soft tissue may result in an asymmetric displacement of the cleft skeletal components. *F,* The medial wall of the displaced cleft segments is, as in the unilateral clefts, superiorly displaced.

dontic treatment is instituted. Clinical and radiographic records, which are invaluable for diagnostic and treatment planning, also serve as data for longitudinal evaluation over periods of growth or treatment.

THE MANDIBLE

Inequality in the growth of the jaws may occur. It may be the result of a genetic potential for continued growth of the mandible or a reduction of maxillary growth. The lower jaw has an inherent potential to develop into a Class I, II, or III skeletal mandible (Ross and Johnston, 1972). This factor in the presence of a hypoplastic maxilla can compound the incidence of facial concavity and resulting prognathism. Orthodontic treatment does not resolve skeletal problems evolving during later states of growth (Converse and associates, 1964), and these problems may be in no way related to the diagnosis and orthodontic treatment plan prescribed. In individuals with clefts of the lip and palate, satisfactory facial appearance is not unusual at an early age, followed by later deterioration in facial contour. Some patients with a cleft lip and palate have the potential for a mandible that may be smaller than that observed in a noncleft population. In this regard, patients with a cleft palate may have a smaller mandible than that of the noncleft palate population (Borden, 1953). In the Pierre Robin sequence one of the three factors making up the clinical triad is mandibular hypoplasia or micrognathia. Growth of the mandible in the presence of a maxillary deformity compounds the problems in the overall treatment objectives from one year to another. It is only with increased knowledge about the growth of the maxilla and mandible in light of the existing deformity that one can become more secure in therapeutic objectives on a continuing basis (Fig. 57–4).

DENTITION

Dental anomalies occur frequently in cleft lip and palate patients (Bohn, 1963). A common example is the *congenital absence of teeth,* particularly the maxillary lateral incisors at the site of the cleft (Fig. 57–5A). An interesting yet inexplicable finding is the *congenital absence of maxillary and/or man-*

dibular second bicuspids (Fig. 57–5B). Since these develop remotely from the site of the cleft and have been found to occur in greater frequency in the cleft palate population, it becomes even more mystifying. One or all four bicuspids may be absent. In addition, the second bicuspids may show an abnormal pattern of calcification and development. Development of the second bicuspids has begun as late as 6 to 8 years of age, i.e., three to five years beyond the normal period of the start of calcification. Clinical examination of such a patient during the mixed dentition stage would lead one to conclude erroneously that these teeth are congenitally missing. Such children must therefore be examined periodically, and treatment plans may have to be modified and often compromised, depending on the severity of the cleft, the growth of the jaws, and the status of the developing deciduous and permanent dentition.

Another common dental aberration is the *presence of supernumerary teeth* (Fig. 57–5C). Cleft palate patients have a greater number of such teeth in contrast to their noncleft counterparts. These teeth are usually located adjacent to the cleft site; some emerge into the oral cavity, while others may remain unerupted within the maxilla. They may vary in size, shape, and location. Some are palatal in position, while others are labial. Many of them are often removed to facilitate the treatment of the remaining dentition. Whenever possible, they may be maintained and used to carry a fixed appliance to expand the palatal segments. They also contribute toward maintaining the integrity of the dental arch and alveolar process. In some patients in whom a lateral incisor is missing, a supernumerary tooth may be retained to take the place of the missing incisor. The maxillary central incisors adjacent to the cleft in the noncleft palate segment in unilateral cases are often found to be severely rotated and poorly calcified (Fig. 57–5D). In bilateral clefts both central incisor teeth may be equally hypoplastic and show varying degrees of rotation. The roots of these teeth may not appear to be normal in their development, and it occasionally appears that there is insufficient supporting alveolar bone. This is especially true in bilateral clefts in which the premaxilla is extremely mobile and there is relatively greater tissue deficiency. Nevertheless, these teeth should be retained and rotated into a normal position as early as possible.

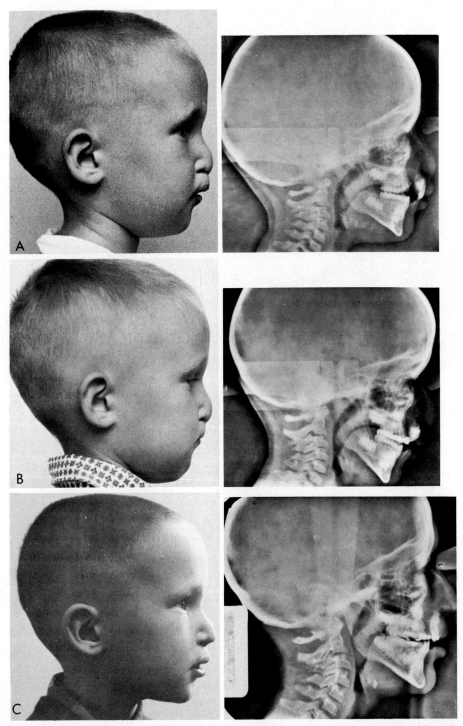

Figure 57–4. Later photographs with matching cephalometric reproductions of a patient with a bilateral cleft lip and palate illustrate changes coincidental with early orthodontic therapy and growth and development of the face. Note change in mandibular size and position, reducing the anteroposterior disparity between the maxilla and mandible. Following the improvements in skeletal relationships, a rhinoplasty was performed, as noted in C.

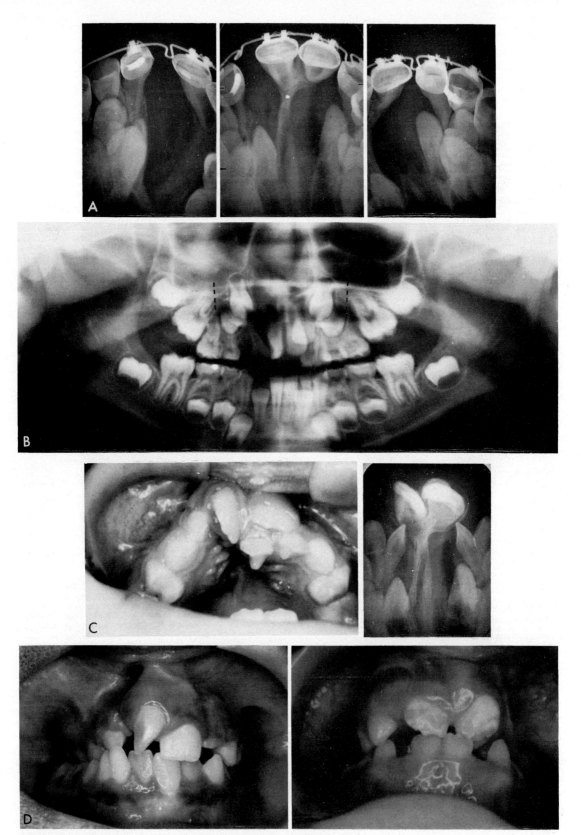

Figure 57–5. Associated dental anomalies. *A,* Periapical radiographs showing the absence of maxillary lateral incisors in a patient with bilateral cleft lip and palate. *B,* Panoramic roentgenogram showing congenital absence of right and left maxillary second bicuspids in a patient with a cleft palate. *C,* Intraoral view showing erupted supernumerary teeth. A periapical radiograph illustrates the presence of unerupted supernumerary teeth. *D,* Examples of severely rotated and poorly calcified maxillary central incisors.

Fixed appliances in the mixed dentition stage are effective in the treatment of rotated teeth. In addition to improving dental relationships within the dental arch and between individual teeth, the appliances establish a more favorable anatomic architecture under the repaired lip. Early management of the rotated teeth contributes toward improved stability of the involved teeth and of the palatal segment in which they are developing (Fig. 57–6). In patients with malpositioned and malformed teeth, early rotation of the teeth is recommended along with a plan to restore and utilize the teeth as additional abutment teeth. Early extraction of such teeth entails loss of part of the dentoalveolar process and the loss of dental units that can serve in expansion procedures to establish a more normal dental arch form.

Other frequently encountered dental abnormalities in cleft lip and palate children are *fused teeth* and *variations in tooth size and location* (Fig. 57–7A). Ectopic teeth are of primary concern, because some decision early in the management of the malocclusion must be made about the disposition of these teeth (Fig. 57–7B,C). Two factors might be at play: one is arch length–tooth material disparity, and the second is the abnormal site of development and eruption of these teeth. They may be palatally posed and completely blocked out of the dental arch; occasionally they may be transposed (Fig. 57–7D). In cleft palate patients such dental aberrations occur in conjunction with the existing maxillary skeletal anomaly, and compel the orthodontist to modify and compromise the treatment objectives. Radiographic, cephalometric, and panoramic films are helpful in diagnosis and treatment planning. Plaster models and photographs should also be taken.

STAGES OF TREATMENT

The Newborn Period

Until recent years orthodontic therapy for the cleft lip and palate child was usually not undertaken until after the eruption of all the

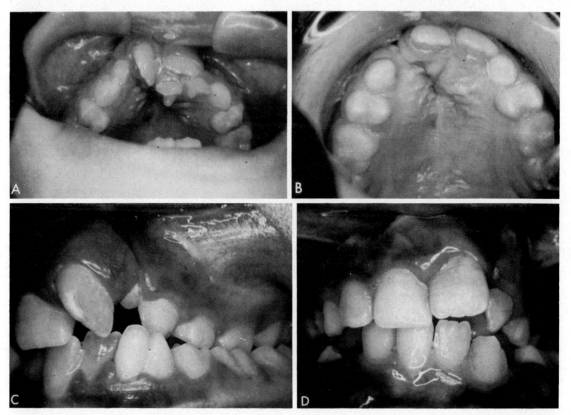

Figure 57–6. Two patients before and after early orthodontic treatment. Note the improvement in the dental alignment and arch form following the removal of supernumerary teeth and the correction of a rotated central incisor. *A, C,* Pretreatment views. *B, D,* Post-treatment views.

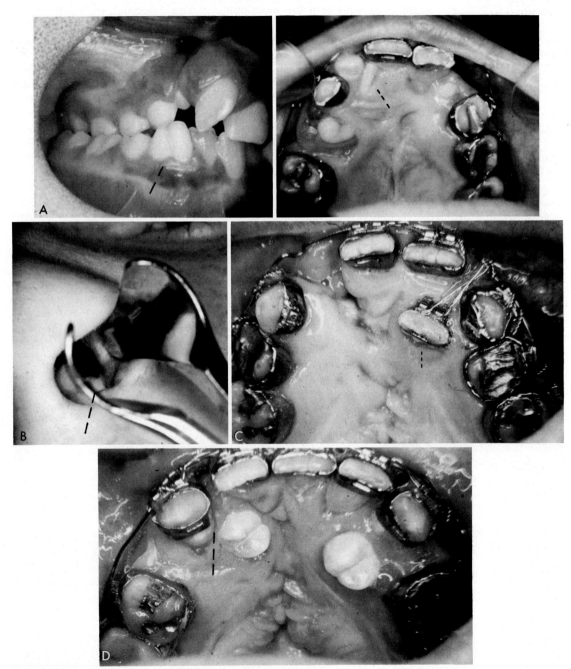

Figure 57–7. Deformities of the dentition. *A,* Lateral and palatal views of fused or "twin teeth" and a severely rotated lateral incisor. Position indicated by the dotted line. *B,* Ectopic tooth in the floor of the nose. *C,* Ectopic tooth in the palate. *D,* Transposed teeth.

deciduous teeth, at approximately 3 years of age. However, in parts of Europe and in the United States some clinicians began to institute correction shortly after birth.

The construction of an expansion prosthesis for infants with bilateral cleft lip and cleft palate was recommended by McNeil (1954), Burston (1958), and Harkins (1960). A bilateral cleft involving the lips, the alveolar process, and the palate is an extensive deformity creating severe esthetic and functional problems. Rehabilitative treatment necessitates the restoration of facial contour and balance, labial mobility, the sublabial space, and the dental arch, and the separation of the oral cavity from the nasal and pharyngeal cavity.

The abnormal position of the infant's premaxilla complicates restorative measures and results. Various surgical methods have been recommended to obtain an adequate repositioning of the premaxilla (see Chap. 53). These methods rely on the pressure of the surgically united lip to retropose the premaxillary process anatomically and functionally. Unfortunately, the desired results are seldom achieved (Harkins, 1960). In many of these cases the surgeon finds it easier to correct the deformity if the premaxilla and maxillary arches are repositioned to a more favorable arch relationship. This treatment objective may be achieved by a split prosthesis that is capable of moving and repositioning the maxillary segments. It may expand or contract the maxillary arch, depending on which direction the forces are applied.

As described by Harkins (1960), the sequence of treatment when an expansion prosthesis is used is as follows:

1. Initial and secondary impressions.
2. Construction of the expansion prosthesis.
3. Resection of the vomer (now seldom done).
4. Placement of the expansion prosthesis in situ.
5. Surgical closure of the lip.
6. Surgical closure of the alveolar process after retroposition of the premaxillary process.
7. Surgical (or prosthetic) restoration of the palate at a later age.

The initial impression is taken, or in some cases specially made acrylic trays from previous models of correct size may be used. From the preliminary impression, a more accurate self-curing acrylic tray is made and used to take a more definitive impression

from which a final working model is made. All safety precautions are followed during the impression taking. The model is studied and designed for the placement of the expansion screws to be used. They are fixed in position, and the mechanism is covered with plaster and waxed to the model. The waxed model is processed in clear acrylic resin. After it has been processed, it is cut through the midline to the expansion screw. The prosthesis when polished is fitted to the patient's palate and the necessary adjustments are made. The prosthesis should not extend too superiorly into the sulcus or too posteriorly or it will irritate the palate.

If the prosthesis is to be used in conjunction with a surgical procedure, it is advisable to pin it in position; alternatively, some surgeons prefer to be able to remove it. To improve the retentive quality of the prosthesis, denture adhesive is used. Rapid expansion is performed. The usual and advisable method is to turn the screw one notch every 12 hours. This is equivalent to a 0.25 mm increase in the width of the appliance with every adjustment. The appliance will not only act as a retainer and prevent maxillary collapse but also stimulate growth. The appliance also alleviates the feeding problem and has a beneficial effect on future speech function. Lindquist (1963) pointed out that the abnormal swallowing pattern, which the baby with a palatal cleft is forced to adopt, may alter the motor action of the nerves to the muscles that are common to speech and deglutition. The resulting patterns of muscular action appear to play a role in maintenance of the typical abnormal speech in some patients despite subsequent and adequate surgical treatment.

Early orthodontic therapy without surgical interference was reported by McNeil in 1956. He used a palatal appliance to keep the palatal segments apart before the palate was repaired (Fig. 57–8A). He believed that constriction of the maxilla could not be avoided after lip surgery. Therefore, he recommended repositioning of the parts before lip surgery; he maintained that his appliance contributed toward bone growth and resulted in a narrowing of the hard palate cleft. McNeil showed that in complete clefts of the primary and secondary palates the involved palatal segments could be moved into satisfactory alignment by using a series of split palatal appliances, specially constructed for the patient at

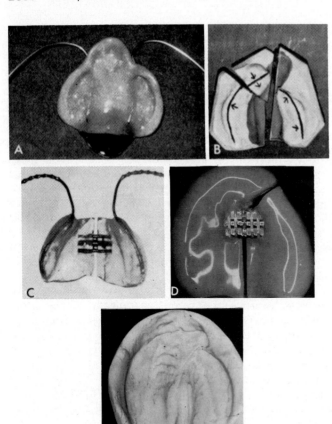

Figure 57–8. Orthodontic therapy in the newborn. *A,* Palatal appliance for the newborn with lateral extensions for external fixation. *B,* Sectioned dental cast with segments in the desired position. *C,* Palatal appliance fabricated on the sectioned dental cast. *D,* Another type of palatal appliance employs a turnbuckle type of expansion device. *E,* Model from which the above appliance (*D*) was made.

specific age intervals. The splints are split in the midline and periodically realigned to move the palatal segments into a more normal anatomic relation. They are constructed by means of a sectioned plaster cast of the palatal segments (Fig. 57–8*B*). The segments are placed into the desired position, and a palatal appliance is constructed (Fig. 57–8*C*). The latter is worn by the neonate in order to move the maxillary segments during the functional activities of sucking and swallowing. Two or three appliances may be required over a period of three months to aid in obtaining the desired correction. After orthodontic repositioning, the cleft lip and nose are surgically repaired, and a gingivoplasty is frequently accomplished.

Burston (1958) described a technique similar to that of McNeil (1956). The new concept of maxillary orthopedics included bone grafting to stabilize the palatal segments in the desired position (see Chap. 55). Forshall, Osborne, and Burston (1964) reported that only about one-third of those treated subsequently maintained adequate form, while one-third showed disappointing results.

Another type of splint employed incorporates the jack screw in the midline for arch expansion (Fig. 57–8*D,E*). An additional variation in the molding force is an extraoral elastic band (Fig. 57–9) used by Desault (1791), and revived by Walker and associates (1966) and Griswold and Sage (1966).

A preliminary lip adhesion was advocated by Johanssen and Ohlssen (1961), Millard (1964), Spina (1964), Randall (1965), and Walker and associates (1966) to bring the maxillary elements into satisfactory alignment before the lip is closed by surgical means (Fig. 57–10).

Georgiade (Georgiade, Mladick, and Thorne, 1968; Georgiade, 1969, 1971) and Latham, Kusy, and Georgiade (1976) proposed the use of pin-retained appliances to expand the collapsed alveolar segments while retracting the premaxilla in the bilateral cleft. This was followed by lip closure and gingivoplasty where possible. Latham (1980) described a pin-retained appliance used to advance the cleft maxillary alveolar segment in the unilateral case (Fig. 57–11). The goal is to correct the retropositioned alveolar proc-

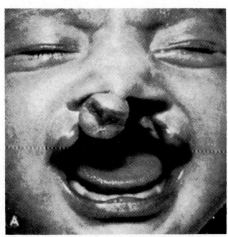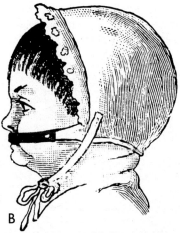

Figure 57–9. Extraoral elastic band. *A,* The protruding premaxilla in a bilateral cleft lip and palate patient. (From Surgical and orthodontic treatment of cleft lip and palate in Denmark. *In* Hotz, R. (Ed.): Early Treatment of Cleft Lip and Palate International Symposium, April 9–11, 1964. University of Zurich–Dental Institute, Bern, Hans Huber, 1964.) *B,* The elastic type of appliance used to retract or rotate the severely procumbent premaxilla. (From Cronin, T., and Penoff, J. H.: Bilateral clefts of the primary palate. Cleft Palate J., *8*:350, 1971.)

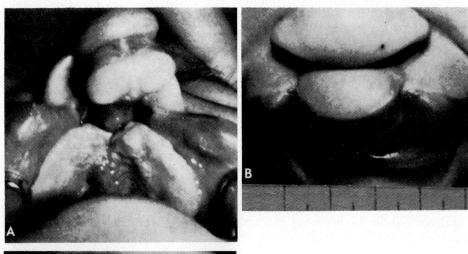

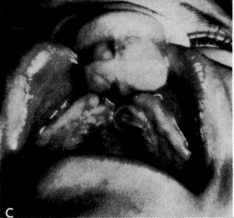

Figure 57–10. Lip adhesion. *A,* Patient with a complete bilateral lip and palate. Note the premaxilla with medially rotated palatal segments. *B,* Appearance of the lip following the lip adhesion procedure. *C,* Reduction of the premaxilla procumbency following the lip adhesion procedure. Note the failure to employ presurgical orthopedic expansion and the medially collapsed posterior alveolar segments. (From Cronin, T., and Penoff, J. H.: Bilateral clefts of the primary palate. Cleft Palate J., *8*:352, 1971.)

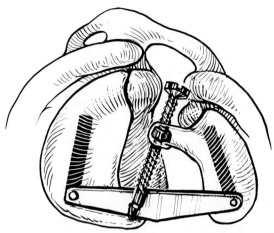

Figure 57–11. The pin-retained appliance of Latham (1980) is used to advance the retropositioned cleft alveolar segment. A screw oriented obliquely to the midsagittal plane is rotated daily to achieve the advancement.

ess and, in so doing, improve support for the alar base on the cleft side (Fig. 57–12). After initial lip and nasal repair and gingivoplasty, the palate is expanded with a fixed, pin-retained appliance and held in place for retention (one to two months). The principle is to correct the reduction in arch circumference that was associated with orthopedic activity before the adoption of gingival, labial, and nasal surgical repair. The goal of postsurgical orthopedic expansion and retention is to overcorrect the presurgically reduced arch width. No bone grafting is done in these procedures. Before closure of the gingival tissue, the periosteum is teased toward the opposite cleft wall in order to encourage primary bone deposition. The pre- and postsurgical orthopedic control of the unilateral cleft palate, as described above, produces an arch that is usually resistant to medial collapse (see p. 2879).

Although it is generally accepted that, in the absence of postsurgical overexpansion, the retention forces exerted by the repaired lip musculature may displace one or both of the maxillary segments medially (Pruzansky and Aduss, 1964), it is also an established fact that early orthodontic treatment can effectively reposition the malposed segments. As a result, not only are the maldeveloped and displaced segments positioned more anatomically but the existing crossbite malocclusion is also corrected (Subtelny and Brodie, 1954; Subtelny, 1966; Coccaro, 1970). Retention appliances are needed in the transition

from deciduous to permanent teeth, and additional periods of fixed appliance therapy are necessary until a full complement of permanent teeth is fully erupted and the teeth are in satisfactory alignment and occlusion (Subtelny, 1966; Coccaro, 1970).

Period of Deciduous Dentition

One of the major clinical features common to many cleft lip and palate patients is the constricted and distorted maxillary arch. McNeil (1956), Nordin (1957), Schrudde and Stellmach (1959), and others believed that a constriction of the maxilla cannot be avoided after lip surgery. Pruzansky and Aduss (1967) showed that other factors are responsible for collapse of the arch. Whether due to the modeling action of the lip after surgery or not, it is a skeletal factor that orthodontists must consider in planning treatment for these patients. Since the alveolar process of the cleft segment may move medially behind the noncleft segment, it should be noted that the character of the cleft tends to influence the form of the maxillary arch. In unilateral cases, the smaller segment (i.e., the cleft segment) is free and unattached to the vomer and nasal septum, while the noncleft segment, which is larger and includes a portion of the premaxilla belonging to the smaller segment, is rotated upward and outward in the premaxillary region. The larger segment is in contact with the vomer and nasal septum and may be influenced in its position by the growth potential of the septum. Therefore, the space between the two segments permits the smaller segment to become impacted by rotating medially, carrying with it the dentoalveolar process and developing dentition. The resulting crossbite is due to skeletal as well as dentoalveolar malpositioning (Fig. 57–13). Early orthodontic correction in the child with a congenital cleft lip and palate has been recommended by many U.S. orthodontists and is initiated after the eruption of all deciduous teeth, when the child is approximately 3½ years of age.

The advantages of early treatment are many, particularly in the areas of function, esthetics, and speech. In addition, a foundation is provided for the support of the surgically reconstructed lip. The dentition must be in satisfactory condition, not only to permit the use of fixed orthodontic appliances but

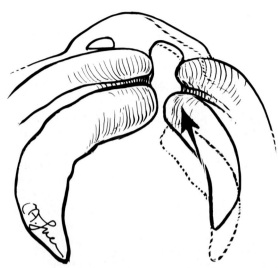

Figure 57–12. Presurgical orthopedic advancement of the cleft alveolar segment along with the basal maxillary bone often improves the bony platform of the alar base before definitive repair.

also to allow prolonged use of retention appliances. The repositioning of the displaced palatal segments of the maxilla is dependent on the presence of teeth, both deciduous and permanent. Since teeth serve to support the orthodontic appliance, dental care of the deciduous teeth is imperative and specialists in pediatric dentistry must be consulted. Cooperation with other professional disciplines helps to fulfill the total rehabilitative needs in cleft lip and palate patients at different age levels coincident with the changing character of the deformity.

The first phase of orthodontic therapy must be directed toward counteracting the adverse muscular forces (Harvold, 1949; Johnston, 1958; Burston, 1958; Glass, 1959). Orthodontic forces must expand (via rotation of cleft palatal segments that are not united because of the cleft) the palatal processes of the maxilla and the accompanying dentoalveolar processes. In the young patient, the bony palatal segments yield to the orthodontic forces employed (Fig. 57–14). By virtue of this maneuver, the unfused palatal segments are moved in a lateral direction. In some bilateral clefts in which the lateral palatal segments are locked behind the premaxillary segment, an advancement of the premaxilla is indicated before an attempt is made to move the constricted palatal segments laterally (Fig. 57–15). The added potential of enhancing maxillary growth is also always

present when malposed and overlapping palatal processes are adequately positioned. If the impacted alveolar segments were allowed to remain overlapping, they would serve to impede growth and contribute toward pressure resorption of the alveolar processes (Fig. 57–16).

Studies have demonstrated that presurgical orthodontics and bone grafting do not necessarily prevent the development of malocclusion (Derichsweiler, 1958; Ross, 1987). Other investigators (Subtelny and Brodie, 1954; Pruzansky and Aduss, 1967; Coccaro, 1970) have found a high percentage of orthodontic collapse, as represented by a crossbite in the deciduous dentition. Collapse of the maxillary arch is a factor in many cleft palate patients, and it was shown to occur in 40 per cent of all cases in one study (Pruzansky and Aduss, 1967). It appears that the problems and the required treatment procedures must be evaluated over a period of time to weigh the effects of time and growth in each individual.

Period of Mixed Dentition

It should be stressed that early orthodontics in the deciduous dentition does not necessarily obviate the need for orthodontics at a later age. Permanent teeth, especially those adjacent to the cleft, are usually malposed and often severely rotated and poorly calcified. Consequently, orthodontic therapy during the period of mixed dentition may be necessary (Fig. 57–17). These abnormalities should be corrected as soon as they become apparent. Banding, bonding, and the use of arch wires appear to be the appliances of choice. The corrections are easily accomplished as soon as these teeth erupt and are maintained in their new position. In addition, the adverse influence of rotated and malpositioned maxillary teeth may be eliminated. It is often impossible to attain a correct midline relationship, a fairly consistent problem. Maxillary teeth may be in an anterior crossbite relationship with the mandibular incisors. In these cases an acrylic inclined plane secured to the mandibular incisors may add to the correction initiated by the bands and arch wire (Fig. 57–18).

Before eruption of the permanent canines in unilateral or bilateral clefts, bone grafts should be placed to provide continuity of the

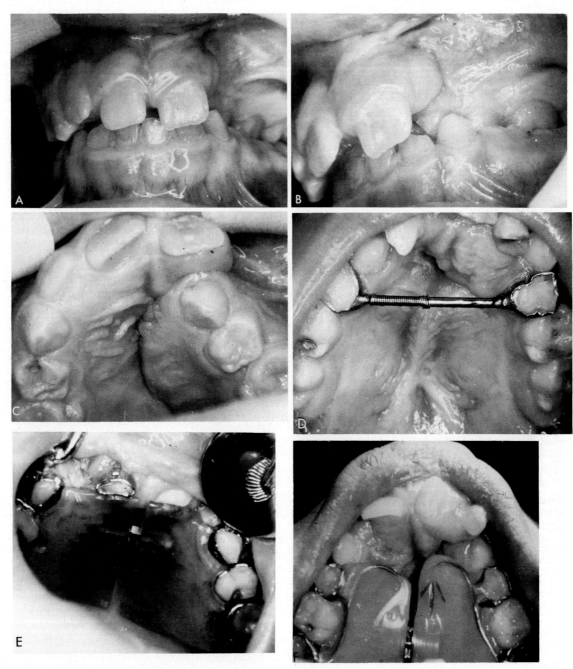

Figure 57–13. Unilateral cleft lip and palate: frontal (*A*), lateral (*B*), and palatal (*C*) views. The severe skeletal and dental abnormalities associated with the congenital defect are apparent. *D* to *F,* Types of expansion appliances used in the early stages of orthodontic treatment. *D* and *F* are fixed, and *E* is removable.

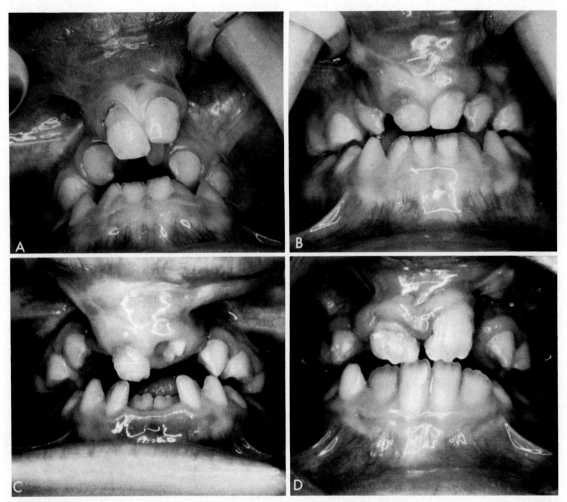

Figure 57–14. Frontal views of the dental occlusion in a patient with a bilateral cleft lip and palate, showing changes associated with orthodontic therapy in the deciduous (*A* and *B*) and mixed dentition (*C* and *D*) stages.

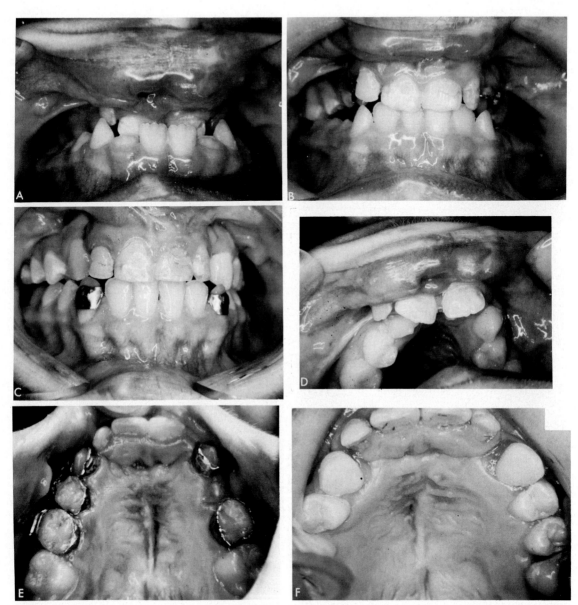

Figure 57–15. Orthodontic therapy in bilateral cleft lip and palate. Sequential frontal (*A* to *C*) and palatal (*D* to *F*) views showing collapse of the maxillary arch and the severity of the accompanying dental malocclusion. Each series depicts the photographic sequence of changes through the early and late stages of orthodontic treatment.

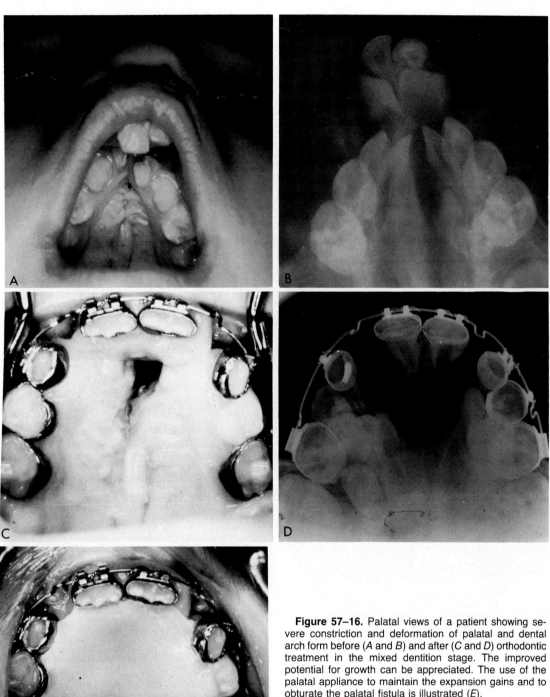

Figure 57–16. Palatal views of a patient showing severe constriction and deformation of palatal and dental arch form before (*A* and *B*) and after (*C* and *D*) orthodontic treatment in the mixed dentition stage. The improved potential for growth can be appreciated. The use of the palatal appliance to maintain the expansion gains and to obturate the palatal fistula is illustrated (*E*).

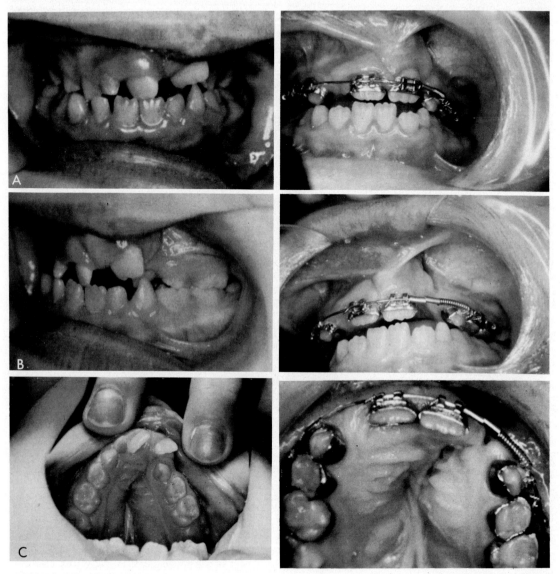

Figure 57–17. Orthodontic therapy during the period of mixed dentition. Frontal (*A*), lateral (*B*), and palatal (*C*) views of a patient with a unilateral cleft lip and palate illustrating the conditions before and after orthodontic treatment in the mixed dentition stage. Fixed appliances (bands on the individual teeth) and arch wires were employed as illustrated.

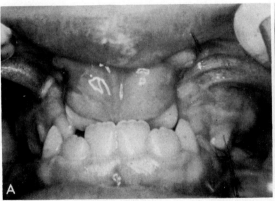
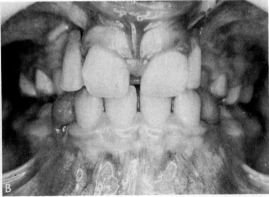

Figure 57–18. Correction of an anterior crossbite during the period of mixed dentition. Pretreatment (*A*) and post-treatment (*B*) frontal views show correction of an anterior crossbite after use of an inclined plane in addition to bands and arch wires.

alveolar arch and a bed of bone and gingival tissue through which the teeth may erupt (see Chap. 55). It is often necessary to expand the clefts orthodontically before placement of bone grafts and closure of the cleft site. The canines may erupt on their own or may be guided down with a surgically placed orthodontic bracket on the canine tooth surface and an elastic or wire ligature to the orthodontic appliances on the dental arch (Fig. 57–19).

Period of Adult Dentition

Close observation of individuals with clefts should be continued until all permanent teeth have erupted into the oral cavity. By late adolescence the final orthodontic positioning of all the permanent teeth should be completed. With the final phases of therapy, it becomes apparent that the early stages of therapy involve moving bony palatal seg-

ments, while the later stages are usually restricted to individual tooth movement. The extraction of teeth may be recommended to establish a balance between the number and size of dental units and the existing available dental arch length. The underdevelopment of the maxilla could be an etiologic factor. Judicious removal of mandibular first bicuspids may be required to obtain an adequate overbite and overjet relationship of the anterior teeth (Fig. 57–20). Secondary bone grafting (see Chap. 55) in the cleft site of the anterior maxillary alveolar process may be indicated after the late stages of orthodontic treatment (Fig. 57–21). It may help to stabilize the segments of the maxillary arch and contribute toward maintaining the final orthodontic results. It also enhances facial appearance, since it adds to the support of the floor of the nose, the alar base, and the lip and minimizes the undesired depressed appearance noted in these areas.

Deficient   anteroposterior   and   vertical

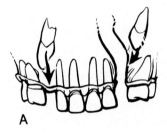
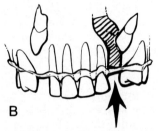
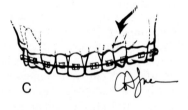

Figure 57–19. *A,* Unilateral cleft before eruption of the maxillary canines (*arrows*). *B,* Bone graft (*shaded*) to the cleft alveolus, providing a bony path through which the canine may erupt. *C,* Eruption of the canine taking a natural position in the dental arch.

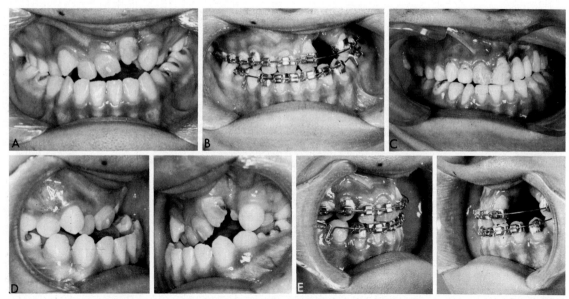

Figure 57–20. Overbite and overjet relationships. *A, B, C,* Serial frontal views of the dental occlusion in a patient with a left-sided cleft lip and palate, showing changes in the occlusion following the extraction of the lower first bicuspids and orthodontic and prosthodontic treatment. *D, E,* Pre- and post-treatment lateral views. Fixed appliances (bands on the individual teeth and arch wires) were used to reposition the palatal segments as well as to correct dental irregularities within each dental arch and between individual teeth.

growth of the maxilla may be seen in the late adolescent or early adult period. If the maxillomandibular discrepancy is great, midface flatness and mandibular prognathism will develop. A complete cephalometric and clinical evaluation is necessary (see Chap. 29). The surgical correction of this abnormality by maxillary advancement and sometimes mandibular set-back requires presurgical orthodontic preparation of the teeth. In this situation the maxillary and mandibular incisors are uprighted and centered over the alveolar ridge. This usually results in an increase in the dental crossbite before surgery. Maxillary and mandibular arch width are also coordinated so that they match correctly upon surgical correction.

Retainer appliances are used at various stages of treatment: (1) after repositioning of the palatal segments, retention is necessary to maintain the newly established palatal positions, otherwise there is a rapid return of the bony segments to their original positions; (2) retainers also serve to obturate a palatal fistula and carry a replacement for missing teeth, and moreover serve to maintain spaces in the dental transitional period; and (3) during the late stages of adolescence, some form of permanent retention appliance must

be inserted to maintain the orthodontic results and often replace a missing tooth in the area of the cleft.

CONCLUSIONS

In the treatment of children with cleft lip and/or palate, the problems associated with growth and development of the skeletal and dentoalveolar processes of the maxilla and the extent of the maxillary involvement by orofacial defects make it difficult to achieve a permanent result during any particular stage of physical development. The need for staged orthodontic therapy to obtain optimal results throughout the formative years becomes more apparent.

The role of the orthodontist in cleft palate rehabilitation, and the need for early orthodontic intervention to unlock impacted palatal segments and permit more normal growth, have long been recognized. Several periods of treatment are necessary, beginning with the newborn infant and extending to the succedaneous teeth; long periods of retention are subsequently required. To unite and create a stable homogenous upper jaw, bone grafting procedures (McNeil, 1956) have been em-

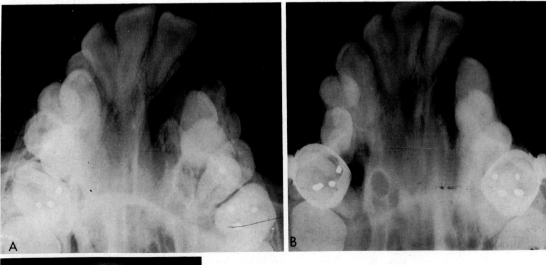

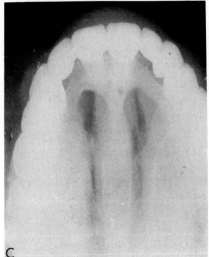

Figure 57–21. Secondary bone grafting. *A,* Palatal view of bone grafts inserted in a unilateral cleft of the primary palate following palatal expansion in the mixed dentition. *B,* Radiograph one year after insertion. *C,* Secondary bone grafting in a patient with a bilateral cleft lip and palate. Bone grafts may be noted bilaterally. A fixed bridge serves to complete the treatment procedure in the incisor region. In addition to serving as a fixed retainer, the fixed bridge permits replacement of missing lateral incisors and full coverage of poorly calcified maxillary central incisors.

ployed in association with retention appliances. The advocates of bone grafting maintain that results cannot be regarded as definitive until a permanent bite has been fully established (Johanssen and Ohlssen, 1961).

Thus, there are three rather important reasons for orthodontic treatment on a continuing basis from childhood through adulthood: (1) to provide symmetry in the dental arch of the infant and bony support for the initial nasal repair, (2) to align the distorted and constricted palatal segments of the maxilla, and (3) to maintain the gains made by expansion and dental alignment procedures.

The ideal method of documentation in these areas is on a longitudinal basis through pho-

tographic and radiographic records (Fig. 57–22). Growth is apparent in malpositioned palatal segments after early orthodontic treatment. Once the impacted segments are free and positioned satisfactorily to reestablish a more normal dental arch, the alveolar and palatal surfaces of the maxilla can manifest more normal growth potentials.

To maintain the gains made in palatal width and in dental arch form, it is essential to use fixed and/or removable retainers. Fixed retainers become obsolete with increasing loss of deciduous units during growth and development. Thus, one must rely upon removable appliances in the transition period.

Maintenance of orthodontic results appears to be difficult even in the presence of retainers

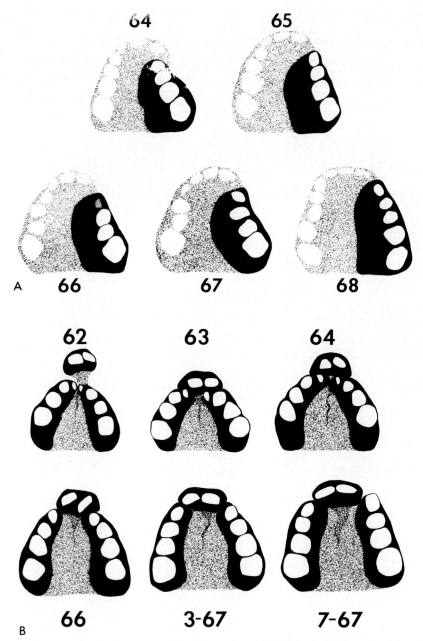

Figure 57–22. Graphic illustrations of palatal and dental arch form. *A,* Unilateral cleft lip and palate with improvement in position of the cleft palatal segment (*darkened area*) following orthodontics in the mixed dentition stage. In the transition period (*66–67*) note the collapse and the final recovery (*68*) following orthodontics in the permanent dentition. *B,* The palatal and dental arch form in a bilateral cleft before and after orthodontic therapy in the deciduous dentition stage. Continued orthodontics in the mixed dentition stage demonstrates improvement in palatal and dental arch form. Note the growth of the palatal segments.

and/or bone grafts, particularly during the formative years of skeletal and dental development. This finding may reflect the adverse impact of soft tissue pull upon palatal segments through the period of adulthood.

It is apparent that palatal and dental relapse is inevitable if the patient is unattended for periods during childhood and adolescence. It is important to offer care at this time to enhance function, growth, and esthetics.

REFERENCES

Bohn, A.: Dental anomalies in hare lip and cleft palate. In Norwegian Monographs on Medical Science. Oslo, Universities for Lagets tryknigssentral, 1963.

Borden, G. H.: Mandibular Growth in the Cleft Palate Infant. University of Illinois, 1953.

Brauer, R., and Cronin, T.: Maxillary orthopedics and anterior repair with bone grafting. Cleft Palate J., 1:31, 1964.

Burston, W. R.: The early orthodontic treatment of cleft palate conditions. Dent. Pract. (Bristol), 9:41, 1958.

Case, C. S.: A practical treatise on the techniques and principles of dental orthopaedia and prosthetic correction of the cleft palate. Chicago, C. S. Case Company, 1921.

Chorin: Sur L'opération d'un bec-de-liévre double, avec fente à la voute du palais. J. Chir. par Desault, 1:97, 1791.

Coccaro, P. J.: Orthodontics in cleft palate children: a continuing process. Cleft Palate J., 6:495, 1970.

Converse, J. M., and Horowitz, S. L.: Facial deformity. In Horowitz, S. L., and Hixon, E. H. (Eds.): The Nature of Orthodontic Analysis. St. Louis, MO, C. V. Mosby Company, 1966.

Converse, J. M., Horowitz, S. L., Guy, C. L., and Wood-Smith, D.: Surgical orthodontic correction in the bilateral cleft lip and cleft palate. Cleft Palate J., 1:153, 1964.

Coupe, T. B., and Subtelny, J. D.: Deficiency or displacement of tissue. Plast. Reconstr. Surg., 30:426, 1962.

Crikelair, G. F., Bom, A. F., Luban, J., and Moss, M.: Early orthodontic movement of cleft maxillary segments prior to cleft lip repair. Plast. Reconstr. Surg., 30:462, 1962.

Cronin, T., and Penoff, J. H.: Bilateral clefts of the primary palate. Cleft Palate J., 8:350, 1971.

Derichsweiler, H.: Some observations on the early treatment of hare lip and cleft palate cases. Trans. Eur. Orthod. Soc., 34:237, 1958.

Desault, P. J.: see Chorin, 1791. Oeuvres Chirurgicales par Xav. Bichat (1830). Vol. II. Paris, Baillière.

Fauchard, M. P.: Le chirurgien dentiste, ou traité des dents. Part II. Paris, Servières, 1786, p. 292.

Forshall, I., Osborne, R. P., and Burston, W. R.: Observations on the early orthopedic treatment of cleft lip and palate conditions. In Hotz, R. (Ed.): Early Treatment of Cleft Lip and Palate. Berne, Switzerland, Hans Huber, 1964, pp. 68–77.

Georgiade, N. G.: The management of premaxillary and maxillary segments in the newborn cleft patient. Cleft Palate J., 7:4, 1969.

Georgiade, N. G.: Improved technique for one stage repair of bilateral cleft lip. Plast. Reconstr. Surg., 48:318, 1971.

Georgiade, N. G., Mladick, R. A., and Thorne, F. L.: Positioning of the premaxilla in bilateral cleft lips by pinning and traction. Plast. Reconstr. Surg., 240:41, 1968.

Glass, D. F.: The orthodontic treatment of cleft lip and palate patients. Ann. R. Coll. Surg. Engl., 25:239, 1959.

Graber, T. M.: A study of the congenital cleft palate deformity. Ph.D. Thesis, Northwestern University, Chicago, 1950.

Grayson, B. H., Bookstein, F., McCarthy, J. G., and Mueeddin, T.: Mean tensor cephalometric analysis of a patient population with clefts of the lip and palate. Cleft Palate J., 24:267, 1987.

Griswold, M. L., and Sage, W. F.: Extraoral traction in the cleft lip. Plast. Reconstr. Surg., 37:416, 1966.

Harkins, C. S.: Principles of Cleft Palate Prosthesis. Philadelphia, Temple University Press, 1960.

Harvold, E.: Principles of the orthodontic treatment of the upper jaw in cases of palate with total cleft on one side. Nor. Tanniaegeforen. Tid., 25:395, 1949.

Hogeman, K. E., Jacobsson, S., and Sarnas, K. U.: Secondary bone grafting in cleft palate: a follow-up of 145 patients. Cleft Palate J., 9:39, 1972.

Johanssen, B., and Ohlssen, A.: Bone grafting and dental orthopedics in primary and secondary cases of cleft lip and palate. Acta. Chir. Scan., 112:122, 1961.

Johnston, M. C.: Orthodontic treatment for the cleft palate patient. Am. J. Orthod., 44:750, 1958.

Kingsley, N.: A Treatise on Oral Deformities. New York., D. Appleton Century Company, 1880, p. 215.

Latham, R. A.: Orthopedic advancement of the cleft maxillary segment: a preliminary report. Cleft Palate J., 17:227, 1980.

Latham, R. A., Kusy, R. P., and Georgiade, N. G.: An extraorally activated expansion appliance for cleft palate infants. Cleft Palate J., 13:253, 1976.

Lindquist, A. F.: Prosthetic and orthodontic procedures for the cleft palate in infants. Int. Dent. J., 13:688, 1963.

McMahon, E. M.: Speech patterns with special reference to cleft palates. Aust. Dent. J., 6:101, 1961.

McNeil, C. K.: Oral and Facial Deformity. London, Pitman, 1954.

McNeil, C. K.: Congenital oral deformities. Br. Dent. J., 101:191, 1956.

Millard, D. R., Jr.: Refinement in rotation-advancement cleft lip technique. Plast. Reconstr. Surg., 37:552, 1964.

Nordin, D. E.: Treatment of primary total cleft palate deformity. Preoperative orthopedic correction of the displaced components of the upper jaw in infants followed by bone grafting to the alveolar process clefts. Trans. Eur. Orthod. Soc., The Hague, 1957.

Pruzansky, S.: Factors determining arch form in clefts of the lip and palate. Am. J. Orthod., 41:827, 1955.

Pruzansky, S.: Pre-surgical orthopedics and bone grafting for infants with cleft lip and palate: a dissent. Cleft Palate J., 1:164, 1964.

Pruzansky, S., and Aduss, H.: Arch form and the deciduous occlusion in complete unilateral clefts. Cleft Palate J., 1:411, 1964.

Pruzansky, S., and Aduss, H.: Prevalence of arch collapse and malocclusion in complete unilateral cleft lip and palate. Trans. Eur. Orthod. Soc., 1:16, 1967.

Randall, P.: A lip adhesion operation in cleft lip surgery. Plast. Reconstr. Surg., *35*:371, 1965.

Ross, R. B.: Treatment variables affecting facial growth in complete unilateral cleft lip and palate. Cleft Palate J., *24*:5, 1987.

Ross, R. B., and Johnston, M. C.: The effect of early orthodontic treatment on facial growth in cleft lip and palate. Cleft Palate J., *4*:157, 1967.

Ross, R. B., and Johnston, M. C.: Cleft Lip and Palate. Baltimore, Williams & Wilkins Company, 1972.

Schrudde, J., and Stellmach, R.: Funktionelle Orthopadishe Gesichtspunkte bei der Osteoplastik der Defekte des Kieferbogens bei Lippenkiefer-Gaumplatten. Fortschr. Kiefer. Orthod., *20*:373, 1959.

Spina, V.: Bilateral harelip surgery, a new concept. *In* Trans. Third Internatl. Congr. Plast. Surg. Baltimore, Williams & Wilkins Company, 1964, pp. 314–323.

Stevens, A. H.: Staphylorraphe or palate suture, successfully performed by A. H. Stevens, Prof. of Surgery in the College of Physicians and Surgeons, New York. N. Am. Med. Surg. J., *3*:233, 1827.

Subtelny, J. D.: Orthodontic treatment of cleft lip and palate: birth to adulthood. Angle Orthod., *36*:273, 1966.

Subtelny, J. D., and Brodie, A. G.: Analysis of orthodontic expansion in unilateral cleft lip and palate patients. Am. J. Orthod., *40*:686, 1954.

Walker, J. C., Collito, M. B., Mancusi-Ungaro, A., and Meijer, R.: Physiologic considerations in cleft lip closure: the C-W technique. Plast. Reconstr. Surg., *37*:552, 1966.

58

David J. David
A. D. Bagnall

Velopharyngeal Incompetence

Key to Symbols

[æ]	as in c<u>a</u>t.	[k]	as in <u>c</u>at.
[ɛ]	as in g<u>e</u>t.	[f]	as in <u>f</u>un.
[i]	as in s<u>ee</u>.	[θ]	as in <u>th</u>in.
[p]	as in <u>p</u>ie.	[s]	as in <u>s</u>un.
[t]	as in <u>t</u>ie.		

ANATOMIC AND FUNCTIONAL CONSIDERATIONS

A competent velopharyngeal sphincter is essential for intelligible speech. The palate is part, but not the whole, of the sphincter, and a cleft palate is but one of the abnormalities affecting the velopharyngeal sphincter and speech. Modern concepts demand that the function of the velopharyngeal sphincter be seen in the context of the function of the whole vocal tract. The object of any surgery performed on the velopharyngeal sphincter is to provide an apparatus that permits the development of normal speech.

"Velopharyngeal incompetence" is the term used when the patient is diagnosed as being unable to close the sphincter completely. The sphincter is situated between the oral and nasal cavities and permits the speaker to separate the nasal from the oral cavity. Closure is achieved by tension in the velum and its elevation toward the posterior pharyngeal wall. At the same time, closure is assisted by the posterior and lateral pharyngeal walls, which move toward the rising velum, thus diminishing the lumen of the pharynx. As the person prepares to speak, the velum is partially raised and held at the ready position before speech begins; it then moves to the closed position as phonation starts. For nasal sounds (i.e., [m], [n], and [ŋ], the sphincter remains open. Complete closure does not always occur on non-nasal sounds, e.g., vowels. However, the ability to close the sphincter is essential for compression of air behind the point of constriction so that the consonants, especially plosives (e.g., [p], [t], and [k]) and fricatives (e.g., [f], [θ], and [s]) can be released with sufficient strength. In general terms, slight opening of the sphincter does not necessarily result in hypernasality. However, for a voice that has quality, richness, and carrying power, and consonants that are clear and precise, the ability to close the sphincter is essential. After normal function is understood, deviation from normal can be analyzed more effectively.

The raising and tensing of the velum, with or without full closure of the sphincter, plays a large part in the production of clear vowels. The size and shape of the pharynx, the degree of opening of the sphincter, and the various degrees of tension in the pillars of fauces and the soft palate are also important variables. The changes that appear in the velopharyngeal sphincter and vocal tract for the vowels [æ], [ɛ], and [i] are demonstrated in Figure 58–1.

Estill (1986) and others have suggested that the precise closure of the velopharyngeal sphincter ensures the efficiency of vocal cord action. Firm closure of the velopharyngeal sphincter makes possible the development of a negative pressure in the pharynx, which, acting as a "back pressure," assists and maintains firm closure of the vocal cords. This ensures adequate compression of the air stream by closely approximated margins of the vocal cords, assisting the production of a clear, strong vocal note. The breathy, weak vocal note emanating from the larynx of the speaker with velopharyngeal incompetence demonstrates this finding. In addition, a speaker who is unable to close this sphincter is handicapped as a communicator. The voice lacks carrying power, richness, warmth, subtlety of light and shade, and above all, esthetic quality. If the vocal note has access to the nasal cavity in excess of what is required for a pleasing tone, hypernasality or excessive nasality result.

The velopharyngeal sphincter has an essential part to play in the production of speech sounds. If air escapes into the nose through an open velopharyngeal sphincter, consonants lack precision and clarity. They may become distorted, may be associated with nasal snorting, or may be substituted for by pharyngeal or glottal sounds. The speaker may develop compensatory habits: excessive tension of the vocal tract; increased breath flow, or articulatory substitutes, which are maladaptive patterns of vocal behavior that further detract from the clarity and quality of speech.

Analysis of the workings of the velopharyngeal sphincter has shown it to be a highly complex and, as yet, only partially understood mechanism. The cerebral cortex, lower neurologic systems, and auditory perceptual monitoring ability of the speaker result in a subtlety of action of the sphincter, which ensures a truly efficient and pleasing voice. It follows, therefore, that the expectations of surgery may be unduly high, considering the complexities of the vocal instrument. It is not yet possible to match the surgery, however

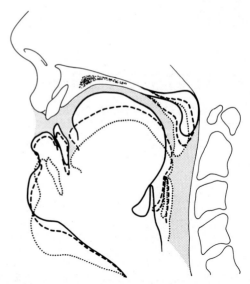

Figure 58–1. Velar elevation. Tracings taken from xeroradiographs in which the velum and tongue are seen in different positions for different cardinal vowels. [æ] = ..., [ɛ] = - - - - -, [i] = ___.

sophisticated and skillful, to the intricacies of the instrument. Progress is being made slowly as the ever more objective tools of investigation are employed to throw more light on the nature and function of the velopharyngeal sphincter. More precise understanding, not only of the mechanism as it presents to the investigator, but also of the changes that result from surgery, subsequent healing, and voice and articulation therapy will ensure the development of more sophisticated and effective treatment. For the present, treatment must be based on precise evaluation of the sphincter deficiency followed by conservative and/or surgical intervention.

Speech analysis is also discussed in Chapter 54.

CAUSES OF VELOPHARYNGEAL INCOMPETENCE

The patient with hypernasal speech or demonstrable nasal air escape may have an incompetent velopharyngeal sphincter. This may have several causes:

1. *Idiopathic insufficiency of the musculature*, in which all elements of the sphincter are working, but a tight seal, i.e., one sufficiently strong to withstand the positive air pressures built up in the oral cavity during speech, is not possible. On oral examination,

no obvious signs of abnormality appear. Patients often complain of vocal fatigue and accusations of mumbling from their family or friends. On closer examination they have some element of excessive hypernasality or nasal air escape. Nasendoscopy and synchronous lateral videofluoroscopy may reveal a slight deficiency in closure of the sphincter. A slit may be seen where the velum approaches the posterior pharyngeal wall but does not quite close the aperture. Conversely, where one or the other lateral wall is not sufficiently active, a gap is seen either unilaterally or (sometimes) bilaterally. These patients may not require surgery. Speech therapy to develop firmer closure may resolve the problem.

2. *Congenital palatal insufficiency* is a condition in which the velum is too short to reach across to the posterior pharyngeal wall. This has been variously termed a short soft palate (Kaplan, Jobe, and Chase, 1969), congenital short palate (Greene, 1964; Morley, 1973), and regional growth and development disturbances (Fletcher, 1960). Conversely, the pharynx has been considered too capacious for the size of the velum. This has been variously described as a "box pharynx" or a congenital large pharynx (Calnan, 1971a). In these cases all elements of the sphincter are working but are disproportionate.

3. *Submucous cleft palate* is a condition in which the soft palate muscles fail to unite in the midline, although the mucous membrane is intact. As the palate elevates, the levators can be seen lifting and pulling the segments of the cleft apart, forming a central furrow or area of translucency (*zona pellucida*). The patient speaks with hypernasality, which may be mild, moderate, or excessive. Submucous cleft palate has been described in various ways, but most investigators agree that it is usually characterized by a bifid uvula, a bony notch in the hard palate, and diastasis of the palatal muscles (Calnan, 1954). In 1977 this concept was supported by Pruzansky (Peterson-Falzone, 1985). However, patients with hypernasal speech without the observable stigmata of submucous cleft palate, as described above, have been reported by Kaplan (1975) as presenting with "occult submucous cleft palate." Kaplan (1975) described the unusual muscle insertions similar to those seen in classic submucous cleft palate, even though oral examination revealed no evidence of submucous cleft

palate. Subsequently, Croft and associates (1978) described the use of nasopharyngoscopy to assist the diagnosis of submucous cleft palate in 20 patients. An absence of the musculus uvulae on the nasal surface of the palate, resembling a V-shaped depression or concavity resulting in a central deficiency on attempted palatal closure, has been described as "occult submucous cleft palate" (Shprintzen, 1979). This lack of muscle bulk is not obvious upon visual inspection or palpation of the oral surface of the velum. Clearly, however, this muscle bulk is essential for velopharyngeal competence. Peterson-Falzone (1985) emphasized that there is considerable disagreement between investigators regarding their criteria when making the diagnosis of submucous cleft palate, and that nasendoscopy can reveal muscular deficiency when other "intraorally visible stigmata" are absent.

4. *Following repair of cleft palate*, velopharyngeal incompetence can occur as a result of anomalies in the movement of the various elements of the closure pattern. Surgery to close the soft palate has, as its major aim, the provision of palatal length, bulk, muscle arrangement, and movement potential sufficient to provide the speaker with full closure of the velopharyngeal port during speech (Morris, 1984). With the nasendoscope, it is sometimes noted that the speaker with a repaired cleft palate has a shortened velum that can never reach the posterior pharyngeal wall. Other patients have satisfactory velar elevation and stretch, but the posterior and lateral pharyngeal walls do not move adequately, leaving a deficit on closure. Yet others close with approximately equal movement of all elements of the sphincter, but there is a central deficit, circular in shape. The shortness of the palate following surgery has been attributed to the original inadequacy of palatal tissue rather than to the inadequacies of the surgery (Greene, 1964).

5. *After pharyngeal flap or pharyngoplasty* a patient may still have velopharyngeal incompetence and hypernasality owing to inadequate flap width, i.e., air escaping on either side. If a pharyngeal flap is so narrow that the lateral ports remain open during speech, there are surgical procedures designed to manage this difficult problem (Cosman and Falk, 1975; Owsley, Lawson, and Chierici, 1976). If a flap is situated too low in the pharynx, beneath the point where the

lateral pharyngeal walls can effect closure, it creates two funnels that aerodynamically promote nasal air escape (Osberg and Witzel, 1981).

6. *After adenoidectomy* a patient may present with velopharyngeal incompetence. Before surgery, he may have been closing the velum against the pad of lymphoid tissue. After adenoidectomy, the velum is unable to close against the posterior pharyngeal wall. Greene (1964) hypothesized a failure in movement of the palate probably due to lack of use, which gradually resolves, although this may take as long as three months. However, Calnan (1971b) stated that speech therapy for this group was without effect, and recommended surgery by a cartilage implant behind the posterior wall of the pharynx to return the speech to normal. Hypernasality that occurs following adenoidectomy has been thought to resolve over time, variously reported as six months to one year (Massengill, 1972) and two to six months (Goode and Ross, 1972). After this time, if speech remains hypernasal, careful evaluation and surgical management may be necessary.

7. *Enlarged tonsils* have also been considered as a cause of velopharyngeal incompetence. When the tonsils restrict the airway in the oropharynx because of their size, the speaker may develop a degree of hypernasality. This results from his awareness of a restricted airway that causes him to open the sphincter (Bloch, 1979). In this situation, a patient may develop a forward tongue carriage in an additional effort to increase the size of the airway. When greatly enlarged, the tonsils may add sufficient weight to the palatopharyngeal arch, such that the speaker has difficulty achieving full closure. In this way, they inhibit velar elevation (Bzoch and Williams, 1979). It is thought that enlarged tonsils interfere with the access of the vocal note to the oral cavity. This impedance leads to the diversion of sound energy into the nasopharynx and nasal cavities, increasing the perceived hypernasality (Subtelny and Koepp Baker, 1956). In this way, enlarged tonsils can have a detrimental effect upon speech, but their precise role, especially with regard to velopharyngeal incompetence, is not fully understood.

8. *After midface advancement*, velopharyngeal incompetence can occur. Patients at risk in this way are those with previously repaired cleft palate and/or those who had demonstra-

ble nasal air escape and hypernasality before surgery. The advancement of the face clearly stresses the sphincter, which subsequently is unable to make full closure (Schwarz and Gruner, 1976; Witzel and Munro, 1977; Schendel and associates, 1979; McCarthy and associates, 1979). It is also important to note that in other cases of midface advancement the sphincter may be disrupted temporarily by the surgery, e.g., subcranial Le Fort III osteotomies in Crouzon's or Apert's syndrome. However, the craniosynostosis patients (with Crouzon's or Apert's syndrome) are generally not at risk of developing velopharyngeal incompetence after Le Fort III advancement osteotomy (McCarthy and associates, 1979).

9. *Neurogenic* conditions give rise to problems of weakness, incoordination, and fatigue affecting the pattern of closure. These include some cases of hemifacial microsomia with unilateral weakness, peripheral neuritis, myasthenia gravis, nuclear lesions, bulbar poliomyelitis, and supranuclear paresis, which is usually congenital and typified by the child with cerebral palsy. Upper and lower motor neuron lesions result in dysarthria, which may include the velopharyngeal sphincter. Velopharyngeal incompetence is a significant element contributing to the speech disturbance of the patient with spastic, flaccid, or mixed dysarthria. The movements of the velopharyngeal sphincter for swallowing are usually affected. Evaluation and management of velopharyngeal incompetence in dysarthria require careful analysis and cooperation between surgeons and speech pathologists (Dworkin and Johns, 1980).

10. *Lack of velopharyngeal sphincter movement for speech.* Some children present with velopharyngeal incompetence of a gross nature, and on nasendoscopy the sphincter has been seen to be immobile. On swallowing, the sphincter appears to be normal. This problem requires further investigation and research, since pharyngoplasty does not resolve their hypernasal speech. In the same way, therapeutic management has also been found to be ineffective. Little is known of this condition, but wide, superiorly based pharyngeal flaps have been performed in order to provide some obturation for these patients (Huskie, 1985).

11. *Functional/hysterical hypernasality* has been found in the presence of a competent speech mechanism. This has been attributed to emotional disturbance (Greene, 1964). In the absence of any organic abnormality, hy-

pernasality does occur (Crikelair and associates, 1964); Porterfield and associates, 1966). Hypernasality can appear in the absence of organic or physiologic abnormalities, e.g., when the individual imitates the speech he perceives in his environment. On nasendoscopy, normal movement and closure of the velopharyngeal sphincter is seen, usually on the production of consonants, a maneuver that requires the development of intraoral air pressure for their precise release. However, the vowels are produced with an open sphincter, imparting hypernasal tone to the voice. Hypernasality is commonly found in the deaf speaker, owing to an inappropriate use of the sphincter. The perception of hypernasality by the listener is dependent on the characteristics of the entire vocal tract and not only on the use of the velopharyngeal sphincter (Curtis, 1968). Hence, *pseudohypernasality*, or *functional hypernasality* presents the greatest challenge in the diagnosis of velopharyngeal

incompetence. Just as no two individuals close their velopharyngeal sphincter in precisely the same way, or position their articulatory organs in precisely the same way, no two individuals have precisely the same voice quality. Issues related to voice quality and the degree of nasality found in the language environment of the speaker, especially in the family, must also be taken into account when deciding when, or if, the velopharyngeal sphincter is incompetent. This understanding is essential when surgery is being considered, as, by definition, the patient with pseudohypernasality does not have velopharyngeal sphincter incompetence, and surgery is, therefore, contraindicated.

HISTORY OF SURGERY

Surgery aimed at correcting velopharyngeal incompetence is not new. In the six-

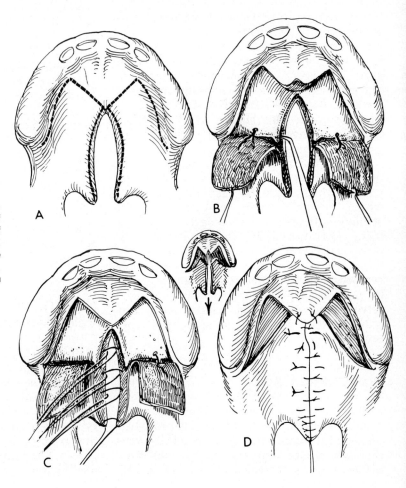

Figure 58–2. The Veau-Wardill-Kilner operation for repair of a cleft of the secondary palate. *A,* Outline of the incision. *B,* The flaps are raised. *C,* Suture of the mucous membrane on the nasal aspect of the palate. *D,* Position of the flaps at the completion of the operation.

teenth century, Pierre Franco (1561) indicated an awareness of the connection between cleft palate and poor speech. During the nineteenth century, surgical procedures were developed that are still being used in modified forms. Following primary cleft palate surgery, secondary techniques for the correction of velopharyngeal incompetence include palatal lengthening procedures; pharyngeal flaps; augmentation of the posterior pharyngeal wall with soft tissue or implants; sphincter reconstruction; and prosthetic obturators.

Palatal Lengthening Procedures
(Fig. 58-2)

Palatal pushback procedures with anterior obturation were reported by Suersen (1869), Passavant (1878), Garel (1894), Kingsley (1897), and Gillies and Fry (1921). These techniques involved dividing the hard and soft palates and placing an obturator in the intervening space. Veau and Ruppe (1922) introduced a technique designed for closure of the hard palate using widely undermined mucoperiosteal flaps that were dependent for their survival solely on the posterior palatine vessels. Ganzer (1917) reported similar flaps, and those operations were subsequently modified by Wardill (1937) and Kilner (1937). This technique may be effectively combined with the intravelar veloplasty of Braithwaite (1964) (Fig. 58-3).

These surgical innovations made possible retrodisplacement and lengthening of the soft palate, which could be used in patients in whom primary palate closure failed to achieve sufficient palate length for competency. Dorrance (1930) had emphasized this point and had also suggested the use of the pushback procedure as a secondary operation. Limberg (1927) advocated removal of the bony posterior palatine shelf to allow greater retrodisplacement of the palate. Many procedures based on the technique have since been described.

Pharyngeal Flaps

The posterior pharyngeal flap was introduced by Passavant (1865). The procedure consisted of the creation of adhesions between the soft palate and the pharyngeal wall, rather than a formal elevation of a full-thickness pharyngeal flap, which was then attached to the palate. Schönborn (1876) and Shede (1889) employed a formal, inferiorly based flap of the posterior pharyngeal wall. Other authors reported such techniques subsequently. Bardenheuer (1892) first suggested a superiorly based pharyngeal flap, which has since been advocated by Sanvenero-Rosselli (1935), Conway (1951), and Stark and DeHaan (1960). Other authors have described variations on this principle.

Augmentation of Posterior Pharyngeal Wall
(Fig. 58-4)

The first operation to correct velopharyngeal incompetence by building up the posterior pharyngeal wall was described by Passavant in 1862, when he developed techniques to accentuate production of the posterior pharyngeal wall muscle ridge. Gersuny (1900) and Eckstein (1904) injected paraffin behind the pharyngeal wall to displace it anteriorly. Perthes (1912) and Hill and Hagerty (1960) inserted cartilage; Halle (1925) and von Gaza (1926) employed fascia implants in the same retropharyngeal site. Blocksma (1963) used Silastic as a retropharyngeal implant, and Ward (1968) used injectable Teflon. Extrusion of the implanted material was common and the level at which it was placed was often ineffective owing to migration, or indeed, to the various levels over which the sphincteric closure takes place, a variable that is dependent on the individual's use of the sphincter. Brauer (1965) advocated seamless Silastic pillows. All these techniques may be used when the deficit in closure is small (less than 0.5 cm).

Reconstruction of Velopharyngeal Sphincter

Browne (1935) attempted to reconstruct the velopharyngeal sphincter anatomically, by placing a constricting suture around the entire oronasal port at the level of Passavant's ridge. McCutcheon (1954) dissected the pharyngeal wall and transposed flaps to the midline from both sides. Braithwaite (1968) reported a technique for the dissection of the medial pterygoid muscles from their origin,

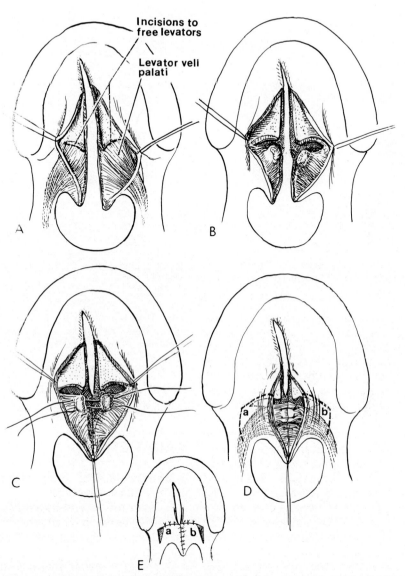

Figure 58–3. Levator transplant procedure (Braithwaite). *A,* In a cleft of the secondary palate, the levator muscles fail to insert into the normal position across the midline. Note the insertion on the posterior maxillary spine. In reconstruction of the soft palate, incisions are made along the posterior border of the hard palate to release the aponeurosis of the levator, allowing it to move posteriorly. *B,* With the incision of the levator aponeurosis and its liberation from the posterior maxillary spine, the levator moves posteriorly and forms a round muscular bundle on each side. *C,* The levator muscle is joined in the midline by suture. Overlap of the muscles at this point, as originally recommended by Braithwaite, may also be performed. *D,* The sutured, reconstructed levator muscle. The levator sling has been reestablished. *E,* When the levator suture is combined with soft palate closure as a primary procedure, there may often be deficiency of mucosa on the soft palate. Small flaps (*a, b*) are formed in closing the midline to aid a difficult soft palate closure.

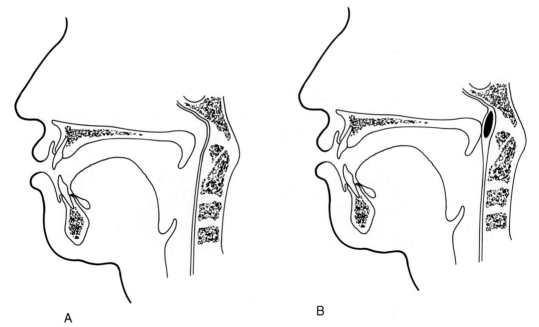

Figure 58–4. *A,* The relative position of the soft palate and the atlas of the spine. *B,* The preferred positioning of the retropharyngeal implant in order to obtain velopharyngeal competence.

allowing them to reorganize more inferiorly and medially. Hynes (1950) transferred the lateral salpingopharyngeal muscles, reflecting them as flaps (Fig. 58–5). The authors, by the use of nasendoscopy, have seen such cases functioning effectively when the lateral wall muscle was maintained in the flap. Orticochea (1968, 1983) advocated the construction of a dynamic muscle sphincter of the pharynx in which the lateral musculo-mucosal flaps are set into a small posterior pharyngeal flap. Modifications were suggested by Jackson and Silverton (1977) (Fig. 58–6) whereby the constructed sphincter provides dynamic and static obturation of the velopharyngeal isthmus. This popular technique awaits long-term assessment of its efficacy compared with the pharyngeal flap technique.

Other Approaches

Combinations of the above procedures have been advocated, including a combined palatal pushback and an inferiorly based flap (Padgett, 1930; Conway, 1951), or a combined pushback operation with a superiorly based flap (Broadbent and Swinyard, 1959; Edgerton, 1962, Buchholz and associates, 1967; Hönig, 1968). In 1954, Hynes reported the combination of his pharyngoplasty with primary pal-

atal repair. Dalston and Stuteville (1975) advocated primary nasopalatal pharyngoplasty.

Prosthetic Obturation

(see Chap. 72)

MANAGEMENT

Management of velopharyngeal sphincter incompetence involves:

1. Evaluation and measurement of the underlying deficiency of the velopharyngeal sphincter and the associated contributing abnormalities.

2. Surgery and/or therapeutic management of the sphincter inadequacy.

3. Modification of the secondary superimposed compensatory habits.

In this way, the speaker with velopharyngeal incompetence can be provided with the potential for normal, acceptable speech.

Evaluation and Measurement

Management of velopharyngeal incompetence and the associated speech distortion involves several choices. Thorough assessment of velopharyngeal incompetence is es-

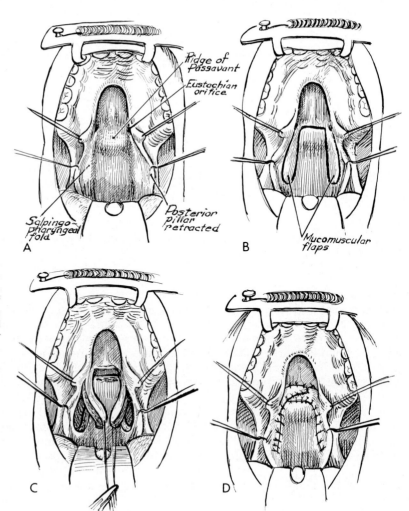

Figure 58–5. The Hynes pharyngoplasty. This procedure, performed as a primary as well as a secondary operation, consists of elevating two superiorly based flaps that envelop most of the salpingopharyngeus muscles. Closure of the donor defects narrows the pharynx, while a medial interpolation and crosslapping of the two flaps produces a horizontal shelf above Passavant's ridge, which brings the posterior pharyngeal "target" closer to the velum. (After Hynes, 1950.)

sential, to avoid inappropriate treatment methods. Initially, it must be determined that the speech distortion is due to the sphincter being unable to close. Second, after it is determined that the sphincter is inadequate in some way, three decisions are possible:

1. The young patient can be observed, reassured at intervals, and, hopefully, with maturity and with satisfactory hearing and speech patterns in his environment, his speech may improve and the velopharyngeal sphincter may eventually be found to be competent. In this way, surgery can be avoided.

2. The patient may receive speech therapy designed to produce firmer, consistent closure of the sphincter and the development of more acceptable speech.

3. The patient may be scheduled for surgery, with or without speech therapy subsequently to develop optimal use of the new mechanism.

As both speech therapy and surgery are costly in terms of time, money, and emotional energy, such decisions must not be made hurriedly. A caring approach to the needs of the individual; thorough investigation; detailed informed discussion with patient, parents, and family; and sensitivity to the specific requirements of the individual speaker are essential. Therapy based on inadequate evaluation of the potential of the velopharyngeal sphincter for change is doomed to failure and can cause much distress. In the same way, careful evaluation before surgery is essential. It follows that for effective treatment, every effort must be made to achieve as objective an analysis of the problem as possible.

Traditionally, the ear of the speech pathologist or surgeon has been the most frequently used assessment tool. Auditory impressions or perceptual measures or ratings are no

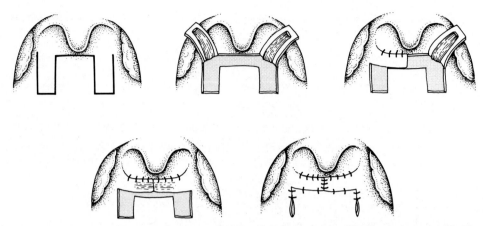

Figure 58–6. The sphincter pharyngoplasty as described by Orticochea and modified by Jackson (1983). The similarity to the Hynes technique is noted.

measure of velopharyngeal incompetence, but they can lead and lend weight to more objective measures. Audio recordings over time can also provide comparisons of gains or changes from surgery or other forms of therapy. There have been attempts to validate auditory perceptual impressions by spectrographic analysis. However, although nasality is immediately perceived by the human ear, the acoustic correlate is difficult to describe and (considering the complexity of the vocal instrument) is of little use as a test of velopharyngeal sphincter competence (van den Berg, 1962). The measurement of oral and nasal sound intensity as a method of analyzing hypernasality was attempted by Fletcher and Bishop (1970). They developed an instrument called TONAR, which is sometimes used to measure velopharyngeal function, but support for this application is lacking (McWilliams, Morris, and Shelton, 1984). The benefits to be gained from TONAR depend on its demonstrated ability to correlate its results with reliable ratings of hypernasality. Although hypernasality related to the individual's ability to close the velopharyngeal port is discussed in relation to TONAR, most of the studies completed with this instrument have been directed toward nasality, rather than to analysis of sphincter closure.

Nasal air flow measures of various types have been used over the years, including pneumotachometers and warm wire flow meters (McWilliams, Morris, and Shelton, 1984). Of particular interest is Warren's PERCI (palatal efficiency rating computed instantaneously) (Warren, 1979). This aeromechanical system was designed to give information

concerning the velopharyngeal mechanism during speech. It displays and records the difference in air pressure in the mouth and in the nose during speech. Differential pressure readings are used to compute the size of the velopharyngeal orifice area. As PERCI is not sensitive to minimal openings in the velopharyngeal sphincter, its use is limited.

Oral/nasal air flow measures have been used by speech pathologists for many years to determine the competence of the velopharyngeal sphincter. A variety of devices, which are indirect methods of assessment, have been used to investigate the sphincter, but do not give detailed analysis of the workings of this mechanism. They range from "cardboard or plastic paddles" (Bzoch, 1979) to a small mirror or mirrored surface, such as the Floxite Detail Reflector (Bloch, 1979). Testing for nasal air emission can also be carried out with a stethoscope held under the nose or against the nares during production of consonants (Bloch, 1979). The Seescape detects nasal air emission during speech; with the tip inserted into the nares, any emission of air causes a float to rise in a rigid plastic tube. In the same way, U-tube manometers, water manometers, ultrasound, and accelerometers provide pressure/flow information concerning nasal air escape. From these data, deductions can be made as to the effectiveness of velopharyngeal closure, but the precise nature of the working of the sphincter cannot be revealed by such devices (McWilliams, Morris, and Shelton, 1984).

Articulation tests have been specifically designed to elicit words containing speech sounds that require oral pressure for correct production. In this way, they assist the speech pathologist to discriminate between speakers who have adequate velopharyngeal closure and those who do not. Such a test is the Iowa Pressure Articulation Test (Morris, Spriestersbach, and Darley, 1961). An articulation test that aims to facilitate identification of articulation errors based on research findings of the characteristic articulation of children 3 to 6 years of age with repaired cleft palate has been designed by Bzoch (Bzoch Error Pattern Diagnostic Articulation Test, 1978). This test aims to delineate the type of substitution or distortion used by these children owing to their difficulty in developing normal articulation related to velopharyngeal incompetence. However, the test makes no objective assessment of velopharyngeal sphincter closure but deduces velopharyngeal incompetence from articulation errors.

Electromyographic studies utilizing bipolar hooked wire electrodes inserted into the velopharyngeal mechanism may give additional information regarding patterns of movement and potential for sphincter closure (Fritzell, 1969; Lubker, Fritzell, and Lindqvist, 1970). When combined with cineradiographic investigation of velar function, additional information is provided (Lubker, 1968). However, this method of investigating velopharyngeal sphincter function can be criticized on the basis that precise placement of the electrodes is difficult, especially for the inexperienced. As the technique is both invasive and somewhat painful, it requires a considerable degree of cooperation from the subject. It is, therefore, problematic for young children. Nevertheless, such studies provide useful information concerning the use of the velopharyngeal sphincter and may throw additional light on its normal function (Bell-Berti, 1983).

More objective information about the velopharyngeal sphincter has been provided by radiology and endoscopy (Pigott, 1979). Lateral pharyngeal radiographs were used to demonstrate the height and position of the velum in relation to the posterior pharyngeal wall, but only in two dimensions. This technique could not provide information concerning the movements of the lateral pharyngeal walls. Cinefluorography and videofluoroscopy followed. It was recognized that there was a need to gather more information from videofluoroscopy than could be provided from the midsagittal view. Multiview videofluoroscopy, a technique that adds a base view to the traditional lateral and frontal projections, was developed by Skolnick (1970). These views, obtained consecutively, are thought to complement each other and are interpreted together. The ability of the observer to retain and recall on observing each of these views what he has gained from the previous one provides the investigator with a three-dimensional understanding of the velopharyngeal sphincter. Clearly, the visual perceptual abilities of the observer and the experience of the radiographer and investigating team play a large part in the usefulness and objectivity of this system. The timing of the speech event, its replication by the patient, and accurate positioning of the patient are crucial to the validity of this system. However, both cine- and videofluoroscopy have added to the understanding of the velopharyngeal sphincter, and have a role in the diagnosis and choice of treatment for the patient with velopharyngeal incompetence (McWilliams, Morris, and Shelton, 1984).

Endoscopy permits observation of the essential elements of the velopharyngeal sphincter as they move in relationship to one another. Over the years, several types of endoscopes have been utilized, but there is general agreement that an endoscope that does not interfere with the movements of the articulatory organs or of the velopharyngeal sphincter is the instrument of choice. At the present time, both flexible and rigid endoscopes are used. The flexible nasopharyngoscope has advantages in respect to its ease of insertion, but many prefer the superior optics of the rigid nasopharyngoscope. For example, the Storz-Hopkins 4.2 × 3.5 mm overall diameter nasopharyngoscope has an angle of 70 degrees, which corresponds closely to the plane of isthmus closure or presumptive plane of closure of the velopharyngeal sphincter in most individuals. Its particular optic system permits more light transmission and greater clarity than other lens or fiberoptic systems. It has an extremely wide field of view encompassing the entire isthmus (Pigott, 1979). However, the nasopharyngoscope provides only a two-dimensional image. The third image, i.e., vertical height of closure, can be provided by a synchronized lateral videofluoroscopic image. When these two images are displayed side by side on a split screen and synchronized with the speech recording, a dynamic view of the changing positions of the various components of closure during different speech events is provided (David and Bagnall, 1984). This technique enables the investigating team to review the examination at will and to compare pre- and post-treatment examinations of the sphincter.

Some concern has been expressed regarding the ease with which a patient, especially a young child, can tolerate and cooperate with the nasendoscopy procedure, especially when the rigid nasopharyngoscope is used. At the South Australian Cranio-Facial Unit, over 1000 nasendoscopies have been performed during the past decade. The Storz rigid nasopharyngoscope with its preferred optical characteristics is used routinely coupled with simultaneous lateral videofluoroscopy and speech recording (David and associates, 1982). The two adjacent images are set on a split screen, permitting instantaneous viewing and video recording. Sixty-five per cent of the nasendoscopies are of adults and adolescents, and 35 per cent of children under 10 years of age. Nasendoscopy of the adults has been almost 100 per cent successful. Of the total patient group, 92 per cent of nasendoscopies were successful, with the patient able to cooperate fully and a precise, clear video recording being obtained for future reference. Twenty-two per cent of nasendoscopies are examinations of younger children, 4 to 6 years of age. This group of children receive one session of orientation to the procedure. It frequently involves the use of a tangible behavior reinforcement game, the child proceeding through each stage of the game, which corresponds with a particular stage of the nasendoscopy procedure. With the use of this tangible reward technique and with careful and thorough preparation, often including some "roleplay," 80 percent of nasendoscopies in this age group are successful at the first attempt. A calm and confident parental attitude, an atmosphere of mutual trust, and an unhurried approach are also essential elements of this success.

CT scans have been proposed as a further investigative tool, especially when combined with endoscopy (Honjo and associates, 1984). Considering the intricacies of sphincter movement and the variable height of closure, the use of 3 mm cuts, as suggested by these researchers, would not provide tomograms capable of delineating the subtleties of closure.

From this overview of the various instruments available for evaluation of the velopharyngeal sphincter, it is apparent that each has its advantages and disadvantages. With more objective diagnostic information, the choice of appropriate patient management is simplified. It is important to remember that impressions gained from evaluating the action of the sphincter during speech production that is in any way contrived have limited value. The most objective investigation results from analysis of movements of the velopharyngeal sphincter during spontaneous speech. Any instrument that permits the patient sufficient freedom to speak at will, while allowing the investigator to observe and analyze every component of the sphincter in view, paves the way for effective treatment.

Choice of Surgery

With the increase of objective, quantitative, preoperative, and postoperative evaluation data, it is possible to approach the problem of treatment choice more rationally. In particular, the information gained from direct viewing with the nasendoscope, together with synchronized lateral videofluoroscopy, provides information to aid the proper choice of surgical technique.

The range of defects of sphincter closure may include:

1. A central defect, small or large, in the velopharyngeal sphincter with satisfactory palatal elevation and lateral wall movement.

2. A flaplike action of the palate with a weak lateral wall component, producing a transverse, slitlike defect in the sphincter. Occasionally a significant posterior pharyngeal wall ridge is observed with this pattern of closure.

3. Poor palatal movement with satisfactory lateral pharyngeal wall movement.

4. Asymmetric gaps with lack of elevation of the palate on one side more than the other, or asymmetric lateral pharyngeal wall movement, as commonly seen in unilateral craniofacial microsomia.

5. Gross failure of all elements of the sphincter.

The challenge presented to the clinician by the use of modern tools of objective assessment is to design the appropriate treatment for the observed deformity. It is clear that *small central defects* with good function of all elements of the sphincter may well respond to a number of different procedures. Such small defects are amenable to treatment by posterior wall implant, or a small, centrally placed superior pharyngeal flap, although the latter treatment also renders the palate immobile. In such cases, the nasendoscope view demonstrates a central muscular deficiency on the upper surface of the palate. Re-repair of the palate with retroposition of the levator mechanism may also be appropriate. Pigott (1986) has suggested that a central augmentation of the area of the musculus uvulae by a local musculomucosal flap, taken from the substance of the oral side of the soft palate and transposed into the midline of the dorsum of the palate, may help.

In cases in which there is *gross failure of all elements of the sphincter*, the situation is much more difficult. Some surgeons use palatal appliances and others prefer a large pharyngeal flap. It is the authors' experience that this rare but unhappy situation cannot be effectively treated by surgery using currently available techniques.

The *asymmetric defects* of the sphincter, which are associated with a lack of elevation of the palate on one side or with an asymmetric lateral pharyngeal wall movement, may be treated by an offset, superiorly based pharyngeal flap or by a unilateral sphincter pharyngoplasty.

If there is a *deficiency in elevation of the palate, but satisfactory lateral wall movement*, the situation is theoretically ideal for a superiorly based pharyngeal flap. The lateral wall movement closes the lateral ports and the tethering of the already deficient palate does not constitute a significant loss of function to the palatal element of the sphincter.

The most common situation in the authors' experience is the finding of a weak lateral wall movement with a stronger palatal function, although there is a great range of variation in the degrees of function of the individual elements of the sphincter. The less prominent the movement of the lateral pharyngeal wall, the less effective is the superiorly based flap. The palate is tethered by the flap and there is incomplete obturation as a result of the limited lateral wall movement. Efforts to overcome this situation have been directed toward adding a pushback procedure to the flap, or making the flap very wide, thus running the risk of nasopharyngeal obstruc-

tion or even sleep apnea. It is in this situation (poor lateral pharyngeal movement) that the sphincter pharyngoplasty may be of more use as a dynamic, or even static, mechanism.

The argument concerning the relative advantages of the superior versus the inferior pharyngeal flap has developed into a challenge to choose the most appropriate operation for the defect based on the findings of videofluoroscopy and nasendoscopy. Jackson (1985) suggested an appropriate matching of surgical procedures to the pattern of sphincter deformity. He preferred to use the sphincter pharyngoplasty to solve the difficult problem of the weak lateral wall movement, as suggested above. Such a procedure allows the dynamic palate to continue moving and it augments the posterolateral aspects of the sphincter with a dynamic mechanism.

In the authors' experience, a vast majority of cases do not show definite lateral wall movement without palatal elevation, or definite failure of lateral wall movement with satisfactory palatal elevation, but a variable mix of relative deficiencies of sphincter components. It is in this group that much energy needs to be expended in evaluating the respective results of the sphincter technique and the superiorly based pharyngeal flap. It is not known how often the palatopharyngeus muscle transposed in the sphincteric operation functions as an integral part of the velopharyngeal sphincter in speech. However, the point is well taken that sphincter pharyngoplasty is not an "end of the line" operation. It is capable of being adjusted and even combined with pharyngeal flap procedures.

Operative Technique

For a superiorly based, lined pharyngeal flap, a videotape of the nasendoscopy and synchronous lateral fluoroscopy is viewed before surgery so that the flap can be tailored to suit the defect as closely as possible (Fig. 58–7).

The operation is begun with oroendotracheal intubation, and an appropriate mouth gag is used to expose the palate and oropharynx. The surgeon sits at the head of the table; a fiberoptic head lamp is a useful aid to visualization. The midline of the palate is injected with 1/80,000 epinephrine in solution of 2 per cent lidocaine, and a small amount of the solution is injected into the posterior

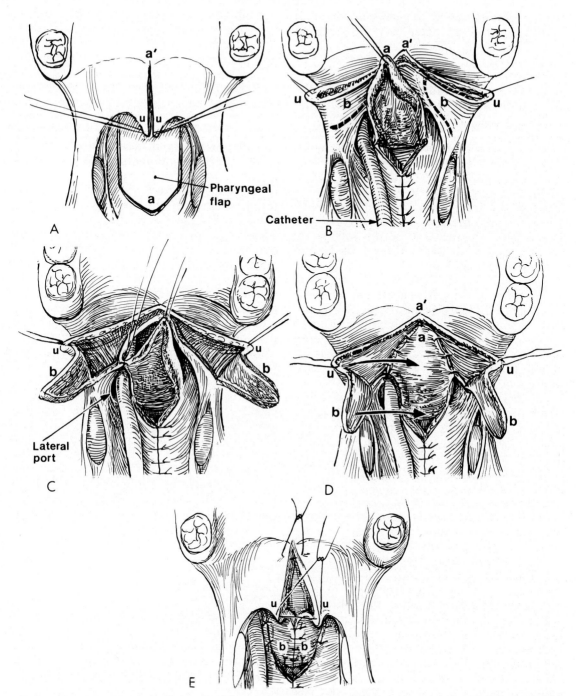

Figure 58–7. Lateral port control pharyngeal flap. *A,* The soft palate is divided and a superiorly based pharyngeal flap is designed, extending the full width of the posterior pharyngeal wall. It is elevated from the prevertebral fascia. *B,* The posterior pharyngeal wall has been closed in the midline with catgut sutures. Closure of the posterior wall should not extend fully to the base of the pharyngeal flap or this will result in a narrowing or tubing of the flap. Alternatively the posterior wall defect can be left open. Development of lining flaps (*b*) on the nasal surface of the soft palate is illustrated. *C,* The lining flaps in the soft palate (*b*) have been elevated and retracted laterally. The catheter is placed in the lateral port on one side of the pharyngeal flap. Suturing of the pharyngeal flap into the mucosa of the soft palate has begun. *D,* The pharyngeal flap has been sutured to the nasal surface of the soft palate; suturing has extended toward the pharyngeal wall snugly around 14 French catheters. The lining flaps (*b*) are about to be rotated over the raw surface of the pharyngeal flap. *E,* The lining flaps have been sutured over the raw surface of the pharyngeal flap in the midline. The oral side of the soft palate is closed, beginning at (*u*) and proceeding anteriorly. (From Hogan, V. M.: A clarification of the surgical goals in cleft palate speech and the introduction of the lateral port control (L.P.C.) pharyngeal flap. Cleft Palate J., *10*:331, 1973.)

pharyngeal wall. The soft palate is divided in the midline, the incision not quite reaching the hard palate. The nasal lining is divided transversely on each side, leaving a fringe attached to the posterior part of the hard palate. The nasal lining distal to the transverse incision is elevated from the underlying musculature. A trapdoor flap is marked on the posterior pharyngeal wall and, within limits, the width of the flap can be tailored to the defect as visualized; e.g., in unilateral craniofacial microsomia, with a unilateral defect in the sphincter, the flap can be constructed mostly on the side of the defect. The flap is elevated from the transverse incision toward the head, separating the mucosa and pharyngeal musculature from the underlying prevertebral fascia. One must be careful not to damage the base of the flap, as the mucosa becomes friable in the area of the adenoids.

The pharyngeal flap, once elevated, is sutured into the fringe of the nasal lining left on the posterior margins of the hard palate. The corners are sutured laterally as far as possible, and one additional suture of 3-0 or 4-0 chromic catgut in the midline is ample. Using finer suture material (4-0 or 5-0 catgut), the nasal lining flaps developed from the dorsal aspect of the soft palate are sutured to the raw surface of the pharyngeal flap. If the pharyngeal flap is relatively narrow, the pharyngeal defect can be closed. Rarely, it is left to heal spontaneously; the posterior wall heals rapidly and the scar contracts the pharyngeal mucosa quickly. The soft palate is closed meticulously in two layers with 4-0 chromic catgut sutures.

The superiorly based pharyngeal flap pharyngoplasty depends on lateral pharyngeal wall movement that is able to close the residual ports. Experience with over 1000 nasendoscopies in ten years has led the authors to the conclusion that the superiorly based flap needs to be positioned sufficiently high to be effective in the area of the pharynx at which the sphincter is operating. The authors have observed a number of flaps that have been of the proper size but malpositioned, so that the pharynx is endeavoring to close at another level. Jackson (1983) made the same point about the Orticochea sphincteric pharyngoplasty, explaining the need to have the flaps inserted higher in the pharynx. Unlined flaps tend to tube and become cordlike and ineffective.

In patients with severe deficiency of the velopharyngeal sphincter, the superiorly based, lined pharyngeal flap can be combined with pushback procedures. The nasal lining attached to the posterior palatal shelf is divided to give additional pushback effect and the lining is used to cover the pharyngeal flap.

Postoperative management involves careful resuscitation and extubation. An intravenous line is maintained for the first 12 hours and intravenous ampicillin is given for this period. Clear fluids only are given for the next 12 hours and the patient may have a soft diet for the next three weeks. Postoperative evaluation follows the preoperative assessment regimen. The results of surgery are evaluated by repeat speech assessment and nasendoscopy with synchronous lateral videofluoroscopy. This evaluation is performed at three months, a period that gives time for adequate healing and permits full evaluation of the capacity of the sphincter.

The pharyngeal flap operation is not without its negative aspects. Some patients develop hyponasality. During the first few weeks after surgery, there is an incidence of snoring that may persist, and a few patients may suffer from sleep apnea. A small number of patients experience an unpleasant taste. Some report halitosis, which may result from retained secretions on the upper surface of the pharyngeal flap; these are often seen during nasendoscopy. In addition, there may be persistent velopharyngeal incompetence.

Postoperative Speech Therapy

Following pharyngoplasty or any surgical procedure to provide a patient with a competent sphincter, it cannot be assumed that a patient will automatically speak clearly without residual resonance or articulation distortion. This is certainly true of a patient who has articulatory distortion or substitution patterns before surgery. After surgery, some patients demonstrate improved or near-normal vocal quality with no need for additional therapeutic intervention (Shprintzen, 1979). However, speech patterns that have been developed in the presence of velopharyngeal incompetence may not automatically change after surgery. Owing to the effect of the speaker's auditory perceptual monitoring, the patient may reproduce the speech he is used to hearing from himself. The pattern of voice use that a speaker favors has been described as the "vocal image" (Cooper, 1971). The speaker with long-standing velopharyngeal incompetence may have identified with the hypernasal vocal tone for so long that after surgery he may reproduce his habitual supralaryngeal adjustments to retain and maintain previous resonant voice quality.

Therapy, after surgery, is begun only after the capacity of the pharyngeal flap or other surgical procedure to provide a competent sphincter has been evaluated. Again, the need is for careful assessment using, if possible, the same measures and instrumentation employed before surgery. After surgery, nasendoscopy and synchronized lateral videofluoroscopy, with the patient duplicating the speech produced at the initial investigation, can determine the need for, and potential success of, speech therapy. After it has been ascertained that the sphincter is capable of closure, sufficient for the production of normal vocal tone and for the necessary development of intraoral air pressure, therapy can be instigated to optimize the results of surgery. Utilizing the techniques of voice therapy, developing the patient's auditory discrimination ability, and encouraging relaxed and slightly more forward tongue carriage, the therapist encourages vocal tone placement or focus to use the supraglottic resonating system in a balanced way. Compensatory habits need to be addressed, such as excessive breath flow, the onset of phonation without firm closure of the vocal cords, tense and constricted laryngopharynx, and retraction of the tongue. The patient learns how to produce his voice without nasal tone, possibly through the use of negative practice, i.e., purposely making the "old" followed by the "new" vowel quality (Van Riper, 1963). He may experience, for the first time, the ability to speak with an efficient vocal tract, in which satisfactory air pressures can be maintained above the level of the larynx, ensuring assistance to the vocal cords in their compression of the air stream. Sucking through a straw closed at its distal end and simultaneously voicing from a nasal phoneme onto a high close vowel, e.g., [i], he may experience the effects of a closed nasopharynx in the form of a bright, clear, ringing voice quality. Modifying the vocal technique in this and other ways, the patient sheds his previous identity

as a nasal speaker and adopts the clear esthetic vocal quality of the speaker with a competent velopharyngeal sphincter. In addition, articulation therapy to eradicate glottal stops and pharyngeal articulation may be required to correct the production of speech sounds.

LONG-TERM RESULTS

The aim of management of velopharyngeal incompetence is to provide the speaker with acceptable speech. To be acceptable, speech must be clearly intelligible. It does not require effort on the part of the speaker and does not have any distortion in its quality that attracts attention to itself.

Speech results after surgery to improve hypernasal speech have been variously reported. Bronsted and associates (1984) reported: "In Copenhagen as in most other cleft palate centers, satisfactory speech results are found in about 80 per cent of cleft palate cases as a result of primary palatoplasty. Another 15 per cent achieve acceptable speech with the aid of speech therapy. The remaining 5 per cent require secondary management because of insufficient velopharyngeal closure." Dalston and Stuteville (1975), who advocated the use of primary nasopalatal pharyngoplasty, found that adequacy of speech varied from less than 50 per cent to 95.8 per cent. Lewin, Heller, and Kojak (1975) reported that after surgical management, 60 per cent of patients presenting without cleft, but with velopharyngeal incompetence, achieved acceptable speech.

However, opinions on what constitutes acceptable speech seem to vary. Speech is variously termed "perfect," "normal," "satisfactory," and "adequate." Different researchers assess the adequacy of speech in various ways. Some have their patients read to them (Bronsted and associates, 1984), some have them perform a variety of speech tasks (Musgrave, McWilliams, and Matthews, 1975), and some make empirical judgments only (Hotz and Gnoinski, 1976). Spontaneous speech is sometimes, but rarely, used (Lewin, Heller, and Kojak, 1975).

In most studies, speech pathologists skilled in the area of cleft palate management assessed the adequacy of speech. A study by Podol and Salvia (1976) threw doubt on the ability of the speech pathologist to remain objective. These authors found that the judgment of unacceptable hypernasality and of the need for speech therapy was made more frequently when listeners (speech pathology students) were presented with visible evidence of cleft palate. A recent study at the South Australian Cranio-Facial Unit addressed the issue of speech acceptability of children with repaired cleft palate, and found that the judgments of untrained naive listeners were in marked variance with those made by a speech pathologist skilled in the treatment of hypernasality. This study used recordings of spontaneous speech elicited at each child's school, and two different modes of assessment. The speech pathologist clearly had a lower expectation of the children's speech. She found that 48 per cent of the cleft subjects were inadequate speakers. In marked contrast, naive listeners, using a rank order, found that 71.5 per cent of the subjects spoke less acceptably than their peers.

Rating scales were the measuring device most commonly favored in most studies. Lewin, Heller, and Kojak (1975) used a five-point scale, 1 being normal voice quality and 5 representing severe hypernasality. The ratings were based sometimes on acceptability, sometimes on a variety of parameters. A rating scale, however, cannot give information as to how the speaker functions in his or her everyday setting. It relates only to an arbitrary standard in the mind of the speech pathologist. Speech standards vary from place to place, from region to region, and certainly across socioeconomic groups. Speakers have to be provided with speech that compares well with that of their peers. Studies of speech acceptability that isolate the speakers from their social and cultural milieu may be less than realistic. Additionally, the judgments of speech acceptability may be more objective if made by those without knowledge of the speaker's history or surgical management.

REFERENCES

Bardenheuer, D.: Vorschlage zu plastischen Operationen bei chirurgischen Eingriffen in der Mundhohle. Arch. Klin. Chir., *43*:32, 1892.

Bell-Berti, F.: The velopharyngeal mechanism. An electromyographic study. A preliminary report. Haskins Laboratories, New Haven, 1983.

Bloch, P. J.: Clinical evaluation for the cleft palate team setting. *In* Bzoch, K. R. (Ed.). Comm. Disord. Re Cleft Lip & Palate, *2*:230, 1979.

Blocksma, R.: Correction of velopharyngeal insufficiency by Silastic pharyngeal implant. Plast. Reconstr. Surg., *31*:268, 1963.

Braithwaite, F.: *In* Gibson, R. (Ed.): Modern Trends in Plastic Surgery. London, Butterworth, 1964.

Braithwaite, F.: The importance of the levator palati muscle in cleft palate closure. Br. J. Plast. Surg., *21*:60, 1968.

Brauer, R. O.: Push-back repair of the cleft palate with nasal mucosal flaps to prevent late contracture; follow up results of the Cronin procedure. Plast. Reconstr. Surg., *36*:529, 1965.

Broadbent, T. R., and Swinyard, C. A.: The dynamic pharyngeal flap: its selective use and electromyographic evaluation. Plast. Reconstr. Surg., *23*:301, 1959.

Bronsted, K., Liisberg, W., Ørsted, A., Prytz, S., and Fogh-Andersen, P.: Surgical and speech results following palatopharyngoplasty operations in Denmark 1959–1977. Cleft Palate J., *21*:170, 1984.

Brown, J. B.: Elongation of the partially cleft palate. Surg. Gynecol. Obstet., *63*:768, 1936.

Browne, D.: An orthopaedic operation for cleft palate. Br. Med. J., *20*:1093, 1935.

Buchholz, R. B., Chase, R. A., Jobe, R. P., and Smith, H.: The use of a combined palatal pushback and pharyngeal flap operation: a progress report. Plast. Reconstr. Surg., *39*:554, 1967.

Bzoch, K. R.: Bzoch Error Pattern Diagnostic Articulation Test. Comm. Disord. Re Cleft Lip & Palate, *2*:168, 1978.

Bzoch, K. R.: Measurement and assessment of categorical aspects of cleft palate speech. Comm. Disord. Re Cleft Lip & Palate, *2*:169, 182, 1979.

Bzoch, K. R., and Williams, W. N.: Introduction, rationale, principles and related basic embryology and anatomy. Comm. Disord. Re Cleft Lip & Palate, *2*:16, 1979.

Calnan, J. S.: Submucous cleft palate. Br. J. Plast. Surg., *6*:264, 1954.

Calnan, J. S.: Congenital large pharynx. A new syndrome with a report on 41 personal cases. Br. J. Plast. Surg., *24*:263, 1971a.

Calnan, J. S.: Permanent nasal escape in speech after adenoidectomy. Br. J. Plast. Surg., *24*:197, 1971b.

Conway, H.: Combined use of the pushback and pharyngeal flap procedures in the management of complicated cases of cleft palate. Plast. Reconstr. Surg., *7*:214, 1951.

Cooper, M.: The vocal image and vocal suicide. Voices: The Art & Science of Psychotherapy, *6*:26, 1971.

Cosman, B., and Falk, A. S.: Pharyngeal flap augmentation. Plast. Reconstr. Surg., *55*:149, 1975.

Crikelair, G. F., Kastein, S., Fowler, E. P., Jr., and Cosman, B.: Velar dysfunction in the absence of cleft palate. N.Y. J. Med., *64*:263, 1964.

Croft, C. B., Shprintzen, R. J., Daniller, A., and Lewin, M. L.: The occult submucous cleft palate and the musculus uvulae. Cleft Palate J., *15*:150, 1978.

Curtis, J. F.: Acoustics of speech production and nasalisation. *In* Spriestersbach, C. (Ed.): Cleft Palate and Communication. New York, Academic Press, 1968.

Dalston, R. M., and Stuteville, O. H.: A clinical investigation of the efficacy of primary nasopalatal pharyngoplasty. Cleft Plate J., *12*:177, 1975.

David, D. J., and Bagnall, A. D.: Evaluation of velopharyngeal closure by CT scan and endoscopy—Honjo et al. Discussion. Plast. Reconstr. Surg., *74*:626, 1984.

David, D. J., White, J., Sprod, R., and Bagwall, A.: Nasendoscopy: significant refinements of a direct-viewing technique of the velopharyngeal sphincter. Plast. Reconstr. Surg., *70*:423, 1982.

Dorrance, G. M.: Congenital insufficiency of the palate. Arch. Surg., 21:185, 1930.

Dworkin, J. P., and Johns, D. F.: Management of velopharyngeal incompetence in dysarthria—a historical review. Clin. Otolaryngol., 5:61, 1980.

Eckstein, H.: Paraffin for facial and palatal defects. Dermatol. Ztschr. (Basel) 11:772, 1904.

Edgerton, M. T.: Surgical lengthening of the cleft palate by dissection of the neurovascular bundle. Plast. Reconstr. Surg., 29:551, 1962.

Estill, J.: Voice Scientist: PhD. program in speech and hearing, The Graduate Center, City University of New York. Personal communication, 1986.

Fletcher, S. G.: Hypernasal voice as indication of regional growth and development disturbances. Logos, 3:3, 1960.

Fletcher, S. G., and Bishop, M. E.: Measurement of nasality with TONAR. Cleft Palate J., 7:610, 1970.

Franco, P.: Traité des Hernies. Lyon, Thibauld Payan, 1561.

Fritzell, B.: The velopharyngeal muscles in speech. An electromyographic and cineradiographic study. Acta Otolaryngol., 250:1, 1969.

Ganzer, H.: Neue Wege des plastischen Verschlusses von Gaumendefekten. Berl. Klin. Wochenschr., 54:209, 1917.

Garel, J.: Deux cas d'anomalie congénitale des piliers antérieurs du voile du palais. Rev. Laryngol. (Bordeaux), 14:489, 1894.

Gersuny, R.: Ueber eine subcutane prosthese. Ztschr. Heilk., 21:199, 1900.

Gillies, H. D., and Fry, W. K.: A new principle in the surgical treatment of "congenital cleft palate," and its mechanical counterpart. Br. Med. J., 1:335, 1921.

Goode, R. L., and Ross, J.: Velopharyngeal insufficiency after adenoidectomy. Arch. Otolaryngol., 96:223, 1972.

Greene, M. C. L.: The Voice and its Disorders. London, Pitman Medical Publishing, 1964, pp. 190, 193.

Halle, M.: Gaumennaht und Gaumenplastik. Arch. Ohr. Nas. Kehlkopfheilk., 12:377, 1925.

Hill, M. J., and Hagerty, R. F.: Efficacy of pharyngoplasty for speech improvement in postoperative cleft palates. Cleft Palate Bull., 10:66, 1960.

Hogan, V. M.: A clarification of the surgical goals in cleft palate speech and the introduction of the lateral port control (L.P.C.) pharyngeal flap. Cleft Palate J., 10:331, 1973.

Hönig, C. A.: Treatment of velopharyngeal insufficiency after palatal repair. Plast. Reconstr. Surg., 41:93, 1968.

Honjo, I., Mitoma, T., Ushiro, K., and Kawano, M.: Evaluation of velopharyngeal closure by CT scan and endoscopy. Plast. Reconstr. Surg., 74:5, 1984.

Hotz, M., and Gnoinski, W.: Comprehensive care of cleft lip and palate in children at Zurich University: a preliminary report. Am. J. Orthod., 70:481, 1976.

Huskie, C. F.: Chief speech therapist, West of Scotland Regional Plastic and Oral Surgery Unit, Canniesburn Hospital, Glasgow, Scotland. Personal communication, 1985.

Hynes, W.: Pharyngoplasty by muscle transplantation. Br. J. Plast. Surg., 3:128, 1950.

Hynes, W.: The primary repair of clefts of the palate. Br. J. Plast. Surg., 7:242, 1954.

Jackson, I. T.: A review of 236 patients treated with dynamic muscle sphincter. Discussion. Plast. Reconstr. Surg., 71:187, 1983.

Jackson, I. T.: Sphincter pharyngoplasty. Clin. Plast. Surg., 12:711, 1985.

Jackson, I. T., and Silverton, J. S.: Sphincter pharyngoplasty as a secondary procedure in cleft palates. Plast. Reconstr. Surg., 59:518, 1977.

Kaplan, E. N.: The occult submucous cleft palate. Cleft Palate J., 12:356, 1975.

Kaplan, E. N., Jobe, R. P., and Chase, R. A.: Flexibility in surgical planning for velopharyngeal incompetence. Cleft Palate J., 6:166, 1969.

Kilner, T. P.: Cleft lip and palate repair technique. St. Thomas Hosp. Rep., 2:127, 1937.

Kingsley, N. W.: Surgery or mechanism in the treatment of congenital cleft palate. N.Y. Med. J., 29:484, 1897.

Lewin, M. A., Heller, J. C., and Kojak, D. J.: Speech results after Millard island flap repair in cleft palate and other velopharyngeal insufficiencies. Cleft Palate J., 12:263, 1975.

Limberg, A.: Neue Wege in der radikalen Uranoplastik bei angeborenen Spaltendeformationen: Osteotomia interlaminaris und pterygomaxillaris, Resectio Marginis Foraminis palatini und neue Plattschennaht. Fissura ossea occulta und ihre Behandlung. Zentralbl. f. Chir., 54:1745, 1927.

Lubker, J. F.: An electromyographic-cinefluorographic investigation of velar function during normal speech production. Cleft Palate J. 5:1, 1968.

Lubker, J. F., Fritzell, B., and Lindqvist, J.: Velopharyngeal function. An electromyographic study. R. Inst. Technol. STL-QPSR, 4:9, 1970.

Massengill, R., Jr.: Hypernasality. Considerations in Causes and Treatment Procedures. Springfield, Charles C Thomas, 1972.

McCarthy, J. G., Coccaro, P. J., Schwartz, M., Wood-Smith, D., and Converse, J. M.: Velopharyngeal function following maxillary advancement. Plast. Reconstr. Surg., 64:180, 1979.

McCutcheon, G. T.: Modified Passavant technic of cleft palate repair. Ann. Surg., 139:613, 1954.

McWilliams, B. J., Morris, H. L., and Shelton, R. L.: Instrumentation for assessing the velopharyngeal mechanism. In McWilliams, B. J., Morris, H. L., and Shelton, R. L. (Eds.): Cleft Palate Speech. St. Louis, MO, C. V. Mosby Company, 1984, p. 152.

Morley, M. E.: Cleft Palate and Speech. Edinburgh & London, Churchill Livingstone, 1973.

Morris, H. L.: Surgical management of clefts. In McWilliams, B. J., Morris, H. L., and Shelton, R. L. (Eds.): Cleft Palate Speech. St. Louis, MO, C. V. Mosby Company, 1984, p. 64.

Morris, H. L., Spriestersbach, D. C., and Darley, F. L.: An articulation test for assessing competency of velopharyngeal closure. J. Speech & Hearing Res., 4:48, 1961.

Musgrave, R. R., McWilliams, B. J., and Matthews, H. P.: A review of the results of two different surgical procedures for the repair of clefts of the soft palate only. Cleft Plate J., 12:281, 1975.

Orticochea, M.: Construction of a dynamic muscle sphincter in cleft palates. Plast. Reconstr. Surg., 41:323, 1968.

Orticochea, M.: A review of 236 cleft palate patients treated with dynamic muscle sphincter. Plast. Reconstr. Surg., 71:180, 1983.

Osberg, P. E., and Witzel, M. A.: Physiologic basis for hypernasality during connected speech in cleft palate patients—a nasendoscopic study. Plast. Reconstr. Surg., 67:1, 1981.

Owsley, J. Q., Jr., Lawson, L. I., and Chierici, G. J.: The re-do pharyngeal flap. Plast. Reconstr. Surg., 57:180, 1976.

Padgett, E. C.: The repair of cleft palates after unsuccessful operations, with special reference to cases with an extensive loss of palatal tissue. Arch. Surg., 20:453, 1930.

Passavant, G.: Ueber die Operation der angeborenen Spalten des harten Gaumens und der damit complicierten Hasenscharten. Arch. Ohr. Nas. Kehlkopfheilk., 3:196, 1862.

Passavant, G.: Ueber die Beseitigung der naeselnen Sprache bei angeborenen Spalten des harten und weichen Gaumens (Gaumensegel, Schlundnaht und Ruecklagerund des Gaumensegels). Arch. Klin. Chir., 6:333, 1865.

Passavant, G.: Ueber die Verbesserung der Sprache nach der Uranoplastik. Dtsch. Gesellsch. Chir., 7:128, 1878.

Perthes, H.: Reported by Hollweg, E. Beitrag zur Behandlung von Gaumenspalten. Dissertation Tübingen, 1912.

Peterson-Falzone, S. J.: Velopharyngeal inadequacy in the absence of overt cleft palate. J. Craniofac. Genet. Dev. Biol. [Suppl.], 1:97, 1985.

Pigott, R. W.: Some physical characteristics of instruments used to investigate palatopharyngeal incompetence. Diag. & Treat. Palatoglossal Malfunction, Monograph 2. London, College of Speech Therapists, 1979.

Pigott, R. W.: Personal communication, 1986.

Podol, J., and Salvia, J.: Effects of visibility of a prepalatal cleft on the evaluation of speech. Cleft Palate J., 13:361, 1976.

Porterfield, H. W., Trabue, J. C., Stimpert, R. D., and Terry, J. L.: Hypernasality in noncleft palate patients. Plast. Reconstr. Surg., 37:216, 1966.

Sanvenero-Rosselli, G.: Divisione palatine e sua cura chirurgica. Atti Cong. Int. Stomatol., 391, 1935.

Schendel, S. A., Oeschlaeger, M., Wolford, L. M., and Epker, B. N.: Velopharyngeal anatomy and maxillary advancement. J. Maxillofac. Surg., 7:116, 1979.

Schönborn, D.: Ueber eine neue Methode der Staphylorrhaphie. Arch. Klin. Chir., 19:527, 1876.

Schwarz, C., and Gruner, E.: Logopaedic findings following advancement of the maxilla. J. Maxillofac. Surg., 4:40, 1976.

Shede, J.: Zur operativen Behandlung der Gaumensplaten. In Predoehl, A. (Ed.) Jahrb. d. Hamburg. Staatskrankenan sta. 274, 1889.

Shprintzen, R. J.: Velopharyngeal insufficiency in the absence of overt or submucous cleft palate. The mystery solved. Diag. & Treat. Palatoglossal Malfunction, Monograph 2. London, College of Speech Therapists, 1979.

Skolnick, M. L.: Videofluoroscopic examination of the velopharyngeal portal during phonation in lateral and base projections—a new technique for studying the mechanics of closure. Cleft Palate J., 7:803, 1970.

Stark, R. B., and DeHaan, C.. The addition of a pharyngeal flap to primary palatoplasty. Plast. Reconstr. Surg., 26:378, 1960.

Subtelny, J. D., and Koepp Baker, H.: The significance of adenoid tissue in velopharyngeal function. Plast. Reconstr. Surg., 17:235, 1956.

Suersen, W.: Ueber die Herstellung einer dentlichen Aussprache durch ein neues System kunstlicher Gaumen bei angeborenen und erworbenen Gaumendefecten. Klin. Wochenschr., 6:110, 1869.

van den Berg, J. W.: Modern research in experimental phonetics. 12th Int. Cong. Logopaedics and Phoniatrics. Folia Phoniatr. (Basel), 14:81, 1962.

Van Riper, C.: Speech Correction. Principles and Methods. Englewood Cliffs, NJ, Prentice-Hall, 1963, p. 296.

Veau, V., and Ruppe, C.: Les résultats anatomiques et foncionnels de la staphylorraphie par les procédés classiques. Rev. de Chir., 60:81, 1922.

von Gaza, W.: Transplanting of free fatty tissue in the retropharyngeal area in cases of cleft palate. Lecture, German Surgical Society, April 9th, 1926.

Ward, P. H.: Uses of injectable Teflon in otolaryngology. Arch. Otolaryngol., 87:637, 1968.

Wardill, W. E. M.: Technique of operation for cleft palate. Br. J. Surg., 25:117, 1937.

Warren, D. W.: PERCI: a method of rating palatal efficiency. Cleft Palate J., 16:279, 1979.

Witzel, M. A., and Munro, I. R.: Velopharyngeal insufficiency after maxillary advancement. Cleft Palate J., 14:176, 1977.

Henry K. Kawamoto, Jr.

Rare Craniofacial Clefts

INCIDENCE

EMBRYOLOGIC ASPECTS

ETIOLOGY

MORPHOPATHOGENESIS

CLASSIFICATION

DESCRIPTION OF CLEFTS

TREATMENT

The cry of a newborn lingers forever when his face is marred by a rare craniofacial cleft. The audible cry is perpetuated as an inner silent grief as the child begins to perceive his misfortune and wanders through life being the subject of crude, curious stares.

Craniofacial clefts exist in a multitude of patterns, varying in degrees of severity. Although they initially appear to be bizarre and to defy description, most craniofacial clefts occur along predictable embryologic lines. Their expression can be unilateral or bilateral. In addition, clefts of different types can occur on opposite sides of the face of an affected individual.

INCIDENCE

The exact incidence of unusual craniofacial clefts is not known, and estimates of their occurrence vary widely. This problem is to be expected, since the cases are rare and the methods of data collection are not standard-

ized. Extensive reviews of congenital malformation by Murphy (1938), Stevenson, Worcester, and Rice (1950), and Ivy (1957) do not categorize facial clefts into specific types.

A general idea of the magnitude of the problem can be drawn from studies of the occurrence of common clefts of the lip and palate. Davis (1935) reported four median clefts of the lip and five oblique facial clefts in a series of 937 examples of common clefts of the lip and palate. Blackfield and Wilde (1950) noted only five lateral (transverse) facial clefts during a period in which they identified 500 clefts of the lip. Burian (1957) reported 97 cases of rare facial clefts in a series of nearly 4000 consecutive common clefts of the lip accumulated during a 40 year period. Fogh-Andersen (1965) detected 48 examples of rare craniofacial clefts among 3988 consecutive cases of facial clefts gathered over a 30 year period. Of the 48 rare clefts, 15 were median clefts of the lip; 12, transverse facial clefts, eight, clefts of the nose; seven, clefts of the scalp; three, oblique facial clefts; and three, atypical clefts. Popescu (1968) reported 14 transverse facial clefts in a series of 1475 patients. Pitanguy (1968) noted 25 patients with rare facial clefts in a group of 736 patients with common clefts. Based on these reports, the occurrence rate of rare craniofacial clefts as compared with common clefts would range between 9.5 per 1000 and 34 per 1000. The true incidence is certainly higher, since some of the reports included only one type of cleft for each patient.

Reviews of birth certificates have also been used in an attempt to determine the incidence of facial anomalies (Ivy, 1957, 1963; Conway and Wagner, 1965). Ivy (1957), however, has cited several inherent problems in using this data collection method for even the common anomalies. Birth certificate reviews are hindered by a lack of standardized nomenclature, the possibilities of an incorrect diagnosis by the clinician, the potential misinterpretation by the reviewer of the reported conditions, and the listing of multiple birth anomalies in the same infant. Furthermore, birth certificates record only malformations occurring in live births.

It has been documented that the intrauterine incidence of facial deformities is greater than that found at birth. Hertig, Rock, and Adams (1956) reported that 40 per cent of the fertilized ova examined during the first 17 days after conception were abnormal; the vast majority of pregnancies involving abnormal ova terminate in spontaneous abortion. Warburton and Frazer (1956) showed that a frequent occurrence of malformations exists in spontaneously aborted and stillborn fetuses. Nishimura (1969) studied material gathered from therapeutic abortions in an attempt to eliminate the built-in sampling bias of studies based on spontaneously aborted and stillborn fetuses. When 13,840 specimens between 3 and 18 weeks of gestational age were examined, nearly 5 per cent had some form of external anomaly. Craniofacial malformations of all types were observed at the rate of 42.5 per 1000.

The possibility exists that more craniofacial clefts will be seen in the future. This speculation is raised because the common clefts of the lip and the palate appear to be increasing in frequency (Gylling and Soivio, 1962; Fogh-Andersen, 1965; Moller, 1965; Tünte, 1969) and also because the development of craniofacial anomalies has directed the attention of the medical community to these problems.

EMBRYOLOGIC ASPECTS

An understanding of the normal events in the embryologic development of the face facilitates the study of rare craniofacial clefts. A detailed discussion of normal embryologic development is presented in Chapter 46. A brief summary of the pertinent events follows.

The embryologic development of the face takes place between the fourth and eighth weeks of gestation (Patten, 1968). The midportion of the face develops immediately anterior to the forebrain by the differentiation of the broad midline frontonasal prominence (Fig. 59–1). Thickened ectodermal plates, the nasal placodes, arise from either side of the frontonasal prominence just above the stomodeum. Progressive elevation of the mesoderm at the margins of the placodes produces a horseshoe-shaped ridge, which is open inferiorly. The limbs of the placodes become the median and lateral nasal processes.

The paired median nasal processes merge with the frontonasal prominence to form the major portion of the frontal process. These structures gradually enlarge to displace the frontonasal prominence in a cephalic direction. The median nasal processes coalesce in the midline during the sixth week. Their caudal prolongations, the globular processes, follow a similar pattern as they expand above the midportion of the stomodeum. The premaxilla, the philtrum of the upper lip, the columella, the nasal tip, the cartilaginous portion of the nasal septum, and the primary palate are derived from the paired median elements. Above them the frontonasal process persists and narrows to form the bridge and root of the nose. The lateral nasal processes form the alar region of the nose.

The mandibular arch lies between the stomodeum and the first branchial groove, marking the caudal limits of the face. Its paired, free ends enlarge and converge ventrally to complete the continuity of the arch during the sixth week. The lower lip and mandible are developed from the mandibular arch. Paired lateral elevations of the pharyngeal surface of this arch unite in the midline to form the anterior portion of the tongue.

During the sixth week three hillocks appear on the caudal border of the first branchial arch (His, 1885). On the cephalic border of the second hyoid arch, three corresponding hillocks can also be identified (Fig. 59–2). The external ear is formed from these elevations. The tragus and the crus of the helix are derived from the first arch, as are the incus and the malleus of the middle ear. The second arch contributes the remainder of the external ear and the stapes of the middle ear.

Budding off the mandibular arch are paired postocular masses of paraxial mesoderm, which constitute the maxillary processes. These triangular mesodermal masses progressively enlarge toward the ventral surface. A deep groove, the naso-optic furrow, marks the superomedial margin of the maxilla from the developing eye and the lateral nasal process. The inferior border of the maxilla separates from the mandibular arch. The maxillary process ultimately coalesces with the mesoderm of the globular processes to form the upper lip. The cheek, the maxilla, the zygoma, and the secondary palate are also derived from the maxillary processes.

The relationship of the various embryonic processes to the adult face is shown in Figure 59–3.

The embryopathogenesis of the craniofacial region is extremely complex. During a short four week period, an extreme demand is placed on the coordination of cell separation, migration, and interaction. The proper amount of tissue must be

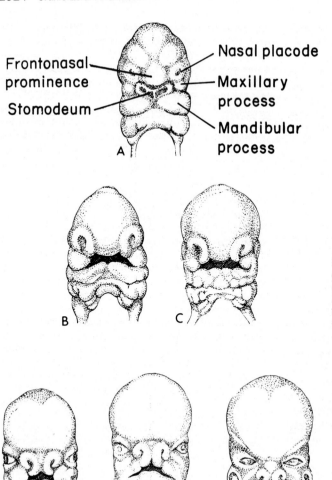

Figure 59–1. Embryonic development of the human face. *A,* Four week embryo (3.5 mm) with designation of facial processes; *B,* five week embryo (6.5 mm); *C,* six week embryo (9 mm); *D,* six and a half week embryo (12 mm); *E,* seven week embryo (19 mm); *F,* eight week embryo (28 mm). (After Patten.)

present at an exact moment in the correct three-dimensional relationship. Precise movement and timing are critical. Any mishap in this intricate program can lead to disastrous consequences. The resulting chasm usually falls along predictable embryonic lines. Some clefts, however, are found in atypical locations that do not correspond to the normal lines of union of the facial processes. Various theories have been proposed to explain the formation of clefts.

Theories of Facial Cleft Formation. Two leading theories of facial cleft formation exist. The classic theory, proposed by Dursy (1869) and His (1892), states that failure of fusion of the facial processes is responsible for the development of the clefts. This concept was questioned by Pohlmann (1910) and Veau and Politzer (1936) as the theory of mesodermal

migration and penetration began to emerge; the investigations of Stark (1954) also supported this challenge.

Although most of the present knowledge is based on the study of cleft lip and palate morphogenesis in nonhuman embryos, it is highly probable that rare craniofacial clefts are produced by similar mechanisms.

The classic concept of fusion pictures the central region of the face as the site of union of the free ends of the facial processes. The face begins to take form as the various processes fuse. Thus, as an example, the upper lip is formed by the union of the finger-like ends of the maxillary processes as they meet and coalesce with the paired globular processes beneath the nasal pits (see Fig. 59–1*D*). After epithelial contact is established, pene-

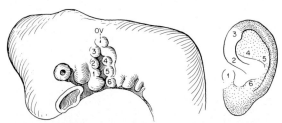

Figure 59–2. Development of the external ear. Hillocks 1 to 3 are from the mandibular arch, 4 to 6 from the hyoid arch. Contribution of the hillocks to the adult ear: 1, tragus; 2, 3, helix; 4, 5, anthelix; 6, antitragus. OV = Otic vesicle. (After Arey.)

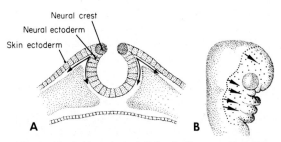

Figure 59–4. Neural crest cells. *A,* Cross section of the neural tube showing the origin and migration pathways of the neural crest cells. *B,* Profile of the embryo showing the dorsoventral migration of the cells. (After Johnston.)

tration by the mesoderm occurs to complete the fusion and the formation of the upper lip and the primary palate. Disruption of this sequence leads to the formation of a cleft.

Proponents of the mesodermal penetration theory believed that the free ends of the facial processes do not exist. Warbrick (1938) and Stark and Ehrmann (1958) showed that separate processes as such are not found in the central portion of the face. According to their work (see Chap. 48), the central portion of the face is composed of a continuous sheet of a bilamellar membrane of ectoderm known as the primary plate. The bilamellar membrane of ectoderm is demarcated by epithelial seams, which delineate the principal "processes." Into this double layer of ectoderm, called "the epithelial wall" (Hochstetter, 1953), mesenchyme migrates and penetrates to smooth out the seams. Caudal to the stomodeum, the lower face and the neck are formed by a series of branchial arches. At first the arches consist of a thin sheet of mesoderm lying between the ectoderm and the endoderm. The craniofacial mesoderm is augmented by neuroectoderm brought in by the migrating neural crest cells.

The importance of the neural crest cells was first recognized by Johnston (1965). The cells arise from the dorsolateral surface of the neural tube and migrate beneath the ectoderm to form a continuous layer that supplements the underlying mesoderm of the frontonasal process and the branchial arches (Fig. 59–4) (see Chap. 48). The craniofacial skeleton is believed to be principally derived from neural crest cells. If penetration by the neuroectoderm does not occur, the unsupported epithelial wall breaks down to form a facial cleft. The severity of the cleft is inversely proportional to the degree of penetration by the neuroectoderm. If penetration fails altogether, a complete cleft is formed as the epithelial wall dehisces; partial penetration leads to the development of an incomplete cleft.

Hoepke and Maurer (1939) borrowed from each of the two leading theories. They suggested that failure of fusion is responsible for facial cleft formation, and they regarded the penetration of the mesoderm as an attempt by the embryo to bridge the gap and thus heal the imperfection. The severity of the cleft would depend on the success of the secondary healing effort.

Many voids remain in the complete understanding of the formation of facial clefts. It is generally agreed that clefts of the secondary palate are formed by failure of fusion. It is principally in the delineation of cleft lip pathogenesis that complete accord of investigators is absent (see Chap. 48). The role of the proposed mechanisms in the formation of rare craniofacial clefts is not precisely defined. Nevertheless, the concepts of fusion and mesodermal penetration enable one to under-

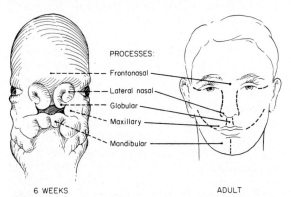

Figure 59–3. Contributions of the embryonic processes to the adult face.

PROCESSES:
Frontonasal
Lateral nasal
Globular
Maxillary
Mandibular

6 WEEKS   ADULT

stand the problems of unusual craniofacial clefts.

Clefts of Midline Craniofacial Structures. The most minor example of a midline facial cleft is that of the median cleft of the upper lip. This lip irregularity can be explained by the imperfect union of the paired globular processes. Increased disruption in the process could lead to the formation of a bifid frenulum, a midline notch of the alveolus, a midline cleft of the palate, or a bifid nose.

Frontonasal dysplasia and a median frontal encephalocele with orbital hypertelorism are examples of major midline developmental failures. Disfigurement of this magnitude occurs when the frontonasal prominence remains in its embryonic location. The forebrain thus retains its low overlying position and interferes with the normal converging movement of the optic placodes toward the midline. Hence, the eyes remain arrested in their "lateralized" embryonic setting (see Fig. 59–1*D*).

At the other end of the spectrum, morphokinetic arrest of the frontonasal prominence can produce monstrous malformations such as cyclopia, ethmocephaly, and cebocephaly (see Chap. 60). The mildest expression of this type of developmental arrest is characterized by the absence of the philtral region of the lip (false median cleft lip) and agenesis of the

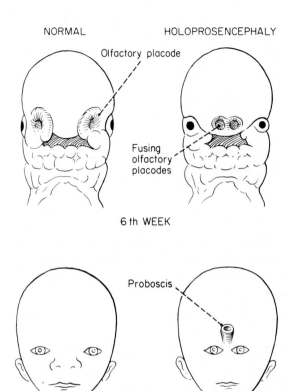

Figure 59–6. Embryonic face with developing holoprosencephaly. Because the development of the frontonasal process is inhibited, the olfactory and optic placodes assume a position closer to the midline. Formation of a proboscis is shown. It is postulated that cyclopia and ethmocephaly are formed by a similar mechanism, depending upon the degree of convergence of the olfactory and optic placodes. (After Cohen and associates.)

primary palate. Cohen and associates (1971a) suggested that the basic mechanism that produces these abnormalities lies in the faulty interaction between the notochordal plate and the neuroectoderm of the brain plate and the oral plate. The notochordal plate in the embryo begins just caudal to the optic plates (Fig. 59–5). When this plate is abnormally short and its cephalic end is caudally displaced, development of the neuroectoderm and frontonasal process is inhibited. Orbital hypotelorism is produced by the failure of the optic anlagen to move in the lateral direction (Fig. 59–6). Because of the intimate association of the frontonasal prominence with the development of the forebrain, the severity of these centrally located craniofacial malformations appears to parallel that of the forebrain defects (Yakovlev, 1956; DeMyer and Zeman, 1963). Therefore the extent of facial

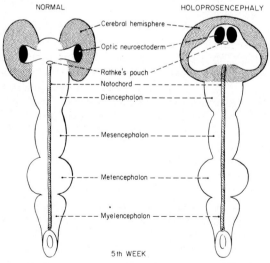

Figure 59–5. Embryonic brain and formation of holoprosencephaly. The notochord falls short of Rathke's pouch and inhibits the development of the neuroectoderm and frontonasal process. The prosencephalon remains "hololistic." (After Cohen and associates.)

disorganization provides a clue to the severity of the developmental arrest of the forebrain: "the face predicts the brain" (DeMyer, Zeman, and Palmer, 1964).

Clefts of Mandibular Process. Interference with the normal union of the paired first branchial arches (mandibular arch) as they converge ventrally results in midline mandibular clefts and anomalies of the anterior two-thirds of the tongue. When the mouth is formed, a notch is present in the midline of the lower lip. As the deformity progresses in severity, clefts of the lip and mandibular symphysis and ankyloglossia can be observed. Cosman and Crikelair (1969) believed that these malformations represent one end of a spectrum of midline branchiogenic syndromes. As the extent of pathologic insult increases, the second, and possibly the third, branchial arch becomes involved. Morton and Jordon (1935) described a 13 day old newborn with a complete form of this midline branchiogenic disorder. The newborn had a cleft of the lower lip and mandible, ankyloglossia, contracture of the neck in the midline, and absence of the hyoid, the manubrium, and the upper portion of the sternum. Without anterior skeletal support, the trachea and the lungs were free to herniate beneath the skin of the neck and anterior chest. Monroe (1966) concluded, after a review of the literature, that midline mandibular clefts were best explained by a failure of mesodermal penetration.

Clefts of Maxillary Process. The maxillary process occupies a key position. Budding off the mandibular arch, the maxillary process is brought into contact with the mandibular process, the median and lateral nasal processes, and the optic placode. Thus, the process has the opportunity to participate in the formation of several facial clefts.

The commissure of the primitive mouth is located at the point of bifurcation of the maxillary and mandibular processes (see Fig. 59–1). This lateral slit is gradually obliterated by the progressive fusion of the processes to form the cheek by the development of the muscles of mastication. By the twelfth week the commissures are formed. Persistence of the furrow between the maxillary and mandibular processes results in a transverse facial cleft, as seen in craniofacial microsomia (see Chap. 62) and Goldenhar's syndrome. A faulty union between the maxillary and globular processes is responsible for the formation of the common clefts of the upper lip.

The naso-optic groove separates the central mass of mesoderm of the frontonasal process from the lateral mesodermal mass of the maxillary process. If the involved masses fail to join properly, the naso-optic groove is transformed into a naso-ocular (nasomaxillary) cleft. The groove contains the future nasolacrimal duct and is confluent with the developing eye. Therefore, associated deformities of these structures are invariably seen. Furthermore, if the maxillary process fails to unite with the globular process, an oronasoocular cleft would result.

Facial clefts within the maxillary process itself are not as easily explained. These malformations, oro-ocular cleft, and the clefts associated with the Treacher Collins syndrome (mandibulofacial dysostosis) do not coincide with any known embryonic seams. These clefts probably reflect a disturbance in the flow of neural crest cells during their dorsoventral migration. The resulting paucity of neuroectoderm within the maxillary process produces a weak point, which can disintegrate to form a cleft. In the case of mandibulofacial dysostosis, Poswillo (1975) was able to produce an animal model by the selective destruction of the neural crest stream. A "vacuum" is created in the region of the otic placode. The neural crest cells destined for the otic placode region are considered "late starters." At the same time that the above derangement occurs, the front-running neural crest cells have presumably already reached the area of the naso-optic furrow. The unsupported area that is subject to a cleft deformity is, therefore, found more proximally in the otomandibular region rather than at the naso-ocular junction. By borrowing from this concept, one can conceive that the destruction of the middle batch of the neural crest cells could produce a mesodermal deficiency in the more ventral section of the maxillary process. A disruption of the weak zone would form the oro-ocular cleft.

Although knowledge of the morphogenesis of rare facial clefts remains incomplete, an even greater gap exists in the understanding of the causal agents of the morphokinetic disturbances.

ETIOLOGY

To be born normal, the newborn must successfully overcome the possible obstacles associated with unfavorable heredity and hostile intrauterine environment (see Chap. 2). Aside from the Treacher Collins and the Goldenhar syndromes, heredity appears to play a minor role in the formation of most rare craniofacial clefts; the majority of atypical clefts occur sporadically (Fogh-Andersen, 1965).

Accumulating evidence from animal and clinical studies supports a multifactorial concept of multiple interacting etiologic factors. The complexity of the problem is underlined by the vast number of teratogenic agents known to produce facial clefts. The study of nonhuman embryos and human statistics has yielded valuable information, but large voids remain in the knowledge of the pathogenesis of rare facial clefts. It should be mentioned that most of the information that is now available is based on studies of the formation of the common clefts of the lip and palate (see Chap. 48). From these investigations, four major categories of environmental factors have been identified: (1) radiation, (2) infection, (3) maternal metabolic imbalances, and (4) drugs and chemicals (Wilson, 1972).

Radiation. Although clefts of the lip and palate can be experimentally produced in animals by the administration of roentgen rays (Warkany and Schraffenberger, 1947; Callas and Walker, 1963; Poswillo, 1968), a similar teratogenic effect in humans has not been verified. An increased incidence of clefts could not be demonstrated in the offspring of Japanese mothers who survived the atomic bombings (Neel, 1958). In a group of 57 women exposed to large doses of radiation during the first 15 weeks of pregnancy, a disproportional rise in the incidence of malformation in their newborns, other than microcephaly, was not observed (Miller, 1969).

Infection. Infectious agents have been implicated in the pathogenesis of congenital malformations in general. In regard to craniofacial malformations, the study of viruses, bacteria, and protozoa has not been particularly rewarding. In animals, the H_1 virus was shown to be capable of producing sporadic occurrences of facial clefts (Ferm and Kilham, 1964). The influenza A_2 virus was also implicated in an epidemiologic study (Leck and associates, 1969). Following an epidemic attributable to this agent, an increased incidence of cleft lip deformities was noted. Although the rubella virus was demonstrated to produce congenital malformation in man, an associated incidence of facial clefts was not documented. In studies of the toxoplasmosis protozoan, a two- to fourfold increase in the rate of infestation with this agent was found in mothers of offspring with facial clefts (Gabka, 1953; Erdelyi, 1957; Jírovec and associates, 1957). Convincing correlations between bacterial infections and facial clefts have not been reported.

Maternal Metabolic Imbalance. Adverse effects on embryologic facial development have been attributed to alterations in maternal metabolism. Tocci and Beber (1970) presented evidence of an abnormal phenylalanine metabolic pathway in some mothers of offspring with cleft lip and palate. Although it has been stated that diabetic mothers have a greater chance of delivering a newborn with a congenital malformation (Pederson, Thigstrop, and Pederson, 1964; Comess, 1969), a higher frequency of craniofacial clefts was not described. Manipulation of the thyroxine levels in animals was shown to influence the frequency of facial clefts. A higher incidence of clefts occurs in the offspring of female rats that had a partial thyroidectomy (Langman and Van Faassen, 1955). Reversal of this phenomenon was demonstrated in mice given supplemental thyroxine (Woollam and Millen, 1960). A collaborative study in humans has not been reported.

Drugs and Chemicals. A considerable effort has been expended in investigating the teratogenic potential of drugs and chemicals (Wilson, 1973). The list of incriminated agents continues to expand. In a parallel fashion, drug consumption by society is ever increasing. Nora and associates (1967) found that a mean of 3.7 potentially teratogenic drugs were taken during the first trimester in a prospective study of 240 pregnancies. The growing list of suspect drugs and the increasing use of these agents might well be responsible for the apparent rise in the number of malformations.

The range of drugs and chemicals known to induce congenital malformations in animals and man is broad. These agents fall into the general categories of anticonvulsants, antimetabolic and alkylating agents, steroids, and tranquilizers.

Anticonvulsants. Several statistical studies showed that mothers who take anticonvulsant medication give birth to a higher number of facially deformed children than do a comparable control population (Janz and Fuchs, 1964; Melchior, Svensmark, and

Trolle, 1967; German, Kowal, and Ehler, 1970; South, 1972; Spidel and Meadow, 1972). The incidence of facial clefts in infants born to women with seizure disorders was reported as approximately 1 per cent (Pashayan, Pruzansky, and Pruzansky, 1971; Erickson and Oakley, 1974). The risk was six times greater than that incurred by children of women without seizure disorders (Erickson and Oakley, 1974). The teratogenic effects of diphenylhydantoin might be related to its antimetabolic effects, since it possesses antifolate properties.

Antimetabolic and Alkylating Agents. The teratogenic activity of these drugs is well established. Except for tretinoin (Accutane), their clinical relevance, however, is limited, since few embryos survive the lethal effects of these agents.

Tretinoin inhibits sebaceous gland function and keratinization and is effective in the treatment of cystic acne. Unfortunately, female patients most likely to be given this medication are of child-bearing age. Braun and associates (1984) were the first to record the craniofacial teratogenic effects of tretinoin in humans. Lammer and associates (1985) conclusively showed potent teratogenic effects of this drug. Of 154 pregnant women who ingested tretinoin 5 to 70 days after the estimated date of conception, 95 had elective and 12 had spontaneous abortions. Of the remaining 47, 26 gave birth to newborns without any major malformations. However, 21 offspring had major malformations, which included anotia, microtia, micrognathia, cleft palate, retinal or optic nerve abnormalities, and central nervous system defects.

Steroids. Many investigators have been able to induce clefts of the palate in animals by the administration of steroids (Frazer and Fainstat, 1951; Harris and Ross, 1955; Murphy, Dagg, and Karnofsky, 1957; Heiberg, Kalter, and Frazer, 1959). Corticosteroids have been shown to reduce the amount of amniotic fluid, which in turn could produce detrimental postural changes in the embryo by limiting the available intrauterine space (Harris, 1964; Walker, 1965; Frazer, Chew, and Verusio, 1967). Restriction of the normal extension of the head could interfere with the normal downward displacement of the tongue, an event that is essential to allow the elevation of the palatal shelves. A decreased synthesis of sulfomucopolysaccharides within the palatal shelves is also caused

by cortisone, and Larsson (1968) explained the formation of clefts on this basis.

Tranquilizers. The tragic history of malformations caused by thalidomide is well known. Ear deformities were documented in the offspring of mothers who ingested thalidomide during pregnancy (Smithells and Leck, 1963; Livingstone, 1965). Kleinsasser and Schlothane (1964) reported a study of women who took the drug during the first six weeks of pregnancy. During the period of use between 1959 and 1962, at least 1000 severe cases of malformations associated with the first and second branchial arches were observed in the offspring. Approximately 2000 less severely deformed children were also noted. Poswillo (1973, 1974b) was successful in reproducing the first and second branchial arch syndrome in primates by administering thalidomide.

Diazepam (Valium), one of the most widely prescribed drugs, was shown by Miller and Becker (1975) to produce cleft palate in animals. Saxén (1975) and Safra and Oakley (1975) documented a higher incidence of cleft lip, with or without a cleft of the palate, in children of mothers who ingested diazepam during the first trimester. Mothers of infants with oral clefts had used diazepam four times more frequently than mothers of infants with other malformations (Safra and Oakley, 1975). On the other hand, subsequent larger studies (Rosenberg and associates, 1983; Shiono and Mills, 1984) showed that the incidence of craniofacial malformations has not increased with its use.

Other Agents. Both thalidomide and triazene, used by Poswillo (1973) to produce an animal model of the first and second branchial arch syndrome, induce a localized hematoma in the otomandibular region. Aspirin and vasopressors are also known to produce hemorrhage in embryos that subsequently develop facial clefts and malformations of the limbs (Warkany and Takags, 1959; Larsson and Boström, 1965; Poswillo and Sopher, 1971; Wilson, 1972; Saxén, 1975). A Treacher Collins–like deformity has also been reproduced in animals given vitamin A (Poswillo, 1975), which can also cause malformations of the brain, the eyes, the ears, and the jaws when administered in varying amounts (Cohlan, 1953; Giroud and Martinet, 1955, 1956, 1957; Poswillo and Roy, 1965; Marin-Padilla, 1966; Morriss, 1972).

The mystery of the cyclopian appearance of

malformed lambs was solved by a series of investigations (Binns and associates, 1959; Binns, Anderson, and Sullivan, 1960; Binns, 1961). The sheepherders called these deformed lambs "monkey-faced." The deformities were found to be caused by a poisonous weed, *Veratrum californicum,* that is found on the grazing lands. Brucker, Hoyt, and Trusler (1963) noted a close resemblance of these face-brain anomalies to the cebocephalic (Gr. *kebos,* monkey) and the holoprosencephalic craniofacial deformity observed in humans.

From this review, it can be appreciated that the intrauterine environment might not be as secure and comforting a milieu for the embryo as one would like to believe. The major part of the face is developed when the mother could be unknowingly pregnant. Thus, even if the teratogenic potential of all drugs were known, malformations might still not be prevented. The embryo might be able to elude the teratogenic effects of a single agent only to have the balance tipped against it by a combination of drugs. Those embryos subject to detrimental genetic factors face an additional handicap.

MORPHOPATHOGENESIS

Several pathways exist through which the various causal elements can exert their detrimental forces. Interference with cell formation, cell replication, or cell migration by the etiologic agent could produce rare craniofacial clefts.

Those who favor the fusion theory explain the morphogenesis of a facial cleft on the basis of failure of the various processes to achieve contact. Any retardation or restriction of movements of the processes could result in spatial misalignment and thereby could physically prevent normal union. Drugs that disturb the metabolic rate and affect the properties of the ground substance could intrinsically alter the normal development and movement of the various processes. Spatial restrictions, such as those imposed by oligohydramnios, could apply an extrinsic restraint on the facial processes and thus mechanically interfere with their normal fusion.

Alterations in the normal equilibrium between cell formation and spontaneous cell death is another possible means of cleft formation. Warbrick (1963) suggested that un-

wanted cells are normally discarded during the fusion procedure. Conceivably, two processes could meet and not coalesce if the programmed death of the epithelial cells does not occur to allow the mesenchyme to stream across. A partial interruption of this turnover cycle could lead to the formation of an incomplete cleft.

The concept of an altered metabolic rate and premature cell death is equally applicable to the mesodermal penetration theory. If the ability of the cell to replicate and migrate is thwarted, weak areas susceptible to cleft formation can be created.

Arrest or turbulence in the dorsoventral flow of neural crest cells is proposed by advocates of the mesodermal penetration theory. Incomplete filling of the epithelial wall caused by these pathologic disturbances would produce an unsupported or fragile zone. Hövels (1953) believed that the early central disorganization of the neural plate or the neural crest is responsible for the Treacher Collins malformation. Subsequently, Johnston (1964) experimentally produced a facial cleft by removing a portion of the neural crest before the cells began their migration. This concept gained additional support from the work of Poswillo (1975). His animal experiments suggested that bilaterally symmetric facial clefts, such as those found in the Treacher Collins syndrome, are best explained by the disorganization of the preotic neural crest cells approximately at the time of their migration into the first branchial arches. The proliferation rate of the neural crest cells has also been implicated. A reduced propagation rate is present in the frontonasal mesenchyme of the mouse embryo with the Dancer gene, and a Waardenburg-like syndrome is produced in these animals (Trasler, 1969). In humans, the white forelock of hair seen in patients with Waardenburg's syndrome can be explained by the patch degeneration of the neural crest cells, since these cells also give rise to melanocytes (Johnston, 1975).

Disturbances in the circulatory system could also reduce the volume of tissue and limit the ability for mesenchymal penetration. Tandler (1903) and Kundrat (1882) are cited by Sanvenero-Rosselli (1953) as being among the first to associate an arterial malformation with a congenital anomaly. An arhinencephalic malformation was described by Kundrat (1882), which he causally linked to a vascular compromise in areas supplied by the anterior cerebral artery. Streeter (1922) postulated "focal fetal deficiencies" to explain congenital malformations. He thought that these deficiencies were due to chromosomal aberrations. Keith (1940a), however, was of the opinion that it was more profitable to explain "Streeter's foetal dysplasia" as a local vascular disturbance. He postulated that the failure of circulatory anastomosis between and within the various facial processes was the responsible underlying pathologic mechanism. Because of the inadequate vascular supply, a "dysplastic crease" or "necrotic groove" was created, and it led to the formation of a partial or complete facial cleft. Frazer (1940) also mentioned the possible detrimental effect of local ischemia during the early phases of embryonic development.

In terms of the ischemic crisis theory, the first and second branchial arch syndrome is the best studied malformation. Lockhard (1929) described an anomaly of the maxillary artery and associated it with deformities of the zygoma, the middle ear, and the muscles of mastication. Braithwaite and Watson (1949) suggested that the ischemic crisis was caused by a maldevelopment or a total absence of the stapedial artery. McKenzie and Craig (1955) elaborated on this theory and pointed out the vulnerability of the stapedial artery. The artery, which is short lived, supplies the first and second branchial arches. After branching off the dorsal aorta of the primitive circulatory system, the artery makes its appearance on the thirty-third day, and seven days later it disappears. The blood supply to the area is then furnished by the external carotid artery, as a transfer of the main arterial trunk occurs from the dorsal aorta to the ventral aorta. An interruption in this orderly transition could lead to a circulatory crisis. The theory of McKenzie and Craig (1955) is based on a postmortem dissection of a 10 week old newborn with Treacher Collins syndrome. The maxillary artery was observed to have "petered out" before it reached the pterygomaxillary fissure. Normal mandibular, posterior superior alveolar, and middle meningeal branches were given off. McKenzie (1958) later used the theory of stapedial artery formation to explain the deformities of the first and second branchial arch syndrome, Pierre Robin se-

quence, cleft lip and palate, orbital hypertelorism, and congenital deaf-mutism. Not all investigators would agree with this expanded application of the stapedial artery theory.

Poswillo (1973) suggested that a localized hemorrhage rather than anomalous development of the stapedial artery best explains the structural malformations found in the first and second branchial arch syndrome. In animal experiments, the hemorrhage occurs in the vicinity of the first and second branchial arches shortly after the formation of the stapedial artery. Depending on the magnitude of local tissue destruction and the extent of delay in differentiation, varying degrees of maldevelopment can be observed.

The role of heredity in the causation of rare craniofacial clefts remains to be clarified. The influence of heredity is most clearly defined in the Treacher Collins syndrome (see Chap. 63). Rogers (1964a) offered some ideas to explain the incomplete and complete forms of this syndrome. The responsible gene is known to have a variable penetration ability. Taking this into consideration, Rogers (1964a) suggested that a "strong" gene exerts its influence early in the course of facial development. Thus, a more comprehensive expression by the aberrant gene occurs, and the complete form of the syndrome is seen. A "weak" gene exerts its inhibitory action at a later stage of embryologic development, hence, an incomplete, mild form of the syndrome is observed. The area of disturbance is thought to be another factor that influences the clinical expression of the anomaly. In the milder forms of the syndrome, the deleterious effects of the offending gene are thought to be confined, more or less, to the maxillary portion of the first branchial arch. Conversely, the complete form of the syndrome involves the maxillary and mandibular portions of the first arch, as well as some of the structures derived from the second branchial arch.

In the final analysis, it can safely be stated that the causal environmental and hereditary factors have potential access to multiple pathways by which to exercise their influences. The teratologist, confronted with the problem of multiple factors acting through numerous channels, assumes an enormous burden when he is asked to explain the formation of a particular cleft. Moreover, the problem is compounded by the lack of a universally accepted classification system.

CLASSIFICATION

The task of classifying rare craniofacial clefts is not a simple one. Several major obstacles must be overcome. Because the clefts are so rare, reviews of the literature are often used to gather descriptive material on the malformations. Unfortunately, descriptions of the individual cases are often incomplete. Furthermore, the diverse groups of specialists involved in the study of these malformations frequently use different terminology for the same deformity. In addition, the observer can be confused by the wide variety of facial clefts that can exist in numerous combinations to distort the face into bizarre forms. Fortunately, the majority of the atypical craniofacial clefts are easily recognized as belonging to a particular group. Although the challenge is admittedly difficult, several attempts have been made to bring order out of chaos.

American Association of Cleft Palate Rehabilitation Classification. In 1962, Harkins and associates proposed a classification system endorsed by the American Association of Cleft Palate Rehabilitation (AACPR). The rare facial clefts are divided into four major groups: (1) mandibular process clefts, (2) naso-ocular clefts, (3) oro-ocular clefts, and (4) oroaural clefts (Fig. 59–7).

Clefts of the lower lip, the mandible, and the lip pits are included in the mandibular process cleft group. The naso-ocular clefts extend from the alar region toward the medial canthus. Clefts of the oro-ocular group connect the oral aperture to the palpebral fissures. This group is subdivided into oro-

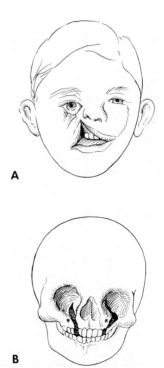

A

B

Figure 59–8. Boo-Chai classification. Type I cleft is shown on the right side of the face, Type II on the left side. The infraorbital foramen is the key landmark. Type I clefts pass medially, and Type II clefts are found lateral to the foramen.

medial canthus and orolateral canthus clefts. The temporal extension from the lateral canthus is included in the orolateral canthus subdivision. The oroaural clefts, which extend directly from the corner of the mouth toward the ear, form the last main group.

The AACPR classification system is lacking in several respects. Conspicuously omitted are the major midfacial clefts and the Treacher Collins malformation. Confusion in terminology is also noted. The oromedial canthus cleft is described in the original text but is illustrated as an oronaso-ocular cleft. Furthermore, the classification is based on the surface anatomy of the malformation and fails to address the underlying skeletal components of the clefts.

Boo-Chai (1970) recognized the deficiencies of the AACPR description of the oro-ocular cleft. Morian (1887) was the first to recognize the anatomic differences between the clefts by drawing attention to the importance of the infraorbital foramen. Using this landmark, Boo-Chai subdivided the oro-ocular clefts into Types I and II (Fig. 59–8). In contrast to the naso-ocular cleft, the oro-ocular clefts do not

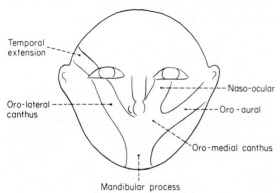

Figure 59–7. American Association of Cleft Palate Rehabilitation (AACPR) classification of facial clefts. (After Harkins and associates.)

Table 59–1. Karfik Facial Cleft Classification

Group A—Rhinencephalic Disorders		
Axial (A 1)	Prolapse	Meningocele
		Glioma
		Dermoid cyst
		Teratoma
	Clefts	Medial nasal (double nose)
		Median cleft of upper lip and premaxilla
	Defects	Coloboma of nostril
		Partial of nose
		Total of nose
		Septal
		Atresia nasi
Para-axial (A 2)	Clefts	Coloboma, iridic or palpebral
		Total or partial para-axial
		Cleft lip, typical
		Lacrimal duct dystopia
Group B—Branchiogenic Disorders		
Lateral otocephalic (B 1)	Clefts	Macrostomia
		Lateral cervical fistula
	Dysostosis	Mandibular (e.g., Pierre Robin)
		Mandibulofacial (e.g., Treacher Collins)
	Defects	Partial or total auricular
		Atresia
Medial axial (B 2)	Clefts	Tongue
		Lower lip
		Mandible
		Fissura colli medialis
		Fissura thoracis medialis
Group C—Ophthalmo-orbital Disorders		
	Malformation	Eyeball: microphthalmia
		anophthalmia
		Lids: blepharophimosis
		epicanthus
		ptosis
		agenesis
	Defect	Orbital
	Clefts	Upper lid coloboma
		Commissural
Group D—Craniocephalic Disorders		
	Malformation	Head and face (e.g., Apert's and Crouzon's diseases)
	Defect	Scalp
		Skull
Group E—Atypical Facial Disorders		
		Oblique facial clefts
		Dysembryoma, parasitic
		Hemifacial atrophy
		Hyperplasia
		Neoplasm, congenital
		Teratoma

violate the piriform aperture. The soft tissue components of the clefts further distinguish the two types.

In the Type I cleft, the fault in the upper lip is seen to begin lateral to the Cupid's bow (Fig. 59–8A). Hence, the departure point is found lateral to that of the common cleft lip. The defect skirts lateral to the nasal ala onto the cheek to end in the medial canthal region. According to Boo-Chai (1970), an extension of the cleft from the lateral canthus can continue into the temporal region. On the facial skeleton (Fig. 59–8B), the Type I cleft begins between the lateral incisor and the canine and does not encroach on the piriform aperture. It continues medial to the infraorbital foramen to enter the inferomedial aspect of the orbit (Fig. 59–8B).

On the other hand, the Type II oro-ocular cleft starts near the corner of the mouth and terminates as a coloboma in the midportion of the lower eyelid or near the lateral canthus. The bony cleft is found in the region of the premolar teeth and takes a path lateral to the infraorbital foramen to enter the inferolateral portion of the orbit (Fig. 59–8*B*).

Karfik Classification. Karfik (1966) proposed a detailed classification of rare craniofacial clefts based on embryologic and morphologic criteria. A revised form of portions of this classification was presented the following year. Five major groups (A to E) are outlined (Table 59–1).

Clefts of Group A are composed of malformations of the "rhinencephalic region." The group is subdivided into axial (Group A 1) and para-axial (Group A 2) malformations. The axial subgroup includes the malformations of the frontonasal prominence derivatives. The para-axial subgroup encompasses the anomalies of the adjacent regions, which are "always combined disorders in the development of the nose and its parts" (Karfik, 1966). The oro-ocular clefts are included in this group, since Karfik (1966) was of the opinion that they begin from "typical lip clefts." However, Boo-Chai (1970) noted that the cleft of the lip associated with this deformity is actually located lateral to the site of the common cleft lip.

Composing the Group B malformations are those deformities related to the first and second branchial arches. In the subdivision of this group, Group B 1 is composed of the "lateral otocephalic" disorders, which include craniofacial microsomia, Pierre Robin sequence, Treacher Collins syndrome, and auricular malformations. The midline mandibular malformation falls in the Group B 2 subdivision.

The Group C malformations are centered in the orbitopalpebral region. Located in the Group D disorders are the "craniocephalic" malformations, such as Apert's syndrome and Crouzon's disease. The final category, Group E, consists mainly of atypical deformities caused by congenital tumors, atrophy, and hypertrophy maldevelopments, which are more closely associated with facial asymmetry problems than with clefts. The oblique facial cleft is also included in this group and is termed by Karfik (1966) a "true oblique cleft," since it cannot be related to any known embryonic facial seam. This cleft is similar to the Type II oro-ocular cleft of Boo-Chai (1970).

Van der Meulen and Associates Classification. Van der Meulen and associates

Table 59–2. Van der Meulen and Associates Classification

Cerebral Craniofacial Dysplasia
  Interophthalmic dysplasia
  Ophthalmic dysplasia
Craniofacial Dysplasia
  Dysostoses
    Frontosphenoid dysplasia
    Frontal dysplasia
    Frontofrontal dysplasia
    Frontonasoethmoid dysplasia
    Internasal dysplasia
    Nasal dysplasia
      Type 1—nasal aplasia
      Type 2—nasal aplasia with proboscis
      Type 3—nasoschizis
      Type 4—nasal duplication
    Nasomaxillary dysplasia
    Maxillary dysplasia
      Medial maxillary dysplasia
      Lateral maxillary dysplasia
    Maxillozygomatic dysplasia
    Zygomatic dysplasia
    Zygofrontal dysplasia
    Zygotemporal dysplasia
    Temporoaural dysplasia
    Zygotemporoauromandibular dysplasia
    Temporoauromandibular dysplasia
    Maxillomandibular dysplasia
    Mandibular dysplasia
    Intermandibular dysplasia
  Synostoses

(1983) attempted to explain the craniofacial clefts on an embryologic basis. The term dysplasia is used instead of cleft, since some of the malformations do not represent true clefts. The defects are labeled by the name of the developmental area or areas (facial processes and bones) that are involved. Those malformations that are caused by *developmental arrest* are believed to occur before or during the fusion of the facial processes, and before the start of ossification, that is, approximately the time of 17 mm crown rump (CR) length of the embryo. In contrast, *differentiation defects* are produced during a later stage and are caused by absence or insufficient outgrowth of the "anlage" of the bone centers. Table 59–2 summarizes the categories in this classification system.

Classification of Median Facial Clefts. Two broad categories of median facial anomalies exist: (1) those in which there is a deficiency of tissue, thereby creating an absence of parts, and (2) those in which the amount of tissue is near normal or in excess, but associated with a malformation.

Tissue Deficiency Malformations. The median facial anomalies with a shortage of

Table 59–3. Types of Holoprosencephaly

Facial Type	Facial Features	Cranium	Brain
I. Cyclopia	Single or partial divided eye in single orbit or anophthalmia; arhinia or single or double proboscis	Microcephaly	Alobar
II. Ethmocephaly	Extreme orbital hypotelorism with separate orbits; arhinia or a single or double proboscis	Microcephaly	Alobar
III. Cebocephaly	Orbital hypotelorism, proboscis-like nose	Microcephaly	Usually alobar
IV. With median cleft lip (premaxillary agenesis)	Orbital hypotelorism; flat nose; absent median portion of upper lip	Microcephaly; sometimes trigonocephaly	Usually alobar
V. With median philtrum- premaxilla anlage	Orbital hypotelorism; bilateral cleft lip; flat nose	Microcephaly; sometimes trigonocephaly	Semilobar or lobar

tissue have been called arhinencephaly malformations. This term was used by Kundrat (1882) to express the absence of the olfactory bulbs and tracts, which were assumed to be the common malformation in this series of brain abnormalities. Investigators subsequently have established that the underlying developmental error is the arrested cleavage of the forebrain (prosencephalon) (Yakovlev, 1959; DeMyer, Zeman, and Palmer, 1964). DeMyer, Zeman and Palmer (1964) proposed the term holoprosencephalon to denote that the prosencephalon tends to remain "holistic" when cleavage does not normally occur. As mentioned above, an intimate relationship exists between the median facial structures and the forebrain. Therefore, the severity of the facial disorganization reflects an equally severe brain anomaly. On the basis of this brain-facial theme, the holoprosencephalic malformations are divided into five types (Table 59–3). The table includes some of the concepts of Cohen and associates (1971a). To emphasize further the brain-facial relationship, Brucker, Hoyt, and Trusler (1963) proposed the term median cerebrofacial dysgenesis.

Near-Normal and Excess Tissue Disorders. In direct contrast to the tissue deficiency disorders, this group of median facial anomalies does not have a high predictive correlation between the distorted face and the underlying brain. The amount of tissue in the midline is near normal or in excess. The spectrum of deformities ranges from a slight midline notch of the upper lip to the severest form of orbital hypertelorism. Between the two extremes, a diverse range of deformities are found.

Median cleft face syndrome is the term favored by DeMyer (1967) for this group of malformations (see Chap. 60). The seven features of the entity are (1) orbital hypertelorism, (2) V-shaped frontal hairline, (3) cranium bifidum occultum, (4) median cleft of the upper lip, (5) median cleft of the premaxilla, (6) median cleft of the palate, and (7) primary telecanthus. DeMyer (1967) concluded that the probability of mental retardation is slight when orbital hypertelorism is combined with one or more of the six remaining features. The chance of mental normalcy diminishes when the hypertelorism is excessive and is the sole facial anomaly or when it is combined with an extracephalic anomaly.

For the same group of anomalies, Sedano and associates (1970) preferred the term frontonasal dysplasia. They consider frontonasal dysplasia and holoprosencephaly malformations to be at opposite ends of the median facial anomaly spectrum. Differences in embryopathogenesis and clinical features form the basis of their reasoning. Although the bifid nose is generally accepted as part of this clinical complex, unilateral and bilateral nasal clefts are included in the frontonasal dysplasia classification system. This is a debatable addition, since the nasal alar clefts are not true midline defects.

Although orbital hypertelorism is frequently associated with the median cleft face syndrome (frontonasal dysplasia), other non-midline malformations can cause an increase in interorbital distance. For a discussion of orbital hypertelorism see Chapter 60.

Tessier Classification. In 1973, Tessier presented a classification of craniofacial clefts. Detailed descriptions of the classification were subsequently published by Tessier (1976) and Kawamoto (1976).

The Tessier classification has several unique features of merit. It is based on the

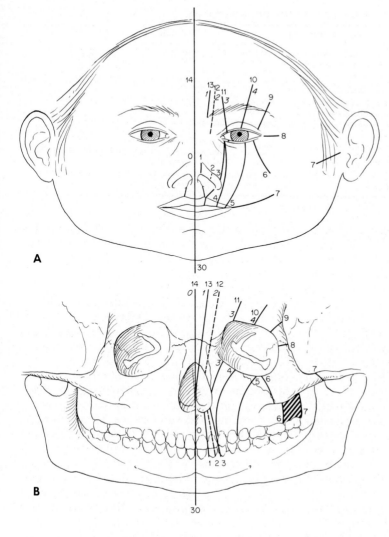

Figure 59–9. Tessier classification of facial clefts. A, Location of the clefts on the face. B, Skeletal pathways. (Courtesy of Dr. P. Tessier.)

extensive personal experience and observation of one investigator rather than on a collection of examples culled from a review of the literature or hospital records. Therefore, the terminology and quality of observations remain uniform. In addition, the classification successfully integrates the clinical examination findings with direct observations of the underlying skeletal deformity at the time of reconstructive surgery. From the standpoint of applicability to treatment, the correlation of the clinical appearance with the surgical anatomic findings increases the value of the classification for the practicing plastic surgeon.

Cleft Numbering System. The clefts are numbered from 0 to 14 and follow constant lines, or axes, through the eyebrows or eyelid,

the maxilla, the nose, and the lip (Figs. 59–9 to 59–11).

The orbit is regarded as the reference landmark, since it is common to both the cranium and the face. Clefts that are located cephalad to the palpebral fissure are directed "northbound" and considered to be mainly "cranial" in nature. The "southbound" clefts pass caudally from the palpebral fissure to become "facial." "Craniofacial" clefts are formed by the combination of northbound and southbound clefts. The craniofacial clefts usually follow the same well-defined "time zones." Thus, the following combinations can be clinically observed: 0 and 14, 1 and 13, 2 and 12, 3 and 11, and 4 and 10. Although the craniofacial clefts tend to coincide with these time zones across the orbit, the vascular supply

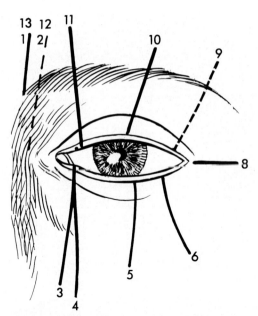

Figure 59–10. Location of the clefts in relation to the eyelids and eyebrow. (Courtesy of Dr. P. Tessier.)

expression of the cleft or be disfigured by a full representation of the defect. The extent of the soft tissue and skeletal components is also variable, and they are seldom affected to an equal degree. Furthermore, although closely related, the soft tissue component of the cleft does not always coincide with the skeletal fault. Therefore, descriptions of the clefts that are based on the bony malformation are more reliable, since the skeletal landmarks tend to be more constant.

Facial clefts located lateral to the infraorbital foramen, as a general rule, have proportionally greater bony disruption than clefts found between the foramen and the midline. Of course, digressions from this general pattern exist, the No. 3 cleft being a good example.

Unilateral or bilateral forms of the clefts are found in varying combinations. The introduction of three-dimensional computed tomography has greatly facilitated diagnosis (David, Moore, and Cooter, 1989).

DESCRIPTION OF CLEFTS

The external features of each of the clefts are readily apparent. It is also important to

and embryonic processes do not necessarily follow the same north-south pathways. Consequently, the embryopathogenesis of some of the rare craniofacial clefts is not easily explained.

It is important to keep the time zone concept in mind during the examination of the patient. The time zone principle disciplines the clinician to search for malformations along the entire axis. Unsuspected and often overlooked soft and bony tissue anomalies will be discovered when an examination is conducted in this methodical manner. For example, the common cleft lip is part of clefts No. 1, 2, and 3. When this relatively common birth defect is encountered, the clinician should be alerted to examine the more cephalic structures with care. Whitaker, Katowitz, and Randall (1974) reported a much higher association of malformations of the nasolacrimal system with common cleft lips than is generally appreciated. Thus, on close inspection one might find a slight caudal orientation of the medial canthus and an absence of an inferior punctum with excessive tearing, features that would represent a "forme fruste" expression of an oronaso-ocular cleft.

Severity of Cleft. The clinical expression of the craniofacial cleft is highly variable. The face can be marred by a faint (microform)

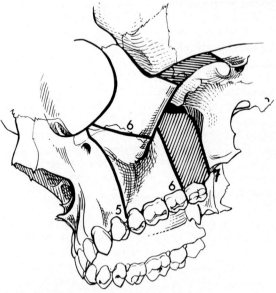

Figure 59–11. Lateral view of the facial clefts on the zygomaticomaxillary skeletal complex. Malformations associated with the No. 6 and 7 facial clefts on the posterior maxilla are located in the shaded zone. An actual cleft of the posterior maxillary alveolus is occasionally observed with a No. 7 facial cleft. With a No. 6 cleft, a cleft per se is not seen, but an area of alveolar hypoplasia can exist. (Courtesy of Dr. P. Tessier.)

consider the variations that exist in the extent of the cleft and the involvement of the embryologically related structures. These factors influence the strategy of treatment and thus should be recognized and appreciated early. The strength of the Tessier classification is that it takes these variables into consideration, emphasizes the underlying skeletal deformity, relates the cleft to the neighboring deformities, and is treatment oriented. Because of the practical nature of this classification, the rare craniofacial clefts will be described using this system.

No. 0 Cleft. The No. 0 cleft is in the midline of the cranium and face (see Fig. 59–9). It includes most of the midline deformities described in the other classification systems: Group A 1 axial cleft (Karfik, 1966), internasal dysplasia (van der Meulen and associates, 1983), median cleft face syndrome (DeMyer, 1967), frontonasal dysplasia (Sedano and associates, 1970), and holoprosencephaly (DeMyer, Zeman, and Palmer, 1964).

The upper lip defect consists of a true or false median cleft lip. In the true median cleft lip defect, similar to the "harelip" seen in rodents, the split occurs between the median globular processes, as opposed to a false median cleft in which there is an agenesis of the globular processes.

The true median cleft lip was first described by Bechard in 1823 according to Galanti (1961). Keith (1909) reported a similar deformity found in a specimen located in the Museum of the Royal College of Surgeons in London. Over 100 examples have subsequently been reported, including those by Davis (1935), Weaver and Ballinger (1946), Braithwaite and Watson (1949), Kazanjian and Holmes (1959), Burian (1960), Fogh-Andersen (1965), Baibak and Bromberg (1966), DeMyer (1967), Scrimshaw (1967), Millard and Williams (1968), and Warkany, Bofinger, and Benton (1973).

Minor degrees of notching of the vermilion border of the lip can be connected to a vertical congenital band extending to the columella, drawing the central portion of the lip cephalad (Fig. 59–12). The cleft often involves the entire vertical dimension of the lip. The labial frenulum is frequently duplicated, and a wide diastema between the central incisors is almost invariably present. The cleft can continue posteriorly in the midline of the premaxilla and less frequently through the secondary palate. When the cleft involves the

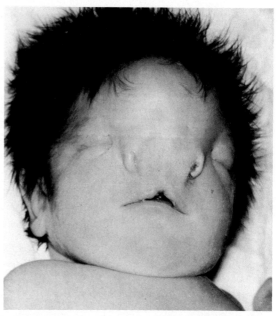

Figure 59–12. No. 0 cleft. A true median cleft of the upper lip associated with a bifid nose, hypertelorism, and a No. 14 cleft.

skeletal framework, a duplication of the anterior nasal spine and angulation of the teeth toward the midline are seen.

The nose is often bifid. Grooving and increased width of the columella are common. The nostrils are intact but can be asymmetrically deformed. The alar and upper lateral nasal cartilages are displaced laterally and are distorted or hypoplastic. The bifid nose is associated with a wide median furrow (see Fig. 59–55). In severe cases, Krikun (1972) described a thick subcutaneous fibromuscular band between the hypoplastic alar cartilages and the frontal bone. The band pulls the columella upward. Early excision of the strip is suggested to allow a more normal development of the nasal tip region.

The skeleton of the nasal bridge is broad and flattened (Fig. 59–13). Studies of the osseous structures by Brejcha and Fára (1971) and Krikun (1972) showed the nasal bones to be large and thick. The nasal septum is thickened, duplicated, or even absent. The frontal processes of the maxilla tend to be well developed. The ethmoid cells are increased in number and enlarged (Converse and associates, 1970); however, the posterior ethmoid cells and the sphenoid sinus are usually not. The cribriform plate is low and is only exceptionally widened. The breadth of the crista

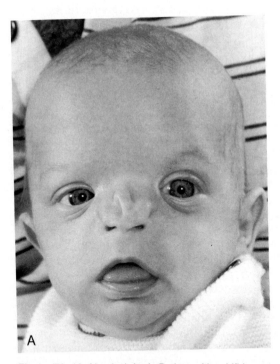
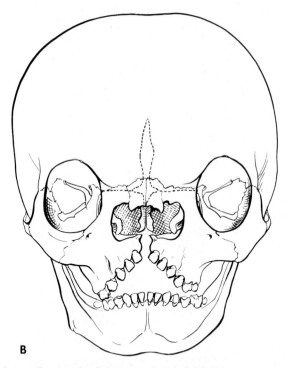

Figure 59–13. No. 0 cleft. *A,* Patient with a bifid nose and a median nasal subcutaneous band. Orbital hypertelorism and midline peak of the frontal hairline are part of the cephalic continuation of the cleft (No. 14 cleft). *B,* Osseous malformation with a cleft between the central incisors, broadening of the nasal framework, and orbital hypertelorism. (*B* courtesy of Dr. P. Tessier.)

galli is exaggerated. The distance between the optic canals is usually within the normal range. Orbital hypertelorism is seen as the cleft encroaches into the interorbital space. The cleft continues into the cranium as the No. 14 cleft (see Fig. 59–9).

If agenesis or hypoplasia is the predominant theme, a false median cleft of the lip is seen. A partial or total absence of the philtrum and premaxilla can occur (Fig. 59–14). The term false median cleft was proposed for this deformity by Braithwaite and Watson (1949). The description of the first reported case is credited by Fogh-Andersen (1965) to Bartholin, who described the deformity 300 years ago. In a review by DeMyer, Zeman, and Palmer (1964), 75 cases were collected from the literature.

The wide central deficiency of the entire height of the upper lip extends into the floor of the nose. The nose fails to develop properly and the columella is absent or rudimentary. The nasal septum is vestigial and unattached to the palate at any point. A cleft of the secondary palate is often present. The nose is depressed and indented at the tip. At the other extreme, the nose may be totally absent or may be represented by a proboscis. The nasal bone and the septal cartilages were noted to be absent in six patients reported by Brucker, Hoyt, and Trusler (1963). The median bony defect extends into the ethmoids to produce orbital hypotelorism (Fig. 59–15) or cyclopia. The cleft is often associated with eye deformities, congenital absence of the skin of the vertex of the scalp, and congenital forebrain deformities, especially in the region of the olfactory bulbs. The associated brain malformation generally limits the life span to infancy. Most of the patients die within the first three months and rarely live to the end of a year. As the severity of deformity decreases, the chance of normalcy improves (Yakovlev, 1956). Those patients with the mildest involvement have the potential to be intellectually near normal (Fig. 59–16) (DeMyer and Zeman, 1963; Converse, McCarthy, and Wood-Smith, 1975).

Median clefts of the lower lip and mandible coincide with the caudal extension of the No. 0 cleft. Although these clefts fall on the No. 0 cleft meridian, Tessier labeled them No. 30

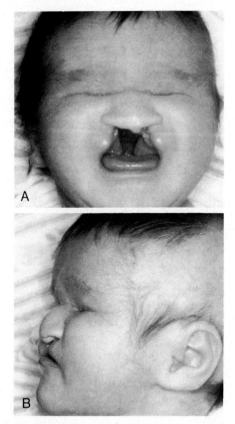

Figure 59–14. No. 0 cleft with agenesis. *A,* Infant with a false median cleft of the upper lip with absence of the philtrum and the premaxilla. The columella is rudimentary, and the nasal septum is vestigial. *B,* Profile view showing the lack of projection of the nose.

clefts. This group would include the mandibular process clefts (AACPR classification), branchiogenic medial axial B 2 clefts (Karfik, 1966), midline branchiogenic syndrome (Cosman and Crikelair, 1969), and intermandibular dysplasia (van der Muelen and associates, 1983).

Couronné (1819) first described the median cleft of the lower jaw. Subsequently approximately 50 cases were reported (Monroe, 1966; Cosman and Crikelair, 1969; Fujino, Yasuko, and Takeshi, 1970).

The cleft of the lower lip can be limited to the soft tissue. In its most minor form, a notch in the lower lip is present. More frequently, however, the cleft extends into the bony mandibular symphysis (Fig. 59–17). As the severity of the malformation increases, the neck structures, the hyoid bone, and even the sternum are progressively involved. The anterior portion of the tongue is often bifid

and is bound to the divided mandible by a dense band of fibrous tissue. The medial margins of the bifid tongue are attached along the length of the cleft of the alveolar ridge (Stewart, 1935). Millard and associates (1971) reported 32 cases associated with ankyloglossia and 10 cases with clefts of the tongue. Total absence of the tongue has also been associated with the mandibular midline clefts (Rosenthal, 1932; Herren, 1964). The cleft of the alveolus is located in the midline and passes between the central incisors.

Although the major deformity is due to the failure of a midline union of the first branchial arch, associated deformities of the neck caused by failure of fusion of the lower branchial arches are not uncommon. The hyoid bone is often absent. Failure of proper development of the thyroid cartilage can also occur. The anterior strap muscles of the neck are atrophic and are replaced by a dense contracted fibrous cord holding the chin in flexion. In addition, bulging at the neck and sternal regions during straining is seen when the structures of the anterior neck are thin and hypoplastic and fail to support the trachea and lungs. In these severe forms, the clavicles are widely spaced, and the manubrium sterni is absent.

By tentatively labeling the mandibular midline deformities as No. 30 clefts, Tessier deliberately kept the classification open. This feature allows for the addition of related deformities of the branchial arches. For example, a patient described by Abramson (1952) had a bilateral paramedian cleft of the

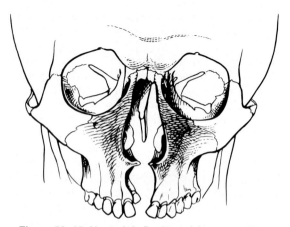

Figure 59–15. No. 0 cleft. Portions of the premaxilla and nasal septum are absent. The supporting structures of the nose are hypoplastic, and the orbits are in a hypoteloric position. (Courtesy of Dr. P. Tessier.)

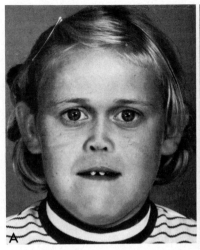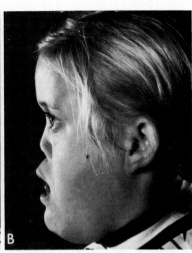

Figure 59–16. No. 0 cleft. Patient with a midline cleft and with the mildest deficiencies of structures. Hypoplasia of the nasomaxillary complex and orbital hypotelorism are present. (From Converse, J. M., McCarthy, J. G., and Wood-Smith, D.: Orbital hypotelorism: pathogenesis, associated faciocerebral anomalies and surgical correction. Plast. Reconstr. Surg., *56*:389, 1975. Copyright © 1975, The Williams & Wilkins Company, Baltimore.)

mandible. A tooth bud was found in the intervening segment of tissue. This is an extremely rare malformation, which, probably in the strictest sense, should not be considered a midline cleft. In 1973, Gardner, Kapun, and Jordan reported a similar case that was confined to one side of the midline. Equally rare deformities such as duplication of the mandible (Fig. 59–18) could be added to this group of clefts.

The mandibular cleft can be associated with deformities of other facial structures. Six mandibular clefts with related deformities of the upper face have been reported. Weyer (1963) and Monroe (1966) described two patients who had clefts of the soft palate.

A stillborn infant reported by Ashley and Richardson (1943) also had a cleft of the upper lip and secondary palate. The case published by Gardner, Kapun, and Jordan (1973) involved a bilateral cleft of the maxillary alveolus. The remaining patients demonstrated a median cleft of the upper lip (Schalbe, 1913), craniofacial microsomia (Braithwaite and Watson, 1949), or a dermoid of the nose (Wolfler, 1890).

Duplication of the midline facial structures is indeed rare. Potter (1975) listed this malformation under the broad category of conjoint twins as a monocephalic partial duplication and illustrated a case. Goulian and Conway (1964) reported a similar facial du-

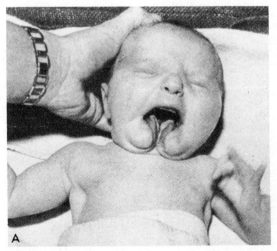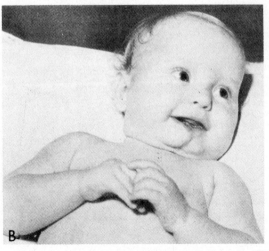

Figure 59–17. No. 30 cleft. Median cleft of the lower lip and mandible. *A,* Preoperative photograph. *B,* Postoperative photograph 9½ months after closure of the defect. (From Stewart, W. J.: Congenital median cleft of the chin. Arch. Surg., *31*:813, 1935.)

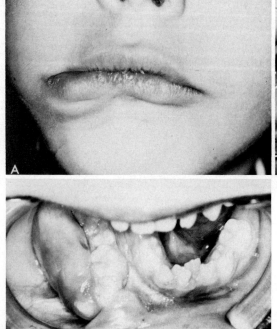

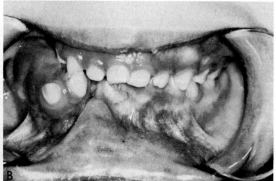

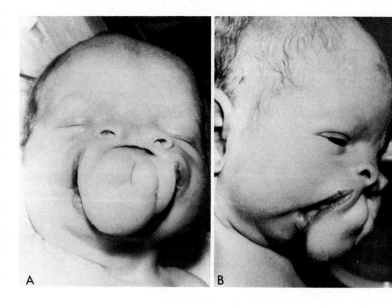

Figure 59–18. Duplication of the mandible. *A,* Patient with duplication of the lower lip. *B,* Intraoral view showing the left maxillary teeth in occlusion with the duplicated portion of the mandible. *C,* Intraoral view of the mandible showing the duplication of the right side of the mandible.

Figure 59–19. Duplication of the midface. *A,* Frontal view. Bulky fleshy mass occupies the macrostomia. Midline opening beneath the broad columella leads to a blind pouch. *B,* Profile view. (Courtesy of Dr. Calaycay and associates.)

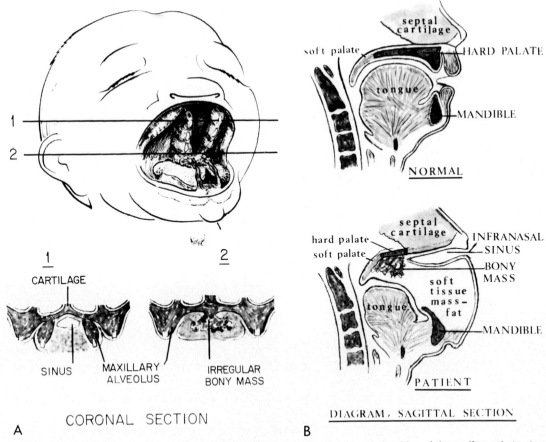

Figure 59–20. Duplication of the midface. *A*, Coronal section showing the relationships of the malformed structures. *B*, Sagittal section comparing the normal anatomy with that found in the patient. (Courtesy of Dr. Calaycay and associates.)

plication in a female infant. The infant also had hydrocephalus and died during the eighth week of life. An autopsy showed hydrocephalus of an advanced degree and severe cerebral atrophy. Duplication of the cranial vault, the brain, or the extrafacial structures was not seen.

The most detailed description of facial duplication is that of Calaycay and associates (1976). Their female patient was the product of a full-term pregnancy and her malformations were limited to the craniofacial region. The most striking was a bulky, protruding mass composed of skin and subcutaneous fat occupying the macrostomia (Fig. 59–19). The hyperteloric eyes were separated by an intervening broad, flat nose. The columella was 3 cm wide. What appeared to be eyelashes were found along the inferior border of a midline infranasal sinus. The sinus terminated in a blind pouch (Fig. 59–20) and was lined with respiratory epithelium.

Bilateral bony struts that traversed the oral soft tissue mass held the jaws apart (Figs. 59–21, 59–22). The duplicated mandible had a W-shaped configuration, as did the maxillary arch. The central limbs of the maxillary alveolar arch each contained three teeth that resembled incisors and canines (Fig. 59–23). An irregular bony mass, which probably represented a rudimentary hard palate or vomer, was observed in the region of the soft palate. The soft palate terminated with four uvulas of variable sizes. The anterior half of the tongue was bifid.

Pneumoencephalography showed an elevated and widened third ventricle, a wide displacement of the lateral ventricles, and agenesis of the corpus callosum (Stiehm, 1972). The fourth ventricle extended from the foramen magnum to the level of the third cervical vertebra, a finding suggesting the presence of Chiari II malformation of the hindbrain.

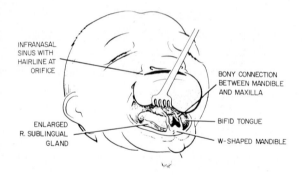

INFRANASAL
SINUS WITH
HAIRLINE AT
ORIFICE

BONY CONNECTION
BETWEEN MANDIBLE
AND MAXILLA

ENLARGED
R. SUBLINGUAL
GLAND

BIFID TONGUE

W-SHAPED MANDIBLE

Figure 59–21. Duplication of the midface. Findings noted at the time of the first operation. (Courtesy of Dr. Calaycay and associates.)

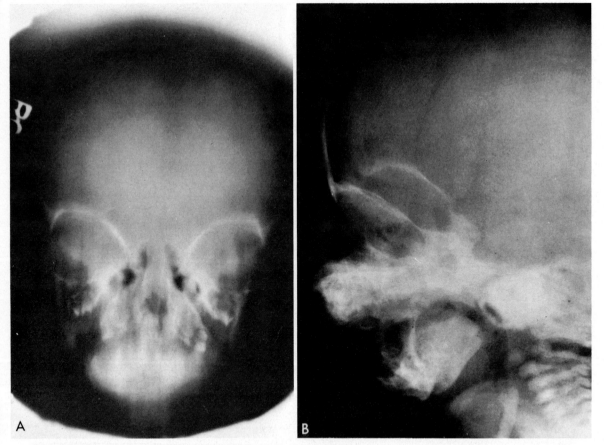

A

B

Figure 59–22. Roentgenograms of the patient with duplication of the midface. *A,* Anteroposterior projection showing the duplicated portions of the maxilla. *B,* Lateral view showing the intermaxillary bony struts. (Courtesy of Dr. Calaycay and associates.)

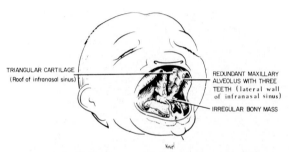

Figure 59–23. Duplication of the midface. Findings noted during the second operation. (Courtesy of Dr. Calaycay and associates.)

No. 1 Cleft. Before Tessier's observation, the No. 1 cleft had not been recognized as a distinct entity. It had been included with median clefts in other classification systems. In the van der Muelen and associates (1983) classification it is known as a Type 3 naso-schizis nasal dysplasia.

The No. 1 cleft begins in the Cupid's bow region, similarly to a common cleft of the upper lip, and passes through the dome of the nostril (see Fig. 59–9). The notching in the dome of the nostril is a distinct feature of the cleft. It occupies a parasagittal position on the nose as it continues northbound into the cranium as a No. 13 cleft (Fig. 59–24). Orbital hypertelorism is often associated.

The skeletal component of this cleft is also unique (Fig. 59–25). The cleft passes between the nasal cavity by traversing the piriform aperture just lateral to the anterior nasal spine. The septum is spared. The cleft is directed through the nasal bone, which in severe cases is absent. An alternate route of the cleft is through the junction of the nasal bone and the frontal process of the maxilla (Fig. 59–26). The cleft does not cross through the frontal process of the maxilla per se, but the process is secondarily displaced and flattened. Contributing to the development of orbital hypertelorism is the involvement of the ethmoid labyrinth.

No. 2 Cleft. This cleft is notably rare. Initially, Tessier (1975) questioned whether this cleft existed as a distinct entity or as a transitional form between clefts No. 1 and 3. The cleft was therefore represented by a dot-

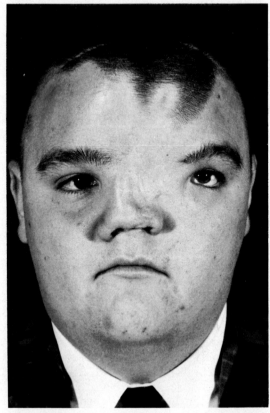

Figure 59–24. No. 1 cleft. The notch of the dome region of the nostril is a distinct feature of this cleft. The cleft is continued onto the cranium as a No. 13 cleft, as shown by the orbital hypertelorism and the paramedian disturbance of the frontal hairline. (Courtesy of Dr. J. M. Converse.)

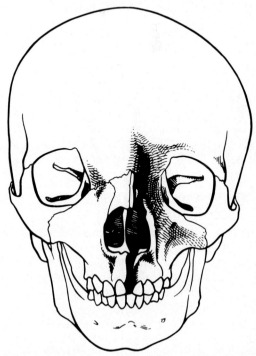

Figure 59–25. No. 1 cleft. Osseous features of the unilateral cleft. Note the paramedian location of the malformation and the compensatory lateral displacement of the orbit of the noncleft side. (Courtesy of Dr. P. Tessier.)

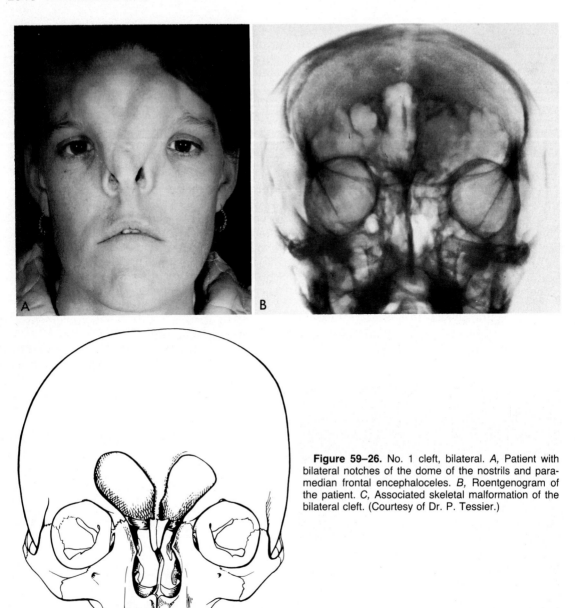

Figure 59–26. No. 1 cleft, bilateral. *A,* Patient with bilateral notches of the dome of the nostrils and paramedian frontal encephaloceles. *B,* Roentgenogram of the patient. *C,* Associated skeletal malformation of the bilateral cleft. (Courtesy of Dr. P. Tessier.)

ted line in Tessier's original drawings (see Fig. 59–9). Nevertheless, the cleft does have unique soft and hard tissue characteristics. Similarly to the No. 1 cleft, this cleft had not been previously described as a separate entity.

When present, the associated cleft of the lip lies in the area of the common cleft of the lip. The location of the deformity on the middle third of the nostril rim is a distinguishing feature of the cleft. The defective area is hypoplastic rather than a true notch,

which contrasts it with the notched dome of the No. 1 cleft and the undermining of the alar region of the No. 3 cleft (Fig. 59–27). On the affected side, the lateral part of the nose is flattened and the nasal bridge is broad (Fig. 59–28). The palpebral fissure is not involved as it is in the No. 3 cleft. Orbital hypertelorism, however, is seen. The medial border of the eyebrow is distorted as the cleft continues into the frontal region as the No. 12 cleft. The location of the eyebrow disturbance also serves to distinguish the cleft.

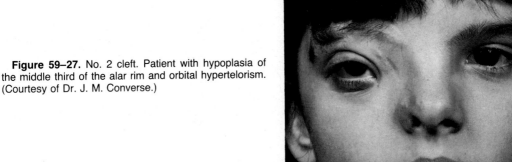

Figure 59–27. No. 2 cleft. Patient with hypoplasia of the middle third of the alar rim and orbital hypertelorism. (Courtesy of Dr. J. M. Converse.)

No. 3 Cleft. Unlike clefts No. 1 and 2, the No. 3 cleft is a well-known entity. Beginning with this cleft in the Tessier classification, the orbit becomes directly involved.

Confusion is created by the various names that have been applied to this malformation. Many authors have given their own interpretation of the deformity and have used the same terminology for similar but distinctly different malformations. The Nomenclature Committee of the AACPR defined the cleft as a naso-ocular cleft, which is "a fissure ex-tending from the nasal region toward the medial angle of the palpebral fissure" (Harkins and associates, 1962). This cleft has also been categorized as a Group A 2 para-axial cleft (Karfik, 1966), a nasomaxillary cleft (Gunter, 1963), an oblique facial cleft (Sakurai, Mitchell, and Holmes, 1966), nasomaxillary dysplasia (van der Muelen and associates, 1983), and more commonly an oronaso-ocular cleft. Tessier (1969a) also used the term oblique facial clefts before proposing his present classification system. The label oblique cleft is particularly ambiguous, since it has been applied to several types of clefts. The designation No. 3 cleft would eliminate the discord in nomenclature.

The first case reported in the literature was by Morian (1887). Subsequently, additional cases were reported by Davis (1935), Gunter (1963), Ergin (1966), Sakurai, Mitchell, and Holmes (1966), Tessier (1969a), Boo-Chai (1970), Dey (1973), and many others.

The cleft lies in the region of the union of median nasal, lateral nasal, and maxillary processes. Various explanations of the deformity include the lack of fusion of the various processes, insufficient mesodermal penetration, and failure of the naso-optic groove to invaginate and form the tubular nasolacrimal system (Mann, 1964). The unilateral, bilateral, complete, and incomplete forms can co-exist.

The cleft of the lip is located in the same regions as the common cleft of the lip (see Fig. 59–9). Thus, this characteristic is shared by clefts No. 1, 2, and 3. In the nasal area, however, the No. 3 cleft changes its course and undermines the base of the nasal ala. A coloboma of the nasal ala represents a mild

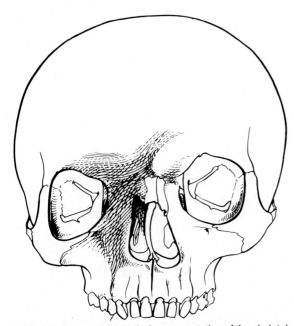

Figure 59–28. No. 2 cleft. A representation of the skeletal malformation of the cleft. The cleft is centered in the region of the junction between the nasal bone and the frontal process of the maxilla. (Courtesy of Dr. P. Tessier.)

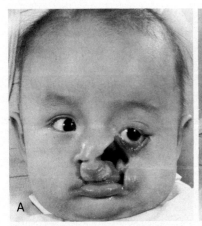
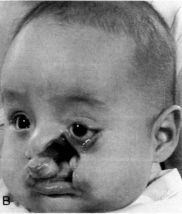

Figure 59–29. *A, B,* No. 3 cleft, unilateral. Patient with a complete form of the cleft. The distance between the nasal ala and the medial canthus is decreased. The medial canthus is displaced inferiorly, and the nasolacrimal system is interrupted.

expression of the malformation. The vertical distance between the alar base and the medial canthus is decreased. The underlying nasolacrimal system is disrupted, leading to a nasolacrimal duct that is blocked and a sac that is prone to repeated infections (Gunter, 1963). The lower canaliculus is malformed and is beyond repair (Tessier, 1969a).

The malformations of the ocular region are usually characteristic. The medial canthus is displaced inferiorly (Fig. 59–29). The colobomas of the lower eyelid are found medial to the punctum. The medial canthal tendon is hypoplastic, and its insertion is inferiorly displaced. Involvement of the eye itself is variable. The problem of restoring facial symmetry is compounded when microphthalmos is present. Damage to a fairly normal eye can occur when it is left unprotected by the associated eyelid defect. The northbound prolongation of the cleft encroaches onto the medial third of the upper eyelid and eyebrows and the forehead as the No. 11 cleft.

The osseous component of the cleft passes through the alveolus between the lateral incisor and the canine (Fig. 59–30). The lateral border of the piriform aperture is involved, and an absence of septation between the nasal cavity and maxillary sinus can occur. In contrast to the No. 2 cleft, the frontal process of the maxilla is disrupted as the No. 3 cleft terminates in the lacrimal groove. Complete absence of the frontal process of the maxilla is often seen. Thus, in the severest form of the cleft, the orbit, the nose, the maxillary sinus, and the mouth are confluent. The facial features are considerably distorted (Fig. 59–31), and the skeletal disruption is extensive (Fig. 59–32) when the cleft is bilateral.

The incidence of the No. 3 cleft is certainly greater than that reported in the literature. This is especially true if the incomplete form, such as a coloboma of the nasal alar base, is also included. It is important for the clinician to recognize the full extent of the mild forms. Search should be made for malformations of the nasolacrimal system and defects of the underlying skeleton.

From analysis of the cases that are described in sufficient detail, the following can be concluded: Nearly equal frequency distribution of the cleft between the sexes is observed. The incidence by side of involvement is also approximately equal, with a third occurring on the right, a third on the left,

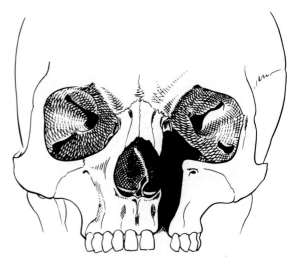

Figure 59–30. No. 3 cleft, unilateral. The cleft passes through the region of the lateral incisor to the lacrimal groove. Septation between the nasal cavity and the maxillary sinus is absent. (Courtesy of Dr. P. Tessier.)

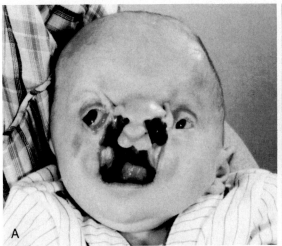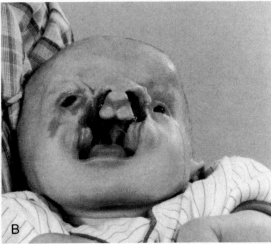

Figure 59–31. *A, B,* No. 3 cleft, bilateral. Patient with full expression of the cleft. The bilateral cleft of the lip and palate is complete. The nasal alae are displaced cephalad above the level of the distorted medial canthi, and a wide coloboma is present in the medial third of the right lower eyelid.

and a third bilaterally. When bilateral involvement is present, a No. 4 or 5 cleft is often seen on the contralateral side.

No. 4 Cleft. Starting with the No. 4 cleft, a departure of the deformity from the median facial structures is noted. The cleft moves onto the cheek and is sometimes called meloschisis (see Fig. 59–9).

The cleft has been classified as an oroocular (AACPR) or oro-ocular type I (Boo-Chai, 1970) cleft, a Group A 2 para-axial cleft (Karfik, 1966), a vertical facial cleft by Tessier in earlier publications (1969a, b), and medial maxillary dysplasia (van der Muelen and associates, 1983). The ubiquitous term oblique facial cleft has also been used for this malformation. As stated above, this term has been loosely applied to several clefts that would correspond to clefts No. 3, 4, and 5 of the Tessier classification.

Boo-Chai (1970) in his comprehensive review article credited the first recorded case to von Kulmus, who described the defect in Latin in 1732. Dick (1837) reported the first case in the English literature. Most of the cases described by Morian (1887) involved stillborn infants. Boo-Chai (1970) found 23 cases in the literature involving infants who survived. Subsequently, other cases were reported by Tessier (1969a), Van der Linden and Borghouts (1970), Dey (1973), Kubaček and Penkava (1974), and Resnick and Kawamoto (in press).

The location of the cleft of the lip differs from that of clefts previously described, and it is found lateral to the Cupid's bow and philtrum (see Fig. 59–9). The cleft rests midway between the philtral crest and the corner of the mouth. It passes lateral to the nasal ala and onto the cheek (meloschisis). The nasal ala is more or less normal. However, in unilateral cases it is often rotated cephalad toward the medial canthus of the involved side (Fig. 59–33). The cleft terminates in the lower eyelid, medial to the punctum. The cranial continuation of the cleft traverses the medial third of the upper eyelid and eyebrow as the No. 10 cleft.

The nasolacrimal canal and the lacrimal sac are usually intact, since the cleft courses lateral to these structures. However, the lower canaliculus lies in the path of the cleft.

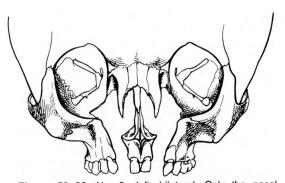

Figure 59–32. No. 3 cleft, bilateral. Only the nasal septum separates the cavities of the midface. On each side, the orbit, the maxillary sinus, the nasal cavity, and the oral cavity are confluent. (Courtesy of Dr. P. Tessier.)

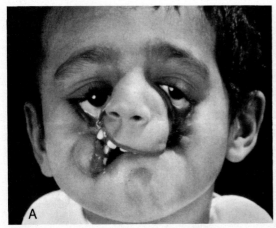

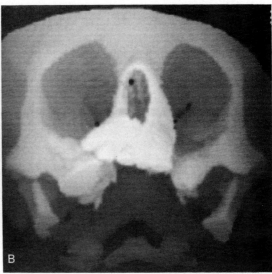

Figure 59–33. No. 4 cleft right and No. 5 cleft left. *A,* The right No. 4 cleft begins lateral to Cupid's bow and passes through the medial third of the lower eyelid; the left No. 5 cleft starts just inside the commissure and ends in the middle third of the eyelid. *B,* Three-dimensional computed tomographic view shows the osseous midfacial disruption with the clefts involving the respective thirds of the orbit. (From David, D. J., Moore, M. H., and Cooter, R. D.: Tessier clefts revisited with a third dimension. Cleft Palate J., *26:*163, 1989.)

The medial canthal tendon is almost normal in respect to its insertion and its direction (Tessier, 1969a). The eye is usually present and functional, but anophthalmos and intermediary forms of development can also occur (Rogalski, 1944).

On the skeleton the cleft is located between the lateral incisor and the canine (Fig. 59–34), similarly to the defect of the No. 3 cleft. The piriform aperture, however, remains intact. The cleft courses lateral to the piriform aperture onto the anterior surface of the maxilla. It continues medial to the infraorbital foramen to terminate in the medial portion of the inferior orbital rim and floor. The contents of the orbit prolapse into the fissure. In depth, the fissure can extend posteriorly as a cleft of the secondary palate. The septation between the maxillary sinus and the nasal cavity remains intact. Often associated with the deformity is a posterior nasal choanal atresia. In the complete form of the cleft, the orbital cavity, the maxillary sinus, and the oral cavity are confluent. In bilateral cases, the premaxilla is in a protrusive position, and the nose appears smaller than normal (Figs. 59–35, 59–36).

An estimate of the distribution of the cleft can be obtained by analyzing the reports cited above. Unfortunately, a complete description of the cases is not recorded in several of these publications. Unilateral cases totaled 33, of which 20 were located on the right side and 13 on the left side (2:1.3 right-to-left ratio). In the unilateral cases, there is a male preponderance with a male-to-female ratio of

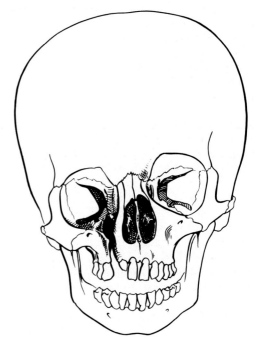

Figure 59–34. No. 4 cleft, unilateral. The cleft passes between the infraorbital foramen and the piriform aperture. The orbit, the maxillary sinus, and the oral cavity are united by the cleft. (Courtesy of Dr. P. Tessier.)

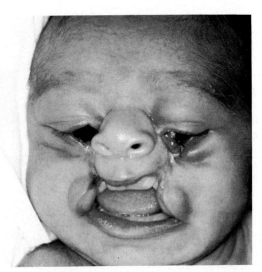

Figure 59–35. No. 4 cleft, bilateral. Note that the cleft of the lip is lateral to the Cupid's bow. The nose is foreshorted with a decreased distance between the alae and the medial canthi. Complete colobomas are present on the lower eyelids, and notches are seen on the upper eyelids; all are located in the medial thirds of the eyelids.

approximately 2.5:1. Nine bilateral cases have been reported. In contrast to the unilateral form, the bilateral cases occurred with equal frequency in both sexes. It should be noted that six of the nine patients had clefts of a different type on the contralateral side. Four patients had a transverse cleft (No. 7 cleft) on the opposite side, three had a closely related No. 5 cleft, and two had a No. 3 cleft on the opposite side.

No. 5 Cleft. Situated more laterally on the face is the No. 5 cleft (see Fig. 59–9). The general term oblique facial cleft has again been used to designate this malformation. Karfik (1966) preferred the term true oblique facial cleft and included it in his Group E, atypical facial disorders. In the AACPR classification, the cleft is included in the oro-ocular group and is called a lateral maxillary dysplasia by van der Muelen and associates (1983). In Boo-Chai's (1970) subdivision of the oro-ocular cleft group, the cleft is called Type II.

Of the oblique facial clefts, the No. 5 cleft is the rarest. Few have been reported in the world literature (Greer, 1961; Pitanguy, 1968; Boo-Chai, 1970; Stewart and associates, 1976). A quarter of the cases were unilateral, another quarter were bilateral, and the remaining half were combined with another rare craniofacial cleft on the contralateral side.

The cleft of the lip is positioned just medial to the corner of the mouth (Figs. 59–35 and 59–37). It courses cephalad across the lateral portion of the cheek (meloschisis) into the area of the medial and lateral thirds of the lower eyelid. The vertical distance between the mouth and the lower eyelid is decreased, and the upper lip and lower eyelid are drawn toward each other. The eye can be microphthalmic.

The path of the skeletal malformation is also distinct. The alveolar portion of the cleft is found posterior to the canine in the premolar region (Fig. 59–38). As pointed out by

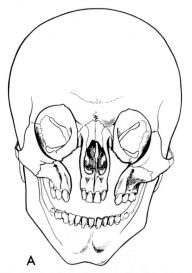

A

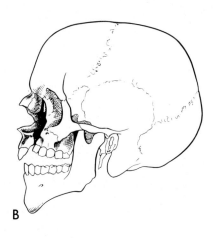

B

Figure 59–36. No. 4 cleft, bilateral. *A,* Frontal view of malformed facial skeleton. *B,* Lateral view showing the protrusion of the premaxilla and nose. (Courtesy of Dr. P. Tessier.)

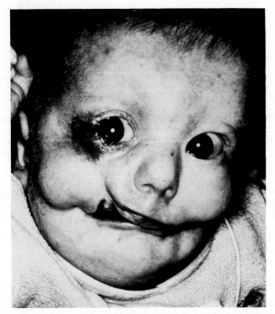

Figure 59–37. No. 5 cleft. Patient with a right No. 5 cleft and bilateral No. 7 clefts. The No. 5 cleft extends from just inside the commissure of the mouth to the middle and lateral thirds of the lower eyelid.

Morian (1887), the cleft passes lateral to the infraorbital foramen, thus distinguishing it from its predecessor, which is located medial to this landmark. The cleft enters the orbit through the middle third of the orbital rim and floor. The orbital contents can prolapse through the gap into the maxillary sinus.

No. 6 Cleft. The incomplete form of the Treacher Collins syndrome is represented by the No. 6 cleft (see Chap. 63). It is designated a maxillozygomatic dysplasia by van der Muelen and associates (1983). Rogers (1964a) believed that the cases originally described

by Treacher Collins were probably of the incomplete type.

The external features of the malformation are less pronounced and extensive when compared with those seen in the complete form (Fig. 59–39). Although the external ear can be near normal or normal, a hearing deficit is often present. The antimongoloid obliquity of the palpebral fissure is milder. The coloboma of the lower eyelid is found in the usual site between the medial and lateral thirds. The cleft is inferiorly directed lateral to the oral commissure and toward the angle of mandible.

It is mainly the osseous deformity that marks the cleft as a distinct entity (Fig. 59–40). In contrast to the situation in the complete form, the malar bone is present but hypoplastic. The continuity of the zygomatic arch remains intact. A bony notch that corresponds to the cleft can be detected by careful palpation of the inferolateral aspect of the orbital rim. The cleft is located in the region of the zygomaticomaxillary suture between the hypoplastic malar bone and the maxilla. An actual cleft of the alveolus is not seen, but a hypoplastic zone is frequently detected in the region of the molars (see Fig. 59–11). The antigonial angle of the mandible is accentuated.

No. 7 Cleft. The No. 7 cleft enjoys the distinction of being the least rare of the atypical craniofacial clefts. A variety of terms have been used to describe this cleft: necrotic facial dysplasia (Keith, 1940a), hemifacial microsomia and microtia (Braithwaite and Watson, 1949), otomandibular dysostosis (Franceschetti and Zwahlen, 1944), unilateral facial agenesis (Ruben, 1967), auricu-

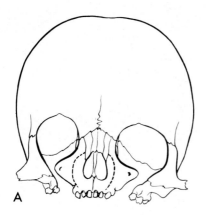

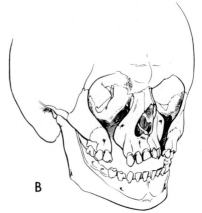

Figure 59–38. No. 5 cleft, bilateral. *A,* The cleft is found in the region of the premolars and traverses the maxilla lateral to the infraorbital foramen to enter the orbit. *B,* Three-quarter view of the facial skeleton. (Courtesy of Dr. P. Tessier.)

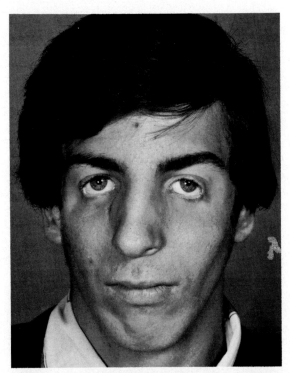

Figure 59–39. No. 6 cleft. Patient with an incomplete form of the Treacher Collins malformation. The antimongoloid obliquity of the palpebral fissures and the colobomas of the lower eyelid are present. The zygomatic eminences are reduced in prominence.

articles were written describing the malformation. Grabb (1965) summarized the findings of a personal series of 102 patients. Converse and associates (1973a) also reported a large personal series of 280 patients.

The statement of Gorlin and Pindborg (1964) that the male is more often affected than the female is confirmed by the statistical analysis of Grabb (1965). The side of involvement is not significant. Bilateral involvement was noted in 12 of 102 patients of Grabb (1965), 15 of 280 cases of Converse and associates (1973a), and eight of 74 cases of Meurman (1957) and was found in a 1:6 ratio in the series reported by Dupertuis and Musgrave (1959).

The birth incidence of the malformation is estimated to be between 1 in 3000 (Poswillo, 1974a) and 1 in 5642 births (Grabb, 1965). The vast majority of cases occur in a sporadic fashion. In the closely related Goldenhar syndrome, an autosomal dominant mode of transmission is reported (Summitt, 1969), but most investigators believe that the pattern is a sporadic one.

The clinical expression of the cleft is highly variable. The "forme fruste" can consist of a lobranchiogenic dysplasia (Caronni, 1971), intrauterine facial necrosis (Greer, 1961), hemignathia and microtia syndrome (Stark and Saunders, 1962), first and second branchial arch syndrome (Longacre, DeStefano, and Holmstrand, 1961), lateral facial clefts, and oromandibuloauricular syndrome. In other classification systems, the cleft has been grouped as an oroaural cleft (AACPR), a Group B 1 lateral otocephalic branchiogenic deformity (Karfik, 1966), and zygotemporal dysplasia (van der Muelen and associates, 1983). The Goldenhar syndrome is closely related and has the additional features of epibulbar dermoids and vertebral anomalies (Goldenhar, 1952; Gorlin and associates, 1963). The first and second branchial arch syndrome (craniofacial microsomia) and its variations are discussed in Chapter 62.

Ballantyne (1894) stated that the earliest recording of the malformation is the cuneiform inscriptions on the teratologic tables written by the Chaldeans of Mesopotamia about 2000 B.C. The first case described in a contemporary language was recorded by Reissmann (1869). Subsequently, countless

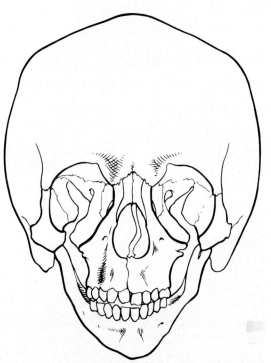

Figure 59–40. No. 6 cleft. The cleft on the facial skeleton is located in the region of the zygomaticomaxillary suture line. The zygoma is present but hypoplastic. (Courtesy of Dr. P. Tessier.)

slight facial asymmetry, minimal malformations of the external ear, and skeletal anomalies detected only on roentgenographic study. Hence, even a seemingly insignificant ear tag should alert the clinician to the need for a careful examination of the child. The oral component varies from a mere broadening of the oral commissure to a complete fissure extending toward the external ear. The cleft, however, rarely extends beyond the anterior border of the masseter. Further extension of the cleft can occur as a deep furrow extending horizontally across the cheek toward or around the superior aspect of the ear (Fig. 59–41). The normal position of the oral commissure can often be established by the characteristic shade of the mucosa lining the cleft, which is slightly lighter than that of the normal vermilion (Boo-Chai, 1969). The

slightly elevated mucocutaneous ridge of the vermilion border also terminates at the normal limit of the lip.

The underdevelopment or maldevelopment of the external ear, the middle ear, the mandible, the maxilla, the zygoma, and the temporal bones has been described by May (1962), Longacre, Stevens, and Holmstrand (1963), Grabb (1965), Powell and Jenkins (1968), and Converse and associates (1973a) (see Chap. 62). On the cleft side, the parotid gland or its duct can be absent. The fifth and seventh cranial nerves and the muscles they serve can also be involved. The ipsilateral soft palate and tongue are often hypoplastic. Parts of the mandibular ramus and condyle and the zygomatic arch can also be absent. When the temporal muscle is involved, corresponding changes of the coronoid process are seen. The

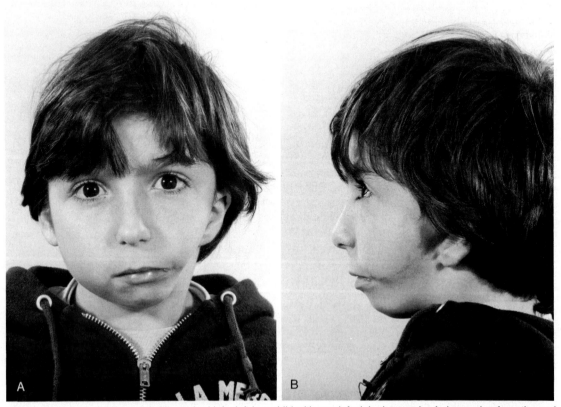

Figure 59–41. *A, B,* No. 7 cleft. Unrepaired left cleft in a child with craniofacial microsomia. A depression from the oral commissure to the ear marks the path of the cleft. The chin deviates toward the hypoplastic mandible. The auricular malformation is mild.

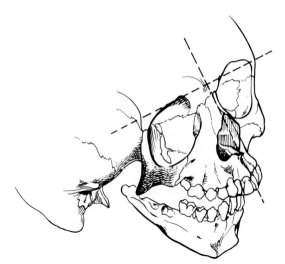

Figure 59–42. No. 7 cleft. A three-quarter view of the complete form of the skeletal malformation. The zygomatic arch and the proximal portion of the mandible are absent. The horizontal line shows the orbital dystopia on the affected side. (Courtesy of Dr. P. Tessier.)

occlusal plane is canted cephalad on the affected side, reflecting the hypoplastic maxilla and the reduced vertical dimension of the ramus. The skeletal malformation of the complete form of the No. 7 cleft is shown in Figure 59–42. Tessier believed that the cleft is centered in the region of the zygomaticotemporal suture (see Fig. 59–9). The zygomatic arch is disrupted and is represented only by small stumps. The descent of the

lateral canthus is caused by the hypoplasia of the zygoma that results in an inferior displacement of the superolateral angle of the orbit. In the severest forms, true orbital dystopia is present. Less frequently, the orbit on the ipsilateral side may actually be elevated.

In a report of 15 patients with bilateral craniofacial microsomia, Converse and associates (1974) described two patients with an unusual supplementary cleft of the maxilla (see Fig. 59–11). In the region of the tuberosity, a distinctly separate segment of bone with supernumerary teeth was found. Stewart and associates (1976) reported two additional patients with a vertical cleft of the posterior maxilla (Fig. 59–43).

No. 8 Cleft. The No. 8 cleft is seldom seen as an isolated malformation. A cleft lip is usually combined with another rare craniofacial cleft. The cleft corresponds to the temporal continuation of the orolateral canthus cleft (AACPR), the commissural clefts of the ophthalmo-orbital disorders (Karfik, 1966), and zygofrontal dysplasia (van der Muelen and associates, 1983).

The No. 8 cleft begins at the lateral commissure of the palpebral fissure and extends into the temporal region (see Fig. 59–9). The lateral commissural coloboma is often occupied by a dermatocele (Fig. 59–44). The osseous component of the cleft lies in the region of the frontozygomatic suture. In this location, a bony notch has also been observed by

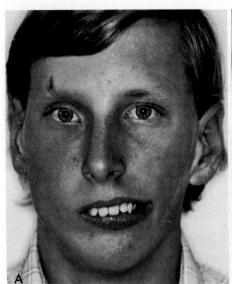
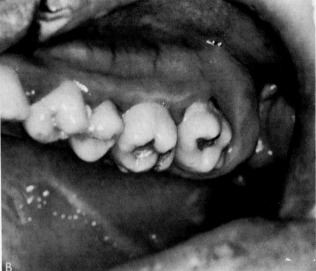

Figure 59–43. Alveolar cleft associated with a No. 7 cleft. *A,* Frontal view of a patient with a macrostomia and a No. 7 cleft on the left side. Note the canthus inversus and the disruption of the eyebrow on the contralateral side. *B,* Cleft of the left posterior maxillary alveolus; the third molar has yet to erupt.

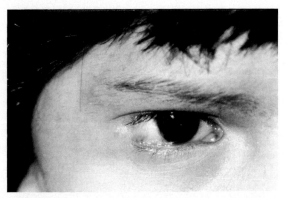

Figure 59–44. No. 8 cleft. The cleft is found in the lateral canthus of the eyelids. Occupying the cleft is a dermatocele. (Courtesy of Dr. B. Zide.)

Tessier (1975) in patients with the Goldenhar syndrome.

Combination of Clefts No. 6, 7, and 8. When rare bilateral craniofacial clefts occur, different combinations of the various clefts are often seen. The bilateral occurrence of a combination of clefts No. 6, 7, and 8 is, however, unique. Tessier (1975) believed that this pattern of clefts best explains the complete form of the Treacher Collins (Franceschetti) syndrome. The three clefts are found in the region of the maxillozygomatic, temporozygomatic, and frontozygomatic sutures (see Fig. 59–9). Tessier (1975) suggested that the sum effect of the three clefts is responsible for the absence of the zygoma. Van der Muelen and associates (1983) included this

malformation in their zygomatic dysplasia and zygotemporoauromandibular dysplasia groups.

On a pre-Colombian terra-cotta statue from the seventh century, the typical Treacher Collins facies can be seen (Poswillo, 1975). Poswillo cited Thomson (1847) as being the first to describe the clinical features of the syndrome. However, Berry (1889) is generally credited with the first description of the malformation. A few years later, Treacher Collins (1900a, b) reported two cases and noted the hypoplasia of the malar bones. Numerous case reports followed. Among the significant articles are those of Lockhard (1929), Franceschetti and Zwahlen (1944), Franceschetti and Klein (1949), and Rogers (1964b) (see Chap. 63).

The absent malar bone is the hallmark of the complete form of the Treacher Collins syndrome (Fig. 59–45). The No. 6 cleft is responsible for the coloboma of the lower eyelid (Fig. 59–46). The medial two-thirds of the eyelashes of the lower eyelid is deficient or absent. Tessier (1975) stated that approximately one-third of the patients do not have an infraorbital foramen. Thus, the infraorbital

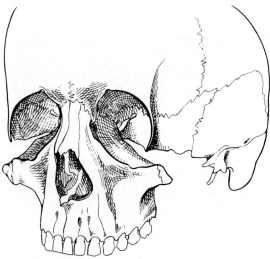

Figure 59–45. No. 6, 7, and 8 clefts, bilateral. The zygomatic bones are absent. The lateral orbital rim is formed by the greater wing of the sphenoid. The deformity has converted the infraorbital foramen into a notch.

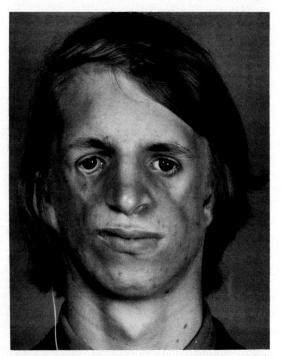

Figure 59–46. Patient with the complete form of the Treacher Collins malformation. The hypoplasia of the soft tissue is in keeping with the absence of the supporting zygoma. Note coloboma on the left lower eyelid.

neurovascular bundle passes from the orbit directly into the subcutaneous tissues. The No. 7 cleft explains the absence of the zygomatic arch, the fusion and hypoplasia of the masseter and temporalis muscles, the ear malformation, the anterior displacement of the sideburns, and the mandibular skeletal deficits. The No. 8 cleft completes the malformation by contributing to the absence of the lateral orbital rim. The lateral border of the deformed orbit is often formed solely by the greater wing of the sphenoid. The inferior displacement of the lateral canthus is responsible for the characteristic antimongoloid slant of the palpebral fissures, because the lateral canthal tendon is without a point of attachment. Additional details of the syndrome are discussed in Chapter 63.

No. 9 Cleft. Beginning with the No. 9 cleft, the superior hemisphere of the orbit is involved. The clefts become the northbound cranial extensions. The No. 9 cleft is found in the superolateral angle of the orbit and affects the underlying superior orbital rim and orbital roof (Fig. 59–47). The eyelid is divided in its lateral third, as is the eyebrow, as the cleft passes into the temporal hairline.

The cleft is extremely rare. The original drawing of this cleft used by Tessier is based on the descriptions of Morian (1887) and Sanvenero-Rosselli (1953). The term fronto-sphenoid dysplasia was used by van der Muelen and associates (1983) to denote this group.

No. 10 Cleft. The No. 10 cleft is centered in the middle third of the orbit and upper eyelid (see Fig. 59–9). The cleft corresponds to the cranial extension of the No. 4 cleft. In the van der Muelen and associates (1983) classification, this malformation falls into the frontal dysplasia group.

A coloboma is present in the middle third of the upper eyelid. A frequent finding is an attempted duplication of the medial third of the upper lid margin that is represented by a transverse split along the lid margin. The cleft continues through the middle third of the eyebrow on its way into the hairline. The osseous structures are cleaved into the midportion of the superior orbital rim, the adjacent orbital roof, and the frontal bones (Fig. 59–48). A fronto-orbital encephalocele often occupies the gap. A secondary lateral and inferior rotation of the orbit occurs. When the displacement is severe, orbital hypertelorism is produced.

No. 11 Cleft. As an isolated deformity, the

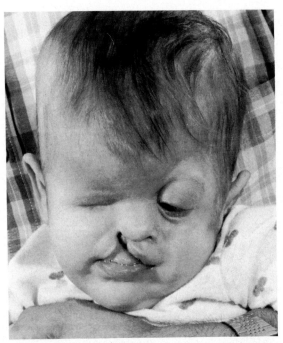

Figure 59–47. No. 9 cleft. The cleft passes through the lateral third of the superior orbital rim and orbital roof, which are absent in this infant. Incidental findings in this particular patient are the right-sided cleft lip and palate and microphthalmos.

No. 11 cleft has not been reported. It is usually found in combination with the southbound No. 3 cleft of the face (see Fig. 59–9). Van der Muelen and associates (1983) included this malformation in their frontal dysplasia group.

The cleft traverses the medial third of the frontal hairline. The cleft takes one of two paths in the region of the frontal process of the maxilla when it is combined with a No. 3 cleft. The first route passes lateral to the ethmoid bone (see Fig. 59–31) to create a cleft in the medial third of the eyebrow and orbital rim. The alternative course is through the ethmoid labyrinth. When this path is taken, orbital hypertelorism is seen.

No. 12 Cleft. The No. 12 cleft is the cranial equivalent of the No. 2 cleft of the face (see Fig. 59–9). Orbital hypertelorism is usually seen. The eyebrow is disrupted just lateral to the medial border (see Fig. 59–27).

On the skeleton, the cleft passes through the frontal process of the maxilla or between this structure and the nasal bone (Fig. 59–49A). The ethmoid labyrinth is involved and is increased in its transverse dimension to account for the associated hypertelorism (Fig.

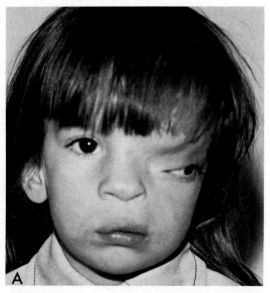 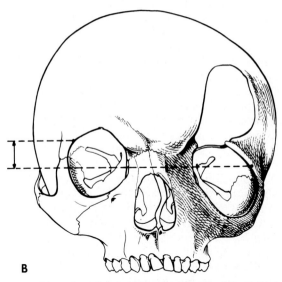

Figure 59–48. No. 10 cleft. *A,* Patient with a cleft that was caused by a frontal encephalocele. Note the inferolateral displacement of the orbit and the resulting orbital hypertelorism. *B,* The osseous malformation and the deformity produced by the frontal encephalocele. Dashed lines show the associated orbital dystopia of the affected side. (*B* courtesy of Dr. P. Tessier.)

59–49*B*). The cleft is located lateral to the olfactory groove. Hence the cribriform plate is of normal width.

No. 13 Cleft. Changes in the cribriform plate are seen beginning with the No. 13 cleft. This cleft corresponds to the cranial extension of the No. 1 cleft of the face (see Figs. 59–9, 59–25).

The hallmark of the No. 13 cleft is the widening of the olfactory groove (Fig. 59–50). The cribriform plate is therefore also increased in its transverse dimension. When a paramedian frontal encephalocele is associated with the malformation, the cribriform plate can also be displaced inferiorly.

Unilateral and bilateral forms exist, as for

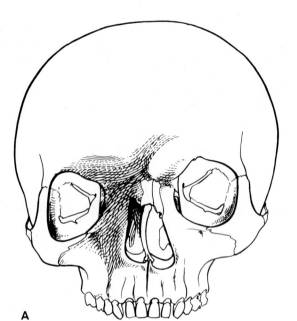 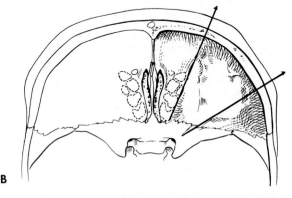

Figure 59–49. No. 12 cleft. *A,* Frontal view showing the broad flattened frontal process of the maxilla and the orbital hypertelorism. Note the notch at the junction of the nasal bone with the frontal process of the maxilla. *B,* Intracranial view of the floor of the anterior cranial vault. The arrows outline the axis of the orbit. The principal deformity is the widening of the ethmoid labyrinth, which is shown by the broken lines. The cribriform plate is of normal width. (Courtesy of Dr. P. Tessier.)

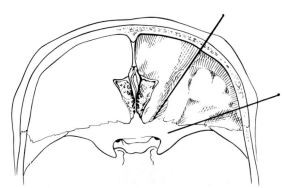

Figure 59–50. No. 13 cleft, bilateral. Intracranial view of the anterior floor of the cranial vault. Arrows outline the laterally displaced orbit. Note the widening of the olfactory grooves, and, hence, the entire cribriform plate. (Courtesy of Dr. P. Tessier.)

most of the craniofacial clefts. When the cleft is bilateral, some of the most extreme degrees of hypertelorism can be seen (Fig. 59–51) (Tessier, 1976). The ethmoid labyrinth is expanded, and extensive pneumatization of the frontal sinus can coexist (Tessier, 1972).

On the external surface, the distinguishing sign of the No. 13 cleft is the dystopia of the hair at the medial end of the eyebrow. A coloboma or notch of the eyebrow per se is not found. The medial end of the eyebrow is actually displaced inferiorly.

No. 14 Cleft. With the No. 14 cleft, the circumferential involvement of the orbit is completed. A return is made to the midline "time zone" that is shared by the No. 0 clefts of the face (see Fig. 59–9). Similar to its facial counterpart, the No. 14 cleft can be produced by agenesis of a part or an overabundance of tissue. When agenesis is the basic theme, orbital hypotelorism is generally seen.

Included in this group of craniofacial malformations are the holoprosencephalic disorders, such as cyclopia, ethmocephaly, and cebocephaly (see Table 59–3). Van der Muelen and associates (1983) included these malformations in their interophthalmic dysplasia subdivision of cerebral craniofacial dysplasias. The cranium is usually microcephalic or occasionally trigonocephalic in shape. A total absence of the usual midline cranial base structures can occur, allowing the orbits to converge in the midline to form a solitary mass, as is seen in cyclopia. Malformations of the intimately related forebrain tend to be proportional to the degree of external facial disorganization. The central nervous system anomalies severely handicap the newborn, and life expectancy is usually limited to hours to several months (see Fig. 59–14).

At the other end of the spectrum is hypertelorism associated with the No. 14 cleft (Fig.

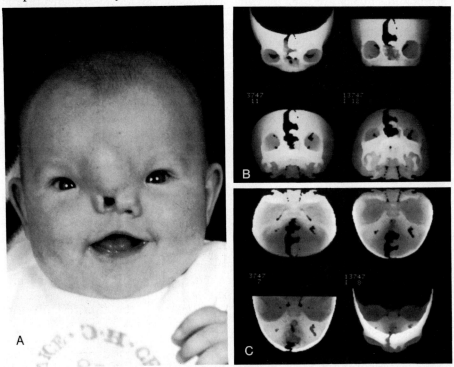

Figure 59–51. No. 1–13 clefts. *A*, the fault begins as a cleft of the dome of the right nostril, and a nasal lipoma extends to the frontal bone and produces hypertelorism. A short paramedian widow's peak disrupts the hairline. *B, C*, Three-dimensional computed tomographic reconstruction shows the bony cleft through the nasal and frontal bones. (From David, D. J., Moore, M. H., and Cooter, R. D.: Tessier clefts revisited with a third dimension. Cleft Palate J., 26:163, 1989.)

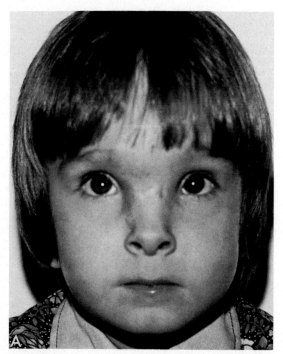 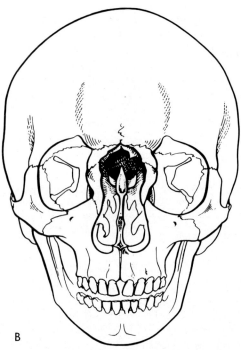

Figure 59–52. No. 14 cleft, *A,* Patient with a midline frontonasal encephalocele and orbital hypertelorism. *B,* Distortion and lateral displacement of the nasal bones, frontal processes of the maxilla, and the medial wall of the orbits by the encephalocele. (*B* courtesy of Dr. P. Tessier.)

59–52). The terms frontofrontodysplasia and frontonasoethmoid dysplasia are used by van der Muelen and associates (1983) to categorize this group. Lateral displacement of the orbits can be produced by cranium bifidum (Fig. 59–53) or a space-occupying mass such as a frontonasal encephalocele or a midline frontal encephalocele (Fig. 59–54). Cohen and associates (1971b) thought that the basic fault in embryologic development lies in the malformation of the nasal capsule. The developing forebrain thus remains in its low-lying position. A morphokinetic arrest of the normal medial movement of the eyes occurs: the orbits remain in their widespread fetal position. The median cranial dysrhaphia is characterized by an increased distance between the olfactory grooves (see Fig. 59–53B). The crista galli is involved and is widened or duplicated in some cases. Occasionally the crista galli is absent (Tessier, 1975). When the crista galli is severely enlarged, preservation of the olfactory nerve is often not possible during the surgical correction of hypertelorism. Prolapse into the enlarged ethmoid labyrinth occurs and leads to an increase in the interorbital space and the orbital divergence. Consequently, the cribri-

form plate, which is normally located 5 to 10 mm below the level of the orbital roof, can be caudally displaced up to 20 mm (Tessier, 1972).

The frontal bone is flattened, giving the glabella an indistinct appearance. When an encephalocele is present, large defects of the frontal bone are often seen (see Fig. 59–54). In a roentgenographic study, Brejcha and Fára (1971) demonstrated absence of typical pneumatization of the frontal bone.

TREATMENT

From the foregoing descriptions, it is evident that each craniofacial malformation is unique. Therefore, treatment plans cannot be standardized. Nevertheless, certain guiding principles can be outlined to plan the sequence and execution of the surgical procedures.

In general, the time of initiating reconstructive surgery varies with the severity of the malformation and any threats that it might pose to vital function. Treatment of milder clefts without associated functional impairment is not urgent. The use of suitable

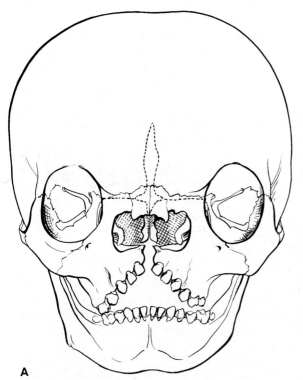

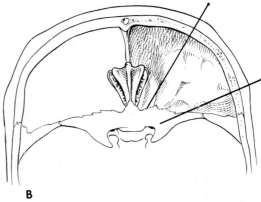

Figure 59–53. No. 14 cleft. *A,* Frontal view of a median craniofacial dysrhaphia with orbital hypertelorism, flattened glabellar region, widened nasal cavities, and a midline cleft of the maxillary alveolus. *B,* Intracranial view of the floor of the anterior cranial fossa. Arrows show the direction of the orbit. Note the increased width of the crista galli. (*B* courtesy of Dr. P. Tessier.)

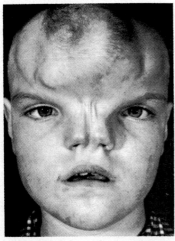

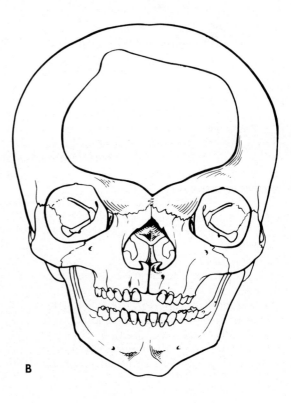

Figure 59–54. No. 14 cleft associated with a midline frontal encephalocele. *A,* Patient with a frontal encephalocele and hypertelorism. *B,* Osseous pattern associated with a midline frontal encephalocele. (From Tessier, P.: Anatomical classification of facial, cranio-facial and latero-facial clefts. J. Maxillofac. Surg., 4:69, 1976.)

delay takes advantage of the rapid physical and physiologic growth of the child. Growth appreciably increases the size of the component structures, facilitates repair, and allows accurate approximation of landmarks. By contrast, when the severity of the malformation imposes physiologic hazards, the initial repair should commence as soon as the infant has adjusted to his environment and has regained his birth weight. In these cases, early intervention improves function and the repaired soft tissues splint and assist molding of the distorted facial skeleton.

The extent of the operative endeavor in early childhood is usually limited to the soft tissue. Interference with any remaining skeletal growth potential by ill-timed operative trauma would not be welcomed. However, the exact effect of surgical manipulation is largely unknown and unpredictable at this time. Patients with severe clefts and hypoplasia of the craniofacial skeleton pose less of a dilemma, since only limited bony growth is expected.

Clefts of the soft tissue generally involve all layers. Any scar interposed within the fissure should be excised to expose normal tissue. Failure to obtain a meticulous layer closure results in loss of anatomic continuity and a depression along the site of repair. When the repair crosses the lines of minimal tension or when there is a loss of length, multiple Z-plasties can be used to advantage. However, anatomic landmarks must be respected or, if displaced by the cleft, returned to normal position.

The esthetic demands of a well-performed repair of the soft tissue deformity cannot be denied. However, the reconstruction of the supporting skeletal framework is equally important. An appreciation and understanding of the skeletal malformation is basic to any reconstructive procedure. Without proper osseous support, the soft tissue correction that appears to be satisfactory at the time of closure is doomed to produce a less than ideal long-term result.

In addition to the principles that apply to all clefts, specific problems arise as the individual clefts are addressed. In the median cleft of the upper lip, repair of the soft tissues of the lip is achieved in layers, with particular attention to accurate alignment of the vermilion border and coaptation of the reoriented muscle layer (Fig. 59–55). Duplication of the frenulum is usually not of functional significance and does not require specific repair. However, the frenulum should be excised if it extends onto the alveolar ridge to produce a diastema between the central incisors. Malposition of the upper central incisors is corrected by orthodontic therapy. Absence of or rudimentary development of the premaxilla creates an instability of the entire maxillary arch. A crossbite is produced as the maxillary segments collapse toward the midline. Protracted orthodontic treatment and bone grafts are often necessary for correction. As an adjunct to orthodontic expansion a horizontal cortical osteotomy in the region of the zygomaticomaxillary buttress expedites the process. Surgical correction of the bifid nose and orbital hypertelorism is reviewed in Chapter 60.

In the median clefts of the lower lip, problems encountered in handling the soft tissue defects are essentially similar to those outlined for the upper lip. A simple V-excision of the cleft with approximation in layers can be performed (see Fig. 59–17). A step closure, staggering the mucocutaneous junction (Millard and associates, 1971), can also be used to prevent notching of the vermilion border. When the tongue is bifid, it is held in an abnormal anterior position by a short frenulum that limits lingual mobility. Lengthening the frenulum is indicated to free the tongue, and a Z-plasty is a satisfactory procedure for this purpose.

Complete clefts of the mandibular symphysis should not be corrected in infancy. Misalignment of the dental arches is always present when the mandible is cleft. Normal interarch relationships cannot be improved by direct approximation of the bone ends, since an actual loss of tissue is involved (Ecker, 1958). The defect can be as great as 3 cm. Restoration of continuity, therefore, requires the insertion of a bone graft. Stabilization of the mandible and graft, even with fixation plates and screws, would be difficult with the soft bone of the infant mandible.

Midline fibrous web contractures of the anterior neck region require early correction to permit adequate growth of the mandible and to restore the cervicomental angle. Simple excision of the contracted fibrous cords of the anterior ribbon muscles fails to provide a permanent cure (Davis, 1950). A Z-plasty is often required (Monroe, 1966) to prevent re-

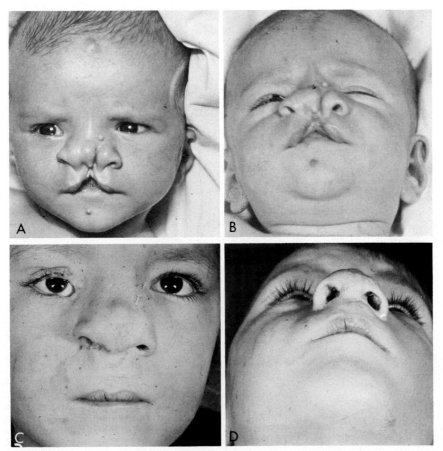

Figure 59–55. Repair of midline cleft of the upper lip and bifid nose. *A, B,* Preoperative views. *C, D,* Postoperative views. The orbital hypertelorism and the coloboma of the right lower eyelid remain untreated.

current contracture. On occasion, introduction of additional soft tissue to the involved area is needed.

The management of a case of partial duplication of the midfacial structures (see Fig. 59–19) by Calaycay and associates (1976) demonstrates what can be achieved by a well-planned, staged approach to an unusual, complex malformation. After the newborn had adjusted to his new environment (at the age of 2 weeks), transection of the oral mass that separated the maxilla from the mandible was performed under local anesthesia to improve the airway (Fig. 59–56A). A gastrostomy was also provided for feeding purposes. During the sixteenth week of life, the entire oral mass with its intermaxillary bony struts was removed under general anesthesia. The second operation also included a palatoplasty and an attempt to repair the cleft of the upper lip (Fig. 59–56B). Unfortunately a dehiscence of the cheiloplasty occurred. When the infant was 9 months old, the bifid tongue was cor-

rected by a Z-plasty, and the redundant portion of the lower lip was excised. Three months later, the lower third of the nose was corrected, and a secondary palatoplasty and upper lip repair were performed (Fig. 59–56C, D).

The No. 3 naso-ocular cleft represents one of the most difficult and challenging malformations for the reconstructive surgeon. The decreased vertical dimension between the ala and the medial canthus can be corrected by a Z-plasty (Fig. 59–57A, B) (Tessier, 1969a, b) or a similar flap (Fig. 59–58) that introduces tissue to increase the distance between the two structures. The restoration of the vertical distance of skin by the local skin flap is accomplished at the expense of the width. Tessier (1969a, b) emphasized the need for wide undermining of the soft tissue over the maxilla and the zygomatic arch to achieve a tension-free soft tissue coverage. Bone grafts are used to support the prolapsed contents of the orbital cavity and to fill the defects of the

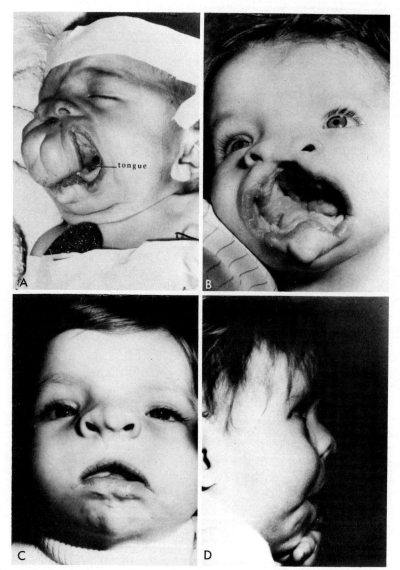

tongue

Figure 59–56. Treatment of duplication of the midface. *A,* First stage. Transection of the oral mass to separate the mandible from the maxilla. *B,* Appearance six months after the second stage. The oral mass and the intermaxillary bony struts have been removed. Three of the four uvulas can be seen. Note the bifid tongue and the remaining redundant lower lip. *C,* Frontal view at the age of 1½ years after the last operative intervention. Cheiloplasty and reconstruction of the nose have been performed. *D,* Profile view at age 1½ years. (Courtesy of Dr. Calaycay and associates.)

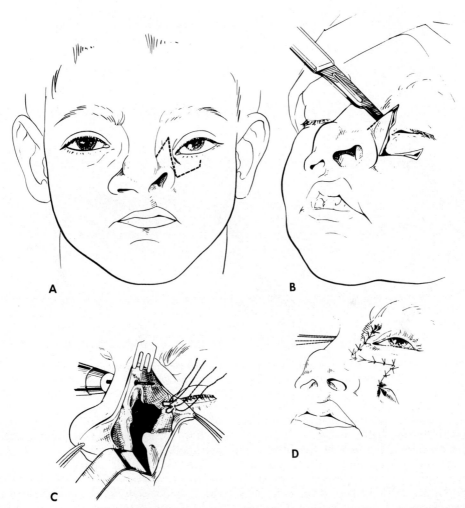

Figure 59–57. Treatment of the No. 3 cleft. *A,* Marking of the Z-plasty used to correct the medial canthal dystopia and to increase the vertical height. *B,* Development of the Z-plasty. *C,* Transnasal approach for the medial canthopexy. *D,* Flaps have been transposed over the bone grafts and the medial canthopexy. (Courtesy of Dr. P. Tessier.)

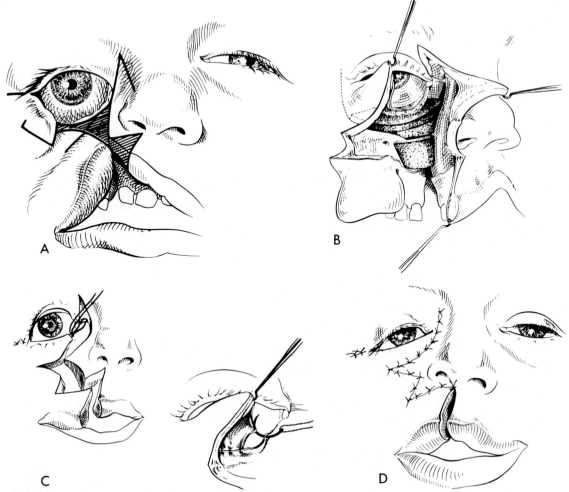

Figure 59–58. Treatment of the No. 4 cleft. *A,* Outline of the skin flaps. *B,* Bone graft in place to restore the facial skeleton. *C,* Transposition of the flaps and closure of the conjunctiva. *D,* Closure of the skin. (Courtesy of Dr. P. Tessier.)

skeleton. Lining is obtained from the mucosa of the nasal floor or septum.

The nasolacrimal system is disrupted by the cleft malformation; the nasolacrimal duct is blocked, and the sac is prone to repeated infection (Gunter, 1963); the lower canaliculus is malformed beyond repair (Tessier, 1969a). Total extirpation of the sac and duct remnants is therefore the treatment of choice. Because the medial canthal tendon is hypoplastic and its insertion is inferiorly displaced, it cannot be relied on for the medial canthopexy. Transnasal wiring must be used to reposition the medial canthus (see Fig. 59–57C). An urgent situation exists when the eye is normal but is unprotected because of the coloboma. Early repair of the coloboma is imperative to prevent corneal ulceration and serious impairment of vision (see Fig. 59–

58). When microphthalmos is present, the problem of restoring facial symmetry is compounded.

The No. 4 cleft spares the nose and the piriform aperture. The cleft begins lateral to the Cupid's bow. Thus, contrary to the principle of saving labial tissue, the tissue lateral to the new philtral column must be discarded (Fig. 59–59). The decrease in vertical dimension occurs between the mouth and the medial third of the lower eyelid. Restoration of soft tissue continuity is achieved with the use of local interdigitating flaps (Tessier, 1969a, b). The nasolacrimal canal and lacrimal sac lie medial to the cleft; the lower canaliculus, however, is disturbed. The medial canthal tendon is also almost normal in respect to its direction and insertion (Tessier, 1969a). Thus the medial canthal tendon stump can be used

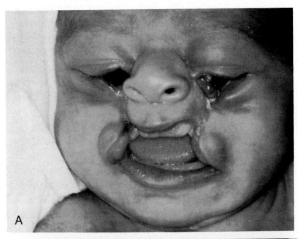

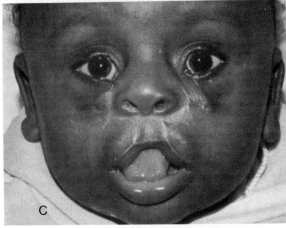

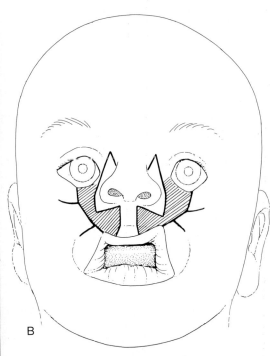

Figure 59–59. Treatment of No. 4 cleft, bilateral. *A,* Preoperative view of an infant whose mother took a drug during the first trimester of pregnancy. *B,* Line drawings of the flaps with shaded areas representing areas of resection. *C,* Postoperative view after the first stage of reconstruction.

when performing a canthopexy. Bone grafts are required to correct the orbital dystopia by rebuilding the orbital rim, orbital floor, and maxilla (Fig. 59–59*B*).

Treatment of the No. 5 cleft is similar to that of the No. 4 cleft. Interlocking small triangular flaps are used to repair the soft tissue cleft (Boo-Chai, 1970). Bone grafts are again employed to restore the underlying skeletal support.

Correction of the No. 6 cleft is similar to that of the Treacher Collins syndrome (see Chap. 63). However, since the soft tissue deficit is less and the zygoma is hypoplastic, rather than absent, the reconstruction is simpler.

There is little disagreement that the soft tissue defects that are associated with the No. 7 cleft should be corrected early. The repair is relatively simple when only the soft tissue is involved. After excision of the margins of the clefts, the soft tissue is approximated in layers. The separated muscles are

identified and carefully approximated. The principle of reorientation and approximation of the orbicularis oris muscle is followed to reconstruct the commissure of the mouth. When the cleft is unilateral, the normal commissure is used as a guide to determine the exact location of the absent commissure. In the case of the bilateral cleft, the site of the future commissure is determined by locating the transition point between the color of the mucosa of the red lip and that of the deeper hue of the buccal mucosa (Boo-Chai, 1969). The actual restoration of the commissure is achieved by the use of a simple Z-plasty (Longacre, DeStefano, and Holmstrand, 1961) or a small Estlander's flap rotated from the lower lip into the upper lip (May, 1962). The pedicle becomes the new commissure. Another method is to construct a broad mucosal vermilion flap along the border of the cleft. The pedicle is based on either lip and is rotated past the new commissure to be inserted into the prepared recipient site of the opposite lip (Stark and Saunders, 1962). The slight "dip in" of the normal commissure can be reproduced by using a small laterally based triangular flap. The tip of this skin flap is transferred inward and is sutured to the mucous membrane lining located just within the commissure. This Y-V procedure is employed as a second stage when a mucosal pedicle has been used to form the commissure during the initial repair. Mansfield and Herbert (1972) suggested the use of a large Z-plasty that transposes the soft tissues of the neck into the depressed area of the lower face.

Correction of the soft tissue defects of the Treacher Collins syndrome depends a great deal on the restoration of the bony architecture (see Chap. 50). It should be recalled that approximately one-third of the patients do not have an infraorbital foramen (Tessier, 1975). In these patients, the infraorbital neurovascular bundle passes from the orbit directly into the subcutaneous tissue. Care must therefore be exercised when the dissection is performed in this area.

When should reconstructive surgery of the facial skeleton begin? There is disagreement. Proponents of early intervention argue that the psychologic consequence of the deformity is less with early repair and that early correction encourages rather than interferes with any growth potential. Although they acknowledge the detrimental psychologic implications, opponents of early osseous reconstruction believe that surgical manipulation interferes with any remaining growth potential.

In the case of the No. 7 cleft (unilateral craniofacial microsomia), Brown, Fryer, and Ohlwiler (1960), Longacre, DeStefano, and Holmstrand (1961), and Stark and Saunders (1962) favor early correction of the problem and have advocated the use of inorganic implants, autogenous cartilage, and bone. Converse and associates (1973b) combined the early use of mandibular osteotomies and orthodontic therapy and have published a series of long-term results. Balancing the early intervention school is the clinical work of Obwegeser (1970, 1974) and the experimental findings of Poswillo (1974b). After the facial skeleton has ceased to increase in size, Obwegeser employs onlay bone grafts to rebuild the deficient skeletal contour, together with sagittal split osteotomies of the mandible and a Le Fort I osteotomy of the maxilla. In animal studies, Poswillo found that hemorrhage in the otomandibular region destroys the developing muscles, ligaments, and bones. The functional matrix (Moss, 1968) thought to be required for growth is obliterated. Thus Poswillo concluded that the results of early reconstructive surgery would be short lived.

On the other hand, in treating the Treacher Collins deformity (clefts No. 6, 7, and 8), Poswillo believed that early intervention is indicated. On the basis of his animal investigations, Poswillo (1974b) suggested that "a degree of functional autonomy sufficient to provide growth of the facial skeleton" is preserved and that the principal deficiency is in the amount of mesenchyme that forms the facial skeleton. Correction of this deficit would restore the functional matrix. The clinical observations of Tessier (1975), however, showed that what is theoretically possible is not often achieved in daily practice. After observing many patients on whom an early operation was performed, Tessier noted that the malformation has an insatiable appetite for bone grafts. Consequently, correction of the skeletal malformation is postponed until adolescence, at which time the resorption of the bone grafts is appreciably less.

Beginning with the No. 9 cleft, the cranium itself becomes involved. Depending on the severity of the deformity, an intracranial or extracranial approach is used. The indications and the surgical techniques of these operations are discussed in Chapter 32.

REFERENCES

Abramson, P. D.: Bilateral congenital clefts of the lower lip. Surgery, 31:761, 1952.

Ashley, L. M., and Richardson, G. E.: Multiple congenital anomalies in a stillborn infant. Anat. Rec., 86:457, 1943.

Baibak, G., and Bromberg, B. E.: Congenital midline defects of the midface. Cleft Palate J., 3:392, 1966.

Ballantyne, J. W.: The teratological records of Chaldea. Teratologia, 1:127, 1894.

Berry, G. A.: Note on a congenital defect (? coloboma) of the lower lid. Roy. Lond. Ophth. Hosp. Rep., 12:255, 1889.

Binns, W.: Poisonous weed causes monkey-faced deformity in lambs. Washington DC, U.S. Department of Agriculture Public Release, June 1961.

Binns, W., Anderson, W. A., and Sullivan, D. J.: Cyclopian-type malformation in lambs. Am. J. Vet. Res., 137:515, 1960.

Binns, W., Thacker, E. J., James, L. F., and Huffman, W. T.: A congenital cyclopian-type malformation in lambs. Am. J. Vet. Res., 134:180, 1959.

Blackfield, H. M., and Wilde, N. J.: Lateral facial clefts. Plast. Reconstr. Surg., 6:68, 1950.

Boo-Chai, K.: The transverse facial cleft: its repair. Br. J. Plast. Surg., 22:119, 1969.

Boo-Chai, K.: The oblique facial cleft: a report of 2 cases and a review of 41 cases. Br. J. Plast. Surg., 23:352, 1970.

Braithwaite, F., and Watson, J.: Three unusual clefts of the lip. Br. J. Plast. Surg., 2:38, 1949.

Braun, J. T., Franciosi, R. A., Mastri, A. R., Drake, R. M., and O'Neil, B. L.: Isotretinoin dysmorphic syndrome (Petter). Lancet, 1:506, 1984.

Brejcha, M., and Fára, M.: Osseous changes in middle clefts of the nose. Acta Chir. Plast. (Praha), 13:141, 1971.

Brown, J. B., Fryer, M. P., and Ohlwiler, D. A.: Study in the use of synthetic materials such as silicone and Teflon as subcutaneous prosthesis. Plast. Reconstr. Surg., 26:264, 1960.

Brucker, P., Hoyt, C. J., and Trusler, H. M.: Severe cleft lip in arrhinencephaly. Plast. Reconstr. Surg., 32:527, 1963.

Burian, F.: Vzácné vrozené vady obličeje a lebky a jejich léčení (Seltene angeborene Defekte d. Gesichts u. d. Schädels u. ihre Behandlung). Acta Universit. Carolinae Praha, 1957.

Burian, F.: Median clefts of the nose. Acta. Chir. Plast. (Praha), 2:180, 1960.

Calaycay, L. A., Gooding, R. A., Brown, R. J., and Herhahn, F. T.: Treatment of a rare facial anomaly. Presented at California Society of Plastic Surgery, 26th Annual Meeting in Anaheim, March 1976.

Callas, G., and Walker, B. E.: Palate morphogenesis in mouse embryos after x-irradiation. Anat. Rec., 145:61, 1963.

Caronni, E. P.: Embryogenesis and classification of branchial auricular dysplasia. In Transactions of the Fifth International Congress on Plastic and Reconstructive Surgery. Melbourne, Butterworth, 1971.

Cohen, M. M., Jr., Jiřasek, J. E., Guzman, R. T., Gorlin, R. J., and Peterson, M. D.: Holoprosencephaly and facial dysmorphia: nosology, etiology and pathogenesis. Birth Defects, 7:125, 1971a.

Cohen, M. M., Jr., Sedano, H. O., Gorlin, R. J., and Jiřasek, J. E.: Frontonasal dysplasia (median cleft face syndrome): Comments on etiology and pathogenesis. Birth Defects, 7:117, 1971b.

Cohlan, S. Q.: Excessive intake of vitamin A as a cause of congenital anomalies in the rat. Science, 117:535, 1953.

Comess, L. J.: Congenital anomalies and diabetes in Pima Indians of Arizona. Diabetes, 18:471, 1969.

Converse, J. M., Coccaro, P. J., Becker, M., and Wood-Smith, D.: On hemifacial microsomia. Plast. Reconstr. Surg., 51:268, 1973a.

Converse, J. M., Horowitz, S. L., Coccaro, P. J., and Wood-Smith, D.: The corrective treatment of the skeleton asymmetry in hemifacial microsomia. Plast. Reconstr. Surg., 52:221, 1973b.

Converse, J. M., Ransohoff, J., Mathews, E. S., Smith, S., and Molenaar, A.: Ocular hypertelorism and pseudohypertelorism. Advances in surgical treatment. Plast. Reconstr. Surg., 45:1, 1970.

Converse, J. M., McCarthy, J. G., and Wood-Smith, D.: Orbital hypotelorism: pathogenesis, associated faciocerebral anomalies and surgical correction. Plast. Reconstr. Surg., 56:389, 1975.

Converse, J. M., Wood-Smith, D. W., McCarthy, J. G., Coccaro, P. J., and Becker, M. H.: Bilateral facial microsomia. Plast. Reconstr. Surg., 54:413, 1974.

Conway, H., and Wagner, K. J.: Congenital anomalies of the head and neck. Plast. Reconstr. Surg., 36:71, 1965.

Cosman, B., and Crikelair, G. F.: Midline branchiogenic syndromes. Plast. Reconstr. Surg., 44:41, 1969.

Couronné, A.: Clin. Soc. Med. Prot., Montpellier, 107, 1819.

David, D. J., Moore, M. H., and Cooter, R. D.: Tessier clefts revisited with a third dimension. Cleft Palate J., 26:163, 1989.

Davis, A. D.: Median cleft of the lower lip and mandible. Plast. Reconstr. Surg., 6:62, 1950.

Davis, W. B.: Congenital deformities of the face. Surg. Gynecol. Obstet., 61:201, 1935.

DeMyer, W.: Cleft lip and jaw induced in fetal rats by vincristine. Arch. Anat. Histol. Embryol. (Strasb.), 48:179, 1964.

DeMyer, W.: The median cleft face syndrome. Differential diagnosis of cranial bifidum occultum, hypertelorism and median cleft nose, lip and palate. Neurology (Minneap.), 17:961, 1967.

DeMyer, W., and Zeman, W.: Alobar holoprosencephaly (arrhinencephaly) with median cleft lip and palate: clinical electroencephalographic and nosologic considerations. Confin. Neurol., 23:1, 1963.

DeMyer, W., Zeman, W., and Palmer, C. A.: The face predicts the brain: diagnostic significance of median facial anomalies for holoprosencephaly (arrhinencephaly). Pediatrics, 34:256, 1964.

Dey, E. I.: Oblique facial clefts. Plast. Reconstr. Surg., 52:258, 1973.

Dick, W.: A case of hyperencephalous monstrosity. Lond. Med. Gaz., 19:897, 1837.

Dupertuis, S. M., and Musgrave, R. A.: Experiences with the reconstruction of the congenitally deformed ear. Plast. Reconstr. Surg., 23:361, 1959.

Dursy, E.: Zur Entwicklungsgeschichte des Kopfes des Menschen und der höheren Wirbeltheire. Tübingen, Verlag der H. Lauppschen-Buchhandlung, 1869, p. 99.

Ecker, H. A.: Medial clefts of the lip. Am. J. Surg., 96:815, 1958.

Erdelyi, R.: The influence of toxoplasmosis on the incidence of congenital facial malformation. Preliminary report. Plast. Reconstr. Surg., 20:306, 1957.

Ergin, N. O.: Naso-ocular cleft: a case report. Plast. Reconstr. Surg., 38:573, 1966.

Erickson, J. D., and Oakley, G. P.: Seizure disorder in mothers of children with orofacial clefts: a case control study. J. Pediatr., 84:244, 1974.

Ferm, V. H., and Kilham, L.: Congenital anomalies induced in hamster embryos with H_1 virus. Science, 145::510, 1964.

Fogh-Andersen, P.: Recent statistics of facial clefts—frequency, heredity, mortality. In Holtz, R. (Ed.): Early Treatment of Cleft Lip and Palate. Bern, Hans Huber, 1964.

Fogh-Andersen, P.: Rare clefts of the face. Acta Chir. Scand., 129:275, 1965.

Fogh-Andersen, P.: Genetic and non-genetic factors in the etiology of facial clefts. Scand. J. Plast. Reconstr. Surg., 1:22, 1967.

Franceschetti, A., and Klein, D.: The mandibulo-facial dysostosis: a new heredity syndrome. Acta Ophthalmol., 27:144, 1949.

Franceschetti, A., and Zwahlen, P.: Un syndrome nouveau: la dysostose mandibulo-faciale. Bull. Schweiz. Akad. Med. Wiss., 1:60, 1944.

Frazer, F. C., Chew, D., and Verusio, A. C.: Oligohydramnios and cortisone-induced cleft palate in the mouse. Nature, 214:417, 1967.

Frazer, F. C., and Fainstat, T. D.: Production of congenital defects in offspring of pregnant mice treated with cortisone. Pediatrics, 8:527, 1951.

Frazer, J. E.: Manual of Embryology. London, Baillière, Tindall & Cox, 1940.

Fujino, H., Yasuko, K., and Takeshi, K.: Median cleft of the lower lip, mandible and tongue with midline cervical cord: a case report. Cleft Palate J., 7:679, 1970.

Gabka, J.: Beitrag zur Atiologie der Lippen-Kiefer-Gaumenspalten unter besonder Berüchsichtigung der Toxoplasmose. Dtsch. Stomatol., 3:294, 1953.

Galanti, S.: Rare congenital malformation of the nose (2 cases of bifid nose). Ann. Laringol., 60:583, 1961.

Gardner, D. G., Kapun, R. N., and Jordan, R. E.: A cleft of the mandible in the lateral incisor cuspid region. Oral Surg., 35:649, 1973.

German, J., Kowal, A., and Ehler, K. H.: Trimethadione and human teratogenesis. Teratology, 3:349, 1970.

Giroud, A., and Martinet, M.: Production d'un excès de liquide aminiotique dans l'anencéphalie. Co. R. Soc. Biol. (Paris), 149:452, 1955.

Giroud, A., and Martinet, M.: Malformations de la face et hypervitaminose A. Rev. Stomatol., 57:454, 1956.

Giroud, A., and Martinet, M.: Morphogénèse de l'anencephalie. Arch. Anat. Microsc. Morphol. Exp., 46:247, 1957.

Goldenhar, M.: Associations malformations de l'oeil et de l'oreille, en particular le syndrome dermoide épibulbaire-appendices auriculaires-fistula auris congenita et ses relations avec la dysostose mandibulo-faciale. J. Génet. Hum., 1243, 1952.

Gorlin, R. J., Jue, K. L., Jacobsen, U., and Goldschmidt, E.: Oculoauriculovertebral syndrome. J. Pediatr., 63:991, 1963.

Gorlin, R. J., and Pindborg, J. J.: Syndromes of the Head and Neck. Chapters 19, 51, 69, 82. New York, McGraw-Hill Book Company, 1964.

Goulian, D., and Conway, H.: A rare case of facial duplication. Plast. Reconstr. Surg., 33:66, 1964.

Grabb, W. C.: The first and second branchial arch syndrome. Plast. Reconstr. Surg., 36:485, 1965.

Greer, W. D.: Malformations of the Face. Edinburgh, Livingstone, 1961.

Gunter, G. S.:Nasomaxillary cleft. Plast. Reconstr. Surg., 32:637, 1963.

Gylling, U., and Soivio, A.: Frequency, morphology and operative mortality in cleft lip and palate in Finland. Acta. Chir. Scand., 123:1, 1962.

Hanhart, E.: Nachweis einer einfach-dominanten, unkomplizierten sowie unregelmassig-dominanten, mit Atresia auris, Palatoschisis und anderen Deformationen verbundenen Anlage zu Ohrmuschelver Kummerung (Mikrotie). Arch. Klaus-Stift. Vererb.-Forsch., 24:374, 1949.

Harkins, C. S., Berlin, A., Harding, R. L., Longacre, J. J., and Snodgrass, R. M.: A classification of cleft lip and cleft palate. Plast. Reconstr. Surg., 29:31, 1962.

Harris, J. W. S.: Oligohydramnios and cortisone-induced cleft palate. Nature, 203:533, 1964.

Harris, J. W. S., and Ross, I. P.: Cortisone therapy in early pregnancy: Relation to cleft palate. Lancet, 1:1045, 1955.

Heiberg, K., Kalter, H., and Frazer, F. C.: Production of cleft palates in offspring of mice treated with ACTH during pregnancy. Biol. Neonate, 1:33, 1959.

Herren, P.: Case depicted in Gorlin, R. J., and Pindborg, J. J.: Syndromes of the Head and Neck. New York, McGraw-Hill Book Company, 1964, p. 38.

Hertig, A. T., Rock, J., and Adams, E. C.: A description of 34 human ova with the first 17 days of development. Am. J. Anat., 98:435, 1956.

His, W.: Die Formentwicklung des ausseren Ohres. In Anatomie Menschlicher Embryonen, Part III. Leipzig. F. C. W. Vogel, 1885, p. 211.

His, W.: Die Entwicklung der Menschlichen und Thierischer Physiognomen. Arch. Anat. Entwicklungsgesch. S., 384, 1892.

Hochstetter, F.: Uber die Entwicklung der Formuerhaltnisse des Menschlichen Antlitzes. Denkschripten Akad. Wiss., 109:1, 1953.

Hoepke, H., and Maurer, H.: Z. Anat. Entwicklungsgesch, 108:768, 1939.

Hövels, O.: Zur Systematik der Missbildungen des 1. Visceralbogens unter besonderer Berücksiehtigung der Dysostosis mandibulo-facialis. Z. Kinderheilkd., 73:532, 1953.

Ivy, R. A.: Congenital anomalies as recorded on birth certificates in Pennsylvania 1951–1955, inclusive. Plast. Reconstr. Surg., 20:400, 1957.

Ivy, R. A.: Congenital anomalies as reported on birth certificates in Pennsylvania 1956–1960, inclusive. Plast. Reconstr. Surg., 32:361, 1963.

Janz, D., and Fuchs, U.: Are antiepileptic drugs harmful when given during pregnancy? Ger. Med. Monthly, 9:20, 1964.

Jírovec, O., Jíra, J., Fuchs, V., and Peter, R.: Studien mit dem Toxoplasmintest. I. Bereitund des toxoplasmins. Zentralbl. Bakteriol., 169:129, 1957.

Johnston, M. C.: Facial malformation in chick embryos resulting from removal of neural crest (abstract). J. Dent. Res., 43:822, 1964.

Johnston, M. C.: The neural crest in vertebrate cephalogenesis. Ph.D. Dissertation, University of Rochester, Rochester, NY, 1965.

Johnston, M. C.: A radioautographic study of the migration and fate of the cranial neural crest cells in the chick embryo. Anat. Rec., 156:143, 1966.

Johnston, M. C.: Morphogenesis and malformation of face and brain. Birth Defects, 11:1, 1975.

Karfik, V.: Proposed classification of rare congenital cleft malformations in the face. Acta Chir. Plast. (Praha), 8:163, 1966.

Karfik, V.: Oblique facial cleft. In Transactions of the Fourth International Congress on Plastic and Reconstructive Surgery. Amsterdam, Excerpta Medica, 1969, p. 105.

Kawamoto, H. K., Jr.: The kaleidoscopic world of rare craniofacial clefts: order out of chaos (Tessier classification). Clin. Plast. Surg., 3:529, 1976.

Kazanjian, V. H., and Holmes, E. M.: Treatment of median cleft lip associated with bifid nose and hypertelorism. Plast. Reconstr. Surg., 24:582, 1959.

Keith, A.: Congenital deformities of the palate, face and neck. Br. Med. J., 2:310, 1909.

Keith, A.: Concerning the origin and nature of certain malformations of the face, head, and foot. Br. J. Surg., 28:173, 1940a.

Keith, A.: Three demonstrations of congenital malformations of the face, head, and foot. Br. J. Surg., 28:173, 1940b.

Kleinsasser, O., and Schlothane, R.: Die Ohrm Bildungen in Rahmen de Thalidomide embryopathie. Z. Laryngol. Rhinol. Otol., 43:344, 1964.

Krikun, L. A.: Clinical features of median cleft of nose. Acta Chir. Plast. (Praha), 14:137, 1972.

Kubáček, V., and Pěnkava, J.: Oblique clefts of the face. Acta Chir. Plast. (Praha), 16:152, 1974.

Kundrat, H.: Arrhinencephalie als typische Art von

Missbildung, von Leuschner and Lubensky, Graz., 1882.

Lammer, E. J., Chen, D. T., Hoar, R. M., Agnish, N. D., Benke, P. J., et al.: Retinoic acid embryopathy. N. Engl. J. Med., 313:837, 1985.

Langman, J., and Van Faassen F.: Congenital defects in rat embryos after partial thyroidectomy of the mother animal: a preliminary report on eye defects. Am. J. Ophthalmol., 40:65, 1955.

Larsson, K. S.: Role of mucopolysaccharide synthesis in embryos with cleft palate. In Longacre, J. J.: Craniofacial Anomalies: Pathogenesis and Repair. Philadelphia, J. B. Lippincott Company, 1968, p. 7.

Larsson, K. S., and Boström, H.: Teratogenic action of salicylate related to the inhibition of mucopolysaccharide synthesis. Acta Paediatr. Scand., 54:43, 1965.

Leck, I., Hay, S., Witte, J. I., and Greene, J. C.: Malformations recorded on birth certificates following A₂ influenza epidemics. Public Health Rep., 84:971, 1969.

Livingstone, G.: Congenital ear abnormalities due to thalidomide. Proc. R. Soc. Med., 58:493, 1965.

Lockhard, R. D.: Variations coincident with congenital absence of the zygoma. J. Anat., 63:233, 1929.

Longacre, J. J., DeStefano, A., and Holmstrand, K.: The early versus the late reconstruction of congenital hypoplasia of the facial skeleton and skull. Plast. Reconstr. Surg., 27:489, 1961.

Longacre, J. J., Stevens, G. A., and Holmstrand, K. E.: The surgical management of first and second branchial arch syndrome. Plast. Reconstr. Surg., 31:507, 1963.

Mann, I.: Development of the human eye. Br. Med. Assoc., London, 1964, p. 259.

Mansfield, O. T., and Herbert, D. C.: Unilateral transverse facial cleft—a method of surgical closure. Br. J. Plast. Surg., 25:29, 1972.

Marin-Padilla, M.: Mesodermal alterations induced by hypervitaminosis. J. Embryol. Exp. Morphol., 15:261, 1966.

May, H.: Transverse facial clefts and their repair. Plast. Reconstr. Surg., 29:240, 1962.

McKenzie, J.: The first arch syndrome. Arch. Dis. Child., 33:477, 1958.

McKenzie, J., and Craig, J.: Mandibulo-facial dysostosis (Treacher-Collins syndrome). Arch. Dis. Child., 30:391, 1955.

Melchior, J. C., Svensmark, O., and Trolle, D.: Placental transfer of phenobarbitone in epileptic women, and elimination in newborns. Lancet, 2:260, 1967.

Meurman, Y.: Congenital microtia and meatal atresia. A. M. A. Arch. Otolaryngol., 66:443, 1957.

Millard, D. R., Jr., and Williams, S.: Median lip clefts of upper lip. Plast. Reconstr. Surg., 42:4, 1968.

Millard, D. R., Jr., Lehman, J. A., Jr., Deane, M., and Garst, W. P.: Median cleft of the lower lip and mandible: a case report. Br. J. Plast. Surg., 24:391, 1971.

Miller, R. P., and Becker, B. A.: Teratogenicity of oral diazepam and diphenylhydantoin in mice. Toxicol. Appl. Pharmacol., 32:53, 1975.

Miller, R. W.: Delayed radiation effects in atomic bomb survivors. Science, 166:569, 1969.

Moller, P.: Cleft lip and palate in Iceland. Arch. Oral Biol., 10:407, 1965.

Monroe, C. W.: Midline cleft of the lower lip, mandible, tongue with flexion contracture of the neck: case report and review of the literature. Plast. Reconstr. Surg., 38:312, 1966.

Morian, R.: Ueber die schräge Gesichtsspalte. Arch. Klin. Chir., 35:245, 1887.

Morriss, G. M.: Morphogenesis of the malformations induced in rat embryos by maternal hypervitaminosis A. J. Anat., 113:241, 1972.

Morton, C. B., and Jordon, H. E.: Cleft of lower lip and mandible. Arch. Surg., 30:647, 1935.

Moss, M. L.: The primacy of functional matrices in orofacial growth. Dent. Pract. Dent. Rec., 19:65, 1968.

Murphy, D. P.: Coincidence of placenta previa and congenital malformation. Am. J. Obstet. Gynecol., 35:653, 1938.

Murphy, M. C., Dagg, C. P., and Karnofsky, D. A.: Comparison of teratogenic chemicals in rats and chick embryos, Pediatrics, 19:70, 1957.

Neel, J. V.: A study of major congenital defects in Japanese infants. Am. J. Hum. Genet., 10:398, 1958.

Nishimura, H.: Incidence of malformations in abortion. In Congenital Malformations (Proceedings of 3rd International Conference, Netherlands, 1969). Amsterdam, Excerpta Medica, 1969, p. 275.

Nora, J. J., Nora, A. H., Sommerville, R. J., Hill, R. M., and McNamara, D. G.: Maternal exposure to potential teratogens. J. A. M. A., 202:1065, 1967.

Obwegeser, H. L.: Zur Korrektur des Dysostosis otomandibularis. Schweiz. Monatsschr. Zahnheilkd., 83:331, 1970.

Obwegeser, H. L.: Correction of skeletal anomalies of otomandibular dysostosis. J. Maxillofac. Surg., 2:73, 1974.

Onizuka, T.: Treatment of deformities of the mouth corner. Jap. J. Plast. Reconstr. Surg., 8:132, 1965.

Ortega, J., and Flor, E.: Incomplete naso-ocular cleft: case report. Plast. Reconstr. Surg., 43:630, 1969.

Pashayan, H., Pruzansky, D., and Pruzansky, S.: Anticonvulsants teratogenic? Lancet, 2:702, 1971.

Patten, B. M.: Human Embryology. 3rd Ed. New York, Blakiston Division, McGraw-Hill Book Company, 1968.

Pederson, L. M., Thigstrop, I., and Pederson, J.: Congenital malformation in newborn children of diabetic women. Lancet, 1:790, 1964.

Pitanguy, I. H. J.: Facial clefts as seen in a large series of untreated adults and their later management. In Longacre, J. J. (Ed.): Craniofacial Anomalies. London, Pitman, 1968, p. 167.

Pohlmann, E. H.: Die embryonale Metamorphose der Physiognomie und der Mundhohle des Katzenkopfes. Morphol. Jahrbuch (Leipzig), 41:617, 1910.

Popescu, V.: Congenital transverse facial clefts. Stomatologia, 15:75, 1968.

Poswillo, D.: The aetiology and surgery of cleft palate with micrognathia. Ann. R. Coll. Surg., 43:61, 1968.

Poswillo, D.: The pathogenesis of the first and second branchial arch syndrome. Oral Surg., 35:302, 1973.

Poswillo, D.: Orofacial malformations. Proc. R. Soc. Med., 67:13, 1974a.

Poswillo, D.: Otomandibular deformity. Pathogenesis as a guide to reconstruction. J. Maxillofac. Surg., 2:64, 1974b.

Poswillo, D.: The pathogenesis of the Treacher Collins syndrome (mandibulofacial dysostosis). Br. J. Oral Surg., 13:1, 1975.

Poswillo, D., and Roy, L. J.: The pathogenesis of cleft palate. An animal study. Br. J. Surg., 52:902, 1965.

Poswillo, D., and Sopher, D.: Malformation and deformation in the animal embryo. Teratology, 4:498, 1971.

Potter, E. L.: Pathology of the Fetus and Infant. 3rd Ed. Chicago, Year Book Medical Publishers, 1975.

Powell, W. J., and Jenkins, H. P.: Transverse facial clefts. Plast. Reconstr. Surg., 42:454, 1968.

Reissmann, H.: Ein Fall Von Makrostoma. Arch. Minerva Chir., *6:*858, 1869.

Resnick, J., and Kawamoto, H. K.: Plast. Reconstr. Surg., 1989, in press.

Rogalski, T.: A contribution to the study of anophthalmia with description of a case. Br. J. Ophthalmol., *28:*429, 1944.

Rogers, B. O.: Rare craniofacial deformities. *In* Converse, J. M. (Ed.): Reconstructive Plastic Surgery. Philadelphia, W. B. Saunders Company, 1964a, p. 1213.

Rogers, B. O.: Berry-Treacher-Collins syndrome: a review of 200 cases. Br. J. Plast. Surg., *17:*109, 1964b.

Rogers, B. O.: Micotic, lop, cup and protruding ears. Four directly inherited deformities? Plast. Reconstr. Surg., *41:*208, 1968.

Rosenberg, L., Mitchell, A. A., Parsells, J. L., Pashayan, H., Louik, C., and Shapiro, S.: Lack of relation of oral clefts to diazepam use during pregnancy. N. Engl. J. Med., *309:*1282, 1983.

Rosenthal, R.: Aglossia congenital: report of a case of the condition combined with other congenital malformations. J. Dis. Child., *44:*383, 1932.

Ruben, A.: Handbook of Congenital Malformations. Philadelphia, W. B. Saunders Company, 1967.

Safra, M. S., and Oakley, G. P.: Association between cleft lip with or without cleft palate and parental exposure to diazepam. Lancet, *2:*478, 1975.

Sakurai, E. H., Mitchell, D. F., and Holmes, L. A.: Bilateral oblique facial clefts and amniotic bands: a report of two cases. Cleft Palate J., *3:*181, 1966.

Sanvenero-Rosselli, G.: Developmental pathology of the face and the dysrhaphia syndromes—an essay of interpretation based on experimentally produced congenital defects. Plast. Reconstr. Surg., *11:*36, 1953.

Saxén, I.: Associations between oral clefts and drugs taken during pregnancy. Int. J. Epidemiol., *4:*37, 1975.

Schalbe, E.: Die Morphologie der Missbildungen des Menschen und der Tiere, Part 3. 1913, p. 119.

Schmid, E.: Zur operativen Behandlung des Angeborenen Hypertelorism. Chir. Plast. Reconstr., *3:*130, 1967.

Scrimshaw, G. C.: Midline cleft lip and nose—true "harelip": two interesting cases. *In* Transactions of the Fourth International Congress on Plastic and Reconstructive Surgery. Amsterdam, Excerpta Medica, 1967, p. 472.

Sedano, H. O., Cohen, M. M., Jr., Jirasek, J., and Koplin, R.: Frontonasal dysplasia. J. Pediatr., *76:*906, 1970.

Shiono, P. H., and Mills, J. L.: Oral clefts and diazepam use during pregnancy (letter). N. Engl. J. Med., *311:*919, 1984.

Smithells, R. W., and Leck, I.: The incidence of limb and ear defects since the withdrawal of thalidomide. Lancet, *1:*1095, 1963.

South, J.: Teratogenic effect of anticonvulsants. Lancet, *2:*1154, 1972.

Spidel, B. D., and Meadow, S. R.: Maternal epilepsy and abnormalities of the fetus and newborn. Lancet, *2:*839, 1972.

Stark, R. B.: The pathogenesis of harelip and cleft palate. Plast. Reconstr. Surg., *13:*20, 1954.

Stark, R. B., and Ehrmann, N. A.: The development of the center of the face with particular reference to surgical correction of bilateral cleft lip. Plast. Reconstr. Surg., *21:*177, 1958.

Stark, R. B., and Saunders, D. E.: The first branchial syndrome: the oral-mandibular-auricular syndrome. Plast. Reconstr. Surg., *29:*299, 1962.

Stevenson, S. S., Worcester, J., and Rice, R. G.: 677 congenitally malformed infants and associated gestational characteristics. Pediatrics, *6:*37, 1950.

Stewart, R., Mulick, J., Kawamoto, H. K., Jr., and Thanos, C.: A syndrome of multiple facial clefts, branchial arch anomalies and Streeter's bands (abstract). J. Dent. Res., *55:*B107, 1976.

Stewart, W. J.: Congenital median cleft of the chin. Arch. Surg., *31:*813, 1935.

Stiehm, W. D.: Facial duplication. Am. J. Roentgenol., *116:*598, 1972.

Streeter, G. L.: Contributions to Embryology. Vol. 14. Washington, DC, Carnegie Institute, 1922, p. 111.

Summitt, R.: Familial Goldenhar syndrome. Birth Defects, *2:*106, 1969.

Tandler, J.: Zur Entwickelungsgeschichte der menschlichen Darmartirien. Anat. Auz. Jena, *23:*132, 1903.

Tessier, P.: Colobomas: vertical and oblique complete facial clefts. Panminerva Med., *11:*95, 1969a.

Tessier, P.: Fente orbito-faciales verticales et obliques (colobomas) complètes et frustes. Ann. Chir. Plast., *14:*301, 1969b.

Tessier, P.: Orbital hypertelorism. 1. Successive surgical attempts, material and methods, causes and mechanisms. Scand. J. Plast. Reconstr. Surg., *6:*135, 1972.

Tessier, P.: Personal communication, 1975.

Tessier, P.: Anatomical classification of facial, craniofacial and latero-facial clefts. J. Maxillofac. Surg., *4:*69, 1976.

Thiersch, J. B.: Therapeutic abortions with a folic acid antagonist, 4-aminopteroylglutamic acid, administered by the oral route. J. Obstet. Gynecol., *63:*1298, 1952.

Tocci, P. M., and Beber, B.: Abnormal phenylalanine loading test in mothers of children with cleft defects. Cleft Palate J., *7:*663, 1970.

Trasler, D. G.: Differences in the face shape of mouse embryos with and without the gene Dance predisposing to cleft lip (abstract). Teratology, *2:*27, 1969.

Treacher Collins, E.: 8. Case with symmetrical congenital notches in the outer part of each lower lid and defective development of the malar bones. Trans. Ophthalmol. Soc. U. K., *20:*190, 1900a.

Treacher Collins, E.: 9. Case with symmetrical congenital notches in the outer part of each lower lid and defective development of the malar bones. Trans. Ophthalmol. Soc. U. K., *20:*191, 1900b.

Tünte, W.: Is there a secular increase in the incidence of cleft lip and cleft palate? Cleft Palate J., *6:*430, 1969.

Van der Linden, F. P. G. M., and Borghouts, H. M. H. M.: Widening a palate by combined surgical and orthodontic procedures. Plast. Reconstr. Surg., *46:*393, 1970.

Van der Meulen, J. C., Mazzola, R., Vermey-Keers, C., Stricker, M., and Raphael, B.: A morphogenetic classification of craniofacial malformations. Plast. Reconstr. Surg., *71:*560, 1983.

Veau, V., and Politzer, J.: Embryologie du bec-de-lièvre. Ann. d'Anat. Path., *12:*275, 1936.

Veau, V.: Bec-de-lièvre. Paris, Masson et Cie, 1938.

Walker, B. E.: Amniotic fluid measurement in cortisone-treated and X-irradiated mice. Proc. Soc. Exp. Biol. Med., *118:*606, 1965.

Walker, B. E., and Frazer, F. C.: The embryology of cortisone-induced cleft palate. J. Embryol. Exp. Morphol., *5:*201, 1957.

Warbrick, J. G.: Early development of the nasal cavity and upper lip in the human embryo. J. Anat., *94:*459, 1938.

Warbrick, J. G.: Aspects of facial and nasal development. Sci. Basis Med., 1963, p. 99.

Warburton, D., and Frazer, F. C.: Genetic aspects of abortion. Clin. Obstet. Gynecol., *2:*22, 1956.

Warkany, J., Bofinger, M. K., and Benton, C.: Median facial cleft syndrome in half sisters. Dilemmas in genetic counseling. Teratology, *8:*273, 1973.

Warkany, J., and Schraffenberger, E.: Congenital malformation induced in rats by roentgen rays. Am. J. Rocntgenol., *57.*455, 1947.

Warkany, J., and Takags, E.: Experimental production of congenital malformations in rats by salicylate poisoning. Am. J. Pathol., *35:*315, 1959.

Weaver, D. F., and Ballinger, D. H.: Bifid nose associated with midline cleft of upper lip. Arch. Otolaryngol., *44:*480, 1946.

Webster, J. P., and Deming, E. G.: Surgical treatment of the bifid nose. Plast. Reconstr. Surg., *6:*1, 1950.

Weyer, H.: Hexadactyly, lower jaw cleft, oligodontia (a new syndrome). Ann. Paediatr., *181:*45, 1963.

Whitaker, L. A., Katowitz, J. A., and Randall, R.: The nasolacrimal apparatus in congenital facial anomalies. J. Maxillofac. Surg., *2:*59, 1974.

Wilson, J. G.: Use of rhesus monkeys in teratological studies. Fed. Proc., *30:*104, 1971.

Wilson, J. G.: Abnormalities of intrauterine development in non-human primates. Acta Endocrinol. (Kbh.) (Suppl.), *166:*261, 1972.

Wilson, J. G.: Present status of drugs as teratogens in man. Teratology, *7:*3, 1973.

Wolfler, A.: Midline cleft of lower lip, tongue and mandible. Arch. Klin. Chir., *40:*795, 1890.

Woollam, D. H. M., and Millen, I. W.: Influence of thyroxine on the incidence of harelip in the "strong A" line of mice. Br. Med. J., *1:*1252, 1960.

Yakovlev, P. I.: Pathoarchitectonic studies of cerebral malformation. III. Arrhinocephalies (holotelencephalies). J. Neuropathol. Exp. Neurol., *18:*22, 1956.

Yakovlev, P. I.: Pathoarchitectonic studies of cerebral malformation. J. Neuropathol. Exp. Neurol., *18:*22, 1959.

60

Joseph G. McCarthy
Charles H. M. Thorne
Donald Wood-Smith

Principles of Craniofacial Surgery: Orbital Hypertelorism

Craniofacial surgery consists of techniques involving the cranial as well as the facial skeletal structures. It includes those surgical procedures employed to correct complex congenital and acquired deformities involving the cranium, orbits, facial bones, and jaws. Surgical osteotomies and advancement or recession of the bones are accomplished either through a combined intra-extracranial approach or through a subcranial (extracranial) approach alone.

The definitive surgical correction of craniofacial deformities initiated by Tessier and associates (1967) is one of the major advances in modern reconstructive plastic surgery. The history of the development of the surgical techniques is detailed in the various sections of the chapter.

ORGANIZATION OF THE TEAM

Before undertaking a program in craniofacial surgery, the plastic surgeon must first organize a multidisciplinary team (Christiansen and Evans, 1973; Munro, 1975; McCarthy, 1976). In addition to the plastic surgeons, the team should be composed of anesthesiologist, geneticist, neurologist, neurosurgeon, ophthalmologist, orthodontist, otolaryngologist, pediatrician and/or internist, physical anthropologist, prosthodontist, psychiatrist, psychologist, radiologist, social worker, and speech pathologist. Such organization not only provides for optimal preparation and care of the patients but also aids in the collection of longitudinal data.

Preoperative Planning. Preoperative planning, discussed later in the chapter, is directed by the plastic surgeon, although the patient is evaluated at a joint multidisciplinary conference by all the members of the team.

The initial ophthalmologic evaluation can include visual acuity, visual fields, exophthalmometry, funduscopic examination, and complete orthoptic evaluation. The study is also repeated in the postoperative period and at six-month intervals thereafter (McCarthy, 1976).

Radiographic studies establish the degree of the deformity and are also helpful in determining the type of surgical correction. As a minimum, cephalograms, panoramic roentgenograms, and routine skull and facial roentgenograms should be available.

The introduction of computed axial tomography (CT scan) has, in the authors' experience, obviated the need for invasive techniques, such as cerebral arteriograms and pneumoencephalograms (Becker and associates, 1976). The introduction of three-dimensional CT scans (Hemmy, David, and Herman, 1983; Marsh and Vannier, 1983) has provided the surgeon with realistic visualization of the craniofacial skeleton (Fig. 60–1), has allowed quantification of various volumes (Dufresne and associates, 1987), and has permitted more precise preoperative planning (Cutting and associates, 1986).

The geneticist is helpful in establishing the diagnosis; he can offer genetic counseling to the families and supervise any chromosomal or genetic studies. A pedigree of the families of patients with congenital deformity is essential.

A discussion of the role of the individual team members is beyond the scope of this chapter.

Designing the Surgical Procedure. After the decision has been made that surgery is indicated, the plastic surgeon works with the orthodontist in designing the actual surgical procedure. In the author's experience, the most valuable factors in the design are clinical and dental examination of the patient, photographs, dental study models, cephalograms (lateral and posteroanterior), and

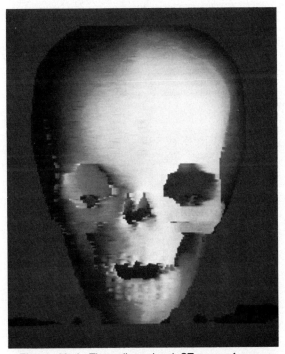

Figure 60–1. Three-dimensional CT scan of a young patient with orbital hypertelorism. Note the orbital asymmetry and the increase in the interorbital distance.

three-dimensional CT scans (Marsh and Vannier, 1985). A cast or montage of the patient's face and a portion of the cranium has been used occasionally for diagnosis and planning of the surgical correction. Polyurethane replicas have been employed by Munro (1975).

Cephalometric studies provide precise two-dimensional analysis of the osseous deformities, facilitate planning of the specific osteotomies, and permit longitudinal growth studies (Firmin, Coccaro, and Converse, 1974; McCarthy, Grayson, and Zide, 1982). The details of cephalometric planning are discussed in the subsequent sections of the chapter.

In addition, the orthodontist makes dental casts (models) if there are associated jaw deformities; the casts are essential in presurgical planning. If intermaxillary fixation is required after surgery, the teeth are individually banded, and preoperative orthodontics is accomplished.

Intraoperative Monitoring. Monitoring during the operation (Fig. 60–2) is the joint responsibility of the plastic surgeon, neurosurgeon, and anesthesiologist. When a combined intracranial-facial route is employed, the following monitoring lines are necessary: (1) a digital pulse oximeter; (2) a central venous pressure line, usually inserted into an antecubital vein; (3) an arterial line inserted percutaneously into the femoral (occasionally the radial) artery and connected to a monitoring device; (4) a peripheral venous line for administration of fluids and colloid; (5) a spinal drainage catheter inserted into the lumbar subarachnoid space and connected to a closed measuring system (approximately 60 ml of spinal fluid is allowed to drain before the catheter is temporarily clamped); (6) a bladder catheter for recording urinary output during the operative procedure; (7) a rectal thermal probe for continuous monitoring of core temperature; and (8) electrocardiographic leads connected to an oscilloscope. Edgerton and associates (1974) advocated monitoring of the intracranial pressure by a pressure screw that enters the posterior cranial subarachnoid space and is left in place for one week postoperatively.

Perioral endotracheal anesthesia is administered unless there are plans for intermaxillary fixation, in which case nasal intubation or a tracheotomy provides an alternative route for the administration of anesthesia; hypotensive anesthesia techniques are pre-

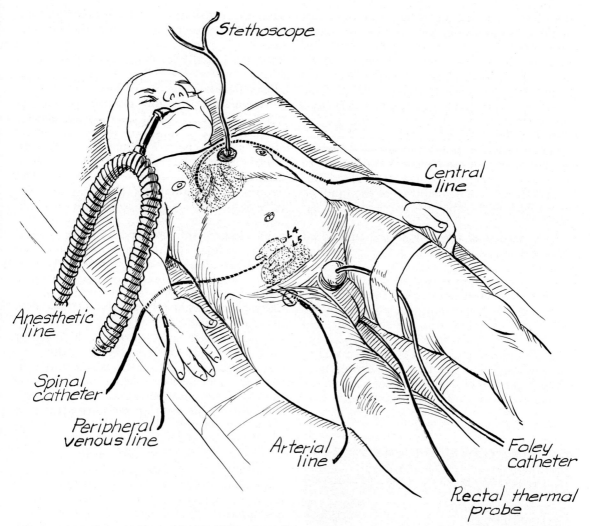

Stethoscope

Central
line

Anesthetic
line

Spinal
catheter

Peripheral
venous line

Arterial
line

Foley
catheter

Rectal thermal
probe

Figure 60–2. Intraoperative monitoring. Patient in position on the operating table. A digital pulse oximeter is not illustrated and the arterial line can also be inserted in the radial artery.

ferred and are associated with a significant diminution of intraoperative blood loss.

The cardiac apex beat and the passage of air into the left main stem bronchus are monitored with a precordial stethoscope.

Mannitol, 1 gm per kg of body weight, is initially given by rapid intravenous infusion. The combination of spinal fluid drainage, hyperventilation technique (calibrated by arterial blood gas monitoring), and mannitol administration ensures improved surgical (intracranial) exposure. Postoperative spinal drainage also aids in sealing any small dural lacerations.

Arterial blood gas levels and hematocrit readings are obtained every 30 minutes during the procedure. Serum electrolytes are monitored every two hours. The coagulation profile, initially documented in the preoperative period, is repeated during the surgical procedure.

Blood is crossmatched in a volume equal to approximately 150 per cent of the patient's estimated blood volume. The author's preference is that replacement be in the form of packed red cells and fresh frozen plasma to ensure coagulability of the blood. All blood transfusions are administered through a blood warmer. The adult patient can donate up to two units before surgery for intraoperative autotransfusion.

Postoperative Period. After a stay of several hours in the recovery room, during which period the anesthesiologist ensures the airway and may remove the endotracheal tube, the patient is transferred to the intensive care unit. At this stage, care of the patient is the joint responsibility of the plastic surgical and neurosurgical services. A wrap-around, moderately compressive head dressing is maintained for approximately two days. If the patient's course is stable, the arterial line is removed by the first postoperative day and the central venous line by the second day. Oral feeding is usually permitted on the first day. Antibiotics, instituted 24 hours before surgery, are continued for ten days and include an antistaphylococcal agent.

After the head dressing is removed, the patient is transferred to the plastic surgical service. Discharge follows the removal of sutures and the restoration of alimentation and a sense of well-being.

CRANIOFACIAL SKELETAL ANATOMY

As a preface to a description of craniofacial deformities, it is important to place emphasis on certain aspects of the skeletal anatomy of the orbits, cranial vault, and maxilla. Two bones, the sphenoid and ethmoid, serve as key structures in this anatomic region.

Sphenoid Bone. The sphenoid bone forms a major part of the cranial, orbital, and nasal cavities, as well as the walls of the temporal, infratemporal, and pterygopalatine fossae (Fig. 60–3). The body of the sphenoid encloses the two large sphenoidal sinuses; the inferior part of each side of the body gives origin to the greater wings and, in part, to the roots of the pterygoid process.

The greater wings spread laterally to form the floor of the middle cranial fossa. There are three surfaces of the greater wings—the cerebral, temporal, and orbital. The orbital surface forms the major portion of the lateral orbital wall; its posterior border forms the lower margin of the superior orbital fissure, while its lower border forms the lateral boundary of the inferior orbital fissure. The anterior edge articulates with the zygomatic bone, while the superior border articulates with the frontal bone.

The lesser wings of the sphenoid project

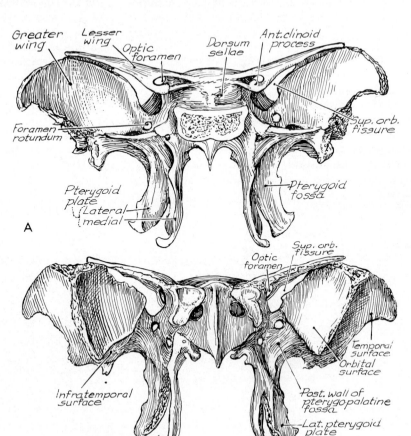

Figure 60–3. Sphenoid bone. *A*, Posterior view. *B*, Anterior view.

laterally from the anterosuperior aspect of the body of the sphenoid, and at their origin from the body of the sphenoid they surround the optic foramen. The upper surface of each lesser wing forms a part of the floor of the anterior cranial fossa, and the posterior border separates the anterior and middle cranial fossae. The lesser wings end medially in the anterior clinoid processes. The inferior surface of the lesser wing forms the most posterior portion of the roof of the orbit and ends as the boundary of the superior orbital fissure; the latter separates the greater and lesser wings.

The body of the sphenoid gives rise to the pterygoid processes, which also partially arise from the root of the greater wing. The lateral and medial pterygoid plates enclose the pterygoid fossa.

Ethmoid Bone. The ethmoid bone, a light and spongy bone situated anterior to the sphenoid, forms the upper part of the nose and the interorbital space, and lies between the two orbits (Fig. 60–4). It is formed of paired lateral masses (ethmoid labyrinths), the cribriform plate, and a central perpendicular plate that forms the skeletal framework of the posterosuperior portion of the nasal septum.

The two lateral masses contain the ethmoidal air cells as small cavities with thin bony walls. The ethmoidal cells are arranged in three groups, anterior, middle, and posterior; the latter articulate with the body of the sphenoid. From a surgical standpoint, it is important to emphasize that the ethmoids occupy the interorbital space. They are enclosed by the medial orbital walls. A thin plate of the ethmoid bone furnishes a major portion of the medial orbital wall posterior to the lacrimal groove: the lamina papyracea. The medial portion of each ethmoidal mass ends inferiorly in a free convoluted structure, the middle turbinate (concha), while near the middle portion of the ethmoidal mass the superior turbinate takes its origin. The ethmoidal cells open into the middle and superior meatus, and occasionally an ethmoidal cell migrates upward below the frontal sinus to form a frontoethmoidal cell.

Cribriform Plate and Olfactory Nerves. The paired cribriform plate, which connects the lateral masses of the ethmoids, forms the central roof of the nose; the roof of each ethmoidal mass, inclined upward from the area of junction with the cribriform plate, completes the roof of the nose and also separates the nasal and anterior cranial cavities (Fig. 60–4).

The perpendicular plate, the upper part of the nasal septum, projects superiorly above the level of the cribriform plate as the crista galli. Each half of the cribriform plate lies between the orbital plate of the frontal bone and the crista galli. The slender olfactory nerves penetrate the deeply grooved cribriform plate on either side of the crista galli to supply the specialized olfactory mucosa of the superior turbinate and part of the adjacent septum.

The olfactory bulb and tract lie beneath the frontal lobes in a midline position (Fig. 60–5). The olfactory nerves are 15 to 20 delicate fibers that arise bilaterally from bipolar cells in the nasal mucosa. They pass through the perforations of the cribriform

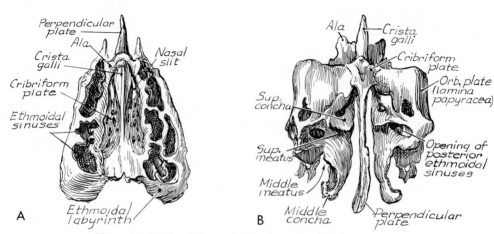

Figure 60–4. Ethmoid bone. *A,* View from above. *B,* Posterior view.

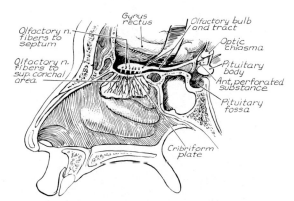

Figure 60–5. Sagittal section through the interorbital space showing the olfactory nerves penetrating the cribriform plate to enter into the olfactory bulb. The cerebral relationship of the olfactory tract is also shown.

plate and enter into the inferior aspect of the olfactory bulb. From the olfactory bulb a slender olfactory tract runs posteriorly to insert into the hemisphere immediately in front of the optic chiasma.

Bony Orbits. The bony orbits have been described as pyramidal in shape (Fig. 60–6). There are, however, some inaccuracies in this analogy. The widest diameter is not located at the orbital rim but approximately 1.5 cm within the orbital cavity. The medial wall of the orbit has a quadrilateral rather than a triangular configuration. Finally, the optic foramen does not lie posterior to the middle point of the base but lies on a more medial and slightly superiorly situated axis. In children, the floor of the orbit is situated at an even lower level in relation to the orbital rim because the maxillary sinus has not reached full development.

Although an artificial division, it is helpful in studying the bony orbit to divide it into four component parts: roof, lateral wall, medial wall, and floor (Fig. 60–6). The *roof of the orbit* is composed mainly of the orbital plate of the frontal bone, but posteriorly it receives a minor contribution from the lesser wing of the sphenoid. The fossa lodging the lacrimal gland is a depression situated along the anterior and lateral aspect under the shelter of the zygomatic process of the frontal bone. The anterior portion of the roof can be invaded by the supraorbital extension of the frontal sinus (Fig. 60–7). The thin roof separates the orbit from the anterior cranial fossa and from the middle cranial fossa in its posterolateral aspect (Fig. 60–8).

The *lateral wall,* which is relatively stout, is formed by the greater wing of the sphenoid, the frontal process of the zygoma, and the lesser wing of the sphenoid lateral to the optic foramen. The superior orbital fissure is a cleft that runs forward and upward from the apex between the roof and lateral wall. The fissure, which separates the greater and lesser wings of the sphenoid, gives passage to the three motor nerves to the extraocular muscles from the middle cranial fossa. The lateral wall of the orbit is related to the temporal fossa (Fig. 60–8), and posteriorly a small part of the wall lies between the orbit and the middle cranial fossa and temporal lobe of the brain—hence the ease and danger of entering the middle cranial fossa in performing an osteotomy through the posterior portion of the lateral orbital wall (Fig. 60–8). Between the floor and lateral wall of the orbit is the inferior orbital fissure, which communicates with the infratemporal fossa.

The *medial wall,* reinforced anteriorly by the frontal process of the maxilla, is relatively fragile and is formed from the frontal bone, the lacrimal bone, the lamina papyracea of the ethmoid, a small extension of the palatine bone, and part of the lesser wing of the sphenoid around the optic foramen (see Fig. 60–6). The lamina papyracea is the largest component and accounts for the structural weakness of the medial wall. The groove for the lacrimal sac is a broad vertical fossa lying partly on the anterior aspect of the lacrimal bone and partly in the frontal process of the maxilla; the anterior and posterior margins

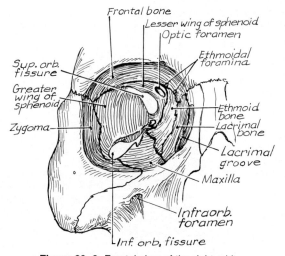

Figure 60–6. Frontal view of the right orbit.

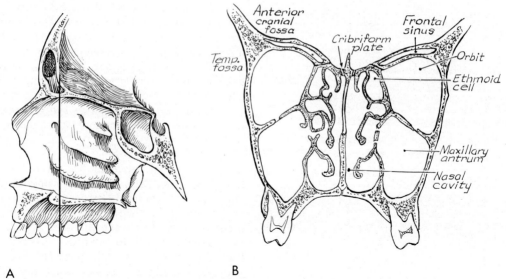

A   B

Figure 60–7. Frontal section showing the relationship of the bony orbits and the interorbital space to the anterior cranial fossa, frontal sinus, temporal fossa, maxillary sinus, and ethmoidal sinus.

of the lacrimal groove form the respective lacrimal crests. The groove is continuous with the nasolacrimal duct at the junction of the floor and medial wall of the orbit, passing into the inferior meatus of the nose. Between the roof and medial wall of the orbit are the anterior and posterior ethmoidal foramina, which lead into canals communicating with the medial part of the anterior cranial fossa.

The *floor of the orbit,* a frequent site of fracture, has no sharp line of demarcation with the medial wall because the orbital floor tilts upward in its medial aspect, while the medial wall has a progressively lateral incli-

nation. It is separated from the lateral wall by the inferior orbital (sphenomaxillary) fissure. The floor of the orbit (the roof of the maxillary sinus) is composed mainly of the orbital plate of the maxilla, a paper-thin structure medial to the infraorbital groove, and partly by the zygomatic bone anterior to the inferior orbital fissure. The infraorbital groove extends across the floor of the orbit beginning at about the middle of the inferior orbital fissure. Anteriorly it penetrates the thick inferior orbital rim as the infraorbital canal, which opens on the anterior surface of the maxilla as the infraorbital foramen.

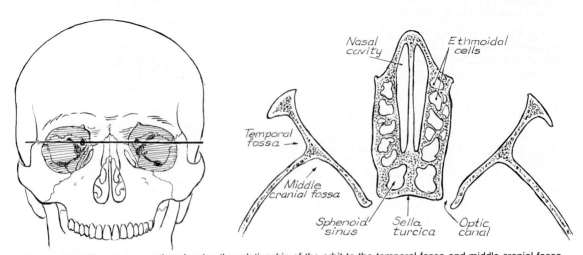

Figure 60–8. Transverse section showing the relationship of the orbit to the temporal fossa and middle cranial fossa.

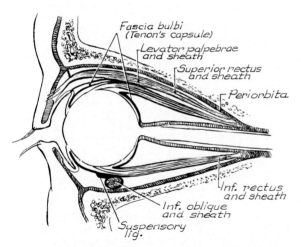

Figure 60–9. Sagittal section through the orbit showing the periorbita and intraorbital contents.

The periosteum of the orbit is designated as the periorbita and is continuous with the dura at those sites where the orbit communicates with the cranial cavity: the optic foramen, the superior orbital fissure, and the anterior and posterior ethmoidal canals (Fig. 60–9). The optic canal, 4 to 10 mm in length,

is the passage through which the optic nerve and ophthalmic artery pass from an intracranial to an intraorbital position. The canal is framed medially by the body of the sphenoid and laterally by the lesser wing, and is thus in close approximation to the sphenoid sinus and the posterior ethmoidal cells.

The reader is referred to Chapters 33 and 34 for additional details of orbital anatomy.

Anterior Cranial Fossa. The anterior cranial fossa supports the frontal lobes of the brain and the olfactory nerves, bulb, and tracts (Fig. 60–10). The floor of the anterior cranial fossa is composed largely of the orbital process of the frontal bone and, to a lesser extent, the cribriform plates of the ethmoid and the sphenoid bone (body and lesser wing). The lesser wing or sphenoid ridge forms a distinct margin between the anterior and middle cranial fossae; it terminates posteromedially in the anterior clinoid process.

Middle Cranial Fossa. The floor of the middle cranial fossa is thicker than that of the anterior cranial fossa. It is formed anteriorly by the greater wing of the sphenoid and posteriorly by the squama and upper surface of the petrous portions of the temporal

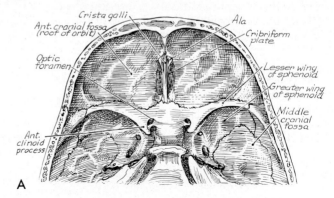

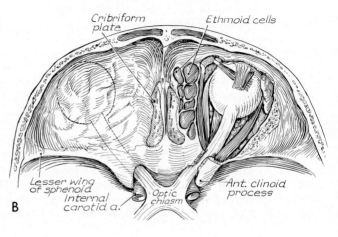

Figure 60–10. A, Superior view of the anterior and middle cranial fossae. B, Close-up view of A with the roof of the orbit and ethmoidal mass removed.

bone. The sella turcica in the body of the sphenoid serves to connect the two sides. Posteromedially, the posterior and middle cranial fossae are separated by the petrous ridges or edges of the petrous pyramids.

Maxilla. The maxilla, formed of paired halves, is relatively cuboidal in shape. It is situated anterior to the pterygoid processes, inferior to the ocular globes, and lateral to the nasal cavities. The maxilla, along with the zygoma, accounts for the prominence of the cheeks and also encloses the maxillary sinuses. The medial wall of the maxillary sinus is completed by the palatine plate, the ethmoidal and maxillary processes of the inferior nasal concha, and the uncinate process of the ethmoid.

The maxilla joins with the orbital, nasal, zygomatic, and palatine structures to form the midfacial skeleton. The frontal process of the maxilla extends upward to form part of the medial orbital wall and base of the nose; the zygomatic process connects with the zygoma in the formation of the cheek prominence; the alveolar process contains the teeth of the upper jaw; and the palatine process forms the major portion of the hard palate. The anterior (approximately) three-fourths of the palate is formed by the palatine processes of the maxilla and the palatine bones.

The piriform aperture of the nose is bounded above by the lower margin of the nasal bones, and laterally and below by the strong frontal processes of the maxilla.

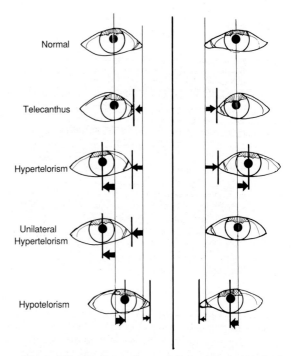

Figure 60–11. Comparison of normal and pathologic orbital anatomy. In telecanthus *only* the medial orbital walls are displaced laterally but the globes are in normal position. In hypertelorism the entire (circumferential) orbits and globes are displaced laterally. The opposite is true in hypotelorism. The vertical lines designate the medial orbital walls (inner) and pupillary planes (outer). (Redrawn from Becker, M. H., and McCarthy, J. G.: Congenital abnormalities. *In* Gonzalez, C., Becker, M. H., and Flanagan, J. (Eds.): Diagnostic Imaging in Ophthalmology. New York, Springer Verlag, 1984.)

ORBITAL HYPERTELORISM

"Ocular" hypertelorism was a term employed by Greig (1924) in his classic paper to describe two cases of congenital facial deformity with a "great breadth between the eyes." The term has been confusing, however, for a variety of reasons. Interpupillary distance can be misleadingly increased by the exotropia, which is so common in these patients. Furthermore, an illusion of hypertelorism results when there is a lateral displacement of the medial canthi (telecanthus), as occurs in a variety of deformities, such as Waardenburg's syndrome, canthus inversus, or blepharophimosis (Fig. 60–11). Patients with these deformities also show epicanthal folds and overlapping of the caruncles and the medial portion of the sclera. The patient in Figure 60–12*A* appears hyperteloric because

of the medial canthal soft tissue deformities, and yet the radiographic interorbital distance is normal. Orbital hypertelorism is, therefore, the preferred term and can be simply defined as an abnormally wide distance between the orbits (Fig. 60–12*B*).

Clinical Findings

Orbital Hypertelorism—Not a Clinical Syndrome. As emphasized by Tessier (1972), orbital hypertelorism is not a syndrome but is a physical finding associated with other cranial and facial malformations. Various prenatal clefts and premature synostoses of the cranial and facial sutures are the principal causes of orbital hypertelorism. Tessier (1974) classified orbital clefts into 15 types, anatomically arranged circumferentially around the orbit (see Chap. 59). Number 0 is

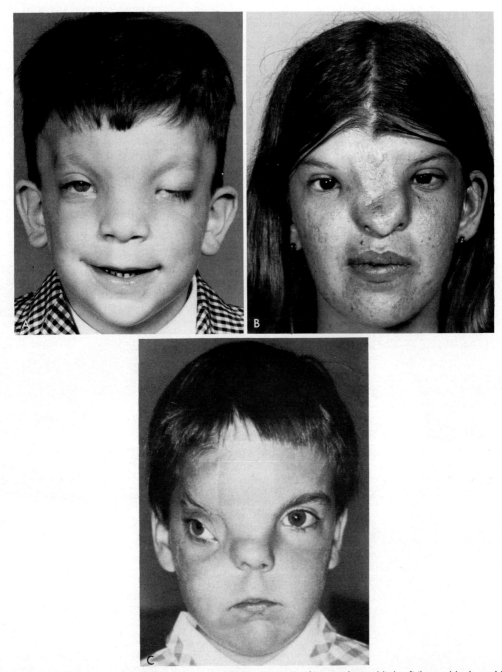

Figure 60–12. *A,* There is an illusion of orbital hypertelorism because of excess interorbital soft tissue, blepharophimosis, and coverage of the caruncles. Note the congenital ptosis of the left upper eyelid. *B,* Adolescent female with midline cleft, bifid nose, and orbital hypertelorism. Note the widow's peak and excess soft tissue in the interorbital area. The patient had undergone multiple operations to resect nasal soft tissue, with little improvement in facial appearance. *C,* The unilateral type of orbital hypertelorism secondary to orbital clefting, characterized by an absence of the lateral orbital wall and lateral rotation of the orbit.

a midline cleft ("median facial dysrhaphia") with bifid nose and orbital hypertelorism (Fig. 60–12B). More laterally situated clefts (numbers 1 to 3) had previously been designated as nasoocular clefts and are usually associated with orbital hypertelorism (Fig. 60–12C). The orbital clefts may involve the supraorbital ridge and frontal bone.

A meningoencephalocele is a congenital herniation of brain and meninges through a craniofacial skeletal defect. Meningoencephaloceles may be subdivided into occipital, parietal, basal, and sincipital. The latter group was further subdivided by Suwanwela and Suwanwela (1972) into frontoethmoidal (nasofrontal, nasoethmoidal, and nasoorbital), interfrontal, and craniofacial clefts. The skeletal and soft tissue morphology of frontoethmoidal meningoencephaloceles was described by David and associates (1984) with three-dimensional CT scan reconstructions. In all cases the cranial end of the defect was a hole in the anterior cranial fossa at the site of the foramen caecum at the junction of the frontal and ethmoid bones. The facial component of the defect determined the subclassification: nasofrontal, nasoethmoidal, or nasoorbital.

In the *nasofrontal type* the facial defect is at the junction of the frontal and nasal bones (Fig. 60–13).

In the *nasoethmoidal type* the facial defect lies between the nasal bones and nasal cartilages (Fig. 60–14).

The *nasoorbital* meningoencephaloceles present on the face through holes on the medial orbital wall (Fig. 60–15) (David and associates, 1984).

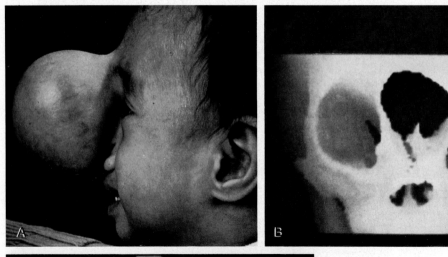

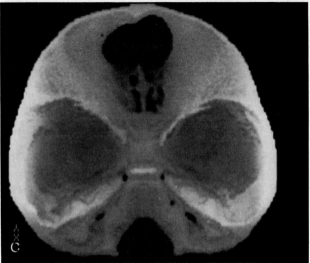

Figure 60–13. Nasofrontal type of frontoethmoidal meningoencephalocele. *A*, Lateral view of a patient with a large meningoencephalocele. *B, C,* Three-dimensional CT views. Note that the cranial end of the defect is at the junction of the frontal and ethmoid bones and the facial defect is at the nasofrontal junction. (Courtesy of Mr. David David.)

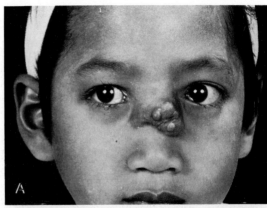

Figure 60–14. Nasoethmoidal type of frontoethmoidal meningoencephalocele. *A*, Frontal view. The facial defect is between the nasal bones and cartilages. *B*, Three-dimensional CT scan showing the cranial end of the defect at the junction of the frontal and ethmoid bones. (Courtesy of Mr. David David.)

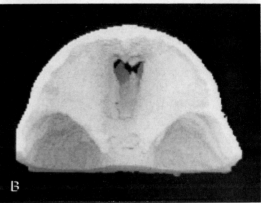

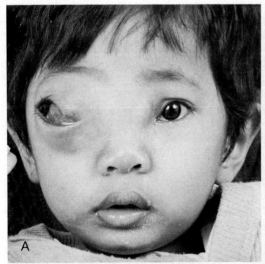

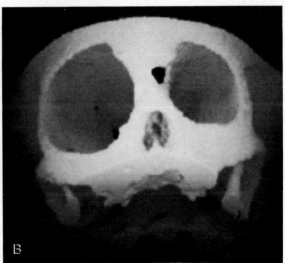

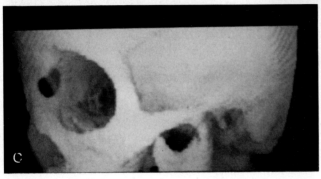

Figure 60–15. Nasoorbital type of fronto-ethmoidal meningoencephalocele. *A*, Frontal view showing the meningoencephalocele and hypertelorism. *B, C*, Three-dimensional CT scans. Note the right megaorbit and the facial defect along the medial orbital wall. There is a smaller defect of the left medial orbital wall. (Courtesy of Mr. David David.)

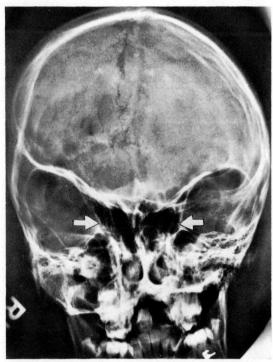

Figure 60–16. Posteroanterior cephalogram of a patient with orbital hypertelorism. Interorbital distance is measured between the two arrows. Note the inferior displacement of the cribriform place and the increase of the horizontal dimension of the ethmoid sinuses.

In all cases the face is elongated and the piriform aperture shorter and wider. Hypertelorism is present in all patients, but is not as severe as that observed in the midline clefts.

Dermoid cysts and glial tumors of the root of the nose result from cranial clefts that can be associated with orbital hypertelorism. Patients with craniofacial synostosis, especially Apert's syndrome, show some element of orbital hypertelorism (Tessier, 1971b), and medial translocation of the orbits, in addition to correction of the midface hypoplasia, is often indicated. Moss (1965) also demonstrated a significantly increased interorbital distance in a radiographic study of a population of patients with cleft lip or palate.

Measurement of Interorbital Distance. Interorbital distance is best measured radiographically. It is recorded as the shortest distance between the medial walls of the orbits at approximately the level of the junction of each medial angular process of the frontal bone with the maxillary and lacrimal bones (Currarino and Silverman, 1960) (Fig. 60–16).

Hansman (1966) documented percentile standards for the measurement of interorbital distances for both sexes from birth through age 25 years. Interorbital distance averages 16 mm at birth and increases to 25 mm by age 12 years. At approximately 13 years, the female curves begin to level off, but males show a continued increase in interorbital distance until approximately age 21. The average adult interorbital distance is 25 mm in females and 28 mm in males.

CT scan evaluation of the medial orbital walls further defines this relationship. As emphasized by Munro (1979), the configuration and shape of the medial orbital walls are variable in orbital hypertelorism, a finding that can influence the efficacy of the orbital translocation.

Pathologic Anatomy of Orbital Hypertelorism. The principal anatomic abnormality associated with the increase in interorbital distance is the horizontal widening of the ethmoid sinuses (Fig. 60–17) (Converse and associates, 1970). The increase in width of the ethmoid sinuses is usually limited to the anterior part of the ethmoid sinuses and does not affect the posterior ethmoidal cells and sphenoid sinus. While the roof of the ethmoid sinus may be enlarged, the cribriform plate usually is not significantly increased in width. It was this observation that made possible a one-stage intra-extracranial procedure for the correction of orbital hypertelorism with preservation of the cribriform plate and olfactory nerves (Converse and associates, 1970). When the roof of each ethmoidal mass is prolapsed, the cribriform plate can be depressed to a point 20 mm below the orbital roof (Tessier, 1972) (the normal is 10 mm) (Fig. 60–18). This anatomic finding serves as the main contraindication to a subcranial or extracranial approach in the surgical correction of the deformity.

The olfactory grooves can be enlarged and rounded, and the crista galli duplicated or absent. The sphenoid bone, including the portion of the lesser wing about the optic foramen, usually shows no abnormalities (Tessier, 1972). It was this latter finding by Tessier and associates (1967)—that the optic canals were in a relatively normal position—that encouraged surgical mobilization of the orbits to within 8 mm of the apex without fear of damage to the optic nerves. However, widely separated optic foramina can occasionally be detected on CT scans.

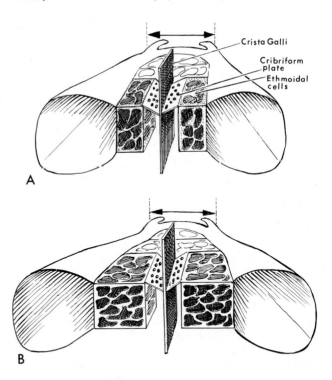

Figure 60–17. Diagrammatic representation of the interorbital space. *A,* Normal relationships between the orbit, the cribriform plate, and the ethmoidal sinuses. *B,* In orbital hypertelorism there is temporal divergence of the orbital cavities with overexpansion of the anterior ethmoidal cells. The posterior ethmoidal cells and the sphenoid sinus are not enlarged, and the distance between the optic foramina is usually not increased. The cribriform plate is usually inferiorly displaced. (From Converse, J. M., Ransohoff, J., Matthews, E. S., Smith, B., and Molenaar, A.: Ocular hypertelorism and pseudohypertelorism. Advances in surgical treatment. Plast. Reconstr. Surg., *45*:1, 1970, Copyright © 1970, The Williams & Wilkins Company, Baltimore.)

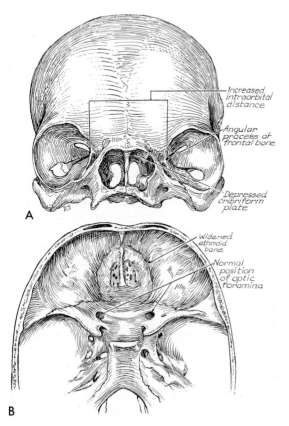

Figure 60–18. Infant skull showing orbital hypertelorism. *A,* Frontal view. Note the increased interorbital distance and depressed cribriform plate. *B,* Cranial view. There is widening of the roofs of the ethmoid labyrinth, but the optic foramina remain in normal position. (Skull supplied by Dr. Paul Tessier.)

The frontal bone is usually affected (Tessier, 1972). The glabella is less prominent and may be the site of a meningoencephalocele defect. Pneumatization of the frontal bone is occasionally quite extensive. Clefting of the frontal bone, as discussed earlier, is not an unusual finding.

The skeletal framework (Fig. 60–18) between the orbits adapts to the enlarged interorbital space and varies in its structure: the nasal bones may be small; the frontal processes of the maxilla are greatly widened; the lateral cartilages are also larger; the nasal bones, lateral cartilages, and nasal septum may be duplicated; and the alar cartilages of the bifid nasal tip are enlarged. Hyperplasia of the subcutaneous layer in the nasoorbital area is a peculiar, yet almost constant, finding.

As a result of the increase of the interorbital distance in orbital hypertelorism, there is a corresponding increase in the divergence of the axis of each orbit from the midsagittal plane (Converse and associates, 1970). The average angle of 25 degrees is increased up to 60 degrees in third degree hypertelorism; in such cases the lateral wall of the orbit is short in its anteroposterior dimension. The bilateral exotropia, so commonly seen in orbital hypertelorism, accentuates the deformity; convergence and binocular vision are not possible in the more severe forms. The extraocular muscle dysfunction associated with craniofacial deformities is discussed later in the chapter.

Whitaker, Katowitz, and Randall (1974) described a variety of lacrimal apparatus abnormalities in patients with orbital hypertelorism. These included nasolacrimal duct obstruction and absent puncta.

Classification of Orbital Hypertelorism. On the basis of Günther's work (1933), Tessier (1972) classified orbital hypertelorism according to the interorbital distance: first degree, 30 to 34 mm; second degree, greater than 34 mm with normal shape and orientation of the orbits; third degree, greater than 40 mm.

Operative Procedures

In orbital hypertelorism the design of the osteotomies and soft tissue surgery depends on decisions made following the clinical and radiologic examinations. A combined intra- and extracranial procedure is usually indicated; a subcranial procedure alone may be indicated in lesser forms of orbital hypertelorism when the cribriform plate is not prolapsed inferiorly into the interorbital space.

The types of osteotomies now being employed are the result of a progressive evolution of techniques over a period of 25 years. A number of palliative procedures had been performed on patients with orbital hypertelorism (Webster and Deming, 1950). These included medial advancement of the eyebrows, elimination of the epicanthal folds, and correction of the nasal bifidity. Converse and Smith (1962) described an operation based on their experience in the treatment of malunited nasoorbital fractures with telecanthus. An osteotomy of the entire medial orbital wall was performed, including the anterior lacrimal crest, thus displacing the medial wall toward the midline. A bone graft or an inorganic implant was placed along the lateral wall to fill the resulting void. The dorsum of the nose was also augmented with an autogenous iliac bone graft. This type of operation was only partly successful, as it failed to achieve any significant displacement of the *functional* orbital volume; Tessier (1972) reported that he attempted a slight modification of this operation without success. These operations failed to give satisfactory results because only a portion of the orbit was mobilized and the periorbita was not adequately elevated. Without mobilization of the *functional* orbital volume there could not be any significant medial displacement of the globe. The first substantive result was obtained by Schmid (1968) in a patient with unilateral orbital hypertelorism; he mobilized the medial orbital wall, the inferomedial portion of the floor, and the orbital roof. The roof osteotomy was possible because the patient had an unusually large frontal sinus.

Development of Intracranial Approach. Tessier and associates (1967) made the major breakthrough when they recognized that an intracranial approach was essential to ensure the safety and efficacy of the definitive corrective procedure. They performed intracranial and extracranial osteotomies of the orbital walls, roof, and floor and resected a central segment from the nasofrontal area and the floor of the anterior cranial fossa. The *functional* orbit on each side was mobilized after a circumferential elevation of the periorbita, respecting the apex of the orbit and the optic nerve as well as the nasolacrimal duct.

Tessier's operative approach consisted of two stages. In a first stage a craniotomy was performed; the frontal lobes were raised from the anterior cranial fossa; the olfactory nerves were severed; and a dermal graft was placed to reinforce the dura and prevent spinal fluid leakage. In a second stage the orbital osteotomies were performed, and a central segment including the cribriform plate and nasal septum was resected. After observing that the cribriform plate was not enlarged in any of the patients examined, Converse and associates (1970) developed a one-stage procedure with osteotomies similar to those of Tessier, except that the cribriform plate and olfactory function were preserved. Long-term studies by McCarthy (1979) demonstrate little change in gustatory or olfactory function after correction of orbital hypertelorism by this technique. Psillakis and associates (1981) modified the Converse technique by leaving a central, T-shaped segment of bone in the nasofrontal region to serve as a bony platform in reconstructing the nose. Edgerton, Udvarhely, and Knox (1970) also emphasized that patients with hypertelorism who have a low cribriform plate require an intracranial approach.

Development of Extracranial (Subcranial) Approach. The original osteotomies of Converse and Smith (1962) and Schmid (1968), involving either the medial orbital wall alone or the medial portions of the roof and floor of the orbit, represented an extension of the type of perinasal osteotomy employed in the treatment of Waardenburg's syndrome or other types of malformations with a lesser increase of the interorbital distance. Mustardé (1971) reported an osteotomy of the medial wall for the correction of orbital hypertelorism of moderate degree. Improved results have been obtained in patients with a moderate degree of orbital hypertelorism by means of a U-shaped osteotomy that involves both walls and the floor but spares the roof of the orbit (Tessier, Guiot, and Derome, 1973).

Surgical Correction of Associated Deformities. Before the combined craniofacial surgical correction of orbital hypertelorism is discussed, mention should be made of the repair of associated deformities. *Frontoethmoidal encephaloceles* can be corrected at the same time that orbital translocation surgery is performed for hypertelorism. The lesion can be adequately exposed through a combined intra- and extracranial route. The dura is opened on each side, the cerebral herniation is exposed under direct vision, and as much is conserved as possible. The neck of the encephalocele is transected; the dural defect is repaired and the orbital translocations are accomplished. The site of exit can be repaired with calvarial bone grafts (Fig. 60–19) (David and associates, 1984).

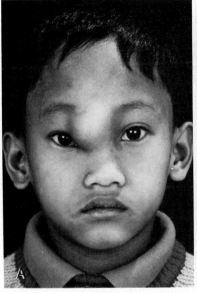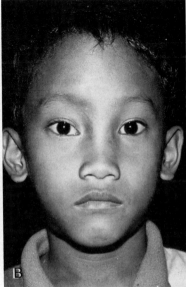

Figure 60–19. Correction of frontoethmoidal meningoencephalocele (nasoorbital type) through a combined craniofacial route. *A,* Preoperative view. *B,* Postoperative view. (Courtesy of Mr. David David.)

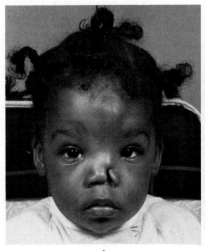
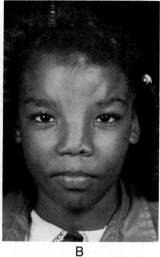

A

B

Figure 60–20. Surgical correction of a nasal cleft and frontal encephalocele. *A,* A 2 year old girl with a cleft involving the alar rim, nasal bone, medial canthus, and frontal bone (Tessier, no. 1). Note the frontal encephalocele and medial canthal dystopia. *B,* Appearance several years after repair of the alar defect with local flaps and closure of the frontal bone defect with an autogenous bone graft.

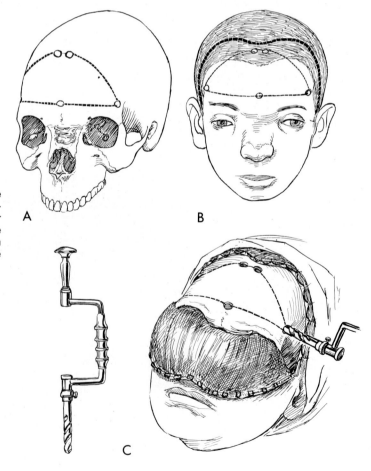

A

B

C

Figure 60–21. The neurosurgical stage of the operative procedure for the correction of orbital hypertelorism. *A,* Site of bur holes preparatory to raising a front bone flap. *B,* Relationship of the scalp incision to the frontal bone flap. *C,* Drilling the frontal bur holes.

Clefts of the nose (Fig. 60–20) (Ortiz-Monasterio, Fuente del Campo, and Dimopulos, 1987) and eyelids (coloboma) should also be corrected at the time of hypertelorism surgery.

TECHNIQUE OF COMBINED INTRA- AND EXTRACRANIAL APPROACH

Neurosurgical Stage. After the patient is prepared and draped, the neurosurgeon begins the operative procedure through a bifrontal scalp incision exposing the frontal bones (Fig. 60–21). A segment of frontal bone of sufficient size to provide exposure of the anterior cranial fossa is removed (Fig. 60–21*A*). The only difficulty that may be encountered is the intimate adherence of the dura and major venous channels penetrating into the inner table of the skull.

Each frontal lobe is raised from the anterior cranial fossa as far posteriorly as the crest of the lesser wing of the sphenoid (Fig. 60–22). The cribriform plate is spared, the raising of each frontal lobe ceasing when the lateral margin of the cribriform plate is reached. The crista galli may be duplicated, and in order to increase exposure it is occasionally necessary to resect it. At any time during the operative procedure, the spinal fluid drainage may be reopened and a small additional amount of mannitol injected to relax the brain and facilitate the exposure of the anterior cranial fossa.

Exposure of Skeletal Framework. At this point in the operation, the neurosurgeon

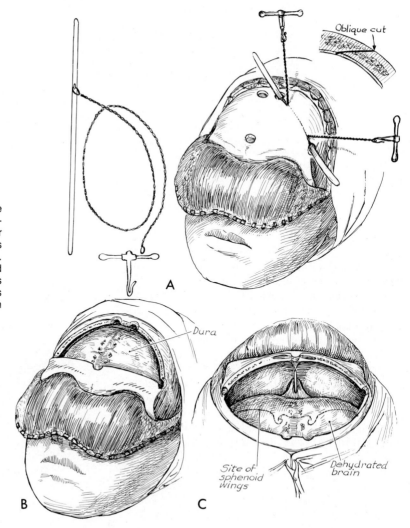

Figure 60–22. *A,* Bur holes are connected by beveled osteotomies made with a Gigli saw (or craniotome). *B,* The bone flap is removed and the dura is exposed. *C,* The frontal lobes are raised from the anterior cranial fossa as far posteriorly as the lesser wings of the sphenoid; the cribriform plate is spared.

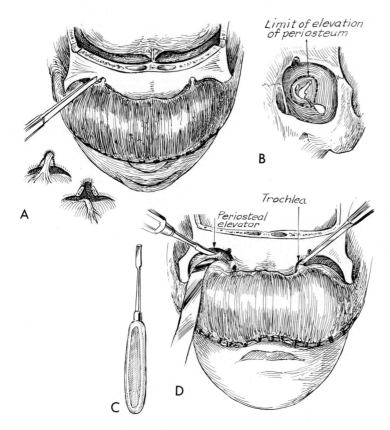

Figure 60–23. *A*, The supraorbital nerves are liberated by resecting the inferior border of the supraorbital foramen. *B*, Dotted lines indicate the posterior limit of the periosteal elevation within the orbit. *C*, Square-ended elevator used in raising the periorbita. *D*, The trochlea is detached subperiosteally.

retires, and the plastic surgeon raises the periorbita and the orbital contents in a subperiosteal plane. The periorbita is freed in a circumferential fashion from the roof and medial and lateral walls of the orbit as far back as the junction of the posterior and middle thirds of the orbit (Fig. 60–23). The apex of the orbit and nasolacrimal duct are thus spared. As the supraorbital ridge is reached, the trochlea of the superior oblique muscle is raised subperiosteally. The supraorbital nerve exits either through a notch in the supraorbital ridge or through a foramen; the nerve is preserved by subperiosteal elevation, leaving it attached to the soft tissues to preserve its continuity. The nerve is liberated from the bone by removing the inferior border of the foramen. The raising of the soft tissues is further continued over the nasal dorsum. Along the medial orbital wall, the medial canthal tendon is detached bilaterally and the lacrimal sac is raised from the lacrimal groove (Fig. 60–24). Its continuity with the nasolacrimal duct is preserved. The subperiosteal elevation of the soft tissues is continued over the lateral orbital walls and extended inferiorly to the level of a projected

line passing horizontally through the base of the piriform aperture. In this way the intraorbital contents are attached to two pedicles: the nasolacrimal duct and the optic stalk.

In some instances, when there is excess nasal soft tissue or when exposure of the distal portion of the nose is required for the

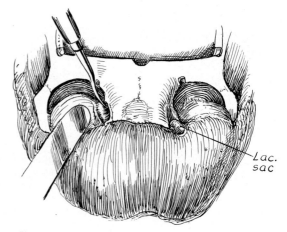

Figure 60–24. The lacrimal sac is raised from the lacrimal groove; its continuity with the nasolacrimal duct is preserved.

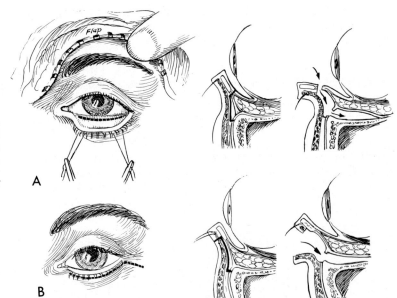

Figure 60–25. *A,* The transconjunctival approach to the orbital floor. Note how the incision is made anterior to the septum orbitale. *B,* The subciliary approach to the orbital floor through an incision near the lower border of the tarsus.

correction of a bifid, foreshortened, or asymmetric nose, it is necessary to make a midline incision along the dorsum to the nasal tip.

At this point a choice must be made as to whether the floor of the orbit should be approached through a subciliary (cutaneous) or transconjunctival incision. The latter approach, extended if necessary by a lateral canthotomy incision (Fig. 60–25*A*) has proved to give limited exposure of the floor of the orbit, the maxilla, and the zygoma. An incision through the lower lid leaves an inconspicuous scar, gives excellent exposure, and is probably easier to execute (Fig. 60–25*B*). The incision, made in a steplike fashion, should be below the tarsus to avoid postoperative shortening of the eyelid. The dissection of the orbital floor is extended in the nasal and temporal directions to join with the previously exposed medial and lateral walls. Subperiosteal elevation of the anterior aspect of the maxilla spares the infraorbital nerve; dissection is continued medially to the margins and base of the piriform aperture joining the previously exposed area of the lateral aspect of the nasal bone and frontal process of the maxilla.

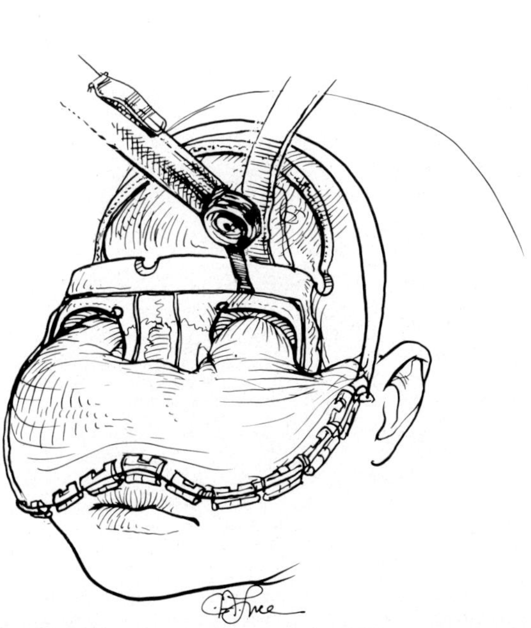

Supraorbital Osteotomy: The Frontal Bar. The first osteotomy is made in the supraorbital region inferior and parallel to the neurosurgeon's horizontal line of osteotomy in order to preserve a frontal bar (Fig. 60–26). The frontal bar, a technique suggested by Tessier, is usually 10 to 12 mm wide, and not only serves as a guide or reference line but also provides an element of stability in the medial translocation of the orbits. The frontal bar is particularly applicable when correction of the orbital hypertelorism requires the translocation of the orbits along a horizontal plane. It is useful as a means of fixation and as a guide in establishing the most anterior position of the orbit. When an upward and lateral rotation of the orbit is

Figure 60–26. The supraorbital osteotomy is made inferior and parallel to the frontal bone flap osteotomy.

indicated to correct antimongoloid slanting or to raise a low-lying orbit, the upward rotation is prevented by the frontal bar unless a segment of bone is removed from the lateral portion of the superior aspect of the mobilized orbit or from the lower edge of the frontal bar itself.

The supraorbital osteotomy line, made with a mechanical saw 1 cm above the roofs of the orbits, extends through the supraorbital ridge above the lateral orbital wall; medially it joins the vertical osteotomies through the bone of the widened interorbital area. The latter osteotomies make possible the resection of a measured section of bone either as a *single median segment* (Fig. 60–27) or as *two paramedian segments* (see Fig. 60–31). The latter technique is preferred for patients in whom the nasal dorsum is adequate and the nasofrontal angle is of normal appearance. When bone grafting is necessary to increase the projection of the nasal dorsum, the preserved central segment also provides a solid recipient site for a bone graft.

Total Mobilization of Lateral Orbital Wall. The lateral orbital wall is usually

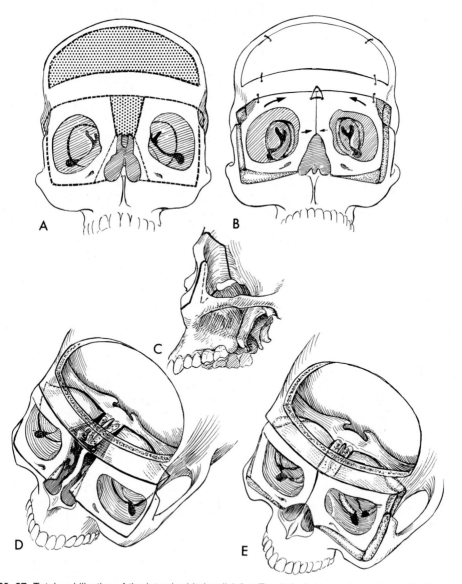

Figure 60–27. Total mobilization of the lateral orbital wall (after Tessier). *A,* Lines of osteotomy. *B,* After translocation of orbits and bone grafting. *C,* The lateral orbital rim only (zygoma) has been split. The remainder of the lateral wall is mobilized after the indicated osteotomy lines have been completed. *D,* Technique of preservation of the cribriform plate (after Converse). *E,* Bone grafting of the lateral orbital wall and anterior aspect of the maxilla.

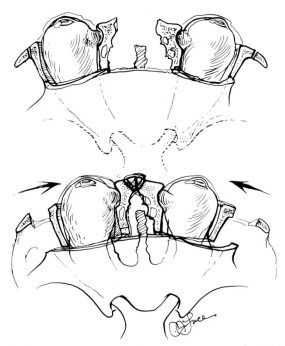

Figure 60–28. Total mobilization of the lateral orbital walls. The osteotomy is made at the junction with the cranium. Note the extent of exenteration of the interorbital space, in order to permit medial mobilization of the orbits. Bone grafts will be placed in the voids between the lateral walls and zygoma.

foreshortened in the sagittal dimension. The full-thickness lateral wall is sectioned at its junction with the cranium following the technique shown in Figure 60–28.

Infraorbital Osteotomy. Through the lower eyelid incision, the anterior aspect of the maxilla is sectioned, the line of osteotomy extending from the lateral osteotomy line horizontally across and below the inferior orbital nerve to the base of the frontal process of the maxilla (Fig. 60–29). This osteotomy line thus reaches the nasal cavity at the base or lateral wall of the piriform aperture. For the most part, the lines of osteotomy are made with the sagittal saw, but the medial extension, because of the thickness of the bone, is completed with an osteotome.

Resection of Median or Paramedian Sections of Bone from Anterior Wall of Interorbital Space and Exenteration of Intranasal Structures. The predetermined measured segment(s) of bone is/are resected, thus exposing the interorbital space (Fig. 60–30A). The enlarged ethmoidal cells are exenterated on each side. If the septum is bifid, the skeletal framework is resected, the mu-

cous membrane lining and the continuity of the lining with the cribriform plate being preserved. The olfactory mucosa contains the end organs of the olfactory nerves; preservation of the cribriform plate alone is not sufficient to preserve olfaction. If the mucosa of the upper portion of the septum and the mucosa over the superior turbinate are sacrificed, olfaction is compromised. Exenteration of the superior and a portion of the middle turbinate should be done in a submucous fashion; the mucosa should be preserved.

When paramedian segments of bone are resected, the resection of bone is continued upward into the cranial fossa on each side of the cribriform plate (Fig. 60–31).

Osteotomies of Anterior Cranial Fossa and Medial and Lateral Orbital Walls. A transverse line of osteotomy is extended across the roof of the orbit approximately 8 to 10 mm anterior to the optic nerve (Fig. 60–32A). The orbital roof osteotomy stops at the cribriform plate and is continued on the other side. The line of osteotomy is extended through the medial wall of the orbit, posterior to the posterior lacrimal crest. Laterally it joins the osteotomy through the lateral orbital wall. An area of bone forming the floor of the anterior cranial fossa, anterior and lateral to the cribriform plate, is outlined by these osteotomies (see Fig. 60–30C) and is resected with a fine-tapered osteotome. The osteotomy may be completed in part along the medial orbital wall by the oscillating saw, but final completion generally requires the use of an osteotome, passed from above obliquely downward.

Osteotomy of Orbital Floor. The floor of the orbit is sectioned through the lower eyelid approach, and the osteotomy traverses the floor of the orbit on each side of the inferior orbital fissure. This osteotomy is performed with the right-angled oscillating saw (Fig. 60–32B).

Mobilization of Functional Orbits. At this point in the operation the sectioned portions of the orbit should be easily movable. If resistance is encountered, it is usually caused by inadequate section of the thick frontal process of the maxilla near its base; this can be completed with an osteotome. Additional resistance can be provided by enlarged middle and inferior turbinates, which can be resected. The details of the osteotomies and orbital translocation are illustrated in Figures 60–28, 60–30, and 60–31.

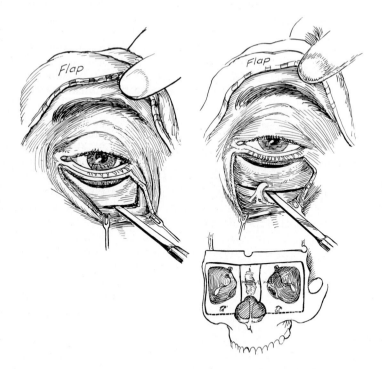

Figure 60–29. The infraorbital osteotomy through the anterior wall of the maxilla.

Figure 60–30. *A,* Resection of a median segment from the anterior wall of the interorbital space. The ethmoid cells and intranasal structures are exenterated. *B,* Osteotomies of the anterior cranial vault with preservation of the cribriform plate. *C,* Bone is resected anterior to the cribriform plate and also along each side of the cribriform plate to permit orbital translocation without impinging upon the olfactory nerves. *D,* The shape of the segments of bone resected from the anterior cranial fossa varies, depending on the type of translocation required to correct the deformity.

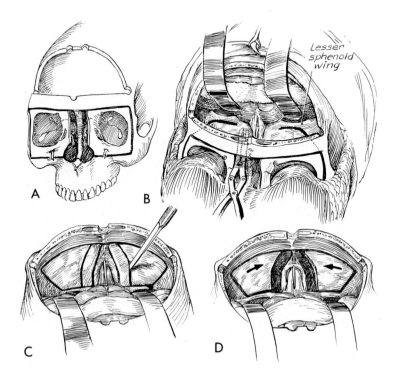

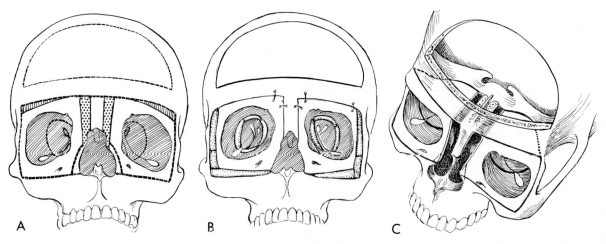

Figure 60–31. Paramedian resection of bone from the interorbital space. *A,* Outline of paramedian segments of predetermined size and shape. When there is a need to rotate the mobilized orbit to correct an antimongoloid slant, bone can be removed from the superolateral aspect of each supraorbital rim. *B,* After completion of the osteotomies, interosseous wiring and bone grafting are accomplished. *C,* The resection of bone is extended from the resected paramedian segments to the anterior cranial fossa on each side of the cribriform plate.

Figure 60–32. *A,* Osteotomy of the orbital roof and the posterior portion of the lateral wall. *B,* The orbital floor is sectioned on each side of the inferior orbital fissure with a right-angled oscillating saw.

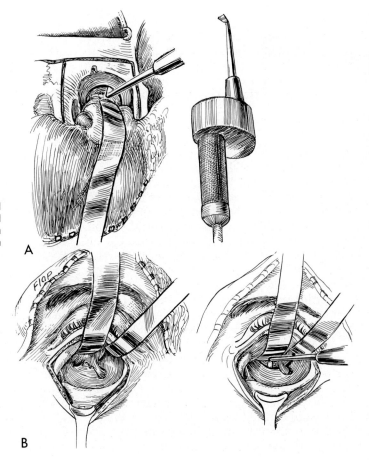

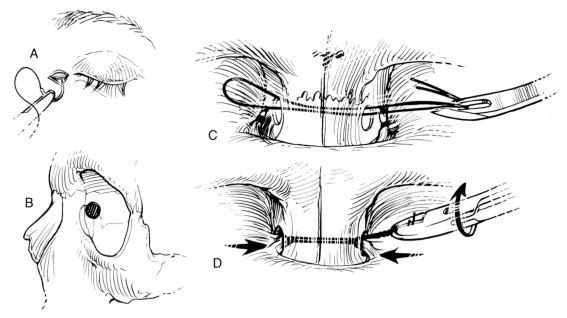

Figure 60–33. Medial canthopexy. *A,* The medial canthal tendon is identified by a small incision and the tendon is labeled with a suture (Munro). *B,* The bony fenestration should be made superior and well posterior to the lacrimal groove. *C, D,* The transnasal wire is sutured to both tendons and twisted under direct vision (on both sides). Note that the tendon is actually drawn into the bony fenestration.

Interosseous Fixation and Bone Grafting. After translocation of the orbits, miniplate fixation or interosseous wiring (No. 26 gauge stainless steel) is established between the mobilized orbits. The frontal bar, if employed, ensures adequate stabilization. Interosseous wire fixation is established at the junction of the frontal bar and medial walls of the mobilized segments (see Fig. 60–31*B*). Bone grafts are wedged into the gap in the lateral orbital wall and the zygoma in order to maintain the medial position of the orbits. Additional onlay bone grafts are placed in a horizontal fashion in the infraorbital region; split rib grafts are particularly suitable for this purpose. If this is not done, there is a resulting infraorbital depression, most noticeable in the profile view.

Medial Canthoplasties. Through sufficiently wide drill holes placed at a point superior and posterior to the lacrimal groove (Zide and McCarthy, 1983), the transnasal wires are passed after they have been inserted into the respective medial canthal tendons (Fig. 60–33). The critical points of a medial canthopexy are (1) identification of the medial canthal tendon for wire insertion, (2) circumferential mobilization of the periorbita for complete mobility of the medial canthal tendon mechanism and orbital contents, and (3) correct placement of the bony fenestration at a point superior and posterior to the lacrimal groove. When twisted, the wires should snug the skin of the canthal area against the nasoorbital skeleton.

Bifid Nose and Bone Grafting. Excess soft tissue must usually be removed along the nasal dorsum. In the bifid nose, a bone graft is placed over the bony dorsum after the tip of the nose has been remodeled by excising excess skin and any reduplicated cartilage.

The bone graft, which extends into the tip of the nose, is secured by lag screws or transnasal wiring. The distal tip of the nasal bone graft is secured under the resculpted alar domes. The nose can be lengthened by either a V-Y advancement or a Z-plasty performed in the nasofrontal angle. An additional benefit of the latter procedure is that it facilitates the redraping of the canthal skin over the nasal bones. In patients in whom the nose is foreshortened, lengthening can also be obtained by means of a skin flap from the glabellar area.

The lateral canthi may also be suspended by means of nylon sutures passed through each lateral canthal raphé and tendon and

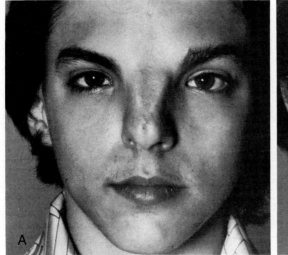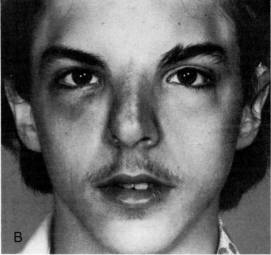

Figure 60–34. An adolescent male with orbital hypertelorism, midline cleft, and widow's peak. *A,* Preoperative view. *B,* Appearance after surgical correction as illustrated in Figure 60–31.

anchored through holes drilled in the lateral orbital rims.

Final Procedures. The dura is inspected for tears and cerebrospinal fluid leakage; tears are repaired by suture. The dura is suspended to the edges of the bony defect, passing the sutures through small drill holes. This procedure is designed to prevent dead space and the development of extradural hematoma. The frontal bone is replaced and secured with wire sutures. A full-head, moderately compressive dressing is placed after the various cutaneous incisions are coapted.

Patients who underwent craniofacial correction of orbital hypertelorism are illustrated in Figures 60–34, 60–35, and 60–36.

A variant of the above described technique for the correction of orbital hypertelorism was described by van der Meulen (1979). It is designed for patients with orbital hypertelorism who also have a midline cleft with an arching of the upper dental arch. The procedure (Fig. 60–37) not only translocates the orbits (and contents) but also levels and expands the maxillary dental occlusion.

Postoperative Treatment. The dressing is changed after 48 hours. Spinal fluid drainage is continued for 48 hours, since this is believed to lessen the risk of cerebrospinal fluid fistulas, which can be expected after such extensive bone and dural surgery. The hematocrit must be observed, inasmuch as it drops continuously for 48 to 72 hours. This is caused by the escape of blood from the naso-

Figure 60–35. Orbital hypertelorism in an adult male. *A,* Preoperative appearance. *B,* After correction by the technique illustrated in Figure 60–30.

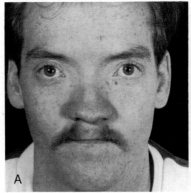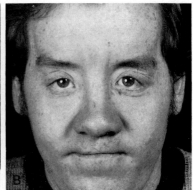

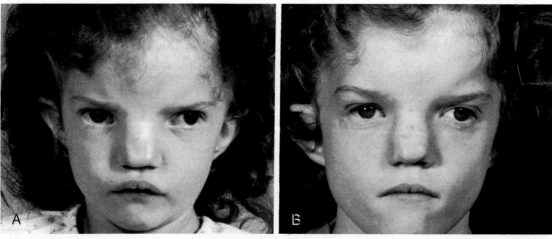

Figure 60–36. A 2 year old girl with orbital hypertelorism and midline cleft. There is also a small, incomplete midline upper lip cleft. *A,* Preoperative view. *B,* After correction of orbital hypertelorism, nasal bone grafting, and medial canthopexy. She awaits left-sided extraocular muscle surgery.

pharynx and from the donor sites of the bone grafts. Blood transfusions are usually necessary in the postoperative period.

Orbital Hypertelorism Surgery in Children. There appear to be a number of advantages to operating at an early age (in the authors' series the youngest patient was 2 years of age) (Fig. 60–36). The surgical procedure is performed with greater ease, and the psychologic advantages of early surgery

are self-evident. However, there is no evidence that either amblyopia or alternating vision is remedied.

The operative procedure is similar to that performed in adults. However, the maxillary portion of the osteotomy is limited by the presence of the follicles of the permanent teeth. The osteotomy through the maxilla should be placed at the level of the infraorbital foramen. The maxillary sinus is situated

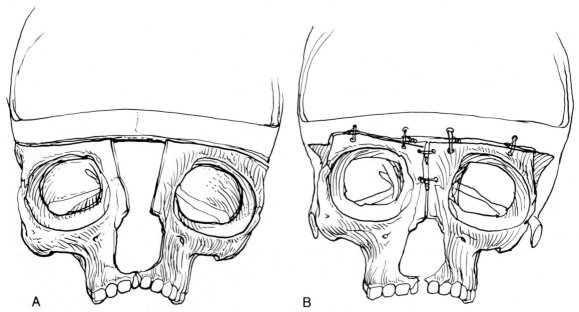

Figure 60–37. Correction of orbital hypertelorism and deformity of the maxillary dental arch. *A,* The maxillary occlusion is arched and constricted and the central nasoorbital segment has been excised. *B,* After medial translocation of the orbits and expansion and leveling of the maxillary arch with a palatal osteotomy (van der Meulen). Rigid skeletal fixation can also be used.

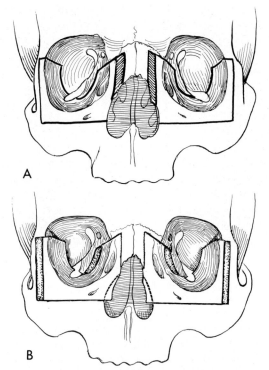

A

B

Figure 60–38. The subcranial approach. A, Lines of osteotomy (U-shaped) and the paramedian bony resection. B, Mobilized orbits with bone grafts.

Bone is resected from the nasal bones and/or frontal processes of the maxilla, either as a median segment or as two paramedian segments. The ethmoidal cells are exenterated in order to permit the medial translocation of the osteotomized portion of each orbit.

Preoperative Planning

In patients with orbital hypertelorism, preoperative radiographic planning (cephalograms and three-dimensional CT scans) provides information concerning the size and shape of the interorbital space, the medial orbital walls, the piriform aperture and the spatial relationships of the bony orbits. Any intracranial abnormalities can also be visualized.

In preoperative planning the interorbital distance should be reduced to 14 mm (Fig. 60–39). The most common causes of dissatisfaction with the postoperative result are incomplete exenteration of the interorbital space (middle and inferior turbinates and ethmoid air cells); inadequate surgical mobilization of the orbits and lateral orbital walls; and a poorly executed medial canthopexy (Hoffman and associates, 1988).

Longitudinal Studies

McCarthy and associates (1979) reported a longitudinal cephalometric study made after surgical correction of orbital hypertelorism. In the series of 18 patients, the age at the time of surgery ranged from 3 to 21 years and the amount of bone resected in the nasoglabellar region averaged 22.1 mm. A remarkable degree of stability of orbital position was demonstrated (Figs. 60–40, 60–41). Significant relapse or lateral drift of the orbits was observed in only three patients, two of whom had undergone surgery at age 4 years and the remaining patient at age 10 years. Nasomaxillary dimensions were normal except in patients who had previously undergone repair of an associated cleft palate or severe orbitofacial cleft. This evidence would indicate that the nasomaxillary dissection/resection, which is part of the hypertelorism correction, does not have a deleterious effect on development of the nasomaxillary complex in the growing child.

in a high position in children, as the final descent of the sinus awaits the eruption of the permanent teeth.

TECHNIQUE OF SUBCRANIAL APPROACH

Most patients in the authors' series have required an intracranial approach, since the cribriform plate descended lower than 10 mm below the superior rim of the orbit as measured on the posteroanterior cephalogram.

An intracranial approach is the only safe approach in the severe form of orbital hypertelorism with a low-lying cribriform plate. In less severe forms, a subcranial approach may be indicated because of the relatively greater simplicity of the operative procedure.

The U-Osteotomy. In patients with an interorbital distance of less than 40 mm, the medial wall, the floor, and the lateral wall of the orbit are mobilized, and the roof of the orbit is left intact (Fig. 60–38). The U-shaped osteotomy permits a medial translocation of each orbit after resection of the required segment of bone from the nasal skeletal area.

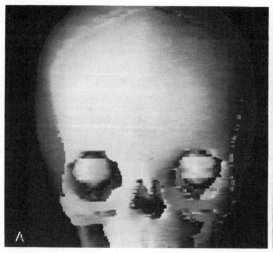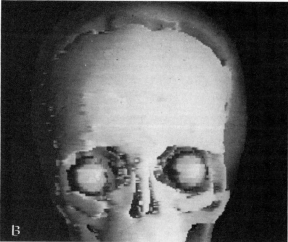

Figure 60–39. Three-dimensional CT evaluation of orbital hypertelorism correction. *A,* Preoperative scan. *B,* After orbital translocation. Note that the globes retain their relationship with the lateral orbital walls. There has been a significant reduction in the interorbital space but the globes are not related to the medial orbital walls.

In a preliminary study of Tessier's young patients who had undergone resection of the whole nasal septum as part of the correction of orbital hypertelorism, Tulasne (1985) reported that there was no evident effect on postoperative maxillary growth. However, he cautioned that there was absence of growth in the region of the anterior nasal spine (only in the anteroposterior dimension).

In a retrospective study of skeletal changes of patients who underwent corrective surgery for hypertelorism (Mulliken and associates, 1986) it was noted that relapse in interorbital distance tended to be related to the most increased preoperative interorbital measurements rather than to the age of the patient at the time of surgery, the orbital configuration, or the diagnosis. The study also suggested that corrective hypertelorism surgery performed in the growing child may interfere with anterior facial growth. There was also long-term resorption or deterioration of the reconstructed nasal complex.

Extraocular Muscle Function

In a study of the New York University patients with orbital hypertelorism who underwent corrective surgery, the majority showed exotropia or exophoria preoperatively (Choy and associates, 1979). There was a trend toward esotropia in the postoperative period. The amount of strabismus appears to

stabilize approximately six months after surgery. Accordingly, corrective strabismus surgery should be deferred for a minimum of six months after the orbital translocation procedure. Similar findings and conclusions were reported by Morax (1985).

ORBITAL HYPOTELORISM

Orbital hypotelorism is defined as a decrease in the distance between the medial orbital walls. Although clinically obvious, orbital hypotelorism is usually more apparent on the facial radiograph. Currarino and Silverman (1960), as mentioned earlier, documented the normal range of the interorbital distance. The mean value ranged from 15 mm in infancy to 23 mm at the age of 12 years.

Clinical Findings and Associated Anomalies

Orbital hypotelorism is an uncommon anomaly; it has been described in patients with trigonocephaly and arhinencephaly, oculodentodigital dysplasia (Gorlin, Meskin, and St. Geme, 1963), chromosome 18p syndrome (DeGrouchy, 1969), trisomy 13 syndrome (Smith, 1970), microcephaly, mongolism (Gerald and Silverman, 1965), and nasomaxillary hypoplasia (Binder, 1962). The

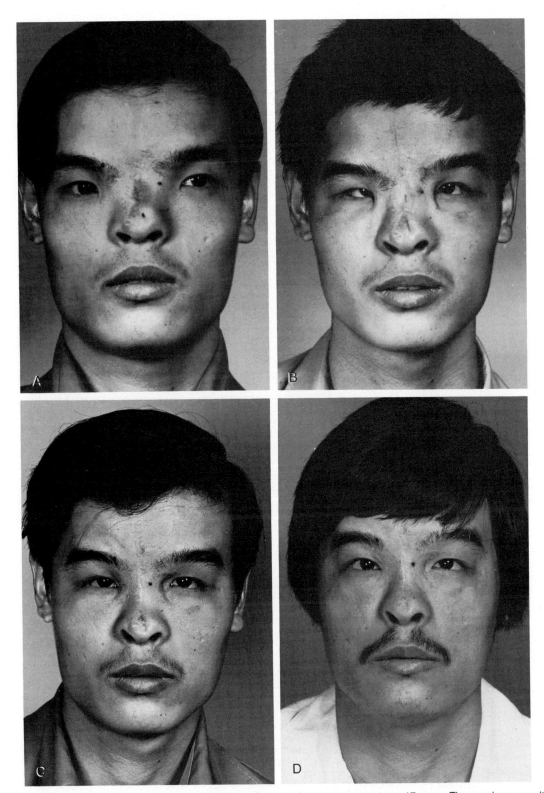

Figure 60–40. Correction of orbital hypertelorism. *A,* Preoperative appearance at age 17 years. The nasal scar resulted from a previous unsuccessful surgical procedure. *B,* Appearance six months after surgery before a secondary medial canthopexy. *C,* One-year postoperatively. *D,* Eight years postoperatively.

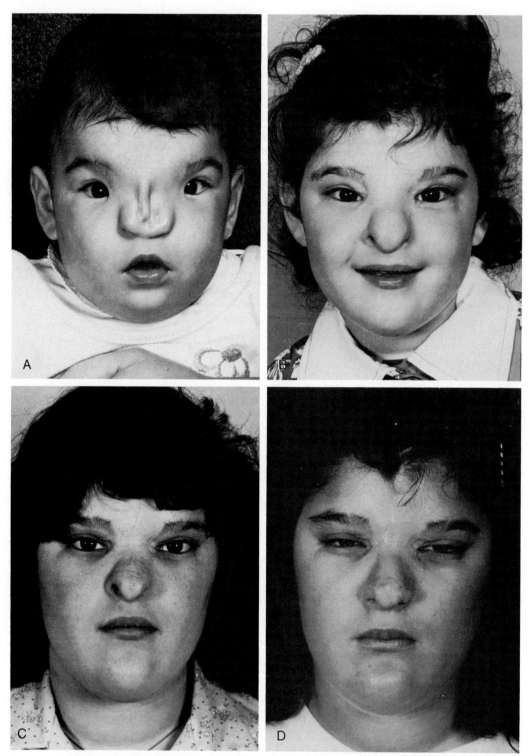

Figure 60–41. Correction of orbital hypertelorism and a midline facial cleft. *A,* Appearance at age 7 months. *B,* At age 4 years. Corrective surgery had been performed at age 2 years. *C,* At age 12 years. *D,* At age 17 years. In the interval the patient had undergone reconstructive nasal surgery, including the insertion of a bone graft and composite graft (auricular) reconstruction of the alar rims and bases.

Table 60–1. Differential Diagnosis of Orbital Hypotelorism

Trigonocephaly
Arhinencephaly
    Midline or lateral lip clefts
    Cebocephaly
    Ethmocephaly
    Cyclopia
    Nasomaxillary hypoplasia (Binder's)
Oculodentodigital dysplasia
Chromosome-18p syndrome
Trisomy 13 syndrome
Mongolism (Down syndrome)
Microcephaly of several types

---

differential diagnosis is outlined in Table 60–1.

Trigonocephaly. Trigonocephaly (see Chap. 61) is a congenital cranial anomaly characterized by a small and pointed forehead and attributed to premature closure of the metopic suture. The resulting decreased transverse dimension of the frontal bone gives a triangular configuration to the cranium. However, there have been reports of trigonocephaly with open metopic sutures (Currarino and Silverman, 1960).

Arhinencephaly. Arhinencephaly, initially described by Kundrat in 1882, represents a complex of faciocerebral malformations in which the olfactory nerves or other parts of the rhinencephalon ("nose brain") are absent. There are several forms. It can also be associated with midline or lateral clefts of the upper lip (McDonald, 1968).

Cebocephaly. Cebocephaly (James and Van Leeuwen, 1970) is a variant of arhinencephaly in which there is a hypoplastic and rudimentary nose with a single nostril but without any septum or columella (Fig. 60–42C). The flat roof of the nose is similar to that of the platyrrhine monkeys from which the name originates. The sphenoid and ethmoid bones are underdeveloped. Associated endocrine abnormalities are not unusual (Haworth, Medovy, and Lewis, 1960).

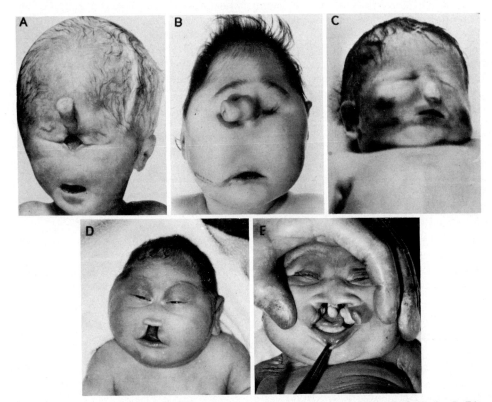

Figure 60–42. Spectrum of facies associated with holoprosencephaly-arhinencephaly. *A,* Cyclopia. *B,* Ethmocephaly. *C,* Cebocephaly. *D,* Orbital hypotelorism with median cleft lip. *E,* Orbital hypotelorism with hypoplastic intermaxillary segment. (Facies *A* is reproduced by permission from Potter, E. L.: Pathology of the Fetus and the Infant. 2nd Ed. Chicago, Year Book Medical Publishers, © 1961. The other four are from DeMyer, W.: Prenatal and developmental defects. *In* Barnett, H., and Einhorn. A. (Eds.): Pediatrics. 15th Ed. New York, Appleton-Century-Crofts, 1972.)

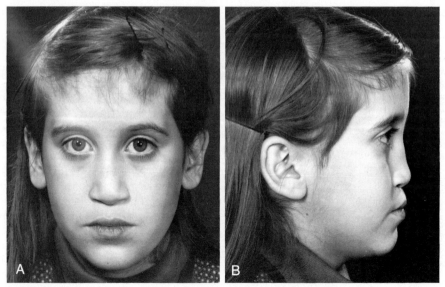

Figure 60–43. Orbital hypotelorism and Binder's syndrome (absence of the anterior nasal spine and nasomaxillary hypoplasia). *A*, Frontal view. *B*, Profile.

Ethmocephaly. Ethmocephaly is a more severe form of arhinencephaly—hypotelorism with accompanying microcephaly and a penis-like proboscis (Fig. 60–42*B*).

Cyclopia. Cyclopia is the most extreme variant of this group of anomalies (Currarino and Silverman, 1960). It is characterized by holoprosencephaly, a supraorbital proboscis, and a single or partly divided eye in a single orbit. Survival of any of these infants is rare (Fig. 60–42*A*).

Binder (1962) described a syndrome of nasomaxillary dysostosis characterized by a hypoplastic nose and maxilla, underdevelopment (absence) of the anterior nasal spine, and atrophy of the nasal mucosa (Fig. 60–43). The columella may be diminutive and there may be an anterior crossbite with Class III malocclusion. It is thought to be a variant of arhinencephaly. The syndrome is discussed in more detail in Chapter 29.

Embryologic Aspects

Any of the above facial configurations should arouse suspicion of severe forebrain maldevelopment. According to De Myer, Zeman, and Palmer (1964), such facies predict a highly characteristic brain anomaly.

In the embryologic development of the brain (Fig. 60–44), there are three distinct zones of demarcation in the cephalic end of the neural axis: the prosencephalon or forebrain, the mesencephalon or midbrain, and the rhombencephalon or hindbrain (Patten, 1968). The prosencephalon subsequently divides into the telencephalon (with its paired cerebral hemispheres) and the diencephalon (with its optic vesicles). Orbital hypotelorism is usually associated with abnormalities of telencephalon differentiation (e.g., holoprosencephaly, fused cerebral hemispheres, and a single ventricular cavity). The cortical areas of the telencephalon are divided into olfactory and nonolfactory areas. The olfactory cortex

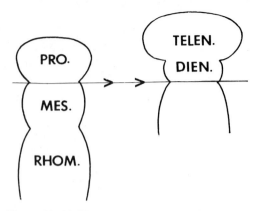

Figure 60–44. The primitive divisions of the brain. There are three zones of demarcation in the cephalic end of the neural axis; the prosencephalon differentiates into the telencephalon and diencephalon (after Patten).

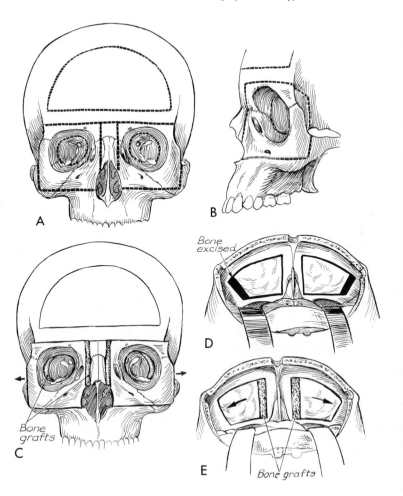

Figure 60–45. The surgical technique employed in the correction of orbital hypotelorism. *A, B, D,* Frontal, lateral, and cranial views showing the lines of the osteotomy and sites of bone excision *(solid black). C, E,* The orbits have been mobilized laterally and the resulting defects have been filled with bone grafts.

and the olfactory bulb and stalk constitute the rhinencephalon ("nose brain").

Yakovlev (1959), in a detailed study of ten specimens of arhinencephaly, showed that the common denominator of these malformations is a failure of evagination of the secondary telencephalic vesicles and of cleavage of the prosencephalon. The significant finding was that the failure of cleavage in the holosphere was complete anteriorly, whereas there were only abortive attempts at cleavage posteriorly.

Forebrain differentiation is induced by the prechordal mesoderm situated around the dorsal lip of the foregut; the hindbrain and spinal cord are induced by the mesoderm of the notochord. Prechordal mesoderm is also the anlage of the median facial bones, defects of which are seen in patients with orbital hypotelorism. The entomesodermal substrate, therefore, determines not only the differentiation of the ectoderm as nervous tissue but also its morphology. The mouth and nose are derived from the entomesoderm of the fore-

gut. Consequently, the development of arhinencephaly and its clinical variants can be attributed to a failure of invagination of the foregut, with secondary deficiency of the induction material in the rostral zone of the prosencephalic plate.

Surgical Correction

Through a bicoronal incision (Converse, McCarthy, and Wood-Smith, 1975a), a flap is raised as far inferiorly as the supraorbital ridges. A segment of frontal bone, sufficient to expose the anterior cranial fossa, is removed as described earlier for the correction of orbital hypertelorism. Through lower eyelid incisions, the orbital walls are exposed by circumferential elevation of the periorbita, as in the correction of orbital hypertelorism. Superior horizontal osteotomies are made approximately 10 mm above the supraorbital margins (Fig. 60–45A). The lines of osteotomy terminate at a point on the lateral orbital wall in the temporal fossa (Fig. 60–45*B*). Vertical components are extended in an inferior direction across the sphenoid and the body of the zygoma. A lower horizontal line of osteotomy traverses the zygoma and anterior maxilla below the infraorbital foramen, and ends at the piriform aperture. Paramedian osteotomies extend through the frontal process of the maxilla on each side and terminate at the superolateral border of the piriform aperture.

With an air driven, right-angled saw, a transverse cut of the orbital roof is made posterior to the anterior two-thirds of the orbit; it is extended down the medial wall posterior to the lacrimal groove. It traverses the floor of the orbit across the inferior orbital fissure to join the osteotomy of the lateral wall. Osteotomies lateral to the cribriform plate connect the superior horizontal and the roof osteotomies.

The orbits are translocated laterally (Fig. 60–45*D*). The resulting defects in the roof and in the nasofrontal areas are filled with bone grafts (Fig. 60–45*E*).

A patient with Binder's syndrome (nasomaxillary dysostosis) (Fig. 60–46) who underwent repair by the above technique (Converse, McCarthy, and Wood-Smith, 1975a) is illustrated.

In addition to orbital hypotelorism, nasomaxillary hypoplasia is a prominent finding in Binder's syndrome. The skeletal deficiency is most noticeable in the piriform aperture and the perinasal aspects of the midface. The nose is recessed and the columella is diminutive and retracted. There may be an anterior crossbite with Class III malocclusion.

In some patients with a satisfactory occlusion and a retruded nose, onlay bone grafting of the nose suffices (see Chap. 29). Additional bone grafts can be placed about the piriform aperture in a subperiosteal plane, and the columella may require lengthening.

If the patient is wearing a maxillary denture the Gillies (1923) nasomaxillary inlay technique (see Chap. 29) can be considered (Fig. 60–46).

Nasomaxillary hypoplasia associated with an anterior crossbite and Class III malocclusion is best corrected by a Le Fort II advancement osteotomy (Jackson, Moos, and Sharpe, 1981) (see Chap. 29).

OTHER INDICATIONS FOR CRANIOFACIAL SURGERY

Tumors of Frontoethmoid Area

As described in Chapter 69, craniofacial techniques can be employed in the en bloc resection of tumors involving the cranium, paranasal sinuses, and orbits.

Fibrous Dysplasia

Orbital displacement and diplopia can result from involvement of the orbit by fibrous dysplasia or the hyperostosis associated with a meningioma (Leeds and Seaman, 1962).

In a series of patients with fibrous dysplasia reported by Georgiade and associates (1955), 10 per cent had ethmoidal and orbital involvement. Of the 46 patients with fibrous dysplasia in another series, the frontal bone was involved in 29, the sphenoid in 19, and the ethmoid in 13 (Leeds and Seaman, 1962). In addition, the initial findings in seven patients were ophthalmologic (decreasing vision, proptosis, scotoma, and epiphora); proptosis was observed in 17 patients. In general, involvement of the cranial bones is much less frequent than that of the mandible and maxilla (Ramsey, Strong, and Frazell, 1968). The histopathology, radiographic appearance, and clinical course of fibrous dysplasia are also discussed in Chapters 33 and 69.

Craniofacial surgical techniques permit repositioning of the affected globe by total or subtotal resection of the lesion, reconstruction of the defect with bone grafts, and translocation of the affected orbit (Tessier, 1977; Munro and Chen, 1981; McCarthy and Zide, 1984).

COMPLICATIONS

In evaluating retrospective analyses of postoperative complications, one must recognize that most of the reported series combine intracranial operations and jaw surgical procedures. The magnitude of the surgical procedure for the former indicates that there would be a higher morbidity/mortality rate if this group were considered alone.

An analysis of the first 50 craniofacial

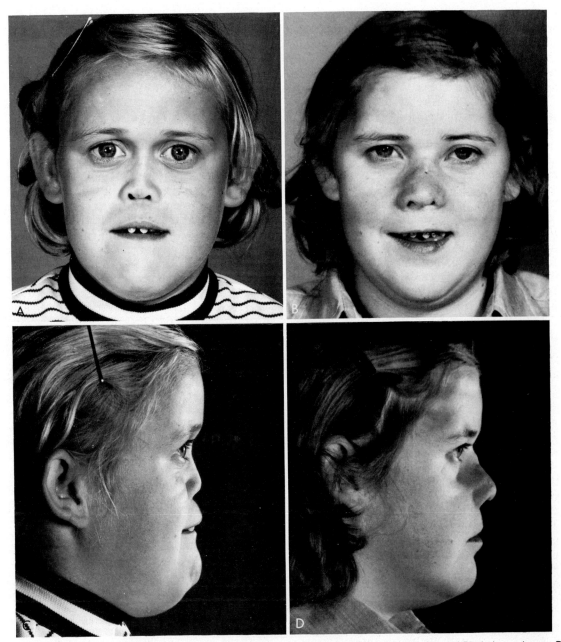

Figure 60–46. *A, C,* Preoperative appearance of a 14 year old girl with orbital hypotelorism and Binder's syndrome. *B, D,* Appearance after the technique illustrated in Figure 60–45 and a subsequent nasomaxillary skin graft inlay (Gillies).

operations (defined as having a craniotomy as part of the procedure) performed at the Institute of Reconstructive Plastic Surgery was reported by Converse, Wood-Smith, and McCarthy (1975b). There was one death in the series due to a combination of inadequate blood replacement and airway problems. Exsanguination and cardiac arrest occurred in another patient when the neurosurgeon encountered unsuspected venous extracranial and intracranial communications while raising the frontal bone plate; the patient was successfully resuscitated.

There were five postoperative neurologic complications, involving three patients with seizures, one with prolonged cerebral edema, and another with an epidural hematoma requiring evacuation. The seizures occurred only in those patients who had a history of intracranial surgery or injury. In the patient with cerebral edema, release of the head dressing, which had caused depression of the frontal bone flap, resulted in cessation of symptoms.

Six infections were recorded. All were local in nature, and staphylococci resistant to penicillin were cultured in all cases. None of the infections caused prolonged morbidity; all responded to antistaphylococcal agents, and surgical drainage procedures were not required.

Three patients had complications relating to the frontal bone: partial resorption of the frontal bone flap in one patient, and small areas of osteitis in two others. The former required bone grafting as a secondary procedure, and curettage and revision of the overlying cutaneous scar were necessary in the patients with chronic sequestration.

Persistent bleeding from the iliac bone donor sites occurred in three patients and necessitated blood transfusion.

There was no loss of visual acuity in any patients. Two had residual exophthalmos after surgical correction of craniofacial dysostosis. In both patients it was felt that surgical expansion of the orbits was inadequate. Postoperative extraocular muscle dysfunction was discussed earlier in the chapter.

Tessier (1974) reported two deaths among 65 patients undergoing surgery for the correction of orbital hypertelorism. Other complications included ulceration of the cornea, sequestration of the nasal or cranial bone graft, resorption of the frontal bone flap, and permanent anesthesia of the infraorbital nerve. Fracture of the cribriform plate was also a complication of the subcranial approach.

Edgerton and associates (1974) reviewed the complications associated with craniofacial surgery performed on 14 children between the ages of 3 weeks and 6 years. There was one death secondary to hypovolemia; one child had permanent brain damage following cardiac arrest during an operation for postoperative stress ulcers. Other complications included pulmonary edema (overhydration), fibrinolysis, and resorption of the cranial bone grafts.

In an international report from six centers, a retrospective analysis was conducted on the records of 793 patients who underwent a craniofacial surgical procedure (Whitaker and associates, 1979). It should be noted that extracranial procedures without an orbital component were also included. There were 13 deaths (1.6 per cent), six of which were of patients under 4 years of age. The causes of death were inadequate blood replacement, cerebral edema, respiratory obstruction, and sepsis. The infection rate was higher (6.2 per cent) after an intracranial procedure. Two patients had decreased vision in one eye. There was no evidence of brain damage but nine patients required an additional operation for cerebrospinal fluid leakage. Other reported problems included loss of bone grafts, excessive blood loss, ectropion, ptosis, nasolacrimal obstruction, and bone donor site morbidity (pneumothorax, contour irregularity, and pain).

A personal experience involving 1092 patients undergoing craniofacial procedures was reported by Munro (1985). The overall mortality was 0.64 per cent. Major complications developed in 14.3 per cent and included infection (6.7 per cent), cerebrospinal fluid leak (4.5 per cent of intracranial operations), blindness in four patients (but temporary in three), seizures in nine patients, and brain damage in one.

REFERENCES

Becker, M. H., McCarthy, J. G., Chase, N., Converse, J. M., and Genieser, N. B.: Computerized axial tomography of craniofacial malformations: a preliminary report. J. Dis. Child., *130*:17, 1976.

Binder, K. H.: Dysostosis Maxillo-Nasalis, ein Arhinencephaler Missbildungskomplex. Dtsch. Zahnaerztl. Z., *17*:438, 1962.

Caronni, E. P. (Ed.): Craniofacial Surgery. Boston, Little, Brown & Company, 1985.

Choy, A. E., Margolis, S., Breinin, G. M., and McCarthy, J. G.: Analysis of preoperative and postoperative extraocular muscle function in surgical translocation of bony orbits: a preliminary report. *In* Converse, J. M., McCarthy, J. G., and Wood-Smith, D. (Eds.): Symposium on Diagnosis and Treatment of Craniofacial Anomalies. St. Louis, MO, C. V. Mosby Company, 1979.

Christiansen, R. L., and Evans, C. A.: Habilitation of severe craniofacial anomalies. The challenge of new surgical procedures. Workshop, National Institute of Dental Research, Besthesda, MD, 1973.

Converse, J. M., McCarthy, J. G., and Wood-Smith, D.: Orbital hypotelorism: pathogenesis, associated faciocerebral anomalies, surgical correction. Plast. Reconstr. Surg., *56*:389, 1975a.

Converse, J. M., McCarthy, J. G., and Wood-Smith, D. (Eds.): Symposium on Diagnosis and Treatment of Craniofacial Anomalies. St. Louis, MO, C. V. Mosby Company, 1979.

Converse, J. M., Ransohoff, J., Mathews, E. S., Smith, B., and Molenaar, A.: Ocular hypertelorism and pseudohypertelorism. Advances in surgical treatment. Plast. Reconstr. Surg., *45*:1, 1970.

Converse, J. M., and Smith, B.: An operation for congenital and traumatic hypertelorism. *In* Troutman, R. C., Converse, J. M., and Smith, B. (Eds.): Plastic and Reconstructive Surgery of the Eye and Adnexa. London, Butterworths, 1962.

Converse, J. M., Wood-Smith, D., and McCarthy, J. G.: Report on a series of 50 craniofacial operations. Plast. Reconstr. Surg., *55*:283, 1975b.

Currarino, G., and Silverman, F. N.: Orbital hypertelorism, arhinencephaly and trigonocephaly. Radiology, *74*:206, 1960.

Cutting, C., Bookstein, F. L., Grayson, B., Fellingham, L., and McCarthy, J. G.: Three-dimensional computer-assisted design of craniofacial surgical procedures: optimization and interaction with cephalometric and CT-based models. Plast. Reconstr. Surg., *77*:877, 1986.

David, D. J., Sheffield, L., Simpson, D., and White, J.: Frontoethmoidal meningoencephaloceles: morphology and treatment. Br. J. Plast. Surg., *37*:271, 1984.

DeGrouchy, J.: The 18p, 18q and 18r syndromes. *In* Bergsma, D. (Ed.): Birth Defects: Original Article Series. Part V. Phenotypic Aspects of Chromosomal Aberrations. White Plains, New York, National Foundation–March of Dimes, 1969, p. 74.

De Myer, W., Zeman, W., and Palmer, C. G.: The face predicts the brain: diagnostic significance of median facial anomalies for holoprosencephaly (arhinencephaly). Pediatrics, *34*:256, 1964.

Dufresne, C. B., McCarthy, J. G., Cutting, C. B., Hoffman, W., and Epstein, F. J.: Volumetric quantification of intracranial and ventricular volume following cranial vault remodeling: a preliminary study. Plast. Reconstr. Surg., *79*:24, 1987.

Edgerton, M. T., Jane, J. A., Berry, F. A., and Fisher, J. C.: The feasibility of craniofacial osteotomies in infants and young children. Scand. J. Plast. Reconstr. Surg., *8*:164, 1974.

Edgerton, M. T., Udvarhely, G. B., and Knox, D. L.: The surgical correction of ocular hypertelorism. Ann. Surg., *172*:3, 1970.

Firmin, F., Coccaro, P. J., and Converse, J. M.: Cephalometric analysis in diagnosis and treatment of craniofacial dysostoses. Plast. Reconstr. Surg., *54*:300, 1974.

Georgiade, N., Masters, F., Horton, C., and Pickrell, K.: Ossifying fibromas (fibrous dysplasia) of the facial bones in children and adolescents. J. Pediatr., *46*:36, 1955.

Gerald, B. F., and Silverman, F. N.: Normal and abnormal interorbital distances with special reference to mongolism. Am. J. Roentgenol., *95*:154, 1965.

Gillies, H. D.: Deformities of the syphilitic nose. Br. Med. J., *29*:977, 1923.

Gorlin, R. J., Meskin, L. H., and St. Geme, J. W.: Oculodentodigital dysplasia. J. Pediatr., *63*:69, 1963.

Greig, D. M.: Hypertelorism: A hitherto undifferentiated congenital craniofacial deformity. Edinburgh Med. J., *31*:560, 1924.

Günther, H.: Konstitutionelle Anomalien des Augenabstandes und der Interorbitalbreite. Virchows Arch. Pathol. Anat., *290*:373, 1933.

Hansman, C. F.: Growth of interorbital distance and skull thickness as observed in roentgenographic measurements. Radiology, *86*:87, 1966.

Haworth, J. C., Medovy, H., and Lewis, A. J.: Cebocephaly with endocrine dysgenesis. J. Pediatr., *59*:726, 1960.

Hemmy, D. C., David, D. J., and Herman, G. T.: Three-dimensional reconstruction of craniofacial deformity using computed tomography. Neurosurgery, *13*:534, 1983.

Hoffman, W. Y., McCarthy, J. G., Cutting, C. B., and Zide, B. M.: Three-dimensional CT analysis of orbital hypertelorism correction. Submitted for publication.

Jackson, I. T., Moos, K. F., and Sharpe, D. T.: Total surgical management of Binder's syndrome. Ann. Plast. Surg., *7*:25, 1981.

James, E., and Van Leeuwen, G.: Familial cebocephaly. Case description and survey of the anomaly. Clin. Pediatr., *9*:491, 1970.

Kundrat, H.: Arhinencephalie als typische Art von Missbildung. Graz, Von Leuschner & Lubernsky, 1882.

Leeds, N., and Seaman, W. B.: Fibrous dysplasia of the skull and its differential diagnosis. A clinical and roentgenographic study of 46 cases. Radiology, *78*:570, 1962.

Marsh, J. L., and Vannier, M. W.: The "third" dimension in craniofacial surgery. Plast. Reconstr. Surg., *71*:759, 1983.

Marsh, J. L., and Vannier, M. W.: Comprehensive Care for Craniofacial Deformities. St Louis, MO, C. V. Mosby Company, 1985.

McCarthy, J. G.: The concept of a craniofacial anomalies center. Clin. Plast. Surg., *3*:611, 1976.

McCarthy, J. G.: A study of gustatory (taste) and olfactory function in craniofacial anomalies. Plast. Reconstr. Surg., *64*:52, 1979.

McCarthy, J. G., Coccaro, P. J., Wood-Smith, D., and Converse, J. M.: Longitudinal cephalometric studies following surgical correction of orbital hypertelorism: a preliminary report. *In* Converse, J. M., McCarthy, J. G. and Wood-Smith, D. (Eds.): Symposium on Diagnosis and Treatment of Craniofacial Anomalies. St. Louis, MO, C. V. Mosby Company, 1979.

McCarthy, J. G., Converse, J. M., Wood-Smith, D., and Casson, P. R.: Other applications of craniofacial surgical techniques. Presented at the American Association of Plastic Surgeons, Atlanta, Georgia, 1976a.

McCarthy, J. G., Converse, J. M., Wood-Smith, D., Choy, D., and Breinin, G. M.: Extraocular muscle function following craniofacial surgery. Transactions of the 6th International Congress of Plastic and Reconstructive Surgery. Paris, Masson, 1976b, p. 177.

McCarthy, J. G., Grayson, B., and Zide, B.: The relationship between the surgeon and orthodontist in orthognathic surgery. Clin. Plast. Surg., *9*:423, 1982.

McCarthy, J. G., and Zide, B. M.: The spectrum of calvarial bone grafting: introduction of the vascularized calvarial bone flap. Plast. Reconstr. Surg., *74*:10, 1984.

McDonald, R.: Median facial cleft with hypotelorism. Am. J. Dis. Child., *115*:728, 1968.

Morax, S.: Changing of the eye position after craniofacial surgery. *In* Caronni, E. P. (Ed.): Craniofacial Surgery. Boston, Little, Brown & Company, 1985.

Moss, M. L.: Hypertelorism and cleft palate deformity. Acta Anat., *61*:547, 1965.

Mulliken, J. B., Kaban, L. B., Evans, C. A., Strand, R. D., and Murray, J. E.: Facial skeletal changes following hypertelorbitism correction. Plast. Reconstr. Surg., *77*:7, 1986.

Munro, I. R.: Orbito-cranio-facial surgery: the team approach. Plast. Reconstr. Surg., *55*:170, 1975.

Munro, I. R.: Improving results in orbital hypertelorism correction. Ann. Plast. Surg., *2*:499, 1979.

Munro, I. R.: An analysis of 12 years of craniomaxillofacial surgery in Toronto. Plast. Reconstr. Surg., *76*:29, 1985.

Munro, I. R., and Chen, Y. -R.: Radical treatment for fronto-orbital dysplasia: the chain link fence. Plast. Reconstr. Surg., *67*:719, 1981.

Mustardé, J. C.: Plastic Surgery in Infancy and Childhood. Edinburgh, E. & S. Livingstone, 1971.

Ortiz-Monasterio, F., Fuente del Campo, A., and Dimopulos, A.: Nasal clefts. Ann. Plast. Surg., *18*:377, 1987.

Patten, B. M.: Human Embryology. New York, McGraw-Hill Book Company, 1968.

Psillakis, J. M., Zanini, S. A., Godoy, R., and Cardim, V. L.: Orbital hypertelorism: modification of the craniofacial osteotomy line. J. Maxillofac. Surg., *9*:10, 1981.

Ramsey, H. E., Strong, E. W., and Frazell, E. L.: Fibrous dysplasia of the craniofacial bones. Am. J. Surg., *116*:542, 1968.

Schmid, E.: Surgical-management of hypertelorism. *In* Longacre, J. J. (Ed.): Craniofacial Anomalies: Pathogenesis and Repair. Philadelphia, J. B. Lippincott Company, 1968, p. 155.

Smith, D. W.: 13 Trisomy syndromes. *In* Recognizable Patterns of Human Malformation. Philadelphia, W. B. Saunders Company, 1970, pp. 42, 43.

Suwanwela, C., and Suwanwela, N.: A morphological classification of sincipital encephalomeningoceles. J. Neurosurg., *36*:201, 1972.

Tessier, P.: The scope and principles, dangers and limitations and the need for special training in orbitocranial surgery. *In* Hueston, J. T.: Transactions of the Fifth International Congress of Plastic and Reconstructive Surgery, Melbourne, 1971. Australia, Butterworth, 1971a, pp. 903–929.

Tessier, P.: The definitive plastic surgical treatment of the severe facial deformities of craniofacial dysostosis, Crouzon's and Apert's disease. Plast. Reconstr. Surg., *48*:419, 1971b.

Tessier, P.: Orbital hypertelorism. 1. Successive surgical attempts, material and methods, causes and mechanisms. Scand. J. Plast. Surg., *6*:135, 1972.

Tessier, P.: Experiences in the treatment of orbital hypertelorism. Plast. Reconstr. Surg., *53*:1, 1974.

Tessier, P.: Reconstitution de l'étage anterieur de la base du crane dans les tumeurs begnignes orbitocraniennes. *In* Rougier, J., Tessier, P., Hervouet, F., Woillez, M., Lekieffre, M., and Derome, P. (Eds.): Chirurgie Plastique OrbitoPalpebrale. Paris, Masson, 1977, Chap. 13.

Tessier, P., Guiot, G., and Derome, P.: Orbital hypertelorism. II. Definitive treatment of orbital hypertelorism by craniofacial or by extracranial osteotomies. Scand. J. Plast. Reconstr. Surg., *7*:39, 1973.

Tessier, P., Guiot, G., Rougerie, J., Delbet, J. P., and Pastoriza, J.: Ostéotomies cranio-naso-orbitales. Hypertélorisme. Ann. Chir. Plast., *12*:103, 1967.

Tulasne, J. F.: Maxillary growth following total septal resection in teleorbitism. *In* Caronni, E. P. (Ed.): Craniofacial Surgery. Boston, Little, Brown & Company, 1985.

van der Meulen, J. C.: Medial faciotomy. Br. J. Plast. Surg., *32*:339, 1979.

Webster, J. P., and Deming, E. G.: Surgical treatment of the bifid nose. Plast. Reconstr. Surg., *6*:1, 1950.

Whitaker, L. A., Katowitz, J. A., and Randall, P.: The nasolacrimal apparatus in congenital facial anomalies. J. Maxillofac. Surg., *2*:59, 1974.

Whitaker, L. A., Munro, I. R., Salyer, K. E., Jackson, I. T., Ortiz-Monasterio, F., and Marchac, D.: Combined report of problems and complications in 793 craniofacial operations. Plast. Reconstr. Surg., *64*:198, 1979.

Yakovlev, P. I.: Pathoarchitectonic studies of cerebral malformations. III. Arhinencephalies (holotelencephalies). J. Neuropathol. Exp. Neurol., *18*:22, 1959.

Zide, B. M., and McCarthy, J. G.: The medial canthus revisited: anatomical basis of medial canthopexy. Ann. Plast. Surg., *11*:1, 1983.

61

Craniosynostosis

Joseph G. McCarthy
Fred J. Epstein
Donald Wood-Smith

Hippocrates provided the first description of craniostenoses in 100 B.C. He noted the variability in appearance of the calvarial deformities and correlated it with the pattern of cranial sutural involvement (Montaut and Stricker, 1977). Celsus (25 B.C. to 50 A.D.) described some skulls without sutures, but failed to give specific details. Oribasios, a Greek physician at the time of the Emperor Julian, reported the presence of cranial deformities in association with palatine deformities. In 1557 Lycosthene described an infant with a deformity of the skull and limbs, the syndrome of acrocephalosyndactyly subsequently described by Apert (1906). Crouzon (1912) described a mother and daughter, both of whom had the same malformation of the face and head, and coined the term "hereditary craniofacial dysostosis." Von Graefe (1866) noted the association of craniostenosis and blindness; Friedenwald (1893) and Meltzer (1908) established the association of craniostenosis and optic atrophy. \
Craniosynostosis is the term that desig-nates premature fusion of one or more sutures in either the cranial vault or cranial base. While most cases of *isolated craniosynostosis* occur in a sporadic fashion, there have been reported examples of autosomal dominant and autosomal recessive inheritance (Gorlin, Pindborg, and Cohen, 1976). In the familial cases the same suture or different single/multiple sutures may be involved in affected individuals. In contrast, there are distinct *craniofacial synostosis syndromes* that share common features such as suture synostoses, midface hypoplasia, and facial and limb abnormalities. In a comprehensive review of the craniofacial synostosis syndromes, Cohen (1975) listed 37, the most common of which are the kleeblattschädel anomaly, Crouzon's disease, Apert's syndrome, Pfeiffer's syndrome, the Saethre-Chotzen syndrome, and Carpenter's syndrome. Table 61–1 outlines the various craniosynostoses.

ETIOPATHOGENESIS

The etiopathogenesis of craniosynostosis remains obscure. Virchow (1851) noted that there is a cessation of growth in a direction perpendicular to that of the affected suture while growth proceeds (with or without overcompensation) in a parallel direction.

The cranial sutures are no longer considered to be sites of primary bone growth; the skull does not grow in response to a multiplication of the suture tissues (Enlow, 1975). Growth or change at the suture area is a secondary, compensatory, and mechanically obligatory event, following the primary growth of the enclosed and protected neural (brain) and facial soft tissue (ocular globes)

Table 61–1. Craniosynostoses and Craniofacial Synostoses Syndromes

| | Craniosynostoses | |
	Suture	Literal Translation
Scaphocephaly	Sagittal	Boat skull
Trigonocephaly	Metopic	Triangle skull
Brachycephaly	Bicoronal	Short skull
Plagiocephaly	Unicoronal	Oblique skull
Acrocephaly/ Turricephaly	Multiple	Topmost/ tower skull
Oxycephaly	Multiple	Sharp skull
Craniofacial Synostoses Syndromes		
Kleeblattschädel anomaly	Multiple	Cloverleaf Skull
Crouzon's disease	Multiple	–
Apert's syndrome	Single or multiple	Acrocephaly
Pfeiffer's syndrome	Single or multiple	Acrocephaly
Saethre-Chotzen syndrome	Single or multiple	
Carpenter's syndrome	Single or multiple	

matrices. The bones of the calvaria are displaced outward by the enlarging brain. Each bone of the domed skull roof responds to the expansion of the brain by depositing new bone at the contact edges of the sutures.

Moss (1959) believed that cranial suture stenosis can be regarded only as an extrinsically influenced event rather than as a primary etiopathogenic factor. He speculated that the architecture of the attached dura plays a major role in cranial suture synosto-

sis. Premature fusion of the metopic suture is associated with an abnormal kyphosis of the cranial base. In premature coronal closure, there is a malrelation of the points of dural attachment at the superior edges of the lesser sphenoid wings, thereby affecting the points of origin of the coronal suture. Similarly, in sagittal synostosis there is a spatial malrelation of the median anterior attachment of the falx cerebri or crista galli at the anterior cranial base. According to this theory, abnormal tensile stresses secondary to abnormalities in the cranial base can be transmitted through the dura to various suture areas to cause premature synostosis. Because of attachment at the cranial sutures the dura-transmitted forces could initiate the osteogenic process, leading to premature synostosis. Investigations have also demonstrated condensations of dural tissue that are direct continuations of the strong cranial base capsule and could therefore be capable of transmitting any abnormal tension directly to the cranial sutures (Blechschmidt, 1976).

In a newborn primate animal model, surgical fusion of the smaller craniofacial sutures (frontozygomatic and sphenozygomatic) with autogenous bone grafts resulted in hypoplasia of the sphenoid and zygomatic bones (McCarthy, Coccaro, and Keller, 1985). A more significant finding was a morphologic change in sutures at a distance from the manipulated suture (Fig. 61–1). There were abnormalities in the topographic relationship of the entire craniofacial skeleton.

There is also clinical evidence supporting

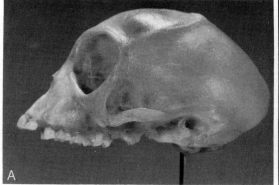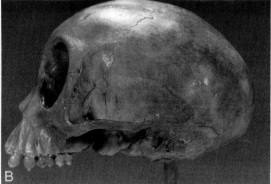

Figure 61–1. Obliteration and fusion (autogenous bone) of the frontozygomatic and sphenozygomatic suture in the newborn monkey resulted in hypoplasia of the sphenoid and zygomatic bone and prominent changes in the coronal, sagittal, and lambdoid sutures. *A,* Experimental skull. *B,* Control skull. (From McCarthy, J. G., Coccaro, P. J., and Keller, A.: Craniofacial suture manipulation in the newborn rhesus monkey. *In* Caronii, E. P. (Ed.): Craniofacial Surgery. Boston, Little, Brown & Company, 1985. Copyright 1985, Little, Brown & Company.)

the concept of Moss (1959) that suture synostosis is only a secondary manifestation of an underlying malformation in the basicranium. A detailed postmortem examination of a stillborn fetus of 24 to 26 weeks' gestation with the classic morphologic stigmata of Apert's syndrome failed to show clinical or histologic evidence of premature fusion of any of the cranial sutures or basilar synchondroses (Stewart, Dixon, and Cohen, 1977). There was, however, shortening of the cranial base in the sagittal dimensions, as well as a steep upward inclination of the anterior cranial fossa and lesser wings of the sphenoid.

An abnormally high incidence of premature cranial stenosis and craniofacial synostosis has been observed in patients with rickets, vitamin D resistant rickets, and other metabolic disorders, such as Hurler's syndrome and achondroplasia, that affect generalized skeletal development (McCarthy and Reid, 1979).

Some of the above-mentioned observations suggest that any pathologic condition interfering with the normal development of the cranial bones can cause a compensatory synostosis of the cranial sutures.

CLINICAL AND RADIOGRAPHIC FINDINGS

The radiographic findings are discussed with each syndrome below.

Scaphocephaly–Sagittal Synostosis. Premature fusion of the sagittal suture is characterized by a narrow, elongated cranial vault and reduced bitemporal dimension (Figs. 61–2, 61–3). Usually, nonfamilial scaphocephaly is the most common of the isolated suture synostoses, and it occurs predominantly in males (Shillito and Matson, 1968).

Trigonocephaly–Metopic Synostosis. There is a triangular-shaped deformity of the anterior cranial fossa and forehead resembling a midline keel (Fig. 61–4) (Marsh and Vannier, 1985). The orbits are medially displaced, with an associated hypotelorism.

Brachycephaly–Bilateral Coronal Synostosis. Fusion of both coronal sutures is associated with a reduction of the anteroposterior dimension of the cranial vault and a compensatory increase in the bitemporal distance (Fig. 61–5). A mild degree of exophthalmos can be observed if the supraorbital rim is recessed. Underdevelopment of the midface is unusual.

Plagiocephaly–Unilateral Coronal Synostosis. Flattening of the forehead and recession and elevation of the brow and superolateral aspect of the orbit are observed on the affected side (Fig. 61–6). On the contralateral side, persistent growth produces frontal bossing, inferolateral orbital dystopia, and bulging of the occipital prominence. The nasal tip is usually deviated to the affected side and the ear on the more affected side can be more superiorly and anteriorly positioned.

The above findings (plagiocephaly) can also be noted in patients without evidence of a coronal synostosis, e.g., those with unilateral

Figure 61–2. Scaphocephaly–sagittal synostosis in an infant. *A,* Frontal view. *B,* Profile.

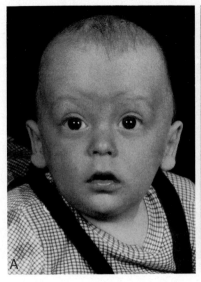
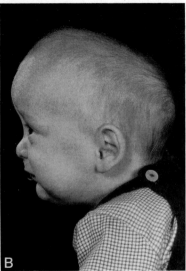

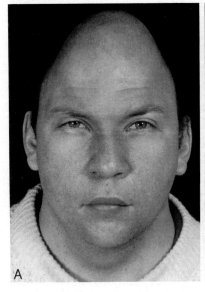
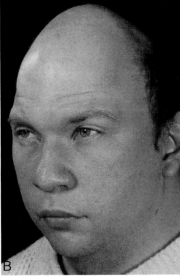

Figure 61–3. Scaphocephaly–sagittal synostosis in an adult. *A,* Frontal view. *B,* Three-quarters view.

Figure 61–4. Trigonocephaly–metopic synostosis in an infant. *A,* Frontal view. Note the orbital hypertelorism. *B,* Superior view. *C,* Three-dimensional CT view of the trigonocephaly forehead deformity and the associated orbital hypotelorism. *D,* Three-dimensional CT intracranial view.

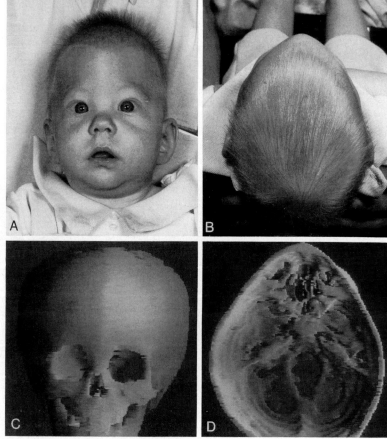

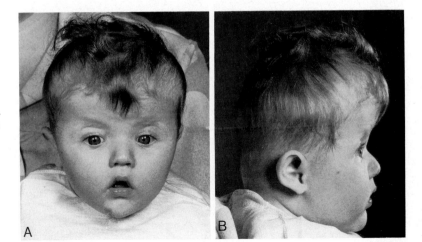

Figure 61–5. Brachycephaly–bilateral coronal synostosis in an infant. *A,* Frontal view. *B,* Profile.

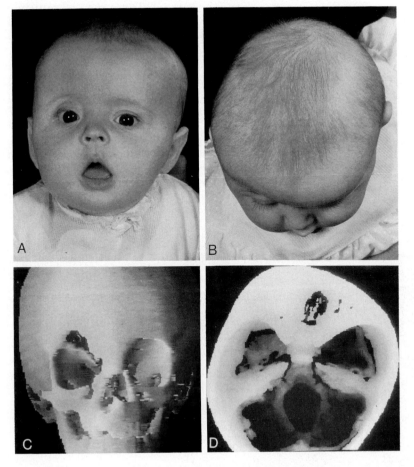

Figure 61–6. Plagiocephaly and unilateral (right) coronal synostosis in an infant. *A,* Frontal view. *B,* Bird's eye view. *C,* Three-dimensional CT frontal view of right-sided plagiocephaly. The defect of the right supraorbital rim is a "pseudoforamen." The "harlequin sign" is apparent on the right orbit. *D,* Three-dimensional CT intracranial view.

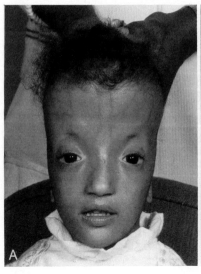
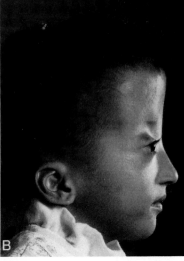

Figure 61–7. Acrocephaly–pansynostosis in a child. *A,* Frontal view. *B,* Profile. Note the vertical elongation of the forehead.

craniofacial microsomia or muscular torticollis.

On radiographic examination the elevation of the lesser wing of the sphenoid on the affected side creates the classic "harlequin" orbital sign.

Acrocephaly (Turricephaly)–Multiple Suture Synostoses. Acrocephaly and turricephaly are terms commonly interchanged to designate a type of untreated brachycephaly with an excess of skull height with a vertical elongation of the forehead ("tower skull") (Fig. 61–7). There may be multiple suture involvement in addition to bicoronal synostoses.

Oxycephaly–Multiple Suture Synostoses. Oxycephaly, literally translated as "pointed head," is characterized by a retroverted forehead, tilted posteroinferiorly on a plane with the nasal dorsum. The forehead is usually reduced in the horizontal dimension and capped by an elevation in the region of the anterior fontanel. There may be multiple suture involvement in addition to bicoronal synostoses.

Kleeblattschädel Anomaly. The Kleeblattschädel anomaly is characterized by a trilobed "cloverleaf" skull with bitemporal and vertex bulging (Fig. 61–8). The spectrum of suture synostosis is wide, and newborns with the deformity can also show no evidence of sutural synostosis.

Crouzon's Disease. Described by a French neurologist in 1912, Crouzon's disease is characterized by craniosynostosis and a froglike facies: exorbitism and midface retrusion (Figs. 61–9, 61–10). The pattern of inheri-

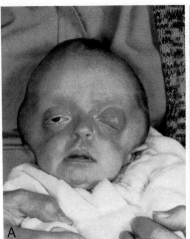
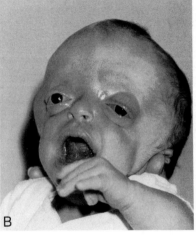

Figure 61–8. Kleeblattschädel anomaly or cloverleaf skull in an infant. *A,* Frontal view. *B,* Oblique view.

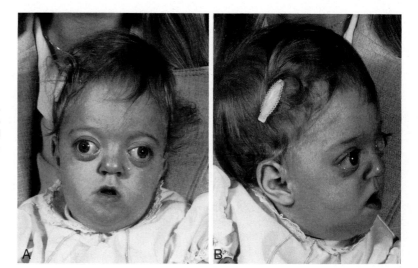

Figure 61–9. Crouzon's disease in an infant. Note the exorbitism, midface hypoplasia, and turricephaly. *A*, Frontal view. *B*, Profile.

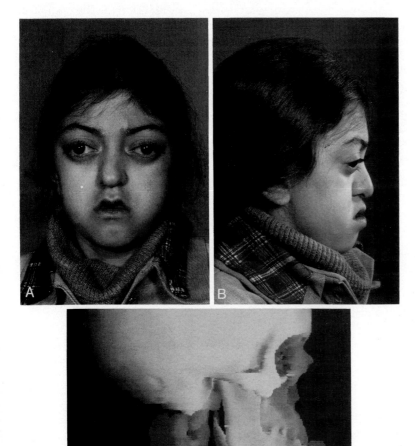

Figure 61–10. Crouzon's disease in a young female. Note the moderate exorbitism and midface hypoplasia. *A*, Frontal view. *B*, Profile. *C*, Three-dimensional CT scan illustrating the degree of midface hypoplasia and anterior crossbite in a patient with craniofacial synostosis.

tance is autosomal dominant with almost complete penetrance. In addition to exorbitism, other ocular findings include nystagmus, strabismus, hypertelorism, and optic nerve atrophy.

In any large series of patients with Crouzon's disease, there is no regular pattern of calvarial deformity; scaphocephaly, trigonocephaly, or oxycephaly can be present, depending on the site of the cranial suture synostosis. The coronal, sagittal, and lambdoid sutures have all been found prematurely synostosed on roentgenographic study; this finding stands in contrast to the simple cranial synostosis (coronal) usually seen in Apert's syndrome (Bertelsen, 1958).

The changes in the cranial vault and orbital cavities represent compensatory changes secondary to the increased intracranial pressures (Fig. 61–11*A*). The sphenoid bone, which delimits the anterior cranial fossa posteriorly, is depressed; thus, the area of transition between the anterior and middle fossae is situated at a lower level (Fig. 61–11*B*). As the greater wings of the sphenoid yield to the increased intracranial pressure, the middle cranial fossa expands anteriorly and inferiorly and comes to lie along the lateral wall of the orbit; the latter may be extremely diminished in its anteroposterior dimension. This forward position of the greater wing of the sphenoid is one of

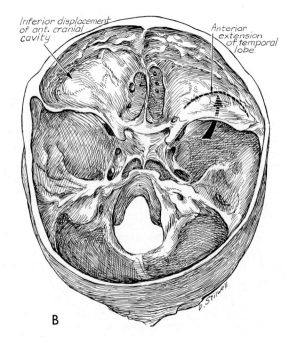

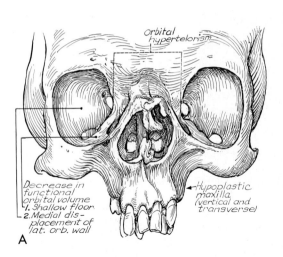

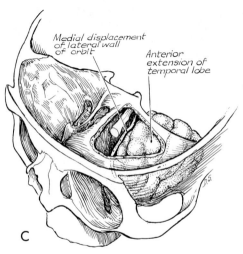

Figure 61–11. Adult skull showing the skeletal features of Crouzon's disease. *A,* Frontal view. Note the increase in the interorbital distance. The maxilla is hypoplastic and there is a decrease in the functional orbital volume. *B,* Cranial view. There is an inferior displacement of the anterior cranial vault and an anterior expansion of the middle cranial fossa. *C,* View showing the middle cranial fossa (and temporal lobe), lying adjacent to and medially displacing the lateral wall of the orbit. (Skull supplied by Dr. Paul Tessier.)

the principal causes of diminished volume of the orbit (Fig. 61–11C). The body of the sphenoid is situated more inferiorly than normal. Consequently, a lordosis of the cranial base develops. Fusion of the coronal suture, which is the principal source of sagittal thrust, results in a shortening of the floor of the anterior cranial fossa in its anteroposterior dimension.

With inferior displacement of the base of the anterior cranial fossa, the posterior portion of the roof of the orbit is situated more inferiorly than normal. In addition to these changes in the roof, the orbits are further shortened by the anterior and medial displacement of the greater wings of the sphenoid secondary to the anteroinferior expansion of the middle cranial fossa. Likewise, the ethmoid labyrinths are displaced laterally by the depression of the cribriform plate (Bertelsen, 1958).

The surface of the floor of the orbit is also shortened as a result of the associated maxillary hypoplasia. Because these changes occur in all dimensions (roof, lateral and medial walls, and floor of the orbit), there is marked reduction in the functional volume of the orbit (see Fig. 61–11A). A reduction of 10 mm in depth results in a 6 ml reduction in volume, and this is exactly the volume of the globe (Tessier, 1971c). Consequently, the pathomechanics of the resulting exorbitism can be easily appreciated: the functional volume of the orbit is too small to accommodate the orbital contents.

The maxilla is hypoplastic in three dimensions (Fig. 61–12), but, as noted by Tessier (1971c), the degree of midfacial skeletal retrusion is distorted by the recession of the frontal bone as well as by the microgenia. The maxillary hypoplasia is reflected in the shallowness of the orbital floor, the narrowness of the upper dental arch, bilateral crossbite, crowded dentition, a high and transversely compressed palate, compression of the zygomatic arch, and a severe narrowing of the pterygomaxillary fossa. The distal and downward tilt of the posterior section of the maxilla and premature occlusion of the molar teeth cause an anterior open bite and a downward and backward rotation of the mandible (Kreiborg, 1981). The chin is usually underdeveloped. Hypoplasia of the zygoma is variable.

Apert's Syndrome. Apert's syndrome, or acrocephalosyndactyly, was described by a

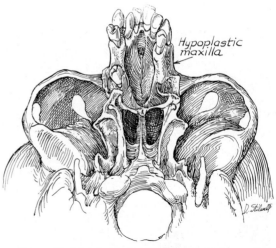

Figure 61–12. Inferior view of the hypoplastic maxilla in Crouzon's disease. The underdevelopment occurs in three dimensions. (Skull supplied by Dr. Paul Tessier.)

French neurologist (1906) and is transmitted by an autosomal dominant (sporadic) mode of inheritance. It is characterized by craniosynostosis, exorbitism, midface hypoplasia, symmetric syndactyly of the hands and feet, and other axial skeletal deformities (Figs. 61–13, 61–14). Brachycephaly and turricephaly are common, with a bulging anterior fontanel in the infant. In association with the maxillary hypoplasia, one can observe a high arched palate, clefts of the secondary palate, crowding of the dental arch, and an anterior open bite.

Although it is the syndactyly of Apert's syndrome that essentially differentiates it from Crouzon's syndrome, Tessier (1971c) listed other findings more characteristic of the patient with Apert's syndrome: acne, submucous clefts hidden in the arched palate, anterior open bite with crossbowing of the upper lip, oculomotor paralysis, asymmetry of the exorbitism, ptosis, and overhanging of the upper frontal area with a transverse frontal skin furrow and enlargement of the ear lobes. Ptosis occurs in Apert's syndrome and, if the zygoma is depressed or hypoplastic, there can be a downward (antimongoloid) slant of the palpebral fissure.

The upper extremities are shortened. The usual hand deformity in Apert's syndrome consists of a bony fusion of the second, third, and fourth fingers, with a single common nail (see Fig. 61–13C). Involvement of the first or fifth digits in this bony mass is variable. There can be a similar deformity involving

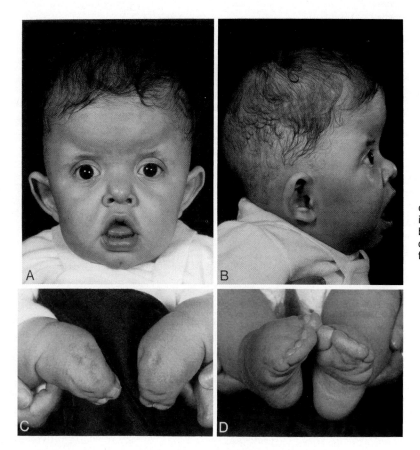

Figure 61–13. Apert's syndrome in an infant. *A,* Frontal view illustrating the acrocephaly, frontal bossing, midface hypoplasia, and open bite. *B,* Profile. *C,* Hand deformities. *D,* Foot deformities.

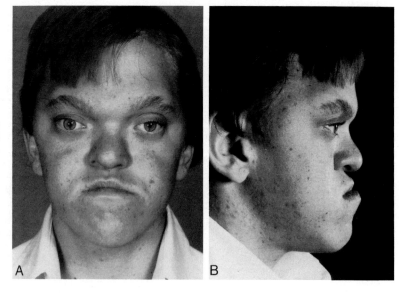

Figure 61–14. Apert's syndrome in an adolescent male. Note the midface hypoplasia and acne. *A,* Frontal view. *B,* Profile.

the foot. The extremity deformities are remarkably symmetric (Blank, 1960).

Pfeiffer's Syndrome. Autosomal dominant in transmission, this syndrome (Pfeiffer, 1964) is characterized by craniosynostosis, enlarged thumbs and great toes, exorbitism (variable), and midface hypoplasia (Figs. 61–15, 61–16). The same ocular and oral findings can be noted as previously described for Crouzon's and Apert's syndromes.

Saethre-Chotzen Syndrome. Described

independently by Saethre (1931) and Chotzen (1932), this syndrome is transmitted as autosomal dominant with full penetrance. Affected individuals show craniosynostosis, low hairline, ptosis, deviated nasal septum, and brachydactyly (Fig. 61–17). Mild exorbitism is associated with retrusion of the brow or supraorbital rim. Maxillary hypoplasia is observed less commonly than in the other craniofacial synostosis syndromes.

Carpenter's Syndrome. Carpenter's syn-

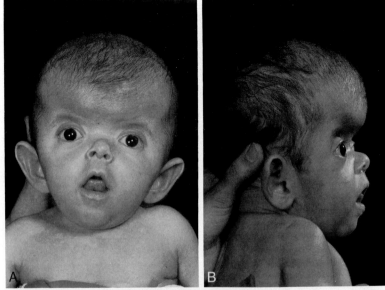

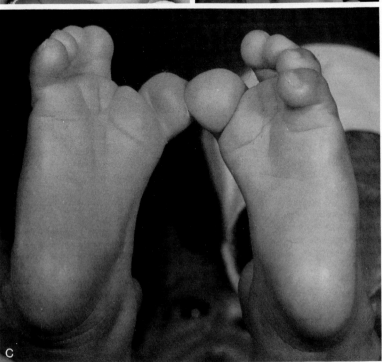

Figure 61–15. Pfeiffer's syndrome in an infant. Note the frontal bossing, midface hypoplasia, and exorbitism. *A*, Frontal view. *B*, Profile. *C*, Feet. Note the large toe.

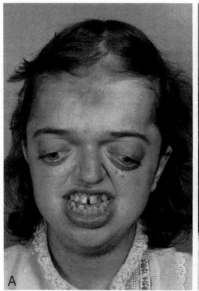
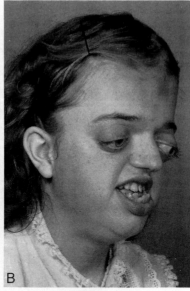

Figure 61–16. Pfeiffer's syndrome in an adolescent female. Note the severe degree of exorbitism, midface hypoplasia, and anterior crossbite. *A*, Frontal view. *B*, Side view. *C*, Feet. Note the large toes.

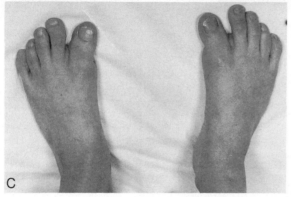

Figure 61–17. Saethre-Chotzen syndrome. Note the low hairline, ptosis of the upper eyelids, retrusion of the brows, and mild exorbitism. There is satisfactory midface development. *A*, Frontal view. *B*, Profile.

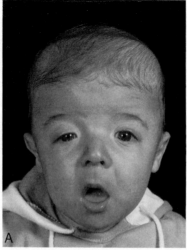
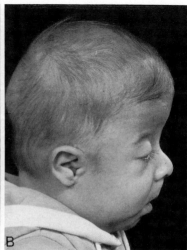

drome is characterized by craniosynostosis, polysyndactyly of the feet, and short hands with variable soft tissue syndactyly. The etiology is autosomal recessive.

FUNCTIONAL ASPECTS

The association of craniosynostosis and blindness was noted by von Graefe in 1866 and the relationship with optic atrophy was documented by Friedenwald in 1893, but a review of most clinical series fails to provide the exact incidence of functional deficits (increased intracranial pressure, mental retardation, and visual disturbances) in the various craniosynostosis syndromes. The reasons are multiple. The literature is replete with individual case reports in which rigorous diagnostic criteria were not employed in defining the absence or presence of a functional defect. The orientation of the investigator also biased the report. For example, a surgical investigator tended to emphasize the reconstructive aspects without documenting the functional deficits.

Increased Intracranial Pressure. It has been assumed that increased intracranial pressure (ICP) is apparent in those cases of craniosynostosis in which there is the greatest disparity between intracranial volume and brain volume. "Thumb-printing" of the calvaria has been regarded as the classical (indirect) radiographic evidence of intracranial pressure.

In an attempt to develop objective assessment of the incidence of increased intracranial pressure in the various craniosynostosis syndromes, Marchac and Renier (1982) recorded intracranial pressure in 121 craniosynostosis patients with an epidural sensor device. Increased intracranial pressure was documented more frequently when several sutures were involved (42 per cent), but was also observed in 13 per cent of patients with only single suture involvement. A reduction in intracranial pressure was noted in patients who underwent cranial vault remodeling.

Hydrocephalus. The development of computed tomography (CT) has provided a noninvasive method of assessing ventricular size. Because of the problems of ascertainment bias listed above, the true incidence of hydrocephalus in the various craniosynostosis syndromes is not known. Both communicating and noncommunicating types of hydrocephalus may be observed (Fishman, Hogan, and Dodge, 1971), but it is thought that the former is more common.

The incidence of hydrocephalus in scaphocephaly and unilateral and bilateral coronal synostosis is lowest. It is highest in multiple suture synostosis, especially the kleeblattschädel deformity in which there is evidence of obstruction of cerebrospinal fluid flow at the level of the fourth ventricle (Angle, McIntire, and Moore, 1967). As in the multiple suture synostoses, hydrocephalus is observed more frequently in patients with Crouzon's disease and Apert's syndrome, but the true incidence is not known.

Mental Retardation. The incidence of mental retardation in the various craniosynostosis syndromes remains speculative. It is certainly not as high as previously assumed, since the diagnosis of mental retardation had been erroneously made because of the facial appearance, and many patients had been relegated at an early age to institutional care with only minimal social-sensory stimulation. In addition there is a paucity of objective psychometric data in the reported series.

The risk of mental retardation is higher than in the general population, and the cause of its presence in craniosynostosis has been attributed to several factors: increased intracranial pressure (unrelieved) with cerebral atrophy, hydrocephalus, associated intracranial anomalies, meningitis, prematurity, or a family history of mental retardation.

The incidence of mental retardation is lowest in patients with involvement of a single suture, except in metopic synostosis, in which it is observed more frequently. It has been attributed to the associated forebrain abnormalities observed in metopic synostosis (trigonocephaly). The highest incidence of mental retardation has been reported in Apert's syndrome and in the kleeblattschädel deformity.

Visual Abnormalities. Optic atrophy and papilledema are not uncommon findings in craniosynostosis. Bertelsen (1958) observed papilledema in 20 children under 7 years of age, in five between the ages of 10 and 17 years, and in one adult under 45 years of age. Papilledema reflects the presence of increased intracranial pressure and tends to be more common in Crouzon's disease, Apert's syndrome, acrocephaly, and oxycephaly; it is rarely seen in plagiocephaly and trigonocephaly (Montaut and Stricker, 1977).

The incidence of optic atrophy has been reported to be more common in brachycephaly, oxycephaly, Crouzon's disease, and Apert's syndrome (Montaut and Stricker, 1977). It is a rare finding in trigonocephaly, plagiocephaly, and scaphocephaly (Montaut and Stricker, 1977). Optic atrophy has been attributed to compression of the nerve by bony overgrowth of the walls of the optic canal (Crouzon, 1912); however, other investigators (Marchac and Renier, 1982) have reported that the diameter of the canal is usually of normal caliber. Alternative theories proposed to explain the presence of optic atrophy include stretching of the nerve, compression by the carotid vessels, or a secondary effect of chronic papilledema and increased intracranial pressure.

In the presence of an associated orbital hypertelorism, the patient may not develop binocular vision, and amblyopia is the result.

Approximately 50 per cent of patients with Crouzon's disease or Apert's syndrome show exotropia in the primary gaze position, and a V pattern associated with overaction of the inferior oblique muscle was demonstrated in two-thirds of these patients (McCarthy and associates, 1976b).

TREATMENT

As noted in Table 61–2, surgical treatment can be employed *early* (within the first year of life) or *late* (after one year). The trend in recent years has been toward early surgery, for obvious reasons. Every effort is made to have the child look as good as possible at as early an age as possible to spare the psychologic and social trauma associated with craniofacial disfigurement.

Early Surgery

The goals of surgery for the newborn with a craniosynostosis are twofold: (1) decompression of the intracranial space (to reduce intracranial pressure, to prevent visual problems, and to permit normal mental development) and (2) achievement of satisfactory craniofacial form.

Before embarking on a description of the various surgical techniques employed, a discussion of craniofacial skeletal growth is indicated.

Table 61–2. Surgical Treatment of Craniosynostosis

Early (before 1 yr of age)
1. Strip craniectomies: limited and extended
2. Frontal bone advancement with or without strip craniectomies
3. Cranial vault remodeling
4. Monobloc or craniofacial advancement
5. Shunt surgery for hydrocephalus

Late (after 1 yr of age)
1. Frontal bone advancement
2. Le Fort III advancement
   a. child
   b. adult
3. Le Fort III and frontal bone advancement
4. Monobloc or craniofacial advancement
5. Le Fort II advancement
6. Maxillary/mandibular/zygomatic surgery

New York University Protocol

Age 6 mos:	Strip craniectomy and/or frontal bone advancement and/or cranial vault remodeling and/or shunt surgery
Age 3–4 yrs:	Le Fort III advancement (if indicated)
Early adolescence:	Jaw surgery (if indicated)

The head and neck region is no longer viewed as a composite consisting of isolated bones, muscles, and glands; rather, it is considered as a number of relatively independent, yet interrelated, units of function. The original concepts of *functional craniology* of Van der Klaaw (1948–1952) began with the recognition that the functions of the head and neck are subserved by "functional cranial components." The latter are formed by all the soft tissues (viscera, such as muscles and glands and visceral spaces, such as the mouth and pharynx, which are related to specific function) and those related skeletal tissues that serve to protect or support the soft tissues. Moss (1962) popularized the concept of the *functional matrix* in which any given bone grows in response to functional relationships representing the sum of all the soft tissues operating in association with the bone.

In the embryologic development of the neurocranium, cartilage is initially laid down in the base of the skull and is eventually replaced by bone. However, dorsal and lateral to the developing brain, chondrification does not occur. Intramembranous bone formation is observed in the frontal, parietal, and intraparietal portions of the occipital and squamous temporal regions. The cranial sutures are no longer considered to be sites of primary growth; the skull does not grow in response to a multiplication of the sutural tissues. Growth or change at the sutural areas is a secondary, compensatory, and mechanically obligatory event, following the primary growth of the enclosed and protected neural and facial soft tissue matrices. The sutures are a type of syndesmosis in which the opposing surfaces of bone are connected by an interosseous ligament.

In contrast, the cartilages at the cranial base grow by *interstitial* or *expansive* growth; the chondrocytes proliferate by mitotic division, form new cartilaginous intercellular substance, and thus spread the cartilage apart. Interstitial or expansive growth, therefore, depends on the division of already differentiated cells, the chondrocytes, to form new cartilaginous intercellular substance. The spheno-occipital synchondrosis is the principal "growth cartilage" of the cranial base during childhood and provides a pressure-adapted bone growth mechanism for elongation of the middle portion of the cranial base.

The bones of the calvarium are displaced outward by the enlarging brain. Each of the bones of the domed skull roof responds to the expansion of the brain by depositing new bone at the contact edges of the sutures. By this mechanism, the perimeter of each calvarial bone is enlarged (Enlow and Azuma, 1975). In addition, bone forms on both the ectocranial (outer) and endocranial (inner) sides of the individual bones. For example, growth of the floor of the anterior cranial fossa and frontal bone is characterized by deposition of bone on the ectocranial side, with resorption of bone from the endocranial side (Enlow and Azuma, 1975). The cranial bones in man are normally separate at birth. There is firm fibrous union between them at age 5 to 6 months, but solid bony union is not complete until the sixth to eighth decades (Matson, 1969).

The cranial base extends from the foramen magnum to the frontonasal junction and consists of the basisphenoid, sphenoid, and cranial surfaces of the ethmoid bones. The growth of the cranial base, which is dependent on that of the brain, is not equal in all of its parts. Growth of that portion of the anterior cranial base between the sella and foramen cecum is complete by 7 years of age; additional growth of the anterior cranial base, however, is expressed anterior to the foramen cecum, with the migration upward and outward of the nasal bones and related growth changes of the frontal bones associated with expansion of the developing frontal air sinuses. The posterior cranial base (sella to basion) continues to grow until adulthood.

Enlargement of the anterior cranial fossa (i.e., the anterior cranial base) is related to the growth of the frontal lobes. Approximately 47 per cent of the adult size of the frontal lobe is attained by 11 months of age and 93 per cent by 7 years of age (Enlow and Azuma, 1975). The relationship between growth of the frontal lobes and enlargement of the anterior cranial base is supported by the fact that the anterior part of the cranial floor has attained 56 per cent of its complete growth by birth and 70 per cent by 2 years of age (Enlow and Azuma, 1975). The overall length of the brain case has completed 63 per cent of its total growth at birth, 82 per cent by the end of the first year, and 89 per cent by 3 years of age (Enlow and Azuma, 1975).

The cranial base is the template on which the upper face develops; consequently, specific characteristics of the face are determined by certain topographic and dimensional aspects of the cranial base (Enlow and Azuma, 1975). The size and alignment of the floor of the anterior and middle cranial fossae are, in turn, determined by the ventral parts of the frontal and temporal lobes, respectively. The nasomaxillary complex is related spatially to the anterior cranial fossa. The posterior boundary of the midface is defined by the posterior margin of the frontal lobes; the portion of the middle cranial fossa anterior to the mandibular condyles is related to the pharyngeal space and airway.

Longitudinal cephalometric studies on patients with Crouzon's disease showed that sagittal maxillary growth was diminished while mandibular growth was unaffected (Kreiborg, 1981).

Because of the relationship between the floor of the anterior cranial fossa and the midface, it was speculated that interference with normal expansion of the cranial base, such as sutural synostosis, could have a secondary effect on development of the midface (McCarthy and associates, 1978). Conversely, any interceptive surgical procedure that would liberate the stenosed craniofacial skeleton and permit sagittal growth of the cranial base and anterior cranial fossa should have a salutary effect on midface development. Brain weight approximately doubles by the

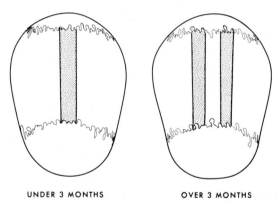

UNDER 3 MONTHS   OVER 3 MONTHS

Figure 61–18. Usual position of strip craniectomies for sagittal synostosis, depending on the age of the patient (Munro, 1977).

age of 6 months and triples by 2 years of age (Blinkov and Glezer, 1968). However, longitudinal studies (McCarthy and associates, 1984a; and Marchac and Renier, 1985) after early surgery demonstrated that, while the long-term results in the fronto-orbital area have been satisfactory, midface hypoplasia still developed in the Crouzon and Apert patient.

Strip Craniectomies. Before the turn of the century, several case reports of strip craniectomies were recorded in the literature (Lane, 1892; Lannelongue, 1890). By the 1920's the technique had found wide clinical acceptance in the United States.

The proper time for neurosurgical strip craniectomies has traditionally been advocated as being before the age of 3 months. While adequate cranial decompression has been obtained, the techniques, except in isolated sagittal synostosis, failed to yield satisfactory results in terms of craniofacial form. Shillito and Matson (1968) reviewed 519 patients with craniosynostosis who had undergone strip craniectomies, and noted that only 52 per cent of them had a satisfactory appearance after surgery; the best results in terms of craniofacial appearance were observed in infants with isolated sagittal sutural synostosis.

In *isolated sagittal synostosis,* either sagittal or parasagittal strip craniectomy (Fig. 61–18) is the treatment of choice.

In *bilateral coronal synostosis,* strip craniectomy (bilateral coronal) has been replaced

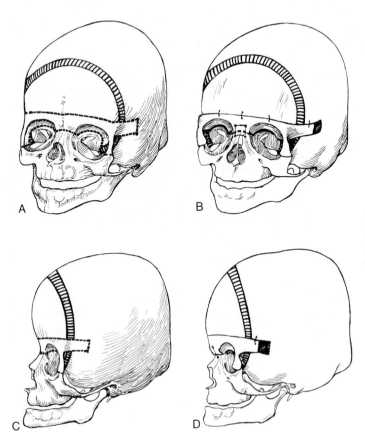

A   B

C   D

Figure 61–19. Frontal bone advancement or fronto-orbital remodeling. *A, C,* Lines of osteotomy-ostectomy. *B, D,* Following advancement and recontouring. The forehead can also be reconstructed with a parieto-occipital bone graft.

in recent years by frontal bone advancement. However, in infants with a mild degree of bilateral coronal synostosis with minimal if any evidence of exorbitism, an extended coronal-sphenozygomatic strip craniectomy (McCarthy and associates, 1978) may be indicated.

The authors have abandoned simple strip craniectomy techniques in the treatment of plagiocephaly, trigonocephaly, or the craniofacial synostosis syndromes (Crouzon's, Apert's).

Frontal Bone Advancement With or Without Strip Craniectomies. In the infant with *bilateral coronal synostosis* and a moderate degree of exorbitism, and in the infant with one of the *craniofacial synostosis syndromes* (Crouzon's, Apert's), the Tessier type of frontal bone advancement is recommended (Tessier, 1971c). In addition, the lines of osteotomy are extended along the lateral orbital wall to encompass wide bony resection in the region of the sphenozygomatic sutures (Fig. 61–19). The procedure, which is performed with more facility in the infant than in the adult, is usually performed at 6 months of age (McCarthy and associates, 1978). The osteotomies are made across the nasofrontal junction, across the roof of the orbit and along the lateral orbital wall. Extensions are made into the temporal fossa to provide a tongue-in-groove arrangement, which obviates the need for bone grafts for fixation purposes. The frontal bone flap is wired to the advanced supraorbital bar, or the forehead is reconstructed by a parieto-occipital bone graft. The frontal bone has been advanced as far as 20 mm, with significant expansion of the orbital volume (Figs. 61–20, 61–21). Closure of the scalp, although difficult after a large degree of frontal bone advancement, can be facilitated by parallel incisions in the galea.

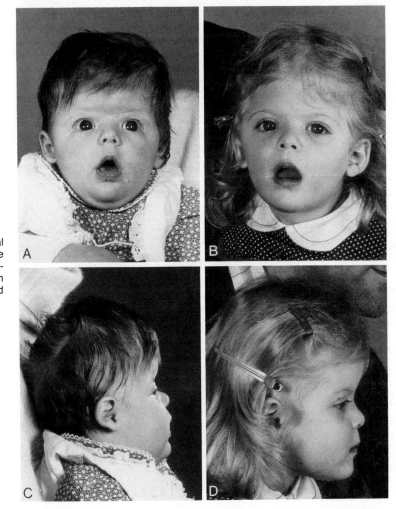

Figure 61–20. Infant with bilateral coronal synostosis, retrusion of the brow, and exorbitism. *A, C,* Preoperative appearance. *B, D,* Eighteen months after the technique illustrated in Figure 61–19.

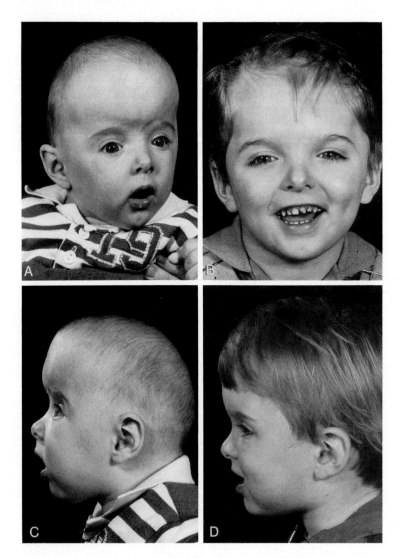

Figure 61–21. Infant male with Crouzon's disease and frontal bossing. *A, C,* Preoperative appearance. *B, D,* Eighteen months after the technique illustrated in Figure 61–19.

Marchac (1978) modified the above technique for use on a patient with oxycephaly by incorporating a lateral temporal spur in the form of a Z-plasty (Fig. 61–22). The technique provides a two-dimensional correction (sagittal and vertical) and permits stabilization of the frontal bone or supraorbital fragment without the need for bone grafts.

Longitudinal three-dimensional CT studies documented significant increases in intracranial and ventricular volume after these techniques (Fig. 61–23) (Dufresne and associates, 1987).

For *unilateral coronal synostosis,* Hoffman and Mohr (1976) described a type of frontal bone advancement that, with modification, is the authors' preferred procedure (McCarthy

and associates, 1978). A supraorbital osteotomy (Fig. 61–24) is made approximately 1.5 cm above the roof of the orbit and carried into the temporal region; bur holes in the middle cranial fossa are usually required to prevent injury to the temporal lobe. A counter osteotomy is made across the nasofrontal junction, halfway up the medial orbital wall, across the roof, and down the lateral wall in a full-thickness fashion. It is essential that the osteotomies be extended across the midline to the unaffected side so that, when the greenstick fracture is accomplished, there is no resulting depression in the midline. Plagiocephaly should be regarded as a bilateral deformity; a bilateral frontal bone advancement (see Fig. 61–19) is often performed and

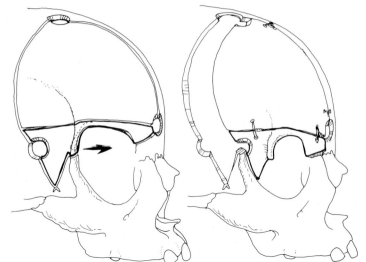

Figure 61–22. Frontal bone advancement (Z-plasty) after Marchac (1978).

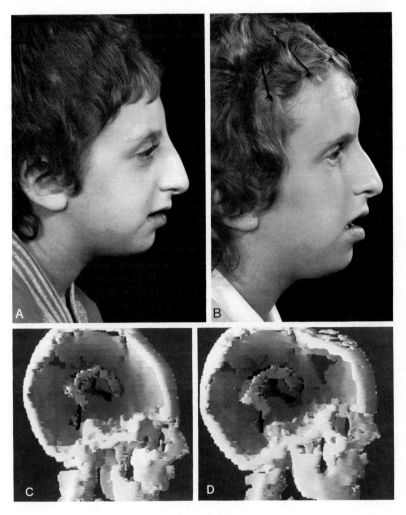

Figure 61–23. Ten year old female with Crouzon's disease and clinical-radiographic evidence of increased intracranial pressure (ICP) without dilated ventricles. *A,* Preoperative profile. *B,* Profile following frontal bone advancement and cranial vault remodeling and enlargement. *C,* Preoperative three-dimensional CT scan. *D,* Postoperative CT scan. Note the enlargement in intracranial and intraventricular volume.

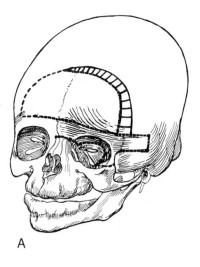 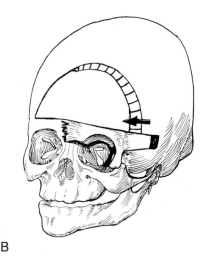

A   B

Figure 61–24. Frontal bone advancement or fronto-orbital remodeling for plagiocephaly (left side). *A*, Lines of ostectomy-osteotomy. In most cases the deformity is treated with bilateral osteotomies (see Figure 61–19). *B*, After advancement of the fronto-orbital segment *(arrow)* and replacement of the forehead with a single-piece calvarial (parieto-occipital) graft.

a single piece calvarial bone graft is used to restore the forehead contour (Figs. 61–25, 61–26).

The affected supraorbital arch is usually flat and lacks the desired convexity. Restoration of contour can be accomplished by bending the mobilized bony segment after making posterior cuts or by placing onlay bone grafts (removed from the frontal bone flap) on the anterior aspect of the supraorbital arch. The segment is then wired in a slightly overcorrected position by placing stainless steel wires between the temporal extension and temporal bone. The resulting gap in the orbital roof does not require bone grafting. Other surgical procedures for use in the infant with plagiocephaly have been re-

ported by Montaut and Stricker (1977) and Marchac (1978).

Metopic Synostosis. Metopic synostosis (trigonocephaly) is usually associated with a supraorbital rim that is recessed in the sagittal dimension. The procedure of Marchac (1978) is used. A supraorbital bar with a greenstick fracture at the midline is advanced as needed, and the forehead is reconstructed by a single piece calvarial bone graft removed from the lateral aspect of the frontal bone flap (Figs. 61–27, 61–28). Albin and associates (1985) reported a series of 33 patients with trigonocephaly operated on by a modification of this technique.

It has been the authors' observation that residual frontal bone defects remaining at

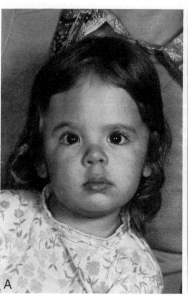 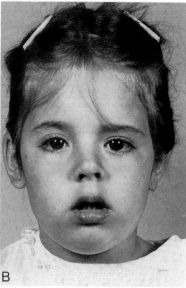

A   B

Figure 61–25. Female child with right-sided plagiocephaly and recession of the brow. *A*, Preoperative view. *B*, Two years after the technique illustrated in Figure 61–24.

Figure 61–26. Newborn male with plagiocephaly–unilateral coronal synostosis. *A,* Preoperative frontal view. Note the right-sided plagiocephaly and recession of the brow. There is frontal bossing with displacement of the globe on the opposite side. *B,* Appearance after the technique illustrated in Figure 61–19. *C,* Preoperative superior view. *D,* Postoperative superior view.

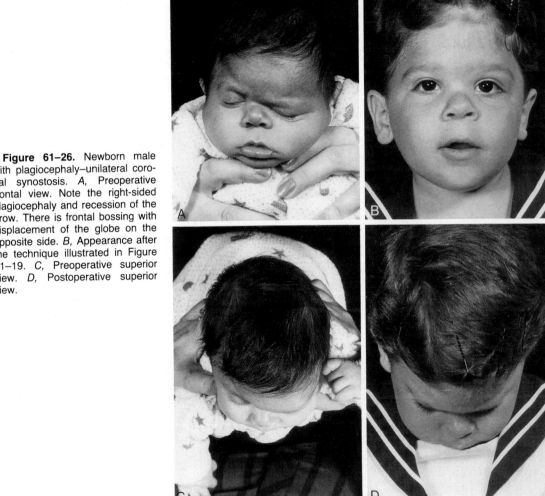

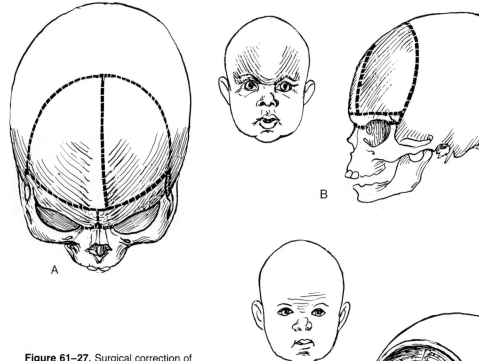

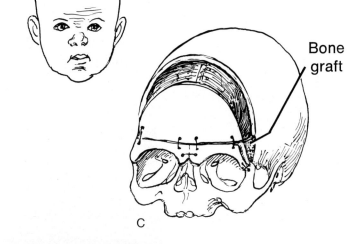

Figure 61–27. Surgical correction of trigonocephaly/metopic synostosis (after Marchac, 1978). *A, B,* Lines of osteotomy. *C,* Following advancement of the frontal bone segment and replacement of the forehead with a single-piece calvarial bone graft. Bone grafts are also wedged in the lateral defects.

Bone graft

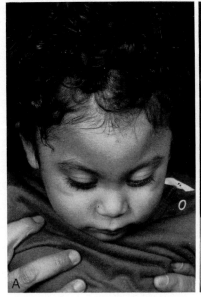

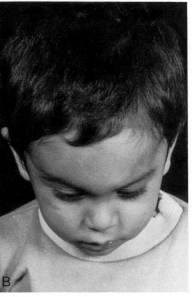

Figure 61–28. Trigonocephaly in an infant male. *A,* Preoperative appearance. Note the keel-like deformity of the forehead and the recessed supraorbital rims. *B,* Appearance after the technique illustrated in Figure 61–27.

the conclusion of surgery in the newborn infant are usually replaced by new bone in the subsequent months (Reid, McCarthy, and Kolber, 1981).

Cranial Vault Remodeling. Additional cranial vault remodeling may be indicated when there is an associated turricephaly. Munro (1977) described a technique in which a frontal bone advancement (Tessier tongue-in-groove) as described above is initially done. A radical calvariectomy is performed bilaterally but a central strip of bone is preserved over the sagittal sinus (Fig. 61–29). A segment of the strip is resected and the strip is then advanced and secured with wire fixation to the previously advanced frontal bone segment (Fig. 61–29C). Consequently there has been a two-dimensional remodeling of the cranial vault: sagittal advancement and a vertical reduction.

An alternative technique for reducing the vertical height of the cranial vault is the "barrel stave" osteotomy reported by Persing and associates (1987). The position of the

patient on the operating table (Fig. 61–30) allows circumferential lowering of the cranial vault.

A patient who underwent cranial vault remodeling is illustrated in Figure 61–31.

Monobloc or Craniofacial Advancement. In infants with a severe variant of a craniofacial synostosis syndrome characterized by midface retrusion, respiratory distress, exorbitism, and corneal exposure, Muhlbauer, Anderl, and Marchac (1983) recommended a monobloc advancement or simultaneous advancement of the forehead, orbits, and midface. In an infant this is a potentially dangerous procedure and should be reserved for the child with combined ocular and respiratory threats. It has been the authors' experience that all cases of craniofacial synostosis and corneal exposure can be successfully managed by frontal bone advancement alone. A tracheotomy can relieve the respiratory distress of the newborn with a severe craniosynostosis syndrome.

Shunt Surgery. The presence or absence

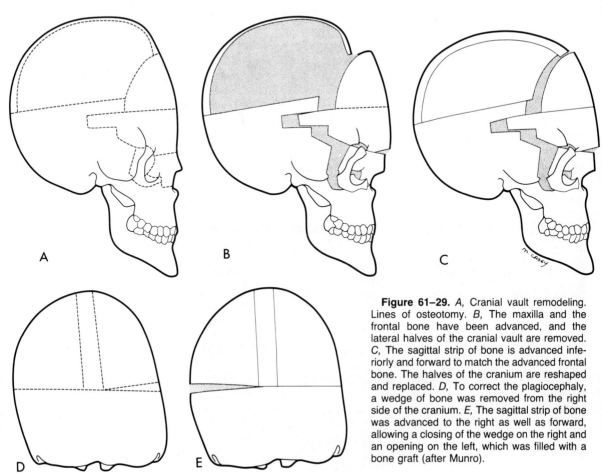

Figure 61–29. *A,* Cranial vault remodeling. Lines of osteotomy. *B,* The maxilla and the frontal bone have been advanced, and the lateral halves of the cranial vault are removed. *C,* The sagittal strip of bone is advanced inferiorly and forward to match the advanced frontal bone. The halves of the cranium are reshaped and replaced. *D,* To correct the plagiocephaly, a wedge of bone was removed from the right side of the cranium. *E,* The sagittal strip of bone was advanced to the right as well as forward, allowing a closing of the wedge on the right and an opening on the left, which was filled with a bone graft (after Munro).

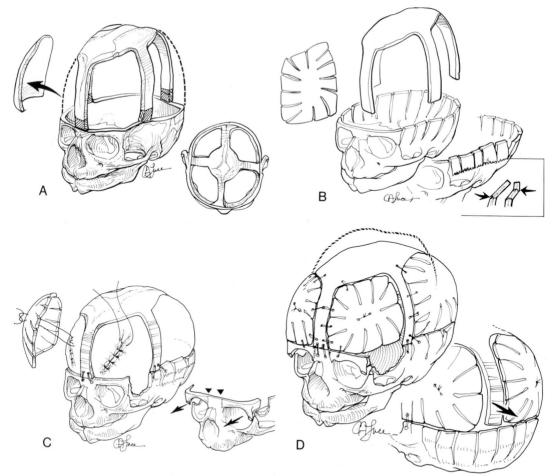

Figure 61–30. Barrel stave osteotomy. *A, B,* Preoperative turricephaly deformity. The cranial vault (circumferential) is removed and lowered *(diagonal lines).* Calvarial quadrants are also removed to be remodeled. *C,* The frontal bone (brow and orbital roof) is advanced to increase the anteroposterior dimension. The dura is plicated and the quadrants are replaced with dural suspension sutures. *D,* Final appearance with reduction of the vertical and increase in the anteroposterior dimensions of the cranial vault. (From Persing, J. A., Edgerton, M. T., Park, T. S., and Jane, J. A.: Barrel stave osteotomy for correction of turribrachycephaly craniosynostosis deformities. Ann. Plast. Surg., *18*:488, 1987.)

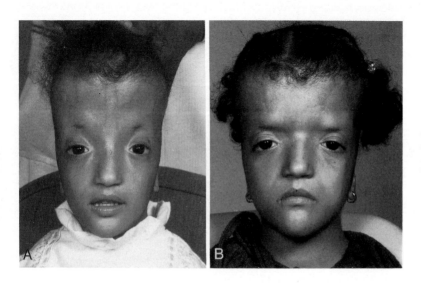

Figure 61–31. Three year old girl with craniosynostosis (pansynostosis). *A,* Preoperative appearance. *B,* After cranial vault remodeling (see Fig. 61–29).

of hydrocephalus and ventricular enlargement can be easily assessed by a CT scan. It is preferable that shunt surgery is done before the craniectomy and cranial vault remodeling.

Late Surgery

Late surgery is defined as surgical procedures performed on the patient with craniofacial synostosis after 1 year of age.

Le Fort III Advancement Osteotomy. Gillies and Harrison (1950–51) reported the first high maxillary (a modified Le Fort III) osteotomy in a patient with craniofacial dysostosis. Through external incisions they performed transverse osteotomies that separated the nasal bones from the frontal bones. The osteotomy of the orbital floor was placed immediately within the infraorbital margin and extended across the floor of the orbit to the medial orbital wall anterior to the lacrimal groove. Osteotomies were also performed through the frontal processes of the maxilla to diminish the width of the nose. The temporal process of the zygoma was divided on each side. An osteotome was then introduced into the pterygomaxillary junction. Anterior to the greater palatine foramen, an incision was made transversely across the mucoperiosteum of the hard palate, extending laterally and posterior to the alveolar ridge. The hard palate was divided, and the line of osteotomy was rejoined at the pterygomaxillary junction. In this way the spatial relationships of the soft palate were undisturbed. The operation was completed by severing the septum with a pair of large scissors introduced through the osteotomy line at the root of the nose. Intermaxillary fixation was established. Although no bone grafting was done, a satisfactory result was reported. Seven and one-half years after this operation, the patient underwent further surgery to correct persistent exorbitism by removal of the medial portion of the orbital floor, and ox cartilage was also placed over the zygoma for contour improvement. The fate of the ox cartilage was not reported.

A considerable advance was made by Tessier and associates (1967), who reported a number of patients operated on by a technique distinctive from that of Gillies and Harrison (1950–51) in that the lines of osteotomy traversing the orbits reproduced the classic Le Fort III lines of fracture. The line of osteotomy traversed the orbital floor and passed obliquely forward behind the lacrimal groove and across the nasofrontal junction, joining with a similar osteotomy on the contralateral side. The lateral wall of the orbit was split sagittally, the line of osteotomy extending downward through the body of the zygoma in a steplike fashion. The pterygomaxillary junction and nasal septum were severed.

Murray and Swanson (1968) performed an osteotomy similar to that performed by Gillies. Jabaley and Edgerton (1969) reported an excellent result in a patient with a midfacial deformity of unknown origin. They performed an osteotomy similar to that of Tessier and associates (1967) by entering the inferior orbital fissure and then passing upward through the lateral orbital wall to the frontozygomatic junction. The osteotomy in the zygomatic area differed, however, in that the osteotomy was done through the zygomatic arch instead of the body of the zygoma. The hard palate was separated from the pterygoid processes, cutting through the posterior wall of the maxillary sinus. Tessier (1971c) subsequently published modifications of his original Le Fort III technique.

Technique of the Le Fort III Advancement Osteotomy Through a Subcranial (Extracranial) Route (Fig. 61–32). Anesthesia is achieved through a transnasal endotracheal tube if the Le Fort III advancement is to be performed without a tracheotomy. The decision depends on the severity of the deformity. If a tracheotomy is not performed, rigid skeletal fixation should be employed and the transnasal endotracheal tube should be left in position for at least 24 hours following surgery; it should be replaced by a soft rubber nasopharyngeal tube to maintain the airway.

When a tracheotomy is indicated, the anesthesia is begun with transoral endotracheal intubation. A tracheotomy is then performed over the endotracheal tube; the anesthesia is administered through the tracheotomy tube.

The exposure of the facial skeleton is obtained through three incisions: (1) scalp (bicoronal), (2) conjunctival or subciliary cutaneous, and (3) buccal vestibular. The eyelid incisions can be avoided but the operation is technically more difficult. The bicoronal incision and the raised scalp flap provide access in a subperiosteal plane to the lateral wall and floor of the orbit, to the root of the nose,

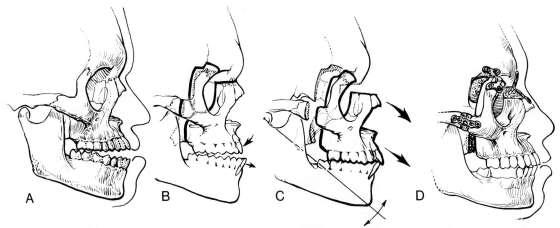

Figure 61–32. Subcranial Le Fort III advancement. *A,* Hypoplastic midface skeleton. *B,* Lines of osteotomy. The goals of preoperative orthodontic therapy are indicated by arrows. *C,* Anteroinferior translation of the osteotomized segment. *D,* Autogenous bone grafts are placed in the nasofrontal junction, lateral orbital wall, zygomatic arch, and pterygomaxillary fissure defects. Fixation is obtained by miniplates.

and to the medial orbital wall. The subperiosteally raised area can then communicate with the area, which will be exposed through the conjunctival or eyelid incision (optional). The latter incisions give access to the inferior orbital rim, the orbital floor, the lower portion of the medial wall, and the medial surface of the lateral orbital wall. Through a buccal, vestibular incision (at the level of the bicuspids), subperiosteal exposure to the pterygomaxillary fissure is obtained.

After the scalp flap is raised, the periorbita is elevated from the roof, the floor, and the lateral and medial orbital walls. The root of the nose and the medial orbital wall are exposed, the medial canthal tendon is left undisturbed, and the lacrimal sac is elevated from the lacrimal groove.

The bony framework of the nose is divided at the nasofrontal junction, the line of section being continued backward across the medial wall of the orbit on each side, downward (behind the lacrimal groove) to the floor of the orbit (Fig. 61–32B). A narrow, tapered osteotome is the most suitable instrument for the section of the delicate lamina papyracea of the ethmoid, which forms the portion of the medial wall of the orbit posterior to the lacrimal bone. A transverse cut is made across the orbital floor and joins the inferior orbital fissure to the lower end of the medial wall osteotomy.

The lateral wall of the orbit is sectioned transversely in the region of the frontozygomatic suture line or above it (Fig. 61–32B).

After retraction of the orbital contents medially and the temporalis muscle laterally, the lateral orbital wall is divided in a full-thickness fashion at its junction with the cranium (Fig. 61–32B). The zygomatic arch is likewise sectioned.

The line of osteotomy through the lateral orbital wall is continued inferiorly and posteriorly to and through the pterygomaxillary fissure (Fig. 61–32B). The pterygomaxillary disjunction is best accomplished with a curved osteotome after the mucoperiosteum has been raised from the tuberosity of the maxilla. A combination of scissors and osteotome is employed to sever the posterior portion of the nasal septum. After all lines of osteotomy are verified, the midfacial skeleton may be loosened with the Rowe disimpacting forceps. Autogenous bone grafts are placed in the defects of the nasofrontal junction, lateral orbital wall, and pterygomaxillary fissure (Fig. 61–32D). Interosseous wiring or miniplate fixation is used at the nasofrontal junction and frontozygomatic sites. Intermaxillary fixation is established after appropriate anterior advancement and inferior tilt of the midfacial segment (Fig. 61–32C). Cranial fixation by wires looped through the frontal bone and secured to the intermaxillary fixation appliance stabilizes the advanced nasomaxillary segment and maintains the mandibular condyle in the glenoid fossa. Alternatively, miniplate fixation can be employed at the nasofrontal, zygomaticotemporal, and zygomaticofrontal osteotomies. A canthopexy is not required since the medial canthal tendons have not been detached from their skeletal attachments.

Tessier described a modification that includes a "vertical spur" of the lateral orbital wall (Fig. 61–33). The method, designed to counteract posterior relapsing forces, represents an advance in surgical technique. Tessier stated that the technique obviates the need for intermaxillary fixation. The use of trephine holes to protect the temporal lobes of the brain ("semiopen method") obviates the need for a craniotomy. Cranial fixation is obtained by direct interosseous wiring at the nasofrontal and lateral orbital wall osteotomies and by circumzygomatic arch suspension wires; bone grafts are inserted in the nasofrontal and pterygomaxillary disjunction area. Split rib onlay grafts are placed over the frontal bone, and a "sleeve" rib graft reunites the divided zygomatic arch.

The patient in Figure 61–34 underwent a Le Fort III osteotomy by the technique illustrated in Figure 61–32. A genioplasty or horizontal osteotomy of the mandible was also performed.

Le Fort III Osteotomy in the Growing Child. Although the Le Fort III osteotomy was once reserved for the adolescent and adult patient, the trend in recent years has been toward performing the operation in young people to improve respiratory function and craniofacial form before the start of formal schooling. McCarthy and associates (1984b) reported a series of 12 patients who underwent Le Fort III advancement at ages ranging from 5 to 12 years (Fig. 61–35). The position of the advanced midface segment was remarkably stable, and any maxillomandibular disharmony demonstrated during the period of follow-up could be attributed to expected mandibular growth. Moreover, in some patients a degree of growth of the maxilla in an anteroinferior direction could be documented after Le Fort III advancement.

Le Fort III Osteotomy Performed Through a Combined Intracranial Approach With Advancement of the Frontal Bone. After the neurosurgeon has removed the frontal bone segment, the supraorbital osteotomy is extended horizontally to the region of the temporal fossa and continued in a stepwise fashion inferiorly toward the base of the skull (Fig. 61–36). A posterior extension is thus outlined, which guides the advancement and maintains bony contact.

In a horizontal direction the osteotomy then transgresses the lateral orbital wall and follows a line through the orbital roof at about the junction of the middle and posterior thirds of the orbit. The procedure is then completed by performing the Le Fort III osteotomy. In this way a horizontal component is also advanced, approximately 2 cm in height, containing the frontal bone, part of the roof, and the lateral wall of the orbit (Fig. 61–37).

Le Fort III Osteotomy Combined With a Le Fort I Osteotomy. This combination

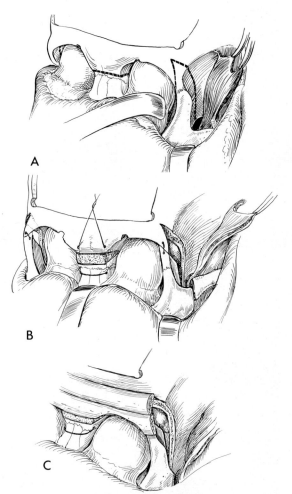

Figure 61–33. Vertical spur osteotomy of the lateral orbital wall (Tessier). *A,* Lines of osteotomy at the nasofrontal junction and lateral orbital wall. The remaining osteotomies follow the classical Le Fort III fracture. *B,* Following inferior displacement and anterior advancement of the midface. Bone grafts are inserted at the site of the nasofrontal dysjunction and in the pterygomaxillary fissure (the latter is not shown). Note the interosseous wires. *C,* Onlay rib grafts are placed over the frontal bone, and a "sleeve" rib graft (not shown) is used to restore continuity of the zygomatic arch.

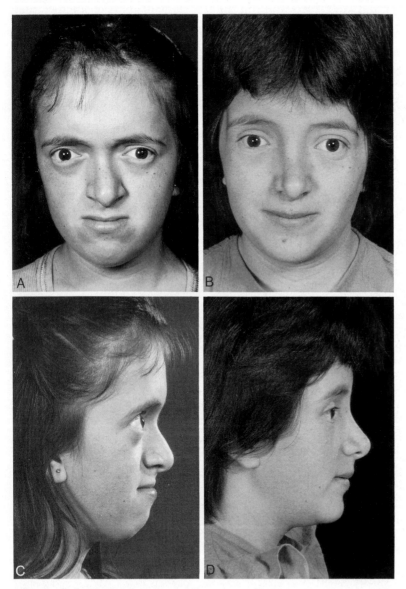

Figure 61–34. Adolescent female with Crouzon's disease. *A,* Preoperative frontal view. Note the midface hypoplasia, exorbitism, and microgenia. *B,* Postoperative frontal view. *C,* Preoperative profile. *D,* Postoperative profile after the technique illustrated in Figure 61–32, as well as horizontal osteotomy of the mandible (genioplasty) and nasalplasty.

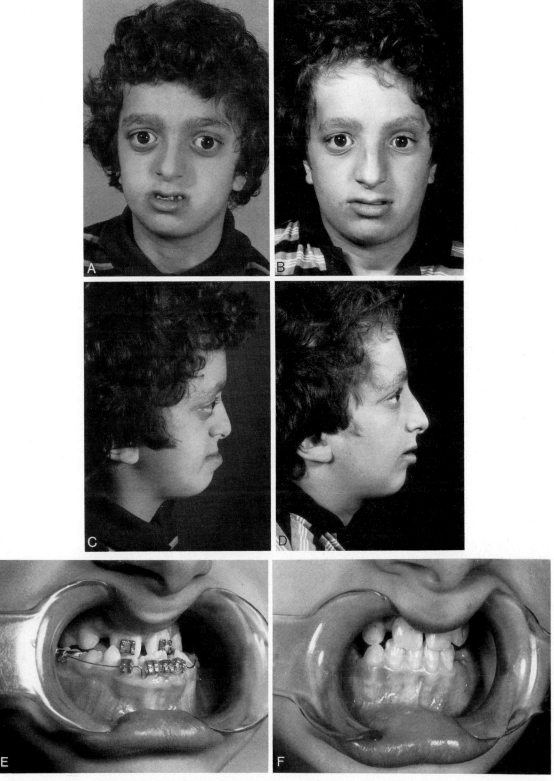

Figure 61–35. Le Fort III advancement in a 9 year old boy. *A, C,* Preoperative views. Note the midface hypoplasia, exorbitism, and lip relationships. *B, D,* Appearance after Le Fort III advancement. *E,* Preoperative occlusion with an anterior crossbite. *F,* Postoperative occlusion.

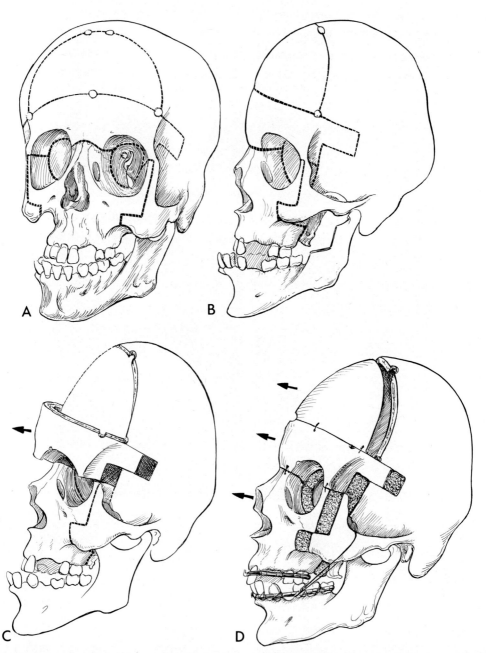

Figure 61–36. Le Fort III/frontal bone advancement osteotomy through a combined craniofacial route (after Tessier). *A,* Lines of osteotomy. *B,* Lateral view of lines of osteotomy. *C,* Frontal bone segment advanced. *D,* Final position after advancement of all bony segments. Bone grafts are wedged into the resulting defects. Stabilization is obtained by intermaxillary wiring or miniplate fixation, and suspension wires to the zygomatic arches (after Tessier.)

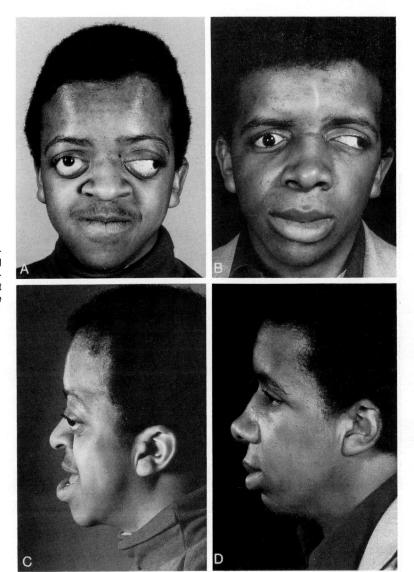

Figure 61–37. Le Fort III advancement combined with a frontal bone advancement. *A, C,* Preoperative views of a young adolescent male. *B, D,* Postoperative views. He awaits extraocular muscle surgery.

(Obwegeser, 1969) is particularly suited for patients in whom the deformity is restricted to the upper aspects of the midface (exorbitism and maxillary hypoplasia) and in whom dental occlusal relationships are within an acceptable range (Fig. 61–38). The line of osteotomy of the Le Fort I procedure is made superior to the apices of the teeth and below the infraorbital nerve. It is continued medially and superiorly to terminate at the upper margin of the piriform aperture. The osteotomy line takes a lateral course, joining the pterygomaxillary fissure, which is divided by means of a curved osteotome after raising the mucoperiosteum around the tuberosity of the maxilla. Intermaxillary fixation is estab-

lished and the upper midline fragment is advanced into the desired position. Bone grafts are placed in the nasofrontal junction, lateral orbital walls, and pterygomaxillary fissures. Miniplate fixation is particularly helpful at the site of the Le Fort I osteotomy (Fig. 61–39).

Monobloc Advancement of Orbits and Midface. To increase the orbital volume for the correction of exorbitism, the subtotal orbits and midface can be advanced as a single skeletal segment. The technique was popularized by Ortiz-Monasterio, Fuente del Campo, and Carrillo (1978). The lines of osteotomy are similar to those previously described for the combined Le Fort III–frontal

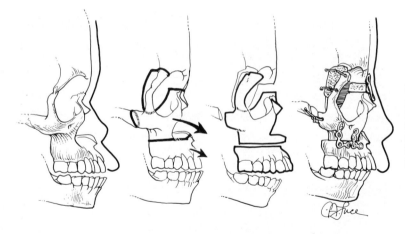

Figure 61–38. The combination Le Fort III–Le Fort I osteotomy offers differential advancement of the mid-face and maxillary segments. Autogenous bone grafts are placed in the defects, and fixation is established with a combination of wires and mini-plates.

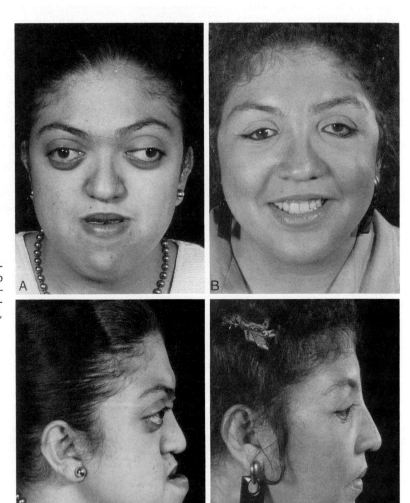

Figure 61–39. Adolescent female with Crouzon's disease who underwent a combined Le Fort III–Le Fort I osteotomy and genioplasty. *A, C,* Preoperative views. *B, D,* Postoperative views.

bone advancement (see Fig. 61–36) except that the nasofrontal junction and frontozygomatic suture are spared of osteotomies (Fig. 61–40).

The technique also has the advantage that a concomitant hypertelorism correction can be done; it suffers the disadvantages of an increased infection rate and limited orbital volume expansion (Firmin, Coccaro, and Converse, 1974).

Le Fort II Advancement. The most common indication for a Le Fort II advancement (Fig. 61–41) is the patient with midface hypoplasia and adequate zygomatic projection. The patient illustrated in Figure 61–42 had craniosynostosis associated with vitamin D resistant rickets.

Zygomatic, Maxillary-Mandibular Osteotomies. As the trend today is toward midface advancements performed in younger patients, it is only logical that jaw surgery will be indicated in adolescent years. As demonstrated in longitudinal studies (McCarthy and associates, 1984b), jaw disharmonies (i.e., anterior crossbite) reflect anticipated mandibular growth after a Le Fort III advancement in a younger child (Fig. 61–43).

In the patient with craniofacial synostosis who has undergone a midface advancement, there is often an obvious microgenia. It has been the authors' experience that most of these patients also require a genioplasty or advancement osteotomy of the anteroinferior border of the mandible (see Chapter 29).

Another useful technique in the years after a Le Fort III osteotomy is a zygomatic advancement in patients in whom orbital and maxillary positions are satisfactory but zygomatic projection is lacking (Figs. 61–44, 61–45).

New York University Protocol for Surgical Treatment of Craniosynostosis. Early surgery is optimally completed by 6 months of age (see Table 61–2). Depending on the diagnosis and associated pathologic condition of the patient, this could include strip craniectomy with or without frontal bone advancement, or cranial vault remodeling.

If by age 3 or 4 years there is evidence of midface hypoplasia with exorbitism and malocclusion, the child is prepared for Le Fort III midface advancement. The orthodontist takes dental impressions and constructs thin occlusal splints made in acrylic and used for fixation purposes.

It is likely that additional jaw surgery (Le Fort I osteotomy) will be required during the period of adolescence. With the eruption of the permanent maxillary teeth, injury to the apices of the teeth will be avoided (see Fig. 61–43).

Text continued on page 3051

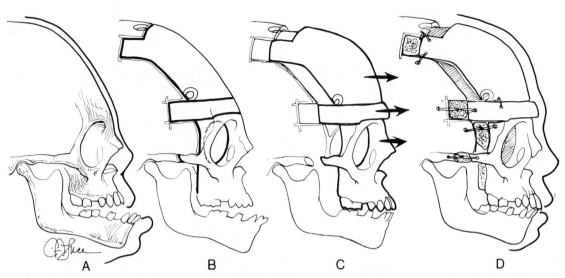

Figure 61–40. Monobloc advancement (after Ortiz-Monasterio and associates, 1978). *A,* Hypoplastic midface and orbitofrontal region. *B,* Lines of osteotomy. Note that the Le Fort III segment also incorporates the roof of the orbits. In addition, the frontal bone is remodeled in two segments. *C,* The three skeletal segments can be advanced to varying degrees. *D,* Final position with bone grafts in position. Rigid skeletal fixation can also be employed.

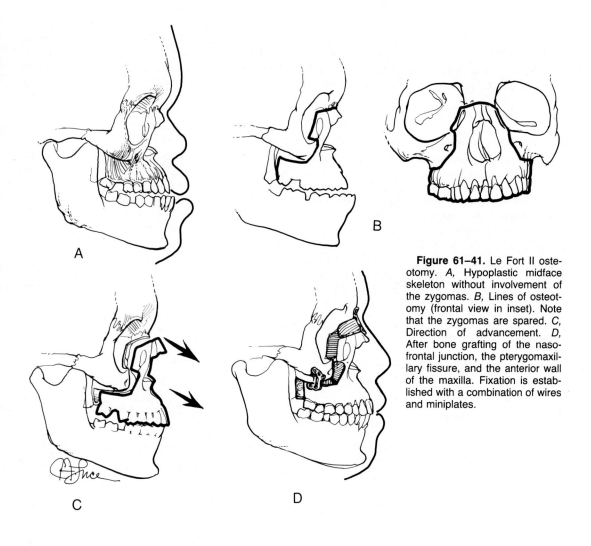

Figure 61–41. Le Fort II osteotomy. *A,* Hypoplastic midface skeleton without involvement of the zygomas. *B,* Lines of osteotomy (frontal view in inset). Note that the zygomas are spared. *C,* Direction of advancement. *D,* After bone grafting of the nasofrontal junction, the pterygomaxillary fissure, and the anterior wall of the maxilla. Fixation is established with a combination of wires and miniplates.

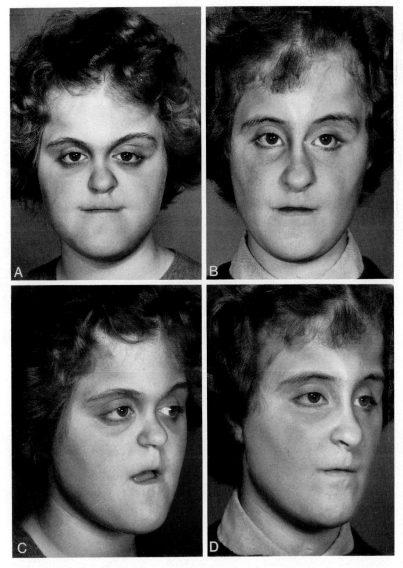

Figure 61–42. Female patient with craniosynostosis associated with vitamin D resistant rickets. *A, C,* Preoperative views. Note the midface hypoplasia and foreshortened nose. *B, D,* After Le Fort II advancement as illustrated in Figure 61–41. (From McCarthy, J. G., and Reid, C. A.: Craniofacial synostosis in association with vitamin D–resistant rickets. Ann. Plast. Surg., *4:*149, 1979.)

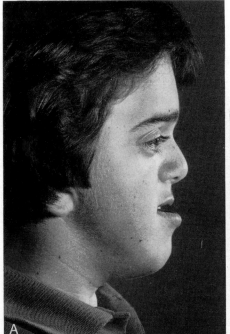

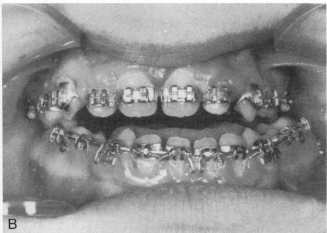

Figure 61–43. Longitudinal study of a male with Pfeiffer's syndrome. *A, B,* Age 14. Note the midface hypoplasia and anterior crossbite.

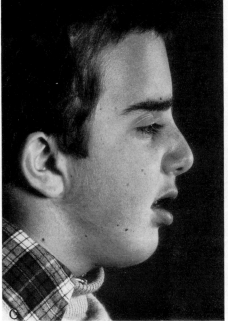

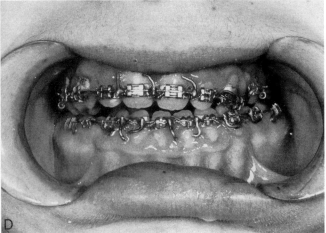

Figure 61–43 *Continued C, D,* Age 15 after Le Fort III advancement. There has been improvement in facial form and the malocclusion has been corrected.

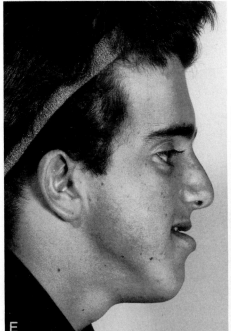

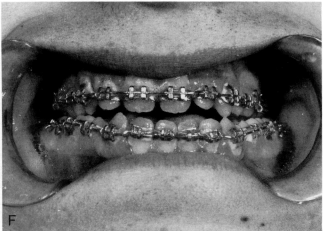

Figure 61–43 *Continued E, F,* Age 17. With expected mandibular growth there is an anterior crossbite with jaw-lip dysharmony.

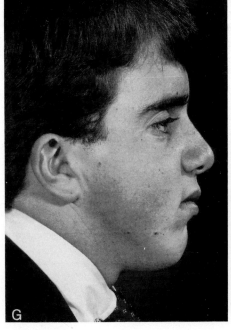

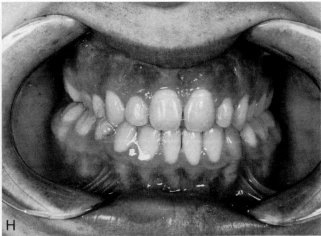

Figure 61–43 *Continued G, H,* Age 18. After a Le Fort I advancement there is a satisfactory jaw-lip relationship and the occlusion is Class I.

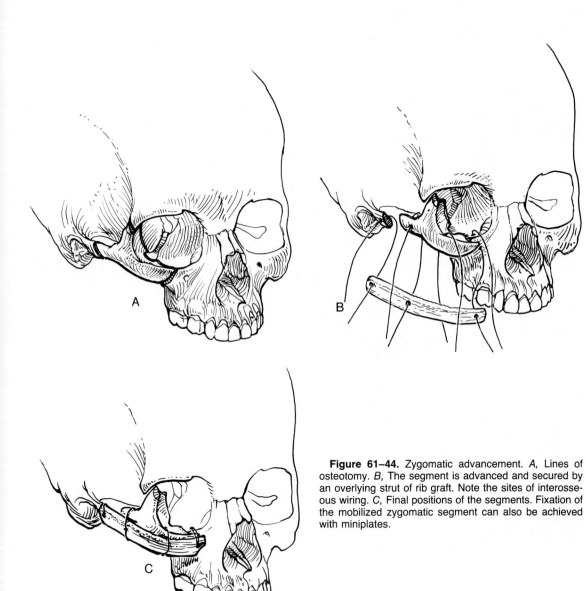

Figure 61–44. Zygomatic advancement. *A,* Lines of osteotomy. *B,* The segment is advanced and secured by an overlying strut of rib graft. Note the sites of interosseous wiring. *C,* Final positions of the segments. Fixation of the mobilized zygomatic segment can also be achieved with miniplates.

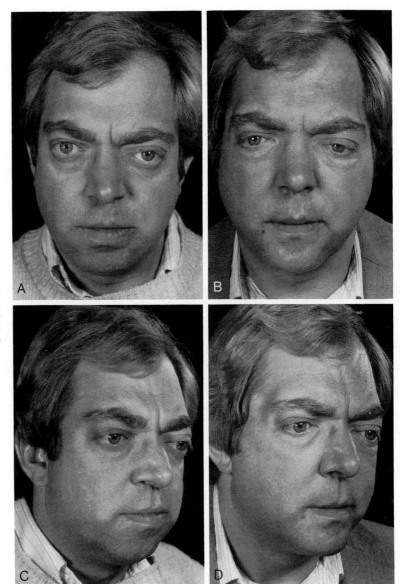

Figure 61–45. Adult male with Crouzon's disease. *A, C,* Preoperative views. Note the zygomatic deficiency and exorbitism. The occlusal relationships are satisfactory. *B, D,* Appearance following zygomatic advancement as illustrated in Figure 61–44. A genioplasty was also performed.

POSTOPERATIVE LONGITUDINAL STUDIES

There is a paucity of longitudinal studies after surgery for craniofacial synostosis. The reports are often subjective and lack strict criteria for the evaluation of craniofacial form, occlusal status, intracranial pressure, or psychosocial function.

In a retrospective analysis of 519 patients with craniosynostosis who had undergone limited strip craniectomies, Shillito and Matson (1968) reported that only 52 per cent showed satisfactory craniofacial form; the most satisfactory results were in those patients with isolated sagittal synostosis.

Several centers have reported their experience with frontocranial remodeling for craniosynostosis (McCarthy and associates, 1984a; Marchac and Renier, 1985). The authors were satisfied with long-term frontoorbital position, especially in the patients with bilateral and unilateral coronal synostosis. In the latter group there was also a correction of the orbitonasal asymmetry with the passage of time. However, in the craniofacial synostoses syndromes (Crouzon, Apert) the desired midface growth was not realized, and many developed an anterior crossbite requiring a midface advancement. Mortality was less than 2 per cent and complications included infection, protruding wires, and contour irregularities or defects.

With the trend toward earlier midface advancements, critical questions have arisen as to the stability and growth of the advanced segment. Preliminary longitudinal data after Le Fort III advancement in the growing child have demonstrated stability of the advanced skeletal segment and there was also evidence of minimal anteroinferior growth of the latter in some patients (McCarthy and associates, 1984b). Any disharmony in jaw relationships could be attributed to expected mandibular growth during the period of postoperative observation (see Fig. 61–43).

Hogeman and Willmar (1974) reported a four-year follow-up of a 14 year old girl after Le Fort III advancement and bone grafting for craniofacial synostosis. During the interval, there was only minimal growth of the midface and upper jaw; because of growth of the mandible, an open bite deformity developed. A degree of exorbitism also recurred. Freihofer (1973) followed nine adult patients for three to 40 months after major midface osteotomies. Five patients showed no change in their occlusal relationships; in three there was relapse; prognathic changes became apparent in two children because of anterior growth of the mandible. The esthetic result, however, was considered satisfactory in eight. In a follow-up (with a range of 10 to 17 years) of six patients who underwent Le Fort III advancement, Tulasne and Tessier (1986) noted that there was no retardation of nasal growth in the patients operated on before puberty. However, in three of the latter patients there was recurrence of the Class III malocclusion. There was also noticeable recession of the advanced zygomatic segments.

REFERENCES

Albin, R. E., Hendee, R. W., O'Donnell, R. S., and Majure, J. A.: Trigonocephaly: refinements in reconstruction. Experience with 33 patients. Plast. Reconstr. Surg., 76:202, 1985.

Angle, C. R., McIntire, M. S., and Moore, R. C.: Cloverleaf skull: kleeblattschädel deformity syndrome. Am. J. Dis. Child., 114:198, 1967.

Apert, E.: De l'acricephalosyndactylie. Bull. Soc. Med. Hop. Paris, 23:1310, 1906.

Bertelsen, T. I.: The premature synostosis of the cranial sutures. Acta Ophthalmol., 51(Suppl.):47, 1958.

Blank, C. E.: Apert's syndrome (a type of acrocephalosyndactyly): observations on a British series of 39 cases. Ann. Hum. Genet., 24:161, 1960.

Blechschmidt, M.: The biokinetics of the basicranium. In Bosma, J. F. (Ed.): Symposium on Development of the Basicranium. DHEW Pub. No. (NIH) 76–989. Bethesda, MD, National Institutes of Health, 1976.

Blinkov, S. M., and Glezer, I. I.: The Human Brain in Figures and Tables: A Quantitative Handbook. New York, Basic Books, 1968.

Caronni, E. P. (Ed.): Craniofacial Surgery. Boston, Little, Brown & Company, 1985.

Chotzen, F.: Unusual familial developmental disturbance of face (acrocephalosyndactylia, craniofacial dysostosis and hypertelorism). Monatschr. Kinderh., 55:97, 1932.

Cohen, M. M., Jr.: An etiologic and nosologic overview of craniosynostosis syndromes. Birth Defects, 11:137, 1975.

Cohen, M. M., Jr. (Ed.): Craniosynostosis. Diagnosis, Evaluation and Management. New York, Raven Press, 1986.

Converse, J. M., and Wood-Smith, D.: An atlas and classification of midfacial and craniofacial osteotomies. Transactions of the Fifth International Congress of Plastic and Reconstructive Surgery. Australia, Butterworth, 1971.

Crouzon, O.: Dysostose, cranio-faciale hereditaire. Bull. Soc. Med. Hop. Paris, 33:545, 1912.

Dufresne, C. R., McCarthy, J. G., Cutting, C. B., Epstein, F. J., and Hoffman, W. Y.: Volumetric quantification of intracranial and ventricular volume following cranial vault remodeling: a preliminary report. Plast. Reconstr. Surg., 79:24, 1987.

Enlow, D. H.: Handbook of Facial Growth. 2nd Ed. Philadelphia, W. B. Saunders Company, 1982.

Enlow, D. H., and Azuma, M.: Functional growth boundaries in the human and mammalian face. Birth Defects, 11:217, 1975.

Firmin, F., Coccaro, P. J., and Converse, J. M.: Cephalometric analysis in diagnosis and treatment planning of craniofacial dysostoses. Plast. Reconstr. Surg., 54:300, 1974.

Fishman, M. A., Hogan, G. R., and Dodge, P. R.: The concurrence of hydrocephalus and craniosynostosis. J. Neurosurg., 34:621, 1971.

Freihofer, H. P.: Results after midface osteotomies. J. Maxillofac. Surg., 1:30, 1973.

Friedenwald, W.: Cranial deformity and optic nerve atrophy. Am. J. Med. Sci., 105:529, 1893.

Gillies, H., and Harrison, S. H.: Operative correction by osteotomy of recessed malar maxillary compound in a case of oxycephaly. Br. J. Plast. Surg., 3:123, 1950–51.

Gorlin, R. J., Pindborg, J. J., and Cohen, M. M.: Syndromes of the Head and Neck. 2nd Ed. New York, McGraw Hill Book Company, 1976.

Hoffman, H. J., and Mohr, G.: Lateral canthal advancement of the supraorbital margin. J. Neurosurg., 45:376, 1976.

Hogeman, K. E., and Willmar, K.: On Le Fort III osteotomy for Crouzon's disease in children. Scand. J. Plast. Reconstr. Surg., 8:169, 1974.

Hoyte, D. A.: Contributions of the sphenoethmoidal complex to basicranial growth in rabbits. In Bosma, J. F. (Ed.): Symposium on Development of the Basicranium. DHEW Pub. No. (NIH) 76–989. Bethesda, MD, National Institutes of Health, 1976.

Jabaley, M. E., and Edgerton, M. T.: Surgical correction of congenital mid-face retrusion in the presence of mandibular prognathism. Plast. Reconstr. Surg., 44:1, 1969.

Kreiborg, S.: Crouzon syndrome. Scand. J. Plast. Reconstr. Surg. (Suppl.), 18:1, 1981.

Lane, L. C.: Pioneer craniotomy for relief of mental imbecility due to premature sutural closure and microcephalus. J.A.M.A., 18:49, 1892.

Lannelongue, J.: De la craniectomie dans la microcephalie. C. R. Acad. Sci., 110:1382, 1890.

Lewin, M. L.: Facial deformity in acrocephaly and its surgical correction. Arch. Ophthalmol., 47:321, 1952.

Marchac, D.: Radical forehead remodeling for craniostenosis. Plast. Reconstr. Surg., 61:823, 1978.

Marchac, D., and Renier, D.: Craniofacial Surgery for Craniosynostosis. Boston, Little, Brown & Company, 1982.

Marchac, D., and Renier, D.: Craniofacial surgery for craniosynostosis improves facial growth: a personal case review. Ann. Plast. Surg., 14:43, 1985.

Marsh, J. L., and Vannier, M. W.: Comprehensive Care for Craniofacial Deformities. St. Louis, C. V. Mosby Company, 1985.

Matson, D. D.: Neurosurgery of Infancy and Childhood. 2nd Ed. Springfield, Charles C Thomas, 1969.

McCarthy, J. G.: The concept of a craniofacial anomalies center. Clin. Plast. Surg., 3:611, 1976.

McCarthy, J. G.: New concepts in the surgical treatment of the craniofacial synostosis syndromes. Clin. Plast. Surg., 6:201, 1979.

McCarthy, J. G., Coccaro, P. J., Epstein, F., and Converse, J. M.: Early skeletal release in the infant with craniofacial dysostosis. The role of the sphenozygomatic suture. Plast. Reconstr. Surg., 62:235, 1978.

McCarthy, J. G., Coccaro, P. J., and Keller, A.: Craniofacial suture manipulation in the newborn rhesus monkey. In Caronni, E. P. (Ed.): Craniofacial Surgery. Boston, Little, Brown & Company, 1985.

McCarthy, J. G., Converse, J. M., Wood-Smith, D., and Casson, P. R.: Other applications of craniofacial surgical techniques. Presented at the American Association of Plastic Surgeons. Atlanta, Georgia, 1976a.

McCarthy, J. G., Converse, J. M., Wood-Smith, D., Choy, D., and Breinin, G. M.: Extraocular muscle function following craniofacial surgery. Transactions of the 6th International Congress of Plastic and Reconstructive Surgery. Paris, Masson, 1976b, p. 177.

McCarthy, J. G., Epstein, F., Sadove, M., Grayson, B., and Zide, B.: Early surgery for craniofacial synostosis: an eight year experience. Plast. Reconstr. Surg., 73:521, 1984a.

McCarthy, J. G., Grayson, B., Bookstein, F., Vickery, C., and Zide, B.: Le Fort III advancement osteotomy in the growing child. Plast. Reconstr. Surg., 74:343, 1984b.

McCarthy, J. G., and Reid, C. A.: Craniofacial synostosis in association with vitamin D-resistant rickets. Ann. Plast. Surg., 4:149, 1979.

Meltzer: Zur Pathengenese der Opticusatrophie und der sogenanten Turnschadels. Zentralbl. Neurochir., 190:27, 1908.

Montaut, J., and Stricker, M.: Dysmorphies craniofaciales: les synostoses prematuries (craniostenoses et faciostenoses). Paris, Masson, 1977.

Moss, M. L.: The pathogenesis of premature cranial synostosis in man. Acta Anat. (Basel), 37:351, 1959.

Moss, M. L.: The functional matrix. In Kraus, B. S., and Riedel, R. A. (Eds.): Vistas of Orthodontics. Philadelphia, Lea & Febiger, 1962.

Muhlbauer, W., Anderl, H., and Marchac, D.: Complete frontofacial advancement in infants with craniofacial

dysostosis. In Williams, B. (Ed.): Transactions of the Eighth International Congress of Plastic Surgery. Montreal, 1983.

Munro, I. R.: Reshaping the cranial vault. In Converse, J. M. (Ed.): Reconstructive Plastic Surgery. 2nd Ed. Philadelphia, W. B. Saunders Company, 1977.

Murray, J. E., and Swanson, L. T.: Mid-face osteotomy and advancement of craniosynostosis. Plast. Reconstr. Surg., 41:299, 1968.

Obwegeser, H. L.: Surgical correction of small or retrodisplaced maxillae. The "dish-face" deformity. Plast. Reconstr. Surg., 43:351, 1969.

Ortiz-Monasterio, F., Fuente del Campo, A., and Carrillo, A.: Advancement of the orbits and the midface in one piece, combined with frontal repositioning, for the correction of Crouzon's deformities. Plast. Reconstr. Surg., 61:507, 1978.

Persing, J. A., Edgerton, M. T., Park, T. S., and Jane, J. A.: Barrel stave osteotomy for correction of turribrachycephaly craniosynostosis deformities. Ann. Plast. Surg., 18:488, 1987.

Pfeiffer, R. A.: Dominant erbliche Akrocephalosyndaktylie. Z. Kinderheilkd., 90:301, 1964.

Reid, C. A., McCarthy, J. G., and Kolber, A. B.: A study of regeneration in parietal bone defects in rabbits. Plast. Reconstr. Surg., 67:591, 1981.

Saethre, H.: Oxycephaly (turmschadel), its neuro-psychiatric symptoms, pathogenesis and heredity. Norsk. Mag. Laegevidensk., 92:392, 1931.

Shillito, J., Jr., and Matson, D. D.: Craniostenosis: a review of 519 surgical patients. Paediatrics, 41:829, 1968.

Stewart, R. E., Dixon, G., and Cohen, A.: Pathogenesis of premature craniosynostosis in acrocephalosyndactyly (Apert's syndrome). Plast. Reconstr. Surg., 59:699, 1977.

Tessier, P.: Relationship of craniostenoses to craniofacial dysostoses, and to faciostenoses: a study with therapeutic implications. Plast. Reconstr. Surg., 48:224, 1971a.

Tessier, P.: The scope and principles, dangers and limitations and the need for special training in orbitocranial surgery. In Hueston, J. T. (Ed.): Transactions of the Fifth International Congress of Plastic and Reconstructive Surgery, Melbourne, 1971. Australia, Butterworth, 1971b, pp. 903–929.

Tessier, P.: The definitive plastic surgical treatment of the severe facial deformities of craniofacial dysostosis, Crouzon's and Apert's disease. Plast. Reconstr. Surg., 48:419, 1971c.

Tessier, P.: Orbital hypertelorism. 1. Successive surgical attempts, material and methods, causes and mechanisms. Scand. J. Plast. Surg., 6:135, 1972.

Tessier, P., Guiot, G., Rougerie, J., Delbet, J. P., and Pastoriza, J.: Osteotomies cranio-naso-orbitales. Hypertelorisme. Ann. Chir. Plast., 12:103, 1967.

Tulasne, J. F., and Tessier, P. L.: Long-term results of Le Fort III advancement in Crouzon's syndrome. Cleft Palate J., 23(Suppl. 1):102, 1986.

Van der Klaaw, C. J.: Size and position of the functional components of the skull. A contribution to the knowledge of the architecture of the skull, based on data in the literature. Arch. Neerl. Zool., 9:1559, 1948–52.

Virchow, R.: Uber den Cretinismus, namentlich in Franken, und uber pathologische Schadelformen. Verhandl. Phys-Med. Gessellschr. Wurzburg., 2:241, 1851.

von Graefe, A.: Uber neuroretinitis und Gervise Fallefulminierende Erbinding. Arch. Ophthalmol., 12:114, 1866.

62

Joseph G. McCarthy
Barry H. Grayson
Peter J. Coccaro
Donald Wood-Smith

Craniofacial Microsomia

Among the congenital otocephalic syndromes, the term "first and second branchial arch syndrome" designates, in the United States, a characteristic congenital malformation that is usually unilateral but occasionally bilateral. In the German literature, the deformity has been termed "dysostosis otomandibularis." Caronni (1971) coined the term "auriculo-branchiogenic dysplasia." Stark and Saunders (1962) referred to a similar clinical association of physical findings as the first branchial arch syndrome or the oral-mandibular-auricular syndrome. Gorlin and Pindborg (1964) reviewed the various names by which the condition has been described and advocated the term "hemifacial microsomia," which implies that the deformity is exclusively unilateral and spares the cranium. Pruzansky (1969) used the term "otocraniocephalic syndromes" to describe aberrations in the development of the first and second branchial arches.

At the Center for Craniofacial Anomalies of the Institute of Reconstructive Plastic Surgery of the New York University Medical Center, the term "unilateral craniofacial microsomia" is preferred for the unilateral form, and the designation "bilateral craniofacial microsomia" is reserved for the bilateral type.

DIFFERENTIAL DIAGNOSIS

The deformity of craniofacial microsomia, whether unilateral or bilateral, is characterized by varying degrees of regional hypoplasia affecting the temporomandibular and pterygomandibular complexes (skeletal and neuromuscular structures). The bilateral form must be distinguished from mandibulofacial dysostosis (Treacher Collins syndrome) (see Chap. 63), which shows a well-defined genetic pattern (Franceschetti and Klein, 1949), the deformity being transmitted in an irregular dominant fashion; the gene is unstable and has a weak degree of penetrance. Tessier (1976) pointed out that craniofacial microsomia has features in common with mandibulofacial dysostosis, such as the temporozygomatic defect and orbital deformities (see Fig. 62–1). Distinguishing characteristics of craniofacial microsomia are the malformations of the mandibular ramus and facial paralysis. Tessier (1976) also described three types of craniofacial clefts that are present in mandibulofacial dysostosis (see Chap. 63).

A jaw malformation similar to that seen in bilateral craniofacial microsomia may be observed in patients who have sustained postnatal trauma or infection that has affected the condylar cartilage and, as a result, mandibular growth. It has been suggested, both experimentally and clinically, by several authors that impaired growth of the condyle may result in an underdevelopment not only of the mandible but also of the craniofacial osseous complex on the affected side (Sarnat and Engel, 1951; Brodie, 1964; Sarnat and Laskin, 1964). Usually, however, it is relatively easy to distinguish postnatal deformities from those resulting from prenatal (genetic or intrauterine environmental) factors.

In postnatal traumatic deformity, the deformity is restricted to the jaws and the auricle is spared; the soft tissues are not deficient, and there is no temporal bone deformity. The earlier the traumatic insult occurs, the more severe is the clinical expression of the deformity, and there is often associated temporomandibular joint ankylosis.

In contrast, in craniofacial microsomia the deformity is more widespread, with involvement of the temporal bone, middle ear, mastoid process, external ear, and base of the skull. Soft tissue hypoplasia is often apparent on the affected side.

Patients with severe orbitofacial clefts (see Chap. 59) and hypoplasia of the maxilla also have an occlusal cant and a shortened mandibular ramus, but the condylar deformity, which is the hallmark of craniofacial microsomia, is lacking.

UNILATERAL CRANIOFACIAL MICROSOMIA

History

Grabb (1965) cited the teratologic tablets written in approximately 2000 B.C. by the Chaldeans of Mesopotamia as the earliest recorded documentation of malformations of the first and second branchial arches in man. Bartholinus (1654) described a child in whom the external auditory canal was absent, and Lachmund (1688) reported a female with microtia and agenesis of the external auditory canal. Thompson (1845) drew attention to the fact that the clinical expression of the syndrome was in structures derived from the first and second branchial arches and the intervening cleft.

In more recent times the publications of Kazanjian (1939), Altman (1951), Meurmann (1957), François (1961), Stark and Saunders (1962), Gorlin and Pindborg (1964), Grabb (1965), Pruzansky (1969), Longacre, De-

Stefano, and Holmstrand (1963), Obwegeser (1970, 1974), Converse and associates (1973a,b, 1974), Munro (1980), Munro and Lauritzen (1985), and Murray and associates (1985) have focused attention on the clinical findings and reconstruction of the individual deformities. Harvold, Vargervik, and Chierici (1983) emphasized the role of a combined functional appliance (orthodontic) surgical treatment program on the developing mandible in this syndrome.

Clinical Spectrum

Incidence. In a study of records at several hospitals in the United States, the birth incidence was determined to be one in 5642 births (Grabb, 1965). Poswillo (1973) cited an incidence of one in 4000. Following the administration of thalidomide to pregnant women in Germany between the years 1959 and 1962, approximately 1000 severe and an additional 2000 less severe cases of first and second branchial arch malformations were reported (Kleinsasser and Schlothane, 1964).

Sex. In the series of 102 patients reported by Grabb (1965), 63 were males and 39 were females.

Unilateral vs. Bilateral. In a series of 74 patients, Meurmann (1957) reported eight patients with bilateral involvement; Dupertuis and Musgrave (1959) noted a unilateral to bilateral incidence of six to one; Grabb (1965) cited bilateral involvement in 12 of 102 patients; and Converse and associates (1974) studied 15 individuals with bilateral craniofacial microsomia out of a total series of 280 patients. However, it should be emphasized that these statistics are misleading. On more thorough clinical and radiographic examination, abnormalities can be detected on the "normal" or "less affected" side—an increased length of the mandibular body, partial facial palsy, orbital dystopia, ear tags, and so forth. The pathologic findings and treatment of bilateral craniofacial microsomia are discussed later in this chapter.

Variations of the Syndrome. The deformity in craniofacial microsomia varies in extent and degree. Because of the heterogeneous nature of craniofacial microsomia, it is difficult to classify the individual deformity (Fig. 62–1).

In the severe form, all the structures derived from the first and second branchial

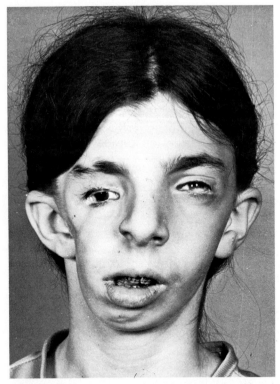

Figure 62–1. Severe craniofacial microsomia with epibulbar dermoids (Goldenhar type), colobomas, preauricular pits, low-set ears, short mandibular rami, micrognathia, deviation of the chin, occlusal cant, and anterior open bite. The skeletal and soft tissue deficiencies are more severe on the right side. (From Converse, J. M., Wood-Smith D., McCarthy, J. G., Coccaro, P. J., and Becker, M. H.: Bilateral facial microsomia. Plast. Reconstr. Surg., *54*:413, 1974. Copyright © 1974, The Williams & Wilkins Company, Baltimore.)

arches are hypoplastic (Fig. 62–2), whereas in other types either the auricular or jaw dysplasias may be predominant.

It is in the latter cases that the associated deformities are less evident. There may be many shades of expression, according to the degree of involvement of the structures derived from the first and second arches and the involvement of the adjacent skeletal structures:

1. The ear deformity may be maximal (Fig. 62–3), while the jaw deformity is not apparent on clinical examination. However, roentgenographic studies, including tomography, demonstrate that all cases of external auditory canal and auricular hypoplasia with middle ear deformity have mandibular changes on the affected side (Fig. 62–4).

2. The ear deformity may be less severe (Fig. 62–5), and the jaw deformity may not

be evident; roentgenographic analysis may show a disparity of the skeletal structures (Fig. 62–6). In these cases of minor jaw deformities, careful clinical examination often shows a slight deviation of the mandible to the affected side. The midsagittal plane extends through the interspace between the upper central incisors (midincisor point), but the lower midincisor point may be off-center in relation to it (Fig. 62–7).

3. The characteristic jaw deformity of unilateral craniofacial microsomia may be present without gross auricular or temporal bone maldevelopment (Fig. 62–8). These cases are difficult to differentiate from postnatal deformities caused by injury, but the diagnosis becomes evident if the deformity was present at birth. This type of deformity may also be complicated by associated malformations such as microphthalmos (see Fig. 62–2). The auricle may be normal in shape, protruding, or low-set, with a normal hearing mechanism.

4. "Formes frustes" or microforms are more frequent than is generally acknowledged. They must be searched for in cases of slight facial asymmetry and in auricular malformations without manifest jaw deformity. The

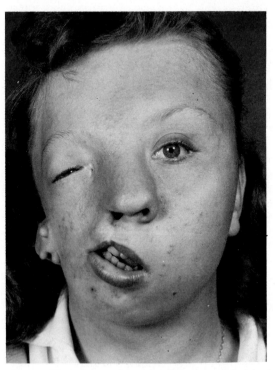

Figure 62–2. Severe form of unilateral craniofacial microsomia with microtia, microphthalmos, and a naso-orbital cleft.

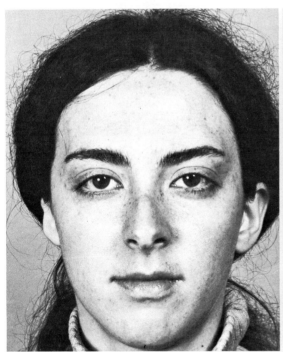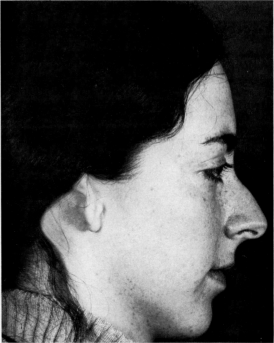

Figure 62–3. Patient with microtia and small auricular remnant: there is no apparent jaw deformity. (From Converse, J. M., Coccaro, P. J., Becker, M., and Wood-Smith, D.: On hemifacial microsomia. Plast. Reconstr. Surg., *51*:268, 1973. Copyright © 1973, The Williams & Wilkins Company, Baltimore.)

patient shown in Figure 62–9*A* is an example of a "forme fruste." The deformity is characterized by a soft tissue deficiency in the right parotid-masseteric area (the parotid gland was hypoplastic), a protruding right auricle (with normal hearing), and a slight degree of macrostomia involving the right oral commissure. The dental occlusal relationships were adequate. Correction was achieved (Fig. 62–9*B*) by insertion of a dermis-fat graft that restored adequate facial contour, a protruding ear operation according to the technique of Converse and associates (1963), and closure of the macrostomia.

Harvold, Vargervik, and Chierici (1983) proposed the following phenotypic classification of *unilateral* craniofacial microsomia:

Type I(A). The classic type characterized by unilateral facial underdevelopment without microphthalmos or ocular dermoids but with or without abnormalities of the vertebrae, heart, or kidneys.

Type I(B). Similar to Type I(A) except for the presence of microphthalmos.

Type I(C). Bilateral asymmetric type in which one side is more severely involved.

Type I(D). Complex type that does not fit Types I(A–C) but does not display limb deficiency, frontonasal phenotype, or ocular dermoids.

Type II. Limb deficiency type—unilateral or bilateral, with or without ocular abnormalities.

Type III. Frontonasal type. Relative unilateral underdevelopment of the face in the presence of hypertelorism, with or without ocular dermoids and vertebral, cardiac, or renal abnormalities.

Type IV(A, unilateral or B, bilateral). Goldenhar type with facial underdevelopment in association with ocular dermoids, with or without upper lid coloboma.

Munro and Lauritzen (1985) proposed an anatomic classification designed to aid in surgical planning (see Fig. 62–36). Other classification systems have been reported by Kaban, Moses, and Mulliken (1988) and David, Mahatumarat, and Cooter (1987).

Embryology

The ear serves as a frame of reference in this syndrome (Pruzansky, 1969) because of

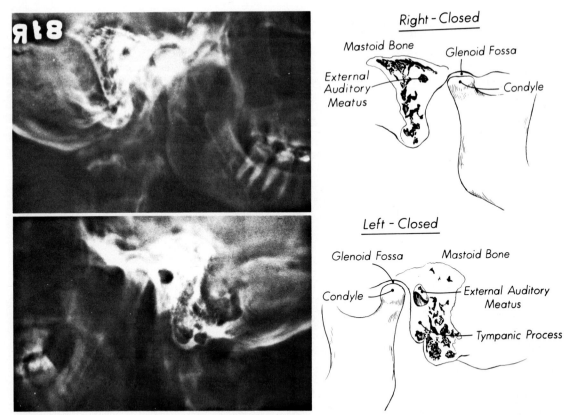

Figure 62–4. *Above,* Tomogram through the right temporomandibular joint (in closed position) of the patient shown in Figure 62–3. The external auditory canal and the mastoid are hypoplastic. Note the change in the morphology of the condyle and glenoid fossa. *Below,* Tomogram of the structures on the left (unaffected side), which more closely represent a normal temporomandibular joint, mastoid, and external auditory canal. (From Converse, J. M., Coccaro, P. J., Becker, M., and Wood-Smith, D.: On hemifacial microsomia. Plast. Reconstr. Surg., *51:*268, 1973. Copyright © 1973, The Williams & Wilkins Company, Baltimore.)

its developmental relationship with the jaw (Table 62–1). A brief review of the phylogeny and ontogeny of the auricle and hearing apparatus is helpful in understanding the embryogenesis of the malformation in the craniofacial microsomia syndrome.

The two principal divisions of the organ of hearing are derived from different embryonic anlagen. The sensory end organ in the inner ear is derived from the ectodermal otocyst, while the sound-conducting apparatus in the external and middle ear comes from the gill structures.

The membranous labyrinth has its beginning in the 3½ week old human embryo (Arey, 1974) as a thickening of the ectoderm on the side of the head—the otic placode (see Chap. 46). This area is enfolded to become the otic pit and is subsequently pinched off to become the otocyst. By means of a series of folds, the otocyst differentiates in the 3

month old fetus into the endolymphatic duct and sac, the semicircular endolymphatic ducts, the utricle, the saccule, and the cochlear duct, which contains the organ of Corti. By the fifth month of fetal life, the sensory end organ of the ear attains adult form and size, as the cartilaginous otic capsule ossifies.

It is speculated that man's piscine ancestors swam in seas not yet as salty as today's oceans and that man's endolymph, entrapped by the enfolding otocyst, closely resembles in chemical composition the dilute salt water of that primeval sea. Our ancient aquatic forebears did not require any special mechanism to transmit sound to the inner ear. As in today's fish, sound was readily transmitted from the sea through the skin to the fluid of the inner ear.

However, when these ancestors struggled out of the seas onto dry land, a new problem appeared. A mechanical device was needed to

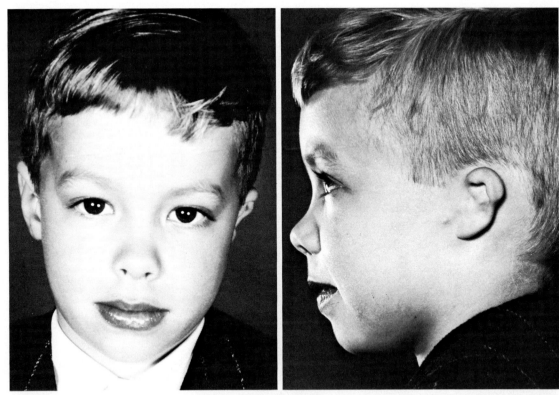

Figure 62–5. Patient with a "mini-ear." The various portions of the auricle are present in a diminutive form. No external auditory canal could be demonstrated. (From Converse, J. M., Coccaro, P. J., Becker, M., and Wood-Smith, D.: On hemifacial microsomia. Plast. Reconstr. Surg., *51*:268, 1973. Copyright © 1973, The Williams & Wilkins Company, Baltimore.)

convert air vibrations of large amplitude and small force into fluid vibrations of small amplitude and large force. The gill structures, no longer needed for breathing, became converted into such a mechanism. The first branchial groove became the external auditory meatus and canal, while the first pharyngeal pouch became the eustachian tube and middle ear. Instead of the branchial groove and pharyngeal pouch connecting to become a gill cleft, a thin intervening layer of tissue remained to form the tympanic membrane.

The mandible, incus, and malleus developed from the cartilage of the first branchial arch (*Meckel's cartilage*), while the stapes (with the exception of the footplate, which originates from the otic capsule), styloid process, and hyoid bone developed from the cartilage of the second branchial arch (*Reichert's cartilage*) (see Table 62–1). The large area of the tympanic membrane, connected by the lever system of the ossicular chain to the small area of the oval window, provided the

ear with an effective mechanism to overcome the sound barrier between air and water.

The gill structures destined to form the sound-conducting apparatus and the jaws are first apparent in the human embryo at 4 weeks, at about the same time as the otic pit.

By the third fetal month, the auricle has been formed from the first and second branchial arches on either side of the first branchial groove; the latter is the primary shallow, funnel-shaped external auditory meatus. From the inner end of the primary meatus, a solid cord of ectodermal cells extends farther inward, with a bulblike enlargement adjacent to the middle ear. It is not until the seventh fetal month that this cord canalizes, beginning medially to form the tympanic membrane and then extending laterally to join with the primary meatus to form the completed external auditory meatus. The external and middle ears, although capable of transmitting sound to the inner ear, are not yet of adult form and size.

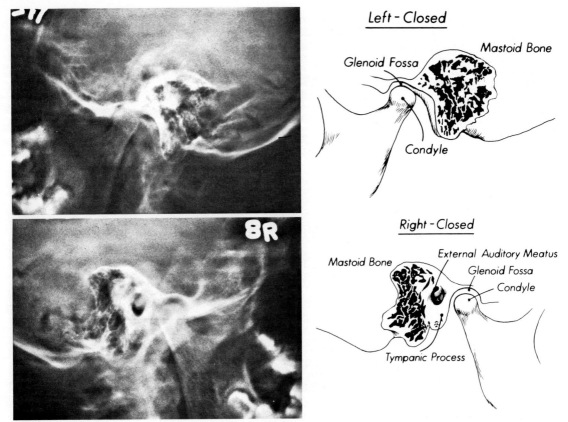

Figure 62–6. *Above,* tomogram through the left temporomandibular joint (in closed position) of the patient shown in Figure 62–5. Note the forward position of the condyle, the shallow glenoid fossa, the absent external auditory canal, and the small mastoid. *Below,* tomogram of the unaffected right side, showing normal anatomic structures in the area of the temporomandibular joint and mastoid. (From Converse, J. M., Coccaro, P. J., Becker, M., and Wood-Smith, D.: On hemifacial microsomia. Plast. Reconstr. Surg., *51:*268, 1973. Copyright © 1973, The Williams & Wilkins Company, Baltimore.)

In the seventh fetal month, pneumatization of the temporal bone begins. At birth the eustachian tube inflates; the fetal mesodermal tissue in the middle ear and antrum continues to resorb until the epithelium lies close to the periosteum, and pneumatization of the temporal bone proceeds.

The external auditory meatus, entirely cartilaginous at birth (except for the narrow incomplete ring of the tympanic bone), deepens by growth of the tympanic bone to form the adult osseous meatus. Except for some pneumatization of the petrous apex, which may continue into adult life, the external and middle ear finally attain adult form and size in late childhood (in contrast to the inner ear, which becomes adult in fetal life). It is generally accepted that the first branchial arch furnishes the anterior part of the auricle (see Table 62–1); the second arch provides the

structures of the remaining external ear (Wood-Jones and Wen-I-Chuan, 1934). The embryology of the external ear is also discussed in Chapter 40.

The maxilla, palatine bone, and zygoma develop from the maxillary process of the first branchial arch; the mandible from the mandibular process. Meckel's cartilage, the primary jaw of lower vertebrates, represents the temporary skeleton of the first pharyngeal arch; the two symmetric cartilaginous bars in early fetal life describe a parabolic arch that serves as a model and guide in the early morphogenesis of the mandible.

Three main regions of Meckel's cartilage should be considered: (1) the distal portion, which becomes incorporated into the anterior part of the body of the mandible; (2) a middle portion, which gives rise to the sphenomandibular ligament and contributes to the my-

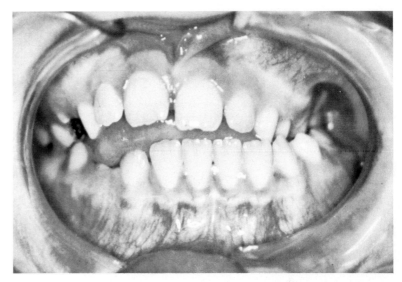

Figure 62–7. Occlusal view of a patient with unilateral craniofacial microsomia. Note that the lower midincisor point (interspace between the central incisors) is off the midsagittal plane. An open bite and lateral crossbite are also present.

lohyoid groove of the mandible; and (3) the proximal or intratympanic portion, which differentiates into the malleus, the incus, and the anterior malleolar ligament.

The embryology of the face is discussed in more detail in Chapter 46.

Etiopathogenesis

Unlike mandibulofacial dysostosis (Treacher Collins syndrome), the genetic component in craniofacial microsomia is ill defined, and there is no evidence of genetic transmission except in a few patients. Grabb (1965) reported that only four of 102 patients studied had one sibling or one parent with evidence of craniofacial microsomia. Hanhart (1949) described a form of inheritable auricular hypoplasia, and Rogers (1968) listed several family studies by other authors that suggested a possible hereditary basis for auricular deformities. Summitt (1969) reported a pedigree of the Goldenhar syndrome that was compatible with autosomal dominant transmission.

Consequently, current etiopathogenic theories favor an intrauterine factor (or factors) that affects the embryo and has the following three characteristics:

1. The factor varies in its intensity and penetrance.

2. The factor strikes at varying periods in the course of prenatal development, from the first to the seventh month.

3. The damage is produced in varying loci along any point of the developing first and second branchial arches, and may be localized (segmental) or widespread.

Table 62–1. Structures Derived From the First and Second Branchial Arches and the Otic Capsule

First branchial arch	
Maxillary process	Maxilla
	Palatine bone
	Zygoma
Mandibular process	Trigeminal nerve
	Anterior part of auricle
	Mandible
	Head of malleus
	Body of incus
	Tympanic bone
	Sphenomandibular ligament
First branchial groove	External auditory meatus
	Tympanic membrane
First pharyngeal pouch	Eustachian tube
	Middle ear cavity
Second branchial arch	Facial nerve
	Posterior part of auricle
	Manubrium of malleus, long process of incus, stapedial superstructure, tympanic surface
	Stapedial artery, styloid process, stylohyoid ligament
	Lesser cornu of hyoid
Otic capsule	Vestibular surface of stapes, internal acoustic meatus
	Inner ear

Modified from Pearson, A. A., and Jacobson, A. D.: The development of the ear. *In* Manual Am. Acad. Ophth. & Otolaryng. Portland, University of Oregon Printing Dept., 1967.

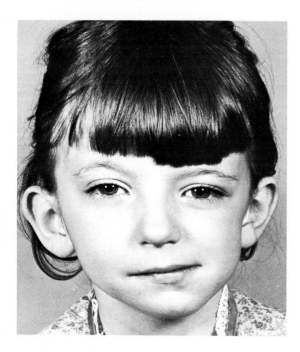

Figure 62–8. Unilateral craniofacial microsomia with the characteristic underdevelopment of the left half of the mandible, upward occlusal cant, hypoplasia of the cheek soft tissue, minimal auricular malformation. The left ear is reduced in size. Note the low-set and protruding position of the right ear. A preauricular pit is also present.

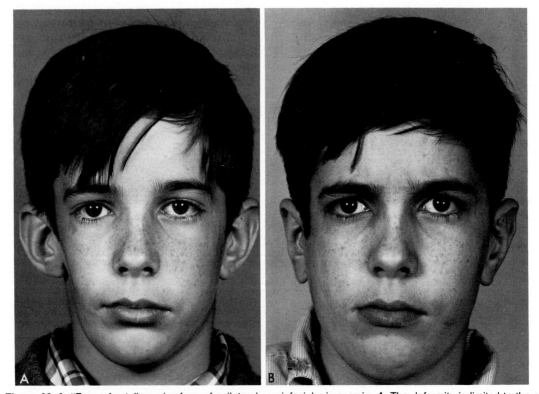

Figure 62–9. "Forme fruste" or microform of unilateral craniofacial microsomia. *A,* The deformity is limited to the soft tissues over the parotid-masseteric area, a protruding auricle (the hearing is normal), tilting of the occlusal plane, and a slight degree of macrostomia of the right oral commissure. *B,* Restoration of the patient's appearance following insertion of a cheek dermis-fat graft and correction of the protruding ear and the macrostomia.

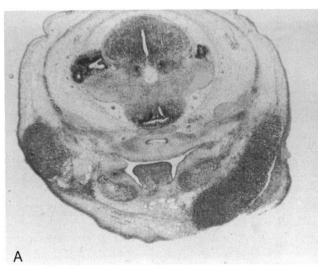

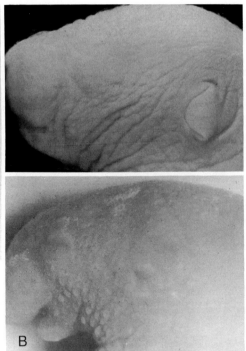

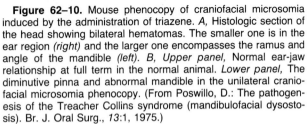

Figure 62–10. Mouse phenocopy of craniofacial microsomia induced by the administration of triazene. *A,* Histologic section of the head showing bilateral hematomas. The smaller one is in the ear region *(right)* and the larger one encompasses the ramus and angle of the mandible *(left). B, Upper panel,* Normal ear-jaw relationship at full term in the normal animal. *Lower panel,* The diminutive pinna and abnormal mandible in the unilateral craniofacial microsomia phenocopy. (From Poswillo, D.: The pathogenesis of the Treacher Collins syndrome (mandibulofacial dysostosis). Br. J. Oral Surg., *13*:1, 1975.)

The theory of mesodermal deficiency as first proposed by Hoffstetter and Veau has been invoked by Stark and Saunders (1962).

Others have suggested that vascular defects of the stapedial artery may account for maldevelopment of the first and second branchial arches (McKenzie and Craig, 1955). The stapedial artery, a temporary vascular supply for the primordia of the first and second branchial arches, appears as a collateral of the hyoid artery and forms anastomosis with the pharyngeal artery; it is ultimately replaced by the finite external carotid system. Willie-Jorgensen (1962) felt that abnormalities of the latter artery were responsible for anomalies of the first and second branchial arches. A decreased heat pattern over the region of the external maxillary artery has also been demonstrated and is interpreted as evidence of a vascular deficiency (Ide, Miller, and Wollschlaeger, 1970).

Poswillo (1973) produced phenocopies of craniofacial microsomia after the administration of triazene to the mouse and thalidomide to the monkey. Embryonic hematoma formation with spreading hemorrhage before the formation of the stapedial artery was dem-onstrated (Fig. 62–10). The extent and size of the hematoma correlated with the size of the anomalous defect. In the mouse experimental model, all the variations found in the human syndrome could be reproduced. The spectrum of defects was broad: a small aural hematoma producing a residual deformity of only the external ear and auditory ossicles; and larger hemorrhagic lesions affecting the condyle, mandibular ramus, and zygoma.

As mentioned earlier, Kleinsasser and Schlothane (1964) reported a large number of newborns with first and second branchial anomalies after the widespread use of thalidomide during pregnancy—presumptive clinical evidence of hematoma formation since thalidomide induces hemorrhages.

Pathology

A characteristic of the syndrome is the variable manifestation of the pathologic findings.

The deformity in craniofacial microsomia usually has the three major features of *auricular, mandibular,* and *maxillary* hypoplasia. The hypoplasia, however, also involves adja-

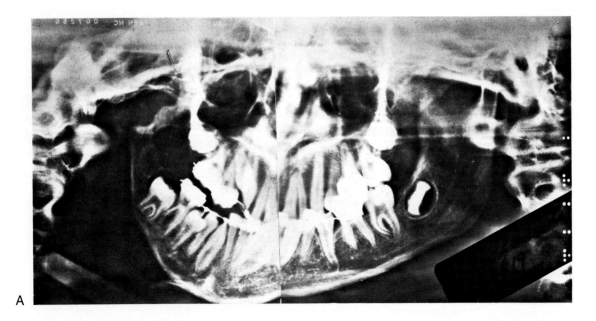

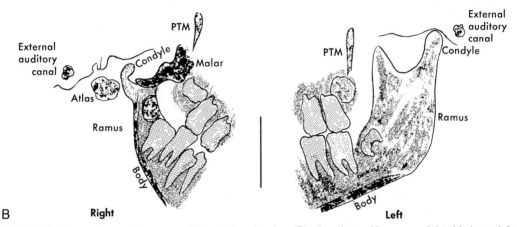

Figure 62–11. Panoramic roentgenogram *(A)* and line drawing *(B)* of patient with severe right-sided craniofacial microsomia. Note the marked reduction in the ramus-condylar process. PTM = pterygomaxillary.

cent anatomic structures: the zygoma, the pterygoid processes of the sphenoid bone, the temporal bone (the middle ear; the mastoid process is small and acellular), the facial nerve and muscles of expression, the muscles of mastication, the parotid, the cutaneous and subcutaneous tissues, and the tongue, soft palate, pharynx, and floor of the nose.

While the jaw and ear deformities are the most conspicuous in the majority of patients, the development of the first and second branchial arches and the structures derived therefrom are intimately interlinked with those of the chondrocranium and membranous bones of the skull; associated deformities of the temporal bone and other cranial bones are

inevitable. In extreme forms of the dysplasia, extensive craniofacial involvement is evident (see Fig. 62–2). As Pruzansky (1969) stated, maldevelopment in one area may trigger a "domino effect," with involvement of the entire craniofacial bone community—microphthalmos, orbital dystopia, and orbitofacial clefts.

JAW DEFORMITY

The most conspicuous deformity of unilateral craniofacial microsomia is the hypoplasia of the mandible on the affected side. The ramus is short or virtually absent (Fig. 62–11), and the body of the mandible curves

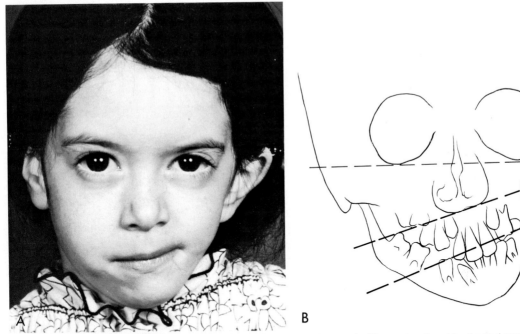

Figure 62–12. *A,* Patient with left-sided unilateral craniofacial microsomia. The occlusal cant is directed upward on the affected side; the chin is deviated to the left side; and the body of the mandible is reduced on the affected side. The gonial angle is increased on the less affected side. *B,* Line drawing of the frontal cephalogram of the patient shown in *A.* The occlusal plane is directed upward on the affected side.

upward to join the short ramus. The chin is deviated to the affected side (Fig. 62–12); the body of the mandible on the "normal" or "less affected" side is also characterized by abnormalities in the skeletal and soft tissue anatomy. The body of the mandible shows increased horizontal length and an increase in the gonial angle (Grayson and associates, 1983a). The increase in length of soft and hard tissue structures on the less affected side may represent compensatory growth, secondary to the growth deficiency on the affected side.

Ramus and condyle malformations vary from minimal hypoplasia of the condyle to its complete absence in association with hypoplasia or agenesis of the ramus. In all patients, condylar anomalies can be demonstrated, and this finding may represent the pathognomonic hallmark of the syndrome. As a consequence, the spatial relationships of the distorted and/or deficient anatomic parts, as well as the associated neuromuscular components, become of paramount importance in the diagnosis and the planning of treatment.

Attempts at classification of the mandibular deformity have been made (Pruzansky, 1969) (Fig. 62–13):

Grade I. Hypoplasia is minimal or slight (see Fig. 62–4).

Grade II. The condyle and ramus are small; the head of the condyle is flattened; the glenoid fossa is absent; the condyle is hinged on a flat, often convex, infratemporal surface; the coronoid process may be absent.

Grade III. The ramus is reduced to a thin lamina of bone, or it is completely absent (see Fig. 62–11).

The posterior wall of the glenoid fossa is partially formed by the tympanic portion of the temporal bone, which provides the bony portion of the external auditory canal in the normally developed ear. When there is hypoplasia of the temporal bone, the posterior wall of the glenoid fossa of the temporomandibular joint may be absent; on occasion, a distinct fossa cannot be identified. The infratemporal surface is flat, and the hypoplastic ramus is often hinged on this flat surface at a point anterior to the contralateral unaffected temporomandibular joint (see Fig. 62–6).

Mandibular growth deficiency usually is closely related to the degree of hypoplasia of the condyle. In the more severe conditions, there is considerable disparity in condylar

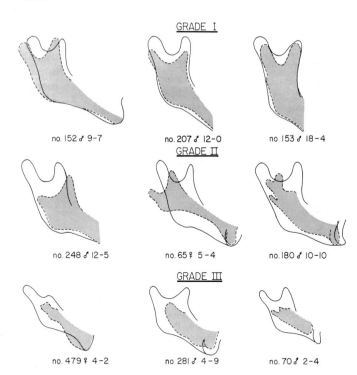

Figure 62–13. Classification of the mandibular anomaly. (Pruzansky, 1969.)

GRADE I

no. 152 ♂ 9-7   no. 207 ♂ 12-0   no. 153 ♂ 18-4

GRADE II

no. 248 ♂ 12-5   no. 65 ♀ 5-4   no. 180 ♂ 10-10

GRADE III

no. 479 ♀ 4-2   no 281 ♂ 4-9   no. 70 ♂ 2-4

growth between the affected and the contralateral sides.

Facial asymmetry increases progressively during the formative years as the growth disparity between the affected and the less affected sides causes the mandible to deviate laterally and upward toward the affected side. The cant of the occlusal plane (higher on the affected side) is caused by the short, hypoplastic ramus and by hypoplasia of the maxilla; the maxillary dentoalveolar process on the affected side is restricted by the short ramus.

The skeletal asymmetry is clinically demonstrated by the high occlusal cant on the affected side (see Fig. 62–12). The floor of the maxillary sinus and of the nose on the affected side is at a higher level; in some patients, it was noted that the base of the skull was elevated on an inclined plane similar to the inclined occlusal plane.

Anteroposterior and superoinferior dentoalveolar and skeletal dimensions are reduced on the affected side. Development and eruption of the molar teeth appear to be latent. Crowded dentition, with a characteristic tilt of the anterior maxillary and mandibular teeth toward the affected side, is often noted.

With growth in the width of the bimastoid and bicondylar areas, it is noted that the associated lateral positioning of the condyle and ramus on the affected side fails to keep pace with the movement laterally of the temporal bone and the glenoid fossa. The medial position of the condyle and ramus places the body and dentoalveolar arch of the mandible in a position lingual to the maxillary arch, with a resulting crossbite.

OTHER SKELETAL DEFORMITIES

Craniofacial bones other than the mandible or maxilla can be involved, especially the tympanic and mastoid portions of the temporal bone; the petrous portion usually is remarkably spared. The styloid process is frequently smaller and shorter on the affected side. The mastoid process can have a flattened appearance, and there can be partial (Fig. 62–14) or complete lack of pneumatization of the mastoid air cells. The petrous portion, which houses the inner ear, might escape underdevelopment because of the protection against spreading hematoma afforded by the precartilaginous otic capsule (Poswillo, 1973).

The zygoma can be underdeveloped in all its dimensions, with flattening of the malar

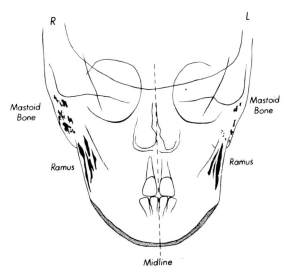

Figure 62–14. Line drawing of a cephalogram showing only partial pneumatization of the mastoid bone in a patient with unilateral craniofacial microsomia. (From Converse, J. M., Coccaro, P. J., Becker, M., and Wood-Smith, D.: On hemifacial microsomia. Plast. Reconstr. Surg., *51*:268, 1973. Copyright © 1973, The Williams & Wilkins Company, Baltimore.)

eminence. A decrease in the span of the zygomatic arch results in a decrease in the length of the canthal-tragal line on the affected side.

Disparities in the vertical axis of the orbit can be seen, with or without microphthalmos. Often in this situation there is a flattening of the ipsilateral frontal bone—an appearance of plagiocephaly without radiographic evidence of coronal synostosis.

Grabb (1965) reported that 11 of the 102 patients in his series had malformations of the vertebrae (hemivertebrae, fused vertebrae, spina bifida, scoliosis) and/or ribs.

The development of three-dimensional CT imaging has permitted precise definition of the craniofacial skeletal pathology (Fig. 62–15).

MUSCLES OF MASTICATION

It is a mistake to consider the deformities of craniofacial microsomia as being only osseous. There is an associated neuromuscular hypoplasia that involves the muscles of mastication—the masseter, medial and lateral pterygoid, and temporalis—with a strong secondary influence on skeletal development (Wolff's law, 1892). Moss (1968) proposed the *functional matrix* concept, in which any given

bone grows in response to its functional relationships, i.e., skeletal growth represents the sum of all the soft tissue and neuromuscular mechanisms operating in association with that bone. It has been experimentally shown that resection of the temporalis muscle in the young animal modifies the architecture of the mandible (Horowitz and Shapiro, 1951).

Muscle function, especially that of the lateral pterygoid muscle, is impaired in many of these patients. The right muscle is responsible for the lateral movement of the mandible to the left, while the left muscle controls movement to the right. Both sides act synergistically in executing protrusive opening movements. In patients with unilateral craniofacial microsomia, a severe limitation of protrusive and lateral movements due to hypoplasia of the lateral pterygoid muscle is observed.

The impact that this factor has both on the developing musculature and on the morphologic character of the attached bones is apparent. An alteration in mandibular movements (opening, lateral, and protrusive) comparable with the degree of mandibular deficiency is often noted.

When the patient opens his mouth, the deviation toward the affected side is produced not only by the skeletal asymmetry but also by the minimal or absent contribution of the ipsilateral medial and lateral pterygoid muscles in countering the opposing actions of the muscles on the unaffected side. The condyle on the less affected side is displaced abnormally downward and laterally when the mandible is depressed, almost to the point of dislocating the condyle. No discernible condylar movement can be elicited on the affected side during opening and protrusive movements of the mandible. Thus, in testing for lateral pterygoid muscle weakness, one finds an absence of ability to shift the jaw laterally toward the unaffected side, and deviation of the midline of the chin toward the affected side during opening and during forceful protrusion.

In many cases, the coronoid process is absent and there is reduction in the size of the temporalis muscle. The associated masseter muscle is also grossly deficient.

EAR DEFORMITY

Auricular malformations are a usual manifestation of the syndrome. Meurmann (1957)

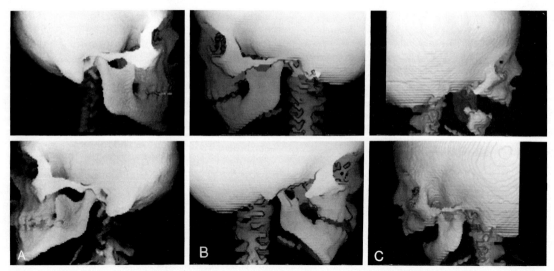

Figure 62–15. Three-dimensional surface reconstructions from CT scans (Vannier-Marsh). *A,* A 17 year old with left unilateral craniofacial microsomia having Pruzansky Grade I mandibular dysmorphology (see Fig. 62–13). Comparison with the unaffected side *(upper panel)* demonstrates hypoplasia of the body of the zygoma, elevation of the zygomatic arch, broadening of the mandibular coronoid process, reduction in the height of the mandibular ramus, and hypoplasia and lateral deviation of the inferior body of the mandible. The stylohyoid ligament is partially calcified on the affected side. *B,* A 4 year old with right unilateral craniofacial microsomia having Pruzansky Grade II mandibular dysmorphology. Comparison with the unaffected side *(upper panel)* demonstrates hypoplasia of the body of the zygoma, hypoplasia of the temporal process of the zygoma, aplasia of the zygomatic process of the temporal bone, hypoplasia of the mandibular coronoid process, reduction in height and width of the mandibular ramus, hypoplasia and lateral deviation of the inferior body of the mandible, and absence of the external auditory meatus. *C,* A 3 month old with right unilateral craniofacial microsomia having Pruzansky Grade III mandibular dysmorphology. Comparison with the unaffected side *(lower panel)* demonstrates hypoplasia of the body of the zygoma; dysmorphology of the temporal process of the zygoma; aplasia of the zygomatic process of the temporal bone; aplasia of the mandibular condyle, coronoid process and ramus; hypoplasia of the mandibular body; and absence of the external auditory meatus. (From Marsh, J. L., and Vannier, M. W.: Computer assisted imaging in the diagnosis, management, and study of dysmorphic patients. *In* Vig, K. W. L., and Burdi, A. R. (Eds.): Craniofacial Morphogenesis and Dysmorphogenesis. Ann Arbor, Center for Human Growth and Development, University of Michigan, 1988, pp. 109–126.)

proposed a classification of the auricular anomalies based on the studies of Marx (1926): Grade I, distinctly smaller malformed auricles with most of the characteristic components (Fig. 62–16*A*); Grade II, vertical remnant of cartilage and skin with a small anterior hook and complete atresia of the canal (Fig. 62–16*B*); and Grade III, auricle almost entirely absent except for only a small remnant, such as a deformed lobule (Fig. 62–16*C*).

In a comprehensive study, Caldarelli and associates (1980), using air and bone conduction audiometry and temporal bone tomography, evaluated 57 patients with craniofacial microsomia. It was observed that the degree of auricular deformity as classified above does not correlate exactly with hearing function. The type of hearing loss, although usually assumed to be conductive in origin,

can be determined only by audiometry. Tomography, not auricular morphology, is the only indicator of middle ear structure. The unaffected ear may also harbor abnormalities in structure and function and should be evaluated. There was, however, a direct relationship between the degree of severity of the auricular malformation and the ipsilateral mandibular deformity (Fig. 62–17). Reconstruction of the auricle and middle ear in patients with craniofacial microsomia is discussed in Chapter 40.

DEFORMITIES OF NERVOUS SYSTEM

Nervous system abnormalities in patients with craniofacial microsomia have received little attention in the medical literature (Gorlin and associates, 1963).

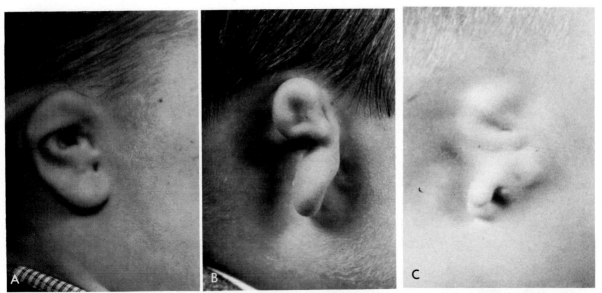

Figure 62–16. Classification of the auricular anomalies (after Meurmann). *A*, Grade I: small, malformed ear with most components present. *B*, Grade II: vertical remnant of skin and cartilage. There is atresia of the external auditory meatus. *C*, Grade III: the auricle is almost entirely absent except for a misplaced lobule and diminutive skin and cartilage remnants.

Cerebral Anomalies. A wide variety of cerebral anomalies exists in craniofacial microsomia and may include ipsilateral cerebral hypoplasia (Aleksic and associates, 1975a), hypoplasia of the corpus callosum (Timm, 1960), hydrocephalus of the communicating type (Timm, 1960; Aleksic and associates, 1975b) and obstructive type (Herrmann and Optiz, 1969), intracranial lipoma (Gaupp and Jantz, 1942; Aleksic and associates, 1975b), and unilateral hypoplasia of the brain stem and cerebellum (Mathies, 1966; Aleksic and associates, 1975b). Other associated abnormalities include mental retardation (Gorlin and associates, 1963), epilepsy, and electroencephalographic findings suggestive of epilepsy (Franceschetti, Klein, and Brocher, 1959; Christiaens and associates, 1966; Aleksic and associates, 1975b).

Cranial Nerve Anomalies. Cranial nerve abnormalities are frequent in unilateral craniofacial microsomia and can range from arhinencephaly of the bilateral type (Virchow, 1864; Timm, 1960) and unilateral type (Aleksic and associates, 1975a) to unilateral agenesis and hypoplasia of the optic nerve with secondary changes in the lateral geniculate body and visual cortex (Aleksic and associates, 1976), congenital ophthalmoplegia and Duane's retraction syndrome (Bowen, Collum, and Rees, 1971), hypoplasia of the trochlear and abducens nuclei and nerves

(Aleksic and associates, 1976), congenital trigeminal anesthesia (Sugar, 1967), and aplasia of the trigeminal nerve and motor and sensory nucleus (Aleksic and associates, 1975b). The most common cranial nerve anomaly is facial paralysis (Fig. 62–18) secondary to agenesis of the facial muscles, aberrant pathway of the facial nerve in the temporal bone (Bellucci, 1972), or hypoplasia of

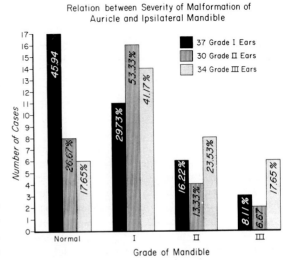

Relation between Severity of Malformation of Auricle and Ipsilateral Mandible

- 37 Grade I Ears
- 30 Grade II Ears
- 34 Grade III Ears

Figure 62–17. Relationship between the malformation of the auricle and the ipsilateral mandible. (Pruzansky, S.: Personal communication, 1971.)

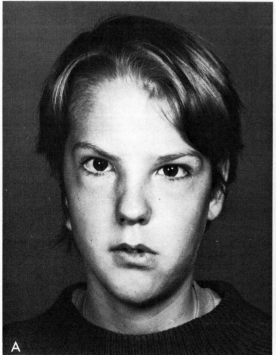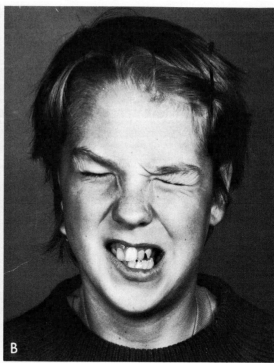

Figure 62–18. Partial right-sided facial nerve palsy in a patient with unilateral craniofacial microsomia. *A,* Repose. *B,* Animation.

the intracranial portion of the facial nerve and facial nucleus in the brain stem (Aleksic and associates, 1975b). Congenital hearing loss may be due to a malformed inner ear (Aleksic and associates, 1976), hypoplasia of the cochlear nerve and brain stem auditory nuclei, or hypoplasia and impaired function of the ninth through the twelfth cranial nerves (Mathies, 1966; Berkman and Feingold, 1968). In conclusion, any cranial nerve can be clinically involved in patients with craniofacial microsomia, and it is likely that hypoplasia or agenesis of a portion of the entire cranial nerve trunk and corresponding brain stem nuclei represents the pathoanatomic substrate of the clinical dysfunction.

Electromyographic abnormalities have been briefly described in the literature (Grabb, 1965). Several of the authors' patients showed diminished or low-normal motor conduction velocity of the facial nerves, usually unilateral, while electromyographic abnormalities ranged from absence of the muscle to long polyphasic potential with incomplete interference pattern on active innervation (Aleksic and associates, 1975b). No cases of fibrillation potentials have yet been documented. The interpretation of the elec-

trodiagnostic data was somewhat hampered by the fact that many patients had undergone earlier surgical procedures in the region of the mandible and auricle.

SOFT TISSUE DEFORMITIES

In addition to the anomalies of the muscles of mastication and nervous system, there is often a generalized soft tissue hypoplasia that involves the skin, the subcutaneous tissue, and the facial muscles of expression. The musculature of the soft palate and of the tongue is occasionally less developed on the affected side. The not infrequent hypoplasia or aplasia of the parotid gland, previously noted by Entin (1958), places the branches of the facial nerve in a superficial and vulnerable position. The latter finding has obvious surgical implications. The deficiency of soft tissues on the affected side is made evident by the shorter distance between the mastoid process and the angle of the mouth or the lateral canthus of the eye. The skin and subcutaneous tissue also show varying degrees of atrophy, particularly in the parotid-masseteric and auriculomastoid areas.

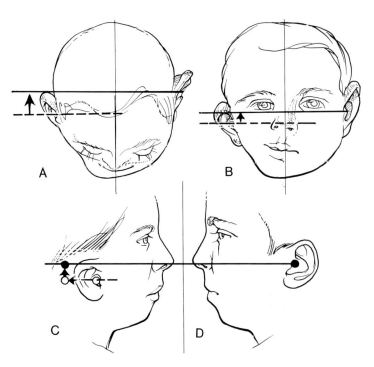

Figure 62–19. Placement of the head in the cephalostat is altered by the fact that in unilateral craniofacial microsomia the ear is displaced down and forward on the affected side. The technician should make a clinical determination of a line perpendicular to the midsagittal plane and use this for the orientation of the head to the ear rods. The x-y coordinates of this geometrically determined porion for the affected side should be recorded directly on the cephalometric film for future reference.

In the series reported by Grabb (1965), 10 per cent of the patients had malformations of the eye and eyelids and/or palate.

Transverse facial clefting (see Fig. 62–50) ranging from macrostomia to a full-thickness defect of the cheek can be present (Converse and associates, 1974). The clefts probably result from failure of the maxillary and mandibular processes to fuse. In embryologic development, the lateral commissure of the oral fissure is initially situated at the point of bifurcation of the maxillary and mandibular processes. With fusion of the latter and development of the muscles of mastication, the original broad mouth is reduced in size. In addition, the parotid glands, originally located near the embryonic oral commissure, grow laterally toward the developing ear, but the parotid duct papillae remain in their more medial position (Converse and associates, 1974).

Preoperative Assessment

Cephalometric Analysis for Description of Craniofacial Asymmetry. In standard cephalometric technique the ear rods of the cephalostat are inserted in the external auditory meatus and the patient's head is placed in the Frankfort Horizontal. The patient with craniofacial microsomia usually has one ear positioned inferior and anterior to the other (Fig. 62–19). If the malpositioned ear is used in this technique, the head is incorrectly oriented to the x-ray beam and the film. The technician should project an imaginary line from the normal ear, perpendicular to the midsagittal plane and passing to the opposite side of the head. The x-y coordinates of this point, in millimeters, should be recorded directly on the cephalogram for future reference. Clinical determination of the midsagittal plane can be made by tipping the head down and observing the gross shape of the calvarium from above.

A considerable amount of cephalometric data is required to define the complex skeletal pathology of craniofacial deformities. In fact, more information is needed than can be provided by the classic lateral-view cephalogram alone. The three-dimensional multiplane cephalometric analysis integrates information from both the posteroanterior and basilar cephalometric radiographs. In order to define and measure facial deformity, especially asymmetries, a method (Grayson, McCarthy, and Bookstein, 1983b) was developed to integrate the findings of the posteroanterior and basilar cephalometric views into the cephalometric analysis (Figs. 62–20, 62–21).

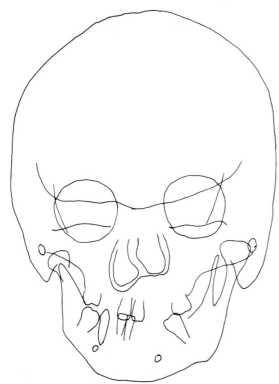

Figure 62–20. Posteroanterior cephalometric tracing. The mandible is deviated toward the affected (right) side and the right orbit is displaced inferiorly. (From Grayson, B., McCarthy, J. G., and Bookstein, F.: Analysis of craniofacial asymmetry by multiplane cephalometry. Am. J. Orthodont., *84*:217, 1983.)

Examination of the posteroanterior cephalogram in a manner to be described enables the observer to visualize distinct regions of the craniofacial complex so as to distinguish the deformation of the structure from symmetry. In practice, three separate acetate tracings are made on the same radiograph, corresponding to structures derived from the lateral view in or near the three planes indicated in Figure 62–22.

When these three tracings (recorded from the posteroanterior cephalogram) are viewed separately, they reveal the degree of asymmetry at each of the three cross sections of the craniofacial complex. A midline is constructed for each view as follows. In the *A* plane (the piriform aperture, orbits, and incisors), the centrum* of each orbit is located (Fig. 62–23*A*), and the point M_{ce} halfway

*The centrum is the midpoint of two midpoints: the midpoint between the most superior and inferior points of the orbit and the midpoint between the most medial and most lateral point on the orbit.

between them is identified. The most lateral point on the perimeter of each piriform aperture is marked, and the point M_p halfway between them is marked. The midpoint M_i between the maxillary and the mandibular central incisors and the gnathion M_g are identified. All four of these points are "on the midline" in some sense. To view the midline, straight lines are constructed connecting M_{ce} with M_p, M_p with M_i, and M_i with M_g. This maneuver results in a segmented construct whose angles express the asymmetry of the structures of this plane.

By the same method, a midline is constructed for the *B* plane (the sphenoid, zygomatic arch, etc.). The points S_i, representing the intersection of the shadows of the greater and lesser wings of the sphenoid, are identified, and their bisector M_{si} is recorded (Fig. 62–23*B*). The midpoints M_z for the centra of the zygomatic arches, M_c for the tips of the coronoid processes, M_x for maxillare† on the left and right zygomas, and M_f for the left and right mental foramina are identified. Vertical line segments are constructed to link

†Maxillare (M_x): Maximal concavity on the contour of the maxilla between the lower contour of the malar bone and the maxillary first molar.

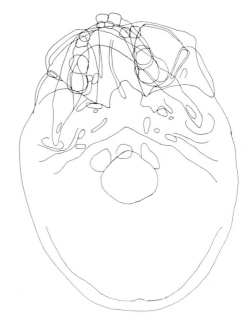

Figure 62–21. Basilar cephalometric tracing. The mandible and the maxilla are deviated toward the right side. (From Grayson, B., McCarthy, J. G., and Bookstein, F.: Analysis of craniofacial asymmetry by multiplane cephalometry. Am. J. Orthodont., *84*:217, 1983.)

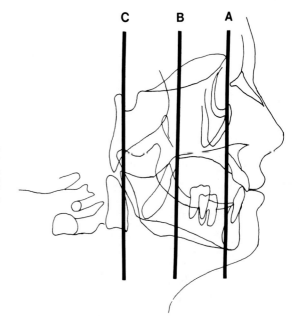

Figure 62–22. The three vertical planes of the face. Separate tracings are made on the same radiograph, corresponding to structures derived from the lateral view in or near the three planes indicated. (From Grayson, B., McCarthy, J. G., and Bookstein, F.: Analysis of craniofacial asymmetry by multiplane cephalometry. Am. J. Orthodont., *84*:217, 1983.)

these points. Finally, in plane C, the heads of the condyles, the innermost inferior points on the mastoid processes, and the gonions yield bisecting points M_d, M_m, M_{go}, and segments M_d–M_m, M_m–M_{go} (Fig. 62–23C).

If the midline constructs of A, B, and C planes are superimposed on the posteroanterior tracing, one can observe a phenomenon termed *warping* within the craniofacial skel-

eton (Fig. 62–24). The midline constructs deviate progressively laterally as one passes from plane C (posterior), through plane B, to plane A toward the anterior of the face. In patients with facial asymmetry, the posterior and middle cranial structures appear less severely affected. For this reason, they are used to guide the observer in the construction of a midsagittal plane. In each of the basilar-

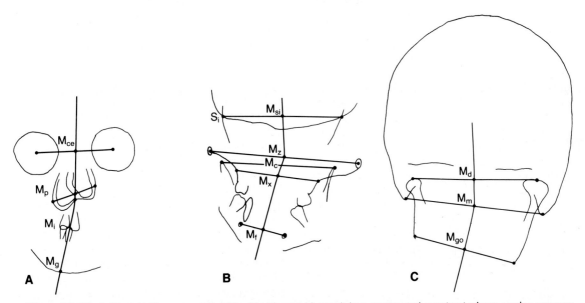

Figure 62–23. *A*, Straight lines connecting M_{ce}, M_p, M_i, and M_g result in a segmented construct whose angles express the asymmetry of structures in this facial plane (see the *A* plane in Fig. 62–22). *B*, Midline construct for the *B* plane. *C*, Midline construct for the *C* plane. (From Grayson, B., McCarthy, J. G., and Bookstein, F.: Analysis of craniofacial asymmetry by multiplane cephalometry. Am. J. Orthodont., *84*:217, 1983.)

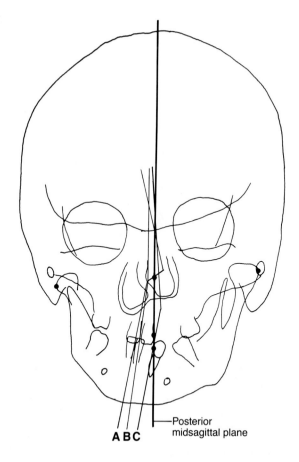

A B C   Posterior
midsagittal plane

Figure 62–24. The midline constructs progressively deviate laterally as one passes from the posterior to the anterior planes of the face. (From Grayson, B., McCarthy, J. G., and Bookstein, F.: Analysis of craniofacial asymmetry by multiplane cephalometry. Am. J. Orthodont., *84*:217, 1983.)

view planes (Fig. 62–25), key triangles are constructed (Fig. 62–26*A,B,C*), each of which may be referred to the primary (posterior) midsagittal plane. Superpositioning of the triangles clearly demonstrates the warping of the craniofacial complex (Fig. 62–27). The craniofacial skeleton is most severely deviated from the midsagittal plane at the level of the mandible; the severity of asymmetry decreases in a cephalic (superior) direction.

By observing the path of the basilar midline over the teeth, piriform aperture, and other structures visible in the posteroanterior cephalogram, the clinician can transfer the midline to the posteroanterior cephalogram.

The basilar midline construct is derived by bisecting the distance between relatively stable bilateral structures on the cranial base level and averaging the mean of the bisects (Fig. 62–28*A*). The following structures were observed to be indicators of the geometric midline: the centers of the left and right occipital condyles, the center of the foramen magnum, and the medial axis (Grayson and

associates, 1985) of the spheno-occipital synchondrosis (Fig. 62–28*B*).

Alternative Method for Determining Midline from Posteroanterior Cephalogram. The petrous portion of the temporal bone is identified (Fig. 62–29). A horizontal line is drawn that averages the horizontal components of this pair of radiographic shadows. A point midway between the medial orbital rims is identified along this line. A perpendicular line is drawn at this point to serve as a guide in establishing the midline of the craniofacial complex.

Planning Correction of Occlusal Cant. The occlusal cant observed in patients with unilateral craniofacial microsomia results from deficient vertical skeletal growth on the affected side in addition to the excess vertical growth on the less affected side. The degree to which vertical growth dysplasia occurs on either side varies greatly among patients. Some cases may also show, superimposed on this growth abnormality, facial findings characteristic of the long face or short face syn-

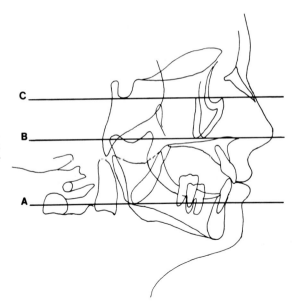

Figure 62–25. The three horizontal planes of the face. (From Grayson, B., McCarthy, J. G., and Bookstein, F.: Analysis of craniofacial asymmetry by multiplane cephalometry. Am. J. Orthodont., *84:*217, 1983.)

drome. Thus, there exist several clinical variations for which the appropriate surgical plan must be chosen. The objectives of surgery are to correct the occlusal cant while at the same time optimizing the lip-incisor relationship and gingival exposure upon smiling. Three common variations of the clinical condition are presented below.

In the first example (Fig. 62–30A), the left side is affected but the soft and hard tissue relationship is normal on this side. In this case, when the patient smiles an excessive amount of teeth and gingivae show on the less affected (right) side. The Le Fort I osteotomy is illustrated as elevated or impacted on the right side only, correcting the cant of

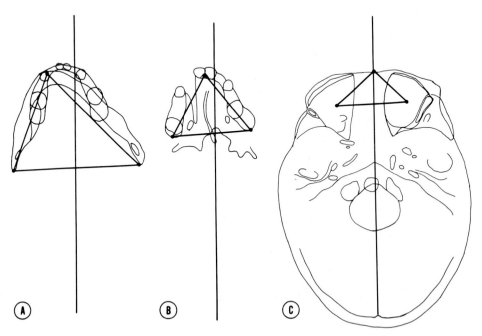

Figure 62–26. Key triangles are constructed in each of the horizontal planes and related to the posterior midsagittal plane. (From Grayson, B., McCarthy, J. G., and Bookstein, F.: Analysis of craniofacial asymmetry by multiplane cephalometry. Am. J. Orthodont., *84:*217, 1983.)

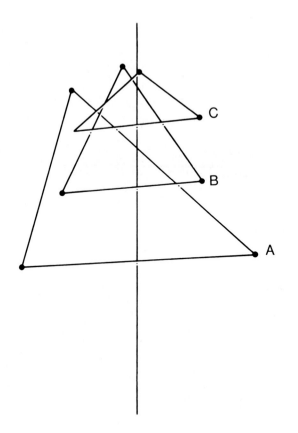

Figure 62–27. Superimposition of the triangles shows that the greatest amount of deviation from the midline occurs at the level of the mandible *(A)*, decreasing in a cephalic direction. *B,* Maxilla. *C,* Cranial base. (From Grayson, B., McCarthy, J. G., and Bookstein, F.: Analysis of craniofacial asymmetry by multiplane cephalometry. Am. J. Orthodont., *84:*217, 1983.)

Figure 62–28. *A,* The midline construct is derived by bisecting the distance between bilateral foramina (f. ovale, f. spinosum, f. lacerum, jugular foramina, carotid canal) and the occipital condyles. A straight line is projected over the linear bisections of each pair of landmarks and the center of the foramen magnum. *B,* The medial axis analysis of the spheno-occipital synchondrosis produces a midsagittal construct. (From Grayson, B., McCarthy, J. G., and Bookstein, F.: Analysis of craniofacial asymmetry by multiplane cephalometry. Am. J. Orthodont., *84:* 217, 1983.)

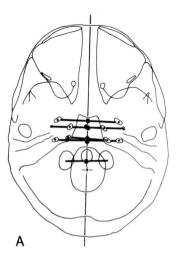

A

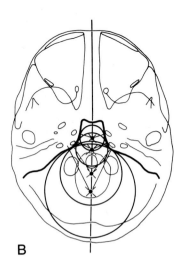

B

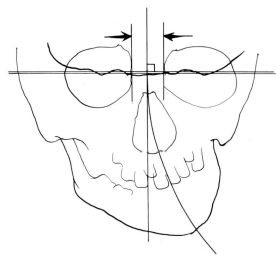

Figure 62–29. The petrous portion of the temporal bone is averaged with a single horizontal line. A perpendicular line is drawn at a point midway between the medial orbital rims. This vertical line serves as a guide in establishing the midline of the craniofacial skeletal complex.

the occlusal plane. In the second case (Fig. 62–30B), the left side is affected and the maxilla is reduced vertically on this side. The patient on smiling shows a normal amount of gingivae and dental structures on the less affected (right) side and a deficient amount of these structures on the affected (left) side. In order to improve the soft and hard tissue relationship on the affected side, the Le Fort

I segment is brought down on the left side only. Note that the center of rotation is located on the right as the occlusal plane is leveled. In the third example (Fig. 62–30C), the patient's left side is affected and the teeth appear slightly above the soft tissue drape of the lips. The right side shows excess hard and soft tissue upon smiling. In this case, correction of the occlusal cant is achieved by rotating the Le Fort I segment around a point located at the midline (impaction on the right, lowering on the left).

Thus far, three alternatives have been presented for the correction of the occlusal cant. The skeletal deformity may also require correction by shifting the Le Fort I segment to the left or right in the horizontal dimension (Fig. 62–30D). Upon evaluation of the lateral view cephalogram, correction of the deformity may require that the segment be rotated superiorly or inferiorly either anteriorly or posteriorly (Fig. 62–30E,F) in combination with advancement or recession of the osteotomized segment (Fig. 62–30G). It is important to understand the impact of these changes on the position of the mandible and soft tissue profile. Decisions regarding the three-dimensional surgical change are facilitated by an understanding of the skeletal deformity in all the three dimensions.

Two-Splint Technique. In the correction of a symmetric deformity when surgery of both jaws is planned for the same operation,

Figure 62–30. Correcting the occlusal cant. *A* to *C,* Vertical changes with the Le Fort I segment (dot = pivot point); dotted lines represent the preoperative position and bold lines the postoperative position of the Le Fort I segment). *D,* Horizontal changes with the Le Fort I segment. *E, F,* Anterior and posterior rotation of the Le Fort I segment in a superior direction. *G,* Anterior advancement. See text for details.

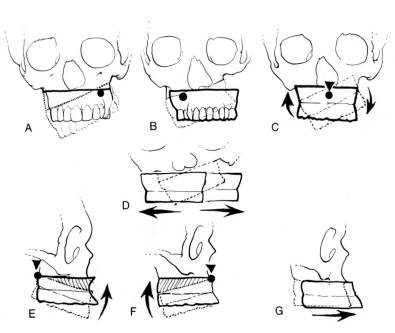

two carefully constructed fixation splints or interocclusal wafers are employed. The first or intermediate splint is used to establish the position of the osteotomized maxillary segment by joining it to the splint and the mandible. The mandible and splinted maxillary segment are rotated around the condyles and mobilized superiorly. The maxilla is fixed into position. The intermediate splint is removed and a second splint is wired to the maxilla. The mandibular osteotomy is completed. At this time the mandible is guided into its planned position as it is wired into the second splint. The two-splint procedure functions only when both condyles and rami are of normal shape and size. This is not the case in unilateral craniofacial microsomia. The unequal bilateral ramus heights and condylar anatomy result in an asymmetric path of closure for the affected mandible. The mandibular body follows a path of opening and closing that is oblique, rather than parallel to the craniofacial midsagittal plane. This complex three-dimensional motion cannot be reproduced on conventional dental articulators. Thus, the intermediate splint does not accurately position the Le Fort I segment when the mandible is rotated upward toward the maxilla.

Establishing the position of the Le Fort I segment is therefore dependent on calculations of the planned change derived from results of mock surgery on articulated study models, mock surgery on the cephalograms and three-dimensional CT or cephalometric data (see Chap. 29), and on careful analysis of the clinical findings. The surgeon must carefully outline and measure the shape and size of the maxillary osteotomy before it is performed. This may be done by scoring or cutting reference landmarks on the surface of the bones.

After the osteotomies have been completed and the segment mobilized, measurement of the change in direction and distance between landmarks indicates the amount in millimeters that the structure has been moved after the osteotomies were made. After the position of the maxilla is established and it is placed in intermaxillary fixation, the mandible may be placed in position by means of a conventionally prepared splint (interocclusal wafer).

Unilateral vs. Bilateral Ramus Osteotomies to Reposition Mandible. The mandible and maxilla in unilateral craniofacial microsomia demonstrate a true bilateral deformity. The primary deformity, by virtue of its effect on altering jaw position and function, induces compensatory shape and size changes on the unaffected or "less affected" side (Grayson and associates, 1983a). This is seen as a bowing out and elongation of the mandibular body and ramus on the less affected side. When the mandible is repositioned by only osteotomizing the affected ramus and rotating around the less affected condyle, the deformity of the less affected side becomes more apparent (Fig. 62–31). When the mandibular midline is centered in this fashion, the less affected side seems to be

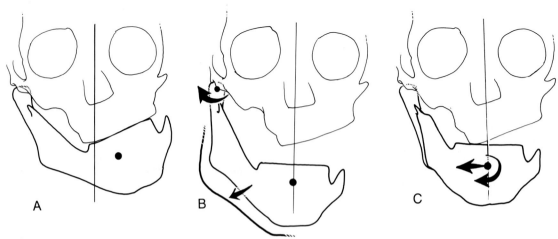

Figure 62–31. Unilateral craniofacial microsomia with underdevelopment of the mandibular ramus and absence of the condyle (left side). *A,* Preoperative appearance. *B,* Unilateral ramus osteotomy and direction of the skeletal segment movement. *C,* Bilateral ramus osteotomies and direction of the skeletal segment movement.

abnormally full and thrust laterally while the affected side continues to appear deficient. The asymmetric bony mandibular anatomy, as well as the associated asymmetric overlying soft tissue, contribute to this effect. The bilateral ramus osteotomy permits repositioning of the mandibular body in a manner that reduces, rather than enhances, the asymmetry. The optimally repositioned mandible results in minimal lateral displacement of the less affected mandibular body while maximal inferior and lateral displacement of the affected side is obtained. This type of mandibular repositioning can usually be achieved by bilateral ramus osteotomies.

Orthodontic Therapy After Combined Surgical Correction. After surgical correction of the mandibular position (without associated maxillary surgery, as in the child), the patient has a unilateral open bite on the affected side. This results from inferior displacement of the affected side of the mandible and its rotation toward the midline. Immediately upon removal of intermaxillary fixation, a unilateral acrylic biteplate is inserted and maintained in position by clasps attached directly to the teeth. The biteplate functions to provide bilateral distribution of occlusal force and balanced stress on the mandible upon mastication and function. Combined with intermaxillary elastics, the plate guides the mandible into the symmetric position achieved through surgery, and relieves excessive stress on the newly placed bone grafts. The biteplate is also used to promote extrusion of teeth and the alveolus in the maxilla on the affected side. This is achieved by removal of the occlusal surface of the biteplate under the most posterior maxillary molar on the affected side. The vertical extrusion of this tooth is enhanced by force applied to it from springs placed on the biteplate itself or through intermaxillary elastics. After the most posterior teeth are brought into occlusion, the adjacent teeth are extruded along with their surrounding alveolar process in the same manner. This process of leveling the maxillary occlusal plane by gradual hypereruption of the posterior teeth on the affected maxillary side may require one year or more. Following this, conventional orthodontic therapy is employed to correct and refine the remaining malocclusion.

Functional Orthopedic Appliance Therapy. Before surgical correction of the maxillary and mandibular deformities, the ortho-dontist may employ functional orthodontic appliances that enhance the neuromuscular environment for the development of these skeletal structures. The objectives of this type of therapy are to increase mandibular and maxillary growth on the affected side, while at the same time expanding the soft tissue envelope for eventual surgical reconstruction (Harvold, Vargervik, and Chierici, 1983). The degree of deformity and the patient's willingness to comply with therapy dictate to a large degree the outcome of functional appliance treatment.

The mechanism for promoting change in the pattern of bone deposition involves controlling the posture of the mandible during function. This is achieved by the use of removable acrylic orthodontic appliances that, with guide planes and shields, force the mandible to follow a symmetric path of closure. The forced posture during function places increased tension on the skeleto-osseous interface of the most deformed bony surfaces. This maneuver is presumed to enhance bone deposition on surfaces in areas that reduce stress and improve the bony anatomy. Functional appliance therapy can be employed only in cases in which the mandible can be mobilized into function. The ankylosed mandible must be surgically released before treatment of this nature is considered.

The appliance is constructed with the mandible advanced in position and directed toward the correct midline. A biteplate is used on the less affected side to permit extrusion of teeth and lengthening of the dentoalveolar structures on the more affected side. The therapy leads to an eventual leveling of the maxillary occlusal plane and results in an open bite on the contralateral or less affected side. The open bite is corrected by a combination of mandibular surgery and orthodontic therapy.

The deformity in unilateral craniofacial microsomia is, to a large degree, manifest in asymmetric development of the soft tissue. The bony deficiency is associated with soft tissue deficiency, just as the compensatory bony excess on the less affected side is associated with soft tissue excess. The soft tissue asymmetry is often revealed more completely upon surgical correction of the bony asymmetry. Correction of the soft tissue deficiency may be approached during the phase of functional appliance therapy. The orthopedic appliance, described above, may be fitted with an acrylic shield suspended in the buccal vestibule on the affected side. The shield may be gradually increased in thickness, plumping out or augmenting the cheek on the affected side. The result is an increase in the soft tissue area and circumference on the affected side. This type of therapy may provide for an increased amount of soft tissue on the affected side postoperatively. The improved appearance offered to the patient by preoperatively increasing the dimension of the tissue has been found to enhance patient compliance with this phase of therapy.

The efficacy of functional appliance therapy awaits the test of time.

Treatment

CORRECTIVE JAW SURGERY

Correction of the jaw deformity in craniofacial microsomia has been attempted either by contour restoration with onlaying of various materials or by osteotomies to change the jaw asymmetry and crossbite.

Contour Restoration Operations. Early augmentation to maintain the contour of the soft tissues on the affected side has been achieved by autogenous rib grafts (Longacre, DeStefano, and Holmstrand, 1963; Longacre, 1968; Munro and Lauritzen, 1985), by allografts of cartilage or bone (Stark and Saunders, 1962), and by preserved cartilage allografts and inorganic implants (Brown, Fryer, and Ohlwiler, 1960).

Other techniques for improvement of contour in the adult include correcting the deficient mandible either with a transplant taken from the lower portion of the unaffected half of the mandible (Gorski and Tarczynska, 1969) or by bone graft onlays (Converse and Shapiro, 1954; Longacre, DeStefano, and Holmstrand, 1963).

Such surgery, however, fails to improve dental occlusion or function and also fails to align the facial skeleton in a position conducive to subsequent growth.

Osteotomies of the Jaws. Correction of the jaw asymmetry and crossbite by osteotomies and bone grafts has been done in children and adults, but the timing of the surgery has been the subject of considerable controversy.

Osteotomies in Adults. Poswillo (1974) cautioned against reconstruction of the facial

bones in patients under the age of 12 years. He felt that the trauma associated with surgery could destroy the functional matrix (Moss, 1968) of the facial skeleton and profoundly interfere with subsequent facial growth.

Correction of the jaw asymmetry and of the crossbite by mandibular osteotomy and bone grafts has been performed in the adult (Limberg, 1928; Converse and Shapiro, 1952; Dingman and Grabb, 1963, 1964).

Obwegeser (1970, 1974) advocated that in severe adult cases the temporomandibular joint should be initially reconstructed with a costochondral rib graft (Fig. 62–32). Any associated hypoplasia of the temporal bone, zygomatic arch, and lateral orbital rim should also be corrected (Fig. 62–33). At a subsequent operation, the lower half of the facial skeleton can be rotated inferiorly and anteriorly by a combination of a Le Fort I osteotomy, a bilateral sagittal split osteotomy of the mandible, and a double-step horizontal advancement osteotomy (Fig. 62–34).

Osteotomies in Children. A metatarsal head transplant, as a substitute for the absent mandibular condyle, has been advocated (Glahn and Winther, 1967). Others who used this procedure earlier found little or no growth of the grafts and no particular improvement in joint function (Dingman and Grabb, 1964; Freeman, 1965).

Converse and Rushton (1957) operated on a 12 year old patient who had the jaw deformity of craniofacial microsomia. A horizontal osteotomy of the ramus was performed above

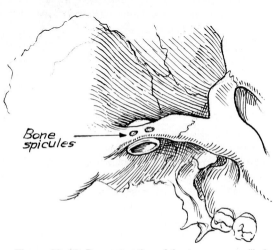

Figure 62–32. Reconstruction of the temporomandibular joint with a costochondral rib graft. (After Obwegeser.)

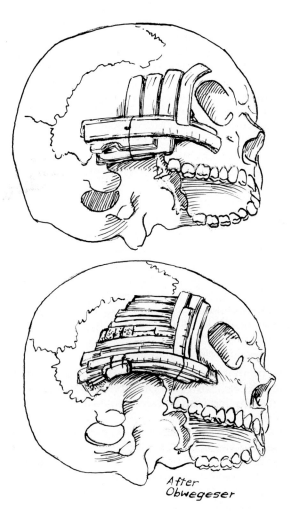

Figure 62–33. Correction of the hypoplasia of the temporal bone, zygomatic arch, and lateral orbital rim with onlay rib bone grafts. This technique has been combined with temporomandibular joint reconstruction by Obwegeser (1974) as illustrated in Figure 62–32.

After Obwegeser

Figure 62–34. Combined Le Fort I maxillary osteotomy, bilateral sagittal split, and horizontal osteotomy of the mandible (after Obwegeser). *A,* The osteotomies are done only in the adult in order to avoid injury to the unerupted maxillary teeth and interference with facial growth. *B,* Bone grafts are placed in the defect following downward rotation of the maxilla on the affected side. The mandible is shifted to the less affected side, and the anteroinferior border of the mandible is rotated and advanced.

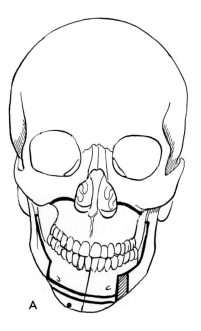

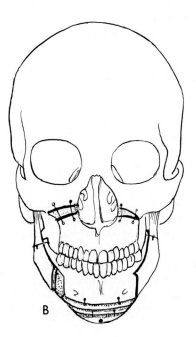

A

B

the inferior alveolar foramen, and an iliac bone graft was inserted between the fragments after the placement of a biteblock to open the occlusion on the affected side.

A similar procedure was performed by Osborne (1964) in patients with craniofacial microsomia and in those with asymmetric growth resulting from injury. Osborne advocated surgery before the age of 6 years in order to give the maxilla an opportunity to develop after the release of the upward pressure exerted on the affected side by the hypoplastic mandible. Longitudinal studies of two of Osborne's cases of congenital origin were made by Knowles (1966), who was able to document maxillary growth.

Delaire (1970) recommended even earlier intervention between the ages of 4 and 6 years. He elongated the shorter ramus with an inverted-L osteotomy and inserted costal bone grafts into the gap formed at the horizontal branch of the L.

Converse and associates (1973b) advocated a two-stage procedure during childhood (period of mixed dentition) to correct the mandibular asymmetry, to allow expansion of the constricted maxilla, and to prevent further contraction of the overlying soft tissue.

Munro and Lauritzen (1985) reconstructed the absent ramus, condyle, and glenoid fossa with a rib costochondral graft and reported considerable elongation and growth of the reconstructed segment. Murray and associates (1985) also recommended mandibular ramus-condyle reconstruction in the growing child.

Restoration of Soft Tissue Contour. Soft tissue hypoplasia is a characteristic feature of the syndrome. The soft tissue hypoplasia is usually not so severe or diffuse as in hemifacial atrophy (Romberg's disease). It is usually most conspicuous in the parotid-masseteric and auriculomastoid areas. Hypoplasia of the facial musculature of expression or congenital facial paralysis caused by agenesis of the facial nerve also results in a generalized deficit in soft tissue contour.

Improvement in the soft tissue deficiency has been obtained by the insertion of a tube flap in the preauricular area (Gillies and Millard, 1957), a deepithelized flap (Brown and McDowell, 1958), or a dermis-fat graft introduced subcutaneously (Davis, 1968). Deepithelized microvascular free flaps of dermis and fat (Fig. 62–35) have been employed by Fujino, Rytinzaburo, and Sugimoto

(1975) to correct severe hemifacial atrophy with deltopectoral tissue, and by Wells and Edgerton (1977) with groin tissue based on the inferior epigastric vessels. Upton and associates (1980) restored the soft tissue contour with microvascular transfers of omentum. The external maxillary vessels were anastomosed to the vessels of the transplanted tissue by microsurgical techniques.

Restoration of hearing and reconstruction of the microtic ear are discussed in Chapter 40.

TREATMENT PROGRAMS

There are two critical variables in the treatment of craniofacial microsomia: the age of the patient and the extent of the skeletal and soft tissue deficiency. In general, the more severe the pathologic condition, the more extensive will be the surgical procedure and it will be commenced at a younger age.

San Francisco Program

In an attempt to provide therapeutic guidelines, the San Francisco group (Harvold, Vargervik, and Chierici, 1983) has advocated the following:

Phase I: Presurgical Treatment (Age 5 to 6 Years). A removable functional appliance is used to reduce the secondary underdevelopment of the maxilla, and to change the force systems on the mandible on the affected side in a direction that will increase bone apposition on the proximal end. A new mandibular closing pattern is also sought.

Phase II: Mandibular Surgery (Age 8 to 10 Years). The mandible is mobilized and elongated with an osteotomy–bone graft. The surgery is performed at an early age in the patient with temporomandibular joint ankylosis or restricted jaw movements. In this situation, the optimal time is after eruption of the deciduous teeth, which allow placement of orthodontic appliances. The family must be forewarned that a second surgical procedure will be indicated when mandibular growth is completed or nearly completed (age 16 to 18 years).

Phase III: Postsurgical Treatment to Induce Bony Replacement of Graft. After eight to ten weeks of intermaxillary fixation, the wires are removed but the splint is rewired to the maxillary arch. Rubber bands, connecting the splint to the lower arch, direct the mandible into the splint for early closure.

The resulting functional pattern of jaw movements protects the bone graft matrix from excessive forces.

Phase IV: Correction of Distorted Maxillary Alveolar Process (Within One Year of Mandibular Procedure). If all the maxillary permanent teeth have erupted, this goal can be achieved with a Le Fort I osteotomy six to nine months after the mandibular procedure. Orthodontic extrusion of the maxillary teeth is an alternative approach in which the maxillary teeth on the affected side

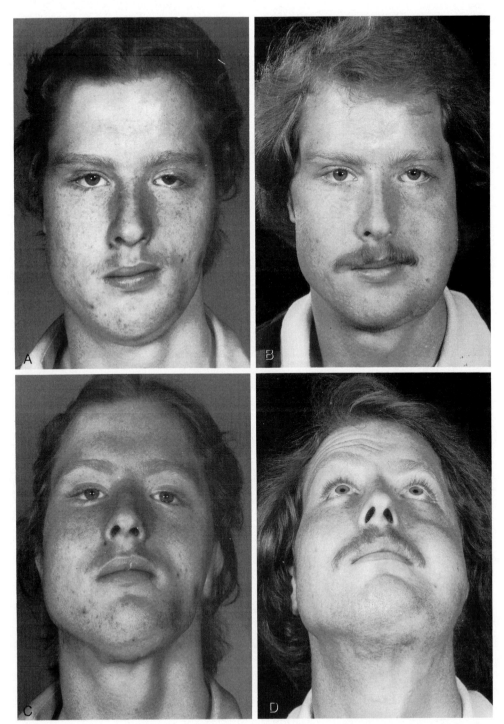

Figure 62–35. Adolescent male with left-sided craniofacial microsomia. *A, C,* Preoperative views. *B, D,* After insertion of a deepithelized microvascular free flap in the parotid-masseteric region. (Courtesy of Dr. Daniel Baker.)

are brought down to the occlusal plane and into contact with the mandibular teeth.

Phase V: Orthodontic Treatment. Conventional orthodontic therapy, often combined with a functional appliance, is employed to align the teeth and balance the occlusion.

Phase VI: Soft Tissue Augmentation (After Age 15 Years). Soft tissue augmentation procedures are postponed until completion of skeletal growth.

Toronto Program

Munro and Lauritzen (1985) proposed an anatomic–pathologic classification of craniofacial microsomia as an aid in designing the surgical procedure (Fig. 62–36). Surgery is preferably performed at age 5 to 6 years for Types II to V. Type V is corrected in two stages to avoid a simultaneous intraoral and intracranial procedure.

Type IA. The facial skeleton is complete

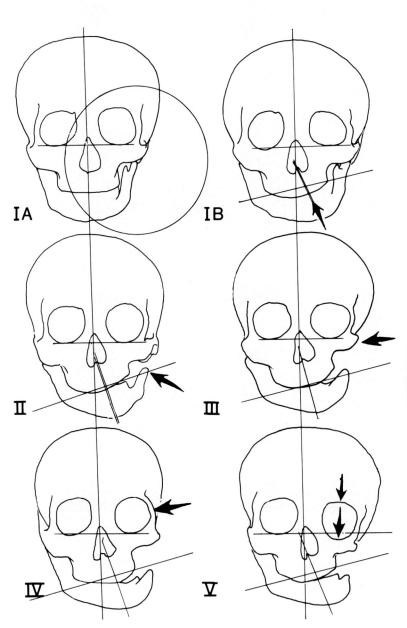

Figure 62–36. Classification of unilateral craniofacial microsomia according to the pathologic skeletal anatomy (After Munro and Lauritzen, 1985). In the upper left panel the circle designates the usual site of skeletal involvement. The midsagittal, midincisor and occlusal planes are illustrated. See text for details.

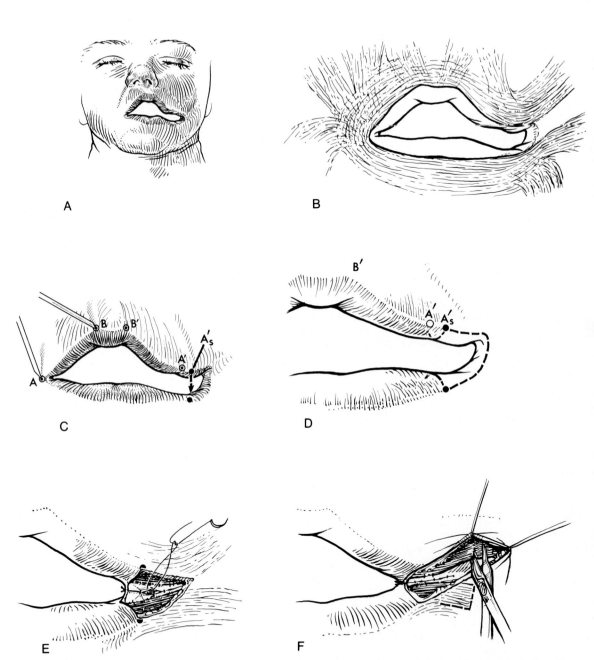

Figure 62–37. Correction of lateral facial cleft. *A,* Preoperative appearance—left-sided lateral facial cleft. *B,* Disruption of the orbicularis sphincter. *C,* Markings are made on the white line with ink: A, oral commissure on unaffected side; B, philtral column; B′, philtral column on affected side; A′, proposed oral commissure (distance = AB); A′s is made the surgical oral commissure because of expected postoperative contraction. A dot is placed opposite on the lower lip. *D,* Proposed vermilion turnover flap (outlined by the interrupted line). *E,* Closure of the oral mucosa. *F,* The upper and lower orbicularis muscle bundles are skeletonized and divided.

Illustration continued on following page

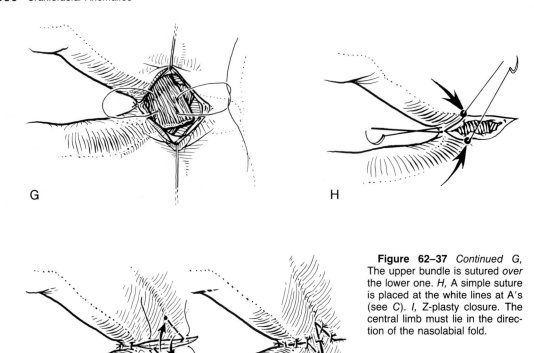

G

H

I

Figure 62–37 *Continued G,* The upper bundle is sutured *over* the lower one. *H,* A simple suture is placed at the white lines at A's (see *C*). *I,* Z-plasty closure. The central limb must lie in the direction of the nasolabial fold.

but hypoplastic. The occlusal plane (and labial fissure) is horizontal. Onlay rib grafts are added to the hypoplastic orbit, zygoma, maxilla, and mandible (see Fig. 62–44).

Type IB. The facial skeleton is hypoplastic but complete. The occlusal plane, however, is tilted. The surgical treatment plan consists of a Le Fort I osteotomy with lowering and rotation of the affected maxilla, bilateral sagittal osteotomies of the mandibular rami, and genioplasty (see Fig. 62–46).

Type II. There is absence of the mandibular condyle and part of the ascending ramus. A Le Fort I osteotomy, unilateral sagittal osteotomy of the remaining mandibular ramus, and genioplasty are employed as in the Type IB patient. A costochondral rib graft (or grafts) is secured to the mandibular remnant on the affected side and directed laterally to the glenoid fossa, to lengthen and reposition the mandible and to increase facial width.

Type III. In addition to the findings in Type II, there is absence of the zygomatic arch and glenoid fossa. The glenoid fossa and zygomatic arch are reconstructed with rib grafts and the surgical procedure is completed as outlined for Type II patients (see Fig. 62–42).

Type IV. This type is uncommon and is characterized by hypoplasia of the zygoma and a posterior and a medial displacement of the lateral orbital wall. Surgical correction consists of a Le Fort III osteotomy of the affected side and a Le Fort I osteotomy on the opposite side. The procedure then proceeds as in a Type III patient.

Type V. The most severe type has either a micro-orbit or inferior displacement of the orbit. In the first surgical stage, performed through an intracranial route, the orbit is translocated as required. In the second stage at least six months later, reconstruction is accomplished as previously described for Types II and III.

New York University Program

Infant Soft Tissue Surgery (Before 1 Year of Age). Within the first year of life ear tags are removed and the lateral facial cleft or macrostomia, if present, is corrected. It is essential that the oral commissure is reconstituted at the orbicularis muscle level (Figs. 62–37, 62–38) (McCarthy and Fulei-han, 1986).

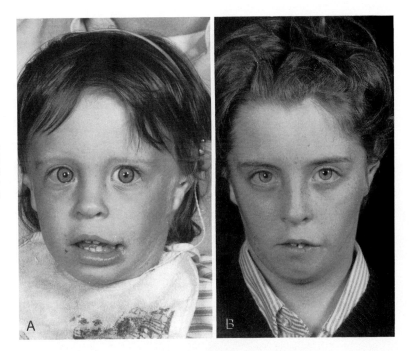

Figure 62–38. A 2 year old boy with left-sided lateral facial cleft and bilateral microtia. *A,* Preoperative appearance. *B,* After correction by the technique illustrated in Figure 62–37.

Surgical Correction of Forehead Deformity or Orbital Dystopia (Under Age 3 Years). In patients with an associated forehead or orbital deformity such as microphthalmos or orbital dystopia (Munro Types IV and V or Harvold Type IB), a combined intracranial approach is employed to restore the skeletal anatomy. The plagiocephaly or forehead deformity and retruded brow can be repaired by the technique developed for the infant with unilateral coronal synostosis and plagiocephaly (Fig. 62–39). Similarly, the orbital dystopia can be corrected in a preliminary stage before reconstructive jaw surgery.

Reconstructive Jaw Surgery–Functional Appliance Therapy (Under Age 6 Years). In the child with Types IB, II, and III deformities (Munro and Lauritzen, 1985), the affected mandibular ramus is lengthened by an interposition (ramus) bone graft (Fig. 62–40).

After the surgical correction of mandibular

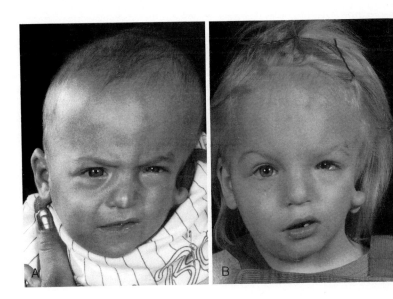

Figure 62–39. Unilateral forehead and cranial vault deformity in a patient with unilateral craniofacial microsomia correction by frontal bone advancement. *A,* Preoperative appearance. *B,* Appearance after frontal bone advancement and cranial vault remodeling (see Chap. 61) and resection of a nasal dermoid. Reconstructive jaw surgery and otoplasty are planned.

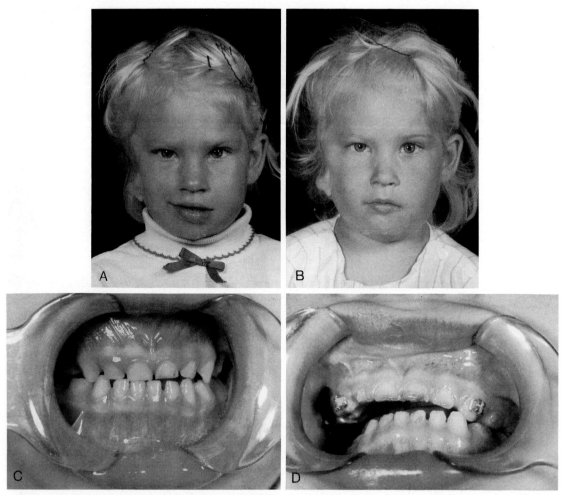

Figure 62–40. A 4 year old girl with right-sided craniofacial microsomia treated by mandibular lengthening (costochondral rib grafts) and reconstruction of the zygomatic arch (see Fig. 62–42*E*). *A,* Preoperative appearance. *B,* Postoperative appearance. Note the improved chin position and improved zygomatic contour on the affected side. *C,* Preoperative occlusion. Note the disparity in the midincisor lines. *D,* Postoperative occlusion. Note the surgically created lateral open bite.

position the patient has a unilateral open bite on the affected side. This results from dropping the affected side of the mandible and rotating it toward the midline. Immediately upon removal of the intermaxillary fixation, a unilateral biteplate is inserted. Combined with intermaxillary elastics, the biteplate guides the mandible into the symmetric position achieved through surgery and relieves excessive stress on the newly placed bone grafts. The biteplate is also used to achieve extrusion of teeth and alveolus in the maxilla on the affected side. The latter goal is achieved by removal of the occlusal surface of the biteplate under the most posterior maxillary molar on the affected side. The vertical extrusion of this tooth is enhanced

by force applied to it from springs placed on the biteplate itself or through intermaxillary elastics. After the most posterior teeth are brought into occlusion, the adjacent teeth are extruded along with their surrounding alveolar process in the same manner (Fig. 62–41).

Reconstructive Jaw Surgery (After Age 7 Years). Reconstructive jaw surgery (after 7 years of age) in the child with a Munro Type II–V deformity consists of costochondral grafts (Obwegeser, 1974; Munro, 1980; Wolfe, 1980) inserted to reconstruct the glenoid fossa, condyle, and zygomatic complex, depending on the pathology. This type of surgical reconstruction (Fig. 62–42) is massive and can exhaust all the available bone graft donor sites. The family must be appraised not

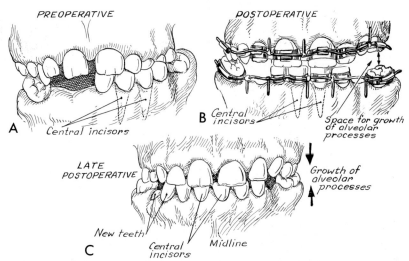

Figure 62–41. Surgical correction of the mandibular anomaly during childhood. *A,* Preoperative occlusion. Note that the lower central incisors are deviated to the affected side, and there is also a crossbite. *B,* After mandibular lengthening the central incisors are in the midline and there is a resulting space for downward growth of the maxillary alveolar process. *C,* Late postoperative view. The maxillary alveolar processes have grown downward and filled the void between the maxillary and mandibular arches.

only of possible complications but also of the need for additional jaw surgery in later years, depending on the pattern of subsequent craniofacial growth (Fig. 62–43).

After an eight week period of postoperative immobilization, functional appliance therapy is begun. The growth behavior of the costochondral graft (MacIntosh and Henny, 1977) must be carefully monitored, since overgrowth of the graft has been reported (Munro and Lauritzen, 1985).

Contour Restoration of Skeletal Deformity With Onlay Bone Grafts (Age 8 Years Upward). In the occasional patient with satisfactory occlusal relationships and absence of an occlusal cant or asymmetry (Munro and Lauritzen Type IA), bone grafting of the deficient mandible, maxilla, and zygomaticoorbital complex is deferred until at least age 8 years when a sufficient amount of bone graft can be harvested (Fig. 62–44).

Reconstructive Jaw Surgery in Adolescence (After Age 12 Years). Reconstructive jaw surgery may be indicated at this age for two reasons. The patient may not have sought surgical correction at an earlier age, or there may be residual deficiency after skeletal surgery performed at an earlier age.

The treatment program is designed according to the pathologic findings. Surgical correction may range from simple autogenous onlay bone grafting (Fig. 62–45) to extensive reconstruction of the zygomatico-orbital com-

plex, maxilla, and mandible as previously described (Figs. 62–46, 62–47). It should be noted that the authors prefer to defer the genioplasty since it can easily be performed on an outpatient basis, and chin symmetry is more easily achieved when the genioplasty is done at a second stage.

Soft Tissue Reconstruction (After Age 6 Years). Soft tissue surgery (auricle, cheek soft tissue) should be deferred until the underlying skeleton is reconstructed. As discussed in Chapter 40, auricular reconstruction is delayed until at least age 6 years when the donor ribs are of adequate size.

Often, restoration of the cheek soft tissue is indicated to complete the facial contour restoration. In more recent years the authors have abandoned nonvascularized dermis-fat grafts in favor of vascularized microvascular deepithelized free flaps (see Fig. 62–35) (Wells and Edgerton, 1977; Upton and colleagues, 1980) or vascularized omental transfers.

On occasion, reconstruction of the paralyzed face may be indicated; the techniques are discussed in Chapter 42.

BILATERAL CRANIOFACIAL MICROSOMIA

There is little mention in the literature of the bilateral form of craniofacial microsomia. *Text continued on page 3096*

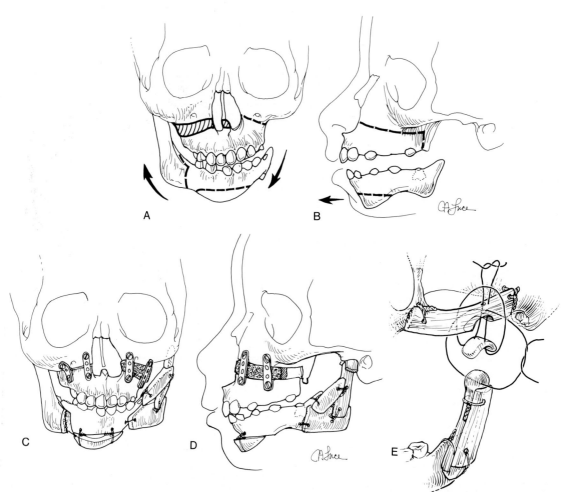

Figure 62–42. Combined Le Fort I, unilateral mandibular ramisection, genioplasty, and costochondral graft reconstruction of the deficient mandible-temporomandibular joint. *A, B,* Preoperative pathology and lines of osteotomy. *C, D,* Postoperative appearance. Note the bone grafts and the combination of interosseous wire–miniplate fixation. Four screws are usually placed in each miniplate. *E,* Details of reconstruction of the temporomandibular joint. A shaving of costal cartilage is placed in a groove on the undersurface of the reconstructed zygomatic arch (costal bone graft) to simulate the glenoid fossa. A costochondral graft is used to replace the ramus and condyle (the cartilage portion simulating the condyle). An absorbable suture temporarily positions the condyle in the reconstructed glenoid fossa (after Munro).

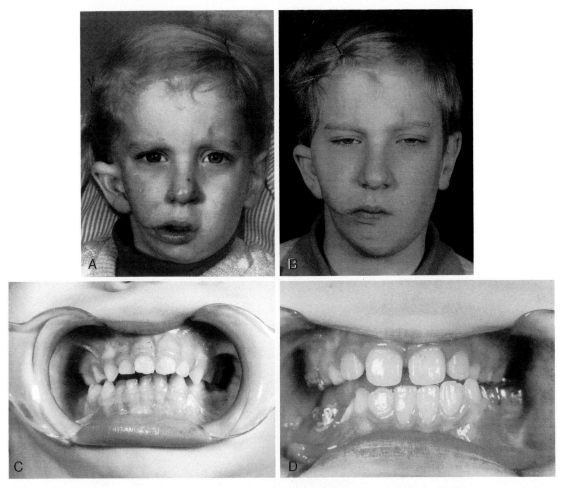

Figure 62–43. A 7 year old male who presented with sleep apnea and right-sided craniofacial microsomia. *A,* Preoperative appearance. *B,* Postoperative appearance. Note the improvement in the chin and oral commissure position. The sleep apnea was relieved. *C,* Preoperative occlusion. Note the disparity in the midincisor lines. *D,* Postoperative occlusion. Note the surgically created open bite and the shift of the mandibular midincisor line (see Fig. 62–42).

Figure 62–44. Extensive onlay bone grafting of the mandible and zygomaticomaxillary and orbital complex in a patient with satisfactory occlusal relationships. Fixation can be accomplished with lag screws.

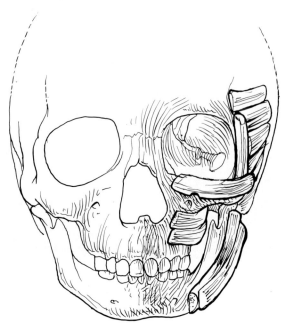

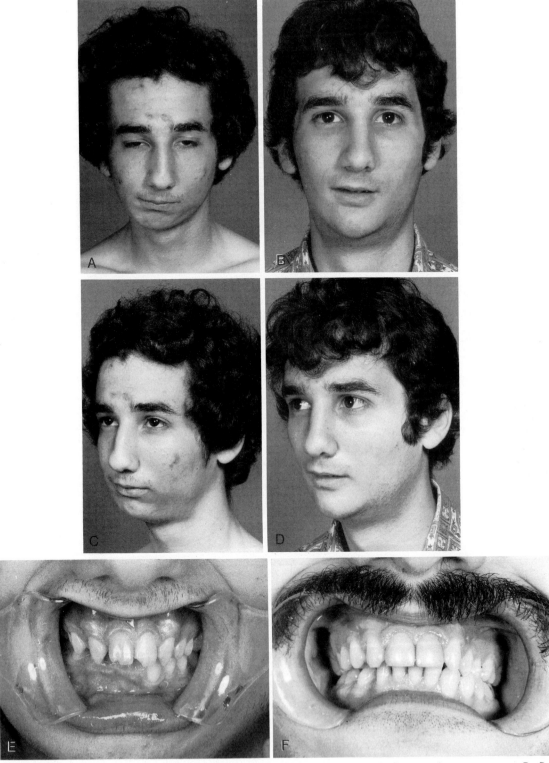

Figure 62–45. Adolescent male with right-sided craniofacial microsomia. *A, C,* Preoperative appearance. *B, D,* Postoperative views after onlay bone grafting, genioplasty, or horizontal osteotomy of the anteroinferior border of the mandible and rhinoplasty. *E,* Preoperative occlusion. *F,* After orthodontic and prosthodontic therapy.

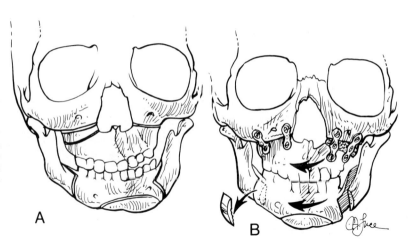

Figure 62–46. Combined Le Fort I osteotomy, bilateral sagittal ramisection of the mandible, and genioplasty. *A,* Lines of osteotomy. Note the wedge resection and impaction of the right maxilla. *B,* Direction of skeletal mobilization. A segment of outer table of the mandible is resected. Miniplate fixation is illustrated. Four screws are generally used with each miniplate.

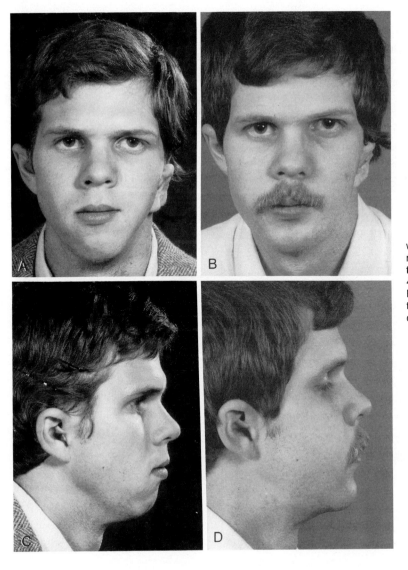

Figure 62–47. A 17 year old male with left-sided unilateral craniofacial microsomia reconstructed by the technique illustrated in Figure 62–46. *A, C,* Preoperative views. *B, D,* Postoperative appearance. Note the improvement in the chin–oral commissure position and contour.

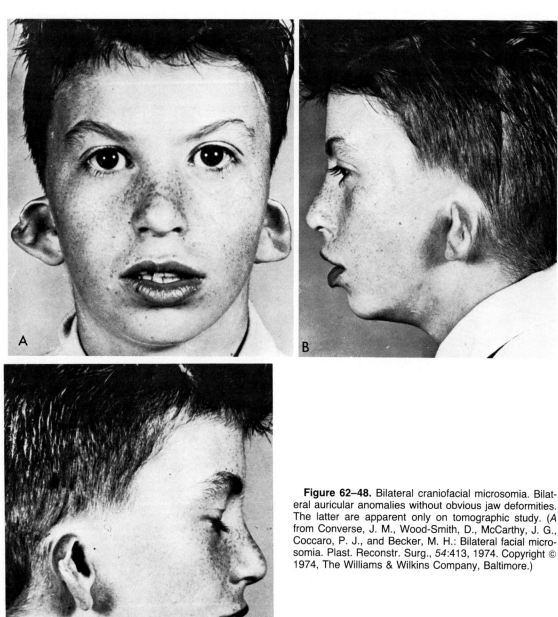

Figure 62–48. Bilateral craniofacial microsomia. Bilateral auricular anomalies without obvious jaw deformities. The latter are apparent only on tomographic study. (*A* from Converse, J. M., Wood-Smith, D., McCarthy, J. G., Coccaro, P. J., and Becker, M. H.: Bilateral facial microsomia. Plast. Reconstr. Surg., *54*:413, 1974. Copyright © 1974, The Williams & Wilkins Company, Baltimore.)

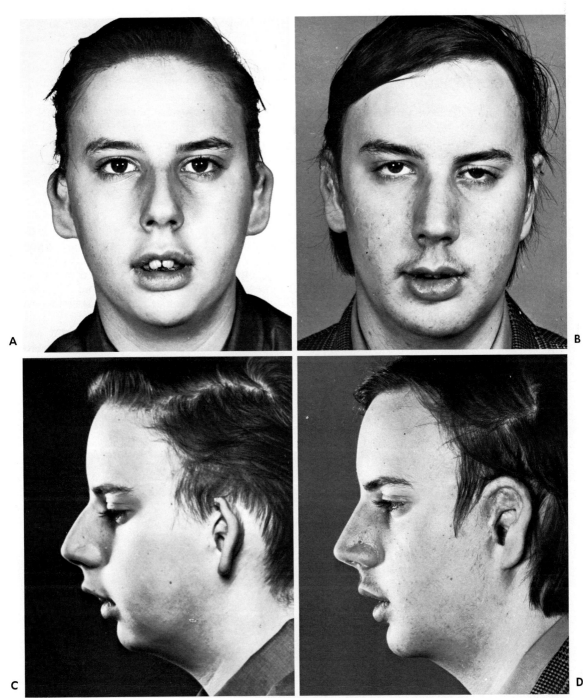

Figure 62–49. Bilateral craniofacial microsomia with microtia and skeletal deformity. *A, C,* Appearance after unsuccessful auricular surgery at another institution. Note the micrognathia-microgenia. *B, D,* After auricular reconstruction, horizontal advancement osteotomy of the lower portion of the mandibular symphysis (see Fig. 62–51C), and corrective rhinoplasty. (From Converse, J. M., Wood-Smith, D., McCarthy, J. G., Coccaro, P. J., and Becker, M. H.: Bilateral facial microsomia. Plast. Reconstr. Surg., *54*:413, 1974. Copyright © 1974, The Williams & Wilkins Company, Baltimore.)

The relative incidence of the unilateral and bilateral types was discussed earlier in this chapter but, as emphasized, the true incidence of bilateral craniofacial microsomia is much higher than previously reported.

Variations of Syndrome

Converse and associates (1974), in a review of 15 patients with bilateral craniofacial microsomia, proposed a classification and noted that the expression of the syndrome was as variable as in the unilateral type.

Some patients show only bilateral microtia without clinically obvious jaw deformities (Fig. 62–48). In this group, however, tomographic studies demonstrated mild condylar blunting or surface irregularities.

Most patients display bilateral microtia, mandibular micrognathia, and a Class II dental occlusal relationship. While the ear deformities may not be symmetric, both halves of the mandible appear equally hypoplastic, and there is an anterior open bite deformity (Fig. 62–49).

In addition to bilateral auricular anomalies and severe mandibular micrognathia, macrostomia or transverse facial clefts are seen in other patients. The clefting can also involve the maxillary alveolus, and "ectopic" dentition is observed. The clefts range from a macrostomia (Fig. 62–50A) to full-thickness buccal clefts extending from the oral commissures to the auricular tragus (Fig. 62–50B). The condition of these patients represents the most complete expression of the bilateral syndrome.

Surgical Reconstruction of Mandible

In the reconstruction of the micrognathic mandible in bilateral craniofacial microsomia, there are three goals: (1) restoration of mandibular size, form, and position; (2) correction of the malocclusion; and (3) correction of the soft tissue and bony deficiency in the mental region.

Restoration of mandibular size and form usually involves increasing the anteroposte-

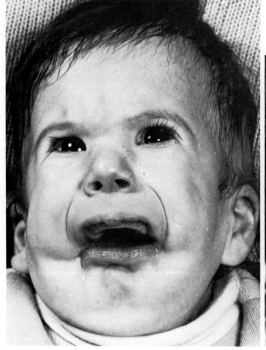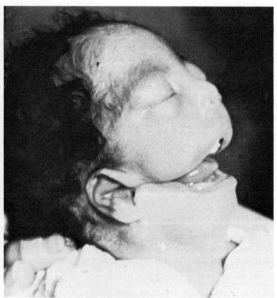

A   B

Figure 62–50. Transverse facial clefts associated with bilateral craniofacial microsomia. *A,* Macrostomia secondary to transverse facial clefts. *B,* Full-thickness clefts extending from the oral commissure to the tragal area. (From Converse, J. M., Wood-Smith, D., McCarthy, J. G., Coccaro, P. J., and Becker, M. H.: Bilateral facial microsomia. Plast. Reconstr. Surg., *54:*413, 1974. Copyright © 1974, The Williams & Wilkins Company, Baltimore.)

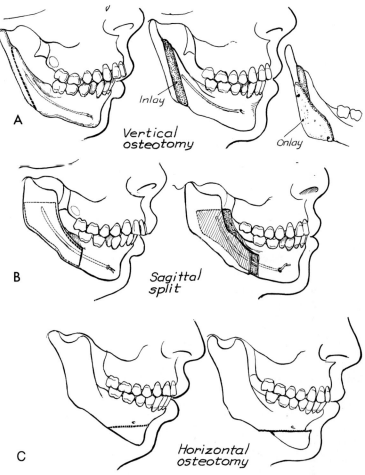

Figure 62–51. Techniques employed for restoration of mandibular size and form in bilateral craniofacial microsomia. *A,* Vertical osteotomy of the ramus with interposition and onlay bone grafts. The technique is suited for the small ramus, as it increases the anteroposterior and vertical dimensions of the underdeveloped ramus. *B,* Sagittal split technique, showing the sites of osteotomy and the resulting increased mandibular projection. This method has been used when the ramus is sufficiently large. *C,* Horizontal advancement osteotomy of the mandible (genioplasty). The technique is employed to obtain projection and/or correct the midline position of the chin (see also Chap. 29). (From Converse, J. M., Wood-Smith, D., McCarthy, J. G., Coccaro, P. J., and Becker, M. H.: Bilateral facial microsomia. Plast. Reconstr. Surg., *54:*413, 1974. Copyright © 1974, The Williams & Wilkins Company, Baltimore.)

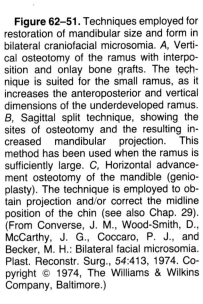

rior dimensions of both mandibular rami. This has been accomplished either by a sagittal split osteotomy or by a vertical osteotomy of the rami with interposition bone grafts, as described by Converse and associates (1974).

Vertical osteotomy (Fig. 62–51A) of the ramus with interposition of bone grafts is particularly suited to increase the anteroposterior dimension of the ramus, and also to add bone grafts to the thin condylar process and underdeveloped mandibular angle. The mandibular body is advanced to the predetermined position, and one can provide for any slight asymmetry requiring more advancement on one side than the other. Intermaxillary fixation is established, the condylar fragments are recessed, and bone grafts are interposed between the fragments and also added as onlay grafts.

When the rami are of sufficient size, the sagittal split technique can be employed (Fig. 62–51B). The wide surface of contact between the split osseous fragments precludes the need for bone grafting.

Horizontal advancement osteotomy of the anteroinferior portion of the mandible (Fig. 62–51C) is usually required to project the mental symphysis. Horizontal advancement osteotomy alone is sufficient to correct the mandibular micrognathia if the dental occlusal relationships are acceptable and additional improvement can be obtained by orthodontic therapy. Refinements of the horizontal osteotomy include the double-tiered osteotomy (Neuner, 1965) or the addition of bone grafts to the osteotomy site. The techniques of the various osteotomies are discussed in Chapter 29.

REFERENCES

Aleksic, S., Budzilovich, G., Choy, A., Reuben R., Randt, C., et al.: Congenital ophthalmoplegia in oculoauriculovertebral dysplasia-hemifacial microsomia (Goldenhar-Gorlin syndrome). A clinicopathologic study and review of the literature. Neurology, *26*:638, 1976.

Aleksic, S., Budzilovich, G., Reuben, R., Laguna, J., Finegold, M., et al.: Unilateral arhinencephaly in Goldenhar-Gorlin syndrome. Dev. Med. Child Neurol., *17*:498, 1975a.

Aleksic, S., Budzilovich, G., Reuben, R., Feigin, I., Finegold, M., et al.: Congenital trigeminal neuropathy in oculoauricovertebral dysplasia–hemifacial microsomia (Goldenhar-Gorlin syndrome). J. Neurol. Neurosurg. Psychiatry, *38*:1033, 1975b.

Altman, F.: Malformations of the auricle and external auditory meatus. Arch. Otolaryngol., *54*:115, 1951.

Arey, L. B.: Developmental Anatomy. 7th Ed. Philadelphia, W. B. Saunders Company, 1974.

Bartholinus, T.: Historiarum Anatomicarium et Medicarum Rariorem. Centuria VI, Historia 36, Hafniae, 1654.

Bellucci, R. J.: Congenital auricular malformations. Indications, contraindications, and timing of middle ear surgery. Ann. Otol. Rhinol. Laryngol., *81*:659, 1972.

Berkman, M. D., and Feingold, M.: Oculo-auriculo-vertebral dysplasia. Oral Surg., *25*:408, 1968.

Bowen, D. I., Collum, M. T., and Rees, D. O.: Clinical aspects of oculo-auriculo-vertebral dysplasia. Br. J. Ophthalmol., *55*:145, 1971.

Brodie, A. G.: Contribution of the mandibular condyle to the growth of the face. In Sarnat, B. G. (Ed.): The Temporomandibular Joint. Springfield, IL, Charles C Thomas, 1964, p. 77.

Brown, J. B., Fryer, M. P., and Ohlwiler, D. A.: Study and use of synthetic materials, such as silicones and Teflon, as subcutaneous prostheses. Plast. Reconstr. Surg., *26*:264, 1960.

Brown, J. B., and McDowell, F.: Skin Grafting. 3rd Ed. Philadelphia, J. B. Lippincott Company, 1958, p. 114.

Caldarelli, D. D., Hutchinson, J. G., Jr., Pruzansky, S., and Valvassori, G. E.: A comparison of microtia and temporal bone anomalies in hemifacial microsomia and mandibulofacial dysostosis. Cleft Palate J., *17*:103, 1980.

Caronni, E. P.: Embryogenesis and classification of branchial auricular dysplasia. In Trans. Fifth Internatl. Congr. Plast. Reconstr. Surg. Melbourne, Australia, Butterworths, 1971.

Christiaens, L. R., Walbaum, J. P., Farriaux, J. P., and Fontain, G.: A propos de deux cas de dysplasie oculoauriculo-vertebrale. Pediatrie (Paris), *21*:935, 1966.

Converse, J. M.: Restoration of facial contour by bone grafts introduced through oral cavity. Plast. Reconstr. Surg., *6*:295, 1950.

Converse, J. M., Coccaro, P. J., Becker, H., and Wood-Smith, D.: On hemifacial microsomia. The first and second branchial arch syndrome. Plast. Reconstr. Surg., *51*:268, 1973a.

Converse, J. M., Horowitz, S. L., Coccaro, P. J., and Wood-Smith, D.: Corrective treatment of the skeletal asymmetry in hemifacial microsomia. Plast. Reconstr. Surg., *52*:221, 1973b.

Converse, J. M., and Rushton, A. M.: In Gillies, H., and Millard, D. R., Jr. (Eds.): The Principles and Art of Plastic Surgery. Vol. I. Boston, Little, Brown & Company, 1957, p. 314.

Converse, J. M., and Shapiro, H. H.: Treatment of developmental malformations of the jaws. Plast. Reconstr. Surg., *10*:473, 1952.

Converse, J. M., and Shapiro, H. H.: Bone grafting in malformations of the jaws. Cephalographic diagnosis in the surgical treatment of malformations of the face. Am. J. Surg., *88*:858, 1954.

Converse, J. M., and Wood-Smith, D.: Technical details in the surgical correction of the lop ear deformity. Plast. Reconstr. Surg., *31*:118, 1963.

Converse, J. M., Wood-Smith, D., McCarthy, J. G., Coccaro, P. J., and Becker, M. H.: Bilateral facial microsomia. Diagnosis, classification, treatment. Plast. Reconstr. Surg., *54*:413, 1974.

David, D. J., Mahatumarat, C., and Cooter, R. D.: Hemifacial microsomia: A multisystem classification. Plast. Reconstr. Surg., *80*:525, 1987.

Davis, W. B.: Reconstruction of hemiatrophy of face. Plast. Reconstr. Surg., *42*:489, 1968.

Delaire, J.: De l'interêt des osteotomies sagittales dans la correction des infragnathies mandibulaires. Ann. Chir. Plast., *15*:104, 1970.

Dingman, R. O., and Grabb, W. C.: Mandibular laterognathism. Plast. Reconstr. Surg., *31*:563, 1963.

Dingman, R. O., and Grabb, W. C.: Reconstruction of both mandibular condyles with metatarsal bone grafts. Plast. Reconstr. Surg., *34*:441, 1964. (Follow-up Clinic, *47*:594, 1971.)

Dupertuis, S. M., and Musgrave, R. H.: Experiences with the reconstruction of the congenitally deformed ear. Plast. Reconstr. Surg., *23*:361, 1959.

Entin, M. A.: Reconstruction in congenital deformity of the temporomandibular component. Plast. Reconstr. Surg., *21*:461, 1958.

Franceschetti, A., and Klein, D.: Mandibulofacial dysostosis. A new hereditary syndrome. Acta Ophthalmol., *27*:143, 1949.

Franceschetti, A., Klein, D., and Brocher, J. E. W.: La dysostose mandibulofaciale dans la cadre des syndromes du premier arc branchial. Schweiz. Med. Wochenschr., *89*:478, 1959.

François, J.: Heredity in Ophthalmology. St. Louis, MO, C. V. Mosby Company, 1961.

Freeman, B. S.: The result of epiphyseal transplants by flap and by free grafts: a brief survey. Plast. Reconstr. Surg., *36*:227, 1965.

Fujino, T., Rytinzaburo, T., and Sugimoto, C.: Microvascular transfer of free deltopectoral dermal-fat flap. Plast. Reconstr. Surg., *55*:428, 1975.

Gaupp, R., and Jantz, J.: Zur Kasuistik der Balkenlipome. Nervenarzt, *15*:58, 1942.

Gillies, H., and Millard, D. R., Jr.: The Principles and Art of Plastic Surgery. Boston, Little, Brown & Company, 1957.

Glahn, M., and Winther, J. E.: Metatarsal transplants as replacement for lost mandibular condyle (3-year follow-up). Scand. J. Plast. Reconstr. Surg., 1:97, 1967.

Goldenhar, M.: Associations malformatives de l'oeil et de l'oreille, en particulier le syndrome dermoide epibulbaire-appendices auriculaires-fistula auris congenita et ses relations avec la dysostose mandibulofaciale. J. Genet. Hum., 1:243, 1952.

Gorlin, R. J., Jue, K. L., Jacobsen, U., and Goldschmidt, E.: Oculoauriculovertebral dysplasia. J. Pediatr., 63:991, 1963.

Gorlin, R. J., and Pindborg, J. J.: Syndromes of the Head and Neck. New York, McGraw-Hill Book Company, 1964.

Gorski, M., and Tarczynska, I. H.: Surgical treatment of mandibular asymmetry. Br. J. Plast. Surg., 22:370, 1969.

Grabb, W. C.: The first and second branchial arch syndrome. Plast. Reconstr. Surg., 36:485, 1965.

Grayson, B., Boral, S., Eisig, S., Kolber, A., and McCarthy, J. G.: Unilateral craniofacial microsomia. Part I—Mandibular analysis. Am. J. Orthod., 84:225, 1983a.

Grayson, B. H., LaBatto, F. A., Kolber, A. B., and McCarthy, J. G.: Basilar multiplane cephalometric analysis. Am. J. Orthod., 88:503, 1985.

Grayson, B., McCarthy, J. G., and Bookstein, F.: Analysis of craniofacial asymmetry by multiplane cephalometry. Am. J. Orthod., 84:217, 1983b.

Hanhart, E.: Nachweis einer einfach-dominanten, unkomplizierten sowie unregelmassig-dominanten, mit Atresia auris, Palatoschisis und anderen Deformationen verbundene Anlage zu Ohrmuschelverkummerung (Mikrotie). Arch. Julius Klaus-Stift., 24:374, 1949.

Harvold, E. P., Vargervik, K., and Chierici, G.: Treatment of Hemifacial Microsomia. New York, A. R. Liss, 1983.

Herrmann, J., and Optiz, J. M.: A dominantly inherited first arch syndrome. First Conference on Clinical Delineation of Birth Defects. Part II. Malformation Syndromes. In Bergsma, D. (Ed.): Birth Defects, Original Article Series, Vol. 2, No. 2, New York, National Foundation—March of Dimes, Baltimore, Williams & Wilkins Company, 1969.

Horowitz, S. L., and Shapiro, H. H.: Modification of mandibular architecture following removal of temporalis muscle in rat. J. Dent. Res., 30:276, 1951.

Ide, C. H., Miller, G. W., and Wollschlaeger, P. B.: Familial facial dysplasia., Arch. Ophthalmol., 84:427, 1970.

Kaban, L. B., Moses, M. H., and Mulliken, J. B.: Surgical correction of hemifacial microsomia in the growing child. Plast. Reconstr. Surg., 82:9, 1988.

Kazanjian, V. H.: Congenital absence of ramus of mandible. J. Bone Joint Surg., 21:761, 1939.

Kleinsasser, O., and Schlothane, R.: Die Ohrmissbildungen im Rahmen der Thalidomid-Embryopathie. Z. Laryngol. Rhinol. Otol., 43:344, 1964.

Knowles, C. C.: Cephalometric treatment planning and analysis of maxillary growth following bone grafting to the ramus in hemifacial microsomia. Dent. Pract. (Bristol), 17:28, 1966.

Lachmund, F.: Occlusion of the right ear. Miscell. Acad. Nat. Curios., 6–7:225, 1688.

Limberg, A. A.: New method of plastic lengthening of the mandible in unilateral micrognathism and asymmetry of the face. J. Am. Dent. Assoc., 15:581, 1928.

Longacre, J. J.: The early reconstruction of congenital hypoplasia of the facial skeleton and skull. In Longacre, J. J., et al. (Eds.): Craniofacial Anomalies, Pathogenesis and Repair. Philadelphia, J. B. Lippincott Company, 1968, pp. 151–159.

Longacre, J. J., DeStefano, G. A., and Holmstrand, K. E.: Surgical management of first and second branchial arch syndromes. Plast. Reconstr. Surg., 31:507, 1963.

MacIntosh, R. B., and Henny, F. A.: A spectrum of application of autogenous costochondral grafts. J. Maxillofac. Surg., 5:257, 1977.

Marx, H.: Die Missbildungen des Ohres. In Denker and Kahler (Eds.): Handbuch des Hals-Nasen-und Ohren-Heilkunde mit Einschluss der Grenzgebiete. Vol. VI. Berlin, Springer-Verlag, 1926.

Mathies, F.: The triad of anotia, facial paralysis and cardiac anomaly not due to thalidomide. J.A.M.A., 195:695, 1966.

McCarthy, J. G., and Fuleihan, N. S.: Commissuroplasty in lateral facial clefts. In Stark, R. B. (Ed.): Plastic Surgery of the Head and Neck. Boston, Little, Brown & Company, 1986.

McKenzie, J., and Craig, J.: Mandibulofacial dysostosis. Arch. Dis. Child., 30:391, 1955.

Meurmann, Y.: Congenital microtia and meatal atresia. Arch. Otolaryngol., 66:443, 1957.

Moss, M. L.: The primacy of functional matrices in orofacial growth. Dent. Pract. Dent. Rec., 19:65, 1968.

Munro, I. R.: One-stage reconstruction of the temporomandibular joint in hemifacial microsomia. Plast. Reconstr. Surg., 66:699, 1980.

Munro, I. R., and Lauritzen, C. G.: Classification and treatment of hemifacial microsomia. In Caronni, E. P. (Ed.): Craniofacial Surgery. Boston, Little, Brown & Company, 1985, pp. 391–400.

Murray, J. E., Kaban, L. B., Mulliken, J. B., and Evans, C. A.: Analysis and treatment of hemifacial microsomia. In Caronni, E. P. (Ed.): Craniofacial Surgery. Boston, Little, Brown & Company, 1985, pp. 377–390.

Nager, F. R., and de Reynier, J. P.: Das Gehororgen bei die angeborenen Kopfmissbildungen. Pract. Otorhinolaryngol. (Basel), 19:1, 1948.

Neuner, O.: Chirurgische Orthodontie. Schweiz. Monatsschr. Zahnheilkd., 75:940, 1965.

Obwegeser, H.: Zur Korrektur der Dysostosis otomandibularis. Schweiz. Monatsschr. Zahnheilkd., 80:331, 1970.

Obwegeser, H. L.: The indications for surgical correction of mandibular deformity by the sagittal splitting technique. Br. J. Oral Surg., 1:157, 1953.

Obwegeser, H. L.: Correction of the skeletal anomalies of otomandibular dysostosis. J. Maxillofac. Surg., 2:73, 1974.

Obwegeser, H. L., Lello, G. E., and Sailer, H. F.: Otomandibular dysostosis. In Bell, W. H., Proffit, W. R., and White, R. P., Jr. (Eds.): Surgical Correction of Dentofacial Deformities. New Concepts. Vol. III. Philadelphia, W. B. Saunders Company, 1985, pp. 639–661.

Osborne, R.: The treatment of the underdeveloped ascending ramus. Br. J. Plast. Surg., 17:376, 1964.

Poswillo, D. E.: The pathogenesis of the first and second branchial arch syndrome. Oral Surg., 35:302, 1973.

Poswillo, D. E.: Otomandibular deformity: pathogenesis as a guide to reconstruction. J. Maxillofac. Surg., 2:64, 1974.

Pruzansky, S.: Not all dwarfed mandibles are alike. Birth Defects, 5:120, 1969.

Rogers, B. O.: Microtic, lop, cup and protruding ears: four directly inheritable deformities? Plast. Reconstr. Surg., *41*:208, 1968.

Sarnat, B. G., and Engel, M. B.: A serial study of mandibular growth after removal of the condyle in the *Macaca* rhesus monkey. Plast. Reconstr. Surg., *7*:364, 1951.

Sarnat, B. G., and Laskin, D. M.: Surgery of the temporomandibular joint. *In* Sarnat, B. G. (Ed.): The Temporomandibular Joint. Springfield, IL, Charles C Thomas, 1964, p. 185.

Stark, R. B., and Saunders, D. E.: The first branchial syndrome: the oral-mandibular-auricular syndrome. Plast. Reconstr. Surg., *29*:229, 1962.

Sugar, H. S.: An unusual example of the oculo-auriculovertebral dysplasia syndrome of Goldenhar. J. Pediatr. Ophthalmol., *4*:9, 1967.

Summitt, R.: Familial Goldenhar syndrome. Birth Defects, *2*:106, 1969.

Tessier, P.: Anatomical classification of facial, craniofacial and latero-facial clefts. J. Maxillofac. Surg., *4*:69, 1976.

Thompson, A.: A description of congenital malformation of the auricle and external meatus of both sides in three persons. Proc. R. Soc. Edinburgh, *1*:443, 1845.

Timm, G.: Zur Morphologie des Auges bei Missbildungen Syndrome. Klin. Monatsbl. Augenheilkd., *137*:557, 1960.

Upton, J., Mulliken, J. B., Hicks, P. D., and Murray, J. E.: Restoration of facial contour using free vascularized omental transfer. Plast. Reconstr. Surg., *66*:560, 1980.

Virchow, R.: Ueber Missbildungen am Ohr und in Berich des erstem Kiembogens. Virchows Arch. [Pathol. Anat.], *30*:221, 1864.

Wells, J. H., and Edgerton, M. T.: Correction of severe hemifacial atrophy with a free dermis-fat flap from the lower abdomen. Plast. Reconstr. Surg., *59*:223, 1977.

Willie-Jorgensen, A.: Dysostosis mandibulo-facialis (Franceschetti). Report of two atypical cases. Acta Ophthalmol. (Kobenhavn), *40*:348, 1962.

Wolfe, S. A.: Lateral facial microsomia with absent temporomandibular joint: constructive tactics. Plast. Reconstr. Surg., *66*:124, 1980.

Wolff, J.: Gesetz der Transformation der Knochen. Berlin, August Hirschwald, 1892.

Wood-Jones, F., and Wen-I-Chuan: The development of the external ear. J. Anat., *68*:525, 1934.

63

Ian R. Munro
Peter P. Kay
Peter Randall
Gregory L. Ruff
John W. Siebert

Craniofacial Syndromes

MANDIBULOFACIAL DYSOSTOSIS (Treacher Collins Syndrome)

Ian R. Munro
Peter B. Kay

Mandibulofacial dysostosis is an inherited disorder transmitted by an autosomal dominant gene. This gene shows variable penetrance and phenotypic expressivity. The genetic defect causes bilateral abnormalities in structures derived from the first and second branchial arches. The various degrees of phenotypic expression vary from a slight antimongoloid slant of the eye fissures to the full spectrum of abnormalities (Fig. 63–1): (1) antimongoloid slant of the palpebral apertures; (2) colobomas of the lower eyelids; (3) absent eyelashes in the medial two-thirds of the lower eyelids; (4) zygomatic and mandibular hypoplasia; (5) auricular defects; and (6) anteriorly displaced sideburns. This variability has, in part, been responsible for the historical debate concerning the correct eponym for this collection of physical findings or deformities.

The earliest report of this condition was by Thompson in 1846 (Gorlin and Pindborg, 1964). In 1889 Berry, a Scottish ophthalmologist, reported two related cases with the characteristic eyelid deformities (Berry, 1889) (Fig. 63–2). In 1900 Collins (1900a,b), an English ophthalmologist, reported two cases of lateral lower lid colobomas and emphasized the associated malar deficiency (Tyrrell, 1903). Coloboma is an almost constant feature of the syndrome, and Treacher Collins' name became widely associated with the deformity (Duke-Elder, 1952).

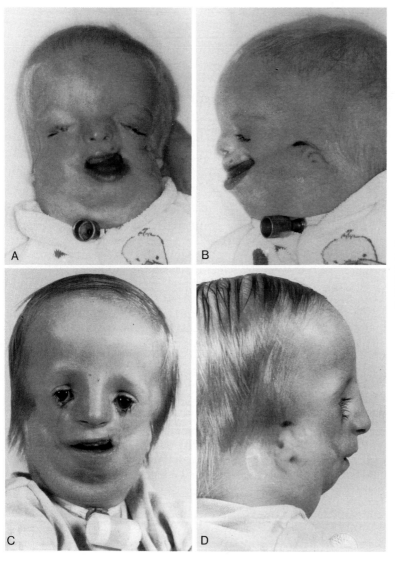

Figure 63–1. *A, B,* A severe form of mandibulofacial dysostosis (MFD) in an infant. Note the absent zygomas, macrostomia, and auricular deformities. *C, D,* A severe form of MFD with absent zygomas and severe mandibular deficiency.

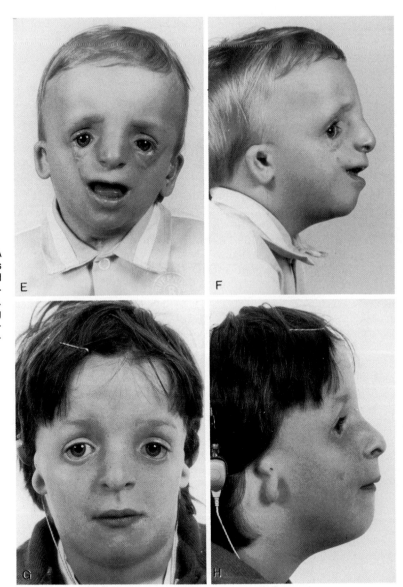

Figure 63–1 *Continued E, F,* A moderate form of MFD. The ears and mandible are less affected and surgery has been attempted to correct the colobomas of the lower lids. *G, H,* A mild form of MFD showing the antimongoloid slant of the palpebral apertures and auricular deformities.

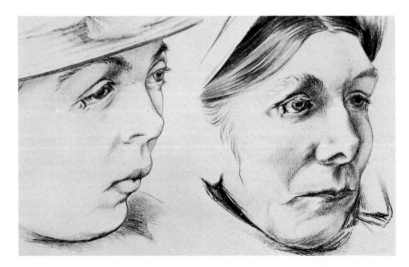

Figure 63–2. Original illustration from Berry's article (1889). *Right,* Mother with symmetric notching deformity of the lower eyelids and left-sided cleft lip. *Left,* Daughter with unilateral notching deformity of the right lower eyelid. The daughter also has a slightly receding chin.

The first fully expressed syndrome was described by Pires de Lima in 1923 (Pires de Lima and Monteiro, 1923). For the first time, researchers emphasized the developmental defects originating in the first and second branchial arches. In 1929 Lockhart reported the anatomic findings from a postmortem dissection of an affected infant (Lockhart, 1929). Franceschetti and Zwahlen in 1944 and Franceschetti and Klein (1949) described the deformities of this syndrome in detail and coined the term mandibulofacial dysostosis (MFD). In the European literature, these three names constitute the common eponym for this syndrome.

The first report of MFD in the American

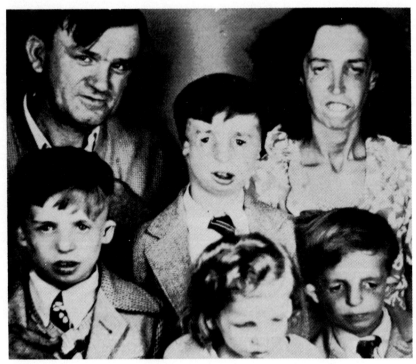

Figure 63–3. Photograph demonstrating the hereditary transmission of mandibulofacial dysostosis in a family in which a mother, her three sons, and one daughter are afflicted with the deformity. (From Straith, C. L., and Lewis, J. R.: Associated congenital defects of the ears, eyelids and malar bones (Treacher Collins syndrome). Plast. Reconstr. Surg., 4:204, 1949. Copyright 1949, The Williams & Wilkins Company, Baltimore.)

literature was by Straith and Lewis (1949), who described a family of five with an affected mother, three sons, and a daughter (Fig. 63–3). Over the years, further information has been added to the spectrum of anomalies making up this syndrome (O'Connor and Conway, 1950; Snyder, 1956; Axellson and associates, 1963; Rogers, 1964a,b; Roberts, Pruzansky, and Aduss, 1975; Rogers, 1976). In 1977 Behrents, McNamara, and Avery reported the microanatomy of a 15-week fetus and described for the first time the mandibular ossification anomalies.

CLINICAL FEATURES AND CLASSIFICATION

There is great variability in the degree of phenotypic expression of this genetic defect, a finding that has resulted in confusion concerning classification. To add to the confusion, other anomalies of the first and second branchial arch have been incorrectly described as variations of this syndrome (McKenzie, 1958; Walker, 1961). Franceschetti and Klein classified the syndrome into five categories dependent on the number of features present (Franceschetti and Klein, 1949). According to Tessier's classification of craniofacial clefts (see Chap. 59), the complete form of the syndrome shows the presence of clefts 6, 7, and 8 (Tessier, 1971). Behrents, McNamara, and Avery (1977) compiled an extensive list of the various physical and radiographic deformities. The obligatory features for diagnosis, as well as frequent and infrequent findings and the approximate embryologic stage at which these occur in the developing embryo, are listed in Tables 63–1 and 63–2 and illustrated in Figure 63–4. With this list of features, the diagnosis of MFD is simple to determine, whether the case be mild, moderate, or severe.

Other abnormalities have been reported in association with MFD. These may not be an integral part of the syndrome but probably reflect the incidence at large of these anomalies: vertebral anomalies (Stovin, Lyon, and Clemmens, 1960; Rubin, 1967); spinal dysplasia (Osebold and Winter, 1982); agenesis of the homolateral lung; frontalis muscle agenesis; club foot; synostosis of the joints; and mental retardation (Hurwitz, 1954). The external, middle, and inner ear deformities are well described in the literature (Sando, He-

Table 63–1. Diagnostic Features of Mandibulofacial Dysostosis

Clinical Features	Frequency	Approximate Age of Development
Cranium		
Flat parieto-occipital bone	Infrequent	8 wks
Midface		
Antimongoloid palpebral fissures	Obligatory	6–8 wks
Colobomas of lower eyelid	Obligatory	7–9 wks
Eyelash (or follicle) malformations	Obligatory	10 wks
Malar defects	Obligatory	7–8 wks
Atresia of lacrimal puncta	Frequent	6 wks
Macrostomia	Frequent	4 wks
Auricular defects	Frequent	5–6 wks
External auditory canal defects	Frequent	7 wks
Preauricular hair displacement	Obligatory	4 mos
High arched palate	Frequent	6–10 wks
Nasal deformity	Frequent	6–7 wks
Preauricular sinuses	Frequent	6–8 wks
Malocclusion	Frequent	After birth
Colobomas of iris and upper eyelid	Infrequent	7–9 wks
Absence of meibomian glands	Infrequent	10 wks
Hypertelorism	Infrequent	6–10 wks
Cleft palate	Infrequent	6–10 wks
Epiglottic underdevelopment	Infrequent	6 wks
Absence of parotid gland	Infrequent	6 wks
Mandible		
Mandibular defects	Obligatory	6 wks
Micrognathia	Obligatory	6 wks
Open bite	Frequent	After birth
Other Features		
"Fishlike" facial appearance	Obligatory	
Deafness (usually conductive)	Frequent	
Skeletal defects	Frequent	
Mental retardation	Infrequent	

menway, and Morgan, 1968; Hutchinson and associates, 1977; Farkas, 1978; Phelps, Poswillo, and Lloyd, 1981).

Sleep apnea and sudden infant death syndrome are of particular significance (Cogswell and Easton, 1974; Lapidot and Ben-Hur, 1975; Johnston and associates, 1981). In 1979 Shprintzen and associates, using flexible fiberoptic nasopharyngoscopy, studied the dimensions of the pharynx and nasopharynx in cases of MFD. They found these areas to be 50 per cent smaller compared with normals.

Table 63–2. Radiographic Features of Mandibulofacial Dysostosis

Diagnostic Features	Frequency	Approximate Age of Development
Cranium		
Hypopneumatization or small mastoids	Frequent	2 mos
Middle ear ossicular defects	Frequent	6–7 wks
Straight nasofrontal angle	Frequent	3 mos
Malformations of styloid process	Infrequent	8–9 wks
Sella turcica defects	Infrequent	After birth
Persistent frontal suture	Infrequent	After birth
Deficient zygomaticotemporal bones	Frequent	7–8 wks
Frontal sinus hypoplasia	Infrequent	4–5 mos
Acute cranial base angle	Infrequent	8–9 wks
Midface		
Deficient zygoma	Obligatory	7–8 wks
Hypoplastic maxilla	Frequent	6–7 wks
Hypoplastic maxillary sinus	Frequent	4–5 mos
Cleft palate	Frequent	6–10 wks
Deficient palatine bones	Infrequent	8 wks
Choanal atresia	Infrequent	6 wks
Inner ear abnormalities	Infrequent	6–7 wks
Mandible		
Hypoplastic mandible	Obligatory	6–7 wks
Short ramus	Frequent	6–7 wks
Short body	Frequent	6–7 wks
Obtuse gonial angle	Frequent	6–7 wks
Antigonial notch on ramus	Obligatory	6–7 wks

Bilateral choanal atresia has been described by Moorman-Voestermans and Vos (1983). In severely affected patients the airway is further compromised by the hypoplastic mandible and glossoptosis. Apart from the catastrophic event of sudden death from sleep apnea, changes in behavior and intelligence quotient have been documented (Cogswell and Easton, 1974). These functions have improved after management of the sleep apnea (Lapidot and Ben-Hur, 1975).

A unilateral form of MFD does not exist. Cases reported as such have usually been variations of unilateral craniofacial microsomia or first and second branchial arch syndromes. The only syndrome that MFD resembles in its facial aspects is Nager's acrofacial dysostosis (Nager and de Reynier, 1948), which is rare and inherited as an autosomal recessive trait (Stuart and Prescott, 1976; Meyerson and associates, 1977). These indi-viduals have the craniofacial features of MFD combined with preaxial reduction defects of the upper and sometimes lower limbs. In the upper limbs there is hypoplasia or agenesis of the thumbs and radius and/or one or more metacarpals. Radioulnar synostosis and elbow joint deformities may also occur. In Nager's acrofacial dysostosis, coloboma of the lower eyelid is less common but cleft palate is more frequent. The mandible tends to be severely hypoplastic in this syndrome (Fig. 63–5) (Bowen and Harley, 1974).

GENETIC CONSIDERATIONS

Evidence of this syndrome dates back to sculptures of pre-Columbian civilizations (600 to 1000 A.D.) (Fig. 63–6). In 1889 Berry was the first to suggest a hereditary factor. It is now thought that the syndrome is transmitted by an autosomal dominant gene with high but variable penetrance and expressivity (Poswillo, 1975). A positive family history is found in at least half of the reviewed cases (Vatré, 1971). This syndrome shows a high intrafamilial variability in phenotypic expression, i.e., between generations, but a low variability among affected siblings of the same generation (Rovin and associates, 1964). The gene appears to be transmitted primarily by the mother (Rovin and associates, 1964; Rogers, 1964a,b). There is some evidence to suggest that the gene may have a lethal or sublethal effect, which increases in severity with each successive generation (Debusmann, 1940; Franceschetti and Zwahlen, 1944; Roussel, 1951; Böök and Fraccaro, 1955; Farrar, 1967). A high incidence of miscarriages in families with a history of MFD is common. Half of the reported cases are patients who have no family history and are thought to have fresh mutations or deformities due to exogenous factors (Balestrazzi and associates, 1953; Szlazak, 1953; Campbell, 1954; McKenzie and Craig, 1955; Cohen, 1973; Poswillo, 1975). Increased paternal age has been implicated as a factor (Jones and associates, 1975). MFD has been reported in all major racial groups (Fig. 63–7) (Leopold, Mahoney, and Price, 1945; Chou, 1960; Kibel, 1960; Fujino, Hiraoka, and Kyoshoin, 1961; Jones and associates, 1975; El-Antably and El-Hoshny, 1976; Sokar and associates, 1980).

No structural genetic defect has been identified in this syndrome; this finding precludes

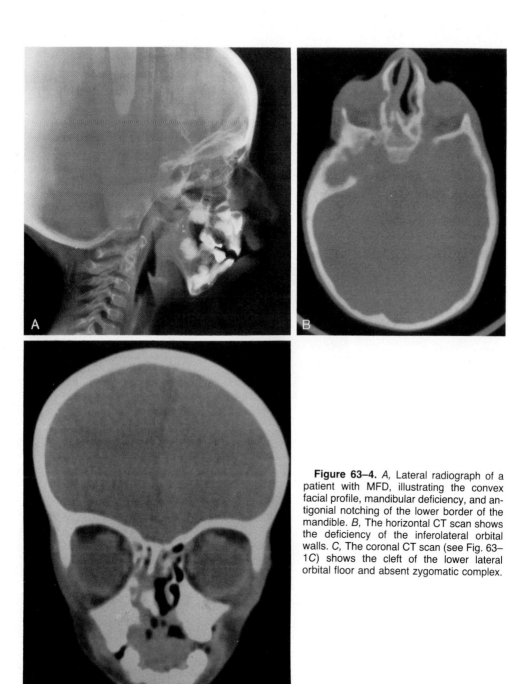

Figure 63–4. *A,* Lateral radiograph of a patient with MFD, illustrating the convex facial profile, mandibular deficiency, and antigonial notching of the lower border of the mandible. *B,* The horizontal CT scan shows the deficiency of the inferolateral orbital walls. *C,* The coronal CT scan (see Fig. 63–1C) shows the cleft of the lower lateral orbital floor and absent zygomatic complex.

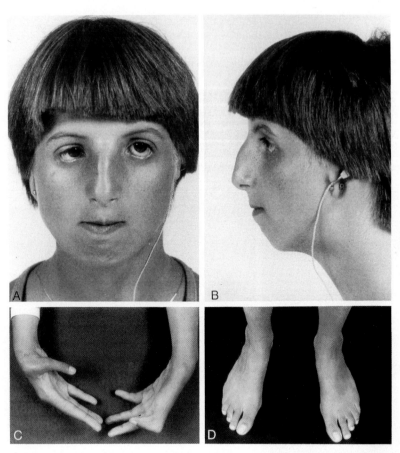

Figure 63–5. Nager's acrofacial dysostosis. The facial features resemble those of MFD, but these individuals also have hand and foot anomalies. In this case, there are four-digit hands and arachnodactyly of the toes. *A,* Frontal view. *B,* Lateral view. *C,* Hands. *D,* Feet.

Figure 63–6. Pre-Columbian terra cotta carving (seventh century) of a typical facies found in MFD. (From Poswillo, D.: The Pathogenesis of the Treacher Collins syndrome (mandibulofacial dysostosis). Br. J. Oral Surg., *13*:1, 1975.)

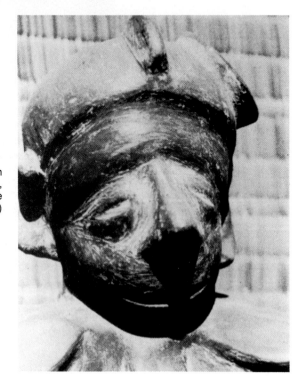

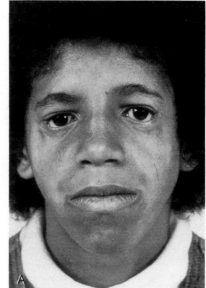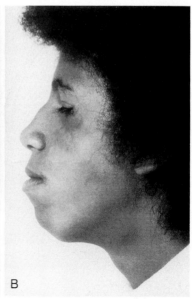

Figure 63–7. Mandibulofacial dysostosis occurring in a black person. Antimongoloid slanting of the palpebral apertures, zygomatic hypoplasia, and mandibular deficiency. *A*, Frontal view. *B*, Lateral view.

chromosomal or biochemical screening for a carrier state. Although variable penetrance and phenotypic expression make genetic counseling difficult, consultation is nonetheless important. In a high risk group of women, Nicolaides reported the use of intrauterine fetoscopy for prenatal diagnosis of this syndrome (Nicolaides and associates, 1984).

PATHOGENESIS

Normal development in the orofacial region depends on the amount of mesoderm in the first and second branchial arches and on the extent and direction of migration (Behrents, McNamara, and Avery, 1977). Much has been written about the specific embryonic area and the time of onset of the defect that results in MFD. Theories include failure of differentiation of the branchial arch mesoderm, defective facial bone ossificiation, and tissue ischemia resulting from stapedial artery hypoplasia (Mann and Kilner, 1943; Briggs, 1952; McKenzie and Craig, 1955; McKenzie, 1958). Rogers (1977) suggested that the variability in the extent of the deformities with this condition is due to the influence of a "strong" or "weak" gene acting at an earlier or later period of the embryo's development. Behrents, McNamara, and Avery (1977) pointed out that all major aspects of MFD are fully expressed by the 15th week of embryonic development.

Current research suggests that the abnormality may occur early as developmental defects of the neural crest cells. The branchial arches are derived from the radial end of the neural crest (Horstadius, 1950; Hövels, 1953). The neural plate begins as a flat, thick bank of ectoderm on the dorsal aspect of the embryo soon after gastrulation. The edges fuse to form a neural tube beneath the ectoderm. Free cells arise from the edge of the plate, forming two projections called the neural crest. These cells migrate into the deeper layers of the embryo (Johnston and Listgarten, 1972), splitting around the optic cup to enter the visceral arches proximally and thereby augment the branchial arch mesoderm. Many of the craniofacial cartilaginous, osseous, dental, and soft tissues are derived from the neural crest ectomesenchyme (Fig. 63–8). Disagreement exists as to whether the neural crest cells are pluripotential or possess fixed predetermined properties that allow them to be independent of local environmental influences (see also Chapters 46 and 48).

Using vitamin A, Poswillo (1975) successfully produced an animal model with the major phenotypic features of MFD. He was able to show that these abnormalities arose when preoptic neural crest cells were damaged, thus producing bilaterally symmetric defects as a result of the central structure being affected. The different degrees of the disorder are explained on the basis of the quantitative and qualitative defects of the

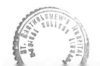

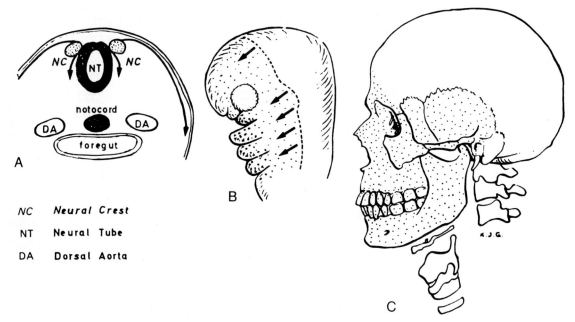

Figure 63–8. *A,* Early development of the neural crest. Arrows indicate the paths of migration of the neural crest cells. *B, C,* The patterns of migration of neural crest cells (broad stippling) derived from a combination of neural crest mesenchyme and lateral plate mesoderm. (From Poswillo, D.: The pathogenesis of the Treacher Collins syndrome (mandibulofacial dysostosis). Br. J. Oral Surg., *13*:1, 1975.)

neural crest cells, and on the degree to which the interacting mesoderm in the arches compensates for this neural crest cell deficiency (Poswillo, 1975).

Pathogenic research concepts have progressed from the gross anatomic to the cellular level; further progress will no doubt be made from research at the chromosomal and subcellular levels.

TREATMENT

Snyder (1956) described MFD as it affects individuals:

Defects and developmental abnormalities of every organ in the human body have been observed and recorded, but none with more pity than those of the face. This exposed area receives the attention of all, and often precipitates psychiatric differences in the child patient and may lead to psychosociologic problems for the parents.

The unusual appearance of the affected individuals, compounded by the physical handicaps of conductive deafness and expressive speech problems, has caused others to regard them as mentally subnormal. The management of craniofacial disorders is more than surgical; the interests of patients are best served with evaluation and management by members of a multispecialty craniofacial team (Munro, 1973, 1975).

From the time of birth, especially in the severely affected individual, the airway must be evaluated and secured. Either positioning alone or tracheotomy in order to prevent sleep apnea or sudden infant death syndrome may be required (Brouillette, Fernback, and Hunt, 1982; Schafer, 1982). To promote normal language development, evaluations by an otolaryngologist, audiologist, and speech pathologist are indicated. Treatment may include a conductive hearing aid to enhance audio stimulation. The parents need counseling on care and feeding procedures by skilled nursing staff. In the case of a child, the assistance of a psychologist, psychiatrist, and medical social worker may be required to help the parents deal with the associated medical and emotional problems.

The spectrum and degree of the deformities related to MFD are extensive. A plan of management needs to be tailored to the patients' specific deformities and timed to take into account their normal facial growth and psychosocial needs. With this disorder, the timing of treatment is important. As a general rule, the bony reconstruction should precede the soft tissue corrections. Modern craniofacial approaches such as bicoronal and intraoral incisions should be used to minimize facial scarring. Autogenous tissues such as split-thickness calvarial grafts, ribs, and costal cartilage should be used. Synthetic materials should be avoided. Anesthetic considerations for these patients are critical, and special techniques are needed for airway management, both during and after surgery (Davies and Munro, 1975; Sklar and Benton, 1976; MacLennan and Robertson, 1981, Roa and Moss, 1984).

Maxillary and Orbital Deficiencies

In the complete form of the syndrome, the bony deficiencies include (1) an oval shape of the orbit with a downward and lateral inclination, (2) a supraorbital ridge sloping downward from medial to lateral, (3) a deficient inferolateral orbital floor (as in the Tessier no. 8 cleft), (4) a rudimentary zygoma often present only as a small spine of bone projecting forward from above the glenoid fossa (as in the Tessier no. 7 cleft), and (5) a laterally and anteriorly positioned maxilla that is flattened and deficient, both in height and width (Fig. 63–9). The soft tissues between the periorbita and the muscles of mastication may be fused across the infraorbital cleft, a finding that makes dissection in this area difficult (Dagys, 1977).

The required bony corrections include reconstruction of a zygomatic arch, zygoma, anterior maxilla, and infraorbital rim; bone grafting of the inferolateral orbital deficiency or cleft; and correction of the downward slope of the superior orbital rim.

Historical Perspective. Correction of the eyelid deformities should be delayed until the hypoplastic zygomaticomaxillary area has been reconstructed. This approach reduces the need for extensive eyelid reconstruction (Marino and Appiani, 1954).

Cartilage has been used to augment the lateral infraorbital depression and reconstruct the zygoma (Straith and Lewis, 1949; Dupertuis, 1950; O'Connor and Conway, 1950; McKenzie and Craig, 1955; Gillies and Millard, 1957). The use of dermal grafts from the infragluteal area placed via a temporal incision has also been described (Snyder, 1956). Longacre, de Stefano, and Holmstrand,

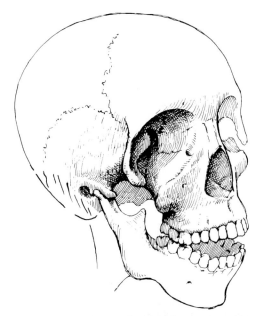

Figure 63–9. Craniofacial skeletal features of MFD with complete absence of the zygomas and zygomatic arch. Note the orbital defect, open bite deformity, and antigonial notching of the inferior border of the mandible.

(1961) reported autogenous split rib as onlay grafts applied to the zygomatic, temporal, orbital, and mandibular areas; their use has been extensively reaffirmed by others (Fig. 63–10) (Tessier, 1971, 1981; Converse and associates, 1974).

The skull as a source of bone graft has been used with increasing frequency in craniofacial surgery. In many respects the calvaria is an ideal donor area because (1) it is in the operative field and is easy to access, (2) it provides grafts of adequate size and contour, (3) it results in minimal postoperative morbidity and discomfort, and (4) the donor scar and site are camouflaged (Tessier, 1982; McCarthy and Zide, 1984). Calvarial bone may be used either full thickness or split thickness (using one of the tables for reconstruction) or as a vascularized bone flap pedicled on the temporalis muscle and fascia (Watson-Jones, 1933; McCarthy and Zide, 1984; van der Meulen and associates, 1984). Zins and Whitaker (1979) demonstrated that a greater volume of grafted membranous cranial bone survives than volume of endochondral rib bone. Edgerton, Jane, and Berry (1974) reported the advantages of correcting many craniofacial deformities in children before the age of 3 years; this philosophy is now routine in most centers. Small calvarial bone

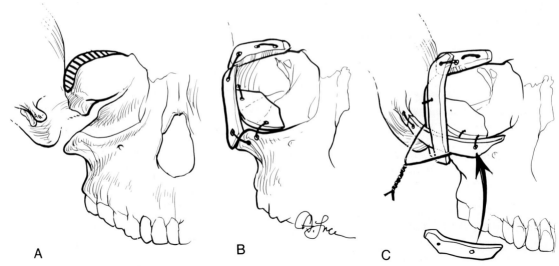

A   B   C

Figure 63–10. Tessier technique for the first stage of the orbital reconstruction. *A,* Hypoplasia of the zygoma. Note the orbital cleft. Bone has been removed in the region of the superolateral orbital rim. *B,* Bone grafts applied to the orbital floor, lateral wall, and inferolateral angle. The inferior orbital fissure is completely obturated. *C,* A second layer of bone graft applied to the infraorbital rim. (Redrawn from Tessier, P., Rougier, J., Hervouet, F., Woillez, M., Lekieffre, M., and Derome, P.: Plastic surgery of the orbit and eyelids. *In* Report of the French Society of Ophthalmology. New York, Masson, 1981, p. 169.)

donor sites may not need reconstruction in this age group because new bone reforms in the defect.

Authors' Preferred Method. The periorbital deformity can be divided into three groups: (1) in the mild deformity there is hypoplasia of the skeleton and soft tissues, (2) in the moderate form the skeletal and soft tissue hypoplasia is more severe, and (3) in the severe group there is absence of part of the zygomatic arch and clefting of the zygoma extending to the inferior orbital fissure. The degree of the antimongoloid slope of the palpebral fissure becomes more severe in relationship to the severity of the skeletal anomaly. The skeleton should be corrected before the age of 5 or 6 years. The more traditional method of Tessier is sufficient for the milder forms, but split cranial bone can be used instead of rib grafts (Tessier, 1981; Jackson and associates, 1982). Figure 63–10 illustrates the surgical technique described for the severe type of deformity with total zygomatic absence.

Through the coronal (scalp) approach an entire subperiosteal stripping of the orbital contents is performed, leaving only the medial area of the lacrimal sac and medial orbital wall and canthus attached. In the posterior direction the dissection reaches the lateral margin of the superior orbital fissure. It is important to separate the soft tissue contents passing through the inferior orbital fissure or cleft from their connection with the soft tissue of the temporal fossa. The lateral part of the superior orbital rim slopes downward (Fig. 63–10A). This bony segment must be raised upward, either by an osteotome or burr (Fig. 63–10B) or by performing an osteotomy and repositioning the segment upward and anteriorly. The lateral superior orbital wall, lateral orbital wall, zygoma, and zygomatic arch are constructed or augmented. The final maneuver is to lay bone grafts across the lateral orbital floor to prevent the orbital contents from displacing into the temporal fossa. This also raises the orbital floor to the horizontal level, thus rotating the orbital contents upward. Figure 63–10 shows the traditional method using split and full-thickness ribs. Rib grafts are easy to use and produce the correct curvature. However, there is a high rate of loss of bony volume (resorption) and most patients need the operation repeated two or three times before a satisfactory long-term result is achieved. Nowadays, it is better to use split-thickness cranial grafts, which, even though harder to obtain and more difficult to shape into the correct curvature, have the advantage of little resorption. Moreover, calvarial flaps (see Fig. 63–11) show minimal resorption tendency.

After the skeleton is adequately corrected (and there is tendency to undercorrect), the lateral canthus must be repositioned. Two drill holes are placed through the lateral margin of the superior orbital rim. A nonabsorbable suture is passed through one drill hole, through the lateral canthus close to the dermis, and then back through the other hole. The entire orbital contents must be transferred upward at the same time as the canthus, and an overcorrection must be created on the operating table as there is always an inferior drift in the postoperative period.

It is rare in this syndrome to have the two sides of the skeleton symmetrically deformed. The degree of soft tissue hypoplasia may also be unrelated to the severity of the skeletal hypoplasia. If the soft tissue coverage of the bone grafts is thin, every small irregularity of the bone grafts will be apparent; to overcome this, a large pericranial flap can be rotated downward to mask these irregularities and produce a softer contour.

In the severe form of MFD (see Figs. 63–1, 63–4, 63–9) there is a complete absence of the zygoma as well as the anterior part of the zygomatic process of the temporal bone. The absence of the zygoma is associated with a lack of lateral orbital wall as far posterior as the sphenoid. The zygomaticofrontal process does not project forward and hangs downward; the zygomatic buttress of the maxilla also does not project forward and is deficient, thus producing a steep downward and backward slope of the orbital floor. It is the deformity of downward sloping of the orbital roof and floor, and lack of lateral orbital wall to support the lateral canthus, which produces the antimongoloid slope to the palpebral fissure.

These severe cases can be treated by the technique shown in Figure 63–10, but large amounts of split-thickness rib or cranium are needed. Although the amount of cranial graft resorption is minimal compared with rib grafts, the long-term survival and growth potential remain uncertain.

From a theoretical point of view, vascularized cranial bone should be better than free grafts. The frontotemporal flap illustrated in Figure 63–11 not only has the advantage of transferring full-thickness vascularized skull, but also provides excellent soft tissue augmentation (McCarthy and Zide, 1984).

A coronal approach is used, but the scalp is elevated in a subfollicular plane lateral to the temporoparietal fascia as inferior as the laterosuperior aspect of the orbital rim. A subperiosteal dissection of the orbit and bone defects is carried out, as in the mild and moderate forms. The defect of the lateral orbital wall, inferior orbital rim, and zygomatic arch forms the shape of a T and its size is measured. This T forms one edge of a square or rectangle that can be marked on the periosteum of the skull anterior to the coronal suture (Fig. 63–11A). The long arm of the T must be lined up with the maximal curvature of the skull at the superior temporal line (Fig. 63–11B). The periosteum is elevated to the margins of the square, as is the periosteum beneath the temporalis inferior to the square. The neurosurgeon can make bur holes and cut the superior, anterior, and posterior margins with a craniotome. The inferior border must be cut with a Gigli saw to avoid damage to the temporalis and periosteal attachment. The bone flap is elevated and the T is redrawn on the inner table. The two residual rectangles of bone have the periosteum stripped to the margins of the T and are removed with a saw (Fig. 63–11B). The laterosuperior orbital rim is also removed (Fig. 63–11B). The T is now rotated downward to form the lateral orbital wall, inferior orbital rim, and zygomatic arch (Fig. 63–11D). Additional split-thickness cranial graft is harvested to construct and elevate the orbital floor. The two residual rectangles of cranial bone are split and used to reconstruct the T defect in the skull (Fig. 63–11E). The superior orbital rim is reattached superiorly and medial to the T (Fig. 63–11F). The lateral canthus is rotated upward and attached to the reconstructed orbital rim.

The timing for this operation is from the age of 2 years and older. By this age the skull is usually thick enough to split to reconstruct the defect resulting from the removal of the T-shaped segment. Any small defects that remain are more likely to reossify than in an older patient. The skull grafts also have a greater degree of malleability than in older people. The technique is, however, too new to make it possible to determine whether there is an advantage or disadvantage related to growth. Figure 63–12 shows an early result of this technique (see also Fig. 63–1C,D).

Eyelid Deformities

Eyelid deformities vary from an antimongoloid obliquity of the palpebral fissure to

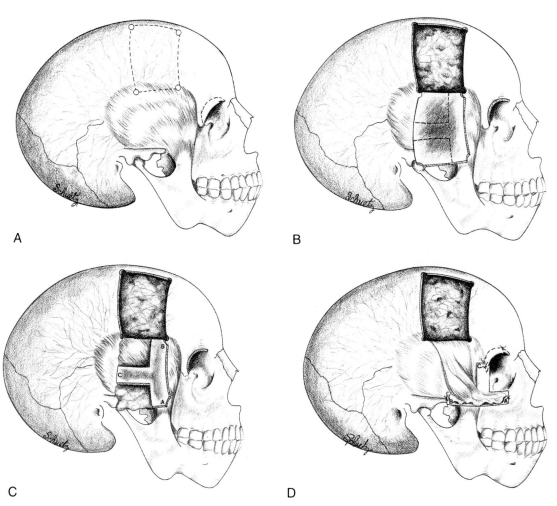

A

B

C

D

Figure 63–11. Calvarial bone flap. *A,* The frontotemporal full-thickness bone flap is raised bilaterally in conjunction with the neurosurgical team. Care is taken to keep the temporalis muscle and pericranium attached to the bone plate. The supraorbital bony rims are removed for superior relocation. *B, C,* The T-shaped bone plate is outlined on the inner cortex of the skull. The redundant squares of bone are removed and split to reconstruct the donor site. *D,* The T-shaped bone is wired into position: point A fixed to the infraorbital rim, B to the zygomatic remnant, and C to the lateral orbital rim.

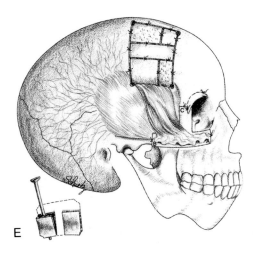

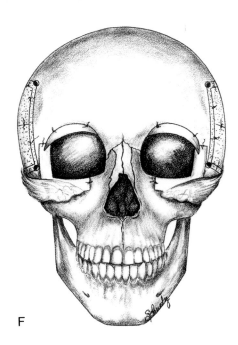

E

Figure 63–11 *Continued E, F,* The donor site is reconstructed with split-thickness calvarial grafts from the bone plate (*see inset*). The supraorbital rims are repositioned superiorly, further correcting the orbital obliquity.

F

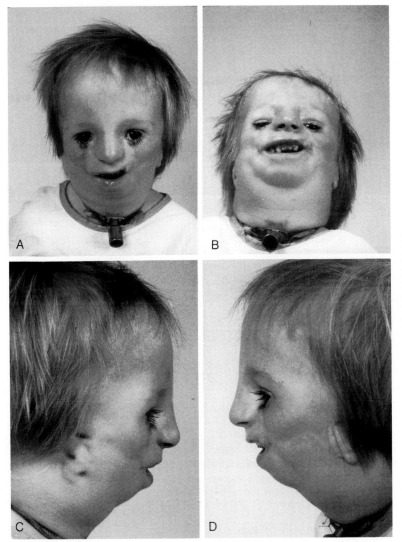

A

B

C

D

Figure 63–12. Child six months postoperatively after the surgical procedure that involved transposing skull bone to the periorbital area, maintaining the temporalis muscle and periosteal attachments, as described in Figure 63–11. See Figure 63–1C and D for preoperative views. A, Frontal view. B, Basilar view. C, D, Profile views.

extensive colobomas lacking skin, tarsal plate, orbicularis oculi muscle, and conjunctiva (Stenström and Sundmark, 1966). In severe cases, colobomas of the upper eyelid may be present, and absence of the lateral canthus has been reported (Bachelor and Kaplan, 1981). These deformities are aggravated by the underlying abnormally shaped orbit; however, the cornea is rarely in danger of exposure damage. The choice of technique to deal with the deformity depends on the extent of the deficiency. Eyelid deformities are the most challenging aspects of this syndrome to correct, as shown by the less than satisfactory results of corrective surgical techniques. The techniques of eyelid reconstruction are discussed in Chapter 34.

Historical Perspective. In 1943 Kilner and Johnstone (Johnstone, 1943) as well as Franceschetti and Klein (1949) reported the transposition of a skin flap from the upper to the lower eyelid that had limited success (McKenzie and Craig, 1955). Previous techniques, in combination or alone, have been used and include full-thickness skin grafts, intermarginal adhesions, the Wheeler operation, the Kuhnt-Szymanowski procedure, Z-plasties, and lateral tarsorrhaphies. A temporalis fascial sling to support the lower lid, combined with a bipedicled flap from the

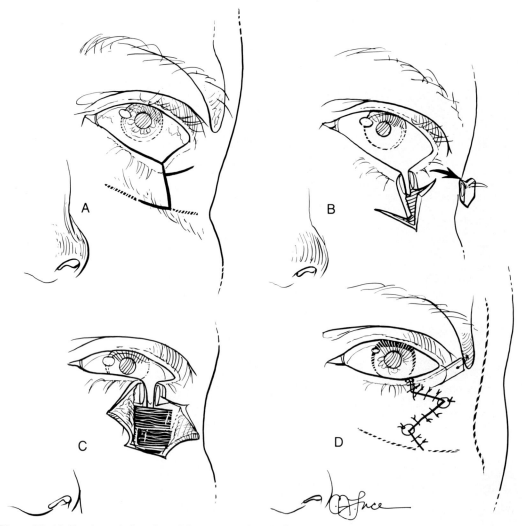

Figure 63–13. Tessier technique for coloboma correction. *A,* Coloboma of the lower eyelid extending into a groove on the cheek. *B,* Marginal excision. Incision for a Z-plasty for cutaneous lengthening. *C,* Overlapping suture of the preseptal orbicularis muscle. *D,* Transposition and suture of the skin flaps with a lateral canthopexy. (Redrawn from Tessier, P., Rougier, J., Hervouet, F., Woillez, M., Lekieffre, M., and Derome, P.: Plastic surgery of the orbit and eyelids. *In* Report of the French Society of Ophthalmology. New York, Masson, 1981, p. 170.)

upper lid, has also been described (Stenström and Sundmark, 1966).

On the basis of their experience with full-thickness reconstruction of lower lid defects, Converse and Smith (1967) advocated the use of a tarsoconjunctival flap followed later by a skin muscle flap transposed from the upper to the lower lid. Jackson and associates (1982) used a full-thickness skin, tarsoconjunctival flap to reconstruct the lower lid deficiency, in combination with a lateral canthopexy. For the more severe colobomas of the lower lid, Tessier's method may be necessary (Fig. 63–13) (Tessier, 1981).

However, all these techniques result in scars on the lower eyelid that are always noticeable and detract from the final correction. The most effective method to correct the antimongoloid slope of the palpebral fissure is reorientation of the orbital shape and its contents, together with a lateral canthopexy (Whitaker, Katowitz, and Jacobs, 1979). Patients with a coloboma in the lateral one-fourth of the lower eyelid (the usual position) can be treated by excision of the lateral eyelid and superior reattachment of the residual lid to the lateral canthus, which avoids any scar on the lower lid (Fig. 63–14).

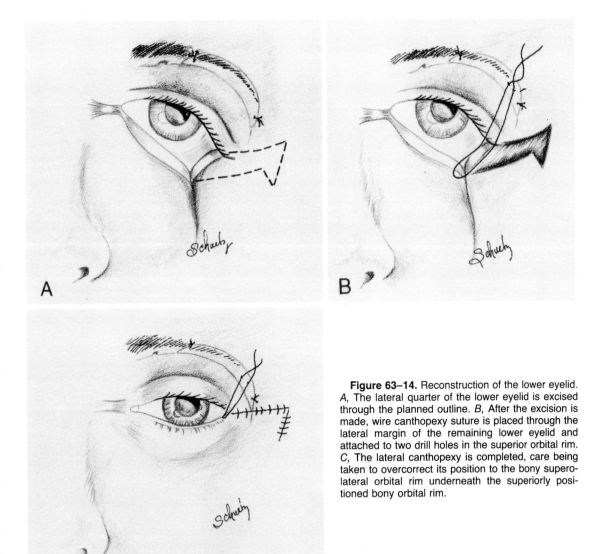

Figure 63–14. Reconstruction of the lower eyelid. *A,* The lateral quarter of the lower eyelid is excised through the planned outline. *B,* After the excision is made, wire canthopexy suture is placed through the lateral margin of the remaining lower eyelid and attached to two drill holes in the superior orbital rim. *C,* The lateral canthopexy is completed, care being taken to overcorrect its position to the bony superolateral orbital rim underneath the superiorly positioned bony orbital rim.

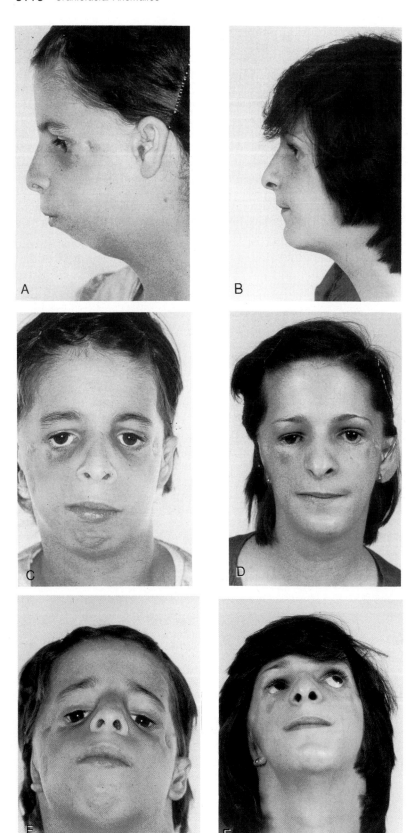

Figure 63–15. *A, C, E,* Preoperative views of a 15 year old girl with MFD. *B, D, F,* Postoperative views after several operations, including bilateral sagittal split osteotomies of the mandible, an advancement genioplasty, and upper and lower dentoalveolar setback osteotomies. Serial split-thickness rib grafts were applied to the orbits in addition to correction of the colobomas.

Mandibular Hypoplasia

Micrognathia and microgenia are consistent features of MFD. The result is a marked lower face retrusion and increased facial convexity on profile. On radiographic study the mandible has a peculiar broad curvature and antigonial concavity (see Fig. 63–4A), considered a diagnostic feature by some (Pruzansky, 1968, 1969). Decreased growth at the condyles results in decreased height and length of the mandibular body. The gonial angle is obtuse, and the condylar heads and coronoid processes are often malformed and deficient (McKenzie and Craig, 1955; Tessier, 1971; Dahl, Kreiborg, and Bjoark, 1975; Behrents, McNamara, and Avery, 1977). In older patients a Class II malocclusion and open bite are common (see Fig. 63–4A). Definitive orthognathic surgery is usually delayed until mandibular growth is complete. This delay is an often frustrating aspect in the overall management of this syndrome, especially when the mandibular micrognathia is contributing to airway compromise. Mandibular reconstruction is discussed in Chapter 29.

Historical Perspective. In 1948 Sanveneroi-Rosselli used onlay bone grafts and fat transplants for mandibular contouring. Cartilage, rib grafts, and iliac bone onlays have been used (Straith and Lewis, 1949; Serson Neto, 1957; Ploner, 1958; Longacre, de Stefano, and Holmstrand, 1961), as well as an osteoperiosteal flap to augment the chin.

Authors' Preferred Method. Before lower facial growth is complete, chin projection can be augmented by costal cartilage or split-thickness cranial graft through a lower buccal sulcus incision. In older patients a variety of methods may be necessary, depending on the degree of deformity. The mandible can be advanced with bilateral sagittal ramus osteotomies (see Chap. 29) and additional chin projection obtained with an advancement and, if necessary, vertical reduction genioplasty. There is often an open bite deformity in association with proclined maxillary and mandibular incisors. These patients can be improved by a combined simultaneous procedure of anterior maxillary setback, anterior mandibular setback, bilateral sagittal ramisection of the mandible, and advancement genioplasty (Fig. 63–15).

If the anterior open bite is severe and cannot be closed by segmental osteotomies, there are two alternatives. The simpler method is to use a Le Fort I osteotomy to lower the posterior maxilla and combine this with bilateral mandibular sagittal split osteotomies and a genioplasty. Anterior maxillary and mandibular segmental osteotomies may be necessary to close the open bite. On occasion the latter can be achieved by extraction of bicuspids and the use of orthodontic therapy.

Many patients with this syndrome have a prominent high-bridged nose and a prominent lower midface. The profile can be improved by a rhinoplasty and anterior maxillary setback

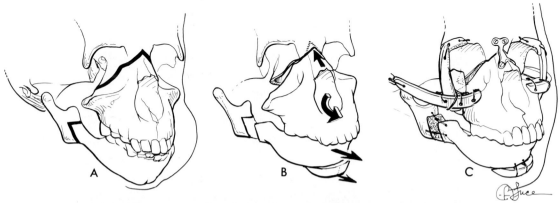

Figure 63–16. Tessier "l'integrale" procedure. *A,* Outline of the midfacial and mandibular osteotomies. Bone grafts are taken from the calvaria to stabilize the fragments and reconstruct the lateral parts of the face. *B,* The midface is sectioned, rotated anteriorly, impacted superiorly and posteriorly, and maintained in position by cranial bone grafts reconstructing the zygomatic arches and zygomas. *C,* Final position of the facial segments. An acrylic splint maintains the advanced mandible in an overcorrected position. The operation is performed under tracheostomy. A genioplasty is performed in a second stage. (Redrawn from Tessier, P., and Tulasne, J.-F.: Cranial surgery update. *In* Habal, M. B. (Ed.): Advances in Plastic and Reconstructive Surgery. Vol. 2. Chicago, Year Book Medical Publishers, 1986, p. 30.)

to close the open bite (Wiflingseder, 1957). Tessier and Tulasne (1986) developed a type of Le Fort II osteotomy that intrudes into the nasofrontal angle and lowers the maxillary tuberosity (Fig. 63–16). This procedure must be combined with a mandibular osteotomy, either of the V type with bone graft as shown by Tessier and Tulasne (1986) or by bilateral sagittal mandibular ramisections. A genioplasty may also be needed.

Auricular Deformities

The auricles may vary from normal to various degrees of structural dysgenesis to agenesis associated with an absent external auditory meatus (Rogers, 1964a,b). Reconstruction of an esthetically acceptable ear is one of the most difficult problems for the plastic surgeon. The techniques for auricular reconstruction are discussed in Chapter 40.

Additional Problems

Many patients have long, anteriorly placed sideburns. These can be transposed backward

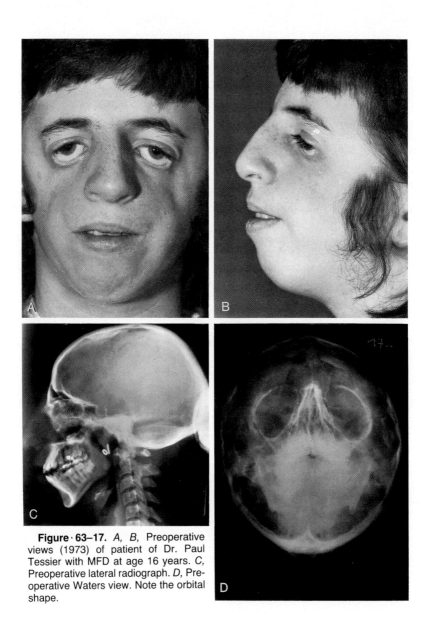

Figure · 63–17. *A, B,* Preoperative views (1973) of patient of Dr. Paul Tessier with MFD at age 16 years. *C,* Preoperative lateral radiograph. *D,* Preoperative Waters view. Note the orbital shape.

Figure 63–17 *Continued E, F,* Postoperative views. *G, H,* Postoperative radiographs five years after the following sequence of seven operations: June, 1973: Orbital reconstruction with iliac and costal bone grafts and genioplasty. December, 1973: Iliac and costal bone grafts to the orbital floors and zygomas. July, 1974: Genioplasty; reduction rhinoplasty; transposition of full-thickness skin flaps from the upper to the lower eyelids; and transposition of the sideburns. June, 1975: Costal bone grafts applied to the superior and inferior orbital rims, the anterior and lateral aspect of the mandible, and the zygoma, combined with septal resection and scar revision. February, 1976: Frontoparietal calvarial bone grafts to the inferior orbital rims and maxilla, combined with reduction of the macrostomia and scar revision. July, 1977: Costal cartilage graft to the right inferior orbital rim, left zygoma, nasal root, and chin, and revision of the lower eyelid colobomas. October, 1978: Scar revision.

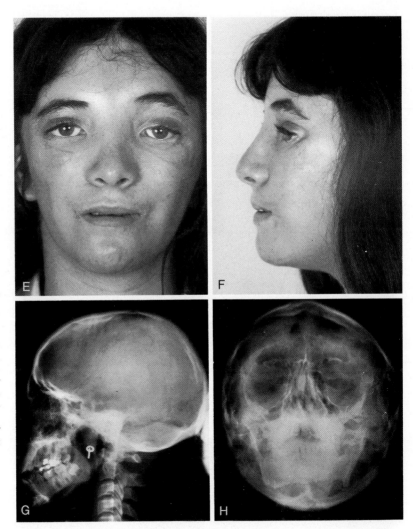

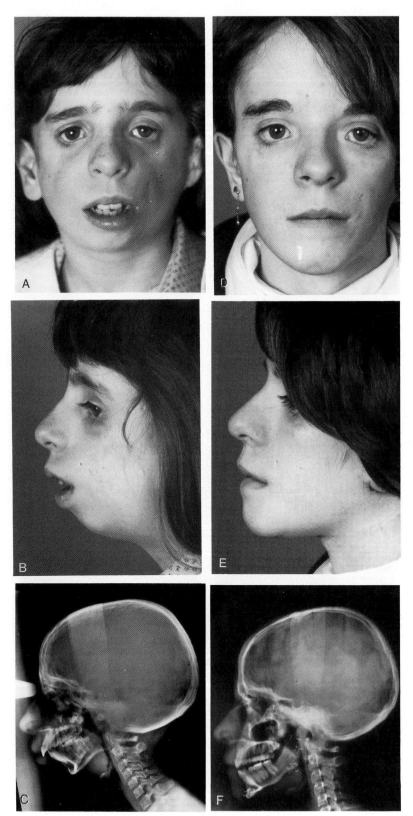

Figure 63–18. Patient of Dr. Paul Tessier with MFD at age 12 years (1981). Preoperative views (*A,* frontal; *B,* profile; *C,* lateral radiograph). Postoperative views (*D,* frontal; *E,* profile; *F,* lateral radiograph) five years later after the following sequence of operations. April, 1982: Modified Le Fort II (see Fig. 63–16) with frontonasal impaction and anterior rotation of the midface; inverted L mandibular ramus osteotomy with anterior mandibular advancement and rotation; reconstruction of the orbits, zygomas, and mandible ramus with calvarial bone grafts; lateral canthopexies; and Z-plasty of the suprahyoid skin. Tracheostomy completed the operation, and intermaxillary fixation was applied for two months. June, 1983: Bone grafts applied to the orbital floors and zygomas; lateral canthopexies; genioplasty; and extraction of four bicuspid teeth. November, 1984: Bone grafts from calvaria and ilium to the inferolateral orbital angles, lateral orbital walls, and zygomas; lateral canthopexy; and repeat genioplasty.

with a flap in male patients or excised in females, but a significant scar remains after both procedures. There is no cosmetically acceptable procedure to replace the absent eyelashes of the lower lid.

The management of MFD is extremely difficult. Many problems have to be corrected, and the older techniques result in a multiplicity of repeat operations owing to bone graft resorption. The use of split-thickness calvarial grafts may diminish resorption, and vascularized calvarial bone flaps may be beneficial for growth. The patients ideally should begin treatment when they are young enough to permit maximal early social acceptance. Even in the best hands, multiple operations are needed to achieve the optimal result. Figures 63–17 and 63–18 illustrate superb clinical results by Tessier from both older and newer techniques. However, the newer techniques still necessitate several operations to augment the periorbital areas.

THE ROBIN SEQUENCE: MICROGNATHIA AND GLOSSOPTOSIS WITH AIRWAY OBSTRUCTION

Peter Randall

When micrognathia (small jaw) and glossoptosis (falling backward of the tongue) occur in the newborn, there is a great danger of upper airway obstruction. These deformities are frequently associated with a cleft of the palate, and the entity is known as the Robin sequence. Robin was far from the first to recognize the anatomic arrangement that bears his name, but he does deserve credit for calling attention to the clinical significance of the problem. He pointed out that in severe cases death was inevitable. In spite of Robin's publications, it has taken many years for this knowledge to become widespread and for an effective method of treatment to be developed (Fig. 63–19) (Robin, 1923a, 1927b, 1928, 1934).

For years this disorder was known as the Pierre Robin syndrome. Gorlin, Pindborg, and Cohen (1976) noted that the condition is not a genetic "syndrome" and preferred the term "Pierre Robin anomalad," an anomalad being described as "a malformation together with its subsequent derived structural changes." More recently the term "sequence" has been used, implying that one condition led to the next and then the next.

DEFINITION

Micrognathia is the term most frequently employed to describe the anomaly of the mandible, although other terms have appeared in the literature, such as hypoplasia of the mandible, mandibular hypotrophy, congenital mandibular atresia, brachygnathia, ateliosis of the mandible, and hypomicrognathia (Lenstrup, 1925; Eley and Farber, 1930; Robin, 1934; Callister, 1937; Weisengreen and Sorsky, 1940; Schwartz, 1940; Llewellyn and Biggs, 1943; Longmire and Sanford, 1949; Beers and Pruzansky, 1955; Benavent and Ramos-Oller, 1958; Oeconomopoulos, 1960).

Retrognathia is a more accurate and more inclusive term inasmuch as several conditions can lead to a posterior displacement of the chin without actually producing an abnormally small jaw. The retroposition of the chin is a finding common in many types of jaw deformities. By positioning the point of the chin posteriorly, the genioglossus muscles are preshortened and are limited in their ability to hold the base of the tongue forward. As a result, the tongue falls backward into the throat (glossoptosis) and produces a ball valve type of inspiratory obstruction. When retrognathia is associated with glossoptosis and respiratory obstruction, it fits Robin's original description.

Retrognathia can be subdivided into several types of anomalies, including those with a normal mandibular size at birth and a posterior displacement of the chin by external

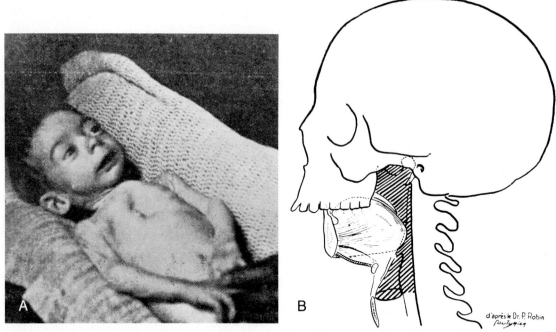

Figure 63–19. *A,* A typical child with the Robin sequence. Note the recessed chin, and the sternal retraction indicating inspiratory obstruction, malnourishment, and cachexia. The airway would be improved by placing the child in the prone position. *B,* Diagram illustrating the retrognathia and the foreshortened genioglossus muscle, allowing the tongue to fall backward (glossoptosis) and produce a ball-valve inspiratory obstruction. (From Robin, P.: La Glossoptose. Paris, Ash & Cie, 1929d.)

pressure. Such a mandible would have an excellent growth potential and is probably the type most frequently seen in the Robin sequence (Fig. 63–20). In addition, some mandibles are reduced in size and have a diminished growth pattern. In other cases, the reduced mandibular growth pattern is associated with diminished growth of the adjacent maxilla and facial bones, and also distortion of the cranial base and cervical spine. In all of these, retrognathia is seen, and in some micrognathia is also noted. However, Ross

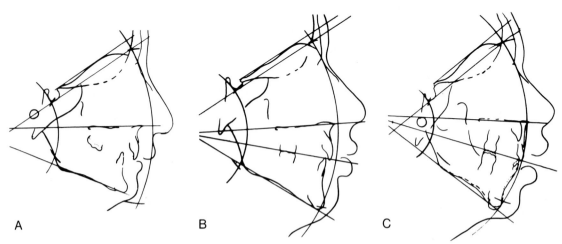

Figure 63–20. Cephalometric studies of three older children showing three different growth patterns (after the Sassouni system of analysis). All children had the Robin sequence at birth. *A,* Age 7 years, 1 month: persistent micrognathia resulting in a severe Class II malocclusion. *B,* Age 7 years, 9 months: underdevelopment of both mandible and maxilla with acceptable occlusion. *C,* Age 4 years, 1 month: satisfactory mandibular and maxillary growth and dental occlusion (Sassouni, 1960; Randall, Krogman and Jahina, 1964, 1965).

(1986) was of the opinion that virtually all the mandibles are small to a greater or lesser degree. Other mandibular problems can be superimposed, but Ross's careful in-depth studies indicated that micrognathia is always present.

HISTORICAL ASPECTS

In 1822 the deformity of micrognathia was reported by Saint-Hilaire, and in 1891 Taruffi subdivided the defect into two categories: hypomicrognathus (small jaw) and hypoagnathus (absence of jaw). In 1891 Lannelongue and Manard reported four patients, two of whom had cleft palates (Eley and Farber, 1930). In 1902 Shukowsky described a surgical adhesion of the tongue to the lip to correct the condition, but the usefulness of this operation was not widely appreciated (Shukowsky, 1911). A further description of this type of mandibular problem was published in 1922 by Gladstone and Wakely.

In 1923 a Parisian stomatologist named Pierre Robin published a paper calling attention to the problems associated with glossoptosis and obstruction of the airway (Robin, 1923a). He said that they were caused by hypoplasia of the mandible and that in 1902 he had first described a prosthetic appliance, which he called a "monobloc" and which he used to restore the relationship between the upper and lower jaws. Robin continued to write profusely on the problems of glossoptosis and "mandibular hypotrophy." He pointed out that glossoptosis in infants could cause episodes of cyanosis and predispose to any of a number of pulmonary complications in the newborn. He further stated: "I have never seen babies live for more than 16 to 18 months who presented hypoplasia such that the lower maxilla was pushed more than 1 cm behind the upper" (Robin, 1934).

He also described in detail the feeding problems of these children and their failure to gain weight, which often was serious and led to death from "athrepsia." Robin, however, became quite carried away by the problem of glossoptosis, its prevalence, and the dire effects that it produced. He thought that it was present in three out of five children and that, if not corrected, it predisposed to "protruding ears, kyphosis, scoliosis, lordosis, strabismus, adenoids, carious teeth, flat feet, harelip, rachitic rosary, cryptorchidism, . . .

appendicitis, constipation and enuresis" (Fig. 63–21) (Robin, 1929b; Schwartz, 1940; Randall, Krogman, and Jahina, 1965). Today, cleft palate is included as part of the Robin sequence, although it really need not be and, indeed, Robin described cleft palate in only one of his many cases.

In 1930 Eley and Farber described three cases and pointed out that "micrognathia" was an important cause of cyanosis during infancy and one which at that time was seldom included in the differential diagnosis of this condition. They treated their patients with a head apparatus designed to force the jaw forward. Since that time, many methods of treatment have been described, leading to the surgical procedures favored today. Perhaps the most significant of these developments was the contribution of Douglas (1946), who showed that many lives could be saved by suturing the tongue forward to the alveolus and lower lip. Through his personal cases and information obtained from an extensive poll of plastic surgeons, Douglas demonstrated an appreciable decrease in the death rate among these infants when the problem was recognized and surgical treatment instituted (Douglas, 1946, 1950, 1956).

Douglas reported having operated only on those patients in whom the condition was more severe. Using his tongue-to-lip and alveolus adhesion, he had one death in 31 patients: a premature infant who died several weeks after surgery and who did not have an airway obstruction at the time of death. The less severe cases were handled by the "conservative" nonsurgical approach, and in 21 patients there was a 65 per cent mortality rate.

ETIOLOGY

The exact cause of retrognathia is not known, and since several different anatomic conditions have been described as being associated with it, it seems likely that there is no single etiologic factor. The possibility that it is inherited has been proposed, and individual case histories have shown a familial tendency in some instances (Kiebel and Mall, 1910; LaPage, 1937; Fraser and Calnan, 1961).

Chapple (1955) pointed out that "the structures involved arise from different anlagen, from different layers at different times. A

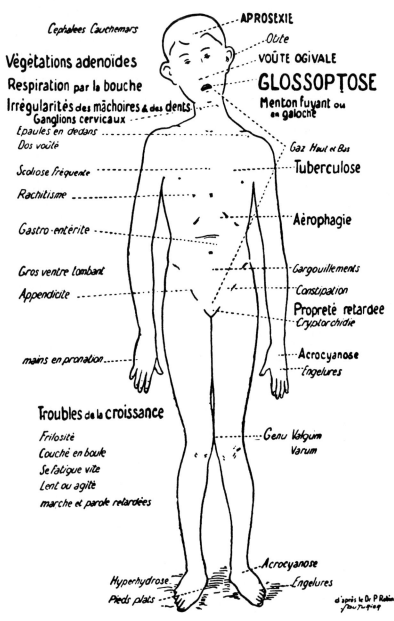

GRANDS SYNDROMES DE LA GLOSSOPTOSE

Céphalées Cauchemars

Végétations adenoïdes

Respiration par la bouche

Irrégularités des mâchoires & des dents
Ganglions cervicaux

Epaules en dedans

Dos voûté

Scoliose fréquente

Rachitisme

Gastro-entérite

Gros ventre tombant

Appendicite

mains en pronation

Troubles de la croissance

Frilosité
Couché en boule
Se fatigue vite
Lent ou agité
marche et parole retardées

APROSEXIE
Otite
VOÛTE OGIVALE

GLOSSOPTOSE

Menton fuyant ou
en galoche

Gaz Haut et Bas
Tuberculose

Aérophagie

Gargouillements
Constipation
Propreté retardée
Cryptorchidie

Acrocyanose
Engelures

Genu Valgum
Varum

Acrocyanose
Engelures

Hyperhydrose
Pieds plats

d'après le Dr P Robin
Boutinnier

Figure 63–21. Robin published this drawing and implied that with inadequate treatment all kinds of problems could be expected. (From Robin, P.: La Glossoptose. Paris, Ash & Cie, 1929d.)

gene covering this odd assortment has no parallel. The structures are in no other way related, to our knowledge, but by their mechanical relationship where the one can so readily affect the other."

There seems to be evidence that intrauterine pressure may well be the most frequent causative factor. The sharply flexed head seen in normal development of the human embryo places the chin up behind the manubrium.

The tongue is normally placed high in the mouth between the vertical palatal shelves. As the cephalic angle straightens and the head is lifted, the chin comes forward, the tongue drops down, and the palatal shelves move up to a horizontal position and fuse from front to back (see Chap. 48). Any delay in the straightening of the cephalic angle would postpone this chain of events and could produce the Robin sequence. Davis and Dunn

(1933) pointed out that the mandibular distortion was probably due more to forcing the angle of the mandible from an obtuse angle to a right angle than to an underdevelopment of the bone itself.

Parmalee (1931) described a number of deformities in infants that could be explained by an abnormal intrauterine position. Such a position can be determined shortly after birth by "folding up" the head and extremities until a "position of comfort" is found. In a baby born by breech delivery, the position of comfort is noted when the legs are sharply flexed at the hips, the knees are straight, and the ankles are placed up by the side of the head. This unusual fetal position for a breech baby is the position of comfort, while the usual fetal position is very uncomfortable for such babies.

Chapple (Chapple and Davidson, 1941; Chapple, 1955) related these data to the problem of retrognathia and found a parallel. He further pointed out that until 6 weeks of age the conformation of the embryo is nearly circular. The head then begins to rise from the cephalic flexion: "In the early life of the embryo, while his head is still on his chest, the tongue lies between the sides of the palatal arch. His head must be lifted from his chest to allow the tongue to fall down into the mouth so that the sides are free to unite into an arch. If it is not raised, the already intact tongue prevents their union, and the tongue grows into the nasopharynx." This would explain the high incidence of cleft palate (Eley and Farber, 1930; Chapple and Davidson, 1941; Chapple, 1950, 1955; Bigotti and d'Agostino, 1959). The flexed position of the head produces all the abnormalities seen in the Robin sequence, and if the head is maintained in this position past the usual time, these abnormalities are likely to persist to a greater or lesser degree and cleft palate is likely to occur.

Cleft palate is frequently seen with micrognathia, cleft lip very rarely, although the usual incidence would be the reverse (Kiskadden and Dietrich, 1953; Benavent and Ramos-Oller, 1958; Bromberg and associates, 1961). Kiebel and Mall (1910) considered the fourth and fifth months of pregnancy the critical period for the occurrence of the deformity. Davis and Dunn (1933), Llewellyn and Biggs (1943), and Sweet and Kemsley (1947) were of the opinion that the weight of the baby on the facial structures in utero should have some bearing on the development of the condition.

Because many of the patients eventually show remarkably good mandibular growth, it seems likely that external pressure on normal structures could indeed account for this sequence of events (Walker, 1961). In some patients the mandible remains hypoplastic, and it may be that in these patients an intrinsic factor causing a reduced mandibular size produces the deformity.

In summary, retrognathia with glossoptosis seems to be caused by one of several factors: (1) normal mandibular facial growth potential, but intrauterine inhibition of mandibular growth probably due to external pressure; (2) local failure of mandibular growth with normal facial bone development; or (3) mandibular failure associated with other craniofacial abnormalities causing a regional failure of growth (Krogman, 1962; Randall, Krogman, and Jahina, 1964).

Robin wrote as follows: "Mandibular hypotrophy is never idiopathic. As a rule it is caused by congenital syphilis or tuberculosis, by hereditary dystrophia from alcoholism or by some other infection. Occasionally, a mild case occurs in the child of parents, one of whom has large jaws and the other, narrow ones: the child has a narrow upper jaw and a broad lower one or vice versa, so that there is a lack of equilibrium between the two and functional troubles appear" (Robin, 1934).

DIAGNOSIS

The child with retrognathia has a characteristic birdlike facies with an undershot chin. When seen, this facial configuration should arouse immediate suspicion of the likelihood of partial or complete airway obstruction, feeding difficulties, and a possible cleft palate. There will be wide variations in the degree of retrognathia, the severity of the airway obstruction, the extent of the feeding difficulties, the age at which these problems arise, and the need for treatment.

Respiratory Obstruction. The difficulty in breathing is caused by the glossoptosis or the falling backward of the tongue into the pharynx causing an inspiratory ball valve type of obstruction. Typical mild to severe retraction of the intercostal spaces, the suprasternal space, and the epigastrium is seen, along with overactivity of the accessory respiratory muscles (Fig. 63–22). In addition, there is an obstructed sound to the baby's breathing, and there may be a history of choking and cyanotic attacks. These findings in the newborn should make one suspect a dangerous airway problem.

The deceptive aspect of the respiratory obstruction is that these children can frequently maintain an adequate airway if they struggle, strain, and cry. They may not even appear to suffer from airway obstruction and the diagnosis may be completely missed. However, whenever the infant relaxes or dozes or tries to sleep, obstruction occurs, he awakens, and he cries again. As a result, he can literally exhaust himself to death unless the obstruction is relieved. Delay in treatment can cause brain injury. The key observation should be to determine whether the infant can rest and sleep and still maintain an adequate airway. If he cannot, immediate treatment is indicated.

Feeding Problems. Because of the abnormal position of the mandible and the tongue, and also the presence of respiratory obstruction and a cleft palate, feeding becomes troublesome. These children are difficult to feed: they eat small amounts, regurgitate readily, and aspirate frequently. Failure to gain weight, malnutrition, exhaustion, and repeated respiratory tract infections may be the only findings, since respiratory obstruction may be obscure or its severity may not always be appreciated.

Other Types of Tongue Displacement. It is not unusual in severe cases associated with cleft palate to see the tongue displaced up into the nasopharynx through the cleft in the hard and soft palate. In this position it is likely to cause considerable airway obstruction and may even be difficult to dislodge. Routledge (1960) pointed out that, when the tongue is in the cleft, obstruction is greater and is likely to increase in severity. In the neonatal period the tongue grows rapidly, and in this abnormal position its disproportionate growth causes the obstruction to become more severe. Even though the infant has no symptoms at the time of birth, the obstruction may become quite severe by the age of 7 or 8 weeks.

The size and position of the tongue vary greatly. Many babies appear to have a microglossus (small tongue). Others, because of the relatively small jaw, are described as having a macroglossus (large tongue). In time, both the large and small tongues apparently approach normal size; the disproportion has not been reported with any regularity in older children. Tongue-tie has been described with micrognathia and even with airway obstruction (Fraser and Calnan, 1961; Bromberg and associates, 1961). When the tongue and the mandible are in the extreme retroposition, the floor of the mouth frequently bulges within the mandibular arches, and the tongue appears to be covering a tumor mass. This deformity usually disappears when the tongue is brought forward.

Other Causes of Respiratory Obstruction. Choanal atresia can also cause respiratory problems in the newborn and has been

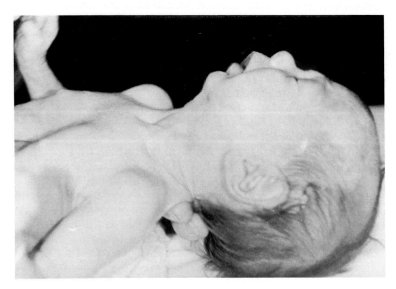

Figure 63–22. Micrognathia and glossoptosis causing severe upper airway obstruction and obvious retraction of the intercostal and suprasternal spaces. Although the infant could maintain an adequate airway with effort, there was obstruction as soon as he relaxed, even in the face-down position. An operation was necessary to relieve the obstruction and to prevent death from exhaustion.

described in association with micrognathia (Bromberg and associates, 1961). It should be looked for in all such patients, and can be ruled out by passing a small catheter through each nostril (see Chap. 37). Tracheoesophageal fistula is another cause of respiratory embarrassment in the newborn; if there is doubt, it should be ruled out by appropriate examinations.

Associated Congenital Defects. The Robin sequence has also been described with laryngomalacia and cervical spine anomalies. A number of other malformations have been reported in patients with micrognathia. In 26 cases of micrognathia, Smith and Stowe (1961) reported nine patients with cardiac murmurs, five of whom died of congenital heart disease; eight patients with anomalies of fingers and toes; three with major ear defects; two with microcephaly and mental retardation; one with hydrocephalus and mental retardation; and nine with major ocular anomalies. It was these authors' recommendation that all patients with micrognathia should have a thorough ophthalmologic examination before the age of 1 year, including ophthalmoscopy and tonometry under anesthesia, to uncover possible lesions that might be unsuspected, although treatable, and sufficiently severe to cause blindness if not treated. The author has not encountered such a high percentage of ophthalmic disease, but Opitz, France, and Herrmann (1972) called attention to the frequency with which Stickler's syndrome is associated with the Robin sequence. Stickler's syndrome, or "hereditary progressive arthro-ophthalmopathy," includes myopia in infancy, retinal detachment, preventable blindness, and cataracts in some cases. This is a mesenchymal dysplasia; it is an autosomal dominant mutation and should be looked for in these patients. Shah, Pruzansky, and Harris (1970) also reported cor pulmonale in a significant number of these patients.

Sadewitz, Goldberg, and Shprintzen (1986) presented several papers on the heterogeneity of the Robin sequence. In general, they described a number of conditions in which various types of airway obstruction are associated with micrognathia and usually palatal clefts with large defects. While it is important to recognize the different conditions producing airway obstruction and to treat them appropriately, one should not forget that the only book Robin published on the subject was simply titled *La Glossoptose* (1929d). Unless glossoptosis is an integral part of the airway obstruction, it does not seem correct to include the entity under the title of Robin sequence.

TREATMENT

The early treatment of retrognathia falls into several categories, depending on the severity of the respiratory difficulties and the feeding problems. No treatment is required if the airway obstruction and feeding difficulties are minimal. In more severe cases, if the baby is placed in the prone position, the tongue and jaw fall forward, and this may be sufficient to overcome a slight respiratory obstruction. As mentioned previously, the most important criterion in determining whether the airway is adequate is to observe whether or not the baby can breathe without obstruction while resting. If the child must struggle, cry, and stay awake in order to breathe, *he will die of exhaustion unless treated.*

If a change to the face-down position does not suffice, the child should be intubated with a nasopharyngeal or an orotracheal tube, or the tongue should be mechanically retracted. Neonatal endotracheal intubation is becoming more available in neonatal nurseries especially as anesthesiologists become more adept at infant intubation. However, two points must be kept in mind. First, these children have short jaws; thus, laryngeal exposure is very difficult. Second, at this point the infant is often exhausted. Awake intubation is advised because the airway will obstruct as soon as the child is anesthetized. Fortunately, the nasopharyngeal airway passed beyond the base of the tongue is a satisfactory temporizing method. Also, if the tongue can be retracted, this maneuver can provide a temporary airway.

A traction suture may be used as a temporary measure; a towel clip accomplishes the same objective and is somewhat easier to apply. In any case, a deep bite in the tongue should be taken well back from the tip. A large safety pin can be used in an emergency.

If a traction suture or towel clip is needed, the patient usually will require later surgery of a more permanent nature to hold the tongue forward, since a traction suture or towel clip causes swelling of the tongue and can be expected to tear through the tongue within a few days. More permanent alleviation of the problem can be achieved in several ways. The tongue can be sutured to the inner side of the lower lip, or a Kirschner wire can be placed through the angles of the mandible, transfixing the base of the tongue in a forward position. Several other methods of achieving the same purpose have been described, but these two techniques appear to be the most dependable. Occasionally, none of these steps is sufficient to ensure an adequate airway and a tracheostomy becomes necessary.

It is appropriate to describe the more important techniques in greater detail. The practice of maintaining the child in the face-down position has gained popularity. This can be done by taping a stockinette to the child's head in the form of a cap and suspending the head face down just clear of the mattress. It can also be accomplished by using a special mattress with a cut-out area for the face. This type of nonsurgical treatment requires vigilant nursing care and often prolonged hospitalization, but with the development of pediatric intensive care units, oxygen saturation, and cardiac monitors, this approach appears to be used more frequently than any other (Takagi, McCalla, and Bosma, 1966). The mortality rate has dropped significantly with satisfactory monitoring, but the monitor is not triggered unless there is a significant drop in oxygenation. However, one again wonders if the "conservative" nonsurgical approach is not subjecting the newborn to repeated episodes of significant cerebral anoxia.

An operation is almost inevitable in a patient with retrognathia, if there is a history of repeated cyanotic episodes or of repeated severe respiratory tract infections, if the mandibular arch is more than 1 cm posterior to the maxillary arch, or if the patient fails to gain weight (Robin, 1934; Benavent and Ramos-Oller, 1958; Routledge, 1960; Bromberg and associates, 1961; Parsons and Smith, 1982). Parsons and Smith (1982) proposed an excellent rule of thumb to help decide when to abandon conservative therapy and proceed with an operation. If after seven days of conservative management the child is still unable to control the airway and has not gained weight, surgery is indicated. If the child is still dependent on an endotracheal tube for an adequate airway after three days of intubation, surgery is indicated.

With the development of polysomnography to study the adequacy of an infant's airway, studies are beginning to evolve on the criteria for conservative (positional) or surgical management of patients with this problem. Pearlman and associates (1987) have presented preliminary data on six patients with the Robin sequence. In four, the transcutaneous O_2, as measured by a noninvasive technique, gave readings that averaged less than 60 mm Hg over an eight hour time frame (minimum) and transcutaneous CO_2 levels of over 50 mm Hg. In addition, these six infants were monitored for sleep apnea for a minimum of 45 minutes, and four had numerous apneic episodes regardless of body or head position. Oxygen saturation values measured by a pulse oximeter were as low as 60 per cent. Surgical tongue-lip adhesions were performed in four patients without further delay and an adequate airway was at once restored. The two infants with the Robin sequence, but without above findings, were treated conservatively by position alone; both improved. These criteria appear to provide a satisfactory objective method of testing airway stability in these patients.

Occasionally the operations designed to hold the tongue forward are not sufficient, and a tracheostomy must be performed. This procedure should not be taken lightly in a newborn child; it is a difficult operation at this age even under the best of conditions. After the tracheostomy tube is in place, there is always an appreciable amount of mucosal edema, and even a millimeter of edema in the tiny trachea of an infant reduces the size of the lumen significantly so that early decanulation is difficult. Care of the tracheostomy at home is important (Oeconomopoulos, 1960; Moyson, 1961; Stool, Campbell, and Johnson, 1968; Bluestone and Stool, 1983).

Many procedures have been suggested that pull or push the mandible forward, but in general they have proved ineffective, cumbersome, undependable, and at times dangerous (Callister, 1937; Longmire and Sanford, 1949; Routledge, 1960). Simple gadgets to be attached to the feeding bottles have been designed to make the child thrust his jaw forward. They may be partly effective, but cannot be relied on to treat respiratory obstruction (Davis and Dunn, 1933; Robin, 1929d). Robin was much concerned with the need for what he termed "orthostatic" feeding; this consisted of holding the baby in a nearly vertical position, particularly while nursing, so that he was forced to push his jaw forward (Robin, 1927b). Gavage may be needed as a temporary measure, particularly if there is a tendency to aspirate.

McEvitt (1968, 1973) reported successful results from passing a nasogastric tube. This tends to hold the tongue a little forward and also allows feeding by gavage, but more important it provides a small but significant airway on either side (laterally) of the tube. The author's experience with this technique is limited and includes several failures.

Burston (1966) favored prolonged hospitalization with a frame to hold the child in the face-down position. This method, as noted above, has achieved a measure of success, but several months' hospitalization are needed.

Robin (1929d) described a "monobloc" to obturate the cleft and to project the tongue and mandible forward. From time to time variations on this approach have been described. Fara (1974) found this technique sufficient in approximately two-thirds of his patients, and emphasized the advantages of preventing the tongue from becoming displaced into the cleft where it obturates the airway. Some authors advocate closure of the palatal cleft as a definitive procedure. This keeps the tongue from being displaced up into the cleft, but does not address the retrognathia and glossoptosis.

Routledge (1960) pointed out that in the Douglas procedure, the undersurface of the tongue, the central portion of the floor of the mouth, the alveolar ridge, the buccal sulcus, and the labial mucosa are denuded to allow the adherence of the tongue and its maintenance in a forward position. The degree of fixation is small, the alveolar mucosa and the submaxillary duct openings are jeopardized, and it is difficult to obtain a satisfactory adhesion. Routledge (1960) proposed a different method of tongue-lip fixation, which has been further modified by the author.

Modified Routledge Procedure. General anesthesia with an endotracheal tube (Rae tube) is preferred if the services of an expert anesthesiologist are available. As pointed out, tracheal intubation in a baby with retrognathia is an extremely difficult procedure and is preferably done with the infant awake, since complete obstruction may occur as soon as relaxation is produced by anesthesia. If tracheal intubation is not successful, anesthesia can be maintained by insufflation with a nasopharyngeal tube *plus* careful use of a tongue suture to maintain an adequate airway. Tracheal intubation over a flexible bronchoscope, or even a tracheostomy, may be needed.

The basis of the procedure is a *horizontal* attachment of the free border of the tongue to the mucosa of the lower lip. When the normal tongue is placed forward against the lower lip, contact is established between the free edge of the tongue and a broad expanse of the lower lip (Fig. 63–23). The two surfaces are incised, after injecting the area with small amounts of lidocaine (1 per cent) and epinephrine (1:100,000) for hemostasis. The inferior edges of the incised mucosa are approximated with a running 5–0 chromic catgut suture everting the mucosal edges.

A deep tension suture of 0 or 00 silk or synthetic material (such as Mersilene) is next placed below the chin pad, brought up anteriorly to the mandibular symphysis, and brought out through the lip incision. A suture carrier or Reverdin needle is used to place this suture through the tongue incision and posteriorly through the substance of the tongue as far as possible. The suture is threaded through a medium-sized button, and is brought back through the tongue and lip and through another button beneath the chin (Fig. 63–23C). A retrieving suture is also placed through the tongue button, brought out through the mouth, and taped loosely to the cheek. The tension suture is the key to holding the tongue forward.

Two or more sutures of 3–0 chromic catgut approximate the muscles of the tongue and lip, on either side of the tension suture, and the superior mucosal edges are approximated with a continuous 5–0 chromic suture everting the edges. Placing the chin button below the chin pad minimizes scarring without losing its effectiveness. The tension suture is left in place for 10 to 14 days and the lip adhesion is maintained for 10 to 18 months. Lower incisor teeth eruption can occur without disruption. When a tongue-tie is present, it usually must be relieved before the tongue can be brought forward adequately. Gavage is used for feeding for the first week postoperatively to minimize tongue movement (Randall and Hamilton, 1971). The modified Routledge operation achieves a secure tongue-to-lip adhesion in a normal position without jeopardizing the alveolar mucosa or the sublingual or submaxillary ducts. The tongue-to-lip adhesion can be maintained for

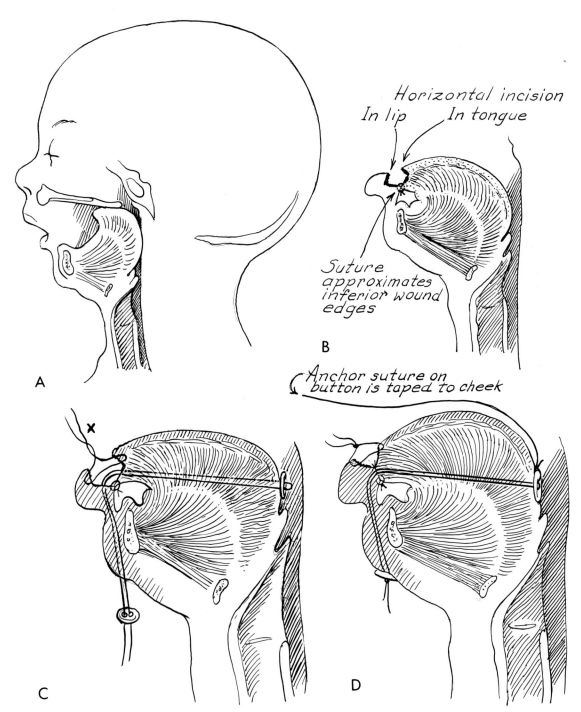

Figure 63–23. Randall modification of the Routledge (1960) tongue to lip adhesion. *A,* An infant with micrognathia, glossoptosis, and upper airway obstruction. With the mentum in retroposition, the genioglossus muscle is unable to hold the tongue forward. When a cleft palate is also present, the tip of the tongue may be displaced into the nasopharynx. *B,* Broad horizontal incisions are made in the tip of the tongue and the labial mucosa, and a suture approximates the inferior wound margins. *C,* A heavy tension suture connects a button beneath the chin to one on the posterior surface of the tongue by way of the lip and tongue incisions. A retrieving suture is tied to the tongue button and brought out through the mouth. A suture (x) is placed on either side of the tension suture to approximate the muscle layer of the lip and tongue. *D,* The superior wound margins are approximated.

a prolonged period with minimal complications even up to the time of eruption of the lower teeth. It can be taken down at three to six or even 18 months and is usually done at the time of the cleft palate repair. If early cleft palate repair (at 3 to 6 months of age) is advocated (the author does not think it appropriate in patients with the Robin sequence), the tongue-to-lip adhesion should be maintained.

Another technique was described by Lewis, Lynch, and Blocker (1968), who used fascia lata as a deep suture passed through the base of the tongue. It was placed through an external incision and used to hold the base of the tongue forward to the symphysis.

Argamasso (1986) was concerned with dehiscence of the Routledge tongue-lip adhesion (which has occurred only rarely in the author's experience) and developed an operation more similar to the Douglas operation, securing the tongue to the mandibular symphysis. However, this could interfere with lower incisor tooth eruption.

To transfix the tongue accurately with a Kirschner wire, Schatten and Tidmore (1966) used insufflation anesthesia administered through a nasopharyngeal tube. A tongue suture is placed. The insufflation tube is withdrawn into the nasopharynx, and the airway is controlled by the tongue suture. The Kirschner wire is inserted through the skin and the mandible superior and anterior to the angle, but care is exercised to avoid the inferior alveolar nerve. The tongue is retracted from the mouth to a position just beyond the point at which it causes obstruction to the airway. The Kirschner wire is placed through the tongue and into the mandible on the opposite side. The tongue suture can then be relaxed to ascertain whether a satisfactory airway can be maintained. If the tongue is pulled too far anteriorly by this technique, swallowing becomes difficult or impossible. The end of the Kirschner wire is left protruding from the skin and protected by adhesive tape, or is cut just short enough to be buried by the skin. It should be long enough to permit a small incision to be made later to allow its withdrawal. Scarring in the cheek can be a disappointing sequela.

Wang and Macomber (1963) described a variation of the Douglas procedure. They raised flaps of mucosa, one from the undersurface of the tongue and the other from the buccal surface of the lip. The flaps were interdigitated, thereby giving a broader surface of contact than is achieved by the Douglas procedure, and at the same time avoiding opening the submaxillary ducts and the need to remove alveolar mucosa.

GROWTH AND DEVELOPMENT

Robin (1926c, 1934) believed that the respiratory insufficiency caused by glossoptosis would lead (1) to physical backwardness and mental retardation and (2) to a child easily angered, difficult to control, and unable to concentrate, with headache, nightmares, and other disturbances persisting into adult life. These complications probably occur only in patients with brain damage.

The growth potential of the micrognathic jaw of the patient with the Robin sequence is inconsistent. A number of authors were of the opinion that the mandible would reach normal proportions in all cases, but a definitely diminished growth potential was demonstrated in some, if not most, patients (see Fig. 63–20) (Randall, Krogman, and Jahina, 1964). Ross (1986), in a careful clinical study, reported that all the mandibles in the patient with the Robin sequence are on the small side.

The cleft palate, when present, almost always involves only the soft palate or the soft palate and the posterior portion of the hard palate. It can be closed in the usual manner. Patients should not be considered for early soft palate repair unless, following the reasoning of Malek, Psaume, and Genton (1985), one is using the soft palate repair to hold the tongue forward. In addition to the obvious cleft, there usually appears to be a severe amount of shortening of the anteroposterior dimension of the palate.

Orthodontic therapy, Silastic chin implants, and repositioning of the mandible by osteotomy may, after the eruption of the permanent dentition, have a place in the late correction of retrognathia and micrognathia (see Chap. 29).

COMPLICATIONS

Possible complications fall into two categories. Some are caused by the respiratory obstruction when it is not treated adequately;

others are the result of the suggested methods of treatment.

In severe cases of the Robin sequence, death from respiratory obstruction can occur immediately if the situation is not recognized and the problem corrected. More likely the respiratory obstruction is partial and can be overcome by the child when he cries and strains. As noted earlier, if the child's airway becomes obstructed when he relaxes, it will be necessary for him to strain in order to breathe, and under these conditions he can literally exhaust himself to death. The downhill course can be quite insidious and the termination abrupt. With lesser degrees of obstruction, the complications can include aspiration with repeated episodes of pulmonary infection and poor eating, and failure to gain weight. The respiratory obstruction is often intermittent and leads to episodes of cyanosis. Procrastination in alleviating this situation can lead to accumulating increments of cerebral anoxia, resulting in permanent brain damage. With today's neonatal intensive care units and monitoring systems, it is easy to respond to multiple episodes of hypoxia. It must be acknowledged that repetition of these events cannot help but produce increasing small increments of brain damage. If conservative steps such as head positioning cannot put a complete stop to these episodes, it is probably safer to carry out an early surgical procedure.

The innumerable possible complications alluded to by Robin (1929,d) were noted earlier under Historical Aspects but seem to be unlikely. It is surprising in recent experience that the problem of respiratory obstruction does not always improve as the child grows. During the first three months of life improvement is usually seen, but the situation can also become steadily worse. This is most often noted in the child in whom airway obstruction is not the most serious problem, but in whom poor nutrition and respiratory infection are the salient features. Occasionally a child is seen in whom a disproportionate growth of the tongue in relationship to the adjacent bony structures occurs, with more growth in the former than in the latter. Under these conditions the degree of respiratory obstruction can gradually worsen.

The face-down position can lead to chronic skin breakdown if not monitored carefully. The suspensory head cap has also been a problem in that occasionally it can constrict the bones of the calvarium and cause overlapping of the edges.

Complications of the surgical techniques have been reported. It should be restated that, if just a traction suture is used in the tongue for more than a day or two, it is likely to cut through the tongue. Should this occur, it is probably best to maintain the airway either with the infant in the head-down position or with the Kirschner wire transfixion technique for the base of the tongue. It is better to let the tissue heal and to perform a secondary repair of the tongue a year or two later.

If the tongue-to-lip adhesion breaks down, it is unlikely that a second surgical attempt in this area will succeed, since the wounds become infected quickly. As a result, one of the other methods of treatment noted above should be employed.

In the Kirschner wire technique through the angles of the mandible, skin breakdown over the wire is a frequent complication and can lead to appreciable scarring in the skin of the cheek. To avoid this, the ends of the wires can be left buried, but it is important to keep the baby from lying on the side of the cheek, a position that could possibly produce pressure over the end of the pin.

It bears repeating that sudden death following exhaustion is a frequent complication of inadequate treatment of the Robin sequence. In addition, repeated episodes of partial airway obstruction with cyanosis unrelieved by conservative (nonoperative) techniques can lead to permanent brain damage (Hoffman, Kahn, and Seitchick, 1965; Randall and Hamilton, 1971; Parsons and Smith, 1982).

PROGRESSIVE HEMIFACIAL ATROPHY: ROMBERG'S DISEASE

Gregory L. Ruff

Although Romberg's eponym prevails by virtue of his detailed report (1846), Parry (1825) was the first to describe the condition afflicting a 28 year old woman who, after the adolescent onset of a mild left hemiplegia, noticed that "the left side of the face began to grow more thin than the right and the eye to become less prominent." Sharply demarcated in the midline, her hair changed from brown to white on the left and this was accompanied by ipsilateral lingual atrophy. In 1871 Eulenburg emphasized the acquired nature of the disease and coined the phrase "progressive facial hemiatrophy."

CLINICAL ASPECTS

Genetic review supports the contention that the disease is not congenital because the vast majority of cases are sporadic; familial cases exhibit no clear mode of transmission but are frequently occasioned by consanguinity (Lewkonia and Lowry, 1983).

The incidence of the condition is unclear. In 1964 Rogers reviewed the 1035 reported cases; of the 772 sufficiently complete to fulfill the diagnostic criteria, he found that women were affected 1.5 times more than men.

Atrophy typically begins before the age of 20 years, affecting the subcutaneous tissue and skin with later involvement of the muscles and osteocartilaginous framework. The immature or developing craniofacial skeleton suffers greater deformity, with delayed dental eruption and atrophic tooth roots (Moss, 1956; Bramley and Forbes, 1960; Crikelair, Moss, and Khuri, 1962). Ipsilateral salivary gland involution may occur.

Unilateral in 95 per cent of the patients with no predilection for either side (Rogers, 1964) the disease may be heralded by pigmentary changes of the hair, skin, or iris. When present, atrophy may originate from the cutaneous stigmata and may become so sharply delimited by the midline that the resultant deformity is called "scleroderma en coup de sabre" (Fig. 63–24). Advanced disease can spread to the contralateral face, skull, neck, or upper extremity.

Other associated abnormalities may share the etiology of the atrophy or simply reflect the natural occurrence of these conditions in a population of approximately 1000 reported cases. Sporadic congenital ear anomalies (Charazinska and Nehrebecka, 1973); ipsilateral renal, adrenal, and ovarian hypoplasia (Steiff, 1933); and ipsilateral amastia (Martin, 1925) may represent the latter category, while ipsilateral ophthalmopathy, noted in more than 10 per cent of patients with Romberg's disease, may represent the former (Rees, 1976). Coloboma of the lids (Smith and Guberina, 1977) and uvea (Streiff, Rosselet, and Jequier, 1955), heterochromia iridis (Ful-

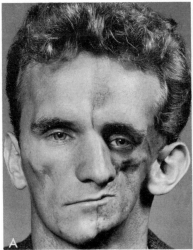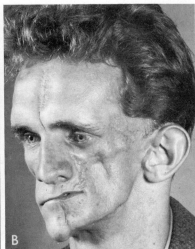

Figure 63–24. *A, B,* Severe left-sided hemifacial atrophy including the left half of the tongue. Note the indentation of the forehead ("coup de sabre").

mek, 1974), or heterochromic cyclitis (Sugar and Banks, 1964), choroidal sclerosis (Moura, 1963), and most commonly, enophthalmos (Muchnick, Aston, and Rees, 1979) were concomitant findings. Contralateral involvement was rare (Johnson and Kennedy, 1969).

Although the disease is reputed to "burn out" after two to ten years, some cases persist for considerably longer periods.

PATHOPHYSIOLOGY

Typified histologically by epidermal keratosis with thinning of the stratum granulosum and rete papillae, and by atrophy of the adnexal elements, Romberg's disease has been distinguished from the chronic inflammation of scleroderma by the selective preservation of elastin in the former (Pešková and Stockar, 1961). Chronic inflammation and scarring characterize the fatty tissue (Pešková and Stockar, 1961).

Muscular function is impaired by tethering to the overlying leathery skin and atrophy of both Type I and Type II fibers (Schwartz and associates, 1981), the latter variously attributed to primary and secondary causes. Masticatory spasm electromyographically consistent with nerve injury was documented in the masseter muscle (Kaufman, 1980); however, no primary muscle or nerve disease was detected by electromyographic study of the extraocular muscles (Le Hunsec and La Porte, 1965). An unusual case in which bone was afflicted much more extensively than soft tissue revealed "degeneration of bone . . . with granulation cells and osteoclasts" (Goldhammer and associates, 1981).

Although the pathologic progression of the disease is descriptively uniform, its etiology is a subject for speculation. Prevailing evidence supports Romberg's original (1846) contention that the cause was a vasomotor trophoneuritis.

Cervical sympathectomy provides the only relevant animal model. Moss and Crikelair (1959) found decreased adipose tissue without bony, muscular, or vascular changes in the 1 month old rat observed for two to four months (Moss and Crikelair, 1959) after sympathectomy. Although sympathetic section in humans fails to induce these changes, the persistent involvement of the adrenergic nervous system, with an associated incidence of neu-

rologic findings in 15.5 per cent of patients (Gorlin and Pindborg, 1964), is too compelling to ignore. Horner's syndrome was found in 22 per cent of the 100 patients reviewed by Franceschetti and Koenig (1952), although Lindemann (1940) noted mydriasis more frequently than miosis. Pupillary dilatation implies sympathetic stimulation, a condition initially proposed by Archambault and Fromm (1932) to result from ablation of the "mixed cervical sympathetic chain." Adjacent trauma, as with thyroidectomy and neck injury, has also been cited. Raynaud's syndrome (Asher and Berg, 1982) and hemiplegic migraine, probably attributed to jacksonian epilepsy (Sagild and Alving, 1985), lend further credence to this hypothesis.

Alternative theories invoke infection, especially measles, and trigeminal neuralgia as inciting causes. While the former could involve the sympathetic nervous system, the latter fails to account for the paucity of hemifacial atrophy after trigeminal neuralgia or section of the sensory root, and the lack of conformity of the area of atrophy with the nerve distribution (Kiskadden and McGregor, 1946).

The evidence thus summarily involves the sympathetic nervous system as a common etiologic pathway in hemifacial atrophy. Although ablation fails to replicate the disease consistently in humans, sympathetic stimulation induces vasoconstriction and lipolysis, findings consistently observed in subcutaneous atrophy.

DIFFERENTIAL DIAGNOSIS

Lipodystrophy manifests only fatty atrophy, which is virtually always bilaterally distributed (Rees, 1976). When confined to the face, upper extremity, or trunk, it is called Barraquer-Simons disease. Generalized lipodystrophy occurs and involves somatic as well as omental and mesenteric fat.

Hemifacial atrophy appears to represent an anatomically defined subset of localized or linear scleroderma. The clinical and family histories are identical, as is the histopathology, except for sparing of elastin in Romberg's disease. Although both can exhibit antinuclear antibodies, Romberg's disease may lack definitive serology. The prognosis and treatment are similar.

TREATMENT

As with lipodystrophy, the site of involvement specifies the pathologic condition; unaffected fat atrophies if placed in the involved area, while tissue removed from that area hypertrophies if placed elsewhere. Thus, most authors recommend foregoing treatment until the disease "burns itself out." Therapy is directed at restoration of the anatomy and preservation of physiology.

Skeletal Reconstruction. Structural support must first be restored. Campbell (1956) promoted onlay grafting for skeletal augmentation with autogenous bone grafts, a technique that remains the standard of comparison. Tantalum mesh (Kiskadden and McGregor, 1946) and irradiated homologous costal cartilage (Schuller, Bardach, and Krause, 1977) provide possible alternatives. While the latter offers little or no resorption, there is the potential for mobility and extrusion. Proplast is readily incorporated by scar, but its use has not been reported for hemifacial atrophy.

Soft Tissue Reconstruction. Most patients require only soft tissue augmentation. Kazanjian and Sturgis (1940) noted less resorption of fascial or dermis grafts than of fat alone (Fig. 63–25). The significance of this problem is underscored by the necessity of regrafting severely involved patients 10 to 15 times (Pešková and Stockar, 1961). Subcutaneous injection with fat obtained by liposuction has been advocated, with a recommended

overcorrection of 50 per cent (Chajchir and Benzaquen, 1986). The period of follow-up was brief, but acute histologic study revealed cystosteatonecrosis and associated inflammation.

Synthetic materials resist resorption but risk extrusion. Woods (discussed in Achauer, Salibian, and Furnas, 1982) deemed the results of a limited clinical study of injectable silicone (Rees, Ashley, and Delgado, 1973) "exceptional" in view of a 5 per cent incidence of significant complications (Fig. 63–26). Despite serial doses of small volume and immediate massage of the injected area, progressive inflammation and extrusion of silicone discouraged the senior investigator (Rees, 1988). It was hoped that Mersilene mesh implanted into the abdominal fat and later placed into the facial defect would prevent reaction (McCollough and Weil, 1979). However, the two-stage procedure, the need to wire the graft to bone for support, and a 10 per cent infection rate are arguments against this technique.

Neumann (1953) hypothesized that vascularized tissue would maintain its volume. Utilizing an abdominal tube flap carried on the wrist, he noted the adherence of the deepithelized dermis to the skin, the disappearance of sebaceous glands, the diminished numbers of hair follicles, and the minimal inflammation. He subsequently needed to reduce the bulk in all transferred flaps (Figs. 63–27, 63–28).

Employing these tenets, many surgeons

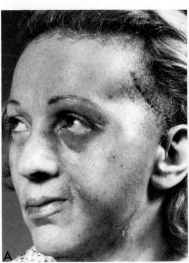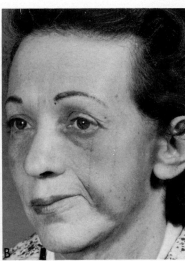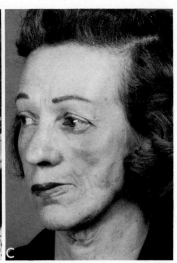

Figure 63–25. *A,* Patient with hemifacial atrophy two weeks after insertion of a large dermis-fat graft. *B,* One year after insertion of the graft. *C,* Two years after insertion of the graft with evidence of considerable resorption.

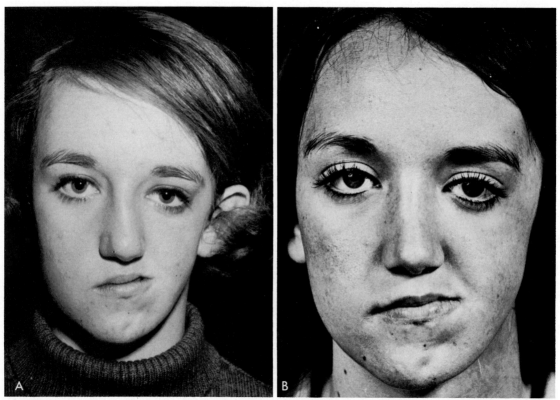

Figure 63–26. Severe Romberg's disease improved by injections totaling 20 ml of silicone fluid during a 12 month period. *A,* Pretreatment. *B,* Four years after the injection. Some soft tissue firmness persists in this patient. (From Rees, T. D., Ashley, F. L., and Delgado, J. F.: Silicone fluid injections for facial atrophy: a 10-year study. Plast. Reconstr. Surg., *52:*118, 1973. Copyright 1973, The Williams & Wilkins Company, Baltimore.)

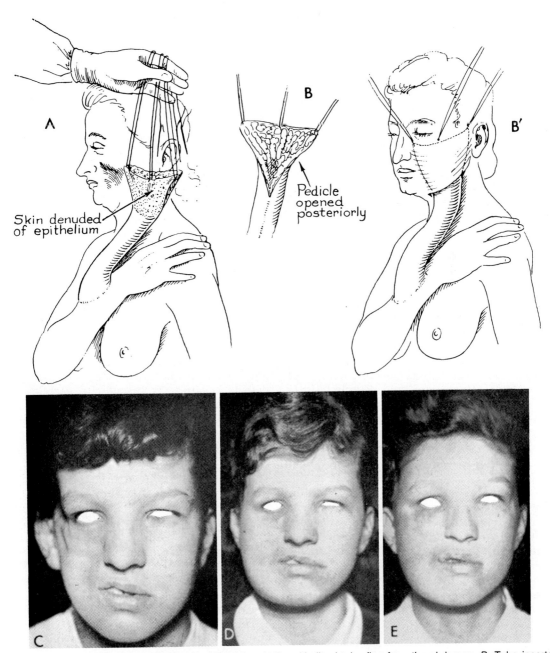

Figure 63–27. Tube flap to provide dermis and fat. *A,* Deepithelized tube flap from the abdomen. *B,* Tube inserted subcutaneously through a submandibular incision. At a later stage the flap is severed, and the submandibular incision is closed. *C,* Right hemifacial atrophy (preoperative), which appeared after slight trauma and radiation therapy. *D,* Postoperative view following subcutaneous insertion of a large abdominal tube flap and reduction in the bulk of the flap one year later *(E).* (From Neumann, C. G.: The use of large buried pedicled flaps of dermis and fat; clinical and pathological evaluation in the treatment of progressive facial hemiatrophy. Plast. Reconstr. Surg., *11*:315, 1953. Copyright 1953, The Williams & Wilkins Company, Baltimore.)

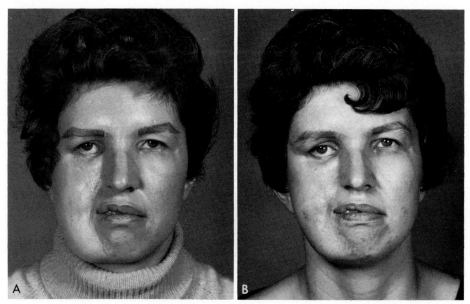

Figure 63–28. *A,* Appearance of the patient in Figure 63–27 19 years after the original surgery. She gained weight, as did the buried dermis-fat transplant. *B,* Appearance of the patient 20 years after the original surgery, following defatting of the transplant and a unilateral face-lifting procedure. (From Converse, J. M., and Betson, R. J., Jr.: A 20 year follow-up of a patient with hemifacial atrophy treated by a buried de-epithelized flap. Plast. Reconstr. Surg., *48:*278, 1971. Copyright 1971, The Williams & Wilkins Company, Baltimore.)

prefer free vascularized dermal-fat transplantation. Deltopectoral (Shintomi and associates, 1981; Harashina and Fujino, 1981), groin (Tweed, Manktelow, and Zuker, 1984) and scapular (Serra, Muirragui, and Tadjalli, 1985) microvascular free flaps have been used; often a skin island is retained to alleviate tension and monitor the circulation in anticipation of a secondary revision (Fig. 63–29). Modified rhytidoplasty and submandibular incisions expose the recipient superficial temporal and facial vessels, respectively. Shintomi and associates (1981) recommended placing the dermis deep in order to anchor the flap to the skeleton, while Tweed, Manktelow, and Zuker (1984) advocated the converse to provide a smooth contour. The authors noted excellent retention of volume, but patients frequently required a second stage for debulking and resuspension of "sagging" flaps as visualized in the upright position.

Wallace and associates (1979) first described the use of free vascularized omentum for hemifacial atrophy, a technique also employed by Jurkiewicz and Nahai (1985) in nine patients, currently the largest series

(Fig. 63–30). Despite the mandatory laparotomy, omentum is recommended for irregular defects because its vascularity permits segmentation of the flap to fill subcutaneous pockets, as designed by Upton and associates (1980). Presumably this same attribute "imparts a healthy glow to the overlying skin" even when omentum is used in patients after subcutaneous extrusion of injected silicone. The propensity of omentum to sag necessitates multiple procedures for suture fixation (Walkinshaw, Caffee, and Wolfe, 1983) or facial slings (Wells and Edgerton, 1979; Achauer, Salibian, and Furnas, 1982) to provide support. Walkinshaw, Caffee, and Wolfe (1983) contended that better facial animation is seen in patients reconstructed with omentum than in those given dermis-fat grafts.

The advantages of vascularized tissue even embrace small defects. Tongue flaps have satisfactorily augmented atrophic lips (Rees, Tabbal, and Aston, 1983), while the galea affords modest bulk when supplied by the posterior auricular and superficial temporal vessels (Avelar and Psillakis, 1981), or only the latter.

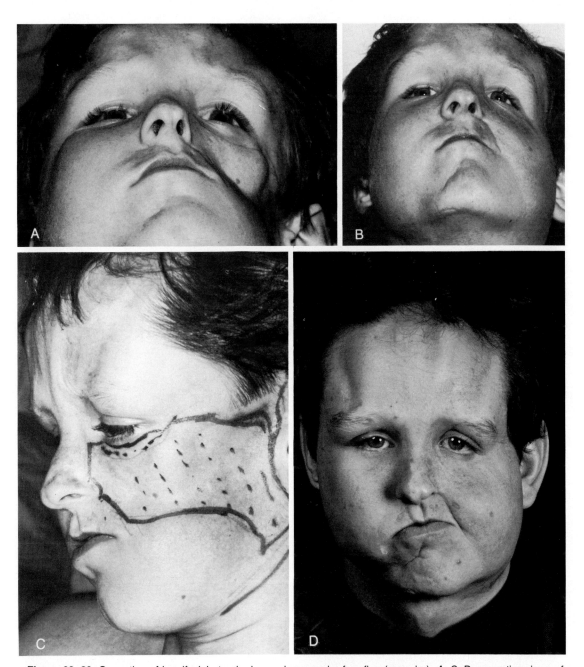

Figure 63–29. Correction of hemifacial atrophy by a microvascular free flap (scapular). *A, C,* Preoperative views of a 14 year old boy with left-sided facial atrophy. *B, D,* Appearance after insertion of a parascapular microvascular free flap in the cheek and jaw areas. (Courtesy of Dr. Barry Zide, Institute of Reconstructive Plastic Surgery, NYU Medical Center.)

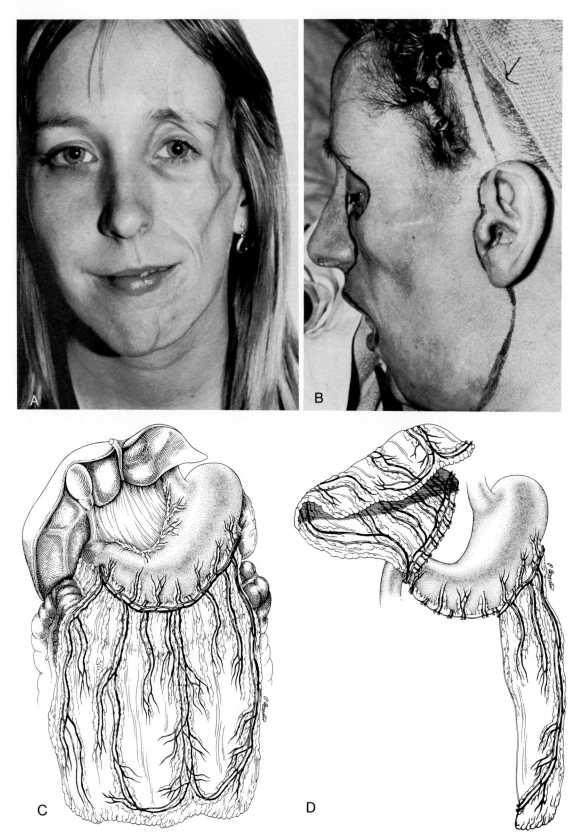

Figure 63–30. Omental flap. *A,* Young woman with hemifacial atrophy. *B,* Outline of the incision. *C, D,* Omental flap based on the right gastroepiploic vessels.

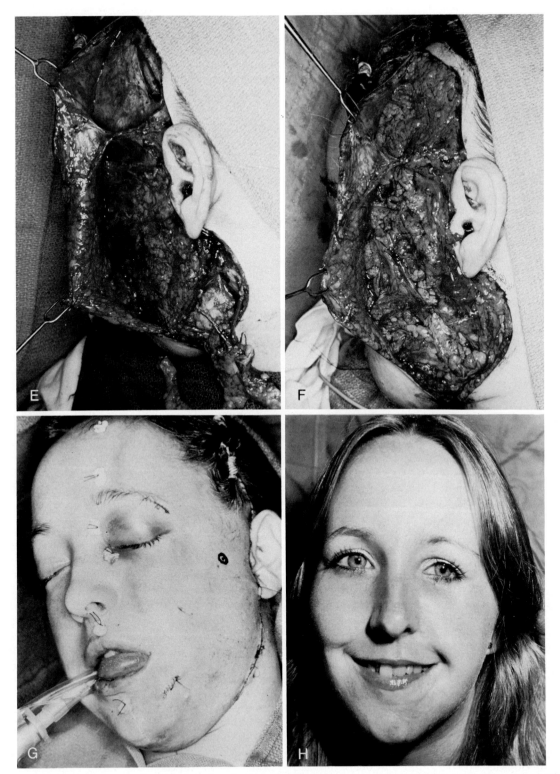

Figure 63–30 *Continued E,* Dissection of a cheek pocket. *F,* Flap in place with extensions to the temporal, cheek, jawline, and neck regions. *G,* The flap is maintained in position with sutures tied over pledgets. *H,* Final appearance. (Courtesy of Dr. Foad Nahai, Emory University.)

KLIPPEL-FEIL SYNDROME

Gregory L. Ruff

In 1912 Klippel and Feil described a French sailor with a low posterior hairline and short, immobile neck who, upon his death from renal disease, was found to have extensive fusion of the cervical vertebrae. Feil (1919) later reported 13 additional patients and defined three radiographic subsets: Type I, massive continuity of the cervical and upper thoracic vertebrae; Type II, involvement of only one or two interspaces occasioned by hemivertebrae, scoliosis, and occipitalization of the atlas; and Type III, fusion of both cervical and lower thoracic or lumbar vertebrae (Feil, 1919). These morphologic distinctions emphasize the etiologic diversity of the Klippel-Feil syndrome (KFS), but are of limited clinical use.

CLINICAL ASPECTS

The complete triad of short neck, low posterior hairline, and painless restriction of cervical motion characterize 52 per cent of patients, the functional limitation being most consistently present (Gray, Romaine, and Skandalakis, 1964). Despite frequent sparing of the atlantoaxial joint, rotation is typically impaired more than flexion and extension, the latter exhibiting a range of over 90 degrees even with only one open disc space (Hensinger, Lang, and MacEwen, 1974).

Rather than overgrowth of the scalp, it is the cervical foreshortening that displaces the hairline and is accompanied by webbing of the neck in over 8 per cent, torticollis in 18 per cent, and scoliosis of over 15 degrees in 60 per cent of patients. Failure of inferior migration of one or both scapulae, Sprengel's deformity, is found in 25 to 35 per cent.

Congenital neurologic disturbances called mirror movements, consisting of involuntary synkinesis of the contralateral, usually upper extremity, are obvious clinically in 15.6 per cent of patients. However, Baird, Robinson, and Buckler (1967) found diagnostic electromyographic changes in 10 of 13 patients with KFS, as opposed to only 1 of 13 controls. Attributed to the absence of the pyramidal decussation in one autopsy, myelographic cervical cord anomalies are associated with agenesis of the corpus callosum. Hair overlying the midline may signify underlying cord anomalies. Mental retardation and motor dysfunction were individually found in 8.75 per cent of patients. The latter may present as Möbius' syndrome involving paresis of the sixth and seventh cranial nerves or as Duane's retraction syndrome, with simultaneous contraction of the medial and lateral recti associated with abducens nuclear hypoplasia (Eisemann and Sharma, 1979). Duane's syndrome was first described by Wildervanck (1952) in conjunction with KFS and hearing loss. As a syndrome (Wildervanck's), it is found in 1 per cent of deaf children. Hearing loss was detected in 19 of 20 ears tested in patients with KFS. As in Wildervanck's syndrome, sensorineural deficiency predominated, as documented in 15 of 19 ears, with conductive losses in four and mixed deficit in one (Windle-Taylor, Emery, and Phelps, 1981). Eleven of 12 ears with severe hearing loss showed inner ear dysplasia on tomography, although primary eighth cranial nerve involvement was not ruled out.

Congenital urinary anomalies in up to 64 per cent of patients with KFS have been reported, with unilateral renal agenesis occurring in 28.2 per cent (Moore, Matthews, and Rabinowitz, 1975). Fourteen cases of KFS and vaginal agenesis have also been described (Willemsen, 1982).

The Klippel-Feil syndrome occurs in one of 42,000 births (Gunderson and associates, 1967) with a statistically significant preponderance of females (54.6 per cent versus 41.0 per cent males) (Helmi and Pruzansky, 1980). The phenotype reflects the severity of the underlying fusion; thus, Type I is reported most frequently in clinical series, while Type II is found 50 times more often at autopsy or radiographically in 7.3 of 1000 Caucasian and black controls (Brown, Templeton, and Hodges, 1964). Hence, Gray, Romaine, and Skandalakis (1964) preferred the phrase "congenital cervical fusion" to the eponym. Convincing genetic evidence supported autosomal dominant (sporadic) transmission with incomplete penetrance and variable expressivity involving the C2–C3 interspace in Type II KFS (Gunderson and associates, 1967), and autosomal recessive inheritance of diffuse involvement of the cervical, upper, and lower thoracic and lumbar spine (Da Silva, 1982).

Diverse ocular defects were found in 20.6 per cent of KFS patients, extraocular movement being most commonly affected.

Speech pathology, predominantly hypernasality, has been documented in 16.9 per cent of patients although control data for a comparable group of hearing deficient patients were not presented. Nevertheless, 18.8 per cent of patients with congenital velopharyngeal incompetence (VPI) displayed cervical vertebral anomalies (Osborne, 1968), including those with increased pharyngeal diameters (Osborne, Pruzansky, and Koepp-Baker, 1971).

Palatal clefts and KFS are more commonly associated with one another than they are in controls. The data reflect the hereditary distinction between patients who have cleft palate alone and those who have cleft lip with or without cleft palate; KFS was found in four of 211 and none of 245, respectively (Fraser and Calnan, 1961). Of 342 cleft palate patients and 800 controls, 8.7 per cent with isolated cleft palate, 2.1 per cent with cleft lip, and 0.75 per cent of controls had cervical vertebral anomalies (Ross and Lindsay, 1965). Osborne's (1968) findings corroborated these with skeletal changes in 7.2 per cent, 2.9, and 1.7 per cent, respectively.

Congenital heart disease occurs in 4.2 per cent, in contrast to the frequency of 0.6 per cent among all live births (Carlgren, 1959). The defects are nonspecific, most commonly ventricular septal defect (Morrison, Perry, and Scott, 1968).

ETIOPATHOGENESIS

Gorlin, Pindborg, and Cohen (1976) noted similar craniocervical relations in Turner's, Noonan's, and Morquio's (mucopolysaccharidosis Type IV) syndromes, as well as in patients with spinal tuberculosis.

Little evidence exists for putative teratogenicity, although the fetal alcohol syndrome and KFS have been reported in three cases (Lowry, 1977; Neidengard, Carter, and Smith, 1978). The former represented the first human association of vertebral anomalies with ethanol intake, although skeletal deformity characterizes the mouse model (Chernoff, 1977).

Although described as a fusion process, the underlying pathologic condition represents faulty segmentation as the mesodermal somites and sclerotomes, having united with those immediately cranial and caudal to form the vertebrae, fail to develop a continuous intervertebral disc. Mesial migration of sclerotomes envelops the notochord by the end of the fourth gestational week (Duncan, 1977).

Two mechanisms have been postulated to inhibit segmentation. Gardner (1979) reviewed the "no-neck" form of KFS distinct from those without axial shortening. He presented one case with iniencephaly and cited similar cases from the literature with associated spina bifida, anencephaly, and hindbrain hernia characterized by "overdistention" of the neural tube. He referred to Weed's (1917) demonstration that upon successive closure of the anterior and posterior neuropores on days 24 and 26 (Moore, 1973), cerebrospinal fluid "factitiously" dissects the subarachnoid space. He thus resurrected the hydrodynamic theory of Morgagni, postulating that overdistention could prevent midline sclerotomal fusion, with resultant hemivertebrae and disruption of the notochord. The latter would impede segmentation. However, Gardner's findings oppose those of Barson (1970). The latter did not include failures of segmentation with dysraphia or spina bifida, which manifests an open neural tube as previously noted by von Recklinghausen. Gardner's (1979) examples also included a much higher incidence of cranial pathology than did other series of KFS. Furthermore, Hensinger, Lang, and MacEwen (1974) noted that the sagittal and transverse diameters of the spinal canal were "generally normal."

Bavinck and Weaver (1986) postulated that disruption of the subclavian artery could create a series of anomalies. If the disruption is distal to the internal thoracic artery, transverse limb bud defects are created; if distal to the vertebral but including the internal thoracic artery, Poland's syndrome; and if proximal to the vertebral artery, KFS. The ascending cervical and deep cervical arteries, respectively, anastomose with the vertebral artery at the C1–C2 and C7–T1 interspaces. These are characteristically spared in KFS, a finding purportedly due to collateral circulation. Bernini and associates (1969) noted anomalous vertebral arteries in 25 per cent of KFS patients (versus 1 per cent of controls). Basilar artery hypoperfusion was invoked to explain involvement of the sixth and seventh cranial nerve nuclei and the vestibulocochlear nerve. Brill and associates (1987) described a patient with Type II KFS and filling of an isolated right subclavian artery via retrograde flow in the ipsilateral vertebral artery.

At 25 to 28 days of gestational age, the pronephric ducts extend cranially to C3–C5. These persist as mesonephric ducts from which ureteral buds emerge and induce formation of the kidneys. The pronephric duct also induces müllerian duct formation, (Duncan, 1977) and therefore the skeletal, neural, and genitourinary primordia most commonly afflicted in KFS are simultaneously adjacent to each other. Thus, vertebral artery disruption in the fourth gestational week offers the most parsimonious explanation of the pathogenesis of KFS.

TREATMENT

Surgical therapy must be individualized. Correction commonly involves the cardiac, palatal, and skeletal defects, and a critical assessment of cervical instability is mandatory prior to intubation. Quadriplegia after minor trauma has been reported (Elster, 1984). Nagib, Maxwell, and Chou (1984) identified those at high risk; of 21 patients, 11 of 12 without neurologic injury had only one unsegmented bone, while the nine with injury had two unsegmented blocks of bone, cervical stenosis on myelography, or cranial involvement. Treatment recommended included a fusion of the unstable segments and decompression of the impingement (Nagib, Maxwell, Chou, 1985).

Esthetic correction of the neck webbing requires resection of the excess skin and subcutaneous tissue and restoration of the posterior hairline. De Bruin (1928) noted that the deformity included the platysma muscle but not the deep muscles or fascia. Chandler (1937) first reported the use of Z-plasty, a technique that necessitates anterior scars. Foucar (1948) described a T incision with a 3

inch vertical and 5 inch transverse limb "hidden in the hair." The flaps were rotated superomedially and the redundancy was removed. Shearin and DeFranzo (1980) divided the vertical limb inferiorly to facilitate mobilization of the lateral flaps. The "butterfly" configuration of the incision was closed with a midline vertical limb, which later required revision because of widening and partial recurrence of the webbing (see Chap. 39). The recommended closure is an X to prevent this complication, although Y to V advancement of the inferior and superior flaps as described sacrifices tissue longitudinally while augmenting the transverse dimension, thereby contravening the purpose of the procedure.

Menick, Furnas, and Achauer (1984) further modified the butterfly excision in order to avoid a midline scar by extending the inferior flap into the scalp. However, neither the flap nor the hairline is elevated. This design consequently displaces the scars laterally and they become visible at the hairline close to the original site of the web, as discussed by Lindsay (Menick, Furnas, and Achauer, 1984).

Agris, Dingman, and Varon (1983) emphasized the procedure of Foucar and attributed his results to a midline elliptic incision (see Chap. 39). Although this design would eliminate the transverse excess, elevation of the hairline necessitates resection of the scalp parallel to this margin. Thus, the most efficient solution employs a V incision to raise the hairline combined with a vertical ellipse to eliminate the webbing. The resultant "Y" minimizes the exposed length of scar, and the obtuse apices of the three resultant flaps resist ischemia. While undermining the platysma, the surgeon must exercise care to avoid injury to the seventh, eighth, and eleventh cranial nerves; the external jugular vein; and the cervical plexus. Positioning the patient in the prone position facilitates operative symmetry (Menick, Furnas, and Achauer, 1984). The techniques are discussed in detail in Chapter 39.

OBSTRUCTIVE SLEEP APNEA

John Siebert

Over the past decade, the clinician has become increasingly aware of the obstructive sleep apnea syndrome (OSAS), particularly in the craniofacial clinic setting. Obstructive sleep apnea remains a therapeutic challenge, despite an increased knowledge of the pathophysiology and the emergence of new forms of treatment.

In 1837, in the "Posthumous Papers of the Pickwick Club," Charles Dickens described an incredibly fat boy named Joe with persistent daytime somnolence. The British physician Caton in 1889 and his French colleague Lamacq in 1897 both observed that "narcoleptics" may suffer from obstructed airways during sleep that lead to "periodic states of suffocation." In 1918 Osler coined the term "Pickwickian," referring to obese, hypersomnolent patients. In 1936 Kerr and Lagen noted that cor pulmonale and cardiac failure could result in patients having such characteristics. Between 1959 and 1962 Alexander, Amad, and Cole (1962) defined a "Joe" type of the pickwickian syndrome, characterized by obesity and hypersomnolence. In 1964 Gastaut, Tassinari, and Duron reported the presence of repetitive obstructive apnea during sleep in the obese "pickwickian" patient. Schwartz and Escande (1967) demonstrated that oropharyngeal collapse occurred in pickwickians, as documented by the first cinematographic study of obstructive apnea. During the following decades, OSAS was further characterized by applying the knowledge of sleep physiology to the syndrome.

Therapeutic attempts were made prior to a complete understanding of the pathophysiology of the condition. Weight loss had been recommended for many years, although Fishman (1972) noted that drastic weight loss does not always solve the problem. In 1969 Kuhlo, Doll, and Franck first reported the effectiveness of tracheostomy in treating OSAS. Kumashiro and associates (1971) described the effective use of tricyclic antidepressant therapy. Today, tracheostomy is still performed along with other surgical options, and tricyclic antidepressants are still recommended for mild to moderate OSAS.

Obstructive sleep apnea patients by definition exhibit persistent and progressively increasing diaphragmatic efforts with no air exchange at the nose and mouth. Sleep apnea secondary to decreased respiratory muscle activity is defined as *central sleep apnea.* *Mixed sleep apnea* is a combination of both. It is obviously imperative that central sleep apnea be differentiated from the obstructive variety before therapy is instituted.

Electromyelographic (EMG) studies and fiberoptic endoscopy have revealed that during both rapid eye movement (REM) and non-REM sleep periods there are episodes of loss of tone in the pharyngeal muscles (Guilleminault, Hill, and Simmons, 1978). The resulting atonia produces a narrowing of or, in pathologic states, collapse of the upper airway that obstructs breathing. These states can be divided into *apnea,* when no air flows from the nostrils or mouth for at least ten seconds, and *hypopnea,* defined as a two-thirds reduction in tidal volume. The narrowing of the upper airway can occur at one or multiple sites, including the soft palate, the base of the tongue, and the lateral pharyngeal wall. These findings may result from local anatomic disproportions or adjacent bone abnormalities such as mandibular or maxillary deficiencies. It must be emphasized that the determinants of airway patency during sleep are multifactorial. Thus, treatment modalities that address single factors such as anatomic anomalies are not uniformly beneficial.

CLINICAL ASPECTS

The incidence and prevalence of sleep apnea are currently unknown. Several studies from around the world report a conservative estimate to be 1 to 1.5 per cent of the population (Franceschi and associates, 1982; Lavie, 1983). These data indicate that the sleep apnea syndrome at least is not an uncommon problem.

The major characteristics of OSAS are male predominance, obesity, hypersomnolence, and excessive snoring. With repetitive apneic events, there are frequent arousals, resulting in excessive daytime sleepiness. Patients suffer deterioration of memory and judgment, irritability, morning headaches, sexual dysfunction, and personality changes involving sudden episodes of inappropriate behavior, jealousy, suspicion, anxiety, or depression. In children it is common to find enuresis, failure to thrive, weight loss, problems in growth, misbehavior, poor school performance, and nightmares.

Physiologic changes involving the cardio-pulmonary system occur and may lead to life-threatening events. Systemic and pulmonary arterial pressures rise. In the early phases of the syndrome, the elevated pressures are seen only during sleep. As the syndrome progresses, patients remain hypertensive when awake. Oxygen desaturation occurs with repetitive episodes of apnea. The amount of desaturation is related to the frequency and duration of apneic episodes, the baseline oxygenation, and coexisting cardiopulmonary disease. Significant cardiac arrhythmias can occur. Sinus bradycardia (heart rate less than 30), sinus arrest, atrioventricular block, premature ventricular contractions (PVC), and tachycardia have been monitored. Cardiopulmonary problems can result in anoxic seizure, cardiac arrest, and sudden death (MacGregor, Block, and Ball, 1972; Kryger and associates, 1974; Guilleminault, 1983).

Obstructive sleep apnea is associated with many conditions. Upper airway allergies, enlargement of lymphoid tissues in the upper airway (resulting from repetitive infections, hemopathy, or Down syndrome), or hormone-related enlargement of the soft tissues of the upper airway (myxedema, pituitary adenoma, corticoadrenal tumors, steroid treatment) can lead to the obstructive sleep apnea syndrome. Obvious mandibular abnormalities, such as observed in acromegaly, Pierre Robin sequence, Crouzon's disease, the Treacher Collins syndrome, and idiopathic micrognathia can be associated with episodes of obstructive sleep apnea and should be investigated when diagnosed.

DIAGNOSIS

The objective should be to identify the site of obstruction so that treatment can be logically directed. Specific parameters should be evaluated at the initial examination since they will determine the treatment selected.

The first parameter to evaluate is obesity and its distribution. Two-thirds of individuals with sleep apnea seen at the Stanford Sleep Disorder Clinic were overweight (over 20 per cent above the ideal weight for age and height) (Guilleminault, 1985). It is important to elicit a history of the patient's eating habits and diet, and the frequency of relapses after weight loss.

Possible aggravating factors producing OSAS must be sought. Alcohol and other central nervous system depressant drugs such as hypnotics and tranquilizers, especially when taken before bedtime, increase the frequency and prolong the duration of complete obstructive episodes. Respiratory allergies, smoking, or a dusty working environment can exacerbate mild obstructive sleep apnea.

Pertinent physical examination includes evaluation of the entire upper aerodigestive tract. The nasal cavity is examined for evidence of significant septal deformity or turbinate enlargement. Macroglossia and deficiencies of the jaw are sought in the oral cavity. In the pharynx a long, soft palate; enlarged tonsils; a large, floppy base of the tongue; and redundant mucosa with fatty infiltration are important findings. It is also mandatory to rule out tumors or masses compromising the airway or vocal cord mobility.

Objective evidence for OSAS begins with *polysomnography*, which includes the electro-encephalogram (EEG), electro-oculogram (EOG), electromyelogram (EMG), and electrocardiogram (ECG, lead V2). Respiration or diaphragmatic function is monitored by plethysmography, and nasal and oral air flow by thermistors. Oxygen saturation is monitored transcutaneously (Rechtschaffen and Kales, 1968; Guilleminault, 1983). Cessation of respiration (obstructive, central, and mixed) and episodes of oxygen desaturation occurring during sleep are recorded. The respiratory disturbance index (RDI), or the number of episodes of apnea and hypopnea per sleep hour, is reported; an RDI greater than five is abnormal. OSAS becomes clinically important when the RDI is greater than 20 and oxygen desaturation falls below 85 per cent.

Radiologic evaluation is by cephalometrics and three-dimensional computed tomography (3D-CT). Standard cephalometric techniques have been described previously (see Chap. 29). Horizontal skeletal discrepancies are important in the diagnosis and management of OSAS. The angles SNA and SNB (Fig. 63–31) have normal mean values of 82 and 80 degrees, respectively. Angles less than the mean suggest a maxillary or mandibular de-

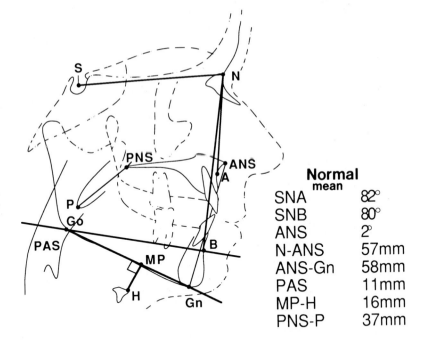

Figure 63–31. Lateral cephalometric roentgenogram with normal measurements.

	Normal mean
SNA	82°
SNB	80°
ANS	2°
N-ANS	57mm
ANS-Gn	58mm
PAS	11mm
MP-H	16mm
PNS-P	37mm

ficiency, respectively. Discrepancies between the maxilla and mandible are evaluated by the angle ANB (mean = 2 degrees). The posterior airway space is evaluated by a line drawn from point B through Go. This line intersects the base of the tongue and posterior pharyngeal wall on the soft tissue outline. The linear measurement between the base of the tongue and posterior pharyngeal wall outlines the posterior airway space (PAS, normal mean = 11.5 mm). The soft palate is evaluated by a line from PNS to the tip of the soft palate contour (P) (PNS-P, mean = 37 mm).

The position of the hyoid bone is determined by a line drawn perpendicular to the mandibular plane (MP) through the hyoid (H) (MP-H, mean = 15 mm). Patients with OSAS have a relatively inferiorly positioned hyoid (MP-H greater than 15) compared to normal subjects. A longer than normal soft palate (PNS-P) and a narrowing of the base of the tongue (PAS) are potential causes of obstruction. Cephalometric radiography is, however, a two-dimensional method of evaluating a three-dimensional area. Thus, its reliability can be advanced by the addition of three-dimensional CT scans. The soft tissue structures of interest are also dynamic struc-

tures; however, their relative static positions provide the clinician with a clue as to the possible pathologic anatomy that will be detected on the dynamic evaluation by fiberoptic endoscopy.

The purpose of fiberoptic endoscopy is to evaluate the nasopharynx, oropharynx, hypopharynx, and larynx sequentially. The nasal cavity and pharynx are anesthetized topically and the endoscope is introduced through the nose. The positions of the soft palate, the base of the tongue, and the lateral pharyngeal wall are noted and photographed. The dynamics of all areas are noted particularly on protrusion of the jaw. A modified Müller maneuver, i.e., inhaling against a closed oral and nasal passage, is performed and close attention is paid to the degree of pharyngeal wall collapse. The larynx is evaluated to rule out any deformities or masses including webs or vocal cord palsies.

NONSURGICAL TREATMENT

As previously stated, a large majority of patients with symptomatic OSAS are substantially overweight. Several reports have documented the resolution of symptoms with weight loss (Hoffmeister, Cabatingan, and McKee, 1978; Sugerman and associates, 1981; Harman, Wynne, and Block, 1982).

Decreased innervation to the genioglossus muscle has also been reported as a possible etiology for OSAS (Onal, Lopata, and O'Connor, 1982). Normalization of genioglossus function (monitored by EMG) with weight loss and resolution of symptoms was reported by Remmers, DeGroot, and Sauerland (1978).

All patients with OSAS should be advised to avoid alcohol and other drugs known to depress the central nervous system. Testosterone should also be avoided, since several studies have linked its use to OSAS (Sandblom and associates, 1983). Clinicians may inadvertently give androgens to patients who complain of impotence. Tricyclic antidepressants have been found to be beneficial in cases of mild to moderate OSAS (Clark and associates, 1979; Brownel and associates, 1982; Conway and associates, 1982; Smith and associates, 1983).

Various devices have been used with varying success in the treatment of OSAS: nasal trumpets, tongue retaining devices, and head position holding apparatuses.

Nasal continuous positive airway pressure (CPAP) effectively reduces the severity of OSAS by "splinting the airway via the creation of positive pressure applied through the nares." This method is successful in reducing or eliminating apnea in the vast majority of patients. However, initial intolerance and poor long-term compliance appear to be drawbacks of this type of therapy (Sullivan and associates, 1981; Rapoport and associates, 1982; Sanders, Moore, and Eveslage, 1983; Sanders, 1984; Berry and Black, 1984).

SURGICAL TREATMENT

Current surgical procedures employed for OSAS include tonsillectomy and adenoidectomy, nasal surgery (septoplasty, partial turbinectomy), tongue reduction, tracheostomy, uvulopalatopharyngoplasty (UPPP), osteotomy advancement of the mandible with hyoid myotomy and suspension, and maxillary, mandibular, and hyoid advancement. Selection of surgical procedure is based on the anatomic site of the obstructive process, the severity of the sleep apnea, the presence of

skeletal abnormality, and evidence of morbid obesity.

The cure rate is excellent with tonsillectomy and adenoidectomy for cases of OSAS associated with tonsillar or adenoidal hypertrophy (Stool and associates, 1977; Eliaschar and associates, 1980; Richardson and associates, 1980; Konno, Hoshino, and Togawa, 1980). Relatively mild tonsillar enlargement may play a role in the pathogenesis of OSAS. Success following tonsillectomy even in cases of mild hypertrophy only raises the question as to whether the size of the tonsil was as important a factor as the altered physiology of the tonsillar area postoperatively.

The nose plays an important role in the etiology of OSAS. Correction of nasal obstruction due to septal deviation and nasal polyps has been associated with surgical cures in cases of mild to moderate OSAS and has played a vital role in the overall management of cases of severe OSAS.

The posterior projection of the tongue onto the posterior pharyngeal wall is another important cause of OSAS. In patients in whom this is found to be a dynamic cause of obstruction, V-shaped wedge reduction of the tongue (anterior to posterior) reduces the absolute tongue size and creates scarring of the base of the tongue, preventing the tongue from falling posteriorly against the pharyngeal wall.

Tracheostomy for OSAS was first performed by Kuhlo, Doll, and Franck (1969). It is curative because it bypasses all the obstructive oropharyngeal sites. However, because of short- and long-term complications as well as obvious adverse psychosocial effects, tracheostomy is reserved only for the most severe cases of OSAS.

Uvulopalatopharyngoplasty (UPPP) was first proposed by Ikematsu (1964) for the treatment of habitual snoring. The goals of surgery are to increase the space in and around the soft palate, tonsillar fossa, and posterior pharyngeal wall in order to decrease upper airway resistance, particularly during sleep. In this technique the posterior margins of the soft palate and the redundant lateral pharyngeal wall mucosa are resected. The area of soft palate resection ranges from 8 to 15 mm, stopping short of the levator palati portion of the palate. The lateral pharyngeal wall is treated by resecting redundant mucosa and developing a flap along the posterior wall. The flap is advanced and sutured to the anterior tonsillar pillar area (Figs. 63–32, 63–33) (Fujita and associates, 1981; Simmons, Guilleminault, and Silvestri, 1983).

The success rate for UPPP in most series of OSAS ranges from 40 to 50 per cent. However, if presurgical evaluation indicates that the obstruction is localized to the soft palate, the success in treating OSAS by UPPP rises to approximately 90 per cent (Riley and associates, 1985). Thus, UPPP is performed in patients who have a long soft palate and redundant or hypertrophic tonsils in the lateral pharyngeal wall.

Reported complications include wound infection (5 to 10 per cent), velopharyngeal insufficiency (approximately 5 per cent) and occasional reflux of liquids into the nose (Simmons, Guilleminault, and Miles, 1984). Hypernasal speech and the refluxing of solid foods has not been reported. Palatal stenosis occurred in 1 per cent of patients.

Because of the intimate relationship between the mandible, base of tongue, pharyngeal wall and hyoid bone by their muscular and ligamentous attachments, Patton and associates (1983) showed that expansion of the hyoid bone results in expansion of the pharyngeal wall and enlargement of the pharyngeal space.

It has also been reported that total mandibular advancement advances the tongue and thereby expands the pharyngeal space (Baer and Priest, 1980; Powell and associates,

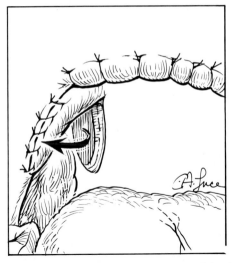

Figure 63–33. Uvulopalatopharyngoplasty. Palatal closure can be aided by a posterior pharyngeal flap that is rotated into the anterior tonsillar area.

1983). In order to avoid intermaxillary fixation and associated orthodontic therapy, Riley, Powell, and Guilleminault (1987) developed the technique of inferior sagittal osteotomy of the mandible with hyoid myotomy and suspension.

The procedures for inferior sagittal osteotomy are outlined in Figures 63–34 and 63–

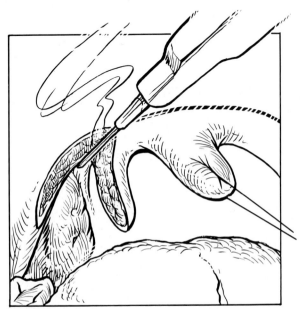

Figure 63–32. Uvulopalatopharyngoplasty. The incision begins at the anterior tonsillar pillar. The resection stops short of the levator palati portion of the soft palate.

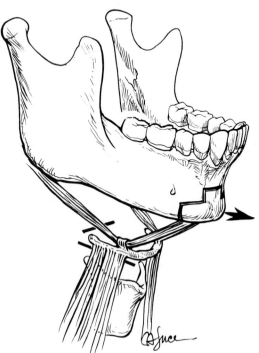

Figure 63–34. Inferior sagittal osteotomy of the mandible with hyoid myotomy and suspension. The level of the osteotomy and muscle transections is shown.

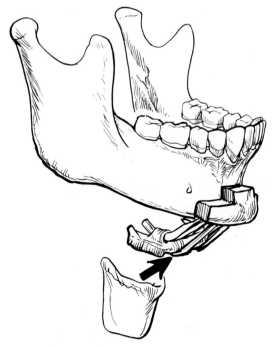

Figure 63–35. The chin point is advanced and the hyoid bone suspended further *(arrow)* with previously harvested fascial strips.

35. The surgical approach is via a submental incision. The mylohyoid and anterior digastric muscles are preserved. The hyoid bone is approached inferiorly. The sternohyoid, thyrohyoid, and omohyoid muscles are divided along the caudal aspect of the hyoid bone, avoiding injury to the superior laryngeal nerve. Strips of fascia harvested from the thigh are sutured to the body of the hyoid. The dissection returns to the mandible where the periosteum of the inferior mandible is reflected. The osteotomy and downfracture of the anteroinferior mandible is completed. The fragment is advanced and secured to the anterior mandible with screw fixation. The hyoid is suspended further from the mandible with the previously placed fascial strips.

Complications have been minimal, including transient mental anesthesia and mandibular fracture in cases in which the osteotomy was continued into the alveolus. Speech and swallowing have not been permanently altered.

Because of reported failures with other surgical techniques, several investigators have revised their views of the indications for seemingly more radical maxillary, mandibular, and hyoid advancement procedures. Orig-

inally, skeletal advancement was recommended only in cases of major skeletal deficiencies. According to Riley, Powell, and Guilleminault (1987), advancement surgery has been successful for patients who have obstruction at the base of the tongue and who fall into one of the following categories: (1) patients with normal skeletal development and severe OSAS (RDI greater than 50, oxygen desaturation less than 70 per cent); (2) morbidly obese patients; (3) patients with severe retro- or micrognathia (SNB less than 74 degrees); and (4) patients who have failed other types of treatment.

REFERENCES

Archambault, L., and Fromm, N. K.: Progressive facial hemiatrophy: report of three cases. Arch. Neurol. Psychiat., 529, 1932.

Achauer, B. M., Salibian, A. H., and Furnas, D. W.: Free flaps to the head and neck. Head Neck Surg., 4:315, 1982.

Agris, J., Dingman, R. O., and Varon, J.: Correction of webbed neck defects. Ann. Plast. Surg., 2:299, 1983.

Alexander, J. K., Amad, H., and Cole, V. W.: Observations on some clinical features of extreme obesity, with particular reference to cardiorespiratory effects. Am. J. Med., 32:512, 1962.

Argamasso, R. V.: An improved technique for glossopexy in the Robin sequence. Presented at the American Cleft Palate Association Meeting, May 16, 1986.

Asher, S. W., and Berg, B. O.: Progressive hemifacial atrophy: report of three cases, including one observed over 43 years ago, and computed tomographic findings. Arch Neurol., 39:44, 1982.

Avelar, J. M., and Psillakis, J. M.: The use of galea flaps in craniofacial deformities. Ann. Plast. Surg., 6:464, 1981.

Axellson, A., Brolin, I., Engstrom, H., and Linden, G.: Dysostosis mandibulofacialis. J. Laryng. Otolaryngol., 87:575, 1963.

Bachelor, E. P., and Kaplan, E. N.: Absence of the lateral canthal tendon in the Treacher Collins syndrome. Br. J. Plast. Surg., 34:162, 1981.

Baer, S. E., and Priest, J. H.: Sleep apnea syndrome: correction with surgical advancement of mandible. J. Oral Maxillofac. Surg., 38:543, 1980.

Baird, P. A., Robinson, G. C., and Buckler, W. S.: Klippel-Feil syndrome. A study of mirror movement detected by electromyography. Am. J. Dis. Child., 113:546, 1967.

Balestrazzi, P., Baeteman, M. A., Mattei, M. G., and Mattei, J. F.: Franceschetti syndrome in a child with a de novo balanced translocation F(5,13)(q11:p11) and significant decrease of hexosaminidase B. Hum. Genet. 64:305, 1953.

Barson, A. J.: Spina bifida: the significance of the level and extent of the defect to the morphogenesis. Dev. Med. Child Neurol., 12:129, 1970.

Bavinck, J. N., and Weaver, D. D.: Subclavian artery supply disruption sequence: hypothesis of a vascular etiology for Poland, Klippel-Feil, and Möbius anomalies. Am. J. Med. Genet., 23:903, 1986.

Beers, M. D., and Pruzansky, S.: The growth of the head of the infant with mandibular micrognathia, glossoptosis, and cleft palate following the Beverly Douglas operation. Plast. Reconstr. Surg., 16:189, 1955.

Behrents, R. A., McNamara, J. A., and Avery, J. K.: Prenatal mandibulofacial dysostosis (Treacher Collins syndrome). Cleft Palate J., 14:13, 1977.

Benavent, W. J., and Ramos-Oller, A.: Micrognathia: report of twelve cases. Plast. Reconstr. Surg., 22:486, 1958.

Bernini, F. P., Elefante, R., Smaltino, F., and Tedeschi, G.: Angiographic study on the vertebral artery in cases of deformities of the occipitocervical joint. Am. J. Roentgenol., 107:526, 1969.

Berry, G. A.: Note on a congenital defect (?coloboma) of the lower lid. Ophthalmol. Hosp. Rep., 12:255, 1889.

Berry, R. B., and Black, A. J.: Positive nasal airway pressure eliminates snoring as well as obstructive sleep apnea. Chest, 85:15, 1984.

Bigotti, A., and d'Agostino, G.: Casistica: un raro caso di glossoptosi congenita senza ipoposia mandibolare: sindrome di Pierre Robin incompleta. Minerva Med., 50:3255, 1959.

Bluestone, C. D., and Stool, S. E. (Eds.): Pediatric Otolaryngology. Vol. 2. Philadelphia, W. B. Saunders Company, 1983.

Boök, J. A., and Fraccaro, M.: Genetical investigation in a North Swedish population: mandibulofacial dysostosis. Acta Genet. (Basel), 5:327, 1955.

Bosma, J. F., Lind, J., and Truby, H. M.: Distortions of upper respiratory and swallow motions in infants having anomalies of the upper pharynx. Acta Paediatr. Scand. (Suppl.), 163:111, 1965.

Bowen, P., and Harley, F.: Mandibulofacial dysostosis with limb malformations (Nager's acrofacial dysostosis). Birth Defects, 10:109, 1974.

Bramley, P., and Forbes, A.: A case of progressive hemiatrophy presenting with spontaneous fractures of the lower jaw. Br. Med. J., 1:1476, 1960.

Briggs, A. H.: Mandibulofacial dysostosis. Br. J. Ophthalmol., 37:71, 1952.

Brill, C. B., Peyster, R. G., Keller, M. S., and Galtman, L.: Isolation of the right subclavian artery with subclavian steal in a child with Klippel-Feil anomaly: an example of the subclavian artery supply disruption sequence. Am. J. Med. Genet., 26:933, 1987.

Bromberg, B. E., Pasternak, R., Walden, R. H., and Rubin, L. R.: Evaluation of micrognathia with emphasis on late development of the mandible. Plast. Reconstr. Surg., 28:537, 1961.

Bromley, D., and Burston, W. R.: The Pierre Robin syndrome. Nursing Times, December, 1966.

Brouillette, R. T., Fernbach, S. K., and Hunt, C. E.: Obstructive sleep apnea in infants and children. J. Pediatr., 100:31, 1982.

Brown, M. W., Templeton, A. W., and Hodges, F. J.: The incidence of acquired and congenital fusions in the cervical spine. Am. J. Roentgen., 92:1255, 1964.

Brownell, L. G., West, P., Sweatman, P., Acres, J. C., and Kryger, M. H.: Protriptyline in obstructive sleep apnea. N. Engl. J. Med., 307:1037, 1982.

Burston, W. R.: Personal communication, 1966.

Callister, A. C.: Hypoplasia of the mandible (micrognathia) with cleft palate: treatment in early infancy by skeletal traction. Am. J. Dis. Child., 53:1057, 1937.

Campbell, R. M.: Unpublished case, 1956.

Campbell, W.: The Treacher Collins syndrome. Br. J. Radiol., 27:639, 1954.

Carlgren, L. E.: The incidence of congenital heart disease in children born in Gothenburg, 1941–1950. Br. Heart J., 21:40, 1959.

Caton, R.: A case of narcolepsy. Br. Med. J., 358, 1889.

Chajchir, A., and Benzaquen, I.: Liposuction fat grafts in face wrinkles and hemifacial atrophy. Aesth. Plast. Surg., 10:115, 1986.

Chandler, F. A.: Webbed neck (pterygium colli). Am. J. Dis. Child., 53:798, 1937.

Chapple, C. C.: Congenital dislocation of the hip in infancy. J. Pediatr., 6:306, 1935.

Chapple, C. C.: Abnormalities of infants resulting from nongenetic factors. Postgrad. Med., 7:323, 1950.

Chapple, C. C.: Possible mechanisms of some congenital defects. Am. J. Obstet. Gynecol., 70:712, 1955.

Chapple, C. C.: A duosyndrome of the laryngeal nerve. A.M.A. J. Dis. Child., 91:14, 1956.

Chapple, C. C.: In Nelson, W. E. (Ed.): Pediatrics. 7th Ed. Philadelphia, W. B. Saunders Company, 1959.

Chapple, C. C., and Davidson, T.: The study of the relationship between fetal position and certain congenital deformities. J. Pediatr., 18:483, 1941.

Charazinska, Z., and Nehrebecka, M.: Hypoplasia of one-half of the face associated with a congenital anomaly of the organ of hearing. Czas. Stomatol., 26:1403, 1973.

Chernoff, G. F.: The fetal alcohol syndrome in mice: an animal model. Teratology, 15:223, 1977.

Chou, Y. C.: Mandibulofacial dysostosis. Chin. Med. J., 80:373, 1960.

Clark, R. W., Schmidt, H. S., Schaal, S. C., Boudoulas, H., and Schuller, D. E.: Sleep apnea: treatment with protriptyline. Neurology, 29:1287, 1979.

Cocke, W. M.: Experimental production of micrognathia and glossoptosis associated with cleft palate (Pierre Robin syndrome). Plast. Reconstr. Surg., 38:395, 1966.

Cogswell, J. J., and Easton, D. M.: Cor-pulmonale in the Pierre-Robin syndrome. Arch. Dis. Child., 49:905, 1974.

Cohen, M. M.: In Bergsma, D. (Ed.): Birth Defects Atlas. Baltimore, Williams & Wilkins Company, 1973, p. 596.

Collins, E. T.: 8. Case with symmetrical congenital notches in the outer part of each lower lid with defective development of the malar bones. Trans. Ophthalmol. Soc. U.K., 20:190, 1900a.

Collins, E. T.: 9. Case with symmetrical congenital notches in the outer part of each lower lid and defective development of the malar bones. Trans. Ophthalmol. Soc. U.K., 20:191, 1900b.

Converse, J. M., and Betson, R. J., Jr.: A 20 year follow-up of a patient with hemifacial atrophy treated by a buried de-epithelized flap. Plast. Reconstr. Surg., 48:278, 1971.

Converse, J. M., and Smith, B.: Surgical treatment of the eyelid defect in the treatment of Treacher Collins syndrome: a preliminary report. Paper read by Wood-Smith, D. In Smith, B., and Converse, J. M. (Eds.): Plastic and Reconstructive Surgery of the Eye and Adnexa. St. Louis, C. V. Mosby Company, 1967.

Converse, J. M., Wood-Smith, D., McCarthy, J. G., and Coccaro, P. H.: Craniofacial surgery. Clin. Plast. Surg., 1:499, 1974.

Conway, W. A., Zorick, F., Piccione, P., and Roth, T.: Protriptyline in the treatment of sleep apnea. Thorax, 37:49, 1982.

Crikelair, G. F., Moss, M. L., and Khuri, A.: Facial hemiatrophy. Plast. Reconstr. Surg., 29:5, 1962.

Cullum, I. M.: An old wives' tale (tongue-tie). Br. Med. J., *2*:497, 1959.

Dagys, A. P.: A cephalometric study of the craniofacial characteristics in mandibulofacial dysostosis. Thesis for diploma course in orthodontics. Faculty of Dentistry, University of Toronto, 1977.

Dahl, E., Kreiborg, S., and Bjoark, A.: A morphologic description of a dry skull with mandibulofacial dysostosis. Scand. J. Dent. Res., *83*:257, 1975.

Da Silva, E. O.: Autosomal recessive Klippel-Feil syndrome. J. Med. Genet., *19*:130, 1982.

Davies, D. W., and Munro, I. R.: The anesthetic management and intraoperative care of patients undergoing major facial osteotomies. Plast. Reconstr. Surg., *55*:50, 1975.

Davis, A. D., and Dunn, R.: Micrognathia: suggested treatment for correction in early infancy. Am. J. Dis. Child., *45*:799, 1933.

De Bruin, M.: Pterygium colli congenitum (congenital webbing). Am. J. Dis. Child., *36*:333, 1928.

Debusmann, M.: Familiare kombinierte Gesichtsmissbildung im Bereich des ersten Viszeralbogens. Arch. Kinderkeilkd., *120*:133, 1940.

Dennison, W. M.: The Pierre Robin syndrome. Pediatrics, *36*:336, 1965.

Dickens, C.: The Posthumous Papers of the Pickwick Club. London, Chapman & Hall, 1837.

Douglas, B.: The treatment of micrognathia associated with obstruction by a plastic procedure. Plast. Reconstr. Surg., *1*:300, 1946.

Douglas, B.: A further report on the treatment of micrognathia with obstruction by a plastic procedure: results based on reports from 21 cities. Plast. Reconstr. Surg., *5*:113, 1950.

Douglas, B.: Treatment of micrognathia with obstruction by a plastic procedure. Lyon Chir., *52*:420, 1956.

Duke-Elder, S.: Text-Book of Ophthalmology. Vol. 5. St. Louis, C. V. Mosby Company, 1952, p. 472.

Duncan, P. A.: Embryologic pathogenesis of renal agenesis associated with cervical vertebral anomalies (Klippel-Feil phenotype). Birth Defects, *13*:91, 1977.

Dupertuis, S. M.: Growth of young human autogenous cartilage grafts. Plast. Reconstr. Surg., *5*:486, 1950.

Edgerton, M. T., Jane, J. A., and Berry, F. A.: Craniofacial osteotomies and reconstructions in infants and young children. Plast. Reconstr. Surg., *54*:13, 1974.

Edwards, J. R., and Newall, D. R.: The Pierre Robin syndrome reassessed in the light of recent research. Br. J. Plast. Surg., *38*:339, 1985.

Eisemann, M. L., and Sharma, G. K.: The Wildervanck syndrome: cervico-oculo-acoustic dysplasia. Otolaryngol. Head Neck Surg., *87*:892, 1979.

El-Antably, S., and El-Hoshny, M.: Mandibulofacial dysostosis. Collins-Franceschetti-Zwahlen syndrome. Bull. Ophthalmol. Soc. Egypt, *69*:735, 1976.

Eley, R. C., and Farber, S.: Hypoplasia of the mandible (micrognathia) as a cause of cyanotic attacks in the newly-born infant: report of four cases. Am. J. Dis. Child., *39*:1167, 1930.

Eliaschar, I., Lavie, P., Halperin, E., Gordon, C., and Alroy, G. Sleep apneic episodes as indications for adenotonsillectomy. Arch. Otolaryngol., *106*:492, 1980.

Elster, A. D.: Quadriplegia after minor trauma in the Klippel-Feil syndrome. J. Bone Joint Surg., *66A*:1473, 1984.

Eulenburg, A.: Lehrbuch der functionellen Nervenkrankheiten. Berlin, 1871.

Fara, M.: Personal communication, 1974.

Farkas, L. G.: Ear morphology in Treacher Collins, Apert's and Crouzon's syndromes. Arch. Otorhinolaryngol., *220*:153, 1978.

Farrar, J. E.: Mandibulofacial dysostosis. Br. J. Ophthalmol., *51*:132, 1967.

Feil, A.: L'absence et la diminution des vertebres cervicales (etude clinique et pathogenique): le syndrome de la reduction numerique cervicale. Theses de Paris, 1–123, 1919.

Fietti, V. G., Jr., and Fielding, W.: The Klippel-Feil syndrome: early roentgenographic appearance and progression of the deformity. A report of two cases. J. Bone Joint Surg., *58A*:891, 1976.

Fishman, A. P.: The syndrome of chronic alveolar hypoventilation. Bull. Physiopathol. Respir., *8*:971, 1972.

Forney, W. R., Robinson, S. J., and Pascoe, D. J.: Congenital heart disease, deafness, and skeletal malformations: a new syndrome? J. Pediatr., *68*:14, 1966.

Foucar, H. O.: Pterygium colli and allied conditions. Can. Med. Assoc. J., *59*:251, 1948.

Franceschetti, A., Brocher, J. E. W., and Klein, D.: Dysostose mandibulofaciale unilatérale avec déformations multiples du squelette (processus paramastoïde, synostose des vertèbres, sacralisation, etc.) et torticolis clonique. Ophthalmologica, *118*:796, 1949.

Franceschetti, A., and Klein, D.: Mandibulo-facial dysostosis: new hereditary syndrome. Acta Ophthalmol., *27*:143, 1949.

Franceschetti, A., and Koenig, H.: L'importance du facteur hérédo-dégéneratif dans l'hémiatrophie faciale progressive (Romberg). J. Genet Hum. *1*:27, 1952.

Franceschetti, A., and Zwahlen, P.: Un syndrome nouveau: la dysostose mandibulo-faciale. Bull. Schweiz. Akad. Med. Wiss., *1*:60, 1944.

Franceschi, M., Zamproni, P., Crippa, D., and Smirne, S.: Excessive daytime sleepiness. A one year study in an unselected inpatient population. Sleep, *5*:239, 1982.

Fraser, G. R., and Calnan, J. S.: Cleft lip and palate: seasonal incidence, birth weight, birth rank, sex, site, associated malformations and parental age. A statistical survey. Arch. Dis. Child., *36*:430, 1961.

Fujino, H., Hiraoka, T., and Kyoshoin, Y.: A case report of Treacher Collins syndrome. Kyushu J. Med. Sci., *12*:343, 1961.

Fujita, S., Conway, W., Zorick, F., and Roth, T.: Surgical correction of the anatomic abnormalities in obstructive sleep apnea syndrome: uvulopalatopharyngoplasty. Otolaryngol. Head Neck Surg., *89*:923, 1981.

Fulmek, R.: Hemiatrophia progressiva faciei (Romberg's syndrome) associated with heterochromia complicata (Fuchs' syndrome). Klin. Monatsbl. Augenheilkd., *164*:615, 1974.

Gardner, W. J.: Klippel-Feil syndrome, iniencephalus, anancephalus, hindbrain hernia, and mirror movements: overdistention of the neural tube. Child's Brain, *5*:361, 1979.

Gastaut, H., Tassinari, C. A., and Duron, B.: Étude polygraphique des manifestations épisodiques (hypniques et respiratoires), diurnes et nocturnes, du syndrome de Pickwick. Rev. Neurol., *112*:568, 1964.

Gillies, H., and Millard, D. R., Jr.: The Principles and Art of Plastic Surgery. Boston, Little, Brown & Company, 1957.

Gladstone, R. J., and Wakely, C. P. G.: Defective development of the mandibular arch; the etiology of arrested development and an inquiry into the question of the inheritance of congenital defects. J. Anat., *57*:149, 1922–1923.

Goldhammer, Y., Kronenberg, J., Tadmor, R., Braham, J., and Leventon, G.: Progressive hemifacial atrophy (Parry-Romberg's disease), principally involving bone. J. Laryngol. Otol., 95:643, 1981.

Gorlin, R.: Personal communication.

Gorlin, R. J., and Pindborg, J. J.: Syndromes of the Head and Neck. 2nd Ed. New York, McGraw-Hill Book Company, 1976.

Gray, S. W., Romaine, C. B., and Skandalakis, J. E.: Congenital fusion of the cervical vertebrae. Surg. Gynecol. Obstet., 118:373, 1964.

Guilleminault, C. (Ed.): Sleeping and Waking Disorders: Indications and Techniques. Menlo Park, CA, Addison-Wesley, 1981.

Guilleminault, C.: Natural history, cardiac impact, and long term follow-up sleep apnea syndrome. In Guilleminault, C., and Lugaresi, E. (Eds.): Sleep/Wake Disorders: Natural History, Epidemiology, and Long-Term Evolution. New York, Raven Press, 1983.

Guilleminault, C.: Obstructive sleep apnea—the clinical syndrome and historical perspective. Med. Clin. North Am., 69:1187, 1985.

Guilleminault, C., Eldridge, F. L., Simmons, F. B., and Dement, W. C.: Sleep apnea in eight children. Pediatrics, 58:23, 1976.

Guilleminault, C., Hill, M. W., and Simmons, F. B.: Obstructive sleep apnea: electromyelographic and fiberoptic studies. Exp. Neurol., 62:48, 1978.

Gunderson, C. H., Greenspan, R. H., Glaser, G. H., and Lubs, H. A.: The Klippel-Feil syndrome: genetic and clinical reevaluation of cervical fusion. Medicine, 46:491, 1967.

Gunderson, C. H., and Solitare, G. B.: Mirror movements in patients with the Klippel-Feil syndrome. Neuropathologic observations. Arch. Neurol., 18:675, 1968.

Hadley, R. C.: Presented at the American Society of Plastic and Reconstructive Surgery, New Orleans, 1961.

Handler, S. D., and Keon, T. P.: Difficult laryngoscopy/intubation: the child with mandibular hypoplasia. Ann. Otol. Rhinol. Laryngol., 92:401, 1983.

Hanson, J. W., and Smith, D. W.: U-shaped palatal defect in the Pierre Robin anomalad: developmental and clinical relevance. J. Pediatr., 87:30, 1975.

Harashina, T., and Fujino, T.: Reconstruction in Romberg's disease with free groin flap. Ann. Plast. Surg., 7:289, 1981.

Harman, E. M., Wynne, J. W., and Block, A. J.: The effect of weight loss on sleep-disordered breathing and oxygen desaturation in morbidly obese men. Chest, 82:291, 1982.

Heaf, D. P., Helms, P. J., Dinwiddie, R., and Matthew, D. J.: Nasopharyngeal airways in Pierre Robin syndrome. J. Pediatr., 100:698, 1982.

Helmi, C., and Pruzansky, S.: Craniofacial and extracranial malformations in the Klippel-Feil syndrome. Cleft Palate J., 17:65, 1980.

Hensinger, R. N., Lang, J. E., and MacEwen, G. D.: Klippel-Feil syndrome; a constellation of associated anomalies. J. Bone Joint Surg., 56A:1246, 1974.

Hoffman, S., Kahn, S., and Seitchick, N.: Late problems in the management of the Pierre Robin syndrome. Plast. Reconstr. Surg., 35:504, 1965.

Hoffmeister, J. A., Cabatingan, O., and McKee, A.: Sleep apnea treated by intestinal bypass. J. Maine Med. Assoc., 69:72, 1978.

Horstadius, S.: The Neural Crest. London, Oxford University Press, 1950.

Hövels, O.: Zur Pathogenese der Missbildungen des 1. Visceralbogens unter besonderer Berücksichtigung der Dysostosis mandibulo-facialis. Z. Kinderheilkd., 73:568, 1953.

Huffman, G. G., and Lorson, E. L.: Treatment of malocclusion in a case of Treacher Collins syndrome. J. Oral Surg., 32:612, 1974.

Hurwitz, P.: Mandibulo-facial dysostosis. Arch. Ophthalmol., 51:69, 1954.

Hutchinson, J. C., Calderelli, D. D., Valvasorri, G. E., Pruzansky, S., and Parris, P. J.: The otologic manifestations of mandibulofacial dysostosis. Trans. Am. Acad. Ophthalmol. Otolaryngol., 84:526, 1977.

Ikematsu, T.: Study of snoring, fourth report: therapy (Japanese). J. Jpn. Otorhinolaryngol., 64:434, 1964.

Ivy, R. H.: Congenital and acquired defects and deformities of the face and jaws: review of literature for 1936. Int. Abstr. Surg., 64:433, 1937.

Ivy, R. H., and Curtis, L.: Some orthopaedic problems of the lower jaw with special reference to unilateral shortening. J. Bone Joint Surg., 10:645, 1928.

Jackson, I. T.: Personal communication, 1984.

Jackson, I. T., Munro, I. R., Salyer, K. E., and Whitaker, L. A.: Atlas of Cranio-maxillofacial Surgery. St. Louis, C. V. Mosby Company, 1982, p. 572.

Jackson, P., Whitaker, L. A., and Randall, P.: Airway hazards associated with pharyngeal flaps in patients who have the Pierre Robin syndrome. Plast. Reconstr. Surg., 58:184, 1976.

Johnson, R. V., and Kennedy, W. R.: Progressive facial hemiatrophy (Parry-Romberg syndrome). Contralateral extraocular muscle impairment. Am J. Ophthalmol., 67:561, 1969.

Johnston, C., Taussig, L. M., Koopmann, C., Smith, P., and Bjelland, J.: Obstructive sleep apnea in Treacher Collins syndrome. Cleft Palate J., 18:39, 1981.

Johnston, M. C., and Listgarten, M.: In Slavkin, H. C., and Bavetta, L. A. (Eds.): Developmental Aspects of Oral Biology. 2nd Ed. New York, Academic Press, 1972, p. 53.

Johnstone, I. L.: A case of deficiency of the malar bones with defect of the lower eyelids. Br. J. Ophthalmol., 27:21, 1943.

Jolleys, A.: Micrognathos: a review of 38 cases treated in the new-born period. J. Pediatr. Surg., 1:460, 1966.

Jones, K. L., Smith, D. W., Harvey, M. A., Hall, B. D., and Quan, L.: Older paternal age and fresh gene mutation. Data on additional disorders. J. Pediatr., 86:84, 1975.

Jurkiewicz, M. J., and Nahai, F.: The use of free revascularized grafts in the amelioration of hemifacial atrophy. Plast. Reconstr. Surg., 76:44, 1985.

Kaufman, M. D.: Masticatory spasm in facial hemiatrophy. Ann. Neurol., 7:585, 1980.

Kazanjian, V. H., and Converse, J. M.: The Surgical Treatment of Facial Injuries. 2nd Ed. Baltimore, Williams & Wilkins Company, 1959.

Kazanjian, V. H., and Sturgis, S. H.: Surgical treatment of hemiatrophy of the face. J.A.M.A., 115:348, 1940.

Kerr, W. J., and Lagen, J. B.: The postural syndrome of obesity leading to postural emphysema and cardiorespiratory failure. Ann. Intern. Med., 10:569, 1936.

Kibel, M. A.: Mandibulofacial dysostosis (Treacher Collins syndrome). Cent. Afr. J. Med., 6:244, 1960.

Kiebel, F., and Mall, F. P.: Manual of Human Embryology. Vol. 1. Philadelphia, J. B. Lippincott Company, 1910, p. 86.

Kiskadden, W. S., and Dietrich, S. R.: Review of the

treatment of micrognathia. Plast. Reconstr. Surg., *12*:364, 1953.

Kiskadden, W. S., and McGregor, M. W.: Report of a case of progressive facial hemiatrophy with pathological changes and surgical treatment. Plast. Reconst. Surg., *1*:187, 1946.

Klippel, M., and Feil, A.: Un cas d'absence des vertebres cervicales avec cage thoracique remontant jusqu'a la base du crane (cage thoracique cervicale). Nouv. Iconogr. Salpet., *25*:223, 1912.

Konno, A., Hoshino, T., and Togawa, K.: The influence of upper airway obstruction by enlarged tonsils and adenoids upon recurrent infection of the lower airway in childhood. Laryngoscope, *90*:1709, 1980.

Kreibos, S., Leth Jensen, B., Dahl, E., and Fogh-Anderson, P.: Pierre Robin sequence: early facial development. Presented at the 5th International Congress on Cleft Palate and Related Craniofacial Anomalies. Monaco, September 3, 1986.

Krogman, W. M.: Personal communication, 1962.

Kryger, M., Quensney, L. F., Holder, D., Gloor, P., and MacLeod, P.: Sleep deprivation syndrome of the obese patients: a problem of periodic nocturnal upper airway obstruction. Am. J. Med., *56*:530, 1974.

Kuhlo, W., Doll, E., and Franck, M. C.: Erfolgreiche Behandlung eines Pickwick-Syndroms durch eine Dauertrachealkanüle. Dtsch. Med. Wochenschr., *94*:1286, 1969.

Kumashiro, H., Sato, M., Hirata, J., Baba, O., and Otsuki, S.: Sleep apnoea and sleep regulating mechanism: a case effectively treated with monochlorimipramine. Folia Psychiatr. Neurol Jpn., *25*:41, 1971.

Lamacq, L.: Quelque cas de narcolepsis. Rev. Med., *17*:699, 1897.

LaPage, C. P.: Micrognathia in the new-born. Lancet, *1*:323, 1937.

Lapidot, A., and Ben-Hur, N.: Fastening the base of the tongue forward to the hyoid for relief of respiratory distress in the Pierre Robin syndrome. Plast. Reconstr. Surg., *56*:89, 1975.

Lavie, P.: Sleep apnea in industrial workers. *In* Guilleminault, C., and Lugaresi, E. (Eds.): Sleep/Wake Disorders: Natural History, Epidemiology, and Long-Term Evolution. New York, Raven Press, 1983.

Le Hunsec, J., and La Porte, B.: Intérêt de l'électromyographie dans les atteintes de la motilité oculaire au cours de la maladie de Parry-Romberg. Bull. Soc. Ophthalmol. Franc., *65*:57, 1965.

Lenstrup, E.: Hypoplasia of mandible as a cause of choking fits in infants. Acta Paediatr., *5*:154, 1925.

Leopold, I. H., Mahoney, J. F., and Price, M. L.: Symmetric defects in the lower lids associated with abnormalities of the zygomatic processes of the temporal bones. Arch. Ophthalmol., *34*:210, 1945.

Lewis, M. B., and Pashayan, H. M.: Management of infants with Robin anomaly. Clin. Pediatr. (Phila.), *19*:519, 525, 1980.

Lewis, S. R., Lynch, J. B., and Blocker, T. G., Jr.: Fascial slings for tongue stabilization in the Pierre Robin syndrome. Plast. Reconstr. Surg., *42*:237, 1968.

Lewkonia, R. M., and Lowry, R. B.: Progressive hemifacial atrophy (Parry-Romberg syndrome): report with review of genetics and nosology. Am. J. Med. Genet., *14*:385, 1983.

Lindemann, H. O.: Interessante Befunde bei Hemiatrophia facialis progressiva. Albrecht von Graefes Arch. Klin. Ophthalmol., *142*:409, 1940.

Llewellyn, J. S., and Biggs, A. D.: Hypoplasia of the mandible: report of a case with résumé of literature and suggestions for modified treatment. Am. J. Dis. Child., *65*:440, 1943.

Lockhart, R. D.: Variations coincident with congenital absence of the zygoma (zygomatic process of temporal bone). J. Anat., *63*:233, 1929.

Longacre, J. J., de Stefano, G. A., and Holmstrand, K.: The early vs. the late reconstruction of congenital hypoplasia of the facial skeleton and skull. Plast. Reconstr. Surg., *27*:489, 1961.

Longmire, W. P., Jr., and Sanford, M. C.: Stimulation of mandibular growth in congenital micrognathia by traction. Am. J. Dis. Child., *78*:750, 1949.

Lowry, R. B.: The Klippel-Feil anomalad as part of the fetal alcohol syndrome. Teratology, *16*:53, 1977.

MacGregor, M. I., Block, A. J., and Ball, W. C., Jr.: Serious complications and sudden death in the pickwickian syndrome. Johns Hopkins Med. J., *126*:279, 1972.

MacLennan, F. M., and Robertson, G. S.: Ketamine for induction and intubation in Treacher Collins syndrome. Anaesthesia, *36*:196, 1981.

Malek, R., Psaume, J., and Genton, N.: New timing and new sequence for operative interventions in CLP patients. Presented at the 5th International Congress on Cleft Palate and Craniofacial Anomalies. Monte Carlo, 1985.

Mann, I., and Kilner, T. P.: Deficiency of the malar bones with defect of the lower eyelids. Br. J. Ophthalmol., *27*:13, 1943.

Marino, H., and Appiani, E.: Disostosis mandibulo-facial. Prensa Med. Argent., *51*:3083, 1954.

Martin, J. P.: A case of facial hemiatrophy with lack of development of the breast on the same side. Brain, *48*:140, 1925.

McCarthy, J. G., and Zide, B. M.: The spectrum of calvarial bone grafting; introduction of the vascularized calvarial bone flap. Plast. Reconstr. Surg., *74*:10, 1984.

McCollough, E. G., and Weil, C.: Augmentation of facial defects using Mersilene mesh implants. Otolaryngol. Head Neck Surg., *87*:515, 1979.

McEvitt, W. G.: Micrognathia and its management. Plast. Reconstr. Surg., *41*:450, 1968.

McEvitt, W. G.: Treatment of respiratory obstruction in micrognathia by use of a nasogastric tube. Plast. Reconstr. Surg., *52*:138, 1973.

McKenzie, J.: The first arch syndrome. Arch. Dis. Child., *33*:477, 1958.

McKenzie, J., and Craig, J.: Mandibulo-facial dysostosis (Treacher Collins syndrome). Arch. Dis. Child., *30*:391, 1955.

Menick, F. J., Furnas, D. W., and Achauer, B. M.: Lateral cervical advancement flaps for the correction of webbed-neck deformity. Plast. Reconstr. Surg., *73*:223, 1984.

Meyerson, M. D., Jensen, K. M., Meyers, J. M., and Hall, B. D.: Nager acrofacial dysostosis: early intervention and long-term planning. Cleft Palate J., *14*:35, 1977.

Monroe, C. W., and Ogo, K.: Treatment of micrognathia in the neonatal period. Plast. Reconstr. Surg., *50*:317, 1972.

Moore, K.: The Developing Human. 4th Ed. Philadelphia, W. B. Saunders Company, 1988.

Moore, W. B., Matthews, T. J., and Rabinowitz, R.: Genitourinary anomalies associated with Klippel-Feil syndrome. J. Bone Joint Surg., *57*:355, 1975.

Moorman-Voestermans, K., and Vos, A.: Bilateral

choanal atresia in two members of one family. J. Pediatr. Surg., *18*:175, 1983.

Morrison, S. G., Perry, L. W., and Scott, L. P., III: Congenital brevicollis (Klippel-Feil syndrome) and cardiovascular anomalies. Am. J. Dis. Child., *115*:614, 1968.

Moss, M. L.: Malformations of the skull base associated with cleft palate deformity. Plast. Reconstr. Surg., *17*:226, 1956.

Moss, M. L., and Crikelair, G. F.: Progressive facial hemiatrophy following cervical sympathectomy in the rat. Arch. Oral Biol., *1*:254, 1959.

Moura, R. A.: Progressive facial hemiatrophia; result of a case showing ocular and neuropthalmologic changes. Am. J. Ophthalmol., *55*:635, 1963.

Moyson, F.: A plea against tracheostomy in the Pierre Robin syndrome. Br. J. Plast. Surg., *14*:187, 1961.

Muchnick, R. S., Aston, S. J., and Rees, T. D.: Ocular manifestations and treatment of hemifacial atrophy. Am J. Ophthalmol., *88*:889, 1979.

Munro, I. R.: The ugly face—deformed but not defective. Can. Fam. Physician, *19*:57, 1973.

Munro, I. R.: Orbito-cranio-facial surgery: the team approach. Plast. Reconstr. Surg., *55*:170, 1975.

Nager, F. R., and de Reynier, J. P.: Das Gehorigen bei den angeboren Kopfmissbildungen. Pract. Otorhinolaryngol., (Suppl 2) *10*:1, 1948.

Nagib, M. G., Maxwell, R. E., and Chou, S. N.: Identification and management of high-risk patients with Klippel-Feil syndrome. J. Neurosurg., *61*:523, 1984.

Nagib, M. G., Maxwell, R. E., and Chou, S. N.: Klippel-Feil syndrome in children: clinical features and management. Child's Nerv. Syst., *1*:255, 1985.

Neidengard, L., Carter, T. E., and Smith, D. W.: Klippel-Feil malformation complex in fetal alcohol syndrome. Am. J. Dis. Child., *132*:929, 1978.

Neumann, C. G.: The use of large buried pedicled flaps of dermis and fat; clinical and pathological evaluation in the treatment of progressive facial hemiatrophy. Plast. Reconstr. Surg., *11*:315, 1953.

Nicolaides, D. K. H., Johansson, D., Donnai, D., and Rodeck, C. H.: Prenatal diagnosis of mandibulofacial dysostosis. Prenatal Diagn., *4*:201, 1984.

O'Connor, G. B., and Conway, M. E.: Treacher Collins syndrome (dysostosis mandibulo-facialis). Plast. Reconstr. Surg., *5*:419, 1950.

Oeconomopoulos, C. T.: The value of glossopexy in the Pierre Robin syndrome. N. Engl. J. Med., *262*:1267, 1960.

Onal, E., Lopata, M., and O'Connor, T.: Pathogenesis of apnea in hypersomnia–sleep apnea syndrome. Am. Rev. Respir. Dis., *125*:167, 1982.

Opitz, J. M., France, T., and Herrmann, J.: The Stickler syndrome (letter to editor). N. Engl. J. Med., *286*:546, 1972.

Osborne, G. S.: The prevalence of anomalies of the upper cervical vertebrae in patients with craniofacial malformations and their effect on osseous nasopharyngeal depth. Ph.D. Dissertation, Southern Illinois University, 1968.

Osborne, G. S., Pruzansky, S., and Koepp-Baker, H.: Upper cervical spine anomalies and osseous nasopharyngeal depth. J. Speech Hear. Res., *14*:14, 1971.

Osebold, W. R., and Winter, R. B.: Spinal dysplasia in Treacher Collins syndrome. A case report. Spine, *7*:516, 1982.

Osler, W.: The Principles and Practice of Medicine. New York, Appleton, 1918.

Parmalee, A. H.: Moulding due to intra-uterine posture; facial paralysis probably due to such moulding. Am. J. Dis. Child., *42*:1155, 1931.

Parry, C. H.: Collections from the Unpublished Medical Writings of the late Caleb Hillier Parry. London, Underwoods, 1825, p. 478.

Parsons, R. W., and Smith, D. J.: A modified tongue-lip adhesion for Pierre Robin anomalad. Cleft Palate J., *17*:144, 1980.

Parsons, R. W., and Smith, D. J.: Rule of thumb criteria for tongue-lip adhesion in Pierre Robin anomalad. Plast. Reconstr. Surg., *70*:210, 1982.

Pasyayan, H. M., and Lewis, M R.: Clinical experience with the Robin sequence. Cleft Palate J., *21*:270, 1984.

Patton, T. J., Thawley, S. E., Waters, R. C., Vandermeer, P. J., and Ogura, J. H.: Expansion hyoidplasty: a potential surgical procedure designed for selective patients with obstructive sleep apnea syndrome (experimental canine results). Laryngoscope, *93*:1387, 1983.

Pearlman, M. A., Brown, A. S., Barot, L. R., and Freed, G.: Polysomnographic indications for surgical intervention in Pierre Robin sequence: acute airway management and follow-up studies after palate repair and take-down of tongue-lip adhesions. Cleft Palate J., accepted for publication, 1987.

Pešková, H., and Stockar, B.: Hemiatrophia faciei progressiva: Romberg's disease. Acta Chir. Plast., *3*:276, 1961.

Pettersson, G.: Surgical treatment of Pierre Robin's syndrome. Acta Chir. Scand., *122*:480, 1961.

Phelps, P. D., Poswillo, D., and Lloyd, G. A. S.: The ear deformities in mandibulofacial dysostosis (Treacher Collins syndrome). Clin. Otolaryngol., *6*:15, 1981.

Pires de Lima, J. A., and Monteiro, H. B.: Aparelho branquial e saas perturbacoes evolutivas. Arq. Anat. e Antrop., *8*:185, 1923.

Ploner, L.: Dysostosis mandibulo-facialis. Fortschr. Kiefer. Gesichts-Chir., *4*:133, 1958.

Poswillo, D.: The pathogenesis of the Treacher Collins syndrome (mandibulofacial dysostosis). Br. J. Oral Surg., *13*:1, 1975.

Powell, N. B., Guilleminault, C., Riley, R. W., and Smith, L.: Mandibular advancement and obstructive sleep apnea syndrome. Bull. Eur. Physiopathol. Respir., *19*:607, 1983.

Pratt. A. E.: The Pierre Robin syndrome. Br. J. Radiol., *39*:390, 1966.

Pruzansky, S.: Postnatal development of craniofacial malformations. J. Dent. Res., *47*:936, 1968.

Pruzansky, S.: Not all dwarfed mandibles are alike. Proceedings of the First Conference on Clinical Delineation of Birth Defects. Part 2, Malformation syndromes. *In* Bergsma, D. (Ed.). Birth Defects, *2*:109, 1969.

Pruzansky, S., and Richmond, J. B.: Growth of the mandible in infants with micrognathia: clinical implications. Am. J. Dis. Child., *88*:29, 1954.

Randall, P., and Hamilton, R.: The Pierre Robin syndrome. *In* Grabb, W. C., Rosenstein, S. W., and Bzoch, K. R. (Eds.): Cleft Lip and Palate. Boston, Little,Brown & Company, 1971.

Randall, P., Krogman, W., and Jahina, S.: Mandibular growth in Pierre Robin syndrome. *In* Transactions of the 3rd International Congress of Plastic Surgery. Amsterdam, Excerpta Medica, 1964, p. 294.

Randall, P., Krogman, W., and Jahina, S.: Pierre Robin and the syndrome that bears his name. Cleft Pal. J., *2*:237, 1965.

Rankow, R. M., and Minervini, F.: Micrognathia in the newborn: Pierre Robin syndrome. Plast. Reconstr. Surg., 25:606, 1960.

Rapoport, D. M., Sarkin, B., Garay, S. M., and Goldring, R. M.: Reversal of the "pickwickian syndrome" by long-term use of nocturnal nasal-airway pressure. N. Engl. J. Med., 307:931, 1982.

Rechtschaffen, A., and Kales, A.: A manual of standardized terminology, techniques and scoring system for sleep stages of human subjects. Brain Information/Brain Research Institution. Los Angeles, University of California, 1968.

Rees, T. D.: Facial atrophy. Clin. Plast. Surg., 3:637, 1976.

Rees, T. D.: Personal communication, 1988.

Rees, T. D., Ashley, F. L., and Delgado, J. P.: Silicone fluid injections for facial atrophy: a ten-year study. Plast. Reconstr. Surg., 52:118, 1973.

Rees, T. D., Tabbal, N., and Aston, S. J.: Tongue-flap reconstruction of the lip vermilion in hemifacial atrophy. Plast. Reconstr. Surg., 72:643, 1983.

Remmers, J. E., DeGroot, W. J., and Sauerland, E. K.: Neural and mechanical factors controlling pharyngeal occlusion during sleep. *In* Guilleminault, C., and Dement, W. (Eds.): Sleep Apnea Syndrome. Vol. 2. New York, Alan R. Liss, 1978, pp. 211–218.

Richardson, M. A., Seid, A. B., Cotton, R. T., Benton, C., and Kramer, M.: Evaluation of tonsils and adenoids in sleep apnea syndrome. Laryngoscope, 90:1106, 1980.

Riley, R., Guilleminault, C., Powell, N., and Simmons, F. B.: Palatopharyngoplasty failure, cephalometric roentgenograms, and obstructive sleep apnea. Otolaryngol. Head Neck Surg., 93:240, 1985.

Riley, R., Powell, N., and Guilleminault, C.: Current surgical concepts for treating obstructive sleep apnea syndrome. J. Oral Maxillofac. Surg., 45:149, 1987.

Rintala, A., Ranta, R., and Stegars, T.: On the pathogenesis of cleft palate in the Pierre Robin syndrome. Scand. J. Plast. Reconstr. Surg., 18:237, 1984.

Roa, N. L., and Moss, K. S.: Treacher Collins syndrome with sleep apnoea; anaesthetic considerations. Anaesthesiology, 60:71, 1984.

Roberts, F. G., Pruzansky, S., and Aduss, H.: An X-radiocephalometric study of mandibulofacial dysostosis in man. Arch. Oral Biol., 20:265, 1975.

Robin, P.: Backward lowering of the root of the tongue causing respiratory disturbances. Bull. Acad. Med., 89:38, 1923a.

Robin, P.: Influence of facio-cranio-vertebral dysmorphosis on health in general. Bull. Acad. Med., 89:647, 1923b.

Robin, P.: De la rééducation respiratoire, chez le nourrisson par la tétée physiologique. Evolution Therap. Med. Chir., 7:521, 1926a.

Robin, P.: Rééducation morpho-fonctionnelle du massif faciocraniovertebral. Evolution Therap. Med. Chir., 7:529, 1926b.

Robin, P.: Deux observations sur la dénutrition des nourrissons atteints de glossoptose congénitale. J. Med. Paris, 45:1052, 1926c. (Also Med. Inf., 33:4, 1927.)

Robin, P.: La glossoptose chez le nourrisson; sa guérison par une nouvelle manière de faire téter. J. Med. Paris, 45:1011, 1926d. (Also Med. Inf., 32:366, 1926.)

Robin, P.: Enfant atteint de glossoptose congénitale en état de dénutrition par insuffisance alimentaire très rapidement ameliorée par la tétée orthostatique. Bull. Soc. Pediatr. Paris, 25:34, 1927a.

Robin, P.: Présentation d'enfants pour démontrer le rôle de la glossoptose dans certains déséquilibres de la vie organovégétative et physique. Bull. Soc. Pediatr. Paris, 25:267, 1927b.

Robin, P.: L'atrésie mandibulaire congénitale et son rôle aggravant dans l'évolution du rachitisme et de l'athrepsie. Bull. Soc. Pediatr. Paris, 26:85, 1928.

Robin, P.: Évolution du reflexe glossique des pronogrades aux orthogrades. Bull. Mem. Soc. Med. Paris, 1:35, 1929a.

Robin, P.: De la physiologie de la tétée au sein et de la forme que doit avoir la tétine du biberon. Bull. Soc. Pediatr. Paris, 27:55, 1929b.

Robin, P.: Evolution du reflexe glossique des pronogrades aux orthogrades. J. Med. Paris, 48:880, 1929c.

Robin, P.: La Glossoptose. Paris, Ash & Cie, 1929d.

Robin, P.: Glossoptosis due to atresia and hypotrophy of the mandible. Am. J. Dis. Child., 48:541, 1934.

Robin, P.: Les déformations maxillo-faciales et les malpositions des dents. Presse Med., 50:259, 1942.

Robin, P.: Obituary. Rev. Stomatol., 51:120, 1950.

Robin, P., and Samana, L.: Lutte contre la glossoptose. Marseille Med., 2:427, 1935.

Robinson, M., and Richardson, E. W.: Surgical orthodontic treatment of Treacher Collins syndrome; report of a case. J.A.D.A., 81:1143, 1970.

Rogers, B. O.: Rare craniofacial deformities. *In* Converse, J. M. (Ed.): Plastic and Reconstructive Surgery. 2nd Ed. Philadelphia, W. B. Saunders Company, 1977, p. 2296.

Rogers, B. O.: Berry-Treacher Collins syndrome: a review of 200 cases (mandibulofacial dysostosis; Franceschetti-Zwahlen-Klein syndrome). Br. J. Plast. Surg., 17:109, 1964b.

Rogers, B. O.: Progressive facial hemiatrophy: Romberg's disease; a review of 772 cases. *In* Transactions of the 3rd International Congress of Plastic Surgery. Amsterdam, Excerpta Medica, 1964c, p. 681.

Rogers, B. O.: The surgical treatment of mandibulofacial dysostosis (Berry syndrome; Treacher Collins syndrome; Franceschetti-Zwahlen-Klein syndrome). Clin. Plast. Surg., 3:653, 1976.

Rogers, B. O.: Mandibulofacial dysostosis. *In* Converse, J. M. (Ed.): Plastic and Reconstructive Surgery. 2nd Ed. Philadelphia, W. B. Saunders Company, 1977, p. 2401.

Romberg, M. H.: Klinische Ergebnisse. Berlin, A. Forstner, 1846, p. 75.

Ross, B.: Personal communication, 1986.

Ross, R. B., and Lindsay, W. K.: The cervical vertebrae as a factor in the etiology of cleft palate. Cleft Palate J., 2:273, 1965.

Roussel, F.: Contribution à l'étude de la dysostose mandibulo-faciale. Ann. Ocul., 184:788, 1951.

Routledge, R. T.: The Pierre Robin syndrome: a surgical emergency in the neonatal period. Br. J. Plast. Surg., 13:204, 1960.

Rovin, S., Dachi, S. F., Borenstein, D. B., and Cotter, W. B.: Mandibulofacial dysostosis; a familial study of 5 generations. J. Pediatr., 65:215, 1964.

Royster, H. P., and Graham, W. P., III: Simplified cervical esophagostomy for long-term extraoral feeding. Surg. Gynecol. Obstet., 125:127, 1967.

Rubin, A.: Handbook of Congenital Malformations. Philadelphia, W. B. Saunders Company, 1967, p. 243.

Ryan, R. F., Longenecker, C. G., Krust, L., and Vincent, R. W.: Anterior fixation of the tongue: a modification of the Douglas and Routledge techniques. Plast. Reconstr. Surg., 32:318, 1963.

Sadewitz, V. L., Goldbery, R. B., and Shprintzer, R. J.: The Robin sequence: an analysis of its heterogeneity. Presented to the American Cleft Palate Association. May 18, 1986.

Sagild, J. C., and Alving, J.: Hemiplegic migraine and progressive hemifacial atrophy. Ann. Neurol., *17*:620, 1985. (letter)

Sandblom, R. E., Matsumoto, A. M., Schoene, R. B., Lee, K. A., and Giblin, E. C.: Obstructive sleep apnea syndrome induced by testosterone administration. N. Engl. J. Med., *308*:508, 1983.

Sanders, M. H.: Nasal CPAP effect on patterns of sleep apnea. Chest, *86*:839, 1984.

Sanders, M. H., Moore, S. E., and Eveslage, J.: CPAP via nasal mask: a treatment for occlusive sleep apnea. Chest, *83*:144, 1983.

Sando, I., Hemenway, W. G., and Morgan, W. R.: Histopathology of the temporal bones in mandibulofacial dysostosis (Treacher Collins syndrome). Trans. Am. Acad. Ophthalmol. Otolaryngol., *72*:913, 1968.

Sanvenero-Rosselli, G.: Die angeborenen Gesichts und Kiefermissbildungen. Dtsch. Zahnarztl. Z., *3*:816, 1948.

Sassouni, V.: The Face in Five Dimensions. Philadelphia, Growth Center Publications, 1960.

Schafer, M. E.: Upper airway obstruction and sleep disorders in children with craniofacial anomalies. Clin. Plast. Surg., *9*:555, 1982.

Schatten, W. E., and Tidmore, T. L., Jr.: Airway management in patients with Pierre Robin syndrome. Plast. Reconstr. Surg., *38*:309, 1966.

Schild, J. A., Mafee, M. F., and Miller, M. F.: Wildervanck syndrome—the external appearance and radiologic findings. Int. J. Pediatr. Otorhinolaryngol., *7*:305, 1984.

Schott, G. D., and Wyke, M. A.: Congenital mirror movements. J. Neurol. Neurosurg. Psychiatry, *44*:586, 1981.

Schuller, D. E., Bardach, J., and Krause, C. J.: Irradiated homologous costal cartilage for facial contour restoration. Arch. Otolaryngol., *103*:12, 1977.

Schwartz, B. A., and Escande, J. P.: Etude cinéradiographique de la respiration hypnique pickwickienne. Rev. Neurol., *116*:677, 1967.

Schwartz, L.: Ateliosis of the mandibular arch; critical comment on glossoptosis, the syndrome of Pierre Robin. Arch. Otolaryngol., *31*:491, 1940.

Schwartz, R. A., Tedesco, A. S., Stern, L. Z., Kaminska, A. M., Haraldsen, J. M., and Grekin, D. A.: Myopathy associated with sclerodermal facial hemiatrophy. Arch. Neurol., *38*:592, 1981.

Serra, J. M., Muirragui, A., and Tadjalli, H.: The circumflex scapular flap for reconstruction of mandibulofacial atrophy. J. Reconstr. Microsurg., *1*:263, 1985.

Serson Neto, D. S.: Disotose mandibulo-facial. O. Hospital, *51*:333, 1957.

Shah, C. V., Pruzansky, S., and Harris, W. S.: Cardiac malformations with facial clefts; with observations on the Pierre Robin syndrome. Am. J. Dis. Child., *119*:238, 1970.

Shearin, J. C., Jr., and DeFranzo, A. J.: Butterfly correction of webbed-neck deformity in Turner's syndrome. Plast. Reconstr. Surg., *66*:129, 1980.

Shintomi, Y., Ohura, T., Honda, K., and Iida, K.: The reconstruction of progressive facial hemi-atrophy by free vascularised dermis-fat flaps. Br. J. Plast. Surg., *34*:398, 1981.

Shprintzen, R. J., Croft, C., Berkman, M. D., and Rakoff, S. J.: Pharyngeal hypoplasia in Treacher Collins syndrome. Arch. Otolaryngol., *105*:127, 1979.

Shukowsky, W. P.: Zur Atiologie des Stridor inspiratorius congenitus. Jahrb. Kinderheilk., *73*:459, 1911.

Simmons, F. B., Guilleminault, C., and Miles, L.: The palatopharyngoplasty operation for snoring and sleep apnea: an interim report. Otolaryngol. Head Neck Surg., *192*:375, 1984.

Simmons, F. B., Guilleminault, C., and Silvestri, R.: Snoring and some obstructive sleep apnea can be cured by oropharyngeal surgery. Arch. Otolaryngol., *109*:503, 1983.

Sjolin, S.: Hypoplasia of the mandible as a cause of respiratory difficulties in an infant. Acta Paediatr., *39*:255, 1950.

Sklar, G. S., and Benton, D. K.: Endotracheal intubation and Treacher Collins syndrome. Anaesthesiology, *44*:247, 1976.

Smith, B., and Guberina, C.: Coloboma in progressive hemifacial atrophy. Am. J. Ophthalmol., *84*:85, 1977.

Smith, J. D.: Treatment of airway obstruction in Pierre Robin syndrome. A modified lip-tongue adhesion. Arch. Otolaryngol., *107*:419, 1980.

Smith, J. L., Cavanaugh, J. J., and Stowe, F. R.: Ocular manifestations of the Pierre Robin syndrome. A.M.A. Arch. Ophthalmol., *63*:984, 1960.

Smith, J. L., and Stowe, F. C.: The Pierre Robin syndrome (glossoptosis, micrognathia, cleft palate). A review of thirty-nine cases with emphasis on associated ocular lesions. Pediatrics, *27*:128, 1961.

Smith, P. L., Haponik, E. F., Allen, R. P., and Bleecker, E. R.: The effects of protriptyline in sleep-disordered breathing. Am. Rev. Respir. Dis., *127*:8, 1983.

Snyder, C. C.: Bilateral facial agenesia (Treacher Collins syndrome). Am. J. Surg., *92*:81, 1956.

Sokar, P., Chamyal, P. C., Kalra, S. K., and Vatwani, V.: Treacher Collins syndrome. J. Ind. Med. Assoc., *75*:221, 1980.

Steiff, A.: About a case of facial hemiatrophy with a dissection report. Z. Ges. Neurol. Psychiat., *147*:573, 1933.

Stenström, S. J., and Sundmark, E. S.: Contribution of the treatment of the eyelid deformities in dysostosis mandibulofacialis. Plast. Reconstr. Surg., *38*:567, 1966.

Stickler, G. B., Belau, P. G., Farrell, F. J., et al.: Hereditary progressive arthro-ophthalmopathy. Mayo Clin. Proc., *40*:433, 1965.

Stool, S.E., Campbell, J. R., and Johnson, D. G.: Tracheostomy in children: the use of plastic tubes. J. Pediatr. Surg., *3*:402, 1968.

Stool, S. E., Eavey, R. D., Stein, N. L., and Sharrar, W. G.: The "chubby puffer" syndrome. Clin. Pediatr., *16*:43, 1977.

Stovin, J. J., Lyon, J. A., and Clemmens, R. L.: Mandibulofacial dysostosis. Am. J. Roentgenol., *74*:225, 1960.

Straith, C. L., and Lewis, J. R.: Associated congenital defects of the ears, eyelids and malar bones (Treacher Collins syndrome). Plast. Reconstr. Surg., *4*:204, 1949.

Streiff, E. B., Rosselet, E., and Jequier, M.: Hemiatrophie faciale progressive (syndrome de Romberg) et colobome de l'uvée. Bull. Mem. Soc. Fr. Ophthalmol., *68*:207, 1955.

Stuart, R. E., and Prescott, G. H. (Eds.): Oral Facial Genetics. St. Louis, C. V. Mosby Company, p. 528, 1976.

Sugar, H. S., and Banks, T. L.: Fuchs' heterochromic cyclitis associated with facial hemiatrophy (scleroderma en coup de sabre). Am. J. Ophthalmol., *57*:627, 1964.

Sugerman, H. J., Fairman, R. P., Lindeman, A. K., Mathers, J. A., and Greenfield, L. J.: Gastroplasty for respiratory insufficiency of obesity. Ann. Surg., *193*:677, 1981.

Sullivan, C. E., Berthon-Jones, M., Issa, F. G., and Eves, L.: Reversal of obstructive sleep apnoea by continuous positive airway pressure applied through the nares. Lancet, *1*:862, 1981.

Sweet, A. M., and Kemsley, M.: Micrognathia. Lancet, *2*:10, 1947.

Szlazak, J.: Treacher Collins syndrome. Can. Med. Assoc. J., *69*:274, 1953.

Takagi, Y., McCalla, J. L., and Bosma, J. F.: Prone feeding of infants with the Pierre Robin syndrome. Cleft Palate J., *3*:232, 1966.

Tessier, P.: Vertical and oblique facial clefts (orbitofacial fissures). *In* Mustardé, J. D. (Ed.): Plastic Surgery in Infancy and Childhood. Edinburgh, Churchill Livingstone, 1971, p. 94.

Tessier, P.: Plastic Surgery of the Orbit and Eyelids. New York, Masson, 1981, pp. 169, 170.

Tessier, P.: Autogenous bone grafts taken from the calvarium for facial and cranial applications. Clin. Plast. Surg., *9*:531, 1982.

Tessier, P., and Tulasne, J-F.: Craniofacial surgery update. *In* Habal, M. B. (Ed.): Advances in Plastic and Reconstructive Surgery. Vol. 2. Chicago, Year Book Medical Publishers, 1986, p. 30.

Trasler, D. G.: Influence of uterine site on occurrence of spontaneous cleft lip in mice. Science, *132*:420, 1960.

Tweed, A. E. J., Manktelow, R. T., and Zuker, R. M.: Facial contour reconstruction with free flaps. Ann. Plast. Surg., *12*:313, 1984.

Tyrrell, F. A. C.: 7. Congenital malformation of the lower lid. Trans. Ophthalmol. Soc. U.K., *23*:263, 1903.

Upton, J., Mulliken, J. B., Hicks, P. D., and Murray, J. E.: Restoration of facial contour using free vascularized omental transfer. Plast. Reconstr. Surg., *66*:560, 1980.

van der Meulen, J. C. H., Hauben, D. J., Vaandrager, J. M., and Birgenhager-Frenkel, D. H.: The use of a temporal osteoperiosteal flap for the reconstruction of malar hypoplasia in Treacher Collins syndrome. Plast. Reconstr. Surg., *74*:687, 1984.

Vatré, J. L.: Étude génétique et classification clinique de 154 cases de dysostose mandibulo-faciale (syndrome de Franceschetti), avec description de leurs associations malformatives. J. Genet. Hum., *19*:17, 1971.

Walker, D. G.: Malformations of the Face. Edinburgh, E. & S. Livingstone, 1961.

Walkinshaw, M., Caffee, H. H., and Wolfe, S. A.: Vascularized omentum for facial contour restoration. Ann. Plast. Surg., *10*:292, 1983.

Wallace, J. G., Schneider, W. J., Brown, R. G., and Nahai, F. M.: Reconstruction of hemifacial atrophy with a free flap of omentum. Br. J. Plast. Surg., *32*:15, 1979.

Wang, M. K. H., and Macomber, W. B.: Personal communication, 1963.

Watson-Jones, R.: The repair of skull defects by a new pedicle bone-graft operation. Br. Med. J., *1*:780, 1933.

Weed, L. H.: Development of cerebro-spinal spaces in pig and in man. Washington, Carnegie Institute, 1917.

Weisengreen, H. H., and Sorsky, E. D.: Congenital hypoplasia of the mandible. J. Pediatr., *16*:482, 1940.

Wells, J. H., and Edgerton, M. T.: Correction of severe hemifacial atrophy with a free dermis-fat flap from the lower abdomen. Plast. Reconstr. Surg., *59*:223, 1979.

Whitaker, L. A., Katowitz, J. A., and Jacobs, W. E.: Ocular adnexal problems in craniofacial deformities. J. Maxillofac. Surg., *7*:55, 1979.

Wiflingseder, P.: Treatment of mandibular facial dysostosis. S. Afr. Med. J., *31*:1296, 1957.

Wildervanck, L. S.: Een geval van aandoening van Klippel-Feil gecombineerd met abducensparalyse, retractio bulbi en doofst omheid. Ned. Tijdschr. Geneeskd., *96*:2752, 1952.

Wildervanck, L. S.: Een cervico-oculo-acusticus syndrome. Ned. Tijdschr. Geneeskd., *104*:2600, 1960.

Willemsen, W. N.: Combination of the Mayer-Rokitansky-Küster and Klippel-Feil syndrome—a case report and literature review. Eur. J. Obstet. Gynecol. Reprod. Biol., *13*:229, 1982.

Windle-Taylor, P. C., Emery, P. J., and Phelps, P. D.: Ear deformities associated with the Klippel-Feil syndrome. Ann. Otol. Rhinol. Laryngol., *90*:210, 1981.

Witzel, M. A.: North American Working Group on Cleft Palate and Craniofacial Anomalies. September 17–19, 1986.

Woolf, R. M., Georgiade, N., and Pickrell, K. L.: Micrognathia and associated cleft palate (Pierre Robin syndrome). Plast. Reconstr. Surg., *26*:199, 1960.

Zins, J. E., and Whitaker, L. A.: Membranous versus endochondral bone autografts: implications for craniofacial reconstruction. Surg. Forum, *30*:521, 1979.

Gottfried Lemperle

Down Syndrome

Langdon Down, in 1866, attempting to categorize mentally retarded persons according to their ethnic background, first proposed the term "mongolism" to describe those individuals with short stature, mental deficiency, and mongolian features. Comprehensive reviews of Down syndrome were provided by Brousseau in 1928 and Øster in 1953. The chronology of mongolism was concisely documented by Smith and Beig in 1976.

The discovery by Lejeune, Turpin, and Gautier in 1959 that Down syndrome was due to a chromosome abnormality, e.g., the presence of 47 chromosomes, has reduced the diagnostic significance of the clinical characteristics. In 91 per cent of cases, an extra small chromosome is present on the 21st pair of chromosomes. This chromosome abnormality is labeled more specifically as trisomy 21 and develops as a result of nondisjunction of two homologous chromosomes during either the first or second meiotic division. Approximately 3 to 4 per cent of individuals also have a chromosomal abnormality known as a *translocation* in which there is breakage of two nonhomologous chromosomes, with subsequent reattachment of the broken pieces to other intact chromosome pairs. The risk of the birth of a second child with Down syndrome to parents who are translocation carriers varies from 2 to 10 per cent, making the risk of recurrence much greater than with the nondisjunction type of trisomy 21. The remaining 4 per cent of cases represent *mosaic* disorders in which some cells within the individual are normal and some are trisomy 21. The children with "mosaicism" tend to be of higher intelligence but still display typical mongoloid features.

Epidemiologic studies have shown that Down syndrome occurs once in every 660 live births. There is an incidence of approximately 1 per 1000 births in the maternal age group up to 35 years, 15 per 1000 in the age group 35 to 39 years, and 35 per 1000 in mothers over 45 years of age (Adams and associates, 1981). Awareness of this fact has accounted for a 26 per cent reduction in the total incidence of Down syndrome and a 43 per cent reduction in the number of cases in the United States since 1960 (Adams and associates, 1981). However, Down syndrome remains the most frequently identified cause of major mental handicap. Of an annual number of approximately 3000 children born with Down syndrome in the United States, 80 per cent are born to mothers under 35 years of age.

While increased maternal age appears to be associated with nondisjunction of the chromosomes, the exact reason for this finding remains speculative. Advanced paternal age has also been implicated as a factor contributing to an increased risk of giving birth to a child with Down syndrome. This aspect, however, can be neglected since subsequent statistics failed to show such a relation (Ferguson-Smith and Yates, 1984). There is no justification at present for using increased paternal age as a sole indication for amniocentesis and prenatal chromosome analysis. Nevertheless, it is important to know that the extra chromosome 21 originates in 25 per cent of cases from the father, independent of his age.

PATHOLOGY

Immunologic Defects

The high mortality rate in infancy is well established. Studies indicate that about 50 per cent of all living neonates with Down syndrome die before the age of 1 year, mainly from respiratory obstruction, pneumonia, and congenital heart disease (Carter, 1958). There have been several studies on the possibility of immunologic deficiency in these children (Barkin and associates, 1980), showing a reduced leukocyte bactericidal capacity, polycythemia, eosinopenia, and sometimes a leukemia-like syndrome. Responsiveness of lymphocytes to phytohemagglutinin (PHA) stimulation is reduced; on the other hand, these children show a high frequency of autoantibodies directed against the pituitary gland.

Before the availability of antibiotic therapy, persons with Down syndrome rarely lived beyond 20 years. They died of tuberculosis, of pneumonia, or in early "midlife" from premature senility, an atrophy of brain cells similar to that observed in Alzheimer's dementia (Jervis, 1948).

Neuropathology

A large number of neuropathologic findings have been described in the literature of Down syndrome (Øster, 1953). An abnormal development of a small brachycephalic skull has been observed. The cranial base is characterized by significant flattening known as "platybasia," a finding similar to that observed in nonhuman primates (Michejda and Menolascino, 1975).

The overall brain weight of individuals with Down syndrome averages 76 per cent of that of normal individuals. The combined weight of the cerebellum and brain stem is proportionately even smaller—an average of 66 per cent of their combined weight in normal individuals (Crome, 1965).

Other gross neuropathologic findings include the more rounded shape of the brains, which may be secondary to the brachycephaly. The brains of infants with Down syndrome also show smaller convolutions than those of normal infants, indicating a relative neurologic immaturity.

Cardiovascular Anomalies

Congenital heart defects are common in individuals with Down syndrome. Cardiac anomalies were present in 60 per cent of those in whom autopsies were performed. The two most common cardiac anomalies were atrioventricular canal defects and ventriculoseptal defects. Most congenital heart defects can be successfully repaired today in these children.

Sensory Deficits

Another common medical problem that may indirectly influence the child's response to educational therapy is hearing loss. In a study of 107 individuals with Down syndrome, binaural hearing loss was noted in 64 per cent of those tested (Balkany and associates, 1979). Otitis media is a frequently recurring medical problem that contributes to hearing deficiencies in these individuals.

Voice quality deviations, as exhibited by breathiness and resonance disability in the form of hypernasality, have been studied by Rolfe and associates (1979). While the velum appeared to make normal closure against the nasopharynx during the production of oral phonemes, structural and possible timing variations of the soft palate may account for the perceived hypernasality. In addition, the mild hearing loss may also affect fine velopharyngeal timing movements (Strome, 1988).

Visual defects are also much more common than in the general population. Strabismus (usually esotropia) was reported in 41.3 per cent of a sample of 75 institutionalized individuals with Down syndrome (Jaeger, 1980). Nystagmus, cataracts, and myopia were also frequently observed. Other ocular findings of less clinical significance were the presence of Brushfield's spots in the iris, and the characteristic upward and outward slanting of the palpebral fissures. The presence of epicanthal folds—a classic clinical diagnostic feature of Down syndrome—was noted in only 17.3 per cent of adults with Down syndrome (Jaeger, 1980), but in up to 60 per cent of children below the age of 10 years.

Farkas, Munro, and Kolar (1985) found short palpebral fissures in 68.8 per cent, a shallow upper third of the face depth in 71.5 per cent, hyperteloric orbits in 40.4 per cent, and disproportionately short noses in 28.9 per cent.

Hypotonia

One of the most prominent diagnostic features at birth is generalized hypotonia. Particularly evident during the early years, the hypotonia is probably a major contributing factor to the significant motor delay characterizing the period of infancy and early childhood in children with Down syndrome.

A number of orthopedic problems such as pes planus and subluxation of the patella, hip, and atlantoaxial joints occurring in these children have been attributed to severe ligamentous laxity.

CORRECTIVE SURGERY

Children with Down syndrome may be unaware of their different appearance and are in general, happy with it. It is the parents who are disturbed by the differences between their child and others and who often approach the plastic surgeon to seek corrective treatment. In addition, the increased life expectation, due to improved health care, has led to new challenges such as vocational training, social integration, and sexual maturation. These factors increase the importance of improving appearance, which is much easier to correct than deficiencies in schoolwork or in sports. There are, however, other areas where plastic surgery can be of help, notably in the functional improvement of the tongue, and therefore of speech.

In the Down syndrome patient there are a number of characteristic facial features (Fig. 64–1) which can be improved or corrected by fairly simple surgical means:

1. Epicanthus (mongoloid fold).
2. Oblique lid axis (slanting eye).
3. Strabismus (unilateral squinting).
4. Hypoplastic nose (saddle nose).
5. Hypoplastic jaw bones (dish face).
6. Macroglossia (large hypotonic tongue).
7. Lip ectropion (hypotonic lower lip).
8. Microgenia (receding chin).

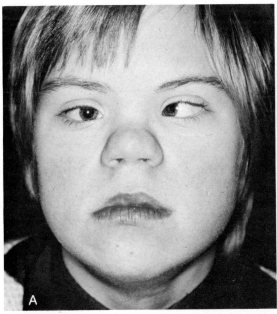 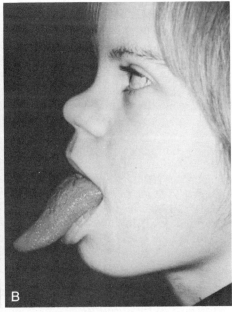

Figure 64–1. Typical features of Down syndrome in a 12 year old girl. *A,* Frontal view. Note the zygomatic hypoplasia, flat nasal dorsum, unilateral esodeviation, and upward slanting of the palpebral apertures. *B,* Lateral view, demonstrating the macroglossia.

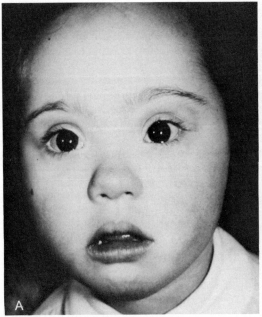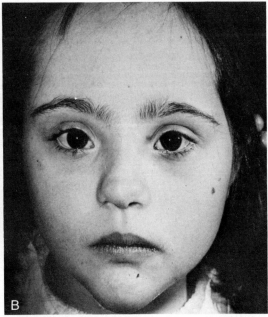

Figure 64–2. Five year old girl with Down syndrome. *A*, Preoperative appearance. *B*, Postoperative view after augmentation of nose and chin with polyethylene implants (Höhler, 1977).

9. Submental fat collection (double chin).
10. Protruding ears (cockleshell ears).

In addition to the congenital mental handicap of varying degrees, these children present a thickset stature, dry skin, generalized muscular hypotonia, hyperextensibility of the joints, the well-known simian palmar crease, and the sandal gap between the first and second toes.

In 1967, Otermin Aguirre (1968) presented the first series of Down syndrome patients who underwent surgical correction. In the same year, Höhler (reported in 1977) reconstructed a child with Down syndrome by augmenting her hypoplastic nose and receding chin with polyethylene implants (Fig. 64–2).

In 1977, Lemperle (Lemperle and Radu, 1980) initiated surgical reconstruction on a larger series of children with Down syndrome (Table 64–1). Reports by Olbrisch (1982), Regenbrecht (1983), Wexler and Peled (1983), and Rozner (1983) followed. The ages of the children ranged from 2 to 22 years, most being between 4 and 8 years of age.

Functional Corrections

Hypotonia of the Tongue. Apart from the associated mental retardation, the delayed speech development of children with Down syndrome may also be caused by the ease with which they become fatigued as well as by the well-known muscular hypotonia. As in patients with muscular dystrophy, the body may try to overcome diminished tongue muscle function by a compensatory muscular hypertrophy. The large tongue of patients with Down syndrome does not form a concave dish with its upper border connecting with the maxillary molars, but lies like a convex loaf of bread in the oral cavity (Fig. 64–3).

Castillo-Morales and associates (1982) developed a palatal device with a central knob 8 mm in diameter and 3 mm in height (Fig. 64–4). The child is forced to move his tongue constantly in an attempt to clear the pros-

Table 64–1. Operations in 276 Children with Down Syndrome (Frankfurt 1977–1985)

		Percentage
Tongue reductions	250	90
Nasal implants	91	33
Epicanthal fold	70	25
Lid axis	53	23
Chin implants	34	12
Malar implants	22	8
Lower lip excisions	16	6
Protruding ears	12	4
Double chin liposuction	3	1

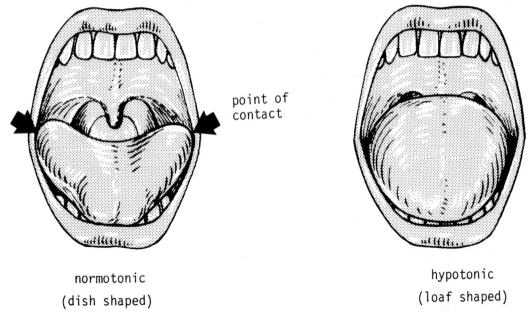

normotonic

(dish shaped)

point of contact

hypotonic

(loaf shaped)

Figure 64–3. Tongue shape in a normal and in a Down syndrome child.

thesis. The palatal plate is worn 24 hours a day, except during meals, for at least one year. It can be applied to infants from the second month of life and can be worn until puberty. It is fitted every three months by the prosthodontist and corrected, when necessary, by appropriate enlarging or repositioning.

Macroglossia. Protrusion of the tongue is a well-known feature of Down syndrome. It tends to improve spontaneously in children with a normal tongue size as they grow older. It is only when the oropharyngeal space is small that the tongue actually protrudes. The typical type of oral hypotonia is characterized by an open mouth, drooling, and cracked lips.

However, at least 50 per cent (Øster, 1953) of patients have true macroglossia, i.e., a broad, flabby, fissured hypotonic tongue that is a handicap in speaking, chewing, and even drinking (Fig. 64–5).

In most patients the protruding tongue has to be reduced by a large rhomboid excision of the anterior third (Fig. 64–6A). In those with a broad-based tongue, the wedge-shaped excision must extend dorsally like a gothic arch to the papillae. Care must be taken that at least 3 cm of the frenulum remains to avoid a roundness of the tongue tip. The patient should be able to reach the entire prolabium with the tip of the tongue to prevent saliva accumulation, crusting, and subsequent chei-

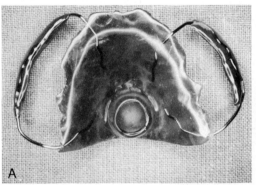
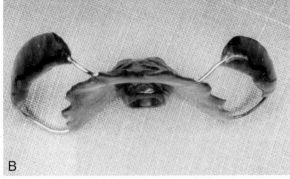

Figure 64–4. *A,* Palatal device according to Castillo-Morales and associates (1982). *B,* The disturbing knob of the palatal plate.

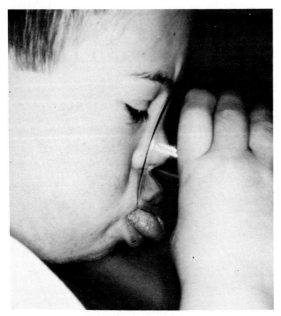

Figure 64–5. Disturbance of drinking by macroglossia.

losis (Fig. 64–6*B*). The various types of tongue reduction procedures are illustrated in Figure 64–7.

After careful hemostasis, the wound margins are coapted in two layers with interrupted sutures, followed by a continuous suture, avoiding any loop at the tip of the tongue. The tongue is initially edematous but will assume its final size only after six to 12 weeks.

The success of the tongue reduction is best documented by the fact that most of the children suddenly keep their mouths closed (Fig. 64–8). It is precisely the open, moist mouth with the protruding and oversized tongue that is the most striking sign of mental deficiency. Moreover, the speech, which previously was slurred and inarticulate, becomes much more intelligible owing to the enlarged intraoral resonance box, which in turn leads to improved communication skills.

If macroglossia is repaired in children before the eruption of the permanent teeth, the surgery can probably help to prevent a later orthodontic problem. Frequently, the mandible is so widened by the oversized tongue that, in conjunction with the hypotonia of the lips, there is an anterior crossbite. However, because of the high rate of malposition of the teeth of these children, and because of their susceptibility to caries resulting from the absence of lip closure, later orthodontic treatment may be unavoidable.

Strabismus. At least one-third of all children with Down syndrome have an obvious unilateral strabismus (see Fig. 64–1). Since this is a rather disturbing feature in communication with any child, one should counsel the parents to seek operative treatment by an ophthalmic surgeon (Jaeger, 1980).

Airway Obstruction. There can be respiratory problems in children with Down syndrome even if the tongue is not enlarged. In some, the maxilla and mandible may be increased in size by the pressure of the tongue. On the other hand, children with macroglossia tend to sleep in the prone or lateral decubitus position: e.g., they bring the back of the tongue forward and widen the pharyn-

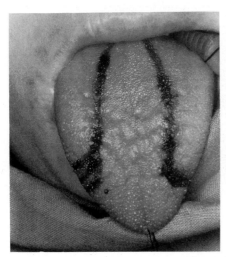
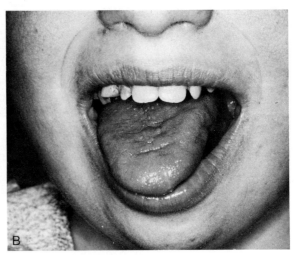

Figure 64–6. *A,* Typical "lingua plicata." Rhomboid excision in the shape of a Gothic arch. *B,* Postoperative result.

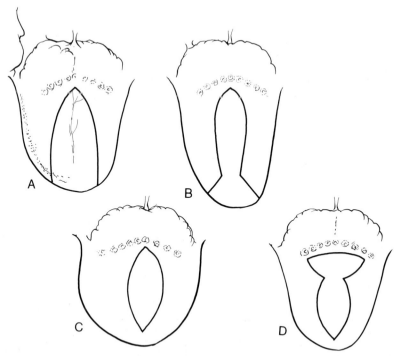

Figure 64–7. Different types of tongue resection. *A,* Standard excision (Bjuggren, Jensen, and Strömbeck, 1968). *B,* Large excision in a long tongue (Egyedi and Obwegeser, 1964). *C,* Type of excision in a broad but short tongue (Edgerton, 1960). *D,* Type of excision in a small tongue (Köle, 1965).

Figure 64–8. Six year old girl with open mouth and protruding tongue. *A,* Preoperative appearance. *B,* Following partial tongue resection, and nasal and chin augmentation. (From Lemperle, G., and Radu, D.: Facial plastic surgery in children with Down's syndrome. Plast. Reconstr. Surg., *66:*337, 1980.)

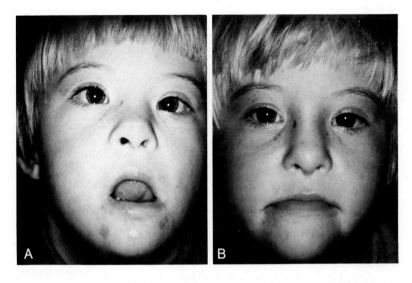

geal airway. In order to relieve possible obstructive sleep apnea, Strome (1988) devised a modified pharyngopalatoplasty for Down syndrome children.

When the adenoids and tonsils are bulky, they should be removed (Ardran, Harker, and Kemp, 1972), thus allowing mouth closure and normal jaw growth.

One can also observe small external nares, hyperplastic turbinates, and occasionally a thickened nasal septum, all of which may further aggravate the airway obstruction caused by an enlarged tongue. Surgical removal of the airway obstructions may also help many of the children to overcome recurrent throat infections.

Esthetic Improvement

The following esthetic corrections can be performed under local or general anesthesia in a single operation.

Saddle Nose. The hypoplastic nasal dorsum can be augmented by insertion of a silicone implant through a vestibular incision (Fig. 64–9). In order to reduce the epicanthus, one tends to insert an oversized implant in smaller children (see Fig. 64–8).

Among 78 children with silicone nasal implants, three could twist their implant around its longitudinal axis. This problem is caused by the typical laxity of connective tissue of these children, but can be solved by a non-

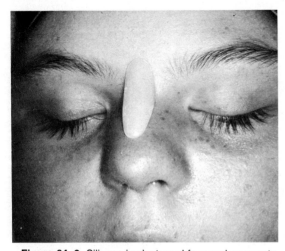

Figure 64–9. Silicone implant used for nasal augmentation. (From Lemperle, G., and Radu, D.: Facial plastic surgery in children with Down's syndrome. Plast. Reconstr. Surg., *66*:337, 1980.)

resorbable fixation suture in the glabellar region. Infected implants, observed in five of 78 children (Lemperle and Spitalny, 1985), must be temporarily removed but can be reinserted four to six weeks later. Alternative implants such as Cialit-preserved allograft cartilage (Olbrisch, 1982), autogenous rib cartilage, or bone graft from the iliac crest are dependent on the individual experience of the surgeon.

Augmentation of the nasal dorsum is also discussed in Chapter 35.

Epicanthus. In most persons with epicanthus, the skin fold appears to be continuous with the tarsal fold when observed in forward gaze. In the true Oriental fold, the epicanthal portion generally remains continuous with the lid fold on downward gaze. However, in Down syndrome the downward gaze often reveals that the fold originates from the orbital portion of the lid, extends in various degrees of curvature to the base of the nose, or blends into the lower lid below the canthus (Fig. 64–10A).

In most cases, the epicanthus is reduced by augmenting the bridge of the nose by a silicone or autogenous implant. Thus, an additional Z-plasty (Fig. 64–10B) above the inner canthus becomes necessary only if the epicanthus is very pronounced or if a nasal implant would greatly impair the profile. However, if the epicanthus extends inferiorly into the lower lid, a more sophisticated Z-plasty according to the technique of del Campo (1984) is the method of choice.

Slanting Palpebral Aperture. The characteristic upward and outward slanting of the palpebral aperture is obvious in more than half of all patients with Down syndrome (Fig. 64–11).

The lateral canthal mechanism is attached to the orbital rim by no more than an ill-defined condensation of connective tissue at the origin of the orbicularis oculi muscles (see Chap. 33). The lateral canthal mechanism contrasts, therefore, with the well-defined medial canthal ligament. In children with Down syndrome there may be an additional shortage of skin and orbicularis muscle in the lateral third of the upper lid, owing to the higher location of the lateral canthal mechanism. By raising a triangular segment of the suspected lateral ligament, one should separate the skin and muscle of the shortened upper lid by subcutaneous blunt dissection until the lateral canthal mechanism is mobile

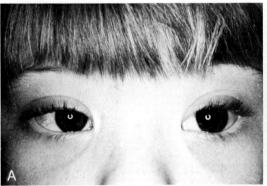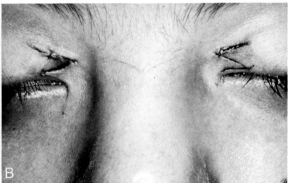

Figure 64–10. Epicanthal fold in a 5 year old boy with Down syndrome. *A,* Preoperative appearance. *B,* After nasal implant and Z-plasty. (From Lemperle, G., and Radu, D.: Facial plastic surgery in children with Down's syndrome. Plast. Reconstr. Surg., *66:*337, 1980.)

(Fig. 64–12). This portion is then sutured to the periosteum of the lower aspect of the orbital rim in a strongly overcorrected position with a nonresorbable 4-0 suture (see also Chap. 33). A more complicated canthoplasty as reported by Marsh and Edgerton (1979) does not seem to be necessary in children with Down syndrome.

Lateral canthoplasty techniques are also discussed in Chapter 33.

Hypoplasia of Malar Bones. Some children with Down syndrome have rather flat zygomas that are complementary to the generalized underdevelopment of the craniofacial skeleton. However, in selected cases an augmentation of the malar bones with silicone implants (Fig. 64–13) improves facial appearance (Hinderer, 1975). A 3 cm incision in the skin of the lower lid is preferred to the oral route, since the subperiosteal pocket prevents any downward movement of the implant. The pocket should be developed by sharp dissection with rasping directly on the bone in order to prevent later mobility. There have been no cases of distortion, infection, or extrusion of the malar implants in the author's series.

Augmentation of the zygomatic complex is also discussed in Chapter 33.

Hypotonia of Lower Lip. A hanging lower lip is almost typical of young children with Down syndrome and is an expression of easy fatigue. As they grow older, this finding disappears spontaneously. The tone of the orbicularis oris muscle can be improved by physiotherapy or speech therapy, or simply by having the patient practice holding a heavy coin between the lips.

If there is a true ectropion of the lower lip, a wedge-shaped excision in the sagittal direction can be performed. In combination with simultaneous tongue reduction and mentoplasty, this technique has resulted in the

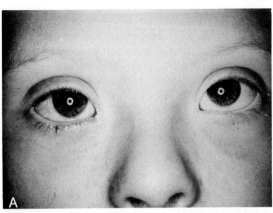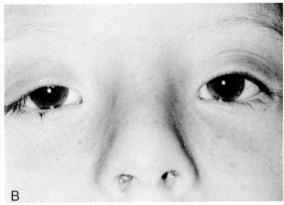

Figure 64–11. Oblique lid axis in a young patient with Down syndrome. *A,* Preoperative view. *B,* After lowering the lateral canthal mechanism.

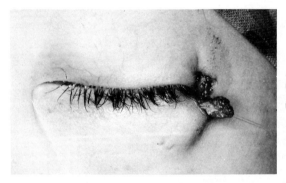

Figure 64–12. Technique of fixation of the lateral canthal mechanism to the orbital rim.

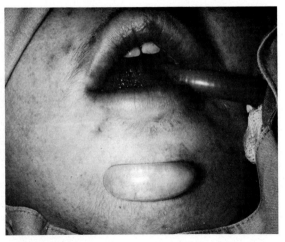

Figure 64–14. Technique of insertion of a chin implant through the labial mucosa. (From Lemperle, G., and Radu, D.: Facial plastic surgery in children with Down's syndrome. Plast. Reconstr. Surg., *66*:337, 1980.)

most significant improvement in some children's facial appearance.

Microgenia. Despite a prognathic jaw relationship, Shapiro (1970) reported that over 60 per cent of children or adults with Down syndrome lack chin projection.

A small chin becomes even more pronounced through the protrusion of teeth. The simplest method to augment it is to insert a commercial silicone implant (Fig. 64–14). Through an incision in the labiogingival fold, the pocket is made subperiosteally by sharp dissection. Frequently this procedure also helps to make the fleshy or thick neck and double chin less conspicuous (Fig. 64–15).

Chin augmentation is also discussed in Chapter 29.

Submental Fat Collection. Some children lack a satisfactory profile relationship be-

tween the chin and the neck. Since the subcutaneous masses in the neck region are not localized, excision of fat is difficult and not advisable. Further improvement, however, may be obtained in the submental and submandibular area by the use of liposuction (see Chap. 81).

Protruding Ears. Approximately 25 per cent of children with Down syndrome have protruding ears. Since most of these children have a rather broad face, the ears are even more conspicuous and tend to make the child look less intelligent. They can be corrected by one of the many available methods (see Chap. 40).

Craniofacial Surgery

The craniofacial skeleton of children with Down syndrome demonstrates certain characteristics. The underdeveloped midface, the flat palatal vault, and the reduced space of the oral cavity are the probable causes of a relative macroglossia.

In a review of the author's first 250 children with Down syndrome, there were only eight cases with obvious exophthalmos, severe malar deficiency, and anterior crossbite that might be corrected with a midface advancement. Tschopp (1983) described a young patient in whom he advanced the midface, with a satisfactory result; the reduced nasopharyngeal space was also expanded. Caronni (1985)

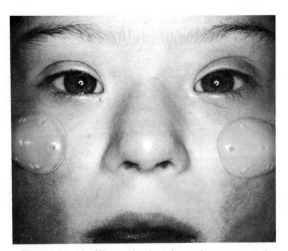

Figure 64–13. Silicone implant for malar augmentation according to Hinderer (1975). (From Lemperle, G., and Radu, D.: Facial plastic surgery in children with Down's syndrome. Plast. Reconstr. Surg., *66*:337, 1980.)

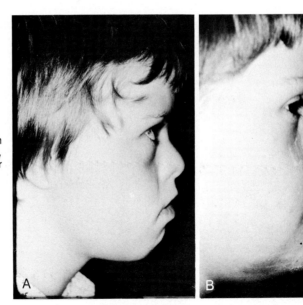

Figure 64–15. Eight year old boy with Down syndrome and a receding chin. *A,* Preoperative profile. *B,* Appearance four days after chin and nasal augmentation.

performed a Le Fort III advancement on a Down syndrome patient with severe exophthalmos and corneal opacification, and achieved satisfactory lid closure. Munro (1988) has treated five older patients among a series of 79 children with Down syndrome by maxillary advancement, with improvement in facial appearance and oral resonance. The use of miniplate fixation in stabilizing the osteotomized segment is a great improvement over intermaxillary fixation, especially in this impaired population.

Whether or not the mental deficiency observed in these children is caused secondarily by premature closure of cranial sutures similar to the condition in Apert's and Crouzon's syndromes (Marchac and Renier, 1982) has yet to be proved. Many children with Down syndrome have a flat skull and a brachycephaly without evidence of increased intracranial pressure. Careful radiographic examination of infants with Down syndrome (Roche, Roche, and Lewis, 1972) reveals some cases that may benefit from surgical expansion of the posterior or anterior cranial fossae (Marchac and Renier, 1982).

Complications

In some children, suture dehiscence occurred at the tip of the tongue between the third and the sixth postoperative days. This requires secondary suturing. The cause may be a severance of the wound edges by the "sawing" sutures and a continuous repulsive mastication by the children. It appears that hypertrophic scarring is extremely rare in children with Down syndrome. In more than 600 operated cases (Olbrisch, 1983; Regenbrecht, 1983; and Lemperle, 1985), only one case of hypertrophic scarring was observed after secondary healing of the tongue.

If after surgery the tip of the tongue is too short to reach the Cupid's bow, a V-Y lengthening of the frenulum should be considered.

Dislocations or infections of autogenous or alloplastic implants may occur and must be treated accordingly. Parents should be warned that the nose or chin implants inserted in early childhood may have to be replaced by larger ones after puberty and craniofacial growth spurts.

Timing of Therapy

The preschool age, between 4 and 6 years, is considered the most favorable time for the above-mentioned surgical repairs. The children are less conspicuous, even in kindergarten, and suffer less from taunts from their schoolmates. It is only at this stage that the speech-related effect of the tongue reduction can be assessed properly. Exceptions to this age rule are, of course, cases of extreme macroglossia, which, for functional reasons, should be repaired when the child is 2 years

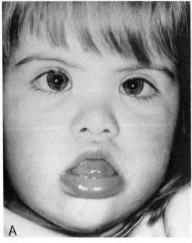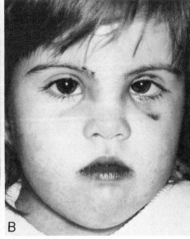

Figure 64–16. Three year old girl with epicanthus, flat nasal dorsum, and open mouth. *A,* Preoperative appearance. *B,* Disappearance of epicanthus six days after nasal augmentation and closure of the mouth following tongue reduction.

old, i.e., before possible assessment of speech. There is, however, no upper age limit if these simple surgical repairs promise significant improvement.

The surgical procedures for the correction of macroglossia, saddle nose, epicanthus, palpebral aperture axis abnormality, and microgenia in children are performed under general anesthesia. They normally require no more than 30 to 60 minutes. Hospitalization for two to six days is recommended.

Longitudinal Studies

There has been considerable discussion as to whether these children benefit from the described operations. The combination of an open mouth, drooling, and a protruding tongue accentuates the expression of Down syndrome (Fig. 64–16). Mearig (1985) as-

sumed that minimized facial characteristics as a result of corrective surgery contribute to better social integration and an improved self-concept. Surgery, when appropriate, should be only one part of a comprehensive program to improve the quality of life of individuals with Down syndrome. Particular emphasis should be placed on the cognitive development of those children who remain with an intelligence quotient of 25 to 50, since they will require supervision within a family or institution in adulthood (Feuerstein, 1982). Numerous examples of parental devotion have proved that the mental development of these children can be greatly fostered through love, patience, and intensive interaction. The reconstructive surgical procedures are intended only to support these efforts (Fig. 64–17).

It would be premature to speculate on the effect of plastic surgery on the mental devel-

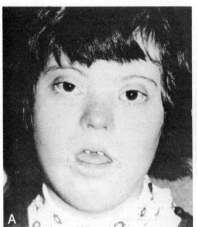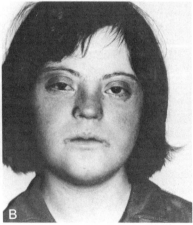

Figure 64–17. Twelve year old girl with characteristic stigmata of Down syndrome. *A,* Preoperative appearance. *B,* Six months after lateral canthoplasty, partial glossectomy, and nose, zygoma, and chin augmentation.

Table 64–2. Parents' Answers to the Question: Would You Send Your Child Again for this Operation?

Answers	Number (%)
Without reservations, yes	93 (78)
With reservations, yes	12 (10)
Don't know	7 (6)
*No	7 (6)

*All seven children had tongue complications.

opment of these children. Ninety per cent of highly critical and committed parents have been satisfied and gratified by the achieved results (Lemperle and Nievergelt, 1983; Olbrisch, 1983; Wexler and associates, 1986).

To date, there are few objective data on speech physiology before and after tongue reduction surgery. Wexler and associates (1986) and Margar-Bacal, Witzel, and Munro (1987) conducted studies on pre- and postoperative audiotapes that were judged by independent teams. While the Jerusalem (Wexler) team documented definite benefits on speech and voice quality, the Toronto study revealed no significant difference in speech intelligibility after partial glossectomy. Additional speech assessment, including evaluation of hypernasality, timing, pitch, and voice quality, as well as spectrographic analysis and normative tongue measurements, needs to be obtained in these patients.

Similar difficulties occur in assessing the longitudinal socioepidemiologic studies, since most parents tend to attribute all normal development in speech and self-esteem to the benefits of surgery. It is the author's conviction that all esthetic improvements on these children are primarily done for the parents (Table 64–2). They bear the burden of their child with Down syndrome throughout their life; they wish to be proud of their child and try to make him or her as presentable as possible.

REFERENCES

Adams, M. M., Erickson, J. D., Layde, P. M., and Oakley, G. P.: Down's syndrome. Recent trends in the United States. J.A.M.A., 246:758, 1981.

Ardran, G. M., Harker, P., and Kemp, F. H.: Tongue size in Down's syndrome. J. Ment. Defic. Res., 16:160, 1972.

Arndt, E. M., Lefebvre, A., Travis, F., and Munro, I. R.: Fact and fantasy: psychosocial consequences of facial surgery in 24 Down syndrome children. Br. J. Plast. Surg., 39:498, 1986.

Balkany, T. J., Downs, M. P., Balkany, D. J., et al.: Hearing problems in children with Down's syndrome. Down Syndr. Pap. Abstr. Profess., 2:5, 1979.

Barkin, R. M., Weston, W. L., Humbert, J. R., and Maire, F.: Phagocytic function in Down's syndrome—I. Chemotaxis. J. Ment. Defic. Res., 24:243, 1980.

Bjuggren, G., Jensen, R., and Strömbeck, J. O.: Macroglossia and its surgical treatment. Indications and postoperative experiences from the orthodontic, phoniatric, and surgical points of view. Scand. J. Plast. Recontr. Surg., 2:116, 1968.

Brousseau, K.: Mongolism. Baltimore, Williams & Wilkins Company, 1928.

Caronni, E. P.: Surgical correction of some defects in mongolism. In Caronni, E. P. (Ed.): Craniofacial Surgery. Boston, Little, Brown and Company, 1985, p. 211.

Carter, C. O.: A life-table for mongols with the causes of death. J. Ment. Defic. Res., 2:64, 1958.

Castillo-Morales, R., Crotti, E., Avalle, C., and Limbrock, G.: Orofaziale Regulation beim Down-Syndrom durch Gaumenplatte. Sozialpädiatrie, 4:10, 1982.

Crome, L.: Pathology of Down's disease. In Hilliard, L. T., and Kirman, B. H. (Eds.): Mental Deficiency. Boston, Little, Brown & Company, 1965.

del Campo, A. F.: Surgical treatment of the epicanthal fold. Plast. Reconstr. Surg., 73:566, 1984.

Down, J. L. H.: Observations on ethnic classification of idiots. Clin. Lect. Reports, London Hospital, 3:256, 1866.

Edgerton, M.: The management of macroglossia when associated with prognathism. Br. J. Plast. Surg., 3:117, 1960.

Egyedi, P., and Obwegeser, H.: Zur operativen Zungenverkleinerung. Dtsch. Zahn Mund Kieferheilk., 41:16, 1964.

Farkas, L. G., Munro, I. R., and Kolar, J. C.: Abnormal measurements and disproportions in the face of Down's syndrome patients: preliminary report of an anthropometric study. Plast. Reconstr. Surg., 75:159, 1985.

Ferguson-Smith, M. A., and Yates, J. R.: Maternal age specific rates for chromosome aberrations and factors influencing them: report of a collaborative European study on 52,965 amniocenteses. Prenat. Diagn., 4:5, 1984.

Feuerstein, R.: Personal communication, 1982.

Gisel, E. G., Lange, L. J., and Niman, C. W.: Tongue movements in 4 and 5 year old Down's syndrome children during eating: a comparison with normal children. Am. J. Occup. Ther., 38:660, 1984.

Hinderer, U.: Malar implants for improvement of the facial appearance. Plast. Reconstr. Surg., 56:157, 1975.

Höhler, H.: Changes in facial expression as a result of plastic surgery in mongoloid children. Aesth. Plast. Surg., 1:245, 1977.

Jaeger, E. A.: Ocular findings in Down's syndrome. Trans. Am. Ophthalmol. Soc., 78:808, 1980.

Jervis, G. A.: Early senile dementia in mongoloid idiocy. Am. J. Psychiat., 105:102, 1948.

Köle, H.: Results, experience, and problems in the operative treatment of anomalies with reverse overbite (mandibular protrusion). Oral Surg., 19:427, 1965.

Lejeune, J., Turpin, R., and Gautier, M.: Le mongolisme, maladie chromosomique (trisomie). Bull. Acad. Nat. Med. (Paris), 143:256, 1959.

Lemperle, G.: Plastic surgery in children with Down syndrome. In Lane, D., and Stratford, B. (Eds.): Current Approaches to Down's Syndrome. Eastbourne, Holt, Rinehart & Winston, 1985, p. 131.

Lemperle, G., and Nievergelt, J.: Plastisch-chirurgische

Korrekturen im Gesicht von Kindern mit Down-Syndrom. *In* Plastische Chirurgie bei Menschen mit Down Syndrom. Lebenshilfe Marburg, *9*:19, 1983.

Lemperle, G., and Radu, D.: Facial plastic surgery in children with Down's syndrome. Plast. Reconstr. Surg., *66*:337, 1980.

Lemperle, G., and Spitalny, H. H.: Long-term experience with silicone implants in the face. *In* Caronni, E. P. (Ed.): Craniofacial Surgery. Boston, Little, Brown & Company, 1985, p. 490.

Marchac, D., and Renier, D.: Craniofacial Surgery for Craniosynostosis. Boston, Little, Brown & Company, 1982.

Margar-Bacal, F., Witzel, M. A., and Munro, I. R.: Speech intelligibility after partial glossectomy in children with Down's syndrome. Plast. Reconstr. Surg., *79*:44, 1987.

Marsh, J. L., and Edgerton, M. T.: Periosteal pennant lateral canthoplasty. Plast. Reconstr. Surg., *64*:24, 1979.

Mearig, J. S.: Facial surgery and an active modification approach for children with Down's syndrome: some psychological and ethical issues. Rehabil. Lit., *46*:72, 1985.

Michejda, M., and Menolascino, F. J.: Skull base abnormalities in Down's syndrome. Ment. Retard., *13*:24, 1975.

Munro, I. R.: Personal communication, 1988.

Olbrisch, R. R.: Plastic surgical management of children with Down's syndrome: indications and results. Br. J. Plast. Surg., *35*:195, 1982.

Olbrisch, R. R.: Plastic Surgery in 250 Children with Down's Syndrome: Indications and Results. Transact. 8 Int. Congr. Plast. Reconstr. Surg. Montreal, I.P.R.S., 1983, p. 702.

Øster, J.: Mongolism. Copenhagen, Danish Science Press Limited, 1953.

Otermin Aguirre, J. A.: Personal communication, 1968.

Patterson, R. S., Munro, I. R., and Farkas, L. G.: Transconjunctival lateral canthopexy in Down's syndrome patients: a nonstigmatizing approach. Plast. Reconstr. Surg., *79*:714, 1987.

Pueschel, S., and Rynders, J. (Eds.): Down Syndrome: Advances in Biomedicine and the Behavioral Sciences. Cambridge, MA, Ware Press, 1982.

Rand, Y., Mintsker, Y., and Feuerstein, R.: Reconstructive plastic surgery in Down's syndrome children and adults: parents' evaluations—follow up data. Jerusalem, Hadassah-Wizo-Canada Research Institute, 1984.

Regenbrecht, J.: Beurteilung unserer Operationsergebnisse durch die Eltern—eine Umfrage. *In* Plastische Chirurgie bei Menschen mit Down Syndrome. Lebenshilfe Marburg, *9*:33, 1983.

Roche, A. F., Roche, P. J., and Lewis, A. B.: The cranial base in trisomy 21. J. Ment. Defic. Res., *16*:7, 1972.

Rolfe, C. R., Montague, J. C., Jr., Tirman, R. M., and Vandergrift, J. F.: Pilot perceptual and physiological investigation of hypernasality in Down's syndrome adults. Folia Phoniatr., *31*:177, 1979.

Rozner, L.: Facial plastic surgery for Down's syndrome. Lancet, *1*:132, 1983.

Shapiro, B. L.: Prenatal dental anomalies in mongolism. Ann. N.Y. Acad. Sci., *171*:562, 1970.

Smith, G. F., and Beig, J. H.: Down's Anomaly. Edinburgh, Churchill Livingstone, 1976, pp. 1–13, 246–263.

Strome, M.: Modified pharyngopalatoplasty for relief of obstructive sleep apnea in Down syndrome children. To be published in Acta Chir. Max.-Fac. *11*, 1988.

Tschopp, H. M.: Psychosoziale Aspekte bei der Planung von plastisch-chirurgischen Operationen am Kopf. *In* Mühlbauer, W., and Anderl, H. (Eds.): Kraniofaziale Fehlbildungen und ihre Operative Behandlung. Stuttgart, Thieme Verlag, 1983, p. 51.

Vogel, J. E., Mulliken, J. B., and Kaban, L. B.: Macroglossia: a review of the condition and a new classification. Plast. Reconstr. Surg., *78*:715, 1986.

Wexler, M. R., and Peled, I.: Plastic surgery in Down's syndrome. Down's Syndrome, *6*:7, 1983.

Wexler, M. R., Peled, I. J., Rand, Y., Mintzker, Y., and Feuerstein, R.: Rehabilitation of the face in patients with Down's syndrome. Plast. Reconstr. Surg., *77*:383, 1986.

Index

Index

Foot
 anatomy of
  for midplantar aspect, 4035, *4036*
  of dorsal surface, 4035, *4036*
  vs. hand anatomy, 5156, *5156–5166*, 5159, 5161–
   5167
 closure of, for great toe to hand transfer, 5175–5176,
  5176, 5177
 cutaneous arteries of, *371*, 373
 dissection of
  for great toe to hand transfer, 5168–5173, *5168–
   5173*
  for thumb reconstruction, 5187–5190, *5187–5190*
 in great toe to hand transfer
  complications of, 5181, *5181*
  postoperative gait analysis for, 5178
 reconstruction of, muscle and musculocutaneous flaps
  for, 401–402, *402*
 soft tissue coverage of, 4080, 4082
  in distal plantar area, 4087
  in dorsal area, 4087–4088
  in weight-bearing heel and midplantar area, 4082,
   4083–4087, 4085, 4087
Foot flap
 fillet type of, for lower extremity reconstruction,
  4052, *4053*
 from first web space, for sensory reconstruction of
  hand, 4862, 4865–4867, *4864, 4866, 4867*
"Football jersey" injury, 4536
Forced duction test, 1062, 1065, *1065*, 1601
Forceps
 Hayton-Williams, 1028, *1029*
 Row disimpaction, 1028, *1029*
Fordyce lesions, 3235, *3236*
Forearm
 cutaneous arteries of, 359, *360, 361*, 362
 longitudinal absence deformities of ulna, clinical
  presentations of, 5275
 muscles of, paralysis of
  in high median nerve injury, *4957*, 4957–4958
  in ulnar nerve paralysis, 4947, *4948*, 4949
 preparation of, for functioning muscle transfer, 4971
 transverse absence of, 5245–5246, *5247*
Forehead
 anatomy of, 2399–2400
 burn injuries of, 2222–2223, *2223*
 flaps of
  for intraoral wounds, 3436, *3437*, 3438
  for nasal lining, 1981
  midline, for nasal reconstruction, 1945, 1948,
   1957–1958, *1950–1964*, 2202, *2203*
 parts of, *1566*, 1567
 reconstruction of, by tissue expansion, 496, *499, 500*
 regional nerve block of, *146*, 146–147
 resurfacing of, 2222–2223, *2223*
Forehead-brow lift
 alternative techniques for, 2410
 anatomical considerations for, 2399–2400
 bicoronal technique for, 2401–2402, 2404–2406,
  2401–2405
 case studies of, *2407–2409*
 complications of, 2406, 2410
 historical perspective of, 2399
 incision for, 2400, *2401*, 2402
 indications for, 2400
 patient evaluation for, 2400–2401
Foreign bodies, in male genitalia, 4236

Forequarter amputation, 4345–4347, *4345, 4346*
Foreskin, reconstruction of, 4238, *4238*
Forked wire extension, for class II mandible fracture,
 in edentulous posterior segment, *951*, 954, *955*
Forward traction test, 1604–1605, *1605*
Frank technique, of intermittent perineal pressure,
 4206
Frankfort horizontal plane, 28, *28*, 1190
Freckles, 3587
Free flap. *See also specific types of free flaps.*
 design of, 277, *277*
 for cheek reconstruction, 2050, *2051*
 for chest wall reconstruction, 3703, 3705, 3707
 for lower extremity reconstruction, 4049–4052, 4054–
  4056, *4050–4053*
 in upper extremity reconstructions, 4459
  advantages of, 4460
  arteriography for, 4460
  composite tissue transfer technique for, 4461–4462
  disadvantages of, 4460
  dorsalis pedis flap as, 4463, 4465, 4467, *4465, 4466*
  gracilis flap as, 4474–4475
  groin flap for, 4462–4463, *4463, 4464*
  historical aspects of, 4459
  indications for, 4460
  lateral arm flaps as, 4471–4472, *4472*
  latissimus dorsi flap as, 4474
  medial arm flaps as, 4469–4471, *4471*
  parascapular flaps as, 4467–4468, *4468*
  posterior calf fasciocutaneous flap as, 4475
  primary vs. delayed coverage of, 4460–4461
  radial artery forearm flaps as, 4472–4474, *4473*
  scapular flaps as, 4467–4468, *4468*
  temporoparietal fascial flaps as, 4468–4469, *4469,
   4470*
  types of, 4459–4460
 microvascular, for neck resurfacing, 2200, *2201*
 neurovascular, donor tissue for, 4861–4862, 4865–
  4868, 4870–4872, *4863, 4864, 4866–4871*
Free muscle transfer. *See* Functioning muscle transfer.
Free tissue transfers, innervated
 in restoration of sensation in hand, 4851
 of hand, 4859
Freeman modification, for lower lip reconstruction,
 2018
Frey's syndrome, 1409, 3314, *3314*
Froment's paper sign, 4272, *4272*
Frontal area fractures, treatment of, 1119–1121, *1120,
 1121*
Frontal bone
 contouring of, 1565
 fractures of, 1107–1108, *1108*
  in children, 1174–1175, 1177, *1174–1177*
 repair and contouring of
  for full-thickness defects, 1562–1564, *1564*
  iliac or cranial vault bone grafts for, 1564–1565,
   1565
  methylmethacrylate implants for, 1561–1562, *1563*
 repositioning of, 1565, 1567, 1570, *1564, 1568–1570*
Frontal lobe, injuries, signs and symptoms of, 1113,
 1113
Frontal nerve paralysis, after forehead-brow lift, 2406,
 2410
Frontal sinus
 fractures of, 1107–1108, *1108*, 1121–1124, *1123–1125*
  in children, 1175, 1177
 postnatal development of, 1147

Genitalia, male *(Continued)*
  burn injuries of, *4234*, 4234–4235
  foreign bodies in, 4236
  injuries of
    anatomic considerations of, 4226–4228
    nonpenetrating, 4228–4229, *4229*
    normal anatomy of, 4156
    normal embryology of, 4153–4154
    penetrating injuries of, 4230–4231
    radiation injuries of, 4235, *4235*
    self-mutilation of, 131
Giant cell tumor
  of hand, 5498, *5498*
  of perionychium, 4512
Giant hairy nevus, malignant melanoma and, 3636–3637, *3637*
Giant pigmented nevus, 3589, 3591
Gigantism
  hemihypertrophic type of, 5365, 5371, *5370–5371*
  hyperostosis type of, 5365, *5368–5369*
  neurofibromatosis type of, 5364–5365, *5366–5367*
  of hand, 5362, 5364–5365, 5371, 5373, *5363, 5366–5372*
    treatment of, 5371, 5373, *5372*
  with nerve-oriented lipofibromatosis, 5362, 5364, *5363*
Gillies, Sir Harold Delf, 8–9, 10, *12*
Gillies fan flap, for lower lip reconstruction, 2021, *2022*
Gilmer technique of intermaxillary fixation, 921, *922*
Gingiva
  attached, 2758
  cysts of, 3337
  of mandible, cancers of, 3451–3452
Gingivoperiosteoplasty, for bilateral cleft lip and palate, 2702, *2703, 2704*
Glabella, 1190
Glabrous skin receptors, 648–651, *648–650*
Glasgow Coma scale, 869, 869*t*, 870
Glass, for alloplastic implants, 717, *717*
Glass transition temperature, 707–708
Glial tumors, of root of nose, 2986
Glioma, neuromas of, 4852–4854, *4853*
Globulomaxillary cyst, 3340
Glomus tumor
  of hand, 5504
  of perionychium, 4510–4511
  pathology of, 3586, *3586*
Glottal stop, 2734
Glottis
  anatomy of, *3416*, 3416–3417
  tumors of, 3466–3467
Glucose, total body stores, in thermal burns, 798
Gluteus maximus flap
  applications for, 4038, *4039*
  for groin and perineum reconstructions, 399
  for pressure sore treatment, 402–403, *403*
  motor innervation of, 4038
  origin and insertion of, 4038
  vascular supply of, 4038
Glycosaminoglycans
  in Dupuytren's contracture, 5057
  in wound healing, 740
Goldenhar's syndrome, 2469, 2491
Golgi tendon organ, 654
Golgi-Mazzoni receptors, 654, 655
Gonorrhea, 5551
Gorlin's cyst, 3338–3339

Gracilis flap
  applications of, 4040, *4042*, 4043
  for free flap transfer, in upper extremity, 4474–4475
  for genital reconstructive surgery, 4128, *4128–4138*, 4136–4137
    advantages of, 4136
    disadvantages of, 4128, 4136
    vs. regional flaps, 4136–4137
  for groin and perineum reconstructions, 398, *398*
  for lower extremity reconstruction, 4052, *4054*
  for pressure sores, 404
  for vaginal construction, after ablative surgery, 4208, *4209*, 4209–4210
  motor innervation of, 4040
  origin and insertion of, 4040
  vascular supply of, 4040
Gracilis muscle
  functioning muscle transfer of, operative technique for, 4972–4974, *4973, 4974*
  microneurovascular transfers, for facial paralysis, 2299–2300, *2300–2303*
  preparation of, for functioning muscle transfer, 4971–4972
Granular cell myoblastoma, 3586–3587, *3587*
Granuloma telangiectaticum, 3584–3585, *3585*
Graves' disease
  orbital pathology in, 1630
  scleral show of, 2327, 2328, 2330, *2328*
Great auricular nerve injury, after facialplasty, of male, 2396–2397
Great toe to hand transfer
  failure of, 5181, *5181*
  historical aspects of, 5153–5154
  indications for, 5154–5156
  operative steps of
    for foot closure, 5175–5176, *5176, 5177*
    for foot dissection, 5168–5173, *5168–5173*
    for hand dissection, 5173–5174
    for transfer and repair, 5174–5175, *5174, 5175*
    in preoperative period, 5167–5168
  postoperative gait analysis for, 5178
  postoperative management for, 5176–5177
  rehabilitation for, 5177–5178, *5177, 5178*
  results from, optimization of, 5181, *5182*, 5183
  secondary procedures for, 5179, *5180*, 5181
Great vessels, development of, 2470–2471
Greater trochanter autografts, 612–613
Greenstick fractures
  nasal, 988
  of mandible, 922, *931*
  radiological evaluation of, 1152–1153, *1152*
Grenz radiation, for superficial basal cell epithelioma, 3600
"Grenz zone," 750, *750, 753*, 756
Groin flap
  anatomy of, 4462, *4463*
  design of, 292, 295, *293, 294*
  disadvantages of, 4452–4453
  for free flap transfer in upper extremity, 4462–4463, *4464*
  for lower extremity reconstruction, 4049–4050, *4050*
  for reconstruction of groin area, 397–399, *398*
  for toe to hand transfer, 5156, 5159, *5157–5159*
Ground substance, 172, 210
Growth, skeletal, concepts of, 2498–2502, *2499–2502*
Growth factors, 179
Growth remodeling, 2499–2500, *2500*

Orbit *(Continued)*
  floor of, osteotomy for, 2995, *2997*
  fractures of. *See* Orbital fractures.
  functional, mobilization of, 2995, *2995–2997*
  growth of, 2509, *2509*
  hemangioma of, 1653, 1655, *1655*
  injuries of, from gunshot, 1127
  lymphangioma of, 1655, *1656*
  neurofibroma of, 1651, *1652,* 1653, *1653,* 3391, *3392–3395,* 3395–3396
  osteotomy-mobilization of, *1629,* 1629–1630
  radiographic techniques for, 1584–1590, *1585, 1587, 1589*
  reconstruction of, for Treacher Collins syndrome, 3111–3113, *3112*
  roof of
    fracture-dislocation or loss of, 1114
    malunited fractures of, 1596–1597
  soft tissues of, injury to, 909
  structures of, innervation of, 1680–1681, *1680–1682*
  surgical approaches to, *1592,* 1593–1594, *1593–1596,* 1596
  surgical principles for, 1590, *1591, 1592,* 1593
  surgical treatment of, 3381–3384, *3382–3384*
  tumors of, 3364, 3366
Orbital apex, 1178
Orbital apex syndrome, 1115, *1115,* 1672
Orbital fat
  anatomy of, 1049, *1049*
  herniated, 2327
    blepharoplasty for, 2320
Orbital fractures, 1043–1044
  anatomic considerations for, 1044–1049, *1045–1048*
  blow-out type of, 1046, 1050–1053, *1052, 1062–1063*
    classification of, 1052*t*
    etiology of, 1052*t, 1053*
    impure, 1057
    in children, 1057–1058, 1169–1170, *1170*
    limitation of oculorotatory movements in, *1064, 1065*
    mechanism of production of, 1053–1055, *1054–1056*
  complications of, 1057, 1057*t,* 1101–1107, *1102, 1104, 1105*
  diplopia in, 1057*t,* 1058–1059
  enophthalmos in, 1057*t,* 1059–1061, *1059, 1060,* 1068–1069, *1069*
  examination and diagnosis of, 1061–1062, *1062*
    limitation of forced rotation of eyeball in, 1062, 1065, *1065*
  impure, 1073, 1075
  in children, 1167–1170, *1168, 1170*
  linear, without blow-out, 1077–1082
    comminuted, of orbital floor, 1078–1079
    of lateral orbital wall, 1080–1081, *1081*
    of medial orbital wall, 1079–1080, *1079, 1080*
    of orbital roof, 1081–1082
  malunion of
    correction of extraocular muscle imbalance in, 1606, 1609
    enophthalmos from, 1600–1601, *1602–1605,* 1604–1606
    in nasoethmoido-orbital fractures, 1610–1611, *1611–1616,* 1614, 1616
    infraorbital nerve anesthesia for, 1609–1610, *1610*
    medial and lateral canthal deformity treatment of, 1609

Orbital fractures *(Continued)*
  malunion of, superior sulcus deformity treatment of, 1609
    surgical treatment for, 1601, 1604–1605, *1604, 1605, 1607–1610*
    vertical shortening of lower eyelid, 1609
    with zygoma fractures, *1664,* 1665, *1665*
  of floor and medial and lateral walls, 1597, *1598*
  of roof, 1107–1108, *1108*
  radiographic evidence of, 1065, *1066–1069,* 1067–1069
  secondary orbital expansion/contraction in, 1057
  sensory nerve conduction loss with, 1069
  surgical pathology of, 1057–1061, *1059, 1060*
  surgical treatment of, 1069–1077
    exposure of orbital floor in, 1071–1073, 1075, *1072–1074*
    operative technique for, 1070–1071, *1071*
    restoration of continuity of orbital floor for, 1075–1077, *1075–1077*
    timing of, 1070
Orbital hypertelorism
  classification of, 2988
  clinical findings in, 2982, 2984, *2984–2986,* 2986
  craniofacial surgery for
    complications of, 3008–3010
    in children, *3000,* 3000–3001
    subcranial approach to, technique for, 3001, *3001*
  design of surgical procedure for, 2975, *2975*
  etiology of, 2926
  operative procedures for, 2988
    combined intra- and extracranial approach to, 2991–2995, *2991–3001,* 2998–3001
    development of extracranial approach to, 2989
    development of intracranial approach to, 2988–2989
    in correction of associated deformities, 2989, *2989, 2990,* 2991
  pathologic anatomy of, 2986, *2987,* 2988
  postoperative extraocular muscle function and, 3002
  postoperative period for, 2976–2977
  preoperative planning for, 3001, *3002*
  surgical correction of, longitudinal studies of, 3001, *3003, 3004*
  terminology for, 2982, *2982, 2983*
  with medial facial clefts, 2540, *2541*
Orbital hypotelorism
  anomalies associated with, 3002, *3005,* 3005–3006
  clinical findings in, 3002, 3005
  differential diagnosis of, 3005*t*
  embryological aspects of, *3006,* 3006–3007
  surgical correction of, *3007,* 3007–3008
Orbital prostheses, 3537, *3537–3540,* 3540–3541
Orbital septum
  anatomy of, 1677–1678, *1678*
  in blepharoplasty, 2324
Orbitale, 28, *28,* 1190
Orbitotomy, marginal, 1601, *1604,* 1606
Orbitozygomatic complex, displaced, *1605,* 1605–1606, *1607*
Orf, 5553
Oriental people. *See* Asian patients.
Oro-aural clefts, 2444
Orofacial-digital syndromes, 2483
Oromandibular cancer, treatment of, 45–46
Oronasal fistula
  after cleft palate surgery, 2747
  closure of, 2754

Polylactic acid (PLA), in suture materials, for alloplastic implants, 720–721

Polymers
for alloplastic implants, 706–714, *707, 708, 710, 711, 713*
in suture materials, for alloplastic implants, 719*t*, 720–721

Polymethylmethacrylate (PMMA), for alloplastic implants, 708*t*, 713–714

Polymorphonuclear cells, migration of, 178

Polyolefin, in suture materials, for alloplastic implants, 721–722

Polypropylene, in suture materials, for alloplastic implants, 719*t*, 721–722, *722*

Polysomnography, 3148

Polytetrafluoroethylene (PTFE), for alloplastic implants, 708*t*, 712–713, *713*

Polyurethane, for alloplastic implants, 708*t*, 709–710, *711*

Popliteal artery
anatomy of, 4034
occlusion of, 4063, *4063*

Porcine xenograft, for thermal burns, 805

Porion, 1190

Port-wine stains
argon laser therapy for, *3667,* 3667–3668
clinical presentation of, 3227, 3229, *3228, 3230,* 3581–3582, *3582*
in newborn, *3233,* 3233–3234
treatment of, 3231–3233, *3232*

Postburn claw deformity, 5458, 5460–5461, *5460*

Posterior calf fasciocutaneous flap, for upper extremity skin coverage, 4475

Posterior interosseous nerve syndrome, 4834–4836, *4835–4837*

Posterior thigh flap, for genital reconstructive surgery, 4141, 4143, *4144–4146*

Postponement of surgery, 47–48

Postural deformities, mechanical origin of, 75

Potter sequence, 75, *76*

Pouce floutant, *5107,* 5107–5108, 5258

Povidone-iodine, 802–803

Preaxial polydactyly, 5121–5125, *5122–5132,* 5129–5130, 5133, 5347

Preaxial polydactyly-triphalangeal thumb, *5131, 5132,* 5133

Precancerous lesions, chemical peeling for, 758

Precorneal film tears, composition of, 1727, *1727*

Pregnancy
anesthesia during, 4303
augmentation mammoplasty and, 3892

Premaxilla
anatomy of, 2726
deformity of
in bilateral cleft lip
closure of clefts one side at a time and, 2658
intraoral traction for, 2659, *2660*
lip adhesion for, 2659, *2660*
repair of, 2656–2657, *2657*
with bilateral clefts, 2653, *2654*
in cleft lip and palate, 2583–2584
malformation of, in bilateral cleft lip and palate, 2581–2583, *2582*
protrusion deformity of, in bilateral cleft lip, surgical setback of, 2659, 2661, *2662*

Premaxilla *(Continued)*
protrusion of
elastic traction for, 2658, *2659*
in cleft lip and palate, causes of, 2587–2588
surgical control of, 2657–2658
retropositioning of, 2887
tilting or retrusion of, 2697

Premaxillary segment, deformities of, in unilateral cleft lip and palate, *2589,* 2589–2590

Premedication
dosages of, 140, 140*t*
for pediatric patient, 156, 156*t*
for regional nerve blocks, 4315

Premolar advancement osteotomy, 1342, *1344–1346,* 1345–1347

Premolar recession osteotomy, 1336–1337, *1338–1341, 1360*

Preoperative interview, psychologic preparation of patient during, 140

Preoperative medication, for rhinoplasty, 1812

Pressure dressings, 52, 54–55

Pressure sores
clinical aspects of, 3806*t*, 3806–3807
clinical studies of, 3803–3804
conservative local treatment of, 3812–3813
etiology of, 3798–3801, *3799*
historical aspects of, 3797
initial treatment of, 3801–3802
pathology of, 3804–3806, *3804, 3805*
spasticity and, 3803
surgical treatment of
complications of, 3834–3835
general principles of, 3814, 3818
in multiple sites, 3827, *3830–3834,* 3834
procedure for, *3815–3817,* 3818–3821, 3819*t, 3820–3826, 3823, 3826–3827, 3828–3834,* 3834–3835
timing for, 3813–3814
ulcer excision as, *3817,* 3819
systemic treatment of, 3807–3812
for relief of pressure, 3809
for relief of spasm, 3808–3809
in cooperation with other services, 3808
treatment of, 3807
type and level of lesion in, 3801–3803, *3802*

Prickle cell epithelioma, 3606–3607, *3607*

Primary Abbé flap, for bilateral cleft lip repair, 2691–2692, *2692*

Primary dye test (Jones I test), 1729

Procerus muscles, 2400

Procollagen, 171

Procollagen peptidase, 180

Prodromal phase, of radiation sickness, 833

Profileplasty, orthopedic, for Asian patients, *2429–2432,* 2431, 2433

Progeria, characteristics of, 2364

Prognathism
mandibular
children and adolescents with, *1257,* 1257–1258
classification of, 1228–1229, *1230, 1231*
clinical presentation of, 1228, *1228*
correction in edentulous patients, 1255–1257, *1255–1257*
etiology of, 1228
intraoral vertical-oblique osteotomy of ramus for, *1244–1245*

Quadriga syndrome, 4331, *4332*, 4558, *4558*
Quadriplegia. *See* Tetraplegia.

Racial differences, in facial morphology, cleft lip/palate
  susceptibility and, 2529–2530
Rad, 832
Radial artery forearm flap
  anatomy of, *4473*, 4473–4474
  for free flap transfer, in upper extremity, 4472–4474,
    4473
  for sensory reconstruction of hand, 4868, *4869*, 4870
Radial bursae, infection of, 5543, *5543*
Radial forearm flap
  fasciocutaneous type of, *297*, 297–298
  for soft tissue coverage, 4457
Radial innervated dorsal skin flap, for soft tissue injuries of thumb, 5100, *5102*
Radial nerve
  anatomy of, 4758–4759
  dorsal branch of, 4280, *4280*
  injuries of, with brachial plexus injuries, 4802
  regional block of, 4323
Radial nerve paralysis, tendon transfers for, 4941–
  4947, *4942, 4944, 4946*, 4963
Radial styloid fractures, 4637–4638, *4638*
Radialization, for longitudinal deficiencies of radius,
  5265
Radiation
  biologic effects of, 832–833
    diagnosis of, 833
    systemic, 833
  chronic, squamous cell carcinoma and, 3630, *3630*
  craniofacial cleft formation and, 2928
  exposure to, basal cell carcinoma and, 3615, *3616*
  historical background of, 831
  immunosuppression by, 195
  ionizing, 831–832
    irradiation injuries and, 5444–5445
Radiation dermatitis, 831
Radiation injuries
  acute, 834, 5445–5446
  chronic, 834, 5446, 5449, *5447, 5448*
  development of, 5443–5444, *5444*
  etiology of, 831–832
  infections in, 835–386, *836, 837*
  ionizing radiation and, 5444–5445
  local effects of, 833–834
  malignant transformation of, 836–838, *837*, 846–847,
    847
  of male genitalia, 4235, *4235*
  osteoradionecrosis and, 838
  subacute, 834
  treatment principles for, 838–842, *839–842*
  ulcers from, 844–846, *845, 846*
Radiation sickness
  latent phase of, 833
  main phase of, 833
  prodromal phase of, 833
Radiation therapy
  for breast cancer, 3899
  for hemangiomas, 3213
  for keloids, 741
  for malignant melanoma, 3652
  for maxillary tumors, 3330
    complications of, 3332–3333

Radiation therapy *(Continued)*
  injury from. *See* Radiation injuries.
  squamous cell carcinoma and, 3629, *3629*
  surgery after, 842–844, *843*
Radicular cysts, 3339
Radioactive microspheres, for flap perfusion assessment, 319*t*, 322
Radiocarpal joint, in rheumatoid arthritis, 4714–4718,
  4715–4717
Radiography
  cephalometric, 1194
  diagnosis of facial injuries by, 882–887, *884–889*,
    893–894, 897–899
  for reconstruction planning, 25–26
  of aerodigestive tract cancers, 3423, 3425, *3423–
    3425*
  of facial injuries, 882–887, 893–894, 897–899, *884–
    889*
  of hand and wrist, 4288–4289
  of maxillary fracture, 1018, *1018*
  of nasoethmoido-orbital fractures, 1090–1091, *1090,
    1091*
  of orbit, 1584–1590, *1585, 1587, 1589*
    for fractures of, 1065, 1067–1069, *1066–1068*
  of zygoma fractures, 997–998, *998*
  panoramic roentgenograms, of mandibular fracture,
    897, 899, *899*
  plain films of
    Caldwell position of, 884–885, *885*
    for axial projection of nasal bones, 886–887, *890*
    for facial injuries, 883–884
    for lateral and profile views of face, 886, *889*
    for nasal bones, 886, *890*
    for occlusal inferosuperior views of mandible, 893,
      893, 894
    fronto-occipital projection of, 885, *886*
    Fuchs position of, 886, *889*
    lateroanterior projection of, 886, *889*
    of mandible, 894, *895, 896*
    of orbit, 1584, *1585*
    of temporomandibular joints, 894, 897, *897, 898*
    optic foramen-oblique orbital position in, 885, *888*
    reverse Waters position in, 885, *887*
    semiaxial projection for, 886, *888*
    submentovertex and verticosubmental positions for
      base of skull, 887, 893, *893*
    superoinferior occlusal views of hard palate, 887,
      891, 892
    Titterington position in, 886, *888*
    Waters position in, 884, *885*
Radionuclide bone scan, 590
  for diagnosis of reflex sympathetic dystrophy, 4904
Radioulnar synostosis
  clinical presentation of, 5309–5310, 5313, *5313*
  treatment of, 5313–5315, *5314*
Radius
  longitudinal absence deformities of, vs. ulnar longitu-
    dinal absence deformities, 5273*t*
  longitudinal deficiencies of
    classification of, 5258, 5260, *5259*
    clinical presentation of, 5258, *5261*
    complications of surgical procedures in, 5265, *5266*,
      5267
    treatment of, 5260, 5262, *5263*, 5264–5265, *5264,
      5266*, 5267
Ranvier, node of, 640
  ultrastructure of, *641*, 641–642